$9

CANCER THERAPEUTICS

CANCER DRUG DISCOVERY AND DEVELOPMENT

Cancer Therapeutics: Experimental and Clinical Agents, edited by
    Beverly A. Teicher, *1997*
Anticancer Drug Development Guide, edited by Beverly A. Teicher, *1997*

CANCER THERAPEUTICS

EXPERIMENTAL AND CLINICAL AGENTS

Edited by

BEVERLY A. TEICHER

Dana-Farber Cancer Institute, Boston, MA

 HUMANA PRESS
TOTOWA, NEW JERSEY

For the beautiful ones
Joseph and Emily

For additional copies, pricing for bulk purchases, and/or information about other Humana titles, contact Humana at the above address or at any of the following numbers: Tel.: 201-256-1699; Fax: 201-256-8341; E-mail: humana@interramp.com

This publication is printed on acid-free paper. ∞
ANSI Z39.48-1984 (American Standards Institute) Permanence of Paper for Printed Library Materials.

Cover illustration: From Fig. 1 in Chapter 14, "Discovery of TNP-470 and Other Angiogenesis Inhibitors," by Donald E. Ingber.

Cover design by Patricia F. Cleary.

Printed in the United States of America. 10 9 8 7 6 5 4 3 2 1

Library of Congress Cataloging-in-Publication Data

Cancer therapeutics: experimental and clinical agents / edited by
   Beverly A. Teicher.
       p. cm. -- (Cancer drug discovery and development)
    Includes index.
    ISBN 0-89603-460-7 (alk. paper)
    1. Antineoplastic agents.   I. Teicher, Beverly A., 1952–   .
II. Series.
    [DNLM: 1. Antineoplastic Agents. QV 269 C2154 1997]
RC271.C5C3228 1997
616.99'4061--dc21
DNLM/DLC
for Library of Congress   96-48083
                                                      CIP

SERIES PREFACE

Cancer drug discovery has been and continues to be a process of ingenuity, serendipity, and dogged determination. In an effort to develop and discover better therapies against cancer, investigators all over the world have increased our knowledge of cell biology, biochemistry, and molecular biology. The goal has been to define therapeutically exploitable differences between normal and malignant cells. The result has been an increased understanding of cellular and whole-organism biology and an increased respect for the flexibility and resiliency of biologically systems. Thus, as some new therapeutic targets have been defined and new therapeutic strategies have been attempted, so have some new biological hurdles resulting from tumor evasion of the intended therapeutic attack been discovered.

Historically, anticancer drugs have originated from all available chemical sources. Synthetic molecules from the chemical industry, especially dyestuffs and warfare agents, and natural products from plants, microbes, and fungi have all been potential sources of pharmaceuticals, including anticancer agents. There is no shortage of molecules; the challenge has been and continues to be methods of identifying molecules that have the potential to be therapeutically important in human malignant disease. "Screening" remains the most important and most controversial method in cancer drug discovery. In vitro screens have generally focused on cytotoxicity and have identified several highly cytotoxic molecules. Other endpoints available in vitro are inhibition of proliferation, inhibition of [^{3}H]thymidine incorporation into DNA and various viability assays, based most frequently on dye exclusion or metabolism. The current National Cancer Institute in vitro screen attempts to take into account both cytotoxic potency and histological selectivity. In vitro screens may be viewed as limited to the discovery of only directly cytotoxic agents, thereby neglecting the fact that cancer is a disease occurring in a host organism.

The discovery of cancer drugs by in vivo screening has traditionally utilized syngeneic transplantable murine tumors. The earliest in vivo screens were the fast-growing murine leukemias (L1210 and/or P388) implanted intraperitoneally and growing as ascites. These tumors, with survival as an endpoint, provided a rapid, reproducible means for identifying potential anticancer drugs. It became evident more than 10 years ago that there were marked similarities in the drugs emerging from the murine leukemia screen. Panels of murine solid tumors and panels of human tumor xenografts were added to or have replaced the murine leukemias as anticancer drug screens. Each of these models has strengths and limitations. Most obviously, xenograft systems are not suitable for testing immunologically active agents or species-specific agents that involve host cell signaling cascades. The endpoints most frequently used with in vivo screens include tumor growth inhibition, tumor growth delay, increase in lifespan, and tumor cell survival.

In vivo systems also allow the opportunity to assess normal tissue damage by prospective agents. Murine dose-limiting toxicities are frequently useful, but studies in larger animals are often done to provide more definitive information on the potential clinically important toxicities of new anticancer agents. Spontaneous tumors in pets (dogs and cats) can provide useful populations in which to test new agents where efficacy and toxicity can be examined.

Having demonstrated activity and with a documented toxicity profile, a new agent enters clinical testing. Initial trials test the tolerance of patients to the drug and try to establish an appropriate dose for the drug in humans. The second phase of clinical testing seeks to demonstrate efficacy of the new drugs as a single agent. The third phase of clinical testing incorporates the new agent into current therapeutic regimens and seeks to demonstrate that the addition of the new agent to the combinations leads to better treatment outcomes than the conventional regimen. Final passage into medical use requires approval from the FDA in the United States and similar regulatory agencies in other countries.

The current volume traces the discovery, preclinical and clinical testing of anticancer agents currently available for routine use as well as the discovery, rationale for, and current status of potentially exciting new agents for cancer therapy. Current screening methods for cancer drug discovery and for determination of the activity of rationally designed agents are discussed with a focus on the strengths and limitations of the methods. The phases of clinical testing of new agents are discussed with a view toward presenting the strengths and limitations of that process. Finally, the requirements for approval of new anticancer drugs are presented.

The time from discovery to the time of approval for a new anticancer agent can be 10 years or more. The survival rate for compounds through this process is small.

We are entering a potentially very exciting period in anticancer agent discovery where the therapeutic focus may expand to include not only agents cytotoxic toward malignant cells, but agents that may be growth controlling, growth inhibitory, activating or deactivating toward stromal cells or malignant cells, or may alter signaling cascades from one cell type to another. At this important time in the development of cancer treatment, *Cancer Drug Discovery and Development* takes stock of what has been accomplished, where experimental therapeutics of cancer are going, and the continuing evolution of the means and methods of cancer drug discovery.

Beverly A. Teicher

PREFACE

The history of modern cancer therapy is contained within the 20th century beginning with the astute observations of physicians treating victims of mustard gas poisoning during World War I. It was the best rational medical and scientific thought that led to the application of nitrogen mustard to the treatment of lymphoma. It was also rational scientific thought toward means to improve on nitrogen mustard that motivated the chemical synthesis programs in Germany and the United States that ultimately produced cyclophosphamide and ifosfamide. The potential of the nitrosoureas first came to light from an early screening program in the 1960s searching for chemicals cytotoxic toward malignant cells and resulted in a large chemical synthesis program intended to improve the antitumor activity of that family of agents by reducing their toxicity. Again in the 1960s, actively searching for natural products with anticancer activity, the anthracyclines were discovered and developed in Italy and France. The antitumor alkylating agents and anthracyclines along with the antimetabolites such as 5-fluoracil formed the basis of medical oncology and are still some of the most widely used anticancer drugs.

The second generation of anticancer drugs included:

1. The fully inorganic molecule cis-diamminedichloroplatinum (II), a well-known inorganic complex championed for use as an anticancer agent by Dr. Barnet Rosenberg;
2. The camptothecins, discovered in the 1950s, whose clinical potential is just now being realized because of the initially unrecognized pH sensitivity of the parent molecule;
3. The epipodophyllotoxins that allowed elucidation of the topoisomerase enzymes; and
4. The taxanes, discovered in the 1960s, whose clinical development was delayed because of the difficulty in formulating these molecules for administration to patients.

Each of the second-generation lead molecules led to the exploration and development of congeners, the clinical potentials of which are still being explored.

In recent years, the scope of the search for anticancer drugs has markedly expanded so that the focus is not only on malignant cell proliferation. Though eradication of all malignant cells remains the goal of anticancer therapy, many new strategies seek to achieve growth control not only of malignant cells, but of endothelial cells and other stromal cells proliferating in response to chemical signals secreted by the malignant cells. Antiangiogenic agents and matrix metalloproteinase inhibitors focus on the inappropriate proliferation of endothelial cells and the inappropriate breakdown of the extracellular matrix that occurs in malignancy. Similarly, the premise for the use of many growth factor inhibitors and many oncogene-directed inhibitors is not only that proliferation of malignant cells will cease, but that the stimulatory signals from the malignant cells to the normal cells supporting growth of the tumor will cease. A greater understanding of the myriad components of the immune system is leading to much more effective use of interferons, cytokines, and immunoconjugates in cancer therapy and may enable the effective use of gene therapy and vaccines in cancer therapy.

This volume covers nearly 100 years of focused effort by scientists and physicians to develop pharmacologic means to cure the many diseases called cancer. This has been, and remains, a successful stepwise progression forward through which we have learned enormous amounts about the complex networks of cells from which we are composed and have steadily decreased the lethality of cancer. Our work is far from completed, but our commitment to the effort remains true to those who came before us.

I wish to thank each of the contributors to this volume for their scholarly efforts in the preparation of these chapters and for their continuing efforts in cancer therapeutics.

Beverly A. Teicher

CONTENTS

CONTRIBUTORS

MARIE-CHRISTINE BISSERY, PhD • *Experimental Therapeutics, Rhône-Poulenc Rorer, Cedex, France*

WALTER A. BLÄTTLER, DrScNat • *Immunogen, Cambridge, MA*

MIGUEL F. BRAÑA, PhD • *Laboratorios Knoll, Madrid, Spain*

MICHAEL J. BRUNDA, PhD • *Department of Oncology, Hoffman-LaRoche, Nutley, NJ*

GIOVANNI CAPRANICO, PhD • *Division of Oncology B, 1st Nazionale per lo Studio e la Cura dei Tumori, Milan, Italy*

RAVI V. J. CHARI, PhD • *Immunogen, Cambridge, MA*

STANLEY T. CROOKE, MD, PhD • *ISIS Pharmaceuticals, Carlsbad, CA*

BEPPINO C. GIOVANELLA, PhD • *Stehlin Foundation for Cancer Research, Houston, TX*

GERALD J. GOLDENBERG, MD, PhD • *Interdepartmental Division of Oncology, University of Toronto, Ontario, Canada*

JILL A. HENDRZAK, PhD • *Department of Oncology, Hoffman-LaRoche, Nutley, NJ*

DONALD E. INGBER, MD, PhD • *Surgical Research, The Children's Hospital, Boston, MA*

MERVYN ISRAEL, PhD • *Department of Pharmacology, University of Tennessee College of Medicine, Memphis, TN*

LLOYD R. KELLAND, PhD • *Department of Biochemical Pharmacology, Institute of Cancer Research, Sutton, Surrey, UK*

JOHN M. LAMBERT, PhD • *Immunogen, Cambridge, MA*

FRANÇOIS LAVELLE, PhD • *Experimental Therapeutics, Rhône-Poulenc Rorer, Cedex, France*

DAN L. LONGO, MD • *Division of Cancer Research, National Cancer Institute–Frederick Cancer Research, Frederick, MD*

DAVID B. LUDLUM, PhD, MD • *Department of Pharmacology, University of Massachusetts Medical Center, Worcester, MA*

MALCOLM J. MOORE, PhD • *Interdepartmental Division of Oncology, University of Toronto, Ontario, Canada*

SUSANNE OSANTO, MD, PhD • *Department of Clinical Oncology, University Hospital, Leiden, The Netherlands*

YVES G. POMMIER, MD, PhD • *Department of Molecular Pharmacology, National Cancer Institute, Bethesda, MD*

CYNTHIA A. ROMERDAHL, PhD • *Oncology, BASF Bioresearch, Worcester, MA*

EDWARD A. SAUSVILLE, MD, PhD • *Division of Cancer Treatment, National Cancer Institute, Rockville, MD*

NINA FELICE SCHOR, MD, PhD • *Division of Pediatrics, Neurology, and Pharmacology, Children's Hospital of Pittsburgh, PA*

PETER I. SCHRIER, PhD • *Department of Clinical Oncology, University Hospital, Leiden, The Netherlands*

JUDITH S. SEBOLT-LEOPOLD, PhD • *Warner-Lambert/Parke-Davis, Ann Arbor, MI*

WILLIAM G. STETLER-STEVENSON, MD, PhD • *Laboratory of Pathology, National Cancer Institute, Bethesda, MD*

TREVOR W. SWEATMAN, PhD • *Department of Pharmacology, University of Tennessee College of Medicine, Memphis, TN*

JOEL E. WRIGHT, PhD • *Dana-Farber Cancer Institute, Boston, MA*
FRANCO ZUNINO, PhD • *Division of Oncology B, 1st Nazionale per lo Studio e la Cura dei Tumori, Milan, Italy*

I

CYTOTOXIC AGENTS:
OLD AND NEW

1
Nitrogen Mustards

Gerald J. Goldenberg, MD, PhD
and Malcolm J. Moore, PhD

CONTENTS

HISTORY
CHEMISTRY AND MECHANISM OF ACTION
MECHANISM OF TRANSPORT
MECHANISMS OF RESISTANCE
CARCINOGENIC ACTIVITY OF THE NITROGEN MUSTARDS
CLINICAL CONSIDERATIONS

1. HISTORY

The use of mustard gas in World War I dramatically demonstrated the biological potential of alkylating agents. In addition to the vesicant action of sulfur mustard to the skin, conjunctiva, and respiratory tract, the myelosuppressive and lymphocytolytic effects were first documented by Krumbhaar and Krumbhaar in 1919 (*1*).

The chemical and biological properties of nitrogen mustards, which are close structural analogs of sulfur mustard, were studied from that time until World War II, and the prototype of this group, nitrogen mustard, was known by the military code name HN2. The pronounced cytotoxic effect of these compounds on lymphoid tissue prompted Gilman, Goodman, Philips, and Dougherty to study the effect of nitrogen mustards against murine lymphosarcoma, and in 1942 patients with neoplastic disease were first treated (*1,2*). In 1946, studies on nitrogen mustards were declassified, and several reports appeared indicating clinical activity in Hodgkin's disease, lymphoma, and chronic lymphocytic and myelocytic leukemia, but not against a wide range of solid tumors (*3–9*). These studies are of historical interest in that they represented the first clear reports of chemical compounds with antitumor activity and ushered in the modern era of cancer chemotherapy.

An intensive search was begun for alkylating agents with more selective cytocidal activity, and these basic and clinical studies were spearheaded by Haddow, Bergel, Ross, Boyland, Timmis, and Galton at the Chester Beatty Research Institute in London, England. The contributions of this group included the synthesis of:

1. Chlorambucil (the phenylbutyric acid derivative of nitrogen mustard), which is relatively stable in aqueous solution, well absorbed from the gastrointestinal tract, and has the distinct advantage over HN2 of being active after oral administration;

From: *Cancer Therapeutics: Experimental and Clinical Agents*
Edited by: B. Teicher Humana Press Inc., Totowa, NJ

2. Melphalan (the phenylalanine derivative of nitrogen mustard), which was synthesized with the objective of achieving selective concentration in tumors, such as multiple myeloma, that are actively engaged in protein synthesis; and

3. Myleran (Busulfan), which was particularly active in chronic myelocytic leukemia.

Although a large number of nitrogen mustard analogs and other alkylating agents have been synthesized with varying degrees of clinical effectiveness, the object of selective cytotoxicity for tumor cells has remained an elusive goal.

2. CHEMISTRY AND MECHANISM OF ACTION

Nitrogen mustards are alkylating agents, which are highly reactive chemically, that dissociate into positively charged carbonium ion intermediates. These electrophilic alkyl groups form covalent bonds with electron-rich nucleophiles, such as sulfhydryl, hydroxyl, carboxyl, acetyl, phosphoryl, amino, and imidazole groups present in normal and neoplastic cells. Thus, nitrogen mustards have the potential to enter into a large variety of chemical reactions with many important biological molecules, including DNA, RNA, and proteins. The mechanism for generation of the carbonium ion intermediate varies with the nature of the alkylating agent. Nitrogen mustards undergo an internal SN1 cyclization to form the highly reactive aziridinum ion (*10,11*):

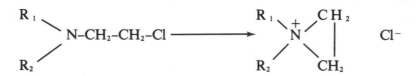

There is considerable evidence linking alkylation of DNA to the cytotoxic, carcinogenic, and mutagenic effects of these agents (*12*). The superiority of bifunctional over monofunctional agents suggests that crosslinking of DNA is critical for cytotoxic activity (*10,13*). The N-7 position of guanine is the most common site of DNA alkylation, with fewer adducts forming at the N-1 and O-6 positions of guanine, the N-1, N-3, and N-7 positions of adenine, the N-3 position of cytosine, and the O-4 position of thymidine (*11*). DNA sequence selectivity for alkylation of the N-7 position of guanine by nitrogen mustard, uracil mustard, and quinacrine mustard has been reported (*14*). DNA extracted from drug-treated cells showed the same base selectivities observed following alkylation of DNA in vitro.

Formation of DNA-interstrand crosslinks has a direct inhibitory effect on DNA replication, repair, and transcription (*15*). Formation of DNA adducts may cause a variety of structural alterations, such as ring openings, base deletions, and strand breaks (*16,17*). Genomic and gene-specific DNA-interstrand crosslinks produced by HN2 were analyzed in the human tumor cell line Colo 320HSR (*18*). Crosslinks were detected in the amplified, overexpressed c-*myc* oncogene, but not in the weakly expressed N-*ras* gene. Furthermore, the crosslinks in the c-*myc* oncogene disappeared more rapidly than total genomic crosslinks. These findings suggested that HN2-induced DNA-interstrand crosslinks are produced and processed in the genome in a nonrandom fashion. Evidence has also been presented that alkylating agents may modulate expression of c-*myc* and c-*fos* with no apparent effect on the steady-state levels of N-*ras* or β-actin (*19*).

Removal of DNA-interstrand crosslinks was postulated as a prerequisite for the outflow of cells from G2 arrest after melphalan treatment (20). Treatment of the RPMI 8226 myeloma cell line with melphalan resulted in cell-cycle arrest, with preferential reduction in the outflow of cells from late S- and G2 phases. As cell arrest abated, all of the DNA-interstrand crosslinks, but only 50% of the DNA-protein crosslinks were removed. No DNA double-strand breaks as measured by neutral elution were formed during the observation period (20). In a study of Burkitt's lymphoma cell lines, no correlation was found between HN2 sensitivity and growth fraction, presence of Epstein-Barr virus, and location of (8,14) translocation breakpoints (21). No simple correlation was detected between HN2 sensitivity and the amount of DNA crosslinks. Evidence was also presented to suggest that HN2-sensitive Burkitt's lymphoma cells may be more susceptible to delay in S phase at a given level of DNA crosslinks and that prolongation of S phase appeared to correlate with apoptotic cell death (21). O'Connor et al. also studied the role of the cdc25C phosphatase in G2 arrest induced by HN2 (22). Evidence was presented that checkpoints guarding against mitotic entry in the presence of unreplicated or damaged DNA suppress formation of the cdc2-cdc25C autocatalytic feedback loop that normally brings about rapid activation of cdc2.

The cytotoxicity, DNA crosslinking ability, and DNA sequence selectivity of the aniline mustards melphalan, chlorambucil, and 4-(bis[2-chloroethyl] amino) benzoic acid were compared (23). The order of cytotoxicity against human colonic adenocarcinoma LS174T and leukemic K562 cell lines was chorambucil > melphalan > the benzoic acid derivative. Simple chemical reactivity or hydrolysis rate was not a good indicator of DNA reactivity or cytotoxicity, whereas DNA-interstrand crosslinking provided a good index of biological activity.

Since the alkylating agents are highly reactive chemically, it is not surprising that reports have appeared describing inhibition of protein synthesis. In a study of the synthesis of histone variants in the HEp-2 cancer cell line, chlorambucil was shown to inhibit histone synthesis with no significant decrease in total protein synthesis (24).

Estramustine chemically can be classified as a nitrogen mustard, since it is a conjugate of nor-nitrogen mustard and estradiol (25). However, the agent accumulates preferentially in cells containing estramustine binding protein and appears to exert its cytotoxic activity as an antimicrotubule agent, not as an alkylator. Accordingly, this compound will not be considered further in this chapter.

3. MECHANISM OF TRANSPORT

3.1. Mechanism of Transport of Nitrogen Mustard

A major complication of many of the early transport studies of alkylating agents was the failure to separate drug transport from alkylation reactions. The latter could result in drug binding to nucleophilic groups within the cell or on the cell membrane, with the formation of apparent cell/medium drug concentration gradients. Using the hydrolyzed derivative of nitrogen mustard HN2-OH, which is inactive as an alkylating agent, we showed that uptake was by an active, carrier mediated mechanism (26). Furthermore, in studies of HN2 and HN2-OH transport, each acted as a mutual and reciprocal competitive inhibitor of the other providing strong evidence that in L5178Y lymphoblasts, both compounds shared the same single transport carrier system.

The chemical specificity of the transport carrier for HN2 was investigated. Strong evidence was obtained that transport of HN2 by L5178Y lymphoblasts was mediated by the transport carrier for choline (*27*). Choline influx in these cells was an active process proceeding "uphill" against a concentration gradient of at least 45-fold and was competitively inhibited by HN2, HN2-OH, ethanolamine, and hemicholinium-3, a specific inhibitor of choline transport. The similarity of K_m and K_i for each of choline, HN2, and HN2-OH suggested that each compound shared the same transport carrier. The relative affinity for the transport carrier was choline > HN2-OH > HN2 consistent with the notion that choline was the preferred transport substrate.

3.2. Mechanism of Transport of Melphalan

Our laboratory provided the first evidence that melphalan uptake was mediated by an active, carrier-mediated process, which was independent of that used by other alkylating agents (*28*). Melphalan transport by LPC-1 Plasmacytoma cells and L5178Y lymphoblasts was mediated by two distinct amino acid transport systems (*29,30*). At high melphalan concentrations, uptake was predominantly by the leucine-preferring System L, which was sodium-independent and inhibited by BCH (DL-β-2-aminobi-cyclo[2,2,1]-heptane-2-carboxylic acid). At low drug concentrations, uptake was by a sodium-sensitive, BCH-independent ASC-like system that also transported the amino acids alanine, serine, and cystine. Vistica et al. (*31,32*) also reported that melphalan and the amino acid leucine share a common transport system in murine L1210 leukemia cells.

The effect of altering the ionic environment was investigated to determine the direct effects of hydrogen and calcium ions on these amino acid transport systems, as well as the indirect effects of modulators of intracellular calcium (*33*). Melphalan transport followed a bell-shaped distribution curve over a pH range from 3.0 to 9.0 with a pH optimum of 4.3 and 4.6 for transport by systems ASC and L, respectively. Agents that cause a decrease in cytosolic calcium, such as the calcium channel blockers verapamil, diltiazem, and nitrendipine, the calcium chelator EGTA and reduction of pH were found to augment melphalan uptake, whereas conditions that elevate intracellular calcium, such as the calcium ionophore A23187, the calcium channel agonist (−) Bay K 8644, the calcium pump inhibitor trifluoperazine, and elevation of extracellular calcium were all found to decrease melphalan uptake. These findings suggested that modification of ionic environment directly or indirectly by agents known to alter intracellular calcium can modulate melphalan uptake.

3.3. Mechanism of Transport of Chlorambucil

The uptake of [^{14}C]chlorambucil by L5178Y lymphoblasts was studied using thin-layer chromatography to identify the various radioactive components that enter or leave cells (*34*). Theoretical calculations predicted that entry of chlorambucil into cells by simple diffusion would be rapid and essentially complete in 45 s or less. Uptake of intact chlorambucil was rapid, reaching a cell/medium ratio of approx 1.5 in < 15 s at both 37 and 4 °C, consistent with a simple diffusion mechanism. In cells treated with [^{14}C]chlorambucil for 60 min, the intracellular level of intact drug decreased with time, and this decay was attributed to hydrolysis and alkylation. The level of intact drug in the medium decreased at a similar rate resulting in a nearly constant cell/medium distribution ratio. Intact chlorambucil in the cells was found to be entirely ethanol- and trichloroacetic acid-soluble. Efflux of intact chlorambucil was very rapid and temperature-insensitive. These findings suggested that chlorambucil efflux, as well as influx, is by a simple diffusion mechanism.

A derivative of chlorambucil was found in ethanol solutions of the drug (34). This derivative, which may be the ethyl ester of chlorambucil, is highly concentrated in cells and may complicate pharmacological studies of the drug. Even minor contamination of chlorambucil solutions by this derivative may interfere with studies, since the derivative is rapidly concentrated by cells. This problem may be avoided by preparing drug solutions immediately before use or by using solvents other than ethanol.

4. MECHANISMS OF RESISTANCE

4.1. The Role of Transport in Resistance to Nitrogen Mustards

4.1.1. THE ROLE OF TRANSPORT IN RESISTANCE TO NITROGEN MUSTARD

Uptake of ^{14}C-labeled HN2 was found to be reduced in drug-resistant L5178Y lymphoblasts (26). In HN2-resistant cells, drug influx was characterized by an increase in K_m and a decrease in V_{max}, suggesting that reduced influx was owing to a decrease in binding affinity, and a reduction in the number of transport sites and/or slower carrier mobility. HN2-resistant cells that were 18.5-fold resistant to HN2 were only two- to threefold resistant to other alkylating agents, including chlorambucil, melphalan, BCNU, mitomycin C, and trenimon (35). However, a major portion of resistance to HN2 was not shared by these alkylating agents. Furthermore, transport of HN2, HN2-OH, and choline was not competitively inhibited by any of these compounds, suggesting that transport of these other alkylating agents was by independent mechanisms.

The sensitivity of L5178Y lymphoblasts to the cytocidal action of HN2 was found to be a function of the proliferative state of the cells (36). Exponentially, dividing cells were approx 2.6-fold more sensitive to HN2 than resting cells. Drug transport was also more efficient in log-phase cells than in resting cells. The more efficient transport was owing to a higher binding affinity between carrier and drug and to a greater number of transport carriers and/or more rapid carrier mobility. The greater sensitivity of log-phase cells to HN2 to a large extent could be accounted for by these differences in drug transport.

4.1.2. THE ROLE OF TRANSPORT IN RESISTANCE TO MELPHALAN

Redwood and Colvin reported decreased melphalan uptake in drug-resistant L1210 cells, which was attributed primarily to a decrease in binding affinity between drug and transport carrier (37). Dantzig et al. (38) isolated a leucine transport mutant of CHO cells that was resistant to melphalan.

Other investigators have not found differences in drug uptake in resistant cells. No difference in melphalan transport was found in human melanoma cell lines that were sensitive (MM253) or resistant (MM253-12M) to melphalan (39). In two clones of melphalan-resistant CHO cells, uptake of [^{14}C]melphalan was not significantly different from that observed in the sensitive parental line, suggesting that the clones were not membrane-altered mutants (40). No difference in drug uptake was observed in a melphalan-resistant human myeloma cell line that was partially cross-resistant to other alkylators and X-irradiation (41). Reduced DNA interstrand crosslinking was noted in the resistant cells, but it was not determined if this was owing to decreased formation or increased rate of removal of the lesion. Conversely, reduced transport of melphalan by system L was reported in melphalan-resistant human breast cancer cells, in which there was no difference in GSH content, GST activity, or expression of pi class GST mRNA (*42*).

4.1.3. THE ROLE OF TRANSPORT IN RESISTANCE TO CHLORAMBUCIL

Since chlorambucil uptake is by a passive diffusion process, one would not expect differences in drug transport between drug-sensitive and drug-resistant cells. In a study comparing untreated and treated resistant patients with chronic lymphocytic leukemia (CLL), no differences in chlorambucil transport or metabolism were detected (*43*).

4.2. The Role of Glutathione and Glutathione-S-Transferases in Resistance to Nitrogen Mustards

4.2.1. THE ROLE OF GLUTATHIONE-S-TRANSFERASES IN DRUG RESISTANCE

Glutathione-*S*-transferases (GSTs) represent a multigene family of enzymes that catalyze the conjugation of glutathione to a broad range of electrophilic xenobiotics and carcinogens (*44–48*). By conjugating glutathione (GSH) to various xenobiotics, GSTs appear to play a role whereby cells develop resistance to antineoplastic agents (*47*). The existence of multiple GST isozymes with overlapping structural and functional features has made it difficult to distinguish among closely related forms and has made the design of a systematic nomenclature a challenge (*49*). Five distinct GST classes or gene families have been identified (*47*). The cytosolic GSTs are abundant and are classified on the basis of isoelectric point as basic (α class), neutral (μ class), and acidic (π class); the other two GST classes are the microsomal isoform and the more recently described θ class (*50*). The π, θ, and microsomal classes each consist of a single gene product, whereas the α and μ classes each contain more than one gene product. Each functional GST enzyme is a homodimer or heterodimer made up of subunits encoded by gene loci from within a given class.

Two major experimental approaches have been followed to establish the role of GSTs in resistance to antineoplastic agents. The first has involved correlative studies in which elevated levels of expression and activity of GSTs have been associated with increased levels of drug resistance (*45,47*). This approach has also included modulation of enzyme activity by inhibitors of GST, such as ethacrynic acid in order to circumvent or reverse drug resistance (*51*). The second approach has used in transfection studies to provide direct functional evidence that GSTs cause drug resistance.

Both approaches, including the more definitive transfection studies, have provided conflicting evidence. Transfection of human GSTπ was reported to increase resistance of Chinese hamster ovary cells (*52*), but not that of NIH-3T3 transfectants (*53*) to the alkylator cisplatinum. More consistently, GSTπ has been associated with resistance to Adriamycin (*53–55*) and GSTα with resistance to alkylating agents (*46*) not only in correlative, but also in transfection studies. Puchalski and Fahl (*56*) reported that GSTα conferred resistance to chlorambucil and melphalan, whereas GSTμ and π conferred resistance to cisplatinum and Adriamycin, respectively, in stably transfected mouse C3H cells and transiently transfected COS cells. Conversely, several attempts to transfect MCF-7 human breast cancer cells with either class π, α, or μ

GST have resulted in overexpression of the gene product and, occasionally, resistance to ethacrynic acid, benzpyrene, or benzpyrene epoxide, but not to antineoplastic agents (57–60).

We undertook a study of the chemical specificity of induction of GST isoforms using two related compounds—the aromatic alkylating agent aniline mustard (AM) and the close structural analog hydrolyzed benzoquinone mustard (HBM) in drug-sensitive and drug-resistant L5178Y murine lymphoblasts (61). The chloroethyl groups in AM make it an active alkylating agent, whereas in HBM, these groups are hydrolyzed and cytotoxicity is owing to the chemically reactive quinone moiety rather than to alkylation. In AM-resistant cells, there was evidence on Northern and Western blot of overexpression of all three cytosolic GST classes π, α, and μ, but with marked predominance of the α class. In HBM-resistant cells, once again there was increased expression of all three classes, but unlike AM-resistant cells, the π isoform was most dominant. These studies provided evidence that induction of GST isoforms in drug-resistant cells may have both a nonspecific as well as a selective component. The difference in isozyme profile between AM- and HBM-resistant cell lines emphasizes how structural differences, in particular, the nature of the electrophilic signal, may influence the pattern of induction of GST isozymes.

Several lines of evidence support a role for GST in resistance to nitrogen mustards:

1. Nitrogen mustards can form GSH conjugates in reactions catalyzed by GSTs (Hall, 1994);
2. Human tumor specimens and cell lines often overexpress GST isozymes;
3. Transient expression of GST genes in cultured cells has resulted in increased resistance to alkylating agents;
4. Transfection of some yeast and mammalian cells with GST isozymes will increase resistance to alkylating agents;
5. GST inhibitors cause sensitization of cultured cells to alkylating agents;
6. Cell-cycle-dependent sensitivity to melphalan correlates with the cell-cycle-dependent expression of GSTs; and
7. Elevation of GST-α occurs within several days of exposure to chlorambucil as part of the normal cellular response (46,48,62–65).

The α, μ, and π classes appear to be the major GST isozymes involved in anticancer drug resistance.

Evidence also exists suggesting that GSTs may not play a major role in drug resistance to nitrogen mustards. As mentioned above, transfection of cells with GST isozymes has not consistently increased the level of resistance to alkylating agents. In some cell lines selected for resistance to alkylating agents, no increase in GST protein or function has been noted (66). In studies of melphalan–glutathione conjugate formation in tumor cells, GST-catalyzed conjugation made only a minimal contribution to the overall rate of conjugation (67). One explanation for the contradictory results of the transfection experiments is that appropriate concentrations of cofactors, such as GSH, might be required to enable GST isozymes to confer resistance (68). Nevertheless, despite these contrary findings, there is reasonable evidence in the literature that high levels of GST isozymes are associated with resistance to the nitrogen mustards. Whether improvements in therapeutic index can be realized by inhibition of GST isozymes has not been clearly established.

4.2.2. The Role of GSH in Drug Resistance

GSH-mediated detoxification pathways play a central role in the inactivation and elimination of xenobiotics, including the nitrogen mustards. γ-Glutamylcysteine synthetase (GCS) catalyzes the rate-limiting step in *de novo* synthesis of GSH. The importance of the GSH pathway in the protection of normal tissue is reflected in its widespread distribution. Increased GSH levels can be related to increased activity of GCS. Studies of the relationship of drug sensitivity to GSH conjugation have examined intracellular GSH, the activity of GCS, and the GSTs. Modulation of GSH conjugation has been accomplished by depletion of cellular GSH using either an inhibitor of GSH synthesis, such as buthionine sulfoximine (BSO), or agents that inhibit the function of one or more GST isoforms. Thiols appeared to play a significant role in resistance, since nonprotein thiols were elevated in resistant cells and resistance dropped on reduction of the thiol content by treatment with BSO (*41*).

In three human prostate carcinoma cell sublines selected for resistance to melphalan, GSH levels were increased 1.7- to 2.8-fold, whereas resistance was increased 2- to 27-fold over the parental lines. However, depletion of GSH to baseline levels in the resistant lines using BSO restored melphalan responsiveness to that of control levels (*66*). A twofold increase in intracellular GSH concentration and a fivefold increase in GST activity were detected in a rat mamary carcinoma cell line selected in vitro for melphalan resistance (*69*). Melphalan responsiveness of these cells, which were cross-resistant to chlorambucil and HN2, was also restored by intracellular depletion of GSH and inhibition of GST. Conversely, resistance was not circumvented in a melphalan-resistant human rhabdomyosarcoma cell line using BSO, despite the presence of elevated GSH levels (*70*). This cell line was crossresistant to other alkylating agents and to topoisomerase I active agents (*70*). Elevated levels of DNA repair enzymes and alterations of topoisomerase I and II were also seen and probably contributed to the resistance phenotype.

Elevated levels of GSH, GCS activity, and of GCS mRNA were observed in melphalan-resistant DU 145 human prostatic carcinoma cells (*71,72*). Nuclear run-on studies established that increased transcription of the GCS mRNA was responsible for the elevation of the steady-state level of the message.

4.2.3. Modulation of Glutathione Conjugation

Depletion of cellular GSH can be achieved using BSO. Several in vitro and in vivo studies have demonstrated that BSO treatment potentiates cytotoxicity induced by alkylating agents in cell lines with acquired drug resistance, as well as in previously untreated cells (*73,74*). In mice treated with BSO and melphalan, toxicity of normal tissue was also increased, but to a lesser extent than that of tumor cells, so that therapeutic index was enhanced (*75*). Although BSO potentiated the effects of melphalan, it did not influence the efficacy of other alkylating agents, such as cyclophosphamide or mitomycin C (*76*). Phase I clinical studies of BSO and melphalan are under way (*77,78*). These have demonstrated that BSO can deplete cellular GSH in mononuclear cells to a variable degree and that increased myelotoxicity is associated with GSH depletion.

A variety of GST inhibitors exist, and some have been tested for their ability to alter the cytotoxicity of alkylating agents. In a chlorambucil-resistant cell line with elevated GSH and GST, cytotoxicity was increased with the use of BSO, and/or the

GST inhibitors ethacrynic acid (EA) or indomethacin (79). Sensitivity could be restored to that of the parental line by a combination of both inhibitors. A chlorambucil-resistant cell line was established in which resistance was solely attributed to a 40-fold increase in GST α (80). Inhibition of GST α by indomethacin, but not by other cyclooxygenase inhibitors restored sensitivity to chlorambucil. EA potentiates the cytotoxicity of melphalan against MCF-7 breast cells when given in combination with BSO (81). In a melanoma cell line, a twofold increase in chemosensitivity to melphalan was observed when EA was given at concentrations sufficient to inhibit GST π, μ, and α by at least 50% (82). This was accompanied by a corresponding increase in DNA crosslinking. Chlorambucil-resistant Yoshida rat ascites hepatoma AH44 and AH66 cells contained higher levels of GSH and greater GST activity than the parental line. Both EA and BSO decreased chlorambucil resistance of AH44 and AH66 cells without influencing the sensitivity of the parental line; sensitivity was not influenced by inhibitors of P-glycoprotein (83).

A patient with chlorambucil-resistant CLL and high GST activity has been reported in whom EA partially circumvented chlorambucil resistance (84). Phase I clinical testing of alkylating agents with the GST inhibitor EA is under way (85,86). O'Dwyer et al. (85) used a schedule of EA orally every 6 h for three doses followed by thiotepa iv 1 h after the second dose of EA. Metabolic abnormalities secondary to the diuretic effects of EA were seen at doses of 75 mg/m², and the recommended dose for further studies was 50 mg/m². This dose reduced GST activity in mononuclear cells to 37% of the baseline level with recovery by 6 h after EA. Plasma concentrations of EA were not measured, and inhibition of specific isozymes was not determined.

4.2.4. DETOXIFICATION BY NONGLUTATHIONE COMPOUNDS

Other sulfhydryl-containing compounds, such as metallothionein, can also form covalent linkages with nitrogen mustards and may assist in intracellular inactivation (87). However, the degree of resistance to HN2 in Chinese hamster ovary cells that had no detectable metallothionein was greater than in a cadmium-resistant variant that overexpressed metallothionein (88).

4.3. The Role of DNA Repair Enzymes in Resistance to Nitrogen Mustards

Alteration of DNA may occur as a result of DNA repair enzymes attacking the DNA adducts, which may either restore DNA integrity or create apurinic sites or DNA strand breaks (89). Apurinic or apyrimidinic endonucleases recognize and excise the defective sites together with neighboring or flanking nucleotides (16,17,89). DNA polymerase fills in the missing gap using the opposite DNA strand as template, and DNA ligase completes the repair process (90). Apurinic sites may persist if the repair process is defective, and result in mutations or chromosomal breakage or rearrangement. Agents that inhibit DNA repair, such as aphidicolin and cytosine arabinoside, have been reported to enhance the cytotoxic activity of melphalan and other alkylating agents (91).

Increased expression of DNA repair enzymes has been reported following treatment with alkylating agents. Overexpression of the ribosomal phosphoprotein PO gene, a putative DNA repair gene, was observed following treatment with HN2, melphalan, and 4-hydroperoxycyclophosphamide (92). Furthermore, constitutive expression of the PO gene in Mer− tumor cell lines, which lack o6-methylguanine methyl-transferase activity, was 30- to 50-fold greater than that in Mer+ cells. These findings suggested that increased expression of the PO gene is linked to DNA repair, and may also compensate for the decreased o6-methylguanine DNA methyltransferase activity in Mer− cells.

DNA repair has been identified as an important component of HN2 sensitivity in other cell lines (93). In cells treated with melphalan, DNA damage is repaired quite rapidly (91,94). Drugs that inhibited DNA repair enhanced cell killing two- to three-fold, although some of the agents, such as cytosine arabinoside, are also cytotoxic. Treatment of human ovarian carcinoma cells A2780 with aphidicolin or hydroxyurea, compounds that inhibit DNA repair, and melphalan alone or in combination with cis-platin or thiotepa, enhanced the cytotoxic action of the alkylators (94).

In patients with CLL, increased activity of the DNA repair enzyme 3-methylade-nine-DNA glycosylase and increased expression of the nucleotide excision repair gene ERCC-1 occur with the development of resistance to the nitrogen mustards, suggest-ing that DNA repair is an important factor in drug resistance (95). In a study of drug resistance in B-lymphocytes of chronic lymphocytic leukemia, the MTT assay was used to measure resistance in vitro to nitrogen mustards and other agents (96). The resistant population was 5.6- and 4.1-fold more resistant to chlorambucil and mel-phalan, respectively. Neither GSH nor GST levels correlated with resistance; how-ever, resistance to nitrogen mustards was associated with enhanced DNA repair. Crossresistance was observed against other alkylating agents, such as mitomycin C and cisplatin drugs that act by forming DNA crosslinks. This group also studied lymphocytes from patients with CLL resistant to chlorambucil and in newly diagnosed untreated patients. The level of DNA interstrand crosslinks in lymphocytes from treated resistant CLL patients was lower than that of untreated patients (97), and a kinetic analysis showed that the rate of removal of the crosslinks was greater in treated resistant than in untreated patients (98). A followup study by the same group of 11 untreated and 12 treated resistant CLL patients showed no difference in the level of expression of the DNA repair enzymes ERCC-1 or ERCC-2 or in expression of DNA polymerase β, GST-α, or topoisomerase I (99). However, two of the resistant patients displayed increased expression of all the DNA repair enzymes examined.

Flow cytometric analysis of cells stained with the monoclonal anti-DNA antibody MoAB F7-26, which binds to single-stranded regions of alkylated DNA, has been used to study DNA damage and repair in drug-resistant cells (100). Development of melphalan resistance in A2780 cells was associated with decreased immunoreactivity of DNA with MoAB F7-26; fluorescence was significantly lower in resistant cells than in sensitive cells. The enhancement of melphalan cytotoxicity by BSO and hyperther-mia in resistant cells was accompanied by a proportional increase of MoAB binding to DNA.

The role of the enzyme poly (adenosine diphosphate-ribose) polymerase (PADPRP) in DNA repair was studied in human HeLa cells treated with PADPRP antisense transcripts under control of a dexamethasone-inducible promoter (101). DNA damage and repair were studied in these cells after dexamethasone induction reduced the level of PADPRP by 90%. Clonal survival studies showed that PADPRP-depleted cells demonstrated increased sensitivity to HN2, but not UV irradiation, suggesting that antisense-induced cells were deficient in DNA repair of HN2-induced lesions.

4.4. Other Factors Contributing to Resistance

The cytotoxicity of melphalan against animal and human tumor cell lines in vitro can be potentiated by acidic and hypoxic conditions (*102*). Although both an acidic microenvironment and cellular hypoxia can increase melphalan uptake, changes in transport were not considered sufficient to account for the observed differences. The combination in vivo of melphalan with agents that reduce intracellular pH has been demonstrated to increase cell kill compared to that observed with melphalan alone (*103,104*). In human A549 adenocarcinoma and mouse KHT sarcoma cells, hypoxia and acidic pH independently increased melphalan cytotoxicity, and the effect was greatest when both conditions were present (*105*). In studies using chlorambucil in vitro at low pH (≤ 7.0), a large potentiation of cytotoxicity was observed, whereas hypoxia alone resulted in minimal change (*106*). A much higher ratio of intracellular/extracellular drug concentration was observed at low pH, which likely accounted for the increase in cytotoxicity.

Mutations of p53 have been associated with resistance not only to nitrogen mustards, but also to a wide range of cytotoxic agents and to radiation therapy (*107*). Mutations of p53 and apoptosis will be considered further below (*see* Section 6.).

4.5. Multifactorial Resistance

We suggested that resistance of L5178Y murine lymphoblasts to nitrogen mustard was multifactorial, since HN2-resistant cells showed elevated sulfhydryl levels, decreased uptake of [^{14}C]HN2, and decreased binding of [^{14}C]HN2 to DNA, RNA, and protein (*26,35,108*). Additional evidence was that cells selected for resistance to HN2 were only partially crossresistant to other alkylating agents, suggesting that some of the factors contributing to resistance were active against alkylating agents generally, whereas other traits, such as transport mechanisms, were agent-specific (*35*).

Our group also provided indirect evidence that chlorambucil resistance in patients with CLL was multifactorial (*109,110*). Although an inverse correlation was observed between chlorambucil-induced DNA crosslinks and GST activity and/or GSH levels, there was no correlation between prior clinical exposure to alkylating agents and DNA crosslink formation (*109*). No correlation was observed between total or protein-bound sulfhydryl (PSH), GSH levels or GST activity, and clinical response to chlorambucil, although a slight positive correlation was noted between the ratio of PSH/GSH and clinical response (*110*). These findings also suggested that resistance to chlorambucil in CLL may be multifactorial.

Inhibition of DNA repair enzymes can in some instances restore sensitivity to nitrogen mustards, but more effective results have been observed with alteration of other resistance factors, such as intracellular GSH (*111*). This finding also supports the notion that multiple factors influence sensitivity to nitrogen mustards (*111*).

5. CARCINOGENIC ACTIVITY OF THE NITROGEN MUSTARDS

The acute effects of the nitrogen mustards are relatively predictable and manageable with appropriate drug dosing and supportive measures. Over the longer term, these drugs can cause permanent gonadal dysfunction and have been demonstrated to be carcinogenic. The nitrogen mustards are DNA-damaging agents that are both mutagenic and carcinogenic in a variety of testing systems. They lead to positive results in the McCann and Ames test, they induce sister chromatid exchanges and other chromosomal changes, they lead to transformation in cell-culture studies, and induce tumors in laboratory animals. Since cohorts of patients treated with nitrogen mustards have now lived for many years following treatment, evidence is accumulating on the risk of development of second tumors. The absolute risk is difficult to determine accurately when based on retrospective analyses where different drug dosages and schedules were used. Often the nitrogen mustards are just one component of a combination chemotherapy regimen that may include other carcinogenic agents. In addition, these drugs may have been used in diseases, such as Hodgkin's disease or myeloma, where an increased incidence of second malignancies is seen regardless of treatment. Nevertheless, there is now sufficient information available in the literature to support the fact that these drugs are associated with a higher risk for the development of second neoplasms.

In patients with ovarian cancer treaated with melphalan, there are a number of different series that have implicated this drug as a cause of secondary acute leukemia (*112,113*). In a review of over 5000 patients with ovarian cancer treated with alkylating agents, predominantly melphalan, chlorambucil, or cyclophosphamide, there was a 36-fold increase in the risk of acute leukemia overall and a 170-fold increase in risk for patients surviving 2 yr following therapy (*114*). Other reviews have confirmed this increased risk of leukemia in women with ovarian cancer, and have suggested that melphalan and chlorambucil are more likely to lead to secondary leukemia than cyclophosphamide (*115,116*). The latency period to develop leukemia after the nitrogen mustards is 4–5 yr, but the risk remains higher than normal for up to 10 yr. There also appears to be a relationship between the dose of melphalan or chlorambucil and the risk of secondary leukemia. In breast cancer where melphalan was used in the earlier adjuvant regimens, there is approximately a fivefold increase in risk of developing leukemia, whereas no such increase in risk has been reported for women receiving adjuvant treatment with cyclophosphamide (*117*). In myeloma, where melphalan is one of the primary drugs used, the risk of developing acute leukemia within 4 yr of therapy is approx 200 times that expected (*118*). An increased risk of secondary leukemia has also been noted in patients treated for Hodgkin's disease. In a large case-control study, the cumulative dose of HN2 appeared to be the most important leukemogenic risk factor (*119*).

The carcinogenic risk of the nitrogen mustards has not been studied as thoroughly as the leukemogenic risk. The latency period for the development of solid tumors may be longer than that for leukemia. In Hodgkin's disease where the largest cohort of patients has been followed for the longest time, there is a higher incidence of solid tumors than would be expected. This has included non-Hodgkin's lymphoma, colon, lung, breast, and thyroid cancer as well as soft tissue sarcomas (*120–122*). Some of this increased risk may be related to the use of radiation therapy, but chemotherapy, and specifically nitrogen mustards, appear to be the most significant factor. Although the increase in relative risk is two- to threefold, which is less than that for acute leukemia, increases in the more common solid tumors account for most of the absolute increase in cancer cases in these patients.

6. CLINICAL CONSIDERATIONS

Alkylating agents remain an integral component of cancer treatment, although the role of the nonoxazaphosphorine nitrogen mustards has diminished somewhat over time. HN2 has been largely replaced by other less reactive agents with the exception of its use in standard regimens to treat Hodgkin's disease. Melphalan is active against breast and ovarian cancer, but is no longer a first-line drug for either of those diseases. Melphalan continues to be an important drug for the treatment of multiple myeloma; whether any treatment has been demonstrated to be superior to melphalan and prednisone in this disease is still a controversial subject despite a large number of randomized trials. Melphalan is also given intra-arterially using limb perfusion for the treatment of melanoma of the extremities (*123*). Melphalan given intrathecally may be useful in the treatment of meningeal carcinomatosis (*124*). Chlorambucil is commonly used in the treatment of low-grade lymphomas and CLL, and has also been used in the treatment of some immunological diseases, such as glomerulonephritis and rheumatoid arthritis.

In CLL, p53 gene mutations are associated with aggressive disease and a high likelihood of resistance to chlorambucil (*125*). Others have found that mutant p53 is associated with resistance not only to nitrogen mustards, but also to a wide range of cytotoxic agents and to radiation therapy (*107*). Chlorambucil may produce its antitumor effect in CLL by inducing apoptosis-associated membrane changes that result in rapid clearance of the apoptotic cells by the immune system (*126*). In cells transfected with bcl-2, HN2 produced only 50% of the cell kill observed in control cells, whereas similar levels of interstrand crosslink formation, DNA repair, and cell-cycle progression were seen in both cell lines (*127*). Transfection with bcl-2 may represent a different mechanism of resistance to nitrogen mustards, which may be mediated by a decrease in drug-induced apoptosis.

Apoptosis has been observed in lymphocytes isolated from patients with CLL and incubated in vitro for 72 h, following a clinical course of chlorambucil (*126*). The level of apoptosis was greater in cells isolated from patients after than before chlorambucil therapy. Because a large increase in drug-induced apoptosis in vitro was followed by a significant decrease in the patient's lymphocyte count, it was suggested that chlorambucil may produce its antitumor activity in CLL by inducing apoptosis-associated membrane changes.

The chemosensitivity of lymphocytes from patients with B-cell CLL was evalutated in vitro using the MTT assay, and patients were arbitrarily designated as "sensitive" or "resistant" to chlorambucil if the IC_{50} was < or > 61 μmol/L, respectively (*125*). The response of "sensitive" patients to a clinical course of chlorambucil therapy was significantly better than that of "resistant" patients, and there was a significant degree of crossresistance between chlorambucil and fludarabine. Mutations of P53 were associated with aggressive disease, a poor prognosis, and resistance to the two drugs. Mutations of p53 have also been associated with resistance of Burkitt's lymphoma and lymphoblastoid cells to HN2, cisplatin, and other agents (*107*).

The effect of melphalan on terminal divisions and self-renewal capacity of acute myeloblastic (AML) progenitors was compared to that of a cyclophosphamide analog (*128*). Melphalan was equally effective in inhibiting terminal divisions and self-renewal as assayed by primary (PE1) and secondary (PE2) colony formation, respectively, whereas the cyclophosphamide analog was less effective in the self-renewal assay. The authors suggested that melphalan might offer a greater potential than cyclophosphamide in the therapy of AML, since chemotherapy should be preferentially directed against the self-renewal of leukemic progenitors.

Owing to the steep dose–response curve of all the nitrogen mustard alkylating agents, they remain an important component of most high-dose autologous or allogeneic bone marrow transplantation regimens. The most common drugs used are melphalan, as well as the oxazaphosphorines cyclophosphamide and ifosfamide (*129,130*). Early myeloablative therapy of multiple myeloma supported by autologous bone marrow transplantation was evaluated in 72 patients with myeloma within 1 yr of their initial therapy (*131*). In patients responding to previous therapy, myeloablative therapy increased the rate of complete remission from 5 to 45%, but with no effect on survival. However, in patients with *de novo* drug resistance, ablative therapy induced remissions in 70% of individuals and prolonged the median survival from 37 to 83%.

REFERENCES

1. Calabresi P, Parks RE Jr. Alkylating agents, antimetabolites, hormones and other antiproliferative agents. In: Goodman LS, Gilman A, eds. *The Pharmacological Bases of Therapeutics.* New York: MacMillan. 1975:1254–1268.
2. Karnofsky DA. Summary of results obtained with nitrogen mustard in the treatment of neoplastic disease. *Ann NY Acad Sci* 1958; 68:899–914.
3. Rhoads CP. Nitrogen mustards in the treatment of neoplastic disease. *J Am Med Assoc* 1946; 131:656–658.
4. Goodman LS, Wintrobe MM, Dameshek W, Goodman MJ, Gilman A, McLennan MT. Nitrogen mustard therapy; use of methyl-bis(beta-chloroethyl)amine hydrochloride and tris (betachloroethyl) amine hydrochloride for Hodgkin's disease, lymphosarcoma, leukemia and certain allied and miscellaneous disorders. *J Am Med Assoc* 1946; 132:126–132.
5. Goodman LS, Wintrobe MM, McLennan MR, Dameshek W, Goodman MJ, Gilman A. The use of methyl-bis(beta-chloroethyl)amine hydrochloride and tris(betachloroethyl)amine hydrochloride ("nitrogen-mustards") in the therapy of Hodgkin's disease, lymphosarcoma, leukemia and certain allied and miscellaneous disorders. In: *Approaches to Tumor Chemotherapy.* Washington, DC. 1947:338–346.
6. Jacobson LO Spurr CL, Guzman-Barron ES, Smith T, Lushbaugh C, Dick GF. Nitrogen mustard therapy: Studies on effect of methyl-bis(beta-chloroethyl)amine hydrochloride on neoplastic disease and allied disorders of hemopoietic system. *J Am Med Assoc* 1946; 132: 263–271.
7. Spurr CL, Jacobson LO, Smith TR, Guzman-Barron ES. The clinical application of methylbis(beta-chloroethyl) amine hydrochloride to the treatment of lymphomas and allied dyscrasias. In: *Approaches to Tumor Chemotherapy.* Washington, DC: Am Assoc Adv Sci. 1947: 306–318.
8. Karnofsky DA, Craver LF, Rhoads CP, Abels JC. Evaluation of methyl-bis(beta-chloroethyl)-amine hydrochloride and tris(beta-chloroethyl)amine hydrochloride (nitrogen mustards) in the treatment of lymphomas, leukemia and allied diseases. In: *Approaches to Tumor Chemotherapy.* Washington, DC: Am Assoc Adv Sci. 1947:319–337.
9. Wilkinson JF, Fletcher F. Effect of beta-chloroethylamine hydrochlorides in leukemia, Hodgkin's disease and polycythemia vera; report on 18 cases. *Lancet* 1947; 2:540–545.
10. Ross WCJ. *Biological Alkylating Agents. Fundamental Chemistry and the Design of Compounds for Selective Toxicity.* London: Butterworths. 1962.
11. Ludlum DB. Alkylating agents and the nitrosoureas. In: Becker F.F, ed. *Cancer, a Comprehensive Treatise,* vol 5. Plenum. 1977:285–387.

12. Ludlum DB. Molecular biology of alkylating agents: An overview, In: Sartorelli AC and Johns DG, eds. *Antineoplastic and Immunosuppressive Agents,* part II. New York: Springer. 1975: 6–17.
13. Goldenberg GJ, Alexander PA. The effects of nitrogen mustard and dimethyl myleran on murine leukemia cell lines of different radiosensitivity in vitro. *Cancer Res* 1965; 25:1401–1409.
14. Hartley JA, Bingham JP, Souhami RL. DNA sequence selectivity of guanine-N7 alkylation by nitrogen mustards is preserved in intact cells. *Nucleic Acids Res* 1992; 20:3175–3178.
15. Lawley PD, Brookes P. Molecular mechanism of the cytotoxic action of difunctional alkylating agents and of resistance to this action. *Nature* 1965; 206:480–483.
16. Hanawalt PC, Cooper PK, Ganesan AK, Smith CA. DNA repair in bacteria and mammalian cells. *Ann Rev Biochem* 1979; 48:783–836.
17. Bohr VA, Philips DH, Hanawalt PC. Heterogeneous DNA damage and repair in the mammaliangenome. *Cancer Res* 1987; 47:6426–6436.
18. Futscher BW, Pieper RO, Dalton WS, Erickson LC. Gene-specific DNA interstrand cross-links produced by nitrogen mustard in the human tumor cell line Colo 32OHSR. *Cell Growth Differ* 1992; 3:217–223.
19. Futscher BW, Erickson LC. Changes in c-myc and c-fos expression in a human tumor cell line following exposure to bifunctional alkylating agents. *Cancer Res* 1990; 50:62–66.
20. Fernberg JO, Levensohn R, Skog S. Cell cycle arrest and DNA damage after melphalan treatment of the human myloma cell line RPMI 8226, *Eur J Haematol* 1991; 47:161–167.
21. O'Connor PM, Wassermann K, Sarang M, Magrath I, Bohr VA, Kohn KW. Relationship between DNA cross-links, cell cycle, and apoptosis in Burkitt's lymphoma cell lines differing in sensitivity to nitrogen mustard. *Cancer Res* 1991; 51:6550–6557.
22. O'Connor PM, Ferris DK, Hoffman I, Jackman J, Draetta G, Kohn KW. Role of the cdc25c phosphatase in G2 arrest induced by nitrogen mustard. *P.N.A.S.* 1994; 91:9480–9484.
23. Sunters A, Springer CJ, Bagshawe KD, Souhami RL, Hartley JA. The cytotoxicity, DNA crosslinking ability and DNA sequence selectivity of the aniline mustards melphalan, chlorambucil and 4-[bis(2-chloroethyl)amino] benzoic acid. *Biochem Pharmacol* 1992; 44:59–64.
24. Sourlingas TG, Aleporou-Marinou V, Pataryas TA, Sekeri-Pataryas KE. Influence of chlorambucil, a bifunctional alkylating agent, on the histone variant biosynthesis of HEp-2 cell, *Biochemica Biophys Acta* 1991; 1092:298–303.
25. Speicher LA, Barone LR, Chapman AE, Hudes GR, Laing N, Smith CD, Tew DK. P glycoprotein binding and modulation of the multidrug resistant phenotype of Estramustine. *JNCI* 1994; 86:688–694.
26. Goldenberg GJ, Vanstone CL, Israels LG, Ilse D, Bihler I. Evidence for a transport carrier of nitrogen mustard in nitrogen mustard-sensitive and -resistant L5178Y lymphoblasts. *Cancer Res* 1970; 30:2285–2291.
27. Goldenberg GJ, Vanstone CL, Bihler I. Transport of nitrogen mustard on the transport carrier for choline in L5178Y lymphoblasts. *Science* 1971; 172:1148–1149.
28. Goldenberg GJ, Lee M, Lam HYP, Begleiter A. Evidence for carrier-mediated transport of melphalan by L5178Y lymphoblasts in vitro. *Cancer Res* 1977; 37:755–760.
29. Goldenberg GJ, Lam HYP, Begleiter A. Active carrier-mediated transport of melphalan by two separate amino acid transport systems in LPC-1 plasmacytoma cells in vitro. *J Biol Chem* 1979; 25:1057–1064.
30. Begleiter A, Lam HYP, Grover J, Froese E, Goldenberg GJ. Evidence for active transport of melphalan by amino acid carriers in L5178Y lymphoblasts in vitro. *Cancer Res* 1979; 39: 353–359.
31. Vistica DT, Toal JN, Rabinowitz M. Amino acids affecting melphalan transport and cytotoxicity in cultured L1210 cells. *Proc Am Assoc Cancer Res* 1977; 18:26.
32. Vistica DT, Rabon A, Rabinowitz M. Interference with melphalan transport and therapy in the L1210 murine leukemia system, its significance and prevention. *Proc Am Assoc Cancer Res* 1978; 19:44.
33. Miller L, Deffie AM, Bose R, Goldenberg GJ. Modulation of melphalan uptake in murine L5178Y lymphoblasts in vitro by changes in ionic environment. *Biochem Pharm* 1992; 43: 1154–1158.
34. Begleiter A, Goldenberg GJ. Uptake and decomposition of chlorambucil by L5178Y lymphoblasts in vitro. *Biochem Pharm* 1983; 32:535–539.

35. Goldenberg GJ. The role of drug transport in resistance to nitrogen mustard and other alkylating agents in L5178Y lymphoblasts. *Cancer Res* 1975; 35:1687–1692.
36. Goldenberg GJ, Lyons RM, Lepp JA, Vanstone CL. Sensitivity to nitrogen mustard as a function of transport activity and proliferative rate in L5178Y lymphoblasts. *Cancer Res* 1971; 31:1618–1619.
37. Redwood WR, Colvin M. Trnasport of melphalan by sensitive and resistant L1210 cells. *Cancer Res* 1980; 40:1144–1149.
38. Dantzig AH, Slayman CW, Adelberg EA. An amino acid transport mutant of Chinese hamster ovary cells resistant to the chemotherapeutic agent melphalan. *Fed Proc* 1981; 40:1894.
39. Parsons PG, Carter FB, Morrison L, SR Regius Mary. Mechanism of melphalan resistance developed in vitro in human melanoma cells. *Cancer Res* 1981; 41:1525–1534.
40. Elliott EM, Ling V. Selection and characterization of Chinese hamster ovary cell mutants resistant to melphalan (L-phenylalanine mustard). *Cancer Res* 1981; 41:393–400.
41. Bellamy WT, Dalton WS, Gleason MC, Grogan TM, Trent JM. Development and characterization of a melphalan-resistant human multiple myeloma cell line. *Cancer Res* 1991; 51: 995–1002.
42. Moscow JA, Swanson CA, Cowan KH. Decreased melphalan accumulation in a human breast cancer cell line selected for resistance to melphalan. *BR J Cancer* 1993; 68:732–737.
43. Bank BB, Kanganis D, Liebes LF, Silber R. Chlorambucil pharmaco-kinetics and DNA binding in chronic lymphocytic leukemia. *Cancer Res* 1989; 49:554–559.
44. Mannervik B, Danielson UH. Glutathione S-transferases-structure and catalytic activity. *CRC Crit Rev Biochem* 1988; 23:283–337.
45. Pickett CB, Lu AY. Glutathione S-transferases:gene structure, regulation and biological function. *Ann Rev Biochem* 1989; 743–764.
46. Waxman DJ. Glutathione S-transferases: role in alkylating agent resistance and possible target for modulation chemotherapy—a review. *Cancer Res* 1990; 50:6449–6454.
47. Waxman DJ, Sundseth SS, Srivastava PK, Lapenson DP. Gene-specific oligonucleotide probes for α, μ, π and microsomal rat glutathione S-transferases: analysis of liver transferase expression and its modulation by hepatic enzyme inducers and platinum and anticancer drugs. *Cancer Res* 1992; 52:5797–5802.
48. Rushmore TH, Pickett CB. Glutathione S-transferases, structure, regulation, and therapeutic implications. *J Biol Chem* 1993; 268:11,475–11,478.
49. Mannervik B, Awasthi YC, Board PG, et al. Nomenclature for human glutathione transferases. *Biochem J* 1992; 282:305–306.
50. Meyer DJ, Coles B, Pemble SE, Gilmore KS, Fraser GM, Ketterer B. θ a new class of glutathione transferases purified from rat and man. *Biochem J* 1991; 274:409–414.
51. Tew KD, Bomber AM, Hoffman SJ. Ethacrynic acid and piriprost as enhancers of cytotoxicity in drug resistant and sensitive cell lines. *Cancer Res* 1988; 48:3622–3625.
52. Miyazaki M, Kohno K, Saburi Y, Matsuo K, Ono M, Kuwano M, Tsuchida S, Sata K, Sakai M, Muramatsu M. Drug resistance to cis-diammine-dichloroplatinum (II) in Chinese hamster ovary cell lines transfected with glutathione S-transferase π gene. *Biochem Biophys Res Commun* 1990; 166:1358–1364.
53. Nakagawa K, Sajo N, Tsuchida S, Sakai M, Tsunokawa Y, Yokota J, Muramatsu M, Sato K, Terada M, Tew KD. Glutathione S-transferase π as a determinant of drug resistance in transfectant cell lines. *J Biol Chem* 1990; 265:4296–4301.
54. Batist G, Tulpule A, Sinha BK, Katki AG, Myers CE, Cowan KH. Over-expression of a novel anionic glutathione transferase in multidrug-resistant human breast cancer cells. *J Biol Chem* 1986; 261:15,544–15,549.
55. Deffie AM, Alam T, Seneviratne C, Beenken SW, Batra JK, Shea TC, Henner WD, Goldenberg GJ. Multifactorial resistance in Adriamycin: relationship of DNA repair, glutathione transferase activity, drug efflux and P-glycoprotein in cloned cell lines of Adriamycin-sensitive- and resistant P388 leukemia. *Cancer Res* 1988; 48:3595–3602.
56. Puchalski RB, Fahl WE. Expression of recombinant glutathion S-transferase π, Ya or Ybl confers resistance to alkylating ageints. *Proc Natl Acad Sci* 1990; 87:2443–2447.
57. Moscow JA, Townsend AJ, Cowan KH. Elevation of π class glutathione S-transferase activity in human breast cancer cells by transfection of the GST π gene and its effect on sensitivity to toxins. *Mol Pharmacol* 1989; 36:22–28.

58. Fairchild CR, Moscow JA, O'Brien EE, Cowan KH. Multidrug resistance in cells transfected with human genes encoding a variant P-glycoprotein and glutathione S-transferase-π. *Mol Pharmacol* 1990; 37:801–809.

59. Leyland-Jones BR, Townsend AJ, Tu CPD, Cowan KH, Goldsmith ME. Antineoplastic drug sensitivity to cytotoxic agents. *Cancer Res* 51; 1991:587–594.

60. Townsend AJ, Tu DP, Cowan KH. Expression of human μ or α class glutathione S-transferases in stably transfected human MCF-7 breast cancer cells: effect on cellular sensitivity to cytotoxic agents. *Mol Pharmacol* 1992; 41:230–236.

61. Stelmack GL, Goldenberg GJ. Increased expression of cytosolic glutathione S-transferases in drug-resistant L5178Y murine lymphoblasts: chemical selectivity and molecular mechanisms. *Cancer Res* 1993; 53:3530–3535.

62. Jungnelius U, Hao XY, Skog S, Castro VM, Mannervik B, Ringborg U. Cell cycle dependent sensitivity of human melanoma cells to melphalan is correlated with the activity and cellular concentration of glutathione transferases. *Carcinogenesis* 1994; 15(1):99–103.

63. Morrow CS, Cowan KH. Glutathione S-transferases and drug resistance. *Cancer Cells* 1990; 2:15–22.

64. Wolf CR, Wareing CJ, Black SM, et al. Glutathione S-transferases in resistance to chemo-therapeutic drugs. In: Hayes JD, Pickett CB, Mantle TJ, eds. *Glutathione S-transferases and Drug Resistance*. London: Taylor & Francis. 1990:295–307.

65. Clapper ML, Kuzmich S, Seestaller LM, Tew KD. Time course of glutathione S-transferase elevation in Walker mammary carcinoma cells following chlorambucil exposure. *Biochem Pharmacol* 1993; 45(3):683–690.

66. Ripple M, Mulcahy RT, Wilding G. Characteristics of the glutathione/glutathione-S-transfer-ase detoxification system in melphalan-resistant human prostate cancer cells. *J Urol* 1993; 150(1):209–214.

67. Guenthner TM, Whalen R, Jevtovic-Todorovic V. Direct measurement of melphalan conjuga-tion with glutathione: studies with human melanoma cells and mammalian liver. *J Pharmacol Exp Ther* 1992; 260(3):1331–1336.

68. Tew KD. Glutathione-associated enzymes in anticancer drug resistance. *Cancer Res* 1994; 54:4313–4320.

69. Alaoui-Jamali MA, Panasci L, Centurioni GM, Schecter R, Lehnert S, Batist G. Nitrogen mus-tard-DNA interaction in melphalan-resistant mammary carcinoma cells with elevated intracellu-lar glutathione and glutathione-S-transferase activity. *Cancer Chemother Pharmacol* 1992; 330(5):341–347.

70. Friedman HS, Dolan ME, Kaufmann SH, Colvin OM, Griffith OW, Moschel RC, Schold SC, Bigner DD, Ali-Osman F. Elevated DNA polymerase alpha, DNA polymerase beta, and DNA topoisomerase II in a melphalan-resistant rhabdomyosarcoma xenograft that is cross-resistant to nitrosoureas and topotecan. *Cancer Res* 1994; 54(13):3487–3493.

71. Bailey HH, Gipp JJ, Ripple M, Wilding G, Mulcahy RT. Increase in gamma-glutamylcysteine synthetase activity and steady-state messenger RNA levels in melphalan-resistant DU-145 human prostate carcinoma cells expressing elevated glutathione levels. *Cancer Res* 1992; 52:5115–5118.

72. Mulcahy RT, Untawale S, Gipp JJ. Transcriptional up-regulation of gamma-cysteine synthe-tase gene expression in melphalan-resistant human prostate carcinoma cells, *Mol Pharmacol* 1994; 46:909–914.

73. Harris AL, Hochhauser D. Mechanisms of multidrug resistance in cancer treatment. *Acta Oncologica* 1992; 31:205–213.

74. Canada A, Herman L, Kidd K, Robertson C, Trump D. Glutathione depletion increases the cytotoxicity of melphalan to PC-3, an androgen-insensitive prostate cancer cell line. *Cancer Chemother Pharmacol* 1993; 32(1):73–77.

75. Kramer RA, Greene K, Ahmad S, et al. Chemosensitization of melphalan by the thiol mod-ulating agent BSO. *Cancer Res* 1987; 47:1593–1597.

76. Siemann DW, Beyers KL. In vivo therapeutic potential of combination thiol depletion and alkylating chemotherapy. *Br J Cancer* 1993; 68(6):1071–1079.

77. O'Dwyer PJ, Hamilton TC, Young RC, et al. Depletion of GSH in normal and malignant human cells in vivo by BSO: clinical and biochemical results. *JNCI* 1992; 84:264–267.

78. Bailey HH, Mulcahy RT, Tutsch KD, et al. GSH levels, GCS activity and BSO pharmaco-

kinetics in patients undergoing phase I treatment with BSO and melphalan. *Proc Am Assoc Cancer Res* 1993; 34:1697.

79. Yang WZ, Begleiter A, Johnston JB, et al. Role of glutathione and glutathione S-transferase in chlorambucil resistance. *Mol Pharmacol* 1992; 41:625–630.

80. Hall A, Robson CN, Hickson ID, et al. Possible role of inhibition of glutathione S-transferase in the partial reversal of chlorambucil resistance by indomethacin in a Chinese hamster ovary cell line. *Cancer Res* 1989; 49:6265–6268.

81. Chen G, Waxman DJ. Role of cellular glutathione and glutathione S-transferase in the expression of alkylating agent cytotoxicity in human breast cancer cells. *Biochem Pharmacol* 1994; 47:1079–1087.

82. Hansson J, Berhane K, Castro VM, Jungnelius U, Mannervik B, Ringborg U. Sensitization of human melanoma cells to the cytotoxic effect of melphalan by the glutathione transferase inhibitor ethacrynic acid. *Cancer Res* 1991; 51(1):94–98.

83. Miyamoto K, Wakabayashi D, Minamino T, Nomura M. Glutathione-S-transferase P-form dependent chlorambucil resistance in Yoshida rat ascites hepatoma cell lines. *Cancer Lett* 1994; 78(1–3):77–83.

84. Petrini M, Conte A, Caracciolo F, Sabbatini A, Grassi B, Ronca G. Reversing of chlorambucil resistance by ethacrynic acid in a B-CLL patient. *Br J Hematol* 1993; 85(2):409–410.

85. O'Dwyer PJ, LaCreta F, Nash S, et al. Phase I study of thiotepa in combination with the GST inhibitor EA. *Cancer Res* 1991; 51:6059–6065.

86. Hantel A, Nelson J, Delknap S, et al. Phase I study of melphalan and the GST inhibitor EA. Minutes of the NCI Phase I working group. 1991:359–379.

87. Yu X, Wu Z, Fenselau C. Covalent sequestration of melphalan by metallothionein and selective alkylation of cysteines. *Biochemistry* 1995; 34(10):3377–3385.

88. Wassermann K, Pirsel M, Bohr VA. Overexpression of metallothionein in Chinese hamster ovary cells and its effect on nitrogen mustard-induced cytotoxicity: role of gene-specific damage and repair. *Cancer Res* 1992; 52(24):6853–6859.

89. Cathcart R, Goldthwait DA. Enzymatic excision of 3-methyladenine and 7-methylguanine by a rat liver nuclear fraction. *Biochemistry* 1981; 20:273–280.

90. Soderhall S, Lindahl T. DNA ligases of eukaryotes. *FEBS Lett* 1976; 67:1–8.

91. Frankfurt OS. Inhibition of DNA repair and the enhancement of cytotoxicity of alklylating agents. *Int J Cancer* 1991; 48:916–923.

92. Grabowski DI, Pieper RO, Futscher BW, Deutsch WA, Erickson LC, Kelley MR. Expression of ribosomal phosphoprotein PO is induced by antitumor agents and increased in Mer-human tumor cell lines. *Carcinogenesis* 1992; 13:259–263.

93. Li Z, Brendel M. Sensitivity to nitrogen mustard in Saccharomyces cerevisiae is independently determined by regulated choline permease and DNA repair. *Mutat Res* 1994; 315(2):139–145.

94. Frankfurt OS, Seckinger D, Sugarbaker EV. Inhibition of DNA repair in cells treated with a combination of alkylating agents. *Anticancer Res* 1993; 13:947–952.

95. Geleziunas R, McQuillan A, Malapetsa A, Hutchinson M, Kopriva D, Wainberg MA, Hiscott J, Bramson J, Panasci L. Increased DNA synthesis and repair-enzyme expression in lymphocytes from patients with chronic lymphocytic leukemia resistant to nitrogen mustards. *J Nat Cancer Inst* 1991; 83(8):557–564.

96. Bramson J, McQuillan A, Aubin R, Alaoui-Jamali M, Batist G, Christodoulopoulos G, Panasci LC. Nitrogen mustard drug resistant B-cell chronic lymphocytic leukemia as an in vivo model for cross-linking agent resistance. *Mutat Res* 1995; 336(3):269–278.

97. Panasci L, Henderson D, Torres-Garcia SJ, Skalski V, Caplan S, Hutchinson M. Transport metabolism and DNA interaction of melphalan in lymphocytes from patients with chronic lymphocytic leukemia. *Cancer Res* 1988; 48:1972–1976.

98. Torres-Garcia SJ, Cousineau L, Caplan S, Panasci L. Correlation of resistance to nitrogen mustards in chronic lymphocytic leukemia with enhanced removal of melphalan-induced DNA crosslinks. *Biochem Pharmacol* 1989; 38:3122–3123.

99. Bramson J, McQuillan A, Panasci LC. DNA repair enzyme expression in chronic lymphocytic leukemia vis-a-vis nitrogen mustard drug resistance. *Cancer Lett* 1995; 90(2):139–148.

100. Frankfurt OS, Seckinger D, Sugarbaker EV. Flow cytometric analysis of DNA damage and repair in the cells resistant to alkylating agents. *Cancer Res* 1990; 50:4453–4457.

101. Stevnsner T, Ding R, Smulson M, Bohr VA. Inhibition of gene-specific repair of alkylation damage in cells depleted of poly(ADP-ribose) polymerase. *Nucleic Acids Res* 1994; 22: 4620–4624.

102. Skarsgard LD, Skwarchuk MW, Vinczan A, Kristl J, Chaplin DJ. The cytotoxicity of melphalan and its relationship to pH, hypoxia and drug uptake. *Anticancer Res* 1995; 15(1): 219–223.

103. Wood PJ, Sansom JM, Newell K, Tannock IF, Stratford IJ. Reduction of tumour intracellular pH and enhancement of melphalan cytotoxicity by the ionophore Nigericin. *Int J Cancer* 1995; 60(2):264–268.

104. Bump EA, Coleman CN, Cerce BA, McGinnis DJ. Sensitization of Chinese hamster ovary cells to melphalan by etanidazole under intermittent hypoxia. *Int J Radiat Oncol Biol Phys* 1992: 22(4):731–735.

105. Siemann DW, Chapman M, Beikirch A. Effects of oxygenation and pH on tumor cell response to alkylating chemotherapy. *Int J Radiat Oncol,Biol, Phy* 1991; 20(2):287–289.

106. Skarsgard LD, Chaplin DJ, Wilson DJ, Skwarchuk MW, Vinczan A, Kristl J. The effect of hypoxia and low pH on the cytotoxicity of chlorambucil. *Int J Radiat Oncol Biol Phys* 1992; 22(4):737–741.

107. Fan S, el-Deiry WS, Bae I, Freeman J, Jondle D, Bhatia K, Fornace AJ Jr, Magrath I, Kohn KW, O'Connor PM. p53 gene mutations are associated with decreased sensitivity of human lymphoma cells to DNA damaging agents. *Cancer Res* 1994; 54(22):5824–5830.

108. Goldenberg GJ. Properties of L5178Y lymphoblasts highly resistant to nitrogen mustard. *Ann NY Acad Sci* 1969; 163:936–953.

109. Johnston JB, Israels LG, Goldenberg GJ, Anhalt CD, Verburg L, Mowat MRA, Begleiter A. Glutathione S-transferase activity, sulfhydryl group and glutathione levels, and DNA cross-linking activity with chlorambucil in chronic lymphocytic leukemia. *JNCI* 1990; 82:776–779.

110. Begleiter A, Goldenberg GJ, Anhalt CD, Lee K, Mowat MRA, Israels LG, Johnston JD. Mechanisms of resistance to chlorambucil in chronic lymphocytic leukemia. *Leukemia Res* 1991; 15:1019–1027.

111. Alaoui-Jamali M, Loubaba BB, Robyn S, Tapiero H, Batist G. Effect of DNA-repair-enzyme modulators on cytotoxicity of L-phenylalanine mustard and cis-diamminedichloroplatinum (II) in mammary carcinoma cells resistant to alkylating drugs. *Cancer Chemother Pharmacol* 1994; 34(2):153–158.

112. Einhorn N. Acute leukemia after chemotherapy (melphalan). *Cancer* 1978; 41:444–447.

113. Sotrel G, Jafari K, Lash AF, et al. Acute leukemi in advanced ovarian carcinoma after treatment with alkylating agents. *Obstet Gynecol* 1976; 47:67S–71S.

114. Reimer PR, Hoover R, Fraumeni JF Jr, et al. Acute leukemia after alkylating-agent therapy of ovarian cancer. *New Engl J Med* 1977; 297:177–181.

115. Greene MH, Harris EL, Gershenson DM, et al. Melphalan may be a more potent leukemogen than cyclophosphamide. *Ann Intern Med* 1986; 105:360–367.

116. Kaldor JM, Day NE, Pettersson F, Clarke EA, Pedersen D, Mehnert W, Bell J, Host H, Prior P, Karjalainen S, et al. Leukemia following chemotherapy for ovarian cancer. *New Engl J Med* 1990; 322(1):1–6.

117. Valagussa P, Tancini G, Bonadonna G. Second malignancies after CMF for resectable breast cancer. *J. Clin Oncol* 1987; 5:1138–1142.

118. Sieber SM, Adamson RH. Toxicity of antineoplastic agents in man, chromosomal aberrations, antifertility effects, congenital malformations, and carcinogenic potential. *Adv Cancer Res* 1975; 22:57–155.

119. van Leeuwen FE, Chorus AM, van den Belt-Dusebout AW, Hagenbeek A, Noyon R, van Kerkhoff EH, Pinedo HM, Somers R. Leukemia risk following Hodgkin's disease: relation to cumulative dose of alkylating agents, treatment with teniposide combinations, number of episodes of chemotharapy, and bone marrow damage. *J Clin Oncol* 1994; 12(5):1063–1073.

120. Sont JK, van Stiphout WA, Noordijk EM, Molenaar J, Zwetsloot-Schonk JH, Willemze R, Vandenbroucke JP. Increased risk of second cancers in managing Hodgkin's disease: the 20-year Leiden experience. *Ann Hematol* 1992; 65(5):213–218.

121. Swerdlow AJ, Douglas AJ, Vaughan Hudson G, et al. Risk of second primary cancers after Hodgkin's disease by type of treatment. *BMJ* 1992; 304:1137–1143.

122. Glanzmann C, Veraguth A, Lutolf UM. Incidence of second solid cancer in patients after treatment of Hodgkin's disease. *Strahlentherapie und Onkologie* 1994; 170(3):140–146.
123. Klaase JM, Kroon BB, van Geel AN, Eggermont AM, Franklin HR, van Dongen JA. A retrospective comparative study evaluating the results of a single-perfusion versus double-perfusion schedule with melphalan in patients with recurrent melanoma of the lower limb. *Cancer* 1993; 71(10):2990–2994.
124. Friedman HS, Archer GE, McLendon RE, Schuster JM, Colvin OM, Guaspari A, Blum R, Savina PA, Fuchs HE, Bigner DD. Intrathecal melphalan therapy of human neoplastic meningitis in athymic nude rats. *Cancer Res* 1994; 54(17):4710–4714.
125. Silber R, Degar B, Costin D, Newcomb EW, Mani M, Rosenberg CR, Morse L, Drygas JC, Canellakis ZN, Potmesil MM. Chemosensitivity of lymphocytes from patients with B-cell chronic lymphocytic leukemia to chlorambucil, fludarabine, and camptothecin analogs. *Blood* 1994; 84(10):3440–3446.
126. Begleiter A, Lee K, Israels LG, Mowat MR, Johnston JB. Chlorambucil induced apoptosis in chronic lymphocytic leukemia (CLL) and its relationship to clinical efficacy. *Leukemia* 8 suppl 1994; 1:S103–S106.
127. Walton MI, Whysong D, O'Connor PM, Hockenbery D, Korsmeyer SJ, Kohn KW. Constitutive expression of human Bcl-2 modulates nitrogen mustard and camptothecin induced apoptosis. *Cancer Res* 1993; 53(8):1853–1861.
128. Demur C, Chiron M, Saivin S, Attal M, Dastugue N, Boussquet C, Galinier JL, Colombies P, Laurent G. Effect of melphalan against self-renewal capacity of leukemic progenitors in acute myeloblastic leukemia. *Leukemia* 1992; 6:204–208.
129. Lazarus HM, Gray R, Ciobanu N, Winter J, Weiner RS. Phase I trial of high-dose melphalan, high-dose etoposide and autologous bone marrow re-infusion in solid tumors: an Eastern Cooperative Oncology Group (ECOG) study. *Bone Marrow Transplantation* 1994; 14(3):443–448.
130. Kergueris MF, Milpied N, Moreau P, Harousseau JL, Larousse C. Pharmacokinetics of high-dose melphalan in adults: influence of renal function. *Anticancer Res* 1994; 14(6A):2379–2382.
131. Alexanian R, Dimpoulos MA, Hester J, Delasalle K, Champlin R. Early myeloablative therapy for multiple myeloma. *Blood* 1994; 84:4278–4282.

2

Phosphoramide and Oxazaphosphorine Mustards

Joel E. Wright, PhD

CONTENTS

1. ANTICANCER ACTIVITY OF MUSTARDS

Phosphoramide mustards and their metabolic precursors, the oxazaphosphorine mustards, belong to the general class of alkylating agents. Some related compounds, the aryl- and alkyl-bis(2-chloroethyl)amines, were covered in the previous chapter. Two oxazaphosphorines, cyclophosphamide and ifosfamide (Fig. 1), are the only phosphorylated mustard compounds ordinarily prescribed for cancer treatment today (*1*). The developmental work that led to their prominent role in medicine and the outgrowth of prospective agents based on their structures and activities will be presented in this chapter.

1.1. Sulfur Mustard

Cyclophosphamide and ifosfamide grew from the original development of sulfur and nitrogen mustards. An early lead compound was 2-chloroethyl sulfide, commonly known as sulfur mustard, a vesicant used as a chemical weapon during World War I. Victims of this notorious aerosol agent suffered rapid reddening and blistering of the skin, blinding eye irritation, violent coughing, and projectile vomiting. Later, some surviving casualties developed bone marrow depression and lymphoid aplasia (*2*).

From: *Cancer Therapeutics: Experimental and Clinical Agents*
Edited by: B. Teicher Humana Press Inc., Totowa, NJ

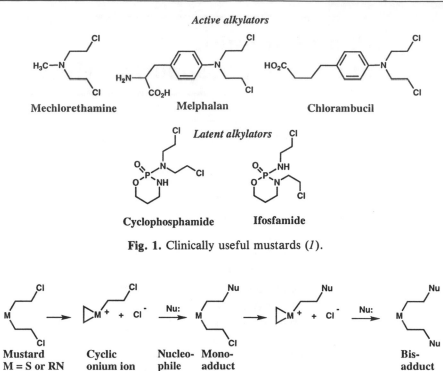

Fig. 1. Clinically useful mustards (*1*).

Fig. 2. Mechanism of action of bifunctional mustards (*5*).

The delayed bone marrow depression caused by sulfur mustard suggested its possible usefulness in low doses for treatment of cancer. Preclinical studies showed that the compound did possess anticancer activity and a clinical trial was conducted, but the therapeutic activity of sulfur mustard proved to be insubstantial and of short duration (*3*).

Seeking to overcome the deficiencies of sulfur mustard, investigators applied the lead drug concept and tested a number of sulfur mustard analogs in the hope that a structurally related compound would succeed where the parent drug had failed (*4*). However, none of the structural variants proved fruitful. Because of the lack of persistent benefit and perhaps the onus of its horrendous history as a chemical warfare agent, interest in sulfur mustard rapidly waned.

1.2. Nitrogen Mustards

As World War II began, research on vesicant mustards resumed. The focus was redirected toward a series of 2-haloethyl amine compounds that had been synthesized almost a half-century earlier. Biological activities superior to those of sulfur mustard were found with bis- and tris(2-chloroethyl)amine, and the mechanism of action was determined (*5*). The delayed systemic effects of sulfur and nitrogen mustards were tied to a chemical reaction that both classes of mustards have in common (Fig. 2), the anchimerically assisted formation of a cyclic onium ion capable of alkylating "a vital cellular constituent." Convincing evidence indicated that the vital constituent was nuclear chromatin. For example, alkylation by mechlorethamine produced inheritable abnormalities in the chromosomes of fruit flies (6). DNA was not specifically mentioned, although its central biological role as the carrier of genetic information had been reported two years earlier (7). Wartime secrecy had delayed publication of the nitrogen mustard data by three years and more. Thus, the two lines of work were approximately concurrent. Prior to 1944, it was widely believed that chromosomal proteins transmitted genetic information (8). When the results of wartime investigations were finally revealed in 1946, the report did not specify which macromolecular species in the nucleus were targeted (6).

Despite severe hematopoietic side effects (9), preclinical results with tris(2-chloroethyl)amine and N-methylbis(2-chloroethyl)amine, now known as mechlorethanime led to a clinical trial (10). Substantial activity was demonstrated against Hodgkin's disease, thus establishing the first beachhead for cancer chemotherapy. Lymphosarcoma and leukemia patients were also treated, but the outcome was less favorable.

Several hundred patients were treated prior to the end of the war in an extensive investigation that uncovered the salient biological characteristics of bi- and trifunctional alkylators (10–14). An early observation was the susceptibility of renewal cell populations, including lymphatics, bone marrow, and gastrointestinal epithelia. This model, the cytokinetic mechanism of selectivity, describes the general behavior of mustards whose alkylating activity is rapid and direct. It is a prodominant mechanism for the three aryl and alkyl mustards commonly used in the clinic today, mechlorethamine, chlorambucil, and melphalan (Fig. 1) (15).

It was soberly concluded that sensitivity to nitrogen mustard treatment varied greatly from tumor to tumor. Furthermore, the clinicians observed a gradual loss of drug sensitivity during retreatment of recurrent disease. This phenomenon was identified as acquired resistance (16). Host toxicity did not vary as much as tumor response, allowing establishment of a maximum tolerated dose (MTD) (17). However, the frequent occurrence of tumors resistant to all reasonable doses was recognized as an inherent problem for drugs whose sole mechanism is cytokinetic selection. This understanding prompted renewed efforts to find exploitable differences between tumor and normal cells that did not depend on their proliferative state.

2. THE RATIONAL ROAD TO SERENDIP

The search for differences between tumor and normal tissues was motivated by the hope of improving selectivity through rational drug development. Historically, this approach has afforded a lower probability of success than other drug development methods, such as random screening of natural or synthetic products (18). The development of oxazaphosphorine anticancer agents was no exception, owing more to large-scale programmatic screening than to *ab initio* reasoning.

2.1. Tumor Phosphoamidase

Arnold Seligman and coworkers in Boston were interested in finding ways to improve selectivity based on differences in hydrolytic enzyme levels of tumor vs normal tissues (19). A method for measuring hydrolysis rates of phosphorus amides had been reported in the 1930s (20) using N-(4-chlorophenyl)diamidophosphoric acid as the substrate (21). Histochemical staining methods had shown apparent phosphoamidase (EC 3.9.1.1) overproduction in 24 tumors of the gastrointestinal tract and in a variety of breast, lung, cervical, testicular, and other carcinomas (22).

Friedman's Precursor [24]

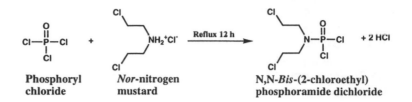

Phosphoryl
chloride

Nor-nitrogen
mustard

N,N-*Bis*-(2-chloroethyl)
phosphoramide dichloride

Latent Phosphorylated Mustards [24, 63]

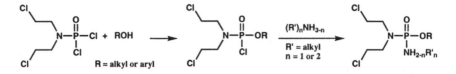

Fig. 3. Synthesis of phosphorylated mustards.

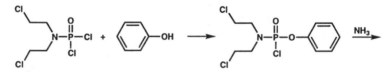

N,N-*Bis*-(2-chloroethyl)
phosphoramide dichloride

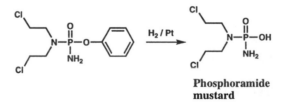

Phosphoramide
mustard

Fig. 4. Synthesis of phosphoramide mustard (*24*).

2.2. Phosphorylated Mustards

In order to exploit differential phosphoamidase levels, Seligman and his colleagues envisioned the synthesis of water-soluble toxagenic substrates whose intracellular hydrolysis would release a cytotoxic product (*19*). Postwar interest in mustards was still high, and this undoubtedly influenced their choice of bis(2-chloroethyl)amine and related compounds as candidate precursors of the hypothetical prodrug (*23*). Since the alkylating activity of a nitrogen mustard depends on the basicity of its β-nitrogen, covalent attachment of an electron-withdrawing phosphoryl group to the nitrogen provided a logical deactivation step (Fig. 3).

Several *N*-phosphorylated secondary nitrogen mustards were synthesized. One of these was phosphoramide mustard, later identified as an important metabolite of cyclophosphamide (Fig. 4) (*24*). Unfortunately, the small academic research group in

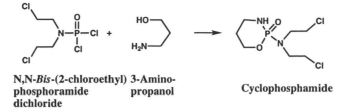

N,N-*Bis*-(2-chloroethyl) **3-Amino-**
phosphoramide   **propanol**
dichloride

Cyclophosphamide

Fig. 5. Synthesis of cyclophosphamide (*27*).

Boston was not able to find the selective, latent agent they were seeking. A very effective phosphorylated mustard compound did soon surface, however, as a result of efforts on a larger scale in Germany.

3. CYCLOPHOSPHAMIDE

Under the leadership of Norbert Brock in Brackwede, Westphalia, the pharmacology department of ASTA-Werke AG had embarked on an anticancer drug discovery program based on biophysical, biochemical, pharmacological, and clinical investigations. The information garnered by these efforts was used to develop a rational approach to the synthesis and testing of new anticancer agents (*25*). In parallel with the ideas of Seligman and coworkers, Hermann Druckrey in Freiberg had proposed that a labile, toxic anticancer agent should be administered in a stable "transport form" to be activated within tumor cells (*26*). Brock's goal was to bring Druckrey's philosophical concept to fruition.

3.1. Discovery

Orrie Friedman, a chemist on Seligman's team, had phosphorylated bis(2-chloroethyl)amine with phosphoryl chloride, yielding *N,N*-bis(chloroethyl)phosphoramide dichloride, a versatile precursor from which straight- and branched-chain alkyl as well as aromatic mono- and diamidophosphate esters could be prepared (Fig. 3) (*24*). ASTA chemists Herbert Arnold and Friedrich Bourseaux recognized that such compounds fulfilled the stability and solubility criteria, but failed the crucial activation requirement (*25,26*). They sought to overcome this defect by a slight modification of the earlier design, incorporating a saturated heterocyclic ring in place of the open-chain substituents. Thus, they prepared Friedman's precursor and condensed it with α,ω-alkanolamines. With 3-aminopropanol, their efficient two-step synthesis (Fig. 5) gave cyclophosphamide (*27*).

3.2. Preclinical Testing

In vivo screening showed that cyclophosphamide had excellent anticancer activity against transplanted rat tumors (*28–31*) and murine leukemia (*32*). Researchers were especially encouraged by the lack of in vivo crossresistance against L1210 cell lines with acquired resistance to the antimetabolites methotrexate, 8-azaguanine, and 6-mercaptopurine (*33,34*).

3.3. Clinical Trials

Immediately after publication of the preclinical studies came a report from Rudolf Gross and Klaus Lambers of the University of Marburg/Lahn on cyclophosphamide's first clinical trial (*35*). Results from 45 patients with a wide variety of tumors indicated that cyclophosphamide had a spectrum of activity similar to those of mechlorethamine and mannitol mustard, but with less severe toxicity. This result was confirmed by worldwide studies (*36–44*) that established the usefulness of cyclophosphamide for treatment of chronic lymphocytic and granulocytic leukemias, acute myelogenous, monocytic and childhood lymphoblastic leukemia, Hodgkin's Burkitt's, and follicular lymphoma, lymphocytic and lymphoblastic lymphosarcoma, reticulum cell sarcoma, multiple myeloma, mycosis fungoides, breast, lung, and cervical carcinoma, neuroblastoma, retinoblastoma, Wilm's tumor, rhabdomyosarcoma, and ovarian adenocarcinoma (*45*). More prescriptions are written today for cyclophosphamide than any other alkylating agent. Indeed, its use may exceed that of any other chemotherapeutic anticancer agent (*46*).

3.4. Tissue Distribution

Why was cyclophosphamide less toxic than mechlorethamine and mannitol mustard in the clinic? One explanation came from the Medical University of Cologne, where investigators were able to demonstrate that cyclophosphamide and/or some of its metabolites selectively accumulated in neoplastic tissues. They prepared tritiated cyclophosphamide and administered it to three moribund patients a few hours before death from metastatic lung carcinoma. Autopsy showed that in all three cases, the highest concentrations of tritiated drug and metabolites (cpm/gm dry wt) had selectively partitioned into the primary tumors and metastases of the liver (2/3 patients), kidneys (2/3), adrenal glands (1/3), and diaphragm (1/3). Lower concentrations were found in normal tissues of the lungs, kidneys, brain, adrenal glands, spleen, lymph nodes, skin, pancreas, skeletal muscle, heart muscle, and testicles (*47*).

These data could be interpreted in various ways. Selective influx into tumor cells or selective efflux from the cells of normal host tissues are two possibilities. Cellular transport studies of cyclophosphamide and a metabolite precursor, 4-hydroperoxycyclophosphamide, were performed with several murine tumor and L929 fibroblast cell lines, but no significant differences in influx or accumulation were seen (*48*). In contrast, the study of cyclophosphamide's metabolism has been an extremely fruitful area of endeavor. The next section is a rough chronology of the effort to uncover the basic features of cyclophosphamide metabolism.

3.5. Metabolism of Cyclophosphamide

Soon after the synthesis of cyclophosphamide, a simple biological experiment overturned the notion of its hydrolysis within tumor cells, as a mechanism of selectivity. Prior to transplantation into rats, Yoshida, Jensen, or Walker tumor cells were incubated with high concentrations (up to 1 mg·mL^{-1}) of cyclophosphamide. Their engraftment and growth did not differ from untreated controls. Since these tumors were sensitive to cyclophosphamide administered directly to the animal, it was obvious that normal cells somewhere in the host must be responsible for the activation (*49*).

3.5.1. ROLE OF THE LIVER

In 1961, the in vivo site of cyclophosphamide activation was established by Foley et al. (*50*). They showed that cyclophosphamide *per se* was inactive against serial cultures of several tumor cell lines, but became cytotoxic on incubation with homogenized mouse liver. Homogenates from other normal tissues or tumors failed to activate cyclophosphamide.

Two years later, the pivotal role of liver in the activation of cyclophosphamide was confirmed in much greater detail by Norbert Brock and Hans-Jürgen Hohorst. They perfused a cyclophosphamide solution through intact rat liver in organ culture and tested the outflow against tumor cells in tissue culture. They also administered cyclophosphamide to hepatectomized rats, harvested their blood serum, and tested that against cultured tumor cells. The serum's cytotoxicity was only one-fourth to one-tenth that of unhepatectomized controls. Using tissue slices, they showed that the remainder of the activity derived from renal cortex and lung. They established that the process did not involve hydrolysis and that bis(chloroethyl)amine was not the primary product of cyclophosphamide activation. Most significantly, they demonstrated that cyclophosphamide activation was an oxidative process requiring NADPH and molecular oxygen. From their results they concluded that the primary activation product was not the effective form, but an intermediate from which the ultimate cytotoxic species was spontaneously generated. They were then unable to characterize the structures of the labile transport form or the subsequent alkylator. However, when these were finally determined, the descriptive conclusions of the ASTA scientists were fully confirmed (51).

The finding that cyclophosphamide is activated in the liver by mixed-function oxidases, rather than by tumor phosphoamidases, appears to undermine the rational hypothesis that predicated its development. A degree of serendipity was surely involved. In spite of this, the rational approach played an essential role in motivating and guiding the inventors of cyclophosphamide (25). As is often the case, discovery resulted from fact and fortune working hand in hand.

3.5.2. MOLECULAR MECHANISM

Well before any firm data had appeared on the molecular structure of cyclophosphamide metabolites, Klaus Norpoth had hypothesized that the mechanism of hepatic oxidation of cyclophosphamide should parallel that of nicotine, as shown in Fig. 6. According to this scheme, the initial step involved hydroxylation of the ring methylene group adjacent to nitrogen. Furthermore, he maintained that subsequent transformations should also resemble those of nicotine (52). Unfortunately, the inability to confirm this hypothesis experimentally using a synthetic standard for the carbonyl derivative, 4-oxocyclophosphamide, led him to an erroneous revision in which cleavage of the cyclophosphamide ring by O-dealkylation was suggested (53).

Although the proposed O-dealkylation of cyclophosphamide later proved incorrect, it did lead to an interesting finding. The structure of Norpoth's putative "primary metabolite" contained a 3-substituted propionaldehyde group. This made it a likely metabolic precursor of acrolein, according to R.A. Alarcon and Johannes Meienhofer of the Children's Cancer Research Foundation. Although its immediate precursor had to be determined later, their experimental evidence for the in vitro production of acrolein from cyclophosphamide with liver microsomes, NADPH, and oxygen (54) received strong confirmation (55).

Evidence that Norpoth's initial proposal had been the correct one came in 1970 from the Southern Research Institute in Birmingham, AL. A metabolite from the urine of a dog treated with [6-^{14}C]cyclophosphamide was isolated and purified by

Metabolism of Nicotine

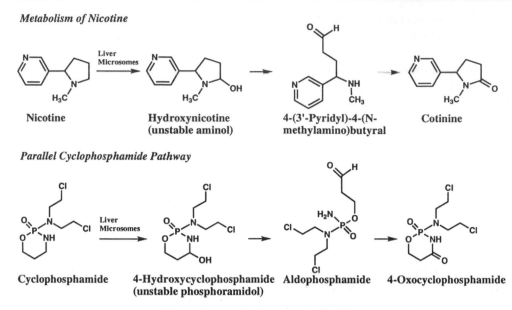

Parallel Cyclophosphamide Pathway

Fig. 6. Norpoth's hypothesis (*52,53*).

chromatography and crystallization. Oxidation adjacent to the ring nitrogen of cyclo-phosphamide was shown by infrared spectrophotometry (IR) and mass spectrometry (MS) to give 4-oxocyclophosphamide. The structure was confirmed by definitive synthesis (*56*). A few months later, 4-oxocyclophosphamide was also identified as a cyclophosphamide metabolite in the urine of sheep who received the drug as part of an experimental defleecing procedure (*57*).

As a consequence of the above reports that empirically defined the position of oxidation of the cyclophosphamide ring and of its *N*-dealkylation, ASTA scientists were able to deduce the basic molecular features of cyclophosphamide activation and detoxification (Fig. 7). As Norpoth had originally suggested, the initial hepatic metabolite was 4-hydroxycyclophosphamide, which was enzymatically detoxified to 4-oxo-cyclophosphamide and eliminated in urine.

The pathway to 4-oxocyclophosphamide was not, however the major metabolic route. A larger portion of the primary 4-hydroxy metabolite was spontaneously converted to its ring-opened tautomer, commonly called aldophosphamide. The most abundant renally excreted metabolite of cyclophosphamide is a product of aldophosphamide oxidation by aldehyde dehydrogenase, commonly known as carboxyphosphamide (*58*).

An additional minor pathway of aldophosphamide metabolism is reduction (*57*), catalyzed by aldose reductase or an unidentified aldo-keto reductase. Consistent with the trivial nomenclature noted above, the product was named alcophosphamide. Formation of alcophosphamide from aldophosphamide is a detoxification pathway, since alcophosphamide possesses little antitumor activity in vivo (*45*).

3.5.3. Metabolite Characterization

The fundamental model of cyclophosphamide metabolism, outlined in Fig. 7, was firmly grounded in basic science, but still required confirmation by synthetic and

Fundamental model (Hohorst, Ziemann and Brock [58])

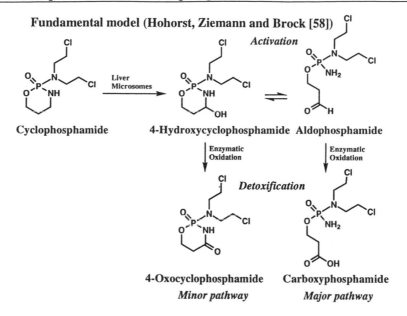

Release of acrolein (Alarcon and Meienhofer [54]) and phosphoramide mustard (Colvin, Padgett and Feneslau [62])

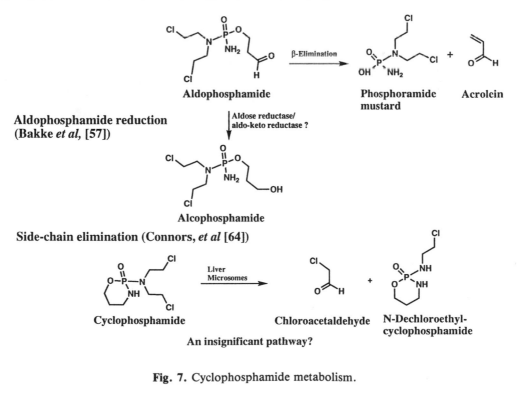

Fig. 7. Cyclophosphamide metabolism.

analytical methods. 4-Oxocyclophosphamide was well established, but more structural evidence was needed for the other three metabolites, 4-hydroxycyclophosphamide, aldophosphamide, and carboxyphosphamide.

A report from the Southern Research Institute provided the needed data for the latter compound. The labile acyclic carboxylic acid metabolite from dog and human urine was stabilized by the reaction with diazomethane and purified by column and thin-layer chromatography. The resulting methyl ester was characterized by IR, MS, and definitive synthesis. The Birmingham group showed that in humans, more than 25% of the cyclophosphamide dose was converted to the open-chain metabolite, carboxyphosphamide, whereas only 1–2% ended up as the ring-carbonyl metabolite, 4-oxocyclophosphamide. Finally, they showed that carboxyphosphamide and 4-oxocyclophosphamide had little or no anticancer activity, and concluded that they were "radically detoxified derivatives of cyclophosphamide" (*59*).

The expected aldehyde precursor of cyclophosphamide, commonly known as aldophosphamide, was converted *in situ* to a semicarbazone derivative by Norman Sladek of the University of Minnesota in 1973 (*60*). Sladek's semicarbazone was purified by thin-layer chromatography, and isolated and characterized by IR and ^{1}H nuclear magnetic resonance spectroscopy (NMR) by Robert Struck in Birmingham (*61*).

Aldophosphamide was shown by Colvin et al. of Johns Hopkins School of Medicine to be the true intermediate from which acrolein derived. Also of great interest was the coproduct of acrolein release, phosphoramide mustard, which they derivatized with diazomethane in order to obtain a mass spectrum (*62*). The synthesis of phosphoramide mustard had been reported 20 years earlier by Orrie Friedman and Arnold Seligman (*24*) and the compound was known to be a potent alkylating agent with good antitumor activity (*63*).

The first metabolite in the framework model was the last to yield the secrets of its physical properties. At the Chester Beatty Research Institute in London, Connors and coworkers tried to characterize the primary metabolite, 4-hydroxycyclophosphamide, but like many before them, found that it was too unstable for direct identification. By their efforts, however, they were able to derivatize it with ethanol and HCl to form 4-ethoxycyclophosphamide, which was then isolated and analyzed (*64*).

3.5.4. Current Perspective

The discussion above has only covered the bare essentials of cyclophosphamide metabolism. In the years since the framework model was pieced together, many new features have been fleshed out. New chemotherapeutic agents are now being developed that owe much to prior metabolism studies (*65*). Further progress will undoubtedly derive from knowledge of oxazaphosphorine metabolites and the enzymes that catalyze their formation and degradation. Toward this goal, recent studies have significantly deepened our understanding of the enzymes that activate and deactivate cyclophosphamide. Other investigations conducted during the last two decades have uncovered additional biochemical pathways and previously unknown metabolites.

The specific cytochrome P450 isozymes responsible for the primary activation of cyclophosphamide have been determined in rats and humans. The IIC6 and IIC11 isozymes are apparently the constitutive forms of importance in rats, but the phenobarbital-inducible IIB1 isozyme appears to be more efficient in response to appropriate pretreatment (*66*). The corresponding human isozymes will be identified in Section 7.1.

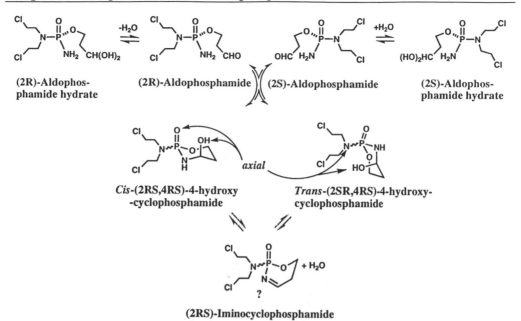

(2R)-Aldophos-   **(2R)-Aldophosphamide**   **(2S)-Aldophosphamide**   **(2S)-Aldophos-**
phamide hydrate   **phamide hydrate**

Cis-(2RS,4RS)-4-hydroxy   *Trans*-(2SR,4RS)-4-hydroxy-
-cyclophosphamide   cyclophosphamide

(2RS)-Iminocyclophosphamide

Fig. 8. Mechanisms of 4-hydroxycyclophosphamide trans-isomerization [*67,68*]).

The determination of active metabolites and exploration of their interconnecting and branching biochemical pathways have continued. The cis- and trans-isomers of 4-hydroxycyclophosphamide were analyzed by ^{31}P, ^{13}C, ^{2}H, and ^{1}H NMR spectroscopy and their equilibrium ratio, approx 2:1, was determined under physiological conditions of pH and temperature (*67*). Interconversion of the two isomers is mediated by ring opening to give aldophosphamide, which may reclose to give either cis- or trans-4-hydroxycyclophosphamide, as shown in Fig. 8. Another possible pathway has also been proposed, the dehydration of 4-hydroxycyclophosphamide to give iminocyclophosphamide. Unselective rehydration of iminocyclophosphamide may given either cis- or trans-4-hydroxycyclophosphamide (*68*).

Branching pathways lead from 4-hydroxycyclophosphamide to a series of thioconjugates in which the mercaptide groups of endogenous compounds, such as reduced glutathione (GSH), replace the 4-hydroxyl group. The reaction is reversible and the thio-conjugates are more stable than 4-hydroxycyclophosphamide. By virtue of these properties, the reversible thio-conjugate family functions as a depot supply of 4-hydroxycyclophosphamide, which would quickly decompose in the absence of a stabilizing mechanism (*67*). Reversible thiol conjugation is illustrated in Fig. 9. Irreversible coupling with GSH is also possible, leading to oxazaphosphorine and phosphoramide mustard detoxification. Reversible and irreversible coupling with thiols will be discussed later, in conjunction with mafosfamide, a useful synthetic analog of the thio-conjugates.

The detailed enzymology of carboxyphosphamide formation has now been elucidated. Aldehyde dehydrogenases in mice (AHD) and humans (ALDH) catalyze the conversion of aldophosphamide to carboxyphosphamide. In the mouse, AHD 2, 8a and 8b are active against pharmacologic concentrations of aldophosphamide (*69*). In humans, ALDH 1 is the isozyme responsible for >80% of the liver's capacity to

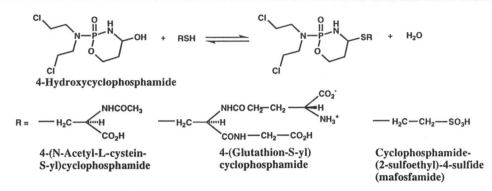

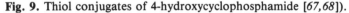

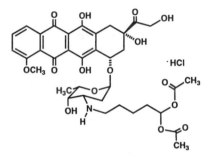

Fig. 9. Thiol conjugates of 4-hydroxycyclophosphamide [67,68]).

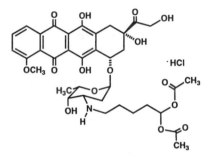

Fig. 10. *N*-(5,5-Diacetoxypent-1-yl)doxorubicin (*71*).

detoxify aldophosphamide (*70*). However, liver may not be the most important site of aldophosphamide detoxification.

Aldehyde dehydrogenase is present in nearly every nonmalignant tissue, but little or none is found in cyclophosphamide-sensitive tumors. The ability of proliferative normal tissues to detoxify aldophosphamide is curtailed in or absent from many tumors. Although other proposed mechanisms may eventually be borne out, at the present time, this the most firmly established explanation for the noncytokinetic selectivity of cyclophosphamide (*45*). Sladek has suggested the design of aldehydes or aldehyde precursors with cytotoxic pharmacophores other than phosphorylated mustard groups, in order to make further use of selective detoxification by aldehyde dehydrogenases. He cites the example of *N*-(5,5-diacetoxypentyl)doxorubicin (Fig. 10), a promising new agent that may operate on this principle (*71*).

4. STRUCTURE–ACTIVITY RELATIONSHIPS

In 1961, three of the principal figures in the development of cyclophosphamide, Arnold, Bourseaux, and Brock published the results of a large study correlating the structures and biological activities of 15 nonphosphorylated mustards and 109 mono-, di-, and triamides of phosphoric and thiophosphoric acid. The nonphosphorylated mustard group included, "the last decade's most important experimentally and clinically established nitrogen-mustard compounds": mechlorethamine, chlorambucil, and melphalan (Fig. 1); uracil mustard, mannitol mustard, and nitromin (Fig. 11).

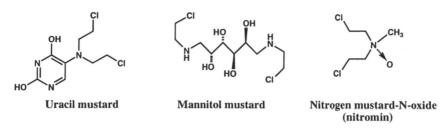

Uracil mustard　　　　Mannitol mustard　　　　Nitrogen mustard-N-oxide
(nitromin)

Fig. 11. Tertiary mustards used clinically in the 1950s (72).

The phosphorylated and thiophosphorylated nitrogen mustards were studied, "as representative compounds selected from nearly 500 synthetic products" (72).

4.1. In Vivo Testing

In keeping with their goal of finding anticancer agents with wider margins of safety, the ASTA scientists evaluated prospective agents against a direct measure of selectivity, the therapeutic index (TI = lethal dose/effective dose in 50% of test animals [73]). For TI determination, they used the Yoshida ascites sarcoma, transplanted in outbred F49 rats (74). They defined the effective dose as that which achieved complete tumor remission lasting 90 d in 50% of the rats. Intraperitoneal treatment was begun 2 h after transplantation and continued for a total of 4 consecutive days. In consideration of the four-injection regimen and the end point, they used the term $DC_{50}(4)$, or *dosus curativa,* to denote effective dose.

All of the mustards from the clinic and many of the new phosphorylated nitrogen mustards "cured" the Yoshida sarcoma, by the 90-d criterion. For speed and economy, the lethal dose was evaluated by a single ip injection followed by 21 d of observation and denoted *dosus lethalis* or $DL_{50}(1)$. The ratio $DL_{50}(1)/DC_{50}(4)$ was calculated as a modified TI and used as the biological end point for evaluation of structure–activity relationships (SAR) (72).

This approach differed from procedures employed elsewhere at the time. For example, the massive US government-sponsored screening program used T/C, a ratio of life-spans for treated vs control animals with transplanted tumors, such as L1210 lymphocytic leukemia grown as an ascites in BDF1, DCBA, or D2BC mice. Several other transplanted murine and a few rat tumor systems were also used (75). Doses were escalated until the maximal increase in median survival time (ILS = [T/C] − 1) was reached. This MTD and associated ILS were reported as indicators of potency and therapeutic effect, but the margin of safety (TI) was not routinely determined (76).

4.2. Congeneric Groups

Because a single change in a lead drug molecule will frequently affect interactions with multiple biological systems, such as cellular transport, metabolism, and target binding, SAR studies of large unrelated groups of compounds have little chance of success (77). Thus, the ASTA compounds were divided into 14 congeneric groups, as shown in Table 1. Group assignments were made on the basis of unifying structural features, e.g., fragments of the molecular skeleton that all members of a group possessed in common. The 14 congeneric groups also included a group of "clinically established" tertiary mustards, eight groups of phosphorylated ring compounds, four

Table 1
Congeneric Groups

Group no.	No. of members	Unifying structural features
1	6	Unphosphorylated tertiary mustards
2	4	Cyclophosphamide analogs with contracted or expanded rings
3	7	Substituted pentacyclic phosphoric diamides
4	14	Oxazaphosphorines, most with alkyl substituents at positions 4, 5, or 6
5	12	*N*-substituted oxazaphosphorines
6	8	Thiophosphoric diamides
7	8	*O*-*n*-alkyl phosphoramide mustards
8	16	*O*-ω-halo-*n*-alkyl phosphoramide mustards
9	12	Cyclic phosphoric or thiophosphoric monoamides
10	7	Ayclic phosphoric monoamides
11	3	Cyclic phosphoric triamides
12	7	Acyclic phosphoric triamides
13	9	Unphosphorylated secondary mustards
14	9	Oxazaphosphorines with one or both chloroethyl side chains altered

groups of phosphorylated acyclic-mustards, and one group of secondary nor-nitrogen mustard analogs with one or two modified side chains.

The unphosphorylated mustards in group 1 were included to show the range of selectivity of the best compounds available prior to cyclophosphamide. Their TI values ranged from 1.8 for uracil mustard to 6.4 for nitromin. The authors maintained that selectivity within this narrow range was inversely related to the rate of ionization of their chloro-substituents in 26 mM bicarbonate buffer, pH 7.5, at 37 °C (incubation assay). Melphalan and nitromin had slower ionization rates than mechloreth-amine, chlorambucil, uracil mustard, and mannitol mustard. This hydrolytic stability was seen as an element of latency, a property believed to confer selectivity. In proper perspective, however, the selectivities of melphalan and nitromin are sorely inadequate. The TI values of cyclophosphamide and some of its congeners are more than threefold greater than those of melphalan and nitromin, yet their margins of safety are also far from ideal.

As an ultimate example of acidic functionalization, the basicities of a series of *N*-acyl derivatives of bis(2-chloroethyl)amine prepared by Preussmann (*78*) were said to have, "practically disappeared" (*72*). They showed nominally no chloride hydrolysis and, as a consequence, were thoroughly inactive pharmacologically. However, between the extremes represented by the labile tertiary alkyl nitrogen mustards and the inert *N*-acylated secondary mustards, a continuum was envisioned from which it might be possible to pick an ideal functional type.

4.3. Limiting the Scope

A numbing range of structural possibilities were presented, even within the particular domain of phosphorylated mustards, owing to the high connectivity of the phosphorus nucleus. However, many of the groups were formed around a common structural feature that conferred decreased selectivity on all members. For example, a ≥ 50% reduction in selectivity, *vis-a-vis* cyclophosphamide, resulted when phosphorus was absent, when any atom geminal to phosphorus was replaced, when the ring size was altered, when N^3 was alkylated, or when either chloroethyl group was extended, branched, or replaced by ethyl. Thus, negative SAR findings characterized all members of the following groups: 1–3, 5, 6, and 9–14.

In the next section, SAR data for all compounds in groups 4, 7, and 8 are presented. This should not imply that that excluded groups represent structural types that hold no promise. Indeed, the authors of the original study did prudently reinvestigate some of them and made a major find, described in Section 5.

4.4. Structural Correlates of Activity and Toxicity

Three of the congeneric groups, a total of 40 compounds, included 11 compounds with TI > 10. The oxazaphosphorines in group 4, with a total of 14 compounds, had 5 members whose TI values ranged from 11.3 (B690)–20 (B618; cyclophosphamide). Group 7, with a total of eight *O-n*-alkyl phosphoramide mustards, and group 8, which contained 16 *O-ω*-halo-*n*-alkyl phosphoramide mustards each contained three highly selective compounds with TI values ranging from 12.8–17.9.

The 11 compounds with the highest activities and selectivities had several structural features in common. They were all phosphorylated monoester-diamides derived from bis(2-chloroethyl)amine. Furthermore, as the original authors of the data observed, "The most favorable derivatives are those with *n*-propylene groups in amide-like linkages with oxygen in the end position. They may be arranged either cyclically. . . (e.g. B 518, B699, B717 and B576) or aliphatically (e.g. B633, B636, B637, B612, B700, B701) " (72).

Among the oxazaphosphoramide group, shown in Table 2, substitution of any of the ring methylenes diminished selectivity. Thus, monomethylation of cyclophosphamide at positions 4, 5, or 6 caused a 28–40% decrease and vicinal 4,5-dimethylation caused a 43.5% decrease in TI. Mono substitutions by alkyl groups larger than methyl or multisubstitution beyond 4,5-dimethylation produced 50–100% reduction in TI (72).

Six of the active, selective compounds in the 1961 SAR study were phosphoramide mustard analogs, shown in Table 3. All possessed an *N*-(3-hydroxy-*n*-propyl) group. In group 7, the ethyl and *n*-propyl esters B633 and B636 were 2.3- to 2.6-fold less potent than cyclophosphamide, but their respective TI values were only 11 and 14% less.

In group 8 (Table 4), the 2-(chloroethyl) ester, B612 was also 2.6-fold less active than cyclophosphamide, but its TI was only 16% less.

These active and selective *N*-(3-hydroxy-*n*-propyl)phosphoramide mustard esters showed little frank alkylating activity and good hydrolytic stability. Four of the compounds, B633, B636, B612, and B702, released only about 15–20 mol% of their available chloride equivalents during the 24-h in vitro incubation assay with 26 m*M* bicarbonate buffer, pH 7.5. In vivo formation of an ionizable phosphoramide mustard from these compounds requires *N*-dealkylation and thus may involve a different kinetic mechanism than the base-catalyzed *O*-dealkylation of aldophosphamide. With such interesting properties, one wonders why they have been left quietly on the shelf for the past 25 years.

Table 2
Structural Correlates of Activity and Selectivity:
Congeneric Group 4: Oxazaphosphorines

ASTA Code Number	Position 4	Position 5	Position 6	DC_{50} (4) mmol/kg	Therapeutic index
Unsubstituted					
B518 (cyclo-phosphamide)	H_3C > H	H > H	H > H	0.03	20.0
Mono-substituted					
B699	H_3C > H	H > H	H > H	0.04	12.5
B717	H > H	H_3C > H	H > H	0.09	14.4
B576	H > H	H > H	H_3C > H	0.04	12.0
Di-substituted					
B690	H_3C > H	H_3C > H	H > H	0.05	11.3
B708	H > H	H_3C > H	H_3C > H	0.28	3.8
B707	H > H	H_3C > H_3C	H > H	inactive	nil
B709	H > H	H_3C > H	C_2H_5 > H	0.33	6.0
B783	H_3C > H	H > H	n-C_3H_7 > H	0.25	3.8
B784	H_3C > H	H > H	i-C_3H_7 > H	0.50	2.5
B785	H_3C > H	H > H	n-C_6H_{13} > H	0.67	1.7
Tri-substituted					
B714	H_3C > H	H > H	H_3C > H_3C	0.10	10.0
B693	H > H	H_3C > H_3C	H_3C > H	1.99	1.0
B617	H_3C > H_3C	H > H	H_3C > H	2.64	0.5
B792	H_3C > H	H_3C > H	n-C_3H_7 > H	0.91	0.7
B787	H_3C > H	H_3C > H	n-C_6H_{13} > H	inactive	nil

Table 3
Structural Correlates of Activity and Selectivity:
Congeneric Group 7: *N*-(*ω*-hydroxy/methoxy-*n*-alkyl)-*O*-*n*-alkyl Phosphoramide Mustards

ASTA code number	R =	m =	n =	DC_{50} (4) mmol/kg	Therapeutic index
B547	H	2	1	1.02	2.7
B635	H	2	2	0.49	4.0
B649	H	2	7	0.55	3.0
B633	H	3	1	0.08	17.2
B636	H	3	2	0.07	17.8
B637	H	3	7	0.05	12.8
B874	CH₃	3	1	0.86	1.3
B634	H	4	1	0.93	2.0

4.5. Stereoisomers

Although stereoisomerism was not discussed in the original paper, in 1982, Gerald Zon, of Washington, DC, reviewed the data for the compounds in group 4. Recognizing the chirality of cyclophosphamide at phosphorus and the additional asymmetric centers of the ring monosubstituted analogs, he pointed out that nongeminal substitution of 1-, 2-, or 3-ring carbon atoms would generate 4, 8, or 16, respective diasteriomers. Figure 12 shows the four stereoisomers of compound(s) B783.

Zon noted that the in vivo environment is chiral; therefore, each asymmetric center could influence the outcome of transport, enzyme metabolism, and perhaps even purely chemical reactions, which may be subject to asymmetric induction. Certainly, he argued, such isomers should possess different therapeutic indices (*79*).

Differential metabolism of stereospecifically deuterated cyclophosphamide had been demonstrated in nontumor-bearing, female Balb/c mice. Analysis of the urine metabolites by MS showed that more of the excreted 4-oxocyclophosphamide was derived from (*R*)-cyclophosphamide than from its antipode (*80*). However in humans, neither enantiomer was therapeutically superior to racemic cyclophosphamide (*81,82*).

5. DEVELOPMENT OF IFOSFAMIDE

In the SAR studies with phosphorylated mustards, a number of congeneric structural types seemed to offer no productive leads. Two examples were analogs of cyclophosphamide in which either of the *N*-(2-chloroethyl) groups was altered or the hydrogen on N³ was substituted. These modifications caused a dramatic loss of cytotoxicity and selectivity, but when both transformations were embodied in a single substance, an important new molecule resulted (*83*). In the design of this molecule, one of the 2-chloroethyl groups was taken from the bifunctional mustard side chain of cyclophosphamide and moved to the ring nitrogen (*84*).

Table 4
Structural Correlates of Activity and Selectivity:
Congeneric Group 8: *N*-Substituted-*O*-(*ω*-halo-*n*-alkyl) Phosphoramide Mustards

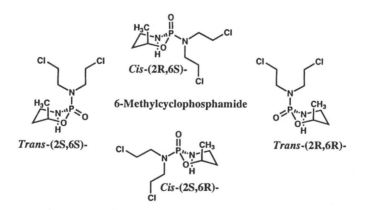

ASTA code number	R =	X =	DC_{50} (4) mmol/kg	Therapeutic index
B711	CH_2CH_3	Cl	0.49	1.0
B643	CH_2NH_2	Cl	0.92	2.0
B640	CH_2OH	Cl	0.61	4.0
B718	CH_2Cl	Cl	0.48	1.3
B612	CH_2CH_2OH	Cl	0.08	16.9
B700	CH_2CH_2OH	Br	0.05	15.0
B701	CH_2CH_2OH	CH_2Cl	0.06	15.0
B698	$CH{<}^{OH}_{CH_3}$	Cl	0.47	3.8
B719	$CH_2CH_2OCH_3$	Cl	0.84	1.0
B861	$CH_2CH_2O_2CCH_3$	Cl	0.52	4.0
B720	$CH_2CH_2N(C_2H_5)_2$	Cl	inactive	nil
B865	$CH_2CH_2O_2C(CH_2)_3Br$	Cl	0.81	2.0
B870	$CH_2CH_2O_2C$—	Cl	inactive	nil
B864	$CH_2CH_2O_2C$ Cl CH—	Cl	0.32	3.8
B664	$CH_2CH_2CH_2OH$	Cl	1.69	0.7
B696	$CH_2CH{<}^{OH}_{CH_3}$	Cl	0.11	5.0

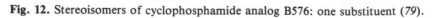

Fig. 12. Stereoisomers of cyclophosphamide analog B576: one substituent (*79*).

Table 5
Ifosfamide and Trofosfamide—Initial Preclinical Results

Common name	R =	R ' =	24-h Hydrolysis Cl^- equiv/mol	DC_{50} (4) mmol/kg	Therapeutic index
Cyclophosphamide	CH_2CH_2Cl	H	0.19	0.032	20
Ifosfamide	H	CH_2CH_2Cl	0.06	0.024	24
Trofosfamide	CH_2CH_2Cl	CH_2CH_2Cl	0.04	0.025	9

The new compound, an isomer of cyclophosphamide, was given the common name ifosfamide. An isostere, trofosfamide, with 2-chloroethyl groups at all available nitrogen valences was also synthesized and received considerable developmental attention, but has subsequently been overshadowed by ifosfamide.

5.1. Preclinical Studies

The techniques used to determine the activity of cyclophosphamide were resurrected, with a slight modification, for characterization of ifosfamide and trofosfamide. The toxicity end point was shortened to 14 d, apparently without affecting the result, since the TI of cyclophosphamide did not differ from the earlier value. Ifosfamide and trofosfamide were shown to be hydrolytically stable prodrugs by incubation at 37°C in 26 mM bicarbonate, pH 7.5 (85).

5.1.1. IN VIVO SCREENING

Against the Yoshida rat sarcoma (Table 5) a single injection of 7.7 mg·kg^{-1} of ifosfamide or 3.9 mg·kg^{-1} of cyclophosphamide gave a 50% cure rate. However, when divided doses were given daily × 4, 50% cures required only 1.58 mg·kg^{-1}·d^{-1} of ifosfamide vs 2.25 mg·kg^{-1}·d^{-1} of cyclophosphamide. This indicated that for ifosfamide, the cumulative therapeutic effect (concentration × time) was particularly important, whereas for cyclophosphamide, achieving a high peak concentration appeared to be more efficacious (86).

A variety of routes and schedules were tested by Abraham Goldin and John Venditti against "early" L1210 leukemic ascites transplant in BDF1 mice (87,88). Three of these regimens were especially informative and will be described here. Single doses of cyclophosphamide and ifosfamide given ip were both highly active (ILS > 300%). As in prior studies, the optimal single dose of ifosfamide, 300 mg·kg^{-1} exceeded that of cyclophosphamide, 180 mg·kg^{-1}. When daily ip doses were divided over 9 d, the optimum dose of ifosfamide, 65 mg·kg^{-1}·d^{-1} still exceeded that of cyclophosphamide, 39 mg·kg^{-1}·d^{-1}. Furthermore, this schedule was inferior to the single dose, since for both drugs, optimal total doses were almost twofold greater and the response much poorer (ILS = 50%). In a third regimen, the doses were divided into 3 ip injections given on days 1, 5, and 9. The optimal dose of ifosfamide was 39 mg·kg^{-1}·d^{-1}, and it gave an ILS of 85%, but that of cyclophosphamide was 108 mg·kg^{-1} giving an ILS of

70%. Therefore, ifosfamide was more potent and therapeutic than cyclophospha-mide on this schedule, but was yet more effective as a single dose, contrary to the Yoshida sarcoma data.

Taken together, the rat sarcoma and mouse leukemia data were inconclusive. Inter-species data did not reveal an unequivocally optimal schedule and probably cannot. For humans, however, a clearer answer to this question did surface, as described below in Section 5.2.

Two additional models studied by Goldin (88) were an advanced L1210 leukemia that was naturally resistant to cyclophosphamide and an L1210 with acquired cyclo-phosphamide resistance developed by treatment over a series of transplant genera-tions. In the naturally resistant system, the optimal single dose of cyclophosphamide, 180 mg·kg^{-1} gave an ILS of 144%. The optimal single dose of ifosfamide, 500 mg·kg^{-1}, gave an ILS of 178%. Thus, ifosfamide was tolerated at a higher dose and was moderately more effective than cyclophosphamide. Goldin did note, however, that the advanced L1210, unlike the early strain, was metastatic at the time treatment began. The subline of L1210 with acquired cyclophosphamide resistance was com-pletely crossresistant to ifosfamide.

Against murine Lewis lung carcinoma, C3H mammary adenocarcinoma, and TA nephroblastoma, ifosfamide was slightly more effective than cyclophosphamide. Against Ridgway osteogenic sarcoma and DS carcinosarcoma, ifosfamide was much more active than cyclophosphamide.

In combination with cisplatin, 5-fluorouracil, cytarabine, camptothecin, or cyclo-cytidine, the activity of ifosfamide against L1210 was greater than additive. It was only additive with cyclophosphamide, lomustine, or semustine (88). Against Yoshida sarcoma, ifosfamide was synergistic with vincristine (89).

5.1.2. PRECLINICAL TOXICOLOGY

Acute, subacute, and chronic toxicity, carcinogenicity, and genotoxicity were mon-itored in mice, rats, dogs, or rabbits. In mice and rats, acute toxicity was determined using oral, iv, and ip administration, and in rats, the sc route was also tested. The dogs and rabbits were given iv injections. Ifosfamide was well tolerated parenterally, and toxicities were milder than expected for a nitrogen mustard.

Acute toxicities included reversible leucopenia, lymphoid depression, cystitis, and alopecia. Acute and subacute urine bladder irritation also occurred. The delayed toxicities were marrow depletion cistitis, enteritis, pneumonia, and testicular atrophy. Chronic lethality was owing to enteritis and pneumonitis.

Rat carcinogenicity assays revealed significant leiomyosarcoma and mammary fibro-adenoma in females. In mice, carcinogenicity testing showed a dose-related increase in malignant lymphomas.

The reproductive toxicology of ifosfamide was evaluated in pregnant mice, rats, and rabbits. Lethal and sublethal embryotoxic effects, e.g., diminished survival, stunting, and craniofacial abnormalities, were seen in all three species (90).

5.2. Early Clinical Trials

Any analog of a highly active agent must be shown to possess distinct advantages over those of the lead drug before it can be introduced into the clinic. One would ex-pect this criterion to be especially stringent in the case of an isomer of the parent compound. In spite of this, a multi-institutional clinical trial in which 49 patients were treated with ifosfamide and 244 with trofosfamide was begun in 1967 (*83*) and results were published early in 1970 (*91*). The latter publication came only three years after the two compounds were first announced to the world at the Fifth International Chemotherapy Congress (*84*). Favorable preclinical screening results with the Yoshida sarcoma apparently accelerated the transition from bench to bedside (*83*). Although some of the initial enthusiasm dampened after reports of severe urothelial toxicity (*92*), development of an effective uroprotector rekindled worldwide interest (*93*).

The early clinical development of ifosfamide went through three stages. The first clinical trial, begun in 1967, used low doses, with disappointing results. For solid tumors, the average dose and duration of treatment were 75 mg·m^{-2}·d^{-1} × 98 d and for systemic disease, 180 mg·m^{-2}·d^{-1} × 63 d (*91*). Next, single doses of 2.9–10 g·m^{-2} were given, resulting in a high remission rate against metastasized solid tumors, but leucopenia, CNS toxicity, and urotoxicity were dose-limiting above 5 g·m^{-2}(*94*). Animal experiments had shown that fractionated doses of ifosfamide had a cumulative therapeutic effect, but toxicity was less cumulative. These findings were incorporated into plans for the third stage of clinical testing.

A large cooperative trial, with 390 patients, were performed with ifosfamide as a single agent. The study compared single vs divided daily doses. A broad spectrum of malignancies were treated, including ovarian, mammary, gastric, pancreatic, colonic, cervical, uterine, and bronchial carcinomas, germ-cell tumors, malignant melanoma, and various sarcomas. The best results were obtained with daily injections of 2.0–2.4 g·m^{-2}·d^{-1} × 5 d (*95*). This finding was confirmed in another cooperative trial with 360 patients, also with a wide variety of solid tumors. Optimum daily doses of 2.4 g·m^{-2}·d^{-1} × 5 d were determined, except for treatment of osteo- or chondrosarcoma, where the schedule was 1.2 g·m^{-2}·d^{-1} × 10 d (*96*).

The dose-limiting urotoxicity that occurred in these early clinical trials had been seen previously with cyclophosphamide, but with an average frequency of only 7% The incidence of urotoxicity with ifosfamide ranged between 20 and 40% (*97*). Development of an effective uroprotector was sorely needed.

5.3. Supportive Care: MESNA and Beyond

Acrolein, formed by β-elimination from aldophosphamide, was identified as the principal etiologic agent of oxazaphosphorine urotoxicity (*93*). Chloroacetaldehyde, a minor metabolite of cyclophosphamide, but a major neurotoxic metabolite of ifosfamide, also contributes to oxazaphosphorine urotoxicity (*98*). The ability of thiol compounds, such as *N*-acetylcysteine, to detoxify acrolein and chloroacetaldehyde was recognized, but when given systemically, *N*-acetylcysteine also conjugated therapeutivally active metabolites. Local instillation of *N*-acetylcysteine into the bladder failed to protect the renal pelvis or ureter (*93*).

A detoxicant was sought for systemic administration that would act only in the urine to protect the whole urinary tract, without compromising therapeutic activity. In 1979, Scheef and associates published preliminary data indicating that 2-mercaptoethanesulfonate, or MESNA, met these criteria (*99*). Subsequent trials have demonstrated that MESNA is the agent of choice for uroprotection because of its effectiveness, ease of administration, and lack of systemic toxicity (*100*).

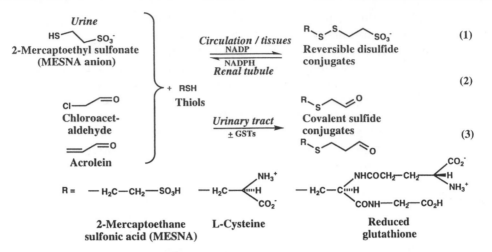

Fig. 13. Chemistry of MESNA and endogenous thiols in vivo (*93,102*).

The MESNA molecule has a negatively charged, water-solubilizing sulfo-group linked by an ethylene spacer to a strongly nucleophilic thiol group. MESNA is capable of inactivating alkylating agents, such as chloroacetaldehyde, or its oxidation product, chloroacetic acid, by covalent replacement of their halogen leaving groups (*101*). When given with cyclophosphamide, MESNA can reversibly sequester 4-hydroxy-cyclophosphamide by substituting the 2-sulfoethanesulfide moiety in place of the hydroxyl. Most importantly, it can detoxify an α, β-unsaturated ketone or aldehyde, such as acrolein, by conjugate addition to the olefinic double bond (*102*). The structure and in vivo chemistry of MESNA are shown in Fig. 13.

After entering the circulation, MESNA is rapidly oxidized to a nonnucleophilic symmetrical disulfide known as diMESNA. More than 90% of the circulating drug is in this form. Unsymmetrical disulfides are also formed by conjugation of MESNA with endogenous thiol compounds, such as cysteine. The disulfide products are incapable of systemic detoxification of acrolein, alkylators, or activated oxazaphosphorines, nor do they affect the activity of other electrophilic anticancer agents, such as cisplatin, nitrosoureas, or doxorubicin (*93*).

In the renal tubule, a large proportion of the disulfides are reconverted to thiol compounds by reduction. The reducing agent is NADPH, and the reaction is catalyzed by GSH. The proposed catalytic cycle is shown in Fig. 14. The reaction takes place during glomerular filtration, and the thiols are released into the urine. Their protective action is present in the renal pelvis, ureter, and bladder (*102*).

The discovery of MESNA was a pivotal step in the development of supportive care. The field is growing, as demonstrated by the development of hematopoietic growth factor (*103*) and stem cell support (*104*).

6. RECENT CLINICAL TRIALS WITH IFOSFAMIDE

Clinical trials of new anticancer agents are ordinarily conducted in sequential phases denoted phase I, II, and III (*105*). Occasionally, phases I and II are combined into a single sequence. Phase IV trials are conducted infrequently, when the need arises to monitor uncommon, idiosyncratic, or delayed complications of drug treatment.

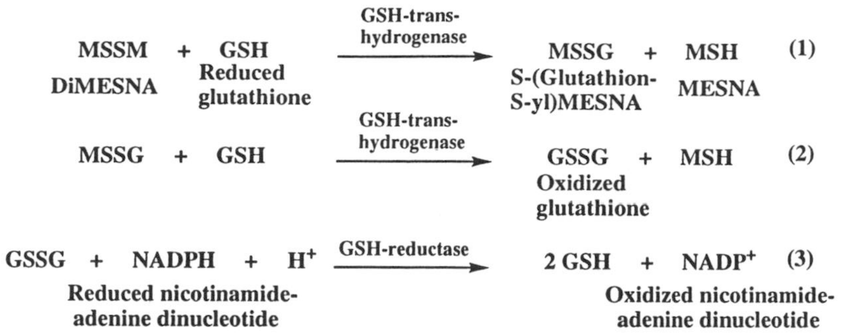

$$\text{MSSM} + \text{GSH} \xrightarrow{\text{GSH-trans-hydrogenase}} \text{MSSG} + \text{MSH} \quad (1)$$

DiMESNA   Reduced glutathione   S-(Glutathion-S-yl)MESNA   MESNA

$$\text{MSSG} + \text{GSH} \xrightarrow{\text{GSH-trans-hydrogenase}} \text{GSSG} + \text{MSH} \quad (2)$$

Oxidized glutathione

$$\text{GSSG} + \text{NADPH} + \text{H}^+ \xrightarrow{\text{GSH-reductase}} 2\,\text{GSH} + \text{NADP}^+ \quad (3)$$

Reduced nicotinamide-adenine dinucleotide   Oxidized nicotinamide-adenine dinucleotide

Fig. 14. MESNA/diMESNA catalytic cycle (*102*).

Phase I clinical trials of anticancer agents have two objectives: providing the best available treatment and determining the optimal treatment dose. The method involves escalation of doses (one drug at a time in combination studies) to a level at which either the desired biologic effect is observed or the limit of tolerability is reached. In the latter case, the penultimate dose is then usually considered the MTD. Since patients with advanced cancer are usually chosen for phase I studies, the toxic end point is most often encountered, rather than the therapeutic. Nonetheless, the therapeutic intent is implicit; studies are not undertaken to see how sick a drug will make someone.

Phase II trials are undertaken to provide a population of patients the most effective diagnosis-specific treatment available, to assess the degree of response of each evaluable patient, and to determine diagnosis-specific response rates and their statistical significance. Although Phase I trials may include diverse and sometimes unusual types of cancer, Phase II trials are more homogeneous and are often specific to one tumor type.

Phase III investigations are comparative trials undertaken to determine whether a new treatment is better than standard therapy or other competitive therapies. Comparative statistical inference requires randomized groups and a large sample. Therefore, Phase III trials are often cooperative studies requiring the joint effort of many hospitals (*106*).

Single-agent clinical regimens were once the rule, but are now the exception. Most current ifosfamide studies include one or more other drugs. Structures of some of the drugs used in combination chemotherapy with ifosfamide are shown in Fig. 15. Several combinations currently under investigation are defined in Table 6.

6.1. Phase I: Defining Doses and Toxicity Limits

The toxicities of cyclophosphamide and ifosfamide are steeply dose-dependent, but for ifosfamide, schedule and route are also important determinants of certain specific toxicities (*89*). Dose-related renal failure was documented in early clinical trials with ifosfamide possibly because of pre-existing renal dysfunction and/or inadequate hydration (*92*). The problem persists, but its incidence is declining as a result of closer monitoring of renal function and improved support. Nonetheless, high-dose continuous infusion of 5.0 or 8.0 g·m^{-2} of ifosfamide produced renal deterioration in 7/40 evaluable patients in a phase II single-agent study. The toxicities occurred despite administration of 400 or 600 mg·m^{-2} of MESNA, before and during chemotherapy. Two of these patients died, and two others suffered renal tubular damage (*107*).

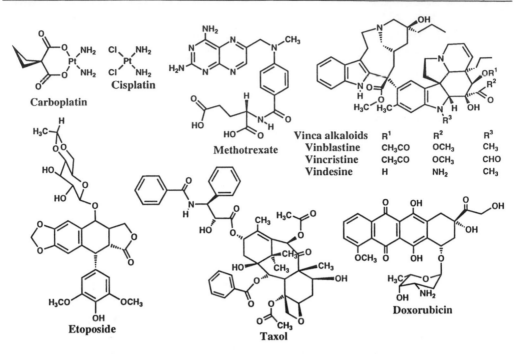

Fig. 15. Anticancer agents used in combination with ifosfamide.

The schedule dependency of ifosfamide toxicity found in preclinical studies and confirmed in early clinical trials has not been ignored in phase I trials. Fractionated single-agent ifosfamide doses of 2.4 g·m^{-2}·d^{-1} × 5 d with MESNA uroprotection have appeared in several reports (*105*).

Intravenous fractionated dosing is labor-intensive, costly, and prone to accidents. These and other motivations have prompted the use of continuous infusions. In a recently published study, marathon 240-h continuous infusions of single-agent ifosfamide were given without stem cell support. The MTD was 1.2–1.3 g·m^{-2}·d^{-1} × 10 d (*108*).

The most important route-dependent side effect of ifosfamide is neurotoxicity associated with oral administration. Symptoms of neurotoxicity occurred in 5/10 patients who received ifosfamide po 1.5 g·m^{-2}·d^{-1} × 5 d and in 4/6 who received ifosfamide po 2.0 g·m^{-2}·d^{-1} × 5 d (*109*).

The neurotoxic side effects of ifosfamide are attributed to overproduction of chloroacetaldehyde. Chloroacetaldehyde is a minor metabolite of cyclophosphamide, but is formed in significant amounts from ifosfamide. In sporadic cases, it is the most abundant ifosfamide metabolite. In two instances, patients who developed encephalopathy during ifosfamide treatment were relieved of their symptoms by treatment with methylene blue (*110,111*), a redox regulator that has been used in the treatment of cyanide poisoning (*112*).

It is frequently noted that, "the optimal doses and schedule of administration of ifosfamide still remain to be defined" (*105*). This may be a repercussion of the attractive array of new treatment options that are now under development, with very specific disease states as targets. Some of these, which utilize ifosfamide-based chemotherapeutic combinations, may require dosage reduction in order to facilitate an overall increase in dose intensity. Other designs may employ up-to-date support measures, such as

Table 6
Ifosfamide-Based Chemotherapeutic Drug Combinations

Acronym	Ifosfamide/MESNA combined with	Application
DI	Doxorubicin	Induction of SCLC, extensive NSCLC, relapsed ALL, advanced soft tissue sarcoma
IF/DDP	Cisplatin	Salvage of Ewing's spindle-cell, osteogenic, and synovial sarcomas, liposarcoma, fibrosarcoma testicular carcinomas
VI	Etoposide	Salvage of Hodgkin's and non-Hodgkin's lymplomas, salvage of testicular cancers
VIP	Etoposide (VP-16) and cisplatin	Induction of salvage of germ-cell tumors, salvage of SCLC, induction of NSCLC
IFF/MTX	Methotrexate	Intensification of SCLC
IFF/VDS	Vindesine	Salvage of SCLC
VIPE	Vincristine, etoposide, and carboplatin	Salvage of germ-cell tumors
VeIP	Vinblastine and cisplatin	Salvage of germ-cell tumors, salvage of SCLC, state IV head and neck carcinoma
ICE	Carboplatin and etoposide	Alternated weekly with DI for induction of SCLC; recurring pediatric solid tumors
VICE	Vincristine, carboplatin and etoposide	Salvage of SCLC
ICE-T	Carboplatin, etoposide and taxol	Phase I lung, breast cancer, sarcoma, adenoid cystic carcinoma
IME	Methotrexate and etoposide	Salvage of non-Hodgkin's lymploma
IMEP	Methotrexate, etoposide, and prednisone	Salvage of non-Hodgkin's lymploma; induction treatment of Hodgkin's disease
MIME	Mitoguazone, methotrexate, and etoposide	Salvage of non-Hodgkin's lymploma
IMV	Methotrexate and vincristine	Advanced malignant lymphoma
MAID	Mesna, doxorubicin, and dacarbazine	Advanced soft-tissue sarcoma
No acronym	Epirubicin and fluorouracil	Advanced breast cancer

administration of autologous hematopoietic progenitor cells, to counterbalance those adjustments (*113,114*). The establishment of "standard" doses, schedules, or routes of ifosfamide administration may be delayed indefinitely because its wide activity spectrum opens up so many avenues of clinical exploration.

Two recent protocols demonstrate the broad range of scheduling that may be applied to a single drug combination. One of these, a 96-h concurrent, continuous, iv infusion of the three-drug ICE combination, with autologous hematopoietic stem cell reinfusion, had an ifosfamide MTD of 4.0 $g \cdot m^{-2} \cdot d^{-1} \times 4$ d (*104*). For another ICE/transplant protocol, divided daily doses of ifosfamide were given by 1-h iv infusion with an MTD of 3.35 $g \cdot m^{-2} \cdot d^{-1} \times 6$ d. In the latter version of ICE, the carboplatin was given 11 h after each ifosfamide dose, by 1-h infusion. Etoposide was administered by 11-h continuous infusion twice daily when the other two drugs were off (*113*). These two studies span the range of possibilities from continuous, concurrent to discontinuous, countercurrent scheduling.

6.2. Phases II and III: Evaluation and Comparison

Depending on the site and type of disease, ifosfamide treatment may be given in any of the following settings: induction, or primary therapy, where the patient is previously untreated and the intent is cure or at least remission; consolidation, treatment given to maintain a complete remission or convert a partial response after induction into a complete remission (also termed intensification); and salvage, treatment given in the hope of re-establishing remission after relapse or to overcome the resistance of a refractory tumor. Neoadjuvant chemotherapy may be given prior to surgery to facilitate complete resection of bulky or otherwise inaccessible disease (*105*).

End point data from different clinical trials need to be determined in a uniform manner, allowing comparison of intertrial results. Therefore, standard response descriptions have been established by the World Health Organization and the International Union Against Cancer. According to their criteria, the number of objective responses in a given clinical trial is the sum of patients exhibiting partial and complete responses. Complete response is the absence of clinical, histological, and biochemical evidence of disease for 2 mo or more. For assessment of partial response, pretreatment measurements are taken in all patients of the longest diameter (D) of each lesion and the widest diameter (d) perpendicular to this. The two measurements of each lesion are multiplied together, and all of these products are summed ($\Sigma = D_1 d_1 + D_2 d_2 + D_3 d_3 + \ldots + D_n d_n$). The measurements are repeated posttreatment for patients who do not have a complete response. If Σ(posttreatment)/Σ(pretreatment) $\leq$ 0.5 and no lesion increases in size and no new lesions are found, this constitutes a partial response (*106*).

Among the malignancies against which ifosfamide/MESNA have been tested, alone or in combination with other agents, we must include pancreatic, head and neck, esophageal, gastrointestinal, colorectal, and renal cell cancers. Data are sparse, but for some of these diagnoses, the outlook is grim (*105*). Against this, there is guarded optimism for the development of ifosfamide/MESNA regimens, with or without other drugs, to combat lung, breast, gynecological and testicular cancers, lymphomas, sarcomas, and pediatric solid tumors.

Within these seven disease categories are found tumors that differ widely in their sensitivity to chemotherapeutic agents. They are therefore subclassified according to prognosis. For example, non-Hodgkin's lymphoma and nonsmall-cell lung cancer (NSCLC) have, on average, poorer treatment outcomes than Hodgkin's disease and small-cell lung cancer (SCLC). Comparative and noncomparative trials usually cover one, and rarely more than two diagnostic subtypes, since the data for each must be analyzed individually (*106*).

6.2.1. LUNG CANCERS

Lung cancers are the most common malignancies and their incidence is increasing (*115*). Although cisplatin or carboplatin in combination with etoposide are the more frequently used regimens for SCLC (*116*), ifosfamide is highly active against this disease (*117*). Against extensive SCLC, single-agent ifosfamide gave an overall response rate of 48% (*118*).

Combination chemotherapy is superior to single-agent treatment for SCLC (*119*). In a randomized trial with 166 patients with previously untreated, extensive SCLC, ifosfamide, etoposide, and cisplatin (VIP), given daily for 4 d, were compared with the standard etoposide/cisplatin regimen. Overall response rates were not significantly different (70% for VIP vs 66% for etoposide/cisplatin), but 1-, 2-, and 3-yr survival rates and toxicity were significantly greater with the three-drug combination (*120*).

For initial chemotherapy of NSCLC, ifosfamide has provided objective response rates of ≥ 20% in single-agent trials with MESNA uroprotection (*121*). However, its inclusion into standard induction therapy (*105*) or high-dose triple or quadruple regimens (*122*), with autologous bone marrow reinfusion, has not improved them significantly. In the neoadjuvant setting, ifosfamide and MESNA have been combined with etoposide and cisplatin (VIP), allowing a 55% complete resection rate (*123*).

6.2.2. BREAST CANCERS

Breast cancers remain the most prevalent malignancies of women, and their incidence appears to be increasing (*124*). Metastatic disease is considered incurable, although high-dose cyclophosphamide-based combination regimens with stem-cell support are now being evaluated in the hope of curing at least some of these patients (*125*). Ifosfamide/MESNA also has substantial activity as a single agent against advanced breast cancer (*126*), and this has prompted its integration into combination protocols (*105*). A trial of ifosfamide/epirubicin/fluorouracil gave a 79% objective response rate and 25% complete responses with 28 evaluable patients (*127*).

6.2.3. GYNECOLOGICAL CANCERS

Primary therapy of advanced ovarian carcinoma with ifosfamide gave a 33% objective response rate. This was viewed as similar to the response rate with conventional alkylating agents. In a Phase II Gynecologic Oncology Group (GOG) trial of ifosfamide for salvage treatment of ovarian carcinoma, there were 3 complete and 5 partial clinical responses among 41 evaluable patients who were refractory to, or had relapsed after cisplatin treatment. In two other salvage trials against advanced ovarian carcinoma, lack of complete crossresistance was observed toward cyclophosphamide (3 objective responses/49 evaluable patients) and chlorambucil (3 objective responses/ 12 chlorambucil refractory patients) (*128*).

Another GOG trial of ifosfamide for salvage treatment of advanced squamous carcinoma of the cervix gave 3 responses, duration 1.8, 2.2, and 3.1 mo in 27 evaluable patients. Two responders had previously relapsed after cisplatin and the third after carboplatin chemotherapy (*129*).

Salvage treatment of advanced or metastatic uterine sarcoma with ifosfamide gave 5 complete and 3 partial responses among 26 patients with about equal numbers of homogeneous and heterogeneous müllerian tumors. Among 28 patients with advanced uterine leiomyosarcomas, 4 partial responses to ifosfamide were seen (*129*).

6.2.4. TESTICULAR CANCERS

About 95% of testicular cancers are seminomatous and nonsemanomitous germ-cell tumors. Approximately 25% of nonseminomatous tumors relapse after standard treatment. Salvage chemotherapy with ICE has achieved a complete remission rate of 25% in a 42 patient study, with 40 evaluable (*130*).

Standard treatment for early seminoma is radiotherapy, but for bulky disease, chemotherapy is the primary treatment modality. In these cases, cisplatin, bleomycin, and either vinblastine or etoposide are used for induction (*131*). Substitution of ifosfamide for bleomycin has given an 87% complete response rate in 24 patients with bulky disease (*132*).

6.2.5. LYMPHOMAS

Induction treatment of Hodgkin's disease by rapidly alternating cycles of two non-crossresistant regimens, such as cyclophosphamide/vincristine/procarbazine/predni-sone (COPP) and doxorubicin/bleomycin/vinblastine/dacarbazine (ABVD), has been supplemented with a third combination, ifosfamide/methotrexate/etoposide/prednisone (IMEP). In the first group of 38 patients to receive IMEP, the complete response rate was 95% (*133*).

A small group of six patients treated with IMV as induction treatment for non-Hodgkin's lymphoma had 67% complete responses. This is about as good as cyclo-phosphamide/doxorubicin/vincristine/prednisone (CHOP), on the best standard induction protocol (*134*).

For late consolidation and salvage treatment of Hodgkin's and non-Hodgkin's lym-phoma, the related combinations IME and MIME are promising additions to the armamemtarium (*134,135*). For salvage and late intensification treatment of non-Hodgkin's lymphoma, MIME has achieved a 60% objective response rate, 24% of which were complete responses in a 208 patient study (*134*).

6.2.6. SARCOMAS

For a group of 105 patients with advanced soft tissue sarcomas, the MAID com-bination achieved a 45% objective response rate. Median survival was 15.5 mo (*136*).

High-dose ifosfamide (4 g $\cdot m^{-2} \cdot d^{-1} \times 3$ d) without stem-cell support was able to overcome resistance to standard-dose ifosfamide (SDI) in a French study. Among 36 evaluable patients, 12 achieved partial responses. Among the responders, five had been refractory to SDI, two were SDI resistant, four were listed as indeterminate SDI sensitive, and only one had not received SDI previously (*110*).

Responding to Phase III results, The Soft Tissue and Bone Sarcoma Group of the European Organization for Research on Treatment of Cancer (EORTC) has deter-mined that ifosfamide is the latent alkylator of choice for soft tissue sarcoma (*105*). This decision was based on a comparative study of ifosfamide/MESNA vs cyclophos-phamide/MESNA that found a statistically significant difference in overall responses of 18 vs 8%, respectively (*136*).

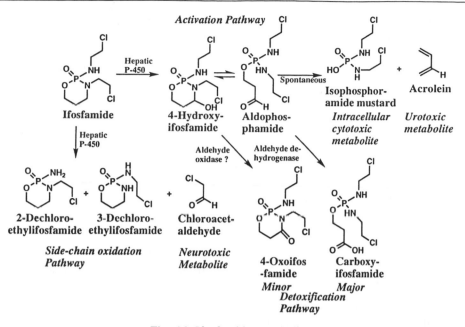

Fig. 16. Ifosfamide metabolism.

6.2.7. PEDIATRIC SOLID TUMORS

Single-agent ifosfamide with MESNA uroprotection has demonstrated activity as salvage treatment against pediatric solid tumors resistant to cyclophosphamide (*105*).

The ICE combination has produced >50% objective response rates against persistent or recurring pediatric solid tumors of various diagnostic types. Investigations of new modalities of supportive care are under way, seeking to enhance recovery and allow greater dose intensification (*137*).

7. OXAZAPHOSPHORINE DISPOSITION

The in vivo dispositions of cyclophosphamide and ifosfamide are qualitatively similar, but quantitatively very different. What structural differences influence their comparative metabolism and pharmacokinetics? In cyclophosphamide, the ring phosphoramide group is secondary and the sidechain phosphoramide group is tertiary. This situation is reversed in ifosfamide. As a consequence, the relative rates of initial activation are not the same, nor are the active/toxic metabolite ratios. These quantitative differences in metabolism lead to dose- and schedule-dependent differences in pharmacokinetic half-life, whole-body clearance, and apparent volume of distribution.

The in vivo activation and degradation of cyclophosphamide and the methods used to characterize its metabolites were described previously. Corresponding studies of ifosfamide are presented here.

7.1. Metabolism of Ifosfamide

Hepatic microsomal hydroxylation of the ifosfamide ring carbon adjacent to N^3 generates the primary activation products (Fig. 16). The C^4-hydroxyl group may occupy axial or equitorial positions on the chair conformers of the four diasterio-mers. Because they are too unstable in aqueous solution for direct isolation, cis- and trans-4-hydroxyifosfamide were derivatized by addition of ethanol during the in vitro microsomal oxidation of the ^{32}P-labeled ifosfamide. The resulting derivatives, cis-and trans-4-ethoxyifosfamide, were separated by thin-layer radiochromatography and characterized by low-temperature ($\leq 100\,°C$) direct insertion MS (*64*).

Akira Takamizawa and coworkers in Osaka, Japan described the synthesis of cis-4-hydroxyifosfamide (mp 74–75 °C) by reduction of cis-4-hydroperoxyifosfamide with triethylphosphite (*138*). Subsequently, they discovered that cis-4-hydroperoxyi-fosfamide could be trans-isomerized in chloroform solution by a catalytic amount of 4-toluenesulfonic acid. They separated the isomers by column chromatography and reduced the trans-4-hydroperoxyifosfamide with triethylphosphite to obtain trans-4-hydroxyifosfamide (mp 49–50 °C) (*139*).

In aqueous solution, the underivatized conformers of 4-hydroxyifosfamide are in rapid pseudo-equilibrium. Their interconversion is mediated by hydrolytic cleavage of N^3—C^4 bond, which generates aldoisophosphamide hydrate. Reannulation may pro-ceed by nonspecific syn- or anti-addition of N^3—H to the carbonyl group, leading to a mixture of isomers. The isomers and their equilibria were characterized by Jila Boal and associates in Washington, DC and Bethesda, MD, using ^{31}P NMR spectroscopy (*140*).

The individual steps involved in ifosfamide metabolism are analogous to those of cyclophosphamide (*45*), but there are important kinetic and thermodynamic differences that must not be overlooked. Although cyclophosphamide and ifosfamide are con-verted to their primary activation products by cytochrome P-450-catalyzed oxidation at positionally and stereochemically analogous ring sites, the human isozymes responsible are not the same. The major constitutive activator of cyclophosphamide is CYP2C9, but that of ifosfamide is the less catalytically efficient CYP3A4 isozyme (*141*).

Interpatient differences in the extent of cyclophosphamide activation have been ascribed to phenotypic polymorphism in the CYP2C cluster (*142*). However, the K_m of ifosfamide for these isozymes is so large that this polymorphism cannot be the reason for the observed variability of ifosfamide activation.

Cyclophosphamide activation rates are enhanced by phenobarbital induction of CYP2B6. Cyclophosphamide metabolism by this inducible form of cytochrome P-450 is more efficient than that of ifosfamide by eightfold, and it makes little (*141*) or no contribution to ifosfamide metabolism (*142*).

Aldehyde dehydrogenases, found in most normal human cells, detoxify aldoiso-phosphamide (*45*). The product, carboxyisophosphamide, is eliminated in the urine. Further oxidation of 4-hydroxyifosfamide probably takes place in the liver, giving 4-oxoifosfamide as a minor detoxification product, which also appears in the urine.

The ability of normal cells to detoxify aldophosphamide is absent or weakly ex-pressed in oxazaphosphorine-sensitive tumor cells. This is a well-defined mechanism of selectivity for cyclophosphamide. It probably works for ifosfamide as well, although the definitive experiments have not yet been performed.

Both carboxyisophosphamide and 4-oxoifosfamide have been found in human urine by Alan Boddy and Jeffrey Idle, of the University of Newcastle upon Tyne. They isolated ifosfamide, carboxyisophosphamide, 4-oxoifosfamide, 2-dechloro-ethylifosfamide, and 3-dechloroethylifosfamide by thin-layer chromatography and identified them by cochromatography of authentic standards (*143*).

T. A. Connors and coworkers originally identified 2- and 3-dechloroethylifosfamide during their characterization of cis- and trans-4-hydroxyifosfamide (*64*). The two dechloroethylated species, account for as much as 48 (*144*) or 50% (*145*) of an administered dose of ifosfamide in some patients. Their in vivo abundance and variability are consequences of the 2-chloroethyl group on the ring nitrogen. Owing to steric hindrance, inductive effects, or both, the N^3-substituted molecule is a poor substrate for the efficient, constitutive CYP2C9 or inducible 2B6 isozymes that rapidly activate cyclophosphamide (*141*). The less-efficient CYP3A isozymes that oxidize ifosfamide are apparently also less regioselective. The hydroxylation responsible for *N*-dechloroethylation of oxazaphosphorine mustards occurs vicinal to chlorine, producing an unstable phosphoramidol that spontaneously eliminates chloroacetaldehyde, a neurotoxic metabolite (*146*) that can also be harmful to kidney function (*147,148*).

Most of an administered dose of ifosfamide is eliminated by the toxification and detoxification reactions described above. Its therapeutic power resides in the small remnant of ring-activated molecules that are converted to aldoisophosphamide, and then avoid further oxidation by entering sites of low aldehyde dehydrogenase activity. These sites lie specifically within tumor tissues. Here the cytotoxic isophosphoramide mustard is released together with acrolein. The *O*-dealkylation of aldophosphamide and aldoisophosphamide is catalyzed by general base (*149*). Acrolein elimination from aldophosphamide may also be catalyzed by enzymes, possibly DNA polymerase-associated 3′,5′-exonucleases (*150*). If so, aldoisophosphamide could, likewise, be a substrate.

Alarcon et al. first demonstrated the release of acrolein from ifosfamide after its microsomal conversion to aldoisophosphamide (*151*). The DNA-binding coproduct, isophosphoramide mustard, was identified by ^{31}P-NMR (*140*).

Cyclophosphamide is an analog of mechloroethamine, but ifosfamide is not. This distinction impacts their metabolism from beginning to end, but particularly at the level of DNA binding. Because cyclophosphamide and mechlorethamine have the same bis(2-chloroethyl)amino pharmacophore, their respective phosphoramide mustard and aziridinium metabolites span similar interhelical DNA crosslinking distances. In contrast, the covalent binding arms of isophosphoramide mustard can connect more widely separated DNA nucleobases (Fig. 17).

In addition to their structural dimensions, there are important kinetic properties that distinguish phosphoramide and isophosphoramide mustards. The 2-chloroethyl groups of isophosphoramide mustard, each occupying its own secondary nitrogen, are capable of cyclizing independently. However, phosphoramide mustard's chloroethyl groups share a single nitrogen and must cyclize in order. In view of these differences, one might expect the first alkylation step of isophosphoramide mustard to be twice as rapid as that of phosphoramide mustard, but it is not. Kinetic experiments have shown that step one is fourfold faster for phosphoramide mustard ($t_{1/2} = 20$ min) than for isophosphoramide mustard ($t_{1/2} = 80$ min). The apparent twofold statistical edge is heavily counterbalanced by the weaker nucleophilicity of isophosphoramide mustard's nitrogens.

The rate difference is even greater in the second alkylation step, since, at this point, both compounds have a single cyclizing group. The $t_{1/2}$ for cyclization of the remaining chloroethyl group of the phosphoramide mustard monoadduct is unchanged, 20 min. For the isophosphoramide mustard monoadduct, it is extended to 170 min. The biological consequences of these rate disparities are not entirely clear, but it has been

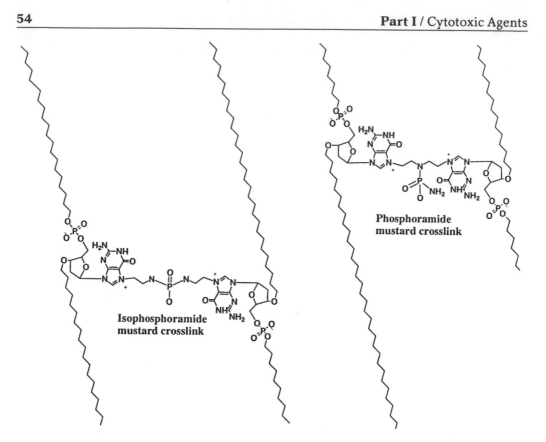

Fig. 17. Arm lengths of phosphoramide and isophosphoramide mustards.

speculated that within the cell, proportionately more isophosphoramide mustard may endure the commute to the nucleus and end up in a DNA crosslink (*140*).

7.2. Pharmacokinetics of Cyclophosphamide and Ifosfamide

In vivo rates of absorption, distribution, and elimination of drugs and their conversion to metabolites are the concern of pharmacokinetics. Three fundamental pharmacokinetic parameters are: elimination half-life ($t_{1/2}$), apparent distribution volume (V_{ap}), and whole-body clearance (Cl_t). They are interrelated according to the expression: $t_{1/2} = (V_{ap}/Cl_t)(\ln 2)$.

Elimination half-life is the time required for clearance of one-half of a bolus dose from the body fluid, blood, or plasma in which it is uniformly distributed. Apparent distribution volume is the volume of the phase in which the drug initially distributes to give a peak concentration, C_{max}. Thus C_{max} is inversely proportional to V_{ap}. Whole-body clearance ($mL \cdot min^{-1}$) is the fractional relationship between the delivered dose, D (millimoles), and the total exposure, AUC ($mmol \cdot mL^{-1} \cdot min$) (*152*).

7.2.1. ANALYTICAL METHODS FOR PHARMACOKINETIC MONITORING

Cyclophosphamide and ifosfamide are rich in nitrogen and phosphorus, and sufficiently volatile for sensitive and rapid gas chromatographic (GC) analysis with thermionic nitrogen-phosphorus (NP) detection. This is an effective method, with one caveat: relative sensitivity to analyte and internal standard can change with detector

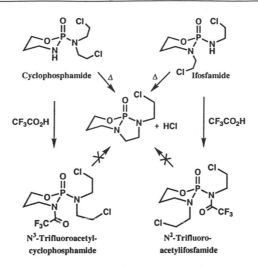

Fig. 18. Thermal cyclization of cyclophosphamide and ifosfamide.

usage. This does not happen if the two compounds have the same percentage content of nitrogen and phosphorus. Therefore, cyclophosphoramide and ifosfamide are ideal internal standards for one another.

Cyclophosphamide exhibits a slight thermal instability at GC injector port temperatures owing to intramolecular alkylation of N^3 by one of its chloroethyl groups (Fig. 18) (*153*). Acylation of N^3 with trifluoroacetic acid prior to GC analysis solves the problem (*154*). Intramolecular alkylation of ifosfamide was also formerly troublesome, requiring protection of the nucleophilic nitrogen. This difficulty was overcome by modifying the GC operating conditions (*155*). However, the new method is not suitable for analysis of underivatized cyclophosphamide. Therefore, trofosfamide is used as the internal standard.

Analytical resolution and quantitation of the stereoisomers of cyclophosphamide, ifosfamide, and their chiral metabolites are important, underutilized capabilities. Efficient separations have been achieved with cellulose-column HPLC (*156*) and capillary GC (*157*) with a bonded cyclodextrin stationary phase.

The indirect analysis of 4-hydroxyoxazaphosphorines/aldo(iso)phosphamide by quantitative acrolein release, derivatization with 3-aminophenol (Fig. 19) and spectrofluorometric quantitation (*54,151*), is subject to approximately twofold enhancement by other fluorogenic substances in blood. Resolution of these fluorochromes by high-performance liquid chromatography (HPLC) appears to be a reliable method for the cyclophosphamide metabolite, assuming subsequent hepatic ring hydroxylation of dechloroethylcyclophosphamide is insignificant (*158*).

Dechloroethylcyclophosphamide and 3-dechloroethylifosfamide are the same substance, although the ratio of enantiomers formed in vivo may differ. 3-Dechloroethylifosfamide is unsubstituted at the N^3 position. Therefore, it may be a good ring hydroxylation substrate for CYP2C9 or CYP2B6, enzymes that have no role in hepatic ifosfamide metabolism (*142*). Because of its greater catalytic efficiency *vis-à-vis* CYP3A4, for which ifosfamide is a substrate, conceivably more acrolein could be released from this inactive metabolite than from the parent drug. If so, 4-hydroxy-

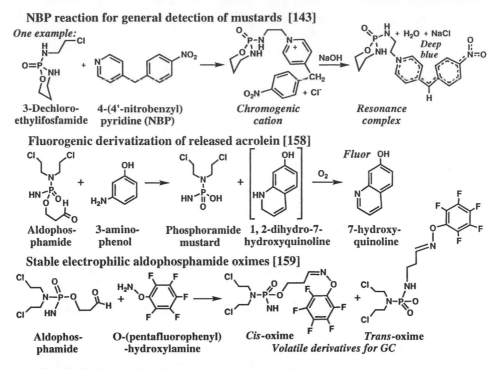

Fig. 19. Derivatization for analytical detection of oxazaphosphorine metabolites.

ifosfamide levels determined by acrolein release assay would be overestimated. Rate and fate determinations in appropriate hepatic or microsomal systems have not been performed with this metabolite, but ought to be done.

The foregoing considerations are a mandate for analysis of intact aldophosphamide/ aldoisophosphamide. A number of aldehyde derivatization reagents have been tried, but elimination of phosphoramide/isophosphoramide mustard during workup or analysis has been a persistent problem. This has been solved recently with the discovery of stable derivatives of aldophosphamide and aldoisophosphamide. The oximes formed by coupling these labile metabolites with pentafluorophenyl hydroxylamine are amenable to GC-MS analysis (Fig. 19). The method is specific, sensitive, and accurate (*159*).

Assays have been developed that are suitable for pharmacokinetic monitoring of phosphoramides and isophosphoramide mustards in human plasma by GC with MS (*160*) and NP detection (*161*), respectively.

For simultaneous determination of cyclophosphamide, carboxyphosphamide, 4-oxocyclophosphamide, phosphoramide mustard, and nor-nitrogen mustard in urine, high-performance thin-layer chromatography with 4-(4′-nitrobenzyl)pyridine staining (Fig. 19) and photodensitometric detection appears to be efficient and reliable. The system has also been used extensively for analysis of 2- and 3-dechloroethylifosfamide, isocarboxyphosphamide, 4-oxoifosfamide, and isophosphoramide mustard in plasma and urine (*143*).

Efficient GC methods for analysis of *N*-dechloroethylated ifosfamide metabolites by GC with NP detection have been reported that allow their determination in the same run with the parent drugs (*155,162*).

Chloroacetaldehyde in human blood has been derivatized with thiourea, isolated by solid-phase extraction, and analyzed by HPLC. The detection limit was 0.5 μM (*163*). Another method uses direct GC with electron capture detection (*155*). The analyte is protected from reactive components in blood or plasma by addition of excess of formaldehyde.

7.2.2. ORAL ABSORPTION

Peak concentrations of cyclophosphamide occur 1 h, and of ifosfamide, 1–2 h after ingestion (*164, 165*). Bioavailability of oral cyclophosphamide and ifosfamide is slightly under 100%. This is owing to first-pass metabolism. Therefore, C_{max} values for the 4-hydroxy metabolites are higher than after iv administration. In view of this, the effective bioavailability is probably total (*45*). Oral cyclophosphamide is well tolerated, but po administration of ifosfamide is avoided, because toxicity is more frequent than by the iv route. The side effects are associated with elevated chloroacetaldehyde levels (*105*).

7.2.3. APPARENT DISTRIBUTION VOLUME

Oxazaphosphorines are polar, water-soluble, nonlipophilic drugs. As a consequence, they distribute uniformly into total body water in nonobese patients. Apparent distribution volumes of cyclophosphamide and ifosfamide (L) are about 2/3 × body mass (kg) of the patient (*166*).

7.2.4. CLEARANCE

Whole-body clearance of cyclophosphamide is approx 82 mL/min, but extremely variable from patient to patient, range 35–200 mL·min^{-1}. For a divided dose of ifosfamide, whole-body clearance on day one is about 70 mL·min^{-1} increasing by day 5 to about 120. Interpatient variability of ifosfamide clearance is similar to that of cyclophosphamide. Renal clearance of cyclophosphamide is approx 10 mL·min^{-1} and that of ifosfamide, 16 mL·min^{-1} (*166–168*).

7.2.5. HEPATIC ELIMINATION

Elimination of cyclophosphamide and ifosfamide are predominantly by hepatic oxidation. Both drugs give large, interpatient differences in elimination half-life. Standard single or divided doses of cyclophosphamide or ifosfamide are eliminated according to first-order kinetics, consistent with a one-compartment, open model. The average elimination half-life of cyclophosphamide is approx 6 h; that of ifosfamide is 7 h (*168*).

Data indicating biexponential elimination of ifosfamide, with $t_{1/2(\beta)}$ = 16 h (*169*), have been cited repeatedly over the years. These data should be re-examined with a view to the method of ifosfamide analysis. [^{14}C]Ifosfamide was administered, and plasma and urine levels assayed as the radioactivity that partitioned into chloroform. Today we can presume that much of the β-phase elimination would represent dechloroethylated species, whose partition coefficients are similar to that of ifosfamide (*77*). At the time the work was performed, little was known of the side chain elimination pathway, and the need for high-resolution separation was not recognized.

The 4.8-fold slower hepatic elimination of ifosfamide vs cyclophosphamide was attributed to its lower affinity for a rat P-450 preparation, in vitro. However, the reported K_m values for ifosfamide and cyclophosphamide, 19.4 and 4.0 mM, respectively, far exceed blood levels attainable in vivo. Identical V_{max} values were seen for the two drugs, 5.4 μmol·g protein^{-1}·h^{-1}. The data need to be reconsidered, in view of the miniscule catalytic efficiencies implied by these quantities (*169*).

From the standpoint of hepatic elimination, the most consequential difference between cyclophosphamide and ifosfamide is the extent of dechloroethylation. For ifosfamide, this is normally 15–23% of an administered dose. However, some patients may eliminate as much as one-half of their ifosfamide dose by side chain metabolism. Ordinarily, 3-dechloroethylifosfamide is found in 2.5-fold greater abundance than 2-dechloroethylifosfamide (*170*). Only about 10% of cyclophosphamide is eliminated by dechloroethylation (*145*).

7.2.6. Renal Elimination

Urine recovery of unchanged cyclophosphamide is about 13% of dose administered. That of ifosfamide varies considerably (14–34% in children [*171*]) and averages 18% (*170*).

7.2.7. Recent Reviews

Additional details are available in recent reviews on pharmacokinetics and metabolism of cyclophosphamide (*45*) and ifosfamide (*105,166*). Despite its title, *Ifosfamide Metabolism and Pharmacokinetics (Review)* includes cyclophosphamide in a comparative discussion (*165*). Lind and Ardiet have described the pharmacokinetics of oxazaphosphorines, chlorambucil, melphalan, BCNU, CCNU, fotemustine, thiotepa, alkylsulfonates, dacarbazine, and procarbazine in a unified presentation (*168*).

In 1982, Gerald Zon prefaced a critical survey of cyclophosphamide analog development, with the observation, "it is rather ironic that the unmodified cyclophosphamide molecule has not yet been displaced from its position of superior therapeutic value." (*79*) In this chapter, we have seen data indicating that ifosfamide has a broader activity spectrum than its prototype, and can induce some cyclophosphamide-resistant sistant tumors to respond. Yet we cannot properly say that ifosfamide is truly superior. Its nonhematopoietic toxicity and 8.5-fold greater cost per dose have raised stern questions about its continued use in the high-dose setting (*145*). Nonetheless, there are instances in which it does afford an appropriate replacement for cyclophosphamide.

Zon's review concluded hopefully, "Assuming that cyclophosphamide continues to attract widespead attention, it seems inevitable that analogues having superior anti-cancer properties will eventually be realized." (*79*) The search goes on.

8. IDENTIFICATION OF NEW AGENTS

In the US, new agent screening protocols developed at the National Cancer Institute (NCI) are designed to uncover patterns of activity against a wide variety of human tumor cell lines. The panel consists of 60 cell lines, including NSCLC, SCLC, breast, central nervous system, ovarian and renal cancers, leukemia, and melanoma (*172*).

Although the NCI's primary screen should be capable of selecting useful preactivated metabolite precursors, it would not be suitable for direct testing of latent prodrugs, such as cyclophosphamide and ifosfamide, which require microsomal activation. However, agents of this class may be properly evaluated by pretreatment with appropriate microsomal preparations prior to dilution and addition to cultures (*173*).

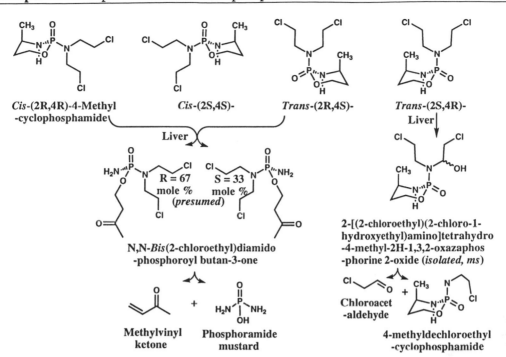

Fig. 20. Stereochemistry of rat cytochrome P450 catalyzed oxidation of 4-methylcyclophosphamide (*175*).

Another possible approach would use recently developed tumor cell lines transfected with oxazaphosphorine-metabolizing CYP genes capable of expressing the required hydroxylating activity (*174*).

8.1. Latent Oxazaphosphorine Analogs

In the aftermath of ifosfamide, most of the new latent phosphorylated mustards have been synthesized strategically, with the goal of identifying substituents, positions of substitution, or stereochemical arrangements that confer desired properties, the foremost being efficient hepatic activation (*79*).

8.1.1. 4-Methyl Analogs

As part of a study of the stereochemistry of CYP hydroxylation, each of the four diasteriomers of 4-methylcyclophosphamide were prepared. They were incubated in vitro with liver microsomes from mice, rats, and rabbits. Rates of disappearance of the four diasteriomers were all similar, but with rat microsomes, only three gave activated products (Fig. 20). The (2*S*,4*R*)-diasteriomer gave chloroacetaldehyde and dechloroethylcyclophosphamide. The phosphorylated metabolites were identified by TLC and MS. Chloroacetaldehyde and the coproduct of 4-hydroxylation, methyl vinyl ketone, were trapped as 2,4-dinitrophenylhydrazones and identified by TLC against authentic standards. The metabolic intermediate prior to dechloroethylation was also isolated and identified as 1′-hydroxy-4-methylcyclophosphamide by chemical ionization MS with deuteroammonia (*175*).

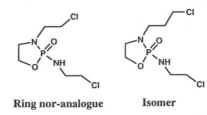

Fig. 21. Inactive ifosfamide pentagonal analog and isomer (*176*).

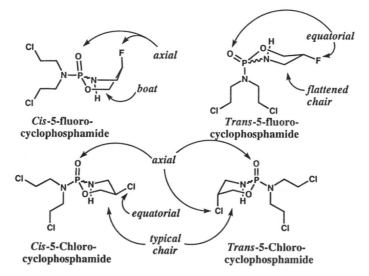

Fig. 22. Conformations of 5-fluoro- and 5-chlorocyclophosphamide epimers.

8.1.2. RING SIZE

Negative results can be revealing, one example being a recent description of two ifosfamide analogs with five-membered rings (Fig. 21). One of these simply had one less methylene in the ring than the parent. The other was an isomer with a ring of methylene transferred to the N^3 side chain, giving a 3-chloropropyl group. Like their elder cousins prepared as cyclophosphamide analogs (*72*), these compounds were inactive against cultured cells and in vivo. The authors concluded that latent precursors of isophosphoramide mustard also require a six-membered ring for initial hepatic activation (*176*).

8.1.3. STERIC AND ELECTRONIC EFFECTS

Other strategic studies have probed steric and electronic effects on the metabolism of cyclophosphamide. Individual cis- and trans-isomers of 5-fluoro- and 5-chloro-cyclophosphamide have been prepared for conformational analysis by ^{13}C and ^{19}F NMR and tested for biological activity in vitro and in vivo (*177*).

The preferred solution conformations of both isomers of 5-fluorocyclophospha-mide were unlike that of cyclophosphamide, for which the chair form with an axial phosphoryl oxygen predominates (Fig. 22). Cis-5-fluorocyclophosphamide appears to be unique among cyclophosphamide analogs, its most stable conformer being the boat form with axial fluorine and phosphoryl oxygen atoms. The corresponding trans-isomer is a flattened chair with an axial fluorine and equatorial phosphoryl oxygen. In contrast, both isomers of 5-chlorocyclophosphamide are conformationally similar to cyclophosphamide.

In vitro rat microsomal activations of coincubated cis- and trans-5-fluorocyclophosphamide were 4 and 46%, respectively, complete after 50 min at 37°C. The corresponding values for cis- and trans-5-chlorocyclophosphamide were 9 and 41%. The assays measured disappearance of the parent compounds by GC of their trifluoroacetylated derivatives.

In vivo, cis-5-fluorocyclophosphamide was inactive against transplanted murine ADJ/PCY plasma cell tumors. Trans-5-fluorocyclophosphamide, cis-5-chlorocyclophosphamide and trans-5-chlorocyclophosphamide gave 90% reductions in tumor weight (ED_{90}), at 37, 9.4, and 6.6 $mg \cdot kg^{-1}$, respectively. The ED_{90} of cyclophosphamide was 2.25 $mg \cdot kg^{-1}$ in this assay. The activity of cis-5-chlorocyclophosphamide, in vivo, was considered surprising by the authors because of its slow activation rate. However, there may be no discrepancy if exposures (AUC) to the active transport metabolite derived from the two isomers are the same. This pharmacokinetic parameter is probably the major determinant of activity (178). AUC should be independent of activation rate if nonhepatic clearance is slow, since the open-chain metabolite enantiomers derived from the two unresolved diasteriomeric pairs are identical.

Several similar strategic studies have been reported, with trifluoromethyl (179), phenyl (180), and other electron withdrawing (and donating) substituents. Some of them are mechanistically informative, but regretably, no latent analog other than ifosfamide has been as active or selective as the lead compound. Reviews by Zon (79) and Wojciech Stec (181) provide ample coverage of these analogs.

8.2. Active Metabolite Analogs

When the site of 4-hydroxylation of cyclophosphamide was found to be the liver, it became apparent that this step was not directly involved in tumor selectivity. This understanding spawned considerable interest in the development of new precursors of 4-hydroxycyclophosphamide, aldophosphamide, and phosphoramide mustard that did not require hepatic activation (139). John Montgomery and Robert Struck have surveyed the synthesis of 80 potential precursors representing all three of these classes and some preactivated analogs (182).

8.2.1. ANALOGS OF 4-HYDROXYCYCLOPHOSPHAMIDE

Efficient syntheses of 4-hydroperoxycyclophosphamide (183) and 4-hydroperoxyifosfamide (184) by Takamizawa and coworkers provided abundant supplies for direct pharmacological study and as convenient precursors of 4-hydroxycyclophosphamide and 4-hydroxyifosfamide. They also developed simple, reliable routes to the individual cis- and trans-isomers of the primary activation products of cyclophosphamide and ifosfamide (Fig. 23) (139).

Preclinical studies of 4-hydroperoxycyclophosphamide given 1 wk after allogeneic transplantation of human MX-1 breast carcinoma in nude mice showed superior activity compared with cyclophosphamide. Furthermore, the difference was greater when treatment was delayed to 3 wk after transplant. Activation studies showed that as the tumor advanced, the ability of the murine liver to activate cyclophosphamide decreased (185).

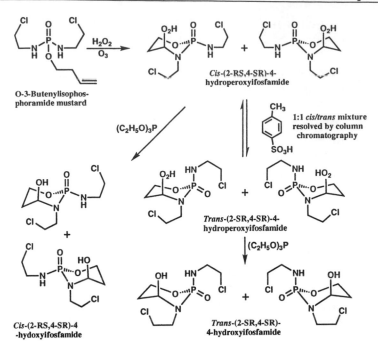

Fig. 23. Preparation of cis- and trans-4-hydroxyifosfamide (*139*).

Clinical studies of iv administration of 4-hydroperoxycyclophosphamide or 4-hydroperoxyifosfamide have not been reported to media accessible by Cancerlit of Medline information retrieval services. Trials of these compounds for purging, aimed at reducing residual disease from re-engrafted marrow or other autologous hematopoietic precursor tissues, appear often and prominently in the literature (*186*). The implication may be that these compounds have gone the way of other rapid metabolite generators, described below.

In addition to their direct use in the clinic and laboratory, 4-hydroperoxycyclophosphamide and 4-hydroperoxyifosfamide are also efficiently reduced to 4-hydroxycyclophosphamide and 4-hydroxyifosfamide, respectively. These in turn may be converted *in situ* to other useful analogs, such as the 4-alkylsulfides (*187*), modeled after the reversible glutathione and cysteine conjugates (*67*). This chemistry, with MESNA as the thiol component, launched the next significant achievement in the field, the synthesis of mafosfamide (*188*).

Mafosfamide is not formed directly from 4-hydroxycyclophosphamide, but as a consequence of its tautomerization to aldophosphamide. Subsequent hydration of the aldehyde group to the gem-diol, its protonation and displacement of water from the oxonium intermediate by MESNA, forms the hemithioacetal. Recyclization, via another round of hydroxyl protonation and displacement of water by the primary phosphoramide give mafosfamide (Fig. 24) (*189*).

In preclinical testing against L1210 ascites in mice, the TI of mafosfamide was comparable to that of cyclophosphamide. Bladder inflammation was examined and the mafosfamide-treated mice showed none, in contrast with the cyclophosphamide-treated animals. Intraperitoneal administration of mafosfamide did cause pericap-

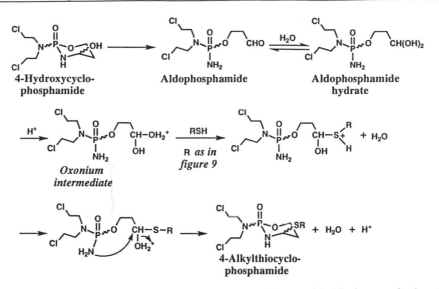

Fig. 24. Mechanism of reversible thiol conjugation (e.g., MESNA) with 4-hydroxycyclophosphamide (*189*).

sular hepatic fibrosis. This was an early warning that local toxicity near the site of injection could present a serious problem for administration of mafosfamide (*190*).

When clinical trials began, mafosfamide was administered intravenously as a single dose given every 3 wk. It had to be administered as a 2–3 h infusion because of severe pain along the injected vein. This side effect limited the dosage to 700 (*191*) or 1000 mg·m^{-2} (*192*). The drug was reformulated as a lysine salt, but this did not ameliorate the pain. The authors concluded that rapid release of active oxazaphosphorine metabolites prior to systemic distribution was clinically untenable. They suggested that derivatives giving low concentrations of active metabolites within the injection vein may be more promising (*191,192*). As in the case of 4-hydroperoxycyclophosphamide, mafosfamide is now widely used for purging (*193*).

A strategic study has pointed the way to regulating the formation of aldophosphamide analogs and release of acrolein and phosphoramide mustard derivatives from 4-hydroperoxy- and 4-(2-sulfoethyl)thiooxazaphosphoranes. Chul-Hoon Kwon and Richard Borch measured the associated rates and equilibria at 37 °C, pH 7.4, in 100 m*M* phosphate. 4-Hydroperoxy and 4-(2-sulfoethyl)thio derivatives of:

1. Cyclophosphamide;
2. 3-Methyl cyclophosphamide;
3. Ifosfamide; and
4. Trofosfamide

were investigated (Fig. 25). Ring opening of the 4-hydroxylated derivatives of these precursors was acid-catalyzed for derivatives of 1 and 2, but base-catalyzed for those of 3 and 4. In contrast with the 4-hydroxy derivatives of 1, 3, and 4, ring opening and subsequent generation of *N*-methyl phosphoramide mustard and acrolein from the 4-hydroxy derivative of 2 were markedly slower. Half-lives for these ring-opening reactions were: 1. 9.9; 2. 23; 3. 6.9; and 4. 3.3 min (*194*).

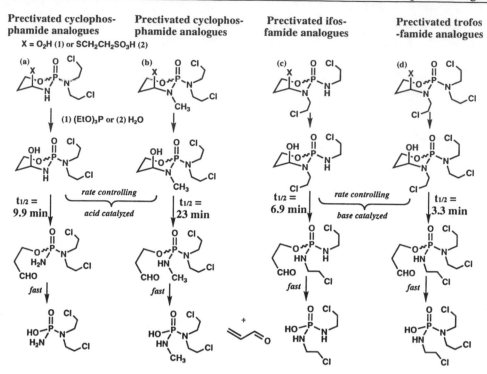

Fig. 25. Kinetics and mechanism: *N*-dealkylation of cis-4-hydroxy analogs (*194*).

8.2.2. ALDOPHOSPHAMIDE ANALOGS

The prototype aldophosphamide precursor was its diethyl acetal (Fig. 26). It was originally prepared as a synthetic precursor from which aldophosphamide would be generated by mineral acid or Lewis acid treatment. However, the reaction did not yield the desired product (*183*). It was later tested against L1210 ascites in mice and was devoid of activity (*182*).

Recognizing that hydrolysis of acyl acetals is spontaneous at pH 7.4, Yu-Qiang Wang and David Farquhar of the M. D. Anderson Cancer Center in Houston, TX, prepared diacetylacetal derivatives of aldophosphamide, four analogs with *N*-substituents (monomethyl, dimethyl, monoethyl, and diethyl), and two with methoxy and ethoxy groups in place of the primary amino group (Fig. 26).

Aldophosphamide diacetylacetal was highly cytotoxic against cultured murine L1210 lymphoblastic leukemia cells with an IC_{50} of 0.9 μM (1-h exposure). The IC_{50} values of the more active analogs were as follows: monomethyl, 39; monoethyl, 28; and diethyl, 78 μM. These values were similar to those of mafosfamide, 42 and 4-hydroperoxycyclophosphamide, 90 μM. The other derivatives were less active, with IC_{50} values ranging from 150 to >300 μM. Half-lives of hydrolysis to form the aldehyde in 0.05M phosphate buffer at 37°C, pH 7.4 ranged between 29 and 42 h. Thus, the compounds were sufficiently stable for preparation of injectable solutions. When they were catalytically hydrolyzed with pig liver carboxylate esterase, half-lives ranged from 36–42 s (*195*). In the case of mafosfamide, such rapid release of cytotoxic products was associated with local toxicity. Available publications on clinical applica-

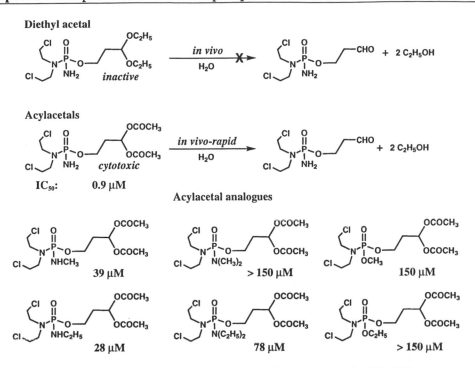

Fig. 26. Aldophosphamide analogs: acetals and acylacetals (*183,195*).

tions describe the suitability of acetaldophosphamide (*196*) and its isomer, acetaldo-ifosfamide, as the compounds are commonly called, for bone marrow purging (*197*).

Eight perhydrooxazine analogs of aldophosphamide were synthesized and characterized by Richard Borch and Ronald Valente (*198*). They invoked an alternative mechanism of intracellular phosphoramide release, initiated by acid-catalyzed opening of the perhydrooxazine ring to form an enamine, shown in Fig. 27. Two of the compounds had pairs of 2-chloroethyl groups on both phosphoramide nitrogens. Sensitivity of wild-type L1210 and P388 cells on tissue culture to 1-h exposure to either of these tetrakis(2-chloroethyl)amidophosphorane oxides was greater than to 4-hydroperoxycyclophosphamide. Against cyclophosphamide-resistant L1210 and P388 cells, they were 6- to 70-fold more effective than 4-hydroxycyclophosphamide.

The presence of mustard groups at all four phosphoramide valences appeared to be an important factor contributing to potency. This aspect of the molecular design was intended to avoid detoxification by ethylene bridging between the two nitrogens, which may occur when a primary or secondary phosphorylated amino group is present.

The perhydrooxazine analogs' low level of cyclophosphamide crossresistance may be owing to absence of substrate activity for aldehyde dehydrogenases. Aldehyde dehydrogenase overproduction is a common mechanism of oxazaphosphorine resistance development (*16*). On the other hand, the in vivo selectivity of oxazaphosphoranes used in the clinic today may depend on their efficient detoxification by aldehyde dehydrogenases in the host's nonneoplastic regenerating cells (*199*), such as those of blood and bone marrow (*200*). The anticancer activity of the perhydrooxazinophosphoramidates against transplanted L1210 ascites cells in mice (T/C ≤ 170%) was substantially lower than that of 4-hydroperoxycyclophosphamide (T/C = 240%) (*198*).

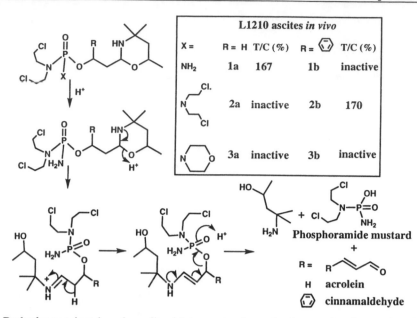

Fig. 27. Perhydrooxazinophosphorodiamidate mustards: activation mechanism and activity (*198*).

These strategic studies emphasize the difficulty of maintaining selectivity while overcoming resistance. Drug resistance development by tumor cells is also a strategic attack against the drug's selectivity mechanisms.

8.2.3. PHOSPHORAMIDE MUSTARD ANALOGS

Phosphoramide mustard, the first active member of its class, was synthesized by Orrie Friedman before the advent of cyclophosphamide. In view of its precedence, phosphoramide mustard is the true prototype, and cyclophosphamide, the second-generation analog. In its preclinical activity spectrum, phosphoramide mustard was better than several clinically approved nitrogen mustards of the time, including some in use today (Fig. 1) (*201*).

Phosphoramide mustard is less active than cyclophosphamide against most transplanted tumors, and less cytotoxic than 4-hydroperoxycyclophosphamide or mafosfamide against most cultured tumor cell lines. Clinically responsive cell types, such as acute lymphocytic pre-B-lymphoblast and T blast II leukemias, Burkitt's B blast I, and histiocytic monoblast lymphoma cell lines are 14- to 26-fold more sensitive in culture to 4-hydroperoxycyclophosphamide than to phosphoramide mustard. Acute and chronic myelocytic leukemia and normal hematopoietic progenitor cells are 6.5-to 7.2-fold more sensitive to 4-hydroperoxycyclophosphamide than to phosphoramide mustard (*45*).

The differences in activity between the aldophosphamide precursors and phosphoramide mustard may be owing, in part, to transport. 4-Hydroxycyclophosphamide/aldophosphamide readily penetrates perfused U937 human histiocytic leukemia cells. The U937 cell membrane is relatively impermeable to phosphoramide mustard influx or efflux. Phosphoramide mustard generated within U937 cells after perfusion of 4-hydroxycyclophosphamide/aldophosphamide is retained after the cells are transferred to drug-free medium. 4-Hydroxycyclophosphamide/aldophosphamide effluxes

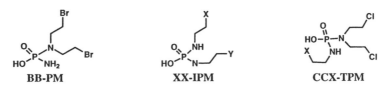

Fig. 28. Halogen-substituted phosphoramide mustard analogs (*205*).

from the cells into drug-free medium (*202*). Similar results have been obtained with Ehrlich ascites (*203*) and P388 cells (*204*).

With another active, phosphorylated mustard, Struck et al. showed that cytotoxicity differences between active and latent phosphorylated mustards involve more than just transport (*205*). The compound in question was synthesized as part of a study of isophosphoramide and triphosphoramide mustards, the cytotoxic metabolites of ifosfamide and trofosfamide, respectively. The parental mustards and eight derivatives, with one or both chlorogroups replaced by bromine or fluorine atoms, were screened against cultured cells and transplanted murine tumors in vivo. Of particular interest was CB-IPM, the chlorobromo derivative of isophosphoramide mustard (Fig. 28). Tested against human ACHN renal and NCI-H23 lung tumor cell lines in tissue culture, CB-IPM was 5- and 50-fold, respectively, more potent than 4-hydroperoxycyclophosphamide. Against SK-MEL28 melanoma and SNB-7 CNS tumor cells, it was 5- and 2.5-fold, respectively, less sensitive than 4-hydroperoxy-cyclophosphamide. Against DLD-1 colon cells, CB-IPM appeared to be inactive.

Halogen substitution on one mustard group is unlikely to alter the steric or electronic properties of isophosphoramide mustard enough to overcome a major transport problem. The panel of five human tumor cell lines described above exhibit a range of sensitivities to other latent and active oxazaphosphorine metabolites. As such, they afford an excellent representation of nature's variety, pertinent to cellular uptake and other cytotoxicity determinants.

A number of in vivo experiments were performed with BC-IPM. Against IP L1210 leukemia in mice, BC-IPM produced 4/6 long-term survivors, as did isophosphamide mustard, vs 2/6 for cyclophosphamide. For BC-IPM, ILS was 388% (2/6 dying mice), compared with 133% for cyclophosphamide (4/6 dying mice). Against subcutaneous, cyclophosphamide-resistant L1210 cells, 2/6 BC-IPM-treated mice were long-term survivors, but CPA was inactive. However, against subcutaneous, wild-type L1210 cells, cyclophosphamide gave 6/6 long-term survivors, compared with 2/6 for BC-IPM. Against subcutaneous murine 16/C mammary tumor, BC-IPM gave a 60% longer tumor growth delay than cyclophosphamide. However, response of the subcutaneous B16 melanoma transplant favored cyclophosphamide by 2.6-fold over BC-IPM, in a tumor growth delay assay (*205*).

Although comparison with ifosfamide would have made the interpretation more definite, the in vivo data for BC-IPM and cyclophosphamide suggest that the selectivities of these model systems may not be based entirely on aldehyde dehydrogenase detoxification. Some of the total cellular burden of 4-hydroxycyclophosphamide is conjugated with GSH (*206*), for which the GSTM1 system is catalytically active. The effect of GSTM1 is not significant for phosphoramide mustard (*207*). GSTM1 is lacking in certain lung and breast cancers (*208*). This system may play a role in determining whether cells are more sensitive to BC-IPM or cyclophosphamide. The

ASTA D-19575: transmembrane carrier strategy

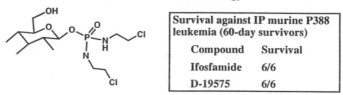

Survival against IP murine P388 leukemia (60-day survivors)	
Compound	Survival
Ifosfamide	6/6
D-19575	6/6

HEX-ALD: Lactate acidosis activation

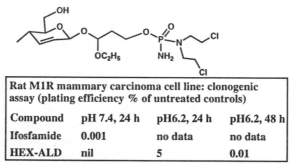

Rat M1R mammary carcinoma cell line: clonogenic assay (plating efficiency % of untreated controls)			
Compound	pH 7.4, 24 h	pH6.2, 24 h	pH6.2, 48 h
Ifosfamide	0.001	no data	no data
HEX-ALD	nil	5	0.01

Fig. 29. Hexose-linked phosphoramide mustards (*212,224*).

deleterious effect of acrolein (*209*) and chloroacetaldehyde (*210*) on glutathione and GST (*211*) levels may limit the tolerated dose of cyclophosphamide or ifosfamide.

In view of evidence that ionized phosphoramide mustards are poorly transported into some tumors, scientists at ASTA Medica AG, Frankfurt am Main, have taken a two-pronged approach to overcome the deficiency. They have masked the ionizing diamidophosphate oxygen of isophosphoramide mustard by esterification with the 1-hydroxyl group of glucose (Fig. 29). In doing so, they hoped to gain the additional benefit of glucose transmembrane transport, since the derivative (D-19575) is an analog of glucose-1-phosphate. The IC_{90} of D-19575 against L1210 and KB cells was 6.3 and 5.2 μM, respectively, in a colony-forming assay. Corresponding values for isophosphoramide mustard were 1.4 and 8.1 μM. Both ifosfamide and D-19575 were curative (6/6 mice) against P388 ascites transplants. The best dose of ifosfamide given QD × 5 was 0.57 mmol·kg^{-1}·d^{-1} × 5 d. That of D-19575 was 0.65 mmol·kg^{-1}·d^{-1} × 5 d. Phlorizin, an inhibitor of the sodium-dependent glucose transporter, decreased cytotoxicity of D-19575 and increased renal recovery of the unchanged drug (*212*).

8.3. Overcoming Drug Resistance with Bioreductive Alkylators

Insensitivity of the hypoxic fraction of neoplastic cells within a tumor to conventional anticancer agents has been recognized as a serious impediment to curative treatment (*213*). There may be a bright side, however, because the disorganized vasculature associated with hypoxia distinguishes tumor cells from their normal counterparts. This distinction may provide a more specific basis for cell killing than proliferation rate, the predominant mechanism of current therapies (*214*). The development of *N*-oxides (*215*), nitroheterocycles (*216*), and quinones (*217*) as bioreducible precursors of toxic metabolites has been widely explored.

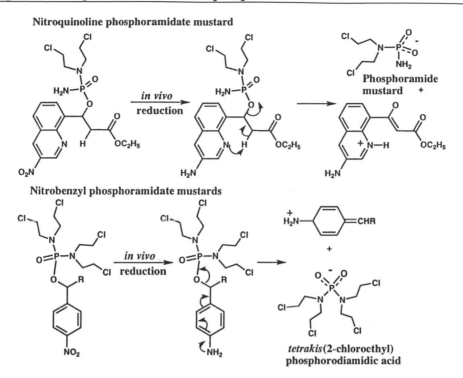

Fig. 30. Bioreductive alkylators.

The cytotoxicity of activated cyclophosphamide was greater against hypoxic than aerobic Chinese hamster V79 cells (*218*) and murine C3H mammary carcinoma (*219*) in tissue culture, but the effect was not reproducible in murine 16/C (*220*) or B16 melanoma (*221*) in vivo.

Juxtaposition of latent drug activation and selective nitro group reduction by hypoxic cells has led to the synthesis of a compound that releases phosphoramide mustard when its nitro group is reduced (Fig. 30). Four hours of exposure to the compound at concentrations between 50 and 300 μM gave >4.5 logs of cell kill against an hypoxic HT-29 human colon carcinoma cell line, but <1 log of cell kill against the same cells in aerobic culture (*222*).

The bioreductive activation of phosphorylated mustards was further elaborated in the synthesis of a series of (4-nitrophenyl)alkanol derivatives esterified with tetrakis(2-chloroethy)diamidophosphoryl chloride. Nitro-reduction was intended to release the tetrakis mustard and various iminoquinone methides. One of these compounds (Fig. 30) was selectively cytotoxic to hypoxic HT-29 cells, giving a 2-log cell kill from a 4-h exposure to 0–25 μM concentrations. Four hours of exposure between 0 and 100 μM killed about 1/2 log–1 log of aerobic HT-29 cells and 1/2 log of aerobic murine bone marrow reticulocyte/macrophage progenitor cells. Four other compounds were cytotoxic toward hypoxic and aerobic cells, indicating that they are activated by processes other than hypoxia-dependent nitro reduction (*223*).

An ancillary cellular consequence of hypoxia is lactate acidosis in response to glucose feeding. Glucose feeding of hypoxic tumor cells readily generates acidosis down to pH 6.2. In vivo blood glucose levels of 20–25 mM are needed to maintain this pH. This effect has been exploited in the design of a selective precursor of aldo-phosphamide. The compound, denoted HEX-ALD, is the acetalglycoside of aldo-phosphamide and 2,3-dideoxy-D-erythro-2-hexenopyranoside (Fig. 29).

Aerobic M1R rat mammary carcinoma cells were exposed to 100 μg/mL HEX-ALD for 72 h at pH 7.4, giving < 1 log of cell kill. After 48 h at pH 6.2, a cell kill of > 4 logs was seen. Although the required exposure time was excessive, the authors indicated that they were preparing new analogs that will hopefully be more acid-labile (224).

9. CONCLUSION

The studies reviewed above show that the selectivity mechanisms of phosphorylated mustards are multifactorial, with governing determinants that vary from tumor to tumor. In terms of drug design and development for the future, a variety of agents with differing transport, cytotoxicity, and selectivity mechanisms are needed. Our vision of the future should include optimizing the administration of these agents on a per-patient basis. Regimen selection based on tumor isozyme expression (GST mRNAs, for instance [225]), and pharmacokinetic dosing, are two steps in this direction.

All anticancer agents, old and new, must be utilized in the safest, most effective ways possible. This calls for an unrelenting commitment to discovery of broader and better supportive care, focused on end-organ protection. The search for new end-organ support modalities is as important as drug development in the overall treatment picture, especially because supportive care impacts on tolerable dose intensity.

Following each defeat of an end-organ toxicity comes a new round of dose rein-tensification (17). Current manifestations of this progress are the high-dose regimens developed in the wake of hematopoietic growth factor (226) and progenitor cell sup-port (227). Every advance across the log-linear dose–response curve leads inevitably toward the one cell limit (228). High hopes are pinned on the reiteration of this cycle to the point of curative treatment with minimal side effects (229).

REFERENCES

1. Colvin M. Alkylating agents and platinum antitumor compounds. In: Holland JF, Frei E III, Bast RC Jr, Kufe DW, Morton DL, Weichselbaum RR, eds. *Cancer Medicine,* 3rd ed. Phila-delphia: Lea & Febiger. 1993:733–754.
2. Krumbhaar EB. Role of the blood and the bone marrow in certain forms of blood poisoning. 1. Peripheral blood changes and their significance. *JAMA* 1919; 72:39–45.
3. Adair FE, Bagg HJ. Experimental and clinical studies on the treatment of cancer by dichloro-ethylsulphide (mustard gas). *Ann Surg* 1931; 93:190–199.
4. Berenblum I. Experimental inhibition of tumor induction by mustard gas and other com-pounds. *J Pathol Bacteriol* 1935; 40:549–558.
5. Salomon G. Kinetics of ring-formation and polymerisation in solution. *Trans Faraday Soc* 1936; 32:153–178.
6. Gilman A, Phillips FS. The biological actions and therapeutic applications of the β-chloroethyl amines and sulfides. *Science* 1946; 103:409–415, 436.
7. Avery OT, MacLeod CM, McCarty M. Studies on the chemical nature of the substance induc-ing transformation of pneumococcal types. Induction of transformation by a deoxyribonucleic acid fraction isolated from Pneumococcus Type III. *J Exp Med* 1944; 79:137–158.
8. Stryer I. *Biochemistry,* 2nd ed. New York: W. H. Freeman and Company. 1981:562.
9. Anslow WP, Karnovsky DA, Val Jager B, Smith HW. The toxicity and pharmacological action of the nitrogen mustards and certain related compounds. *J Pharmacol Exp Ther* 1947; 91: 224–235.

10. Gilman A. The initial clinical trial of nitrogen mustard. *Am J Surg* 1963; 105:574–578.

11. Rhoads CP. Nitrogen mustards in the treatment of neoplastic disease. *JAMA* 1946; 131:656–659.

12. Goodman LS, Wintrobe MM, Dameshek W, Goodman MJ, Gilman A, McLennan MT. Nitrogen mustard therapy. *JAMA* 1946; 132:126–131.

13. Jacobson LO, Spurr CL, Guzman Barron ES, Smith T, Lushbaugh C, Dick GF. Nitrogen mustard therapy. *JAMA* 1946; 132:263–271.

14. Gilman A. Therapeutic applications of chemical warfare agents. *Fed Proc* 1946; 5:285–292.

15. Golomb FM. Agents used in cancer chemotherapy. *Am J Surg* 1963; 105:579–590.

16. Sladek NE. Oxazaphosphorine-specific acquired cellular resistance. In: Teicher BA, ed. *Drug Resistance in Oncology*. New York: Marcel Dekker. 1993:375–410.

17. Frei III E, Canellos GP. Dose: a critical factor in cancer chemotherapy. *Am J Med* 1980; 69:585.

18. Narayanan V. Development of new chemotherapeutic agents. In: Magrath I, ed. *New Directions in Cancer Treatment*. Berlin: Springer-Verlag. 1987:227–242.

19. Seligman AM, Nachlas MM, Manheimer LH, Friedman OM, Wolf G. Development of new methods for the histochemical demonstration of hydrolytic intracellular enzymes in a program of cancer research. *Ann Surg* 1949; 130:333–341.

20. Ichihara M. Über die phosphamidase. *J Biochem* 1933; 18:87–106.

21. Rorig K. *N*-(*p*-chlorophenyl-)diamidophosphoric acid. *J Am Chem Soc* 1949; 71:3561,3562.

22. Gomori G. Histochemical demonstration of sites of phosphamidase activity. *Proc Soc Exp Biol Med* 1948; 69:407–409.

23. Seligman AM, Milden M, Friedman OM. A study of the inhibition of tumor growth in mice and rats with 10-methyl-1,2-benzanthracene and derivatives related to the nitrogen and sulfur beta-chloroethyl vesicants. *Cancer* 1949; 2:701–706.

24. Friedman OM, Seligman AM. Preparation of *N*-phosphorylated derivatives of bis β-chloroethylamine. *J Am Chem Soc* 1954; 76:655–661.

25. Brock N. Oxazaphosphorine cytostatics: past-present-future. *Cancer Res* 1989; 49:1–7.

26. Druckrey H. Esperimentelle Grundlagen des Krebses. *Dtsch Med Wochenschr* 1952; 77:1534–1537.

27. Arnold H, Bourseaux F. Synthese und abbau zytostatisch wirksamer zyklischer *N*-phosphamidester des bis-(chloroethyl)-amins. *Angew Chem* 1958; 70:539–544.

28. Arnold H, Bourseaux F, Brock N. Neuartige krebs-chemotherapeutika aus der gruppe der zyklischen N-lost phosphoramidester. *Naturwiss* 1958; 45:64–66.

29. Brock N, Wilmanns H. Wirkung eines zyklisches N-lost-phosphoramidesters auf experimentell erzeugte tumoren der ratte. *Deutsch Med Wschr* 1958; 83:453–458.

30. Arnold H, Bourseaux F, Brock N. Chemotherapeutic action of a cyclic nitrogen mustard phosphamide ester (B518-ASTA) in experimental tumors of the rat. *Nature* 1958; 181:931.

31. Brock N. Zur pharmakologischen characterisierung zyklischer N-lost-phosphamid-ester als krebs-chemotherapeutica. *Arzneim-Forsch* 1958; 8:1–9.

32. Lane M. Some effects of cyclophosphamide (cytoxan) on normal mice and mice with L1210 leukemia. *JNCI* 1959; 23:1347–1357.

33. Venditti JM, Humphreys SR, Goldin A. The effectiveness of cytoxan against mouse leukemia L1210 and resistant sublines. *Cancer Chemother Rep* 1959; 3:6–8.

34. Venditti JM, Humphreys SR, Goldin A. Investigation of the activity of cytoxan against leukemia L1210 in mice. *Cancer Res* 1959; 19:986–995.

35. Gross R, Lambers K. Erste erfahrungen in der behandlung maligner tumoren mit einem neuen N-lost-phosphamidester. *Dtsch Med Wochenschrft* 1958; 83:458–462.

36. Coggins PR, Ravdin RG, Eisman SH. Clinical pharmacology and preliminary evaluation of cytoxan (cyclophosphamide). *Cancer Chemother Rep* 1959; 3:9–11.

37. Foye LV Jr, Chapman CG, Willet FM, Adams WS. Cyclophosphamide a preliminary study of a new alkylating agent. *Cancer Chemother Rep* 1960; 6:39,40.

38. Haar H, Marshall GJ, Bierman H, Steinfeld JL. The influence of cyclophosphamide upon neoplastic diseases in man. *Cancer Chemother Rep* 1960; 6:41–51.

39. Bethall FH, Louis J, Robbins A, et al. Phase II evaluation of cyclophosphamide a study by the midwest cooperative chemotherapy group. *Cancer Chemother Rep* 1960; 6:112–115.

40. Bergsagel DE, Levin WC. A prelusive clinical trial of cyclophosphamide. *Cancer Chemother Rep* 1960; 6:120–134.
41. Korst DR, Johnson FD, Frenkel EP, Challener III WL. Preliminary evaluation of the effect of cyclophosphamide on the course of human neoplasms. *Cancer Chemother Rep* 1960; 7:1–12.
42. Nissen-Meyer R, Hoest H. A comparison between the hematologic side effects of cyclophosphamide and nitrogen mustard. *Cancer Chemother Rep* 1960; 9:51–55.
43. Hoest H, Nissen-Meyer R. A preliminary clinical study of cyclophosphamide. *Cancer Chemother Rep* 1960; 9:47–50.
44. Papac R, Petrakis NL, Amini F, Wood DA. Comparative clinical evaluation of two alkylating agents mannitol mustard and cyclophosphamide (cytoxan). *JAMA* 1960; 172:1387–1391.
45. Sladek NE. Metabolism and pharmacokinetic behaviour of cyclophosphamide and related oxazaphosphorines. In: Powis G, ed. *Anticancer Drugs, Reactive Metabolism and Drug Interactions.* Newcastle upon Tyne: Pergamon. 1955:79–156.
46. Colvin M. Cyclophosphamide and analogues. In: Crooke ST, Prestayko AW, eds. *Cancer and Chemotherapy,* vol. III. New York: Academic. 1981:25–36.
47. Bolt W, Ritzl F, Toussaint R, Nahrmann H. Verteilung und ausscheidung eines cytostatisch wirkenden, mit tritium markierted N-lost derivatives beim krebskranken menschen. *Arzneim-Forsch* 1961; 11:170–175.
48. Draeger U, Hohorst H-J. Permeation of cyclophosphamide (NSC-26271) metabolites into tumor cells. *Cancer Chemother Rep* 1976; 60:423–427.
49. Arnold H, Bourseaux F, Brock N. Chemotherapeutic action of a cyclic nitrogen mustard phosphoramide ester (B 518-ASTA) in experimental tumors of the rat. *Nature* 1958; 181:931.
50. Foley GE, Friedman OM, Drolet BP. Studies on the mechanism of action of cytoxan. Evidence of activation in vivo and in vitro. *Cancer Res* 1961; 21:57–63.
51. Brock N, Hohorst H-J. Über die aktivierung von cyclophosphamide in vivo und in vitro. *Arzneim-Forsch* 1963; 13:1021–1031.
52. Norpoth K. Untersuchungen zur oxidativen umzetzungen von endoxan® in vivo und in vitro [Habilitationsschrift]. Münster (Westf.):Fach Physiologische Chemie, Westfälischen Wilhelms Universität, 1969.
53. Norpoth K, Golovinsky E, Rauen HM. Untersuchungen an hypothetischen metaboliten des 2-[bis(2-chloroäthyl)amino]tetrahydro-2H-1,3,2-oxazaphosphorine-2-oxids (cyclophosphamid). *Z Physiol Chem* 1970; 351:377–383.
54. Alarcon RA, Meienhofer J. Formation of the cytotoxic aldehyde acrolein during in vitro degradation of cyclophosphamide. *Nature New Biol* 1971; 233:250–252.
55. Sladek NE. Therapeutic efficacy of cyclophosphamide as a function of its metabolism. *Cancer Res* 1972; 32:535–542.
56. Hill DL, Kirk MC, Struck RF. Isolation and identification of 4-ketocyclophosphamide, a possible active form of the antitumor agent cyclophosphamide. *J Am Chem Soc* 1970; 92:3207,3208.
57. Rakke JE, Feil VJ, Zaylskie RG. Characterization of the major sheep urinary metabolites of cyclophosphamide, a defleecing chemical. *J Agric Food Chem* 1971; 19:788–790.
58. Hohorst H-J, Ziemann A, Brock N. 4-Ketocyclophosphamide, a metabolite of cyclophosphamide. *Artzneim-Forsch* 1971; 21:1254–1257.
59. Struck RF, Kirk MC, Mellett LB, El Dareer S, Hill DL. Urinary metabolites of the antitumor agent cyclophosphamide. *Mol Pharmacol* 1971; 7:519–529.
60. Sladek N. Evidence for an aldehyde possessing alkylating activity as the primary metabolite of cyclophosphamide. *Cancer Res* 1973; 33:651–658.
61. Struck RF. Isolation and identification of a stabilized derivative of aldophosphamide, a major metabolite of cyclophosphamide. *Cancer Res* 1974; 34:2933–2935.
62. Colvin M, Padgett CA, Fenselau C. A biologically active metabolite of cyclophosphamide. *Cancer Res* 1973; 33:915–918.
63. Friedman OM, Boger E, Grubliauskas V, Somer H. Synthesis of N-phosphorylated derivatives of nitrogen mustards with latent cytotoxicity. *J Med Chem* 1963; 6:50–58.
64. Connors TA, Cox PJ, Farmer PB, Foster AB, Jarman M. Some studies of the active intermediates formed in the microsomal metabolism of cyclophosphamide and isophosphamide.

Biochem Pharmacol 1974; 23:115–129.

65. Borch RF, Valente RR. Synthesis, activation and cytotoxicity of aldophosphamide analogues. *J Med Chem* 1991; 34:3052–3058.
66. Clarke L, Waxman DJ. Oxidative metabolism of cyclophosphamide: identification of the hepatic monooxegenase catalysts of drug activation. *Cancer Res* 1989; 49:2344–2350.
67. Zon G, Ludeman SM, Brandt JA, et al. Nmr spectroscopic studies of intermediary metabolites of cyclophosphamide. A comprehensive kinetic analysis of the interconversion of *cis*- and *trans*-4-hydroxycyclophosphamide with aldophosphamide and the concomitant partitioning of aldophosphamide between irreversible fragmentation and reversible conjugation pathways. *J Med Chem* 1984; 27:466–485.
68. Feneslau C, Lehman JP, Myles A, et al. Iminocyclophosphamide as a chemically reactive metabolite of cyclophosphamide. *Drug Metab Dispos* 1982; 10:636–640.
70. Dockham PA, Lee M-O, Sladek NE. Identification of the human liver aldehyde dehydrogenases that catalyze the oxidation of aldophosphamide and retinaldehyde. *Biochem Pharmacol* 1992; 43:2453–2469.
71. Cherif A, Farquhar D. *N*-(5,5-diacetoxypent-1-yl)doxorubicin: a new intensely potent doxorubicine analogue. *J Med Chem* 1992; 35:3208–3214.
72. Arnodl H, Bourseaux F, Brock N. Über beziehungen zwischen chemischer konstitution und cancertoxischer wirkungen in der reihe der phosphamidester des bis-(β-chloräthyl)-amins. *Arzneim-Forsch* 1961; 11:143–158.
73. Goldstein A, Arownow L, Kalman SM. *Principles of Drug Action.* New York: Harper & Row. 1969:351.
74. Ishidate M, Kobayashi K, Sakurai Y, Sato H, Yoshida T. *Proc Japan Acad* 1951; 27:493–500.
75. Skipper H E, Schmidt LH. A manual on quantitative drug evaluation in experimental tumor systems. Part I. Background, description of criteria, and presentation of quantitative therapeutic data on various classes on drugs obtained in diverse experimental tumor systems. *Cancer Chemother Rep* 1962; 17:1–143.
76. Goldin A, Venditti JM. A manual on quantitative drug evaluation in experimental tumor systems. Part II. Quantitative assessment of various classes of agents employing advanced leukemia L1210 in mice. *Cancer Chemother Rep* 1962; 17:145–178.
77. Reinhoudt DN, Connors TA, Pinedo HM, van den Poll KW, eds. *Structure–Activity Relationships of Anti-tumor Agents.* The Hague: Martinius Nijhoff Publishers, 1983.
78. Preussmann R. Chlor-abspaltbarkeit und wirksamkeit von N-lost-verbindungen. *Arzneim-Forsch* 1958; 8:9,10.
79. Zon G. Cyclophosphamide analogues. In: Ellis GP, West GB, eds. *Progress in Medicinal Chemistry.* Amsterdam: Elsevier Biochemical. 1982:205–246.
80. Cox PJ, Farmer PB, Foster AB, et al. Application of deuterium labelling mass spectrometry in a study of the metabolism of the enantiomers of cyclophosphamide. *Biomed Mass Spectrom* 1977; 4:371–375.
81. Farmer PB. Enantiomers of cyclophosphamide and ifosfamide. *Biochem Pharmacol* 1988; 37:145–148.
82. Holm KA, Kindberg CG, Stobaugh JF, Slavik M, Riley CM. Stereoselective pharmacokinetics and metabolism of the enantiomers of cyclophosphamide. *Biochem Pharmacol* 1990; 39:1375–1384.
83. Burkert H. Ifosfamide: European perspective. *Semin Oncol* 1982; 9(suppl 1):28–35.
84. Arnold H. Über die chemie neuer zytostatisch wirksamer N-chlor-aethyl-phosphorsäuresterdiamide. Vortrag auf dem V. Internat. Kongreb für Chemotherapie; 1967 Jun 26–Jul 1; Wien. Verlag der Wiener Medizinische Akademie Abstr A IV-1a/5.
85. Brock N. Nouveau esters phosphamidés de moutarde azotée et leur activité cytostatique. *Laval Médical* 1968; 39:696–701.
86. Brock N. The oxazaphosphorines. *Cancer Treatment Rev* 1983; 10:3–15.
87. Venditti JM. Treatment schedule dependency of experimentally active antileukemic (L1210) drugs. *Cancer Chemother Rep* (Part 3) 1971; 2:35–59.
88. Goldin A. Ifosfamide in experimental tumor systems. *Semin Oncol* 1982; 9(suppl 1):14–23.
89. Zalupski M, Baker LH. Ifosfamide. *JNCI* 1988; 80:556–566.

90. Barnett D. Preclinical toxicology of ifosfamide. *Semin Oncol* 1982; 9(suppl 1):8–13.
91. Drings P, Allner R, Brock N, et al. Erfahrungen mit neuartigen N-lost-phosphoramidestern. *Dtsch Med Wochenschrft* 1970; 95:491–497.
92. van Dyk JJ, Falkson HC, van der Merwe. Unexpected toxicity in patients treated with iphosphamide. *Cancer Res* 1972; 32:921–924.
93. Munshi NC, Loehrer PJ, Williams SD. Uroprotection in patients receiving cyclophosphamide and ifosfamide. In: Muggia FM, ed. *New Drugs, Concepts and results in Cancer Chemotherapy.* Boston: Kluwer Academic Publishers. 1992:119–126.
94. Drings P, Fritsch H. Ifosfamide in higher single doses for treatment of metastasized solid tumors. *Veh Deut Ges Inn Med* 1972; 78:166–169.
95. Schnitker J., Brock N, Burkert H, Fichter E. Evaluation of a cooperative clincal study of the cytostatic agent ifosfamide. *Arzneim-Forsch* 1976; 26:1783–1793.
96. Hoefer-Janker H, Scheef W, Gunther W, Hüls W. Erfahrungen mit der fraktionierten ifosfamide-stoβtherapie bei generalisierten malignen tumoren. *Med Welt* 1975; 26:972–979.
97. Brade WP, Herdrich K, Varini M. Ifosfamide, pharmacology, safety and therapeutic potential. *Cancer Treatment Rev* 1985; 12:1–47.
98. Pohl J. Stekar J, Hilgard P. Chloroacetaldehyde and its contribution to urotoxicity during treatment with cyclophosphamide or ifosfamide. *Arzneim-Forsch* 1989; 39:704,705.
99. Scheef W, Klein HO, Burkert H, et al. Controlled clinical studies with an anitidote against the urotoxicity of oxazaphosphorines: preliminary results. *Cancer Treatment Rep* 1979; 63: 501–505.
100. Brock N, Pohl J, Stekar J. Studies on the urotoxicity of oxazaphosphorine cytostatics and its prevention. 2. Comparative study on the uroprotective efficacy of thiols and other sulfur compounds. *Eur J Cancer* 1981; 17:1155–1163.
101. Colvin M. The comparative pharmacology of cyclophosphamide and ifosfamide. *Semin Oncol* 1982; 9(suppl 1):2–7.
102. Brock N, Pohl J. The development of mesna for regional detoxification. *Cancer Treatment Rev* 1983:33–43.
103. Crawford J, George M. The role of hematopoietic growth factors in support of ifosfamide/carboplatin/etoposide chemotherapy. *Semin Oncol* 1995; 22(suppl 7):18–22.
104. Elias AD, Ayash LJ, Wheeler C, et al. High-dose ifosfamide/carboplatin/etoposide with autologous hematopoietic stem cell support: safety and future directions. *Semin Oncol* 1994; 21 (suppl 12):83–85.
105. Dechant KL, Brogden RN, Pilkington T, Faulds D, Ifosfamide/Mesna. A review of its antineoplastic activity, pharmacokinetic properties and therapeutic efficacy in cancer. *Drugs* 1991; 42:428–467.
106. Freireich EJ, Bodey GP. Evaluating new agents: planning, execution and evaluation of clinical studies. In: Kuemmerle HP, ed. Berkarda B, Karrer K, Mathé G, coeds. *Clinical Chemothertherapy,* vol. III, *Antineoplastic Chemotherapy.* New York: Thieme-Stratton. 1984:115–138.
107. Stuart-Harris R, Harper PG, Kaye SB, Wiltshaw E. High-dose ifosfamide by infusion with mesna in advanced soft tissue sarcoma. *Cancer Treatment Rev* 1983; 10(suppl A):163,164.
108. Keizer HJ, Ouwerkerk J, Welvaart K, van der Velde CJH, Cleton FJ. Ifosfamide treatment as a 10-day continuous intravenous infusion. *J Cancer Res Clin Oncol* 1995; 121:297–302.
109. Lewis LD. Ifosfamide pharmacokinetics. *Invest New Drugs* 1991; 9:305–311.
110. Le Cesne A, Antoine E, Spielmann M, et al. High-dose ifosfamide: circumvention of resistance to standard dose ifosfamide in advanced soft tissue sarcomas. *J Clin Oncol* 1995; 13: 1600–1608.
111. Küpfer A, Aeschlimann C, Wermuth B, Cerny T. Prophylaxis and reversal of ifosfamide enencepalopathy with methylene blue. *Lancet* 1994; 343:763,764.
112. Zullian GB, Tullen E, Maton B. Methylene blue for ifosfamide associated encepalopathy. *New Eng J. Med* 1995; 332: 1239,1240.
113. Fields KF, Elfenbein GJ, Lazarus HM, et al. Maximum tolerated doses of ifosfamide, carboplatin, and etoposide given over 6 days followed by autologous stem-cell rescue: toxicity profile. *J Clin Oncol* 1995; 13:323–332.
114. Sledge GW, Antman KH. Progress in chemotherapy for metastatic breast cancer. *Semin Oncol* 1992; 19:317–332.

115. Wingo PA, Tong T, Bolden S. Cancer statistics, 1995. *CA* 1995; 45:8–30.
116. Henwood JM, Brogden RN. Etoposide: a review of its pharmacodynamic and pharmacokinetic properties, and therapeutic potential in combination chemotherapy of cancer. *Drugs* 1990; 30:438–490.
117. Ettinger DS. The place of ifosfamide in chemotherapy of small cell lung cancer: The eastern oncology group experience and a selected literature update. *Semin Oncol* 1995; 22(suppl 2): 23–27.
118. Warenius HM, Hurman DC, Cottier B. High-dose ifosfamide in small cell lung cancer [letter]. *Br J Cancer* 1986; 54:216.
119. Hanson HH. Management of small cell cancer of the lung. *Lancet* 1992; 339:846–849.
120. Nichols CR. The role of ifosfamide in germ cell tumors and non-small cell lung cancer. *Semin Oncol* 1995; 22(suppl 7):13–17.
121. Miller VA, Rigas JR, Grant SC, Pisters KMW, Kris MG. New chemotherapeutic agents for non-small cell lung cancer. *Chest* 1995; 107:306S–311S.
122. Gomm SA, Thatcher N, Cuthbert A, et al. High dose combination chemotherapy with ifosfamide, cyclophosphamide or cisplatin, mitomycin C and mustine with autologous bone marrow support in advanced non-small cell lung cancer. A phase I/II study. *Br J Cancer* 1991; 63: 293–297.
123. Pujol J-L, Rossi J-F, Le Chevalier T, et al. Pilot study of neoadjuvant ifosfamide, cisplatin, and etoposide in locally advanced non-small cell lung cancer. *Eur. J Cancer* 1990; 26:798–801.
124. Miller BA, Feuer EJ, Hankey BF. The significance of the rising incidence of breast cancer in the United States. In: DeVita VT, Hellman S, and Rosenberg SA, eds. *Important Advances in Oncology 1994*. Philadelphia: J.B. Lippencott. 1994:193–207.
125. Ayash LJ, Wheeler C, Fairclough D, et al. Prognostic factors for prolonged progression-free survival with high-dose chemotherapy with autologous stem cell support for advanced breast cancer. *J Clin Oncol* 1995; 13:2043–2049.
126. Sanchiz F, Milla A. High-dose ifosfamide and mesna in advanced breast cancer. A phase II study. *Cancer Chemother Pharm* 1990; 26(suppl):S91,S92.
127. Ghavamzadeh A. Treatment of metastatic breast cancer with the combination of ifosfamide, epirubicin and fluorouracil. *Cancer Chemother Pharm* 1990; 26(suppl):S66–S68.
128. McGuire, Rowinsky EK. Old drugs revisited, new drugs, and experimental approaches in ovarian cancer therapy. *Semin Oncol* 1991; 18:255–269.
129. Sutton GP, Blessing JA, Photopulos G, Berman ML, Homesley HD. Gynecologic oncology group experience with ifosfamide. *Semin Oncol* 1990; 17(suppl 4):6–10.
130. Motzer RJ, Cooper K, Geller NL, et al. The role of ifosfamide plus cisplatin-based chemotherapy as salvage therapy for patients with refractory germ cell tumors. *Cancer* 1990; 66:2476–2481.
131. Einhorn LH. Testicular cancer as a model for curable neoplasm: the Richard and Hilda Rosenthal Foundation award lecture. *Cancer Res* 1981; 41:3275–3280.
132. Clemm C, Hartenstein R, Willich N, Ledderose G, Wilmanns W. Combination chemotherapy with vinblastine, ifosfamide and cisplatin in bulky seminoma. *Acta Oncol* 1989; 28:231–235.
133. von Kalle A-K, Schaadt M, Diehl V. European experience with ifosfamide in lymphomas. *Semin Oncol* 1989; 16(suppl 3): 73–77.
134. Cabanillas F. Experience with ifosfamide combinations in malignant lymphomas. *Semin Oncol* 1989; 16(suppl 3):78–81.
135. Enblad G, Glimelius B, Hagberg H, Hindemalm C. Methyl-GAG, ifosfamide, methotrexate and etoposide (MIME) as salvage therapy for Hodgkin's disease and non-Hodgkin's lymphoma. *Acta Oncol* 1990; 29:297–301.
136. Elias A, Ryan L, Aisner J, Antman KH. Mesna, doxorubicin, ifosfamide, dacarbazine (MAID) regimen for adults with advanced sarcoma. *Semin Oncol* 1990; 17(suppl 4):41–49.
137. Cairo MS. The use of ifosfamide, carboplatin and etoposide in children with solid tumors. *Semin Oncol* 1995; 22(suppl 7):23–27.
138. Takamizawa A, Matsumoto S, Iwata T, et al. Synthesis and metabolic behavior of the suggested active species of isophosphamide having cytostatic activity. *J Med Chem* 1974; 17: 1237–1239.
139. Takamizawa A, Iwata T, Yamaguchi K, et al. Stereochemistry, metabolism, and antitumor

activity of 4-hydroperoxyisophosphamide (NSC-227114) and its stereoisomer. *Cancer Treatment Rep* 1976; 60:361–368.

140. Boal JH, Williamson M, Boyd V, Ludeman SM, Egan W. 31P nmr studies of the kinetics of bisalkylation by isophosphoramide mustard: comparisons with phosphoramide mustard. *J Med Chem* 1989; 32:1768–1773.

141. Chang TKH, Weber GF, Crespi CL, Waxman DJ. Differential activation of cyclophosphamide and ifosfamide by cytochromes P-450 2B and 3A in human liver microsomes. *Cancer Res* 1993:5629–5637.

142. Walker D, Flinois J-P, Monkman S, et al. Identification of the major human hepatic cytochrome P-450 involved in inactivation and *N*-dechloroethylation of ifosfamide. *Biochem Pharmacol* 1994; 47:1157–1163.

143. Boddy AV, Idle JR. Combined thin-layer chromatography-photography-densitometry for the quantification of ifosfamide and its principal metabolites in urine, cerebrospinal fluid and plasma. *J Chromatogr* 1992; 575:137–142.

144. Norpoth K. Studies on the metabolism of ifosfamide (NSC-109724) in man. *Cancer Treatment Rep* 1976; 4:437–443.

145. Kamen BA, Frenkel E, Colvin OM. Ifosfamide: should the honeymoon be over? [letter] *J Clin Oncol* 1995; 13:307–309.

146. Goren MP, Wright RK, Pratt CB, Pell FE. Dechloroethylation of ifosfamide and neurotoxicity. *Lancet* 1986; 2:1219,1220.

147. Skinner R, Sharkey IM, Pearson ADJ, Craft AW. Ifosfamide, mesna and nephrotoxicity in children. *J. Clin Oncol* 1993; 11:173–190.

148. Zamlauski-Tucker MJ, Morris ME, Springate JE. Ifosfamide metabolite chloroacetaldehyde causes fanconi syndrome in the perfused rat kidney. *Toxicol Appl Pharmacol* 1994; 129:170–175.

149. Low JE, Borch RF, Sladek NE. Further studies on the conversion of 4-hydroxyoxazaphosphorines to reactive mustards and acrolein in inorganic buffers. *Cancer Res* 1983; 43:5815–5820.

150. Hohorst HJ, Bielicki L, Voelcker G. The enzymatic basis of cyclophosphamide specificity. *Adv Enzyme Reg* 1986; 25:99–122.

151. Alarcon RA, Meienhofer J, Atherton E. Isophosphamide as a new acrolein-producing antineoplastic isomer of cyclophosphamide. *Cancer Res* 1972; 32:2519–2523.

152. Gibaldi M, Perrier D. *Pharmacokinetics*. 2nd ed. New York: Marcel Dekker, 1982.

153. Pantarotto C, Martini A, Belvedere G, Donelli MG, Frigerio A. Studies on the disposition of cyclophosphamide (NSC-26271) in tumor bearing mice by means of gas chromatography-chemical ionization-mass fragmentography. *Cancer Treatment Rep* 1976; 60:493–500.

154. Juma FD, Rogers HJ, Trounce JR. The pharmacokinetics of cyclophosphamide, phosphoramide mustard and nor-nitrogen mustard studied by gas chromatography in patients receiving cyclophosphamide therapy. *Br J. Clin Pharmacol* 1980; 10:327–335.

155. Kurowski V, Wagner T. Comparative pharmacokinetics of ifosfamide, 4-hydroxyifosfamide, chloroacetaldehyde and 2- and 3-dechloroethylifosfamide in patients on fractionated intravenous ifosfamide therapy. *Cancer Chemother Pharm* 1993; 33:36–42.

156. Masurel D, Wainer IW. Analytical and preparative high-performance liquid chromatographic separation of the enantiomers of ifosfamide, cyclophosphamide and trofosfamide and their determination in plasma. *J Chromatogr* 1989; 490:133–143.

157. Granvil CP, Gehrcke B, Konig WA, Wainer IW. The determination of the enantiomers of ifosfamide and its 2- and 3-*N*-dechloroethylated metabolites in plasma and urine using enantioselective gas chromatography with mass spectrometric detection. *J. Chromatogr* 1993; 622:21–31.

158. Wright JE, Tetyakov O, Ayash L, Elias A, Rosowsky A, Frei E III. Analysis of 4-hydroxycyclophosphamide in human blood. *Anal Biochem* 1995; 224:154–158.

159. Anderson LW, Ludeman SM, Colvin OM, et al. Quantitation of 4-hydroxycyclophosphamide/aldophosphamide in whole blood. *J Chromatrogr* 1995; 667:247–257.

160. Chan KK, Hong PS, Tutsch K, Trump DL. Clinical pharmacokinetics of cyclophosphamide and metabolites with and without SR-2508. *Cancer Res* 1994; 54:6421–6429.

161. Bryant BM, Jarman M, Baker MH, Smith IE, Smyth JF. Quantification by gas chromatog-

raphy on *N,N'*-di-(2-chloroethyl)-phosphoramidic acid in the plasma of patients receiving iso-phosphamide. *Cancer Res* 1980; 40:4734–4738.

162. Kurowski V, Cerny T, Küpfer A, Wagner T. Metabolism and pharmacokinetics of oral and intravenous ifosfamide. *J Cancer Res Clin Oncol* 1991; 117(suppl IV):S148–S153.

163. Kaijser GP, Beijnen JH, Jeunink EL, et al. Determination of chloroacetaldehyde, a metabolite of oxazaphosphorine cytostatic drugs, in plasma. *J Chromatogr* 1993; 614:253–259.

164. Moore MJ. Clinical pharmacokinetics of cyclophosphamide. *Drug Dispos* 1991; 20:194–208.

165. Kaijser GP, Beijnen JH, Bult A, Underberg WJM. Ifosfamide metabolism and pharmaco-kinetics. *Anticancer Res* 1994; 14:517–532.

166. Lind MJ, Margison JM, Cerny T, Thatcher N, Wilkinson PM. Comparative pharmacokinetics and alkylating activity of fractionated intravenous and oral ifosfamide in patients with bronchogenic-carcinoma. *Cancer Res* 1989; 49:753–757.

167. Lewis LD. Ifosfamide pharmacokinetics. *Invest New Drugs* 1991; 9:305–311.

168. Lind MJ, Ardiet C. Pharmacokinetics of alkylating agents. *Cancer Surveys* 1993; 17:157–188.

169. Allen LM, Creaven PJ, Nelson RL. Studies on the human pharmacokinetics of ifosfamide (NSC-109724). *Cancer Treatment Rep* 1976; 60:451–458.

170. Thomas Wagner, Ifosfamide clinical pharmacokinetics. *Clin Pharmacokinet* 1994; 26: 439–456.

171. Boos J, Welslau W, Ritter J, Blaschke G, Schellong G. Ifosfamid und die metabolite der seitenkettenoxidation-ausscheidung im urine bei verschiedenen pädiatrischen therapieproto-kollen. *Klin Pädiatr* 1992; 204:299–305.

172. Grever MR, Schepartz SA, Chabner BA. The National Cancer Institute: cancer drug discovery and development program. *Semin Oncol* 1992; 19:622–638.

173. Brock N. Oxazaphosphorine cytostatics: structure-activity relationships. Selectivity and metabolism, regional detoxification. In: Reinhoudt DN, Connors TA, Pinedo HM, van den Poll KW, eds. *Structure–Activity Relationships of Anti-Tumor Agents*. The Hague: Martinius Nijhoff Publishers. 1983:239–267.

174. Chen L, Waxman DJ. Intratumoral activation and enhanced chemotherapeutic effect of oxa-zaphosphorines following cytochrome P-450 gene transfer: development of a combined chemotherapy/cancer gene therapy strategy. *Cancer Res* 1995; 55:581–589.

175. Abel G, Cox PJ, Farmer PB, et al. Isolation and identification of a metabolic intermediate in the selective dechloroethylation of one of the four stereoisomers of 4-methylcyclophospha-mide. *Cancer Res* 1978; 38:2592–2599.

176. Kutscher B, Niemeyer U, Engel J, et al. Synthesis and antitumor activity of two ifosfamide analogs with a five-membered ring. *Arzneim-Forsch* 1995; 45:323–326.

177. Foster AB, Jarman M, Kinas RW, et al. 5-Fluoro- and 5-chlorocyclophosphamide: synthesis, metabolism, and antitumor activity of the cis and trans isomers. *J Med Chem* 1981; 24: 1399–1403.

178. Ayash LJ, Wright JE, Tretyakov O, et al. Cyclophosphamide pharmacokinetics: Correlation with cardiac toxicity and tumor response. *J. Clin Oncol* 1992; 10:995–1000.

179. Farmer PB, Cox PJ. Synthesis and antitumor activity of 6-trifluoromethylcyclo-phosphamide and related compounds. *J Med Chem* 1975; 18:1106–1110.

180. Ludeman SM, Boyd VL, Regan JB, Gallo KA, Zon G, Ishii K. Synthesis and antitumor activ-ity of cyclophosphamide analogues. 4. Preparation, kinetic studies, and anticancer screening of "phenylketophosphamide" and similar compounds related to the cyclophosphamide metabolite aldophosphamide. *J Med Chem* 1986; 29:716–727.

181. Stec WJ. Cyclophosphamide and its congeners. *J Organophosphorus Chem* 1982; 13:145–174.

182. Montgomery JA, Struck RF. Synthesis and structure-activity relationships of pre-activated analogs of cyclophosphamide (NSC-26271). *Cancer Treatment Rep* 1976; 60:381–393.

183. Takamizawa A, Matsumoto S, Iwata T, et al. Studies on cyclophosphamide metabolites and their related compounds. 2. Preparation of an active species of cyclophosphamide and related compounds. *J Med Chem* 1975; 18:376–383.

184. Takamizawa A, Matsumoto S, Iwata T, et al. Synthesis and metabolic behavior of the suggested active species of isophosphamide having cytostatic activity. *J Am Chem Soc* 1973; 95:985,986.

185. Kubota T, Hanatani YH, Tsuyuki K, et al. Antitumor effect and metabolic activation of cyclo-phosphamide and 4-hydroperoxycyclophosphamide in the human breast carcinoma (MX-1)-nude mouse system. *Gann* 1983; 74:437–444.

186. Jones RJ. Purging with 4-hydroperoxycyclophosphamide [review]. *J Hematother* 1992; 1: 343–348.

187. Peter G, Wagner T, Hohorst H-J. Studies on 4-hydroxycyclophosphamide (NSC-18185): a simple preparation method and its application for the synthesis of a new class of "activated" sulfur-containing cyclophosphamide (NSC-26271) derivatives. *Cancer Treatment Rep* 1976; 60:429–435.

188. Niemeyer U, Engel J, Scheffler G, et al. Chemical characterization of ASTA Z 7557 (INN mafosfamide, CIS-4-sulfidoethylthio cyclophosphamide), a stable derivative of 4-hydroxycyclophosphamide. *Invest New Drugs* 1984; 2:133–139.

189. Kwon C-H, Borch RF, Engel J, Niemeyer U. Activation mechanisms of mafosfamide and the role of thiols in cyclophosphamide metabolism. *J Med Chem* 1987; 30:395–399.

190. Klein HO, Wickramanye PD, Christian E, Coerper C. Preclinical evaluation of toxicity and therapeutic effacy of a stabilized cytostatic metabolite of cyclophosphamide (ASTA Z 7557, INN mafosfamide). *Invest New Drugs* 1984; 2:191–199.

191. Abele R, Aapro MS, Haeflinger JM, Alberto P. Phase I study of cyclohexylamine and lysine salt of mafosfamide. *Cancer Chemother Pharm* 1986; 16:182,183.

192. Bruntsch U, Groos G, Hiller TA, Wandt, Tigges FJ. Phase-I study of mafosfamide-cyclohexylamine (ASTA-Z-7557, NSC 345 842) and limited phase-I data on mafosfamide-lysine. *Invest New Drugs* 1985; 3:293–296.

193. Laporte JP, Douay L, Lopez M, et al. One hundred twenty-five adult patients with primary acute leukemia autografted with marrow purged by mafosfamide: a 10-year single institutional experience. *Blood* 1994; 84:3810–3818.

194. Kwon C-H, Borch RF. Effects of *N*-substitution on the activation mechanisms of 4-hydroxycyclophosphamide analogues. *J Med Chem* 1989; 32:1491–1496.

195. Wang Y, Farquhar D. Aldophosphamide acetal diacetate and structural analogues: synthesis and cytotoxicity studies. *J Med Chem* 1991; 34:197–203.

196. Beran M, Borje SA, Wang Y, McCredie KB, Farquhar D. The effects of acetaldophosphamide, a novel stable aldophosphamide analogue, on normal human and leukemic progenitor cells in vitro: implications for use in bone marrow purging. *Cancer Res* 1988; 48:339–345.

197. Andersson BS, Wang Y-Q, McCredie KB, Farquhar D. Suitability of a new stable acetal analogue of aldoifosfamide for purging leukemic cells from human bone marrow. *Leukemia* 1990; 4:435–440.

198. Borch RF, Valente RR. Synthesis, activation and cytotoxicity of aldophosphamide analogues. *J Med Chem* 1991; 34:3052–3058.

199. Sladek NE, Dockham PA, Lee M-O. Human and mouse hepatic aldehyde dehydrogenases important in the biotransformation of cyclophosphamide and the retinoids. *Adv Exp Med Biol* 1990; 284:97–104.

200. Sahovic E, Colvin M, Hilton L, Ogawa M. Role for aldehyde dehydrogenase in survival of progenitors for murine blast cell colonies after treatment with 4-hydroperoxycyclophosphamide in vitro. *Cancer Res* 1988; 48:1223–1226.

201. Friedman OM, Wodinsky I, Myles A. Cyclophosphamide (NSC-26271)-related phosphoramide mustards-recent advances and historical perspective. *Cancer Treatment Rep* 1976; 60:337–346.

202. Boyd VL, Robbins JD, Egan W, Ludeman SM. ^{31}P Nuclear magnetic resonance spectroscopic observation of the intracellular transformations of oncostatic cyclophosphamide metabolites. *J Med Chem* 1986; 29:1206–1210.

203. Lenssen U, Hohorst HJ. Zur frage der permiabilität von *N,N*-bis(2-chloräthyl)-phosphorsäurediamid in tumorzellen. *J Cancer Res Clin Oncol* 1979; 93:161–164.

204. Sonawat H, Liebfritz D, Engel J. Hilgard P. Biotransformation of mafosfamide in P388 mice leukemia cells: intracellular ^{31}P-nmr studies. *Biochim Biophys Acta* 1990; 1052:36–41.

205. Struck RF, Schmid SM, Waud WR. Antitumor activity of halogen analogs of phosphoramide, isophosphoramide and triphosphoramide mustards, and cytotoxic metabolites of cyclophosphamide, ifosfamide, and trofosfamide. *Cancer Chemother Pharm* 1994; 34:191–196.

206. Yuan Z-M, Smith PB, Brundrett RB, Colvin M, Fenselau C. Glutathione conjugation with phosphoramide mustard with cyclophosphamide. A mechanistic study using tandem mass spectrometry. *Drug Metab Dispos* 1991; 19:625–629.

207. Dirven HAAM, van Ommen B, van Bladeren PJ. Involvement of human glutathione S-trans-

ferase isozymes in the conjugation of cyclophosphamide metabolites with glutathione. *Cancer Res* 1994; 54:6215–6220.

208. Vaury C, Lane é R, Noguiez P, et al. Human glutathione S-transferase M1 null genotype is associated with a high inducibility of cytochrome P450 1A1 gene transcription. *Cancer Res* 1955; 55:5520–5523.

209. Meier T, Allenbacher A, Mueller E, et al. Ifosfamide induced depletion of glutathione in human peripheral blood lymphocytes and protection by mesna. *Anti-cancer Drugs* 1994; 5:403–409.

210. Lind MJ, McGown AT, Hadfield JA, Thatcher N, Crowther D, Fox BW. The effect of ifosfamide and its metabolites on intracellular glutathione levels *in vitro* and *in vivo*. *Biochem Pharmacol* 1989; 38:1835–1840.

211. Insittoris E, Tretter L, Gaal D. Severe depletion of cellular thiols and glutathione-related enzymes of a carmustine-resistant L-1210 strain associates with collateral sensitivity to cyclophosphamide. *Cancer Chemother Pharm* 1993; 33:85–88.

212. Pohl J, Bertram B, Hilgard P, Nowrousian MR, Stüben J, Weißler M. D-19575-A sugar-linked isophosphoramide mustard derivative exploiting transmembrane glucose transport. *Cancer Chemother Pharm* 1995; 35:364–370.

213. Coleman CN. Hypoxia in tumors: a paradigm for the approach to biochemical and physiological heterogeneity. *JNCI* 1988; 80:310–317.

214. Kennedy KA, Teicher BA, Rockwell S, Sartorelli AC. The hypoxic tumor cell: a target for selective cancer chemotherapy. *Biochem Pharmacol* 1980; 29:1–8.

215. Bickel MH. The pharmacology and biochemistry of N-oxides. *Pharmacol Rev* 1969; 21:325–355.

216. Adams GE, Stratford IJ, Wallace RG, Wardman P, Watts. Toxicity of nitro compounds towards hypoxic mammalian cells in vitro: dependence on reduction potential. *JNCI* 1980; 64:555–560.

217. Moore HW, Czerniak R. Naturally occurring quinones as potential bioreductive alkylating agents. *Med Res Rev* 1981; 1:249–280.

218. Begg AC, Shrieve DC, Smith KA, Terry NHA. Effects of hypoxia, pH and growth stage on cell killing in Chinese hamster V79 cells *in vitro* by activated cyclophosphamide. *Cancer Res* 1985; 45:3454–3459.

219. Grau C, Bentzen SM, Overgaard J. Cytotoxic effects of misonidazole and cyclophosphamide on aerobic and hypoxic cells in a C₃H mammary carcinoma. *Br J Cancer* 1990; 61:61–64.

220. Tannock I. Response of aerobic and hypoxic cells in a solid tumor to adriamycin and cyclophosphamide and interaction of the drugs with radiation. *Cancer Res* 1982; 42:4921–4926.

221. Hill RP, Stanley JA. The response of hypoxic B16 melanoma cells to in vivo treatment with chemotherapeutic agents. *Cancer Res* 1975; 35:1147–1153.

222. Firestone A, Mulcahy RT, Borch RF. Nitroheterocycle reduction as a paradigm for intramolecular catalysis of drug delivery to hypoxic cells. *J Med Chem* 1991; 34:2933–2935.

223. Mulcahy RT, Gipp JJ, Schmidt JP, Joswig C, Borch RP. Nitrobenzyl phosphorodiamidates as potential hypoxia-selective alkylating agents. *J Med Chem* 1994; 37:1610–1615.

224. Tietze LF, Neumann M. Möllers T, et al. Proton-mediated liberation of aldophosphamide from a nontoxic prodrug: a strategy for tumor selective activation of cytocydal drugs. *Cancer Res* 1989; 49:4179–4184.

225. Waxman DJ, Sundseth SS, Srivastava PK, Lapenson DP. Gene-specific oligonucleotide probes for alpha, mu, pi, and microsomal rat glutathine S-transferases: analysis of liver transferase expression and its modulation by hepatic enzyme inducers and platinum anticancer drugs. *Cancer Res* 1992; 52:5797–5802.

226. Antman KS, Griffin JD, Elias A, et al. Effect of recombinant human granulocyte-macrophage colony-stimulating factor on chemotherapy-induced myelosuppression. *New Engl J Med* 1988; 319:593–598.

227. Antman K, Eder JP, Frei E III. High-dose chemotherapy with bone marrow support for solid tumors [review]. *Imp Adv Oncol* 1987:221–235.

228. Wilcox WS. The last surviving cancer cell: the chances of killing it. *Cancer Chemother Rep* 1966; 50:541–542.

229. Frei E III. Curative cancer chemotherapy [review]. *Cancer Res* 1985; 45:6523–6537.

3 Development of the Nitrosoureas

David B. Ludlum, PhD, MD

CONTENTS

1. INTRODUCTION

Several of the most important principles in cancer drug development are illustrated by the discovery of the nitrosoureas as antitumor agents: the success of random screening in finding new agents; the importance of the assay system in evaluating new agents; the use of structure–activity relationships in developing more active agents when a lead compound is discovered; and the understanding and further developments that arise from mechanism of action studies. These contributions are all discussed in the following chapter. Additionally, since the nitrosoureas are still under active investigation, it is reasonable to hope that further advances in basic research may lead to additional improvements in the clinical use of these agents.

2. INITIAL DISCOVERY AND ANALOG SYNTHESIS

In the 1950s, after the alkylating agents had become established as useful chemotherapeutic agents, the National Cancer Institute organized a comprehensive screening program to discover new compounds with antitumor activity (*1*). Several animal tumors were investigated for use in the screening assay, and the L1210 murine leukemia line was chosen for much of the testing; literally thousands of synthetic and naturally occurring compounds were tested for activity against this tumor. In 1960, Greene and Greenberg reported that the synthetic compound, *N*-methyl-*N*'-nitro-*N*-nitrosoguanidine (MNNG), resulted in a moderate increase in the life-span of mice carrying intraperitoneal L1210 cells (*2*). As discussed in Section 3, the choice of this animal species for screening purposes probably favored the discovery of the nitrosoureas—the therapeutic index is high in rodents because these animals have high

From: *Cancer Therapeutics: Experimental and Clinical Agents*
Edited by: B. Teicher Humana Press Inc., Totowa, NJ

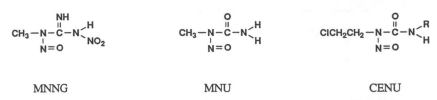

Fig. 1. Structures of MNNG, MNU, and CENU. CENUs in clinical use in this country include: BCNU (R = chloroethyl), CCNU (R = cyclohexyl), and MeCCNU (R = methylcyclohexyl).

levels of a DNA repair enzyme, O^6-alkylguanine-DNA alkyltransferase, which protects normal cells from some of the DNA damage caused by the nitrosoureas.

Since MNNG represented a new class of compounds, the National Cancer Institute decided to investigate its activity further and to synthesize analogs of MNNG in an attempt to find more active derivatives. A synthetic program was started at the Southern Research Institute in Birmingham, AL, and new compounds were tested for activity against L1210 cells (*3,4*).

One of the first congeners tested, *N*-methyl-*N*-nitrosourea (MNU), whose structure is shown in Fig. 1, proved to be significantly more active against ip injected L1210 cells than MNNG (*5*). Even more importantly, given the scarcity of agents effective against central nervous system malignancies, this compound was active against intracerebrally implanted L1210 cells as well (*5*).

These findings led to a systematic study of the effects of varying the structure of MNU on the antitumor activity of this compound; *see* Fig. 1. Replacing the methyl group in the N-position with alkyl groups that did not contain a halogen atom had little effect on activity (*6*). However, replacing this group with a 2-chloroethyl or a 2-fluoroethyl group resulted in a major increase in activity (*3,4,6,7*). Compounds with a 2-bromoethyl group in this position were less active than the 2-chloroethyl derivatives, and compounds with a 2-iodoethyl group were inactive. 2-Chloroethyl derivatives were chosen for development over 2-fluoroethyl derivatives, because the latter can give rise to the toxic metabolite, 2-fluoroacetic acid (*4*).

The compound containing two 2-chloroethyl groups, *N,N'*-bis(2-chloroethyl)-*N*-nitrosourea (BCNU), proved to be especially active; it cured mice that had been injected with a lethal dose of L1210 cells either intraperitoneally or intracerebrally (*7*). Ultimately, this compound was the first nitrosourea to be chosen for clinical trial.

With the advantage of 2-chloroethyl substitution at the N-position established, attention was paid to the effects of varying substituents at the N'-position. By varying the hydrophobicity of this group, it was possible to change the lipid solubility of the entire molecule. This was important because the activity of the nitrosoureas against intracerebrally implanted L1210 was attributed to their fat solubility allowing them to penetrate cell membranes by passive diffusion. A compound bearing the hydrophobic cyclohexyl group at the N'-position, *N*-(2-chloroethyl)-*N'*-cyclohexyl-*N*-nitrosourea (CCNU), was especially effective against intracerebrally implanted L1210 cells and was chosen for further development on this basis (*8*). Hansch and his colleagues established the relationship between lipid solubility and antitumor activity for a wide range of nitrosoureas (*9,10*).

An additional objective of the synthetic program was to find nitrosoureas that would be effective against solid tumors. To this end, nitrosoureas were tested for

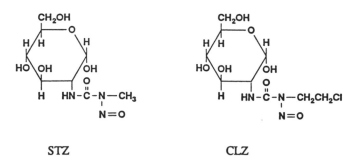

Fig. 2. Structures of STZ and CLZ.

activity against a panel of solid animal tumors and human tumor xenografts (*11*). *N*-(2-chloroethyl)-*N'*-(trans-4-methylcyclohexyl)-*N*-nitrosourea (MeCCNU) proved to be more active than BCNU or CCNU against one of these, the Lewis lung carcinoma, and was chosen for further development for this reason (*11*).

At about the same time that the synthetic nitrosoureas were being developed, a naturally occurring methylnitrosourea derivative, streptozotocin (STZ), was also found to have antitumor activity (*12*). This interesting compound, whose structure is shown in Fig. 2, had less bone marrow toxicity than MNU. This observation led Montgomery and his colleagues to synthesize the chloroethyl analog of STZ, chlorozotocin (CLZ), whose structure is also shown in Fig. 2. (*13*)

3. INITIAL CLINICAL TRIALS

Because of their activity against animal tumors, clinical trials of the *N*-(2-chloroethyl)-*N'*-alkyl-*N*-nitrosoureas (CENUs) were begun with great enthusiasm. Especially encouraging were the results obtained in the treatment of brain tumors. In keeping with animal data showing that CENUs could cure mice that had been injected intracerebrally with L1210 cells, these agents had moderate activity against CNS neoplasms in humans (*14–16*). Both BCNU and CCNU were effective, but the more lipid-soluble CCNU had no clear superiority over BCNU. The responses were more modest than hoped for, but they were nevertheless definite, and the CENUs remain one of the few classes of drugs effective against gliomas and other CNS tumors.

The CENUs also had activity against Hodgkin's and non-Hodgkin's lymphoma, malignant melanoma, tumors of the gastrointestinal tract, and some other solid tumors (*17*), and are currently used in combination with other agents in the treatment of these malignancies (*18*). Nevertheless, it was disappointing that the CENUs were not more active in the clinic in view of their high activity in animal models (*19*). As described below, the probable explanation for this is that levels of the DNA repair enzyme, O^6-alkylguanine-DNA alkyltransferase, are higher in the normal tissues of rodents than in humans, thus enhancing the therapeutic ratio in the animal models that were used to evaluate the CENUs.

The naturally occurring nitrosourea, STZ, was also introduced into clinical trials in the 1970s. This compound had previously been shown to be diabetogenic in animals (*20*) and, consistent with that finding, had activity against islet cell carcinomas in humans (*21*). Furthermore, STZ was found to be less toxic to the bone marrow than

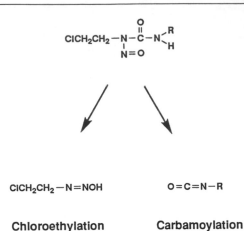

Fig. 3. Decomposition of a CENU. Chloroethylation results from the production of a chloroethylating species like chloroethyl diazonium hydroxide, and carbamoylation results from the production of an isocyanate.

the CENUs. As discussed below, the presence of the sugar moiety on STZ prevents protein carbamoylation by this compound, and it was anticipated that other nitrosoureas containing the same sugar would not be myelosuppressive. Unfortunately, however, the chloroethyl analog of STZ, chlorozotocin, was found to have bone marrow toxicity (*22*).

4. MECHANISM OF ACTION STUDIES

Early investigations of the nitrosoureas suggested that they were in a different category from the "alkylating agents," a group of compounds that are known to react with DNA and that are thought to produce their therapeutic effects through DNA modification. Not only did the nitrosoureas have a different chemical structure from the classical alkylating agents, many of which are related to nitrogen mustard, but their spectrum of activity in animal models was different and even their bone marrow toxicity in humans differed from that of the nitrogen mustards, being slower in onset.

It became apparent early in the investigation of the nitrosoureas that these compounds decomposed rapidly in aqueous solution, and that they had the capacity both to alkylate DNA and to carbamoylate proteins (*23*). The decomposition scheme shown in Fig. 3 accounted for this; the chloroethyl diazonium hydroxide moiety shown at the left could alkylate DNA and the isocyanate moiety shown at the right could carbamoylate proteins (*23*). The ability to carbamoylate proteins clearly distinguished the nitrosoureas from the mustards at a molecular level.

An alternate or additional point of view was that the DNA modification produced by the nitrosoureas was qualitatively different from that produced by the mustards and that differences in biological activity reflected this difference. In studying the reactions of MNU with DNA, Lijinsky et al. had shown that a fully deuterated methyl group was transferred intact from MNU to DNA (*24*). We reasoned that an analogous transfer of a chloroethyl group from a CENU would confer alkylating ability on the DNA itself and would lead to secondary reactions, including DNA crosslinking (*25*). The first indication that such reactions occurred came from the isolation of a

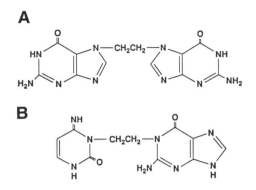

Fig. 4. DNA crosslinks formed by the CENUs. **A.** 1,2-bis(7-guanyl)-ethane; **B.** 1-(3-cytosinyl),2-(1-guanyl)ethane.

derivative of cytosine, $3, N^4$-ethanocytosine, that had evidently been formed by an initial transfer of a chloroethyl group to a base N, followed by an intramolecular condensation reaction (*25,26*).

Kohn then showed that DNA modified by CENUs underwent reversible denaturation, indicating that interstrand crosslinks had indeed been formed (*27*). This, of course, led to a search for the nature of the crosslink. Ultimately, the two crosslinked entities shown in Fig. 4, 1,2-bis(7-guanyl)ethane and 1-(3-cytosinyl),2-(1-guanyl)ethane, were isolated from DNA treated with BCNU (*28,29*). For steric reasons, it seemed probable that 1,2-bis(7-guanyl)ethane (the "GG crosslink") was intrastrand in nature and that 1-(3-cytosinyl),2-(1-guanyl)ethane (the "GC crosslink") was responsible for interstrand crosslinking, but this has never been firmly established.

It seemed probable that 1,2-bis(7-guanyl)ethane was formed by the sequential attachment of a chloroethyl group to the N-7 position of one guanine followed by its reaction with the N-7 position of a second guanine. Neither of the base positions that are connected by the $-CH_2CH_2-$ bridge in 1-(3-cytosinyl), 2-(1-guanyl)ethane is very reactive, however, and it was not immediately clear how this crosslink was formed.

Meanwhile, in an important discovery, Erickson et al. had shown that the sensitivity of human tumor cells to the nitrosoureas was inversely related to their ability to remove alkyl groups from the O^6- position of guanine; cells that had higher levels of O^6-alkylguanine-DNA alkyltransferase ("alkyltransferase") were resistant to the action of the nitrosoureas (*30*). Consequently, we proposed the scheme shown in Fig. 5 to explain both the formation of the GC crosslink and the role of alkyltransferase in conferring resistance to the action of the nitrosoureas (*29*).

The first step in the crosslinking reaction shown in Fig. 5 is the transfer of a chloroethyl group from the CENU to the O^6-position of guanine in DNA. This is followed by an intramolecular condensation to form the intermediate, $1,O^6$-ethanoguanine, which ultimately reacts with the N-3 position of cytosine to form the GC crosslink. However, alkyltransferase can remove the chloroethyl group from the O^6-position of guanine before crosslinking can occur. If this happens, the DNA is truly repaired; the modified O^6-chloroethyl guanine is restored to its original unmodified form, and the cell is protected from toxicity. Alkyltransferase also recognizes the second intermediate in this pathway, $1,O^6$-ethanoguanine, but in this case, the protein becomes

Cytotoxic Reaction   Resistance Mechanism

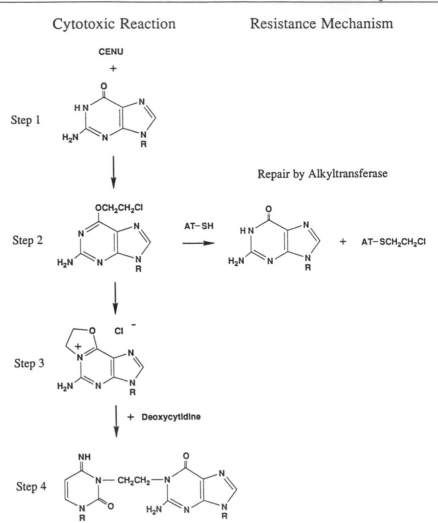

Fig. 5. Reaction of a CENU with guanine in DNA. The attachment of a chloroethyl group to the O^6-position of guanine leads to a crosslink in a four-step reaction. However, this process can be interrupted by alkyltransferase, which causes resistance by removing the chloroethyl group before crosslinking can occur. R = deoxyribose contained in the DNA structure.

bound to DNA, and additional steps are necessary to restore the DNA to its original condition (*31*).

The formation of the O^6-chloroethyl guanine in DNA was finally demonstrated by Parker et al. (*32*), and the other steps shown in Fig. 5 have been fully established (*33*). GC crosslinks are depleted in cells that are resistant to the action of CENUs (*34*), and the evidence that GC crosslink formation is cytotoxic is altogether convincing. In fact, the GC crosslink is probably the first crosslink whose formation has been directly linked to cytotoxicity. This information is now being put to use, since inhibitors of alkyltransferase are being tested for their ability to restore the sensitivity of tumor cells to CENUs (*see* Section 5).

However, formation of the GC crosslink is not essential for antitumor activity, because the methylating agents, MNU and STZ, are also active. These agents methylate the O^6-position of guanine, which suggests that O^6-alkylation itself is cytotoxic (*35*). Nevertheless, the CENUs produce a variety of other DNA modifications, and it seems probable that some of these modifications that do not involve the O^6-position of guanine also contribute to their cytotoxicity.

Some evidence for this was obtained several years ago in studies of adapted *Escherichia coli* (*36*). When either *uvrA*-deficient or *recA*-deficient mutants were adapted by growth in MNNG, they became more resistant to the cytotoxic action of MNNG and to *N*-ethyl-*N*-nitrosourea, but they remained sensitive to BCNU. More recently, Wu et al. have investigated the effects of transfecting alkyltransferase into wild-type and excision repair-deficient Chinese hamster ovary (CHO) cells (*37*). Both of these cell lines are deficient in alkyltransferase and are sensitive to MNNG, but the excision repair-deficient strain is more sensitive to *N*-(2-chloroethyl)-*N*1-nitrosourea (CNU) than is the wild type. When human alkyltransferase is transfected into either cell line, sensitivity to MNNG is greatly diminished. However, the transfected excision repair-deficient cells are still more sensitive to CNU than are the transfected wild-type cells. The authors suggest that this difference represents the ability of the excision repair mechanism to recognize a CNU-induced GG intrastrand crosslink that is cytotoxic to these cells (*37*).

Other studies have suggested that purine glycosylases may also play a role in the resistance phenomenon. HPLC profiles of the DNA modifications present in resistant glial cells that have been treated with CNU show that several adducts besides the GC crosslink are absent or diminished in amounts in comparison with the amounts present in sensitive cells (*34*). Since both alkyltransferase and 3-methyladenine DNA glycosylase II are upregulated in the *E. coli* adaptive response to methylating agents (*38*), it seems likely that glycosylases may also participate in the resistance of mammalian cells to DNA-modifying agents. Bacterial 3-methyladenine DNA glycosylase II, has in fact, been shown to act on all of the CNU-modified bases in Fig. 6 (*39,40*) At least two of these, 1,2-bis(7-guanyl)ethane and N^2,3-ethanoguanine, probably disrupt the DNA structure in a way that may be cytotoxic. Furthermore, biochemical assays have shown that glycosylase levels are elevated in a resistant glial cell line that is apparently depleted in some of the modified bases shown in Fig. 6 (*41*).

In summary, the haloethylnitrosoureas exert their cytotoxic action by modifying DNA. The formation of one lesion, 1-(3-cytosinyl),2-(1-guanyl)ethane, is clearly a lethal event, and it is likely that other DNA modifications are cytotoxic as well. At the same time, DNA repair is an important cause of resistance: one repair enzyme, alkyltransferase, prevents the formation of the lethal GC crosslink, and other repair enzymes probably act on other DNA modifications that are cytotoxic.

Our understanding of the mechanism of action of these agents is not complete, however. For example, the first step in DNA modification, transfer of the chloroethyl group to a DNA base, is more complicated than indicated in Fig. 3. By a mechanism that is not yet fully established, the carbon-halogen bond in the CENU is broken during alkylation, and the carbon that was originally attached to the halogen becomes the one that attaches to the DNA base (*42,43*). Also, one would expect that the distribution of DNA adducts would be the same for different CENUs if the agents acted

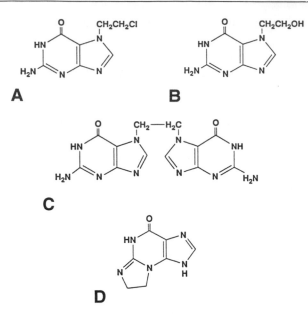

Fig. 6. Modified bases released from CENU-treated DNA by bacterial 3-methyladenine DNA glyco-sylase II. **A**. 7-(2-chloroethyl)guanine; **B**. 7-(2-hydroxyethyl)guanine; **C**. 1,2-bis(7-guanyl)ethane; **D**. N^2,3-ethanoguanine.

by generating a common alkylating intermediate as shown in Fig. 3, but the distribution is actually different for different agents (*44*).

Also not explained by a simple alkylation mechanism is the observation that these agents have a preference for guanine-rich sequences in DNA (*45*). Clearly, neighboring bases affect the alkylation sites, and this raises the possibility that CENUs could be targeted to specific regions, perhaps increasing their toxicity to tumor cells more than to normal cells.

Finally, the role of carbamoylation is not completely elucidated. CENUs with carbamoylating activity inhibit several enzymes involved in DNA repair, presumably by reacting with proteins involved in the repair process. Thus, it is possible that the ability of some CENUs to damage DNA and, at the same time, to inhibit repair may contribute to their antitumor activity (*46*).

5. FURTHER DEVELOPMENTS

Since alkyltransferase activity is closely linked to CENU resistance, attention has turned to methods of inhibiting this enzyme as a means of restoring sensitivity (*47*). Inhibition is favored by the fact that the reaction is stoichiometric. A single molecule of alkyltransferase has the ability to remove just one alkyl group from an O^6-alkylguanine in DNA; the alkyl group that is removed is transferred to the alkyltransferase, which is thereby inactivated.

Two approaches to inactivation have been used. In one approach, STZ is given somewhat before the CENU; in the interval before CENU administration, alkyltransferase is consumed in repairing the DNA methylation caused by STZ (*48,49*). In the second approach, a low-mol-wt inhibitor is given to inactivate the alkyltransferase directly (*50,51*). Both approaches have been shown to work, but the latter seems to be particularly promising and is being pursued actively at the present time.

The use of low-mol-wt inhibitors began with the observation that exposure of mammalian cells to O^6-methylguanine and certain other O^6-alkylguanines caused a major decrease in cellular alkyltransferase activity (*50,51*). O^6-Methylguanine was shown to be a substrate for alkyltransferase, although it is a very poor substrate in comparison with O^6-methylguanine in DNA (*50*). Relatively high concentrations of O^6-methylguanine were required to produce inhibition, and a search for more effective inhibitors was initiated.

O^6-Benzylguanine was found to be much more active than O^6-methylguanine, producing as much inhibition at a concentration of 2.5 μM as O^6-methylguanine did at 0.2 mM (*52*). Other O^6-alkylguanine inhibitors have been synthesized, and their ability to inactivate alkyltransferase has been tested; compounds having easily displaced allyl or benzyl groups are most active (*53,54*). Research in this area is being pursued actively, and the critical question will be whether the alkyltransferase inhibitors sensitize tumor cells to the cytotoxic action of the CENUs more than they sensitize normal cells.

Meanwhile, the search for more active CENUs continues. Derivatives that include carrier steroid or amino acid groups that may target the CENU to particular tumor cell populations have been synthesized as reviewed recently (*55*). At a molecular level, attempts have been made to increase the sequence specificity of these agents by linking them to peptides that bind in the minor groove of DNA (*56,57*). Although these agents do show a different specificity of reaction, they have not yet shown any increase in antitumor activity.

6. SUMMARY

As mentioned in Section 1., the development of the nitrosoureas has illustrated several important aspects of cancer drug discovery. First, the lead compound was discovered by a random screening process that focused attention on a chemical structure different from any that had been used previously in the treatment of cancer. Careful synthetic work combined with an ongoing evaluation of antitumor activity led to the development of significantly more active compounds.

Both the initial screening and the drug development program emphasize the importance of the choice of assay system for evaluating antitumor activity. In this case, the major role of alkyltransferase in both causing tumor resistance and protecting normal cells from toxicity illustrates the problems that may arise from testing compounds in a model that has different DNA repair capabilities from those found in human cells. As an aside, this particular problem might now be avoided by engineering animal tumor models with human DNA repair genes.

Finally, mechanism of action studies have helped greatly in understanding the limitations of the CENUs and, perhaps, in overcoming them. Study of the CENUs has provided us with a specific example of a cytotoxic DNA modification whose formation can be prevented by a particular cellular enzyme. At the same time, indications that other CENU-induced DNA modifications may be cytotoxic suggest that effective antitumor agents may produce a variety of DNA modifications that depend on different repair modalities to produce complete resistance.

ACKNOWLEDGMENTS

The author would like to express his appreciation for the contributions of his many colleagues to the work from our laboratory that is reviewed here. Support by grant CA-44499 from the National Cancer Institute, Department of Health, Education and Welfare is also gratefully acknowledged.

REFERENCES

1. Schepartz SA. Early history and development of the nitrosoureas. *Cancer Treatment Rep* 1976; 60:647–649.
2. Greene MO, Greenberg J. The activity of nitrosoguanidines against ascites tumors in mice. *Cancer Res* 1960; 44:1166–1171.
3. Montgomery JA. Chemistry and structure–activity studies of the nitrosoureas. *Cancer Treatment Rep* 1976; 60:651–664.
4. Montgomery JA. The development of the nitrosoureas: A study in congener synthesis. In: Prestayko AW, Crooke ST, Baker LH, Carter SK, Schein PS, eds. *Nitrosoureas: Current Status and New Developments*. New York: Academic. 1981:3–8.
5. Skipper HE, Schabel FM Jr, Trader MW, Thomson JR. Experimental evaluation of potential anticancer agents. VI. Anatomical distribution of leukemic cells and failure of chemotherapy. *Cancer Res* 1961; 21:1154–1164.
6. Johnston TP, McCaleb GS, Montgomery JA. The synthesis of antineoplastic agents. XXXII. N-nitrosoureas. I. *J Med Chem* 1963; 6:669–681.
7. Johnston TP, McCaleb GS, Oplinger PA, Montgomery JA. The synthesis of potential anticancer agents. XXXVI. N-nitrosoureas. II. Haloalkyl derivatives. *J Med Chem* 1966; 9: 892–910.
8. Schabel FM Jr. Nitrosoureas: A review of experimental antitumor activity. *Cancer Treatment Rep* 1976; 60:665–698.
9. Hansch C, Smith N, Engle R, and Wood, H. Quantitative structure-activity relationships of antineoplastic drugs: Nitrosoureas and triazenoimodazoles. *Cancer Chemother Rep* 1972; 56: 443–456.
10. Hansch C, Leo A, Schmidt C, Jow PY, Montgomery JA. Antitumor structure-activity relations. Nitrosoureas vs. L-1210 leukemia. *J Med Chem* 1980; 23:1095–1101.
11. Goldin A. Historical overview of nitrosourea development. In: Serrou B, Schein PS, Imbach J-L, eds. *Nitrosoureas in Cancer Treatment*. Amsterdam: Elsevier. 1981:3–11.
12. Evans JS, Gerritsen GC, Mann KM, Owen SP. Antitumor and hyperglycemic activity of streptozotocin (NSC-37914) and its cofactor, U-15,774. *Cancer Chemother Rep* 1965; 48:1–6.
13. Johnston TP, McCaleb GS, Montgomery JA. Synthesis of chlorozotocin, the 2-chloroethyl analog of the anticancer antibiotic streptozotocin. *J Med Chem* 1975; 18:104–106.
14. Levin VA. Chemotherapy of recurrent brain tumors. In: Prestayko AW, Crooke ST, Baker LH, Carter SK, Schein PS, eds. *Nitrosoureas: Current Status and New Developments*. New York: Academic. 1981:259–268.
15. Rosenstock JG. Lipid-soluble nitrosoureas in the management of children with primary and recurrent brain tumors. In: Prestayko AW, Crooke ST, Baker LH, Carter SK, Schein PS, eds. *Nitrosoureas: Current Status and New Developments*. New York: Academic. 1981:269–276.
16. Walker ME. Adjuvant therapy of brain tumors with nitrosoureas. In: Prestayko AW, Crooke ST, Baker LH, Carter SK, Schein PS, eds. *Nitrosoureas: Current Status and New Developments*. New York: Academic. 1981:277–284.
17. Carter SK, Schabel FM Jr, Broder LE, Johnston TP. 1,3-Bis(2-chloroethyl)-1-nitrosourea (BCNU) and other nitrosoureas in cancer treatment: A Review. *Adv Cancer Res* 1972; 16: 273–332.
18. Colvin M. Alkylating agents and platinum antitumor compounds. In: Holland JF, Frei III E, Bast RC Jr, Kufe DW, Morton DL, Weichselbaum RR, eds. *Cancer Medicine,* 3rd ed. Philadelphia: Lea & Febiger, 1993:733–754.

19. Wasserman TH, Slavik M, Carter SK. Clinical comparison of the nitrosoureas. *Cancer* 1975; 36: 1258–1268.

20. Rakieten N, Rakieten ML, Moreshwar V. The diabetogenic action of streptozotocin (NSC-37917). *Cancer Chemother Rep* 1963; 29:91–98.

21. Byrne PJ, Schein PS. Streptozotocin. In: Prestayko AW, Crooke ST, Baker LH, Carter SK, Schein PS, eds. *Nitrosoureas: Current Status and New Developments.* New York: Academic. 1981:367–377.

22. Hoth DF, Duque-Hammershaimb L. Chlorozotocin: clinical trials. In: Prestayko AW, Crooke ST, Baker LH, Carter SK, Schein PS, eds. *Nitrosoureas: Current Status and New Developments.* New York: Academic. 1981:387–398.

23. Wheeler GP. Mechanism of action of nitrosoureas. In: Sartorelli AC, Johns DG, eds. *Handbook of Experimental Pharmacology*, vol. XXXVII/2. New York: Springer-Verlag, 1975:65–84.

24. Lijinsky W, Garcia H, Keefer L, Loo J, Ross AE. Carcinogenesis and alkylation of rat liver nucleic acids by nitrosomethylurea and nitrosoethylurea administered by intraportal injection. *Cancer Res* 1972; 32:893–897.

25. Ludlum DB, Kramer BS, Wang J, Fenselau C. Reaction of 1,3-bis-(2-chloroethyl)-1-nitrosourea with synthetic polynucleotides. *Biochemistry* 1975; 14:5480–5485.

26. Kramer BS, Fenselau CC, Ludlum DB. Reaction of BCNU (1,3-bis[2-chloroethyl]-1-nitrosourea) with polycytidylic acid. Substitution of the cytosine ring. *Biochem Biophys Res Commun* 1974; 56:783–788.

27. Kohn KW. Interstrand cross-linking of DNA by 1,3-bis-(2-chloroethyl)-1-nitrosourea and other 1-(2-haloethyl)-1-nitrosoureas. *Cancer Res* 1977; 37:1450–1454.

28. Tong WP, Ludlum DB. Formation of the cross-linked base, diguanylethane, in DNA treated with N,N'-bis(2-chloroethyl)-N-nitrosourea. *Cancer Res* 1981; 41:380–382.

29. Tong WP, Kirk MC, Ludlum DB. Formation of the cross-link, 1-[N^3-deoxycytidyl],2-[N-deoxyguanosinyl]-ethane, in DNA treated with N,N'-bis(2-chloroethyl)-N-nitrosourea (BCNU). *Cancer Res* 1982; 42:3102–3105.

30. Erickson LC, Laurent G, Sharkey NA, Kohn KW. DNA cross-linking and monoadduct repair in nitrosourea-treated human tumour cells. *Nature* 1980; 288:727–729.

31. Gonzaga PE, Brent TP. Affinity purification and characterization of human O^6-alkylguanine-DNA alkyltransferase complexed with BCNU treated, synthetic oligonucleotide. *Nucleic Acids Res* 1989; 17:6581–6590.

32. Parker S, Kirk MC, Ludlum DB. Synthesis and characterization of O^6-(2-chloroethyl)guanine: a putative intermediate in the cytotoxic reaction of chloroethylnitrosoureas with DNA. *Biochem Biophys Res Commun* 1987; 148:1124–1128.

33. Ludlum DB. DNA alkylation by the haloethylnitrosoureas: nature of modifications produced and their enzymatic repair or removal. *Mutat Res* 1990; 233:117–126.

34. Bodell WJ, Tokuda K, Ludlum DB. Differences in DNA alkylation products formed in sensitive and resistant human glioma cells treated with N-(2-chloroethyl)-N-nitrosourea. *Cancer Res* 1988; 48:4489–4492.

35. Bennett RA Pegg AE. Alkylation of DNA in rat tissues following administration of streptozotocin. *Cancer Res* 1981; 41:2786–2790.

36. Kacinski BM, Rupp WD, Ludlum DB. Repair of haloethylnitrosourea-induced DNA damage in mutant and adapted bacteria. *Cancer Res* 1985; 45:6471–6474.

37. Wu Z, Chan C-L, Eastman A, Bresnick E. Expression of human O^6-methylguanine-DNA methyltransferase in a DNA excision repair-deficient Chinese hamster ovary cell line and its response to certain alkylating agents. *Cancer Res* 1992; 52:32–35.

38. Lindahl T, Sedgwick B, Sekiguchi M, Nakabeppu Y. Regulation and expression of the adaptive response to alkylating agents. *Annu Rev Biochem* 1988; 57:133–157.

39. Habraken Y, Carter CA, Sekiguchi M, Ludlum DB. Release of N^2,3-ethanoguanine from haloethylnitrosourea-treated DNA by *Escherichia coli* 3-methyladenine DNA glycosylase II. *Carcinogenesis* 1991; 12:1971–1973.

40. Habraken Y, Carter CA, Kirk MC, Ludlum DB. Release of 7-alkylguanines from N-(2-chloroethyl)-N'-cyclohexyl-N-nitrosourea-modified DNA by 3-methyladenine DNA glycosylase. *Cancer Res* 1991; 51:499–503.

41. Matijesevic Z, Bodell WJ, Ludlum DB. 3-Methyladenine DNA glycosylase activity in a glial cell line sensitive to the haloethylnitrosoureas in comparison with a resistant cell line. *Cancer Res* 1991; 51:1568–1570.

42. Parker S, Kirk MC, Ludlum DB, Koganty RR, Lown JW. Reaction of 1,3-bis-(2-chloroethyl) -1-nitrosourea (BCNU) with guanosine: Evidence for a new mechanism of DNA modification. *Biochem Biophys Res Commun* 1986; 139:31–36.

43. Naghipur A, Ikonomou MG, Kebarle P, Lown JW. Mechanism of action of (2-haloethyl)- nitrosoureas on DNA: Discrimination between alternative pathways of DNA base modification by 1,3-bis-(2-fluoroethyl)-1-nitrosourea by using specific deuterium labeling and identification of reaction products by HPLC/tandem mass spectrometry. *J Am Chem Soc* 1990; 112: 3178–3187.

44. Tong WP, Kohn KW, Ludlum DB. Modifications of DNA by different haloethylnitrosoureas. *Cancer Res* 1982; 42:4460–4464.

45. Hartley JA, Gibson NW, Kohn KW, Mattes WB. DNA sequence specificity of guanine-N7 alky- lation by three antitumor chloroethylating agents. *Cancer Res* 1986; 46:1943–1947.

46. Kann HE Jr. Carbamoylating activity of the nitrosoureas. In: Prestayko AW, Crooke ST, Baker LH, Carter SK, Schein PS, eds. *Nitrosoureas: Current Status and New Developments*. New York: Academic, 1981:95–105.

47. Pegg AE. Mammalian O^6-alkylguanine-DNA alkyltransferase: Regulation and importance in response to alkylating carcinogenic and therapeutic agents. *Cancer Res* 1990; 50:6119–6129.

48. Futscher BW, Micetich KC, Barnes DM, Fisher RI, Erickson LC. Inhibition of a specific DNA repair system and nitrosourea cytotoxicity in resistant human cancer cells. *Cancer Commun* 1989; 1:65–73.

49. Gerson SL. Modulation of human lymphocyte O^6-alkylguanine-DNA alkyltransferase by streptozotocin *in vivo*. *Cancer Res* 1989; 49:3134–3138.

50. Dolan ME, Morimoto K, Pegg AE. Reduction of O^6-alkylguanine-DNA alkyltransferase activ- ity in HeLa cells treated with O^6-alkylguanines. *Cancer Res* 1985; 45:6413–6417.

51. Karran P, Williams SA. The cytotoxic and mutagenic effects of alkylating agents on human lymphoid cells are caused by different DNA lesions. *Carcinogenesis* 1985; 6:789–792.

52. Dolan ME, Moschel RC, Pegg AE. Depletion of mammalian O^6-alkylguanine-DNA alkyltrans- ferase activity by O^6-benzylguanine provides a means to evaluate the role of this protein in pro- tection against carcinogenic and therapeutic alkylating agents. *Proc Natl Acad Sci USA* 1990; 87:5368–5372.

53. Moschel RC, McDougall MG, Dolan ME, Stine L, Pegg AE. Structural features of substituted purine derivatives compatible with depletion of human O^6-alkylguanine-DNA alkyltransferase. *J Med Chem* 1992; 35:4486–4491.

54. Chae MY, McDougall MG, Dolan ME, Swenn K, Pegg AE, Moschel RC. Substituted O^6-benzylguanine derivatives and their inactivation of human O^6-alkylguanine-DNA alkyltrans- ferase. *J Med Chem* 1994; 37:342–347.

55. McCormick JE, McElhinney RS. Nitrosoureas from chemist to physician: Classification and re- cent approaches to drug design. *Eur J Cancer* 1990; 26:207–221.

56. Chen FX, Zhang Y, Church KM, Bodell WJ, Gold B. DNA crosslinking, sister chromatid ex- change and cytotoxicity of N-2-chloroethylnitrosoureas tethered to minor groove binding pep- tides. *Carcinogenesis* 1993; 14:935–940.

57. Gold B, Church KM, Wurdeman RL, Zhang Y, Chen FX. Control over the sequence specificity of DNA alkylation: syntheses and reactions with ^{32}P-end-labelled DNA of N-alkyl-N-nitro- soureas linked to minor groove binding lexitropsins. *IARC Sci Publications* 1991; 105:439–442.

4

Platinum Complexes

Lloyd R. Kelland, PhD

CONTENTS

1. HISTORICAL ASPECTS

It is now over 20 years since the platinum-based drug cisplatin (cis-diamminedichloro platinum [II]) was added to the armamentarium available to the oncology physician. Interestingly, the chemical identity of cisplatin was first established in the mid-19th century (and known as Peyrone's chloride) and, were it not for the well-documented serendipitous observations of Barnett Rosenberg while performing experiments investigating the effects of electric fields on bacteria, its antitumor properties may have remained undiscovered (*1*). Cisplatin has long been accepted to confer significant antitumor activity against a variety of neoplasms; in particular, as a result of the introduction of cisplatin-containing chemotherapy regimes, over 80% of men presenting with testicular cancer are now cured of their disease (*2*). Initial studies at the Royal Marsden Hospital (London) by Wiltshaw and Carr also established that cisplatin conferred promising activity against ovarian cancer (*3*). Combination regimens including cisplatin (typically with cyclophosphamide) generally produce clinical complete remissions in approx 50% of patients with advanced disease. Moreover, long-term followup studies in patients with advanced ovarian cancer have shown that combination chemotherapy containing cisplatin enhanced survival by at least 10% at 5 and 10 yr postdiagnosis compared to the accepted best available drugs of the pre-cisplatin era (*4*). In addition to these dramatic effects on the long-term survival of cancer sufferers, cisplatin also offers substantial palliative benefit to patients with small-cell lung, bladder, cervical, and head and neck carcinomas (*2*).

In spite of demonstrable dramatic efficacy against these neoplasms, from early days, cisplatin was observed to suffer from two major drawbacks: (1) its particularly severe normal tissue toxicities, and (2) the propensity of many tumors to be resistant *ab initio* or to acquire resistance to its tumor inhibitory properties. Therefore, there has been substantial effort to discover and develop analogs of cisplatin that address

From: *Cancer Therapeutics: Experimental and Clinical Agents*
Edited by: B. Teicher Humana Press Inc., Totowa, NJ

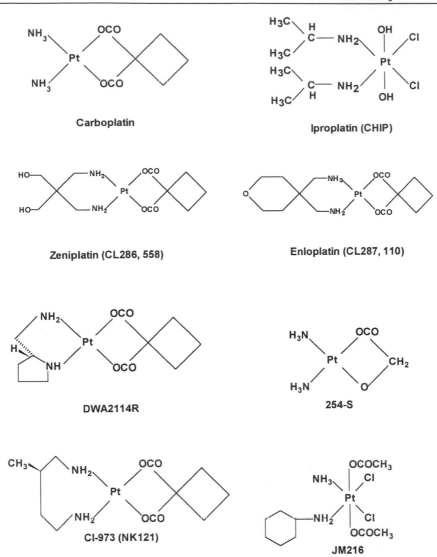

Fig. 1. Structures of analogs designed principally to reduce the toxicity of platinum-based chemotherapy.

these two limitations. This chapter summarizes early efforts to improve on cisplatin, the current clinical status of analog development (a total of 13 platinum complexes are currently undergoing or have recently undergone clinical trial), and future prospects for the discovery of new platinum-based anticancer drugs, particularly with respect to the circumvention of resistance mechanisms known to limit the efficacy of cisplatin.

2. THE STATUS OF DEVELOPMENT OF CISPLATIN ANALOGS

2.1. Analogs Developed to Reduce the Toxicities of Cisplatin

In contrast to the circumvention of tumor resistance to cisplatin (*see* Section 2.2.), efforts to ameliorate the drug's severe adverse effects (predominantly nephro-, gastrointestinal-, and neurotoxicities) have met with considerably more success (Fig. 1).

Table 1
Dose-Limiting Toxicities of Cisplatin Analogs

Analog	Dose-limiting toxicity	Other notable toxicity
Carboplatin	Thrombocytopenia	
Iproplatin	Thrombocytopenia	Diarrhea
Zeniplatin	Neutropenia	Nephrotoxicity
Enloplatin	Neutropenia	Nephrotoxicity
DWA2114R	Leukopenia	
254-S	Leukopenia, thrombocytopenia	Nephrotoxicity
CI-973	Neutropenia	
JM216	Leukopenia, thrombocytopenia	
Tetraplatin	Neuropathy	
Oxaliplatin	Neuropathy	
Lobaplatin	Thrombocytopenia	
Cycloplatam	Myelosuppression	
L-NDDP	Neutropenia, thrombocytopenia	

A summary of the dose-limiting toxicities of these analogs is shown in Table 1. To date, the most successful advance has been provided by carboplatin (cis-diammine-1, 1-cyclobutane dicarboxylato platinum [II]; Paraplatin), which remains the only cisplatin analog to have been licensed worldwide and to have entered routine clinical practice (5).

2.1.1. CARBOPLATIN

From the initial clinical trials with carboplatin in the early 1980s, it was clear that the drug was substantially less toxic than cisplatin, not only in terms of nephrotoxicity, but also in terms of nausea, vomiting, and neurotoxicity. Myelosuppression, primarily thrombocytopenia (see Table 1) is dose-limiting (6). Today, the main area of contention with carboplatin revolves around whether this less toxic analog should replace cisplatin as the first-line treatment for patients where cisplatin-based therapy has proven efficacy (i.e., those presenting with ovarian or testicular cancer). Numerous randomized trials (especially in patients with advanced ovarian cancer) have been performed; overviews of these trials have also been published (7). Conclusions drawn from such studies should bear in mind that:

1. Accrual to some of the larger studies did not include early stage (IC,II) good prognosis groups;
2. The median followup of some of the studies is still at too early a stage to comment on comparative effects on long-term survival; and
3. The doses of cisplatin and carboplatin have varied from trial to trial (it is generally accepted that carboplatin is approximately fourfold less dose-potent than cisplatin; thus doses of 400 vs 100 mg/m^2, respectively, should be compared).

Nonetheless three major conclusions may be drawn (7):

1. Carboplatin is less toxic to the kidneys, nerves, and gastrointestinal system than cisplatin;
2. Response rates in ovarian cancer are broadly comparable; and

3. Survival rates among similar prognostic groups at comparable doses (*see above*) are similar.

Recently published long-term followup results of the first randomized trial of cisplatin (100 mg/m² q 4 wk for 5 courses and 30 mg/m² for another 5 courses) vs carboplatin (400 mg/m² q 4 wk for 10 courses), performed at the Royal Marsden Hospital, London, between October 1981 and June 1984 in 131 patients with advanced epithelial ovarian cancer, have shown that the two drugs produce similar long-term survival (*8*). With a median followup of 9 yr, 5-yr survival rates were 15% (95% confidence interval [CI], 8–26%) for cisplatin (median survival duration of 19.5 mo) and 19% CI, 11–30%) for carboplatin (median survival duration of 13 mo); none of these differences were statistically significant (*8*).

Although these analyses have led some to propose that the less toxic carboplatin rather than cisplatin should currently be considered the standard choice of platinum compound in the first-line treatment of advanced ovarian cancer (typically in combination with cyclophosphamide, e.g., *9*), this view has not yet gained universal acceptance. Similarly, carboplatin has been shown to possess equivalent activity to cisplatin in germ-cell tumors of the testis and is less toxic (*10*).

A further advantage of carboplatin might be in studies of dose intensity (*see* Section 3.2.2.), since the drug largely lacks nonhematological toxicity (thus allowing high doses to be given with hematologic support by growth factors). Second, as developed by Calvert and colleagues, dosage calculations in terms of the area under the plasma concentration vs time curve (AUC) based on pretreatment renal function are applicable (*11*); dose (mg) = AUC × (glomerular filtration rate + 25). Carboplatin AUC values of 5 mg/mL × min for previously untreated patients were recommended.

Carboplatin undoubtedly offers patients a more acceptable level of morbidity compared to cisplatin, but clinical data suggest that the two agents share crossresistance. For example, in the above-described Royal Marsden Hospital randomized trial (*8*), where the study design allowed crossover between the two arms, patients who crossed over from one platinum to the other owing to progressive or nonresponding disease exhibited a low (14.3%; 95% CI, 4.8–30.25%) response rate to the other platinum compound.

2.1.2. IPROPLATIN (CHIP)

Similarly to carboplatin, iproplatin (JM9, CHIP, [cis-dichloro-trans-dihydroxo-bis {isopropylamine} platinum {IV}) (Fig. 1) was developed on the basis of a favorable preclinical toxicity profile to that of cisplatin with accompanying retention of antitumor efficacy (*12*). To date, iproplatin is the only platinum analog in addition to carboplatin to have undergone extensive phase II/III evaluation. The results of these trials, including large randomized trials with carboplatin, support the following conclusions (*13–15*):

1. As with carboplatin, the dose-limiting toxicity of iproplatin is thrombocytopenia.
2. Iproplatin is active in cisplatin-responsive disease (e.g., ovarian cancer), but shares crossresistance with cisplatin and carboplatin, and thus does not offer significant activity in cisplatin refractory disease. In patients with ovarian cancer, previously treated with either cisplatin or carboplatin, response rates to iproplatin were 12% in 60 patients resistant to cisplatin and 11% in 18 patients resistant to carboplatin (*14*).

3. In randomized trials of iproplatin vs carboplatin in ovarian (*14*) (120 patients) and cervical (*15*) (394 patients) cancers, iproplatin was more toxic (especially in terms of gastrointestinal effects) and less active than carboplatin. In the ovarian trial, median survival was 114 wk for patients in the carboplatin arm (400 mg/m² q 28 d) and 68 wk for patients receiving iproplatin (300 mg/m² q 28 d) ($p = 0.008$).

Based on such clinical data, iproplatin appears to offer no advantage over carboplatin, and therefore, its future use would appear to be limited.

2.1.3. OTHER ANALOGS

Since the introduction of carboplatin and iproplatin in the early to mid-1980s, several other analogs designed mainly to reduce the toxicity of cisplatin-based chemotherapy have entered clinical trial (Fig. 1). Many of the complexes (e.g., zeniplatin, enloplatin, and the Japanese-based DWA2114R and CI-973) possess identical leaving group chemistry (oxygenated leaving groups conferring good aqueous solubility and greater stability) to carboplatin. However, and perhaps surprisingly, both zeniplatin and enloplatin caused some nephrotoxicity in patients while in phase I clinical trial. Their future clinical role would appear to be limited. In addition, another analog, 254-S (cis-diammine [glycolato] platinum, synthesized in Japan) has also produced one severe episode of renal toxicity. 254-S is currently undergoing phase II/III trials in Japan, generally using a schedule of 100 mg/m² q 4 wk (*16*). In a phase II trial in patients ($n = 15$) with advanced germ-cell testicular cancer, prostatic cancer ($n = 16$), or transitional-cell carcinoma of the urinary tract ($n = 35$), objective response rates were 80, 18.8 and 28.6%, respectively. DWA2114R in phase II trials has also shown response rates broadly comparable to that observed for cisplatin, e.g., a 44% response rate was observed in patients ($n = 34$) with advanced ovarian cancer (*17*).

In addition to studies based in Japan, CI-973 was evaluated in a five-daily dose schedule phase I at the Fox Chase Cancer Center, Philadelphia (*18*). In common with the Japanese phase I, neutropenia was dose-limiting, and in contrast to carboplatin, thrombocytopenia was infrequent. No responses were recorded; the recommended phase II dose of CI-973 was 30 mg/m²/d for 5 d. In another US-based phase I study using a bolus q 28-d schedule, similar results were reported; granulocytopenia was dose-limiting, no responses were observed, and recommended phase II doses were 230 and 190 mg/m² for previously untreated and treated patients, respectively (*19*).

2.1.4. ORALLY ACTIVE PLATINUM DRUGS: JM216

The success of carboplatin is testimony to the importance of considering patient quality of life issues in cancer chemotherapy. Since cisplatin and carboplatin require iv administration, scientists at the Institute of Cancer Research, London, in conjunction with the Johnson Matthey Technology Centre and Bristol Myers Squibb, have attempted to facilitate patient comfort and convenience further during platinum-based chemotherapy through the discovery and development of platinum complexes capable of oral administration. Moreover, through potential treatment on an outpatient basis, hospitalization costs may be substantially reduced. Such studies have led to the introduction of the first clinically used orally administrable platinum complex: bis-acetato-ammine-dichloro-cyclohexylamine platinum (IV) (JM216) (Fig. 1). Preclinically, JM216 possesses several encouraging properties (*20,21*):

1. Rodent toxicology resembled carboplatin rather than cisplatin; myelosuppression was dose-limiting;
2. Ferret emesis studies showed that JM216 was substantially less emetic than cisplatin;
3. Orally administered JM216 showed antitumor activity broadly comparable to intravenously administered cisplatin/carboplatin in murine tumor and human ovarian carcinoma xenograft models;
4. JM216 exhibited greater antitumor activity using a daily × 5 schedule q 21 d compared to administering the same total dose as a bolus q 21 d; and
5. In vitro, JM216 showed evidence of circumvention of acquired cisplatin resistance, especially in tumor cells where resistance was attributable to reduced drug transport.

JM216 entered phase I clinical trial at the Royal Marsden Hospital, London, in August 1992. Two phase I trials have now been completed; a single dose q 21 days and a schedule of daily administration on days 1–5, q 21 d. In agreement with preclinical rodent studies, myelosuppression (including both leukopenia and thrombocytopenia) was the dose-limiting toxicity. Emesis has been controllable, and no nephro- or neurotoxicity has been observed. A partial response and a reduction in the ovarian tumor marker CA125 were observed in a patient with ovarian cancer, which recurred after treatment with cisplatin (22). In late 1994, JM216 entered phase II trials in Europe and North America in patients with ovarian and lung carcinomas.

2.2. Analogs Designed Principally to Circumvent Tumor Resistance

As stated above, compared to efforts aimed at reducing the side effects of platinum-based chemotherapy, progress in overcoming tumor resistance to cisplatin has, thus far, met with little success in the clinic. Thus, circumvention of resistance remains the major goal in current platinum drug discovery programs.

2.2.1. 1,2-DIAMINOCYCLOHEXANE (DACH) PLATINUM COMPLEXES

The earliest lead to compounds that might offer clinical utility against cisplatin resistance arose over 20 years ago in studies by Burchenal and colleagues through their discovery of so-called DACH containing platinum complexes (23). Notably, these complexes exhibited activity in murine L1210 leukemia tumor models possessing acquired resistance to cisplatin. However, since this observation has not been translated to all other murine or human acquired cisplatin-resistant tumor models (e.g., in our own studies using the murine ADJ-PC6 plasmacytoma [24] and various human ovarian carcinoma xenografts [25]), doubt has been cast on the predictive utility of this mouse leukemia for human malignancies. Following formulation difficulties with early DACH complexes selected for clinical trial (e.g., JM82, PHIC), two more water-soluble derivatives have recently undergone phase I clinical trial: tetraplatin and oxaliplatin (Fig. 2; Table 1) (26–28). Disappointingly, in the phase I trials of both tetraplatin (26,27) and oxaliplatin (28), severe neurotoxicity has proven a limitation to their therapeutic efficacy. At this time, it is uncertain whether tetraplatin (where severe neurotoxicity was observed in patients receiving a cumulative dose above 200 mg/m² using a day 1, day 8 q 28 d schedule [26] and above 165 mg/m² using a daily × 5 schedule [27] will be progressed to phase II evaluation.

Oxaliplatin has also exhibited neurotoxicity during a phase I trial (28). Comprehensive phase II data for single-agent oxaliplatin have not yet been reported. However, four partial responses were observed in the phase I study (in patients with eso-

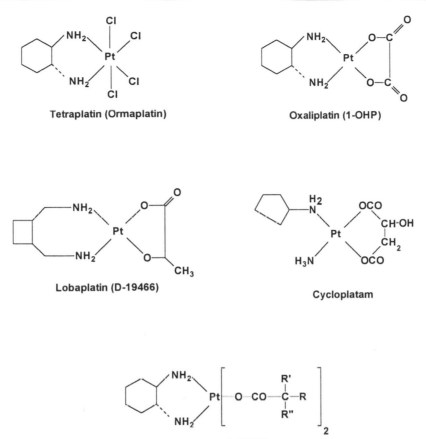

Fig. 2. Structures of analogs designed principally to circumvent tumor resistance.

phageal [2 cases], lung [1], and urothelial cancer [1]) (28). In addition, oxaliplatin (20 mg/m²/d for 5 d q 21 d) has been used in a randomized chronomodulated vs fixed infusion rate chemotherapy regime along with 5-fluorouracil (600 mg/m²/d for 5 d q 21 d) and folinic acid (leucovorin) (300 mg/m²/d for 5 d q 21 d) in patients with colorectal cancer metastases (29). In 47 patients, drug delivery was kept constant, whereas in 45 patients it was chronomodulated (5 fluorouracil and leucovorin at 0400 h and oxaliplatin at 1600 h). Whereas peripheral sensitive neuropathy was dose-limiting in the chronomodulated arm (attributed to the oxaliplatin), a significantly higher (and encouraging) objective response rate (53%, 95% CI = 38–68% compared to 32%; 95% CI = 18–46%) was observed in the chronomodulated arm. However, the contribution of oxaliplatin to the activity of this complex treatment protocol is difficult to ascertain.

Another approach to the clinical evaluation of DACH complexes has been provided through liposomal preparations of DACH complexes. A phase I trial with L-NDDP has reported dose-limiting toxicities of neutropenia and thrombocytopenia (30). However, drug stability formulation, and delivery problems remain to be overcome before this approach can be fully evaluated.

2.2.2. OTHER ANALOGS (FIG. 2)

Two other platinum analogs that, at least from preclinical data, may offer some utility against acquired cisplatin resistance, are in early clinical trials. Lobaplatin (D-19466) has completed phase I evaluation in Germany and the Netherlands (*31,32*). Thrombocytopenia was dose-limiting; responses (one partial, one complete) occurred in two patients with ovarian cancer (both pretreated with cisplatin and carboplatin) in the 5-d trial (*31*), and one partial response was observed in another ovarian cancer patient pretreated with platinum in a trial using a schedule of 72-h infusion every 4 wk (*32*). The results of phase II trials using this interesting complex are awaited. As with carboplatin, resulting plasma AUCs following administration of lobaplatin appeared to be dependent on renal function.

To date, clinical trials with cycloplatam have been conducted only in Russia and await full reporting.

3. FUTURE PROSPECTS

Tumor resistance remains the major factor that limits the clinical effectiveness of cisplatin/carboplatin. Various strategies to circumvent clinical resistance, based largely on increasing knowledge of how cisplatin exerts its cell killing effects and of mechanisms of resistance, may be envisaged. These include:

1. Development of analogs of cisplatin;
2. Dose intensification of cisplatin/carboplatin:
3. Pharmacological modulation of resistance mechanisms; and
4. Combination with other active anticancer drugs with nonoverlapping toxicities and mechanisms of resistance.

3.1. Mechanisms of Resistance to Cisplatin

Cisplatin reacts primarily by stepwise exchange of its two labile chlorides (leaving ligands) for water or hydroxyl ions (Fig. 3). The final positively charged, highly reactive, diaquo species (which is the same for cisplatin and carboplatin) is then capable of reacting with nucleophilic sites on DNA, RNA, or proteins. The presence of high chloride ion concentrations in extracellular fluid (approx 100 mM) suppresses the aquation reactions and allows the uncharged complex to penetrate cell membranes. However, on entering a cell, where the cytoplasmic chloride concentration is much lower (as low as 4 mM), the chloride ligands begin to exchange. Replacement of the two chloride ligands of cisplatin by the bidentate cyclobutane dicarboxylic acid (CBDCA) ligand in carboplatin results in a complex more than 100-fold resistant to the above aquation reactions; in chloride-free phosphate buffer, pH 7.0, cisplatin had a half-life of 2.4 h compared to a half-life of 268 h for carboplatin (*33*).

The cell killing effects of cisplatin appear to be the result of the formation of an assortment of stable bifunctional adducts on DNA, which then block replication and/or inhibit transcription (*34,35*). The most common adduct (60–65%) involves binding of platinum to the nitrogen on position 7 of the imidazole ring of adjacent deoxyguanosines along the same strand of DNA (the GpG 1,2-intrastrand adduct). In addition, ApG (20–25%) and GpXpG and ApXpG (5–6%; where X is any base) 1,3-intrastrand adducts, monofunctional adducts (2–3%), DNA–protein crosslinks, and G-G interstrand crosslinks (ISCs, 2%) are also found. Moreover, recent evidence

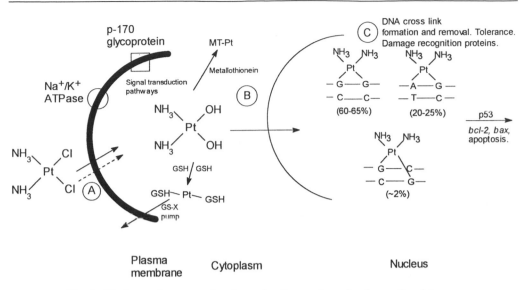

Fig. 3. Platinum drugs: mechanism of action and mechanisms of resistance.

measuring the sequence specificity of cisplatin DNA binding in the N-*ras* gene from cells exposed to cisplatin suggests that a novel adduct in the sequence 5′-TACT-3′ may also be formed (*36*). However, controversy still remains regarding the relative role of each of the various DNA adducts induced by cisplatin (especially intra- vs interstrand adducts) in mediating cell killing. On the one hand, there is supportive evidence emphasizing the importance of 1,2 intrastrand adducts. The inactive transplatin (*37*) is sterically unable to form the major GpG and ApG 1,2-intrastrand adducts formed by cisplatin. Instead, a high proportion of DNA monoadducts are formed (up to 85% of adducts following a 1–2 h drug incubation with DNA (*38*). These are mainly detoxified through rapid reaction with glutathione. A minority slowly rearrange to form bifunctional 1,3 or 1,4 G-G ISCs or DNA ISCs. Furthermore, the GpG intrastrand adduct has been shown to be poorly repaired compared to GpXpG and monofunctional adducts (*39,40*). Interestingly, both the G-G and A-G intrastrand adducts unwind DNA by 13°, whereas the G*X*G (*1,3*) intrastrand adduct unwinds DNA by 23°; bending of the DNA double helix is similar (32–35°) for all three adducts (*41*).

Although they represent only approx 2% of total adducts formed by cisplatin, other findings suggest that ISCs may be important determinants of cytotoxicity. Early studies in L1210 leukemia cells, using cis- and trans-platinum, showed a relationship between cell killing and levels of ISCs (*42*); although both isomers produce ISCs in naked DNA, only cisplatin produces substantial ISCs in whole cells. Moreover, two independent studies determining repair at the level of individual genes in paired cisplatin-sensitive and cisplatin-resistant human ovarian carcinoma cell lines have shown a marked increase in the gene-specific removal of ISCs in resistant lines, but no difference between sensitive and resistant lines in the removal of intrastrand adducts (*43,44*). Recent data have also indicated that the nature of the ISCs formed by transplatin and cisplatin in purified DNA differs with cisplatin favoring crosslink formation between guanines and transplatin between guanine and complementary cytosines (*45*).

Table 2
Genes/Proteins That May Play a Role
in Determining Tumor Sensitivity/Resistance to Cisplatin

Gene/protein	Comment	Reference
CPR²⁰⁰	Increased drug efflux	52
SQM1	Decreased drug accumulation	53
ERCC1	Increased DNA repair	79,80
HMG domain proteins (including HMG1 and 2)	Increased repair(?)/shielding from repair(?)	73–76; 79,80
c-Ha-*ras*	Increased drug resistance Decreased uptake/increased MT	81
c-*myc*	Increased drug resistance	82
c-*fos*	anti-*fos* ribozyme reverses resistance	83
HSP60	Heat-shock protein, chaperonin	87
p53	Mutations associated with drug resistance Cell-cycle checkpoint control/DNA repair	60,86,88

The type of crosslinks that eventually lead to death of the cell following exposure to cisplatin and how they bring about cell death are unknown. However, it appears likely that a programmed cell death, or apoptosis, is triggered in a variety of cell types (*46*), including in our own panel of human ovarian carcinoma cell lines (*47*).

Largely through the use of in vitro murine and human tumor cell lines, three major mechanisms of resistance to cisplatin have been identified:

1. Decreased intracellular transport of drug;
2. Increased cytoplasmic detoxification through increased levels of thiol-rich species, such as glutathione and/or metallothioneins; and
3. Enhanced removal of platinum-induced adducts from DNA and/or increased tolerance to platinum-DNA adducts (Fig. 3A, B, and C) (*see 48* for a review).

In addition, a number of genes and proteins (some directly associated with the three main cellular mechanisms of resistance described above) have been shown to be involved in determining the cellular sensitivity of tumor cells to cisplatin. These are summarized in Table 2.

3.1.1. DECREASED DRUG TRANSPORT

Many (but not all) acquired cisplatin-resistant cell lines (including our own 41McisR human ovarian carcinoma) (*49*) exhibit a decrease in platinum accumulation (typically two- to fourfold) compared to their respective parent line (*see 50* for a review). However, the mechanism by which platinum drugs enter cells remains unclear, with supportive laboratory evidence for roles for both passive diffusion (e.g., the uptake of cisplatin is not saturable) and active transport (e.g., uptake can be modulated by a variety of pharmacological agents including the Na$^+$/K$^+$-ATPase inhibitor, ouabain). This has led some to postulate that cisplatin may enter cells by both passive diffusion and partly through facilitated transport via a gated channel (*50*). In contrast to the increased efflux of drug observed in tumor cells with multiple resistance to other commonly used anticancer drugs (such as doxorubicin, paclitaxel, etoposide, and the vinca alkaloids, mediated through 170- and/or 190-kDa membrane glycoproteins), cisplatin resistance mediated at the level of the plasma membrane appears to occur mainly through reduced drug influx (*50*). None of our own acquired cisplatin-resistant human ovarian carcinoma cell lines exhibit increased levels of P-glycoprotein (*51*).

Although at least two studies have reported changes in membrane proteins that appear to be associated with decreased drug uptake (*52, 53*; Table 2), these proteins (a 200-kDa glycoprotein and a 46-kDa protein, SQM1) have not, as yet, been identified in additional cell lines. Further, it is not yet clear whether reduced drug uptake also plays a role in determining clinical resistance to platinum drugs.

3.1.2. Increased Cytoplasmic Detoxification

As with reduced drug accumulation, many (but again, not all) in vitro studies have provided evidence for a role for the cytoplasmic thiol-containing tripeptide glutathione (GSH) in mediating platinum drug resistance (e.g., *54*). In our own studies using eight human ovarian carcinoma cell lines exhibiting a 100-fold range in intrinsic sensitivity to cisplatin, GSH (but not glutathione *S*-transferase [GST]) levels showed a significant correlation with cisplatin sensitivity; the most resistant line possessing fourfold higher GSH levels than the most sensitive (*55*). Evidence for a direct interaction between cisplatin and GSH inside tumor cells involving 2 mol of GSH complexed with 1 mol of platinum to form bis(glutathionato)-platinum has also been reported (*56*). Elimination of this complex from tumor cells has been proposed to occur via an ATP-dependent glutathione *S*-conjugate export pump (the GS-X pump, which has recently been shown to be functionally overexpressed in acquired cisplatin-resistant HL-60 human leukemia cells [*57*] and has been linked to another efflux protein, multidrug resistance related protein (MRP), associated with a form of multidrug resistance [*58*]). Cytoplasmic detoxification of platinum-based drugs may also occur through binding to metallothioneins (MT), a class of cysteine-rich, low-mol-wt isoproteins. Increased levels of MT have been reported in at least some acquired cisplatin-resistant cell lines (*59*).

A number of studies have attempted to correlate clinical platinum resistance of ovarian cancer to increased levels of GST (*60–63*) or MT (*64*). However, apart from one study (*62*), which used a semiquantitative intensity of staining method and reported a higher intensity of staining for GST π in resistant tumors, these results do not support a role for either GST or MT in clinical platinum drug resistance.

3.1.3. Increased DNA Repair/Tolerance

Studies using both bacterial enzymes (*Escherichia coli* UVRABC nuclease [*65*]) and mammalian cell extracts [*66*] indicate that platinum-DNA adducts are removed from DNA by nucleotide excision repair. The *E. coli* UVRABC nuclease has been shown to incise the eighth phosphodiester bond 5′ and the fourth bond 3′ to G-G intrastrand crosslinks, thereby excising an oligomer containing the adduct [*65*]. Resistance to cisplatin in many acquired resistant cell lines, including our own studies, appears to be owing to either an enhanced repair/removal of platinum adducts from DNA or an increased tolerance to such adducts (*67,68*). Moreover, the possible relevance of DNA repair in determining responses to platinum-based therapy in ovarian cancer patients has been highlighted in studies measuring RNA levels encoding for the ERCC1 human DNA repair gene (*69,70*). Patients who were clinically resistant to cisplatin- (or carboplatin)-based therapy had a 2.6-fold significantly higher expression level of ERCC1 in their tumor biopsy than did patients who responded to that therapy. There is some evidence to suggest that the hypersensitivity of testicular cancer cell lines, which correlates with the clinical sensitivity of this tumor, might also be related to defective removal of platinum-DNA adducts (71,72).

3.1.4. OTHER PROTEINS/GENES

Over recent years, proteins, termed structure-specific recognition proteins (generally of approx 28 and 80–100 kDa), have been identified in mammalian cell extracts that bind specifically to the two major types of cisplatin-induced DNA 1,2,-intrastrand crosslinks and do not bind to adducts induced by transplatin (73,74). These proteins have been shown to possess high mobility group (HMG) domain motifs (e.g., SSRP1) (74); in addition, HMG1 and HMG2 themselves (proteins of 28.5 and 26.5 kDa, respectively) can recognize and bind to DNA platinated with cisplatin (75,76). The exact function of these damage recognition proteins, however, is presently unknown. Models have been proposed for their involvement in promoting the repair of cisplatin-damaged DNA or, in contrast, in blocking access of repair enzymes to damaged DNA. Support for the model involving shielding of ISCs from DNA repair enzymes has arisen from studies in yeast mutants where deletion of the HMG domain protein, lxr1, led to a twofold decrease in sensitivity to cisplatin (77). In addition, HMG domain proteins have recently been shown to inhibit specifically the repair of cisplatin-induced 1,2-intrastrand crosslinks by human excision nuclease (78). Alternatively, some support for the repair supposition is provided by observations that some (but not all) cisplatin-resistant tumor cell lines (some of which have an increase in DNA-repair capacity) also exhibit an increase in levels of damage recognition proteins (73,79). In addition, a damage recognition protein complex, B1, has been shown to contain a protein involved in an early stage of mammalian excision repair, human single-stranded binding protein (HSSB) (80).

Other genes/proteins that may have an involvement in determining cellular sensitivity to platinum drugs include various oncoproteins (e.g., p21*RAS*, *MYC*, *FOS/JUN*, and *BCL2/BAX/BCLx*), the p53 tumor suppressor gene, and a 60-kDa mitochondrial chaperonin heat shock protein (HSP60) (*see* Table 2) (81–88). Transformation of mouse fibroblasts with *ras* oncogenes produced a four- to eightfold increase in cisplatin resistance associated with a 40% decrease in accumulation and a 3.3-fold elevation in MT levels (81). Cisplatin has been shown to induce cell death through a programmed death pathway (apoptosis); at least some pathways of cell death appear to be activated through the wild-type p53 gene (84). Interestingly, testicular tumors (which are hypersensitive to cisplatin) have been reported rarely to exhibit p53 mutations, whereas tumors less responsive to chemotherapy commonly acquire p53 mutations (85). Moreover, p53 mutations have recently been shown to be associated with decreased sensitivity of human lymphoma cells to DNA-damaging agents, including cisplatin (86), and nuclear immunoreactivity of p53 in ovarian carcinomas has been associated with shorter overall survival in at least some studies (e.g., 60). Elevated constitutive levels of HSP60 have been observed to correlate with clinical resistance of ovarian cancer (87). Modulation of various intracellular signal transduction pathways (e.g., those mediated by protein kinase C or via the epidermal growth factor) may also influence sensitivity and resistance to cisplatin (89). Intriguingly, there is also evidence suggesting that some forms of resistance to cisplatin may only be operative in vivo and may not be apparent in two-dimensional tissue-culture systems (90).

3.2. Circumvention of Resistance

3.2.1. PLATINUM ANALOGS

In addition to the many platinum analogs currently in clinical trial (*see* Section 2.), including the DACH-containing complexes tetraplatin and oxaliplatin, and lobaplatin and JM216, which all circumvent cisplatin resistance in at least some (typically L1210 leukemia) preclinical models, further analog development is ongoing. Since cisplatin and carboplatin both possess symmetrical diammine carrier ligands, our efforts in collaboration with chemists at the Johnson Matthey Technology Centre, have centered on asymmetric ammine/amine (or mixed amine) platinum complexes (e.g., JM216) (*see* Section 2.1.4.), which may bind to DNA in a different manner to that of cisplatin (e.g., to differing sequences of DNA or to produce a differing spectrum of adducts). Consequently, recognition by the HMG domain damage recognition proteins and/or repair proteins might differ. Moreover, in additional efforts to design novel platinum complexes which should bind to DNA in a manner distinct from that of cisplatin (and carboplatin) we, and others, have pursued the idea of activating the trans geometry of platinum complexes (*91–93*), whereas Farrell and colleagues have synthesized a series of novel neutral bis(platinum) complexes where two cis-diammine platinum groups are linked by an alkyldiamine of variable length (*94*).

The realization that some trans platinum complexes are as active as their cis counterparts in vitro and, moreover, for the trans ammine(amine) dichlorodihydroxo platinum(IV) complexes, in vivo (*92*), contravenes the original structure–activity rules for platinum complexes based on cis and transplatin (*37*). Our studies have centered on JM335 (trans ammine [cyclohexylamine]dichlorodihydroxo platinum[IV]), which is the first transplatinum complex to demonstrate marked in vivo activity against both murine (including two acquired cisplatin-resistant models) and human (ovarian carcinoma) subcutaneous tumors. Other recently reported novel synthetic approaches include the demonstration of in vivo antitumor activity (P388 leukemia) for platinum(II) organoamides, which do not possess a hydrogen substituent on any nitrogen donor atom (general formula; $Pt(NRCH_2)_2L_2$ where R = polyfluorophenyl and L = pyridine or substituted pyridine) (*95*) and for a series of 2-substituted-4,5-bis(aminomethyl)-1,3-dioxolane platinum(II) complexes (*96*).

3.2.2. DOSE INTENSIFICATION OF CISPLATIN/CARBOPLATIN

In recent years, attempts have been made to increase the doses of cisplatin administered to patients in the hope of achieving improved response rates. Although the renal and gastrointestinal toxicities of cisplatin may be ameliorated through iv hydration and forced diuresis and 5HT3 inhibitor antiemetics, respectively, disabling neurotoxicity has proven to be dose-limiting (*97*). Carboplatin may be better suited to such studies (especially in combination with hematological support with growth factors) (*98*), since the main toxicities of carboplatin are hematological and dosage calculations based on kidney function are applicable (*11*). However, although a randomized trial of high- (100 mg/m²) vs low- (50 mg/m²) dose cisplatin in advanced ovarian cancer (both administered with cyclophosphamide every 21 d) has shown a clear survival advantage for the higher dose schedule (*99*), results with carboplatin (particularly for doses producing AUC values higher than 5–7 mg/mL × min) are presently less clear (*100*). Further clinical trials, including comparison of carboplatin AUC values of 6 vs 12, are ongoing. Thus, it remains an area of controversy concerning whether increased doses above a certain level will be reflected in improved patient survival. Our own data, using a panel of human ovarian carcinoma cell lines, have shown a difference in intrinsic cellular sensitivity to carboplatin and cisplatin of 30- and 100-fold, respectively (*101*), and, typically, acquired cisplatin-resistant cell lines are 5- to 10-fold resistant (*48,102*). Thus, dose escalations of a similar magnitude may be necessary in the clinic. In addition, attempts have been made to increase the dose intensity of platinum in patients by combining platinum drugs with generally nonoverlapping toxicities (e.g., as recently reported for carboplatin and oxaliplatin [*103*]).

3.2.3. MODULATION OF PLATINUM RESISTANCE MECHANISMS

To date, attempts at the modulation of platinum resistance mechanisms have generally been conducted in preclinical models and have not reached the stage of clinical trials. However, a diverse range of agents has shown promise (*see 104* for a review), and at least some may reach clinical trial in the near future. Examples include modulation at the level of the plasma membrane using the antifungal agent, amphotericin B, reduction of GSH levels using buthionine sulfoximine (which is already undergoing clinical trial with the nonnephrotoxic bifunctional alkylating agent, melphalan), and inhibition of DNA repair using aphidicolin.

3.2.4. COMBINATIONS WITH OTHER ANTICANCER AGENTS: PACLITAXEL

Although the vast majority of currently available anticancer drugs do not exhibit significant activity against ovarian tumors that are, or have become, resistant to cisplatin, in recent years, paclitaxel (taxol), a natural tubulin binding taxane extracted from the bark of the Pacific Yew, has shown a promising level of activity (*105*). Response rates in the region of 20–30% have been reported in platinum refractory ovarian cancer; clinical studies combining cisplatin and paclitaxel and, more recently, carboplatin and paclitaxel, are also ongoing.

4. SUMMARY

While much has been achieved in making platinum-based chemotherapy more acceptable to the patient (principally through the introduction of carboplatin) the key issue of circumvention of tumor resistance to cisplatin has, disappointingly, met with limited clinical success. In particular, the thorough clinical evaluation of platinum complexes possessing the DACH ligand appears to be precluded at present owing to dose-limiting neurotoxicity. Other attempts to develop analogs to reduce the toxicity of cisplatin (e.g., iproplatin, zeniplatin, 254-S) have shown no clear advantages over carboplatin. However, laboratory-based studies have shed significant light in recent years on the underlying mechanisms by which tumors acquire resistance to cisplatin; this should guide the way toward either improved platinum drugs targeted against particular mechanisms of resistance or pharmacological modulation of resistance mechanisms by nonplatinum drugs.

ACKNOWLEDGMENTS

Studies described from the CRC Centre for Cancer Therapeutics at the Institute of Cancer Research were supported by grants from the UK Cancer Research Campaign, the Medical Research Council, the Johnson Matthey Technology Center (JMTC), and Bristol Myers Squibb Oncology. Thanks are owed to Barry Murrer (JMTC) and my colleagues Ken Harrap, Mark McKeage, Ian Judson, Florence Raynaud, Prakash Mistry, and Sarah Morgan for numerous constructive discussions, and Swee Sharp and Jeff Holford for preparation of figures and proofreading.

REFERENCES

1. Rosenberg B. Fundamental studies with cisplatin. *Cancer (Phila)* 1985; 55:2303–2316.
2. Loehrer PJ, Einhorn LH. Cisplatin. *Anna Intern Med* 1984; 100:704–713.
3. Wiltshaw E, Carr B. *Cis*-platinumdiamminedichloride. In: Connors TA, Roberts JJ, eds. *Platinum Coordination Complexes in Cancer Chemotherapy.* Heidelberg: Springer-Verlag. 1974:178–182.
4. Neijt JP, ten Bokkel Huinink WW, van der Burg MEL, van Oosterom AT, Willemse PHB, Vermorken JB, van Lindert ACM, Heintz APM, Aartsen E, van Lent M, Trimbos JB, de Meijer AJ. Long-term survival in ovarian cancer. *Eur J Cancer* 1991; 27:1367–1372.
5. Harrap KR. Preclinical studies identifying carboplatin as a viable cisplatin alternative. *Cancer Treat Rev* 1985; 12:21–33.
6. Calvert AH, Harland SJ, Newell DR, Siddik ZH, Harrap KR. Phase I studies with carboplatin at the Royal Marsden Hospital. *Cancer Treat Rev* 1985; 12:51–57.
7. Williams CJ, Stewart L, Parmar M, Guthrie D. Meta-analysis of the role of platinum compounds in advanced ovarian carcinoma. *Semin Oncol* 1992; 19:120–128.
8. Taylor AE, Wiltshaw E, Gore ME, Fryatt I, Fisher C. Long term follow up of the first randomised study of cisplatin versus carboplatin for advanced epithelial ovarian cancer. *J Clin Oncol* 1994; 12:2066–2070.
9. Alberts DS, Canetta R, Mason-Liddil N. Carboplatin in the first-line treatment of ovarian cancer. *Semin Oncol* 1990; 17:54–60.
10. Horwich A, Mason M, Dearnaley DP. Use of carboplatin in germ cell tumors of the testis. *Semin Oncol* 1992; 19:72–77.
11. Calvert AH, Newell DR, Gumbrell LA, O'Reilly S, Burnell M, Boxall FE, Siddik ZH, Judson IR, Gore ME, Wiltshaw E. Carboplatin dosage: prospective evaluation of a simple formula based on renal function. *J Clin Oncol* 1989; 7:1748–1756.
12. Foster BJ, Harding BJ, Wolpert-DeFilippes MK, Rubinstein LY, Clagett-Carr K, Leyland-Jones B. A strategy for the development of two clinically active cisplatin analogs:CBDCA and CHIP. *Cancer Chemother Pharmacol* 1990; 25:395–404.
13. Sessa C, Vermorken J, Renard J, Kaye S, Smith D, Huinink WTB, Cavalli F, Pinedo H. Phase II study of iproplatin in advanced ovarian carcinoma. *J Clin Oncol* 1988; 6:98–105.
14. Trask C, Silverstone A, Ash CM, Earl H, Irwin C, Bakker A, Tobias JS, Souhami RL. A randomized trial of carboplatin versus iproplatin in untreated advanced ovarian cancer. *J Clin Oncol* 1991; 9:1131–1137.
15. McGuire WP, Arseneau J, Blessing JA, DiSaia PJ, Hatch KD, Given FT Jr, Teng NNH, Creasman WT. A randomized comparative trial of carboplatin and iproplatin in advanced squamous carcinoma of the uterine cervix: A Gynecologic Oncology Group Study. *J Clin Oncol* 1989; 7:1462-1468.
16. Akaza H, Togashi M, Nishio Y, Miki T, Kotake T, Matsumura Y, Yoshida O, Aso Y. Phase II study of *cis*-diammine(glycolato)platinum, 254-S, in patients with advanced germ cell testicular cancer, prostatic cancer and transitional-cell carcinoma of the urinary tract. *Cancer Chemother. Pharmacol.* 1992; 31:187–192.
17. Majima H. Clinical studies with cisplatin analogues, 254-S, DWA2114R and NK121, In: Howell S, ed. *Platinum and Other Metal Coordination Compounds in Cancer Chemotherapy.* New York: Plenum. 1991:345–355.
18. O'Dwyer PJ, Hudes GR, Walczak J, Schilder R, LaCreta F, Rogers B, Cohen I, Kowal C, Whitfield L, Boyd RA. Phase I and pharmacokinetic study of the novel platinum analogue CI-973 on a 5-daily dose schedule. *Cancer Res* 1992; 52:6746–6753.
19. Theriault RL, Cohen IA, Esparza L, Kowal C, Raber MN. Phase I clinical evaluation of [SP-4-3(R)]-[1,1-cyclobutanedicarboxylate(2-)](2-methyl-1,4-butanediamine-N,N¹) platinum in patients with metastatic tumors. *Cancer Chemother Pharmacol* 1993; 31:333–337.

20. Kelland LR, Abel G, McKeage MJ, Jones M, Goddard PM, Valenti M, Murrer BA, Harrap KR. Preclinical antitumor evaluation of bis-acetato-ammine-dichloro-cyclohexylamine platinum(IV): an orally active platinum drug. *Cancer Res* 1993; 53:2581–2586.

21. McKeage MJ, Kelland LR, Boxall FE, Valenti MR, Jones M, Goddard PM, Gwynne J, Harrap KR. Schedule dependency of orally administered bis-acetato-ammine-dichloro cyclohexyl-amine-platinum (IV) (JM216) *in vivo. Cancer Res* 1994; 54:4118–4122.

22. McKeage MJ, Mistry P, Ward J, Boxall FE, Loh S, O'Neill C, Ellis P, Kelland LR, Morgan SE, Murrer BA, Santabarbara P, Harrap KR, Judson IR. A phase I and pharmacokinetic study of oral bis-acetato-ammine-dichloro cyclohexylamine platinum(IV) (JM216) on a single dose (q21day) administration schedule. *Cancer Chemother Pharmacol* 1995; 36:451–458.

23. Burchenal JH, Kalaher K, Dew K, Lokys L. Rationale for development of platinum analogs. *Cancer Treat Rep* 1979; 63:1493–1498.

24. Goddard PM, Valenti MR, Harrap KR. The role of murine tumour models and their acquired platinum-resistant counterparts in the evaluation of novel platinum antitumour agents: a cautionary note. *Ann Oncol* 1991; 2:535–540.

25. Harrap KR, Jones M, Siracky J, Pollard L, Kelland LR. The establishment, characterization and calibration of human ovarian carcinoma xenografts for the evaluation of novel platinum anticancer drugs. *Ann Oncol* 1990; 1:65–76.

26. Schilder RJ, LaCreta FP, Perez RP, Johnson SW, Brennan JM, Rogatko A, Nash S, McAleer C, Hamilton TC, Roby D, Young RC, Ozols RF, O'Dwyer PJ. Phase I and pharmacokinetic study of Ormaplatin (Tetraplatin, NSC 363812) administered on a day 1 and day 8 schedule. *Cancer Res* 1994; 54:709–717.

27. O'Rourke TJ, Weiss GR, New P, Burris HA III, Rodriguez G, Eckhardt J, Hardy J, Kuhn JG, Fields S, Clark GM, von Hoff DD. Phase I clinical trial of ormaplatin (tetraplatin, NSC 363812). *Anticancer Drugs* 1994; 5:520–526.

28. Extra JM, Espie M, Calvo F, Ferme C, Mignot, L, Marty M. Phase I study of oxaliplatin in patients with advanced cancer. *Cancer Chemother Pharmacol* 1990; 25:299–303.

29. Levi FA, Zidani R, Vannetzel J-M, Perpoint B, Focan C, Faggiulo R, Chollet P, Garfi C, Itzhaki M, Dogliotti L, Iacobelli S, Adam R, Kunstlinger F, Gastiaburu J, Bismuth H, Jasmin C, Misset J-L. Chronomodulated versus fixed infusion-rate delivery of ambulatory chemotherapy with oxaliplatin, fluorouracil, and folinic acid (leucovorin) in patients with colorectal cancer metastases: a randomized multi-institutional trial. *J Natl Cancer Inst* 1994; 86:1608–1617.

30. Perez-Soler R, Lopez-Berestein G, Lautersztain J, Al-Baker S, Francis K, Macias-Kiger D, Raber MN, Khokhar AR. Phase I clinical and pharmacological study of liposome-entrapped *cis*-Bis-neodecanoato-*trans*-R,R-1,2-diaminocyclohexane platinum(II). *Cancer Res* 1990; 50: 4254–4259.

31. Gietema JA, de Vries EGE, Sleijfer DTH, Willemse PHB, Guchelaar H-J, Uges DRA, Aulenbacher P, Voegeli R, Mulder NH. A phase I study of 1,2-diamminomethyl-cyclobutane-platinum (II) lactate (D-19466; lobaplatin) administered daily for 5 days. *Br J Cancer* 1993; 67: 396–401.

32. Gietema JA, Guchelaar H-J, deVries EGE, Aulenbacher P, Sleijfer Dth, Mulder NH. A phase I study of lobaplatin (D-19466) administered by 72h continuous infusion. *Anticancer Drugs* 1993; 4:51–55.

33. Knox RJ, Friedlos F, Lydall DA, Roberts JJ. Mechanism of cytotoxicity of anticancer platinum drugs: Evidence that cisdiamminedichloro platinum(II) and cisdiammine(1,1-cyclobutanedicarboxylato) platinum (II) differ only in the kinetics of their interaction with DNA. *Cancer Res* 1986; 46:1972–1979.

34. Fichtinger-Schepman AMJ, van der Veer JL, den Hartog JHJ, Lohman PHM, Reedijk J. Adducts of the antitumor drug cis-Diamminedichloroplatinum(II) with DNA: formation, identification and quantitation. *Biochemistry* 1985; 24:707–713.

35. Eastman A. Reevaluation of interaction of cis-dichloro(ethylenediamine) platinum(II) with DNA. *Biochemistry* 1986; 25:3912–3915.

36. Grimaldi KA, McAdam SR, Souhami RL, Hartley JA. DNA damage by anti-cancer agents resolved at the nucleotide level of a single copy gene: evidence for a novel binding site for cis-platin in cells. *Nucleic Acids Res* 1994; 22:2311–2317.

37. Connors TA, Cleare MJ, Harrap KR. Structure–activity relationships of the antitumor platinum coordination complexes. *Cancer Treat Rep* 1979; 63:1499–1502.

38. Eastman A, Barry MA. Interaction of trans-diamminedichloroplatinum(II) with DNA: formation of monofunctional adducts and their reaction with glutathione. *Biochemistry* 1987; 26: 3303–3307.

39. Page JD, Husain I, Sancar A, Chaney SG. Effect of the Diaminocyclohexane carrier ligand on platinum adduct formation, repair, and lethality. *Biochemistry* 1990; 29:1016–1024.

40. Szymkowski DE, Yarema K, Essigmann JM, Lippard SJ, Wood RD. An intrastrand d(GpG) platinum crosslink in duplex M13 DNA is refractory to repair by human cell extracts. *Proc Natl Acad Sci USA* 1992; 89:10,772–10,776.

41. Bellon SF, Coleman JH, Lippard SJ. DNA unwinding produced by site-specific intrastrand cross-links of the antitumor drug *cis*-Diamminedichloroplatinum(II). *Biochemistry* 1991; 30: 8026–8035.

42. Zwelling LA, Anderson T, Kohn KW. DNA-protein and DNA interstrand cross-linking by cis- and trans- platinum(II) Diamminedichloride in L1210 mouse leukemia cells and relation to cytotoxicity. *Cancer Res* 1979; 39:365–369.

43. Johnson SW, Perez RP, Godwin AK, Yeung AT, Handel LM, Ozols RF, et al. Role of platinum-DNA adduct formation and removal in cisplatin resistance in human ovarian cancer cell lines. *Biochem Pharmacol* 1994; 47:689–697.

44. Zhen W, Link CJ Jr, O'Connor PM, Reed E, Parker R, Howell SB, Bohr VA. Increased gene-specific repair of cisplatin interstrand cross-links in cisplatin-resistant human ovarian cancer cell lines. *Mol Cell Biol* 1992; 12:3689–3698.

45. Brabec V, Leng M. DNA interstrand cross-links of trans-diamminedichloroplatinum(II) are preferentially formed between guanine and complementary cytosine residues. *Proc Natl Acad Sci USA* 1993; 90:5345–5349.

46. Eastman A. Activation of programmed cell death by anticancer agents: cisplatin as a model system. *Cancer Cells* 1990; 2:275–280.

47. Ormerod MG, O'Neill CF, Robertson D, Harrap KR. Cisplatin induces apoptosis in a human ovarian carcinoma cell line without concomitant internucleosomal degradation of DNA. *Exp Cell Res* 1994; 211:231–237.

48. Andrews PA, Howell SB. Cellular pharmacology of cisplatin: perspectives on mechanisms of acquired resistance. *Cancer Cell* 1990; 2:35–43.

49. Loh SY, Mistry P, Kelland LR, Abel G, Murrer BA, Harrap KR. Reduced drug accumulation as a major mechanism of acquired resistance to cisplatin in a human ovarian carcinoma cell line: circumvention studies using novel platinum(II) and (IV) ammine/amine complexes. *Br J Cancer* 1992; 66:1109–1115.

50. Gately DP, Howell SB. Cellular accumulation of the antitumour agent cisplatin: a review. *Br J Cancer* 1993; 67:1171–1176.

51. Sharp SY, Rowlands MG, Jarman M, Kelland LR. Effects of a new antioestrogen, idoxifene, on cisplatin- and doxorubicin-sensitive and -resistant human ovarian carcinoma cell lines. *Br J Cancer* 1994; 70:409–414.

52. Kawai K, Kamatani N, Georges E, Ling V. Identification of a membrane glycoprotein overexpressed in murine lymphoma sublines resistant to cis-diamminedichloroplatinum(II). *J Biol Chem* 1990; 265:13,137–13,142.

53. Bernal SD, Speak JA, Boeheim K, Dreyfuss AI, Wright JE, Teicher BA, Rosowsky A, Tsao SW, Wong YC. Reduced membrane protein associated with resistance of human squamous carcinoma cells to methotrexate and cis-platinum. *Mol Cell Biochem* 1990; 95:61–70.

54. Godwin AK, Meister A, O'Dwyer PJ, Huang CS, Hamilton TC, Anderson ME. High resistance to cisplatin in human ovarian cancer cell lines is associated with marked increase of glutathione synthesis. *Proc Natl Acad Sci USA* 1992; 89:3070–3074.

55. Mistry P, Kelland LR, Abel G, Sidhar S, Harrap KR. The relationships between glutathione, glutathione-S-transferase and cytotoxicity of platinum drugs and melphalan in eight human ovarian carcinoma cell lines. *Br J Cancer* 1991; 64:215–220.

56. Ishikawa T, Ali-Osman F. Glutathione-associated *cis*-diamminedichloroplatinum(II) metabolism and ATP-dependent efflux from leukemia cells. *J Biol Chem* 1993; 268:20,116–20,125.

57. Ishikawa T, Wright CD, Ishizuka H. GS-X pump is functionally overexpressed in *cis*-Diamminedichloroplatinum(II)-resistant human leukemia HL-60 cells and down-regulated by cell differentiation. *J Biol Chem* 1994; 269:29085–29093.

58. Muller M, Meijer C. Zaman GJR, Borst P, Scheper RJ, Mulder NH, et al. Overexpression of

the gene encoding the multidrug resistance-associated protein results in increased ATP-dependent glutathione S-conjugate transport. *Proc Natl Acad Sci USA* 1994; 91:13,033–13,037.

59. Kelley SL, Basu A, Teicher BA, Hacker MP, Hamer DH, Lazo JS. Overexpression of metalliothionein confers resistance to anticancer drugs. *Science* 1988; 241:1813–1815.

60. van der Zee AGJ, Hollema H, Suumeijer AJH, Krans M, Sluiter WJ, Willemse PHB, Aalders JG, de Vries EGE. Value of P-glycoprotein, glutathione S-transferase pi, c-*erb*B-2, and p53 as prognostic factors in ovarian carcinomas. *J Clin Oncol* 1995; 13:80–78.

61. Murphy D, McGown AT, Hall A, Cattan A, Crowther D, Fox BW. Glutathione S-transferase activity and isoenzyme distribution in ovarian tumour biopsies taken before or after cytotoxic chemotherapy. *Br J Cancer* 1992; 66:937–942.

62. Green JA, Robertson LJ, Clark AH. Glutathione S-transferase expression in benign and malignant ovarian tumours. *Br J Cancer* 1993; 68:235–239.

63. van der Zee AG, van Ommen B, Meijer C, Hollema H,, van Bladeren PJ, de Vries EG. Glutathione S-transferase activity and isoenzyme composition in benign ovarian tumours, untreated malignant ovarian tumours, and malignant ovarian tumours after platinum/cyclophosphamide chemotherapy. *Br J Cancer* 1992; 66:930–936.

64. Murphy D, McGowan AT, Crowther D, Mander A, Fox BW. Metallothionein levels in ovarian tumours before and after chemotherapy. *Br J Cancer* 1991; 63:711–714.

65. Beck DJ, Popoff S, Sancar A, Rupp WD. Reactions of the UVRABC excision nuclease with DNA damaged by diamminedichloroplatinum(II). *Nucleic Acids Res* 1985; 13:7395–7412.

66. Hansson J, Wood RD. Repair synthesis by human cell extracts in DNA damaged by cis- and trans- diammine dichloroplatinum(II). *Nucleic Acids Res* 1989; 17:8073–8091.

67. Shellard SA, Hosking LK, Hill BT. Anomalous relationship between cisplatin sensitivity and the formation and removal of platinum-DNA adducts in two human ovarian carcinoma cell lines in vitro. *Cancer Res* 1991; 51:4557–4564.

68. O'Neill CF, Orr RM, Kelland LR, Harrap KR. Comparison of platinum binding to DNA and removal of total platinum adducts and interstrand crosslinks in three human ovarian carcinoma cell lines sensitive and resistant to cisplatin. *Cell Pharmacol* 1995; 2:1–7.

69. Dabholkar M, Bostick-Bruton F, Weber C, Bohr VA, Egwuagu C, Reed E. ERCC1 and ERCC2 expression in malignant tissues from ovarian cancer patients. *J Natl Cancer Inst* 1992; 84:1512–1517.

70. Dabholkar M, Vionnet J, Bostick Bruton F, Yu JJ, Reed E. Messenger RNA levels of XPAC and ERCC1 in ovarian cancer tissue correlate with response to platinum-based chemotherapy. *J Clin Invest* 1994; 94:703–708.

71. Kelland LR, Mistry P, Abel G, Freidlos F, Loh SY, Roberts JJ, et al. Establishment and characterization of an in vitro model of acquired resistance to cisplatin in a human testicular nonseminomatous germ cell line. *Cancer Res* 1992; 52:1710–1716.

72. Hill BT, Scanlon KJ, Hansson J, Harstrick A, Pera M, Fichtinger-Schepman AMJ, et al. Deficient repair of cisplatin-DNA adducts identified in human testicular teratoma cell lines established from tumours from untreated patients. *Eur. J Cancer* 1994; 30:832–837.

73. Chu G, Chang E. Cisplatin-resistant cells express increased levels of a factor that recognizes damaged DNA. *Proc Natl Acad Sci USA* 1990; 87:3324–3328.

74. Bruhn SL, Pil PM, Essigmann JM, Housman DE, Lippard SJ. Isolation and characterization of human cDNA clones encoding a high mobility group box protein that recognizes structural distortions to DNA caused by binding of the anticancer agent cisplatin. *Proc Natl Acad Sci USA* 1992; 89:2307–2311.

75. Hughes EN, Engelsberg BN, Billings PC. Purification of nuclear proteins that bind to cisplatin-damaged DNA: identity with high mobility group proteins 1 and 2. *J Biol Chem* 1992; 267:13,520–13,527.

76. Pil PM, Lippard SJ. Specific binding of chromosomal protein HMG1 to DNA damaged by the anticancer drug cisplatin. *Science* 1992; 256:234–237.

77. Brown SJ, Kellett PJ, Lippard SJ. lxr1, a yeast protein that binds to platinated DNA and confers sensitivity to cisplatin. *Science* 1993; 261:603–605.

78. Huang J-C, Zamble DB, Reardon JT, Lippard SJ, Sancar A. HMG-domain proteins specifically inhibit the repair of the major DNA adduct of the anticancer drug cisplatin by human excision nuclease. *Proc Natl Acad Sci USA* 1994; 91:10,394–10,398.

79. Chao CC-K, Huang S-L, Lee L-Y, Lin-Chao S. Identification of inducible damage-recognition proteins that are overexpressed in HeLa cells resistant to cis-diamminedichloroplatinum(II). *Biochem J* 1991; 277:875–878.

80. Clugston CK, McLaughlin K, Kenny MK, Brown R. Binding of human single-stranded DNA binding protein to DNA damaged by the anticancer drug cis-diamminedichloroplatinum (II). *Cancer Res* 1992; 52:6375–6379.

81. Isonishi S, Hom DK, Thiebaut FB, Mann SC, Andrews PA, Basu A, Lazo JS, Eastman A, Howell SB. Expression of c-Ha-ras oncogene in mouse NIH 3T3 cells induces resistance to cisplatin. *Cancer Res* 1991; 51:5903–5909.

82. Sklar MD, Prochownik EV. Modulation of cis-platinum resistance in Friend erythroleukemia cells by *c-myc. Cancer Res* 1991; 51:2118–2123.

83. Scanlon KJ, Jiao L, Funato T, Wang W, Tone T, Rossi JJ, Kashani-Sabet M. Ribozyme-mediated cleavage of *c-fos* mRNA reduces gene expression of DNA synthesis enzymes and metallothionein. *Proc Natl Acad Sci USA* 1991; 88:10,591–10,595.

84. Lowe SW, Ruley HE, Jacks T, Housman DE. p53-dependent apoptosis modulates the cytotoxicity of anticancer agents. *Cell* 1993; 74:957–967.

85. Peng H, Hogg D, Malkin D, Bailey D, Gallie BL, Bulbul M, et al. Mutations of the p53 gene do not occur in testis cancer. *Cancer Res* 1993; 53:3574–3578.

86. Fan S, El-Diery WS, Bae I, Freeman J, Jondle D, Bhatia K, Fornace AJ Jr, Magrath I, Kohn KW, O'Connor PM. p53 gene mutations are associated with decreased sensitivity of human lymphoma cells to DNA damaging agents. *Cancer Res* 1994; 54:5824–5830.

87. Kimura E, Enns RE, Alcaraz JE, Arboleda J, Salmon DJ, Howell SB. Correlation of the survival of ovarian cancer patients with mRNA expression of the 60-kD heat shock protein HSP-60. *J Clin Oncol* 1993; 11:891–898.

88. Smith ML, Chen I, Zhan Q, Bae I, Chen C, Gilmer TM, et al. Interaction of the p53-regulated protein GAdd45 with proliferating cell nuclear antigen. *Science* 1994; 266:1376–1380.

89. Howell SB, Isonishi S, Christen RC, Andrews PA, Mann SC, Hom D. Signal transduction pathway regulation of DDP sensitivity. In: Howell SB, ed. *Platinum and Other Metal Coordination Compounds in Cancer Chemotherapy*. New York: Plenum. 1991:173–179.

90. Teicher BA, Herman TS, Holden SA, Wang YY, Pfeffer MR, Crawford JW, et al. Tumor resistance to alkylating agents conferred by mechanisms operative only in vivo. *Science* 1990; 247:1457–1461.

91. Farrell N, Kelland LR, Roberts JD, Van Beusichem M. Activation of the *trans* geometry in platinum antitumor complexes: a survey of the cytotoxicity of *trans* compounds containing planar ligands in murine L1210 and human tumor panels and studies on their mechanism of action. *Cancer Res* 1992; 52:5065–5072.

92. Kelland LR, Barnard CFJ, Mellish KJ, Jones M, Goddard PM, Valenti M, Bryant A, Murrer BA, Harrap KR. A novel *trans*-platinum coordination complex possessing in vitro and in vivo antitumour activity. *Cancer Res* 1994; 54:5618–5622.

93. Coluccia M, Nassi A, Loseto F, Boccarelli A, Mariggio MA, Giordano D, et al. A trans-platinum complex showing higher antitumor activity than the Cis congeners. *J Med Chem* 1993; 36:510–512.

94. Farrell N, Qu Y, Hacker MP. Cytotoxicity and antitumor activity of bis(platinum) complexes. A novel class of platinum complexes active in cell lines resistant to both cisplatin and 1,2-diaminocyclohexane complexes. *J Med Chem* 1990; 33:2179–2184.

95. Webster LK, Deacon GB, Buxton DP, Hillcoat BL, James AM, Roos IAG, et al. cis-Bis(pyridine) platinum(II) organoamides with unexpected growth inhibition properties and antitumor activity. *J Med Chem* 1992; 35:3349–3353.

96. Kim D, Kim G, Gam J, Cho Y, Kim H, Tai J, et al. Synthesis and antitumor activity of a series of [2-substituted-4,5-bis(aminomethyl)-1,3-dioxolane] platinum(II) complexes. *J Med Chem* 1994; 37:1471–1485.

97. Ozols RF, Ostchega Y, Myers CE, Young RC. High-dose cisplatin in hypertonic saline in refractory ovarian cancer. *J Clin Oncol* 1985; 3:1246–1250.

98. Calvert AH, Newell DR, Gore ME. Future directions with carboplatin: Can therapeutic monitoring, high-dose administration, and hematologic support with growth factors expand the spectru compared with cisplatin? *Semin Oncol* 1992; 19:155–163.

99. Kaye SB, Lewis CR, Paul J, Duncan ID, Gordon HK, Kitchener HC, Cruickshank DJ, Atkinson RJ, Soukop M, Rankin EM, Cassidy J, Davis JA, Reed NS, Crawford SM, MacLean A, Swapp GA, Sarkar TK, Kennedy JH, Symonds RP. Randomised study of two doses of cisplatin with cyclophosphamide in epithelial ovarian cancer. *Lancet* 1992; 340:329–333.
100. Jodrell DI, Egorin MJ, Canetta RM, Langenberg P, Goldbloom EP, Burroughs JN, Goodlow JL, Tan S, Wiltshaw E. Relationships between carboplain exposure and tumor response and toxicity in patients with ovarian cancer.*J Clin Oncol* 1992; 10:520–528.
101. Hills CA, Kelland LR, Abel G, Siracky J, Wilson AP, Harrap KR. Biological properties of ten human ovarian carcinoma cell lines: calibration *in vitro* against platinum complexes. *Br J Cancer* 1989; 59:527–534.
102. Kelland LR, Mistry P, Abel G, Loh SY, O'Neill CF, Murrer BA, Harrap KR. Mechanism-related circumvention of acquired cis-diamminedichloroplatinum(II) resistance using two pairs of human ovarian carcinoma cell lines by ammine/amine platinum(IV) dicarboxylates. *Cancer Res* 1992; 52:3857–3864.
103. Llory JF, Soulie P, Cvitkovic E, Misset JL. Feasibility of high-dose platinum delivery with combined carboplatin and oxaliplatin. *J Natl Cancer Inst* 1994; 86:1098–1099.
104. Timmer Bosscha, H., Mulder, N.H., and de Vries, E.G. Modulation of cis-diamminedichloro-platinum(II) resistance: a review. *Br J Cancer* 1992; 66:227–238.
105. Trimble EL, Adams JD, Vena D, Hawkins MJ, Friedman MA, Fisherman JS, et al. Paclitaxel for platinum-refractory ovarian cancer: Results from the first 1,000 patients registered to national Cancer Institute Treatment Referral Center 9103. *J Clin Oncol* 1993; 11:2405–2410.

5 Anthracyclines

Trevor W. Sweatman, PhD and Mervyn Israel, PhD

CONTENTS

1. INTRODUCTION: DAUNORUBICIN AND DOXORUBICIN: PROTOTYPICAL ANTHRACYCLINES

The clinical activity of actinomycin D against Wilm's pediatric kidney tumor and choriocarcinoma in the early to mid-1950s resulted in a widespread effort to discover other antibiotic substances for potential use in the treatment of malignancies. As a result, cancer chemotherapy was altered immeasurably more than 30 years ago by the independent discoveries by Grein (*1*), Dubost (*2*), and their colleagues of an anthracycline antibiotic, derived from a *Streptomyces* soil mold, with significant experimental activity against leukemias. Structurally this intensely red product whose common name, daunorubicin, reflects both its Italian (daunomicina) and French (rubidomycine) origins, consists of a planar anthraquinone attached to a daunosamine sugar; the latter has been shown to stabilize intercalation of the molecule with DNA, which for many years was considered to be the principal mechanism of anthracycline action (*3*). Subsequently, although not necessarily through DNA interaction, this structural requirement has proven essential for the multiple potential mechanisms of action now identified for anthracyclines, including inhibition of DNA topoisomerase I (*4*) and II (*5*), inhibition of helicases (*6*), generation of toxic free radicals (*7*), alteration of membrane structure and function (*8–10*), and endonucleolytic cleavage (*11*).

Encouraging early activity data for daunorubicin (*12–14*) prompted a search for other anthracyclines with improved therapeutic activity, a quest that continues to the present day. In 1969, DiMarco and colleagues (*15*) reported that doxorubicin (Adriamycin®), a closely related (14-hydroxy) analog of daunorubicin (Fig. 1), possessed superior preclinical activity to daunorubicin, with a broad spectrum of activity against leukemias, lymphomas, and solid tumors (*16*). Notwithstanding more recent clinical data supporting daunorubicin activity against a variety of solid tumors (*17–19*),

From: *Cancer Therapeutics: Experimental and Clinical Agents*
Edited by: B. Teicher Humana Press Inc., Totowa, NJ

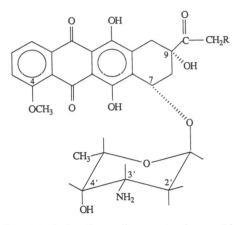

Fig. 1. Structure of prototypical anthracycline agents, daunorubicin and doxorubicin.

daunorubicin has become associated more closely with combination chemotherapy of leukemia, where it is considered to be less toxic than doxorubicin (*20*). By contrast, doxorubicin is employed not only as a single agent, but also as an important component of many combination chemotherapy regimens for the treatment of lymphoma, breast, and small-cell lung carcinoma, and sarcomas (*21*). Despite these successes, doxorubicin has proven ineffective against many tumors, including colon cancer, melanoma, chronic lymphocytic leukemias, CNS tumors, and renal cancer.

2. LIMITATIONS TO ANTHRACYCLINE THERAPY

2.1. Toxicities

In common with most anticancer agents that possess a narrow therapeutic index, early reports of anthracycline clinical activity (*12–14*) documented acute toxicities against rapidly dividing cells, e.g., myelosuppression, gastrointestinal toxicity (nausea and vomiting), alopecia, and stomatitis. Indeed, leukopenia is the dose-limiting toxicity with all clinically tested anthracyclines. Of equal importance was the recognition of the acute and chronic effects of doxorubicin and daunorubicin on the heart. Electrocardiographic changes have been documented during anthracycline administration (*22*), although the significance of these phenomena are equivocal (*23,24*). However, it is the insidious dose-dependent cardiomyopathy produced by these agents that has the greatest impact on their clinical utility. Cardiac tissue that, as a result of mitochondrial multiplicity and low antioxidant levels (*25*), appears particularly susceptible to lipid peroxidation (*26*), undergoes progressive dose-related irreversible vacuolization and myocyte necrosis in response to doxorubicin and daunorubicin exposure. Correlation of drug exposure with overt signs of congestive heart failure have led to the now familiar recommendations of 450–550 mg/m² being placed on total doxorubicin and daunorubicin dose exposure (*22,27*). However, this "safe" dose may be illusory; combination chemotherapy and thoracic irradiation are both known to exacerbate myocardial damage at lower cumulative anthracycline levels (*28*); Lipschultz and coworkers (*29,30*) have identified cardiac abnormalities in patients who have received total doxorubicin doses as low as 45 mg/m². In addition, the aging of large numbers of long-term cancer survivors has produced increasing evidence of heart failure many years following doxorubicin or daunorubicin exposure (*31–35*). Thus, the dilemma for the oncologist is how best to administer these highly active antitumor agents while at the same time minimizing the potential for the cancer-free patient to subsequently succumb to late heart failure. To provide for greater safety in the continued use of daunorubicin and doxorubicin, there has been active research interest in the areas of dose schedule optimization, drug formulation, and antioxidant co-administration.

Despite almost three decades of use, optimal dosage regimens have yet to be fully defined (*36,37*). In consideration that drug fractionation or drug infusion reduces peak plasma anthracycline levels without reducing overall drug exposure (as measured by the area under the concentration time curve; AUC), a marked reduction in cardiotoxicity has been reported following weekly (*27,38*) or 48–96 h doxorubicin infusions (*39,40*). However, in demonstrating a correlation between high peak serum anthracycline concentrations and therapeutic response (*41–43*), others have suggested better tumor drug penetration by higher drug levels (*38,44–46*). Given the wide interpatient variability in anthracycline pharmacokinetics and the relatively small number of subjects in the studies conducted to date, deValeriola (*36*) has advocated larger prospective studies to validate these data.

Although liposomes remain a controversial area, following initial problems with physicochemical stability and marked extravasation of liposomes into the reticuloendothelial system, their potential value in reducing anthracycline cardiotoxicity has not been overlooked (*47*). Initial experimental studies with liposomal drug encapsulation have documented superior activity to the corresponding free agent (*48–51*). Among the number of clinical trials of liposomal encapsulated doxorubicin presently under way, significant antitumor activity and reduced toxicity of liposomal daunorubicin (DaunoXone®) have been demonstrated against Kaposi's sarcoma (*52,53*). Conversely, liposomal doxorubicin (Lipodox®) produced no evidence of activity against advanced renal cell carcinoma (*54*). The ultimate potential utility of liposomal drug formulations must await the outcome of such clinical trials.

Implication of intracellular free iron in complexing with the planar anthraquinone portion of the anthracycline molecule to liberate free radicals and produce cardiomyopathy (*55*) had led to the evaluation of a number of iron-chelating agents, principally those related to edetic acid (EDTA), as cardioprotective agents. Dexrazoxane (ICRF-187; Zinecard®) has undergone the most extensive preclinical and clinical evaluation. It has proven effective in reducing experimental free radical generation (*56,57*) and in reducing clinical cardiotoxicity of breast cancer therapy (*58–60*), although at the expense of a slight increase in myelotoxicity. However, the effects of this chelator on antitumor efficacy remain equivocal (*61,62*); for this reason, Zinecard, which has recently received FDA approval for use in conjunction with doxorubicin against metastatic breast cancer, is presently limited to use in patients who have already received > 300 mg/m^2 doxorubicin (*63*).

2.2. Drug Resistance

Inability to achieve cytotoxic drug concentrations in the tumor with consequent treatment failure may relate, in part, to pharmacokinetic considerations of drug sanctuary or metabolism to inactive products, but more than likely to problems associated with the development of cellular drug resistance in subpopulations of tumor cells.

Since the first reports of in vitro drug resistance in 1968 (*64*) and 1970 (*65*), experimental investigation of mammalian cells has highlighted the many ways in which drug cytotoxicity can be circumvented. Of the numerous potential resistance mechanisms that have been identified, only two, the multidrug resistance (MDR) phenotype and the multidrug resistance-associated protein (MRP), have demonstrated some correlation with clinical drug resistance. Thus, the well-characterized MDR phenotype, with a membrane-associated P-glycoprotein (P-gp) encoded in human cells by the MDR 1 gene (*66,67*), confers crossresistance to a broad spectrum of natural product drugs, including the anthracyclines. Although distribution of P-gp in secretory cells of the kidney, liver, pancreas, jejunum, and colon suggests some physiological role in normal tissue, it is now recognized that overexpression of MDR 1 mRNA or P-gp is associated with poor prognosis in human tumors, e.g., acute leukemia (*68*). A further membrane-associated efflux mechanism, the MRP pump, has now been characterized (*69,70*) with the ability to extrude natural product drugs from the cell against the concentration gradient. Unlike P-gp, whose function can be interrupted by MDR-reversing agents, such as verapamil or cyclosporin A, MRP action is not significantly affected by these reversing agents (*71,72*). In common with P-gp, overexpression of MRP has demonstrated some clinical correlation with disease prognosis, e.g., for leukemias (*73*) and neuroblastoma (*74*). Both of these resistance mechanisms have received extensive literature reviews.

Although these membrane protein pumps confer on the tumor cell the ability to reduce intracellular drug concentrations, for anthracyclines there is a further potential mechanism of resistance that does not involve drug trafficking, but rather altered intracellular topoisomerase I and II enzyme levels. These essential nuclear enzymes, which are intimately involved in cell division by controlling the topology of the DNA during strand separation and replication, catalyze the relaxation/supercoiling and catenation/decatenation of DNA. In common with a number of anticancer agents, such as the epipodophyllotoxins, aminoacridines, and mitoxantrone, daunorubicin and doxorubicin inhibit cell division through formation of stable drug–DNA–topoisomerase II complexes (*75*). There is also evidence that some of the morpholinylanthracycline analogs produce the same effect through an interaction with topoisomerase I rather than topoisomerase II. Such agents differ from actinomycin D (Dactinomycin), which acts against both enzymes, by demonstrating no apparant interaction with topoisomerase II. In consequence of these drug–enzyme interactions, the inhibited religation of DNA is manifest as protein-associated single- and double-strand breaks (*76*). Resistance to topoisomerase-directed drugs is imparted by a decrease in the topoisomerase protein and/or a decline in catalytic activity (*77*). Although topoisomerases remain a fertile research area, with extensive literature citation, at the present time there is no convincing correlation between altered topoisomerase activity and clinical drug resistance.

Two approaches have been used to circumvent drug resistance clinically, combination chemotherapy, and resistance modifying agents. As noted above, the P-gp pump confers crossresistance on the cell, thereby negating combination chemotherapy involving other natural product drugs. A number of agents have shown the ability to competitively inhibit P-gp activity in vitro; these include steroids, nonimmunosuppressive cyclosporin A derivatives, and calcium channel antagonists, such as verapamil. Unfortunately, verapamil has itself proven toxic at the clinical levels required for

Table 1
Comparison of Anthracycline Analog
Clinical Activity with that of Doxorubicin

Analog	Clinical findings
Older agents	
Carminomycin	No advantage over doxorubicin
Esorubicin	Inferior to doxorubicin
Marcellomycin	Toxicity
Quelamycin	Toxicity
Rubidizone	Toxicity
Current agents	
Aclarubicin	No advantage over doxorubicin
Pirarubicin	Comparable activity (less myelosuppression)
Epirubicin	Comparable activity (less toxicity)
Idarubicin	Activity data equivocal

reversal of drug resistance. Additionally, interaction of calcium channel antagonists with cardiotoxicity has been demonstrated experimentally by an increase in doxorubicin-induced myocyte damage in neonatal rat myocytes exposed to verapamil (78). Clinical trials are presently under way with other resistance modifiers.

3. NEWER ANTHRACYCLINE DRUG DEVELOPMENT

Although anthracyclines are of significant clinical utility in chemotherapy, cardiotoxicity and tumor drug insensitivity (natural or acquired) are clearly major impediments to optimal clinical prognosis. Historically, the development of new anthracycline antitumor agents has focused primarily on improving the spectrum of clinical activity, reducing the cardiotoxicity, and overcoming known mechanisms of clinical drug resistance. Approaches to new anthracycline analogs include primarily isolation and evaluation of fermentation-derived antibiotic substances and semisynthetic modification of parental antibiotics. Relatively little of clinical utility has come from the former approach, the most significant contributions being represented by carminomycin (Table 1) and aclacinomycin (*vide infra*). Many more significant leads have come from structure–activity relationship studies of synthetically derived products. However, despite the considerable promise of this class of antitumor agents and the extensive research conducted to date, there have been no new anthracyclines yet introduced to the marketplace whose clinical activity is superior to that of doxorubicin or daunorubicin. Based on these facts, a recent review article by Weiss (79) posed the question, "Will we ever find a better doxorubicin?"

Of necessity, many of the earlier anthracycline analogs were developed for clinical trials at a time when our understanding of drug resistance was in its infancy. Selection of potential therapeutic agents was based initially on in vitro activity, usually against P388 leukemia cells. Use of such tools failed to provide detailed knowledge of the structure–activity relationships of the various analogs relative to drug resistance and, as a consequence, many interesting leads may have been overlooked (80). However, the field of drug resistance has now matured to the extent that many mammalian cell lines that are drug resistant through a variety of well-defined mechanisms, e.g., cells expressing the MDR, MRP, and altered topoisomerase II (at-MDR) phenotypes, are now available as research tools. These are proving invaluable in the preclinical evaluation of new anthracycline analogs and in a more rigorous evaluation of the structure–activity relationships.

3.1. The First Wave of Second-Generation Analogs

Over the 30-yr span since the original discovery of doxorubicin and daunorubicin, several dozen anthracycline analogs have achieved the milestone of clinical evaluation as a result of promising preclinical studies (Table 1). Consistent with the then prevailing mechanistic view for anthracyclines, the earliest analogs were all based on the paradigm of avid DNA complexation. In general, these agents failed to show significant therapeutic advantage over the prototypical antibiotics, and trials with some were discontinued. However, as indicated below, several of the agents are currently marketed in various regions of the world. These appear to offer comparable antitumor activity, but somewhat lesser toxicity than the parental agent; none of them has demonstrated any clear therapeutic advantage over doxorubicin, especially against anthracycline-resistant tumors.

3.2. Clinically Approved Analogs

Aclacinomycin (Aclarubicin®), originally developed in Japan, is presently available in France, although studies in the US have failed to demonstrate any therapeutic advantage over doxorubicin and daunorubicin (79). Likewise, tetrahydropyranyldoxorubicin (Pirarubicin®) is marketed in France and Japan and has undergone clinical trials in the U.S. Data for this agent, recently reviewed (81), have demonstrated only comparable antitumor activity to doxorubicin. The major difference between them appears to be one of lesser acute toxicity (leukopenia, alopecia, nausea, vomiting) and, possibly, risk of cardiotoxicity (up to 700 mg/m²) for Pirarubicin. However, these differences do not appear to provide a compelling case for further trials of this agent in the US.

4'-Epidoxorubicin (Epirubicin), presently marketed worldwide with the exception of the US, was originally selected on the basis of reduced experimental cardiotoxicity compared to doxorubicin (82). Clinical trials with this agent have confirmed that when doxorubicin and epirubicin are compared on a equimolar basis, the latter does indeed demonstrate less acute and cardiotoxicity (83,84), primarily as a result of pharmacokinetic differences between the two agents. Epirubicin has a much faster conversion to its 13-carbinol metabolite (4'-epidoxorubicinol), with extensive glucuronide conjugation facilitating the excretion process (85). However, when the two agents are compared on an equi-myelosuppressive basis, their acute toxicity is comparable (86) and epirubicin clearly produces fatal cardiotoxicity (87,88), the cumulative dose limit for this agent being 900–1000 mg/m² (about 9 mo of therapy). Thus, epirubicin shows some advantage in terms of toxicity, but in common with many of the clinically approved analogs, its spectrum of clinical activity is not sufficiently different from that of doxorubicin that this analog represents an therapeutic advantage against anththracycline-insensitive tumors.

4-Demethoxydaunorubicin (idarubicin; Idamycin®) is presently the only anthracycline analog that is marketed worldwide, being active against leukemias and breast carcinoma both by iv and oral administration, although the latter formulation is not marketed in the US. In contrast to daunorubicin and doxorubicin, whose principal metabolic products, the respective 13-carbinol species, are less cytotoxic than the parental agent, 4-demethoxydaunorubicinol (idarubicinol) has demonstrated equipotency with idarubicin in cell-culture systems (*89*). However, this difference does not appear to have provided a significant advantage, since idarubicin demonstrates no clear-cut advantage over doxorubicin in terms of toxicity (*79*) or antitumor activity. Some iv drug studies demonstrate an advantage, whereas others fail to substantiate these findings (*90,91*). Comparison of oral idarubicin with iv doxorubicin has highlighted problems of variation in bioavailability (12–49%) of oral administered drug (*92*), resulting in lower response rates by this route (*93–95*). Data on in vitro activity against drug-resistant tumors are also equivocal, with some studies showing a lack of crossresistance between idarubicin and daunorubicin in MDR leukemic cell lines (*96*) and others finding crossresistance in relapsed tumor samples from children with acute lymphoblastic leukemia (*97*). Certainly in clinical trials, idarubicin produced best antitumor activity in patients who had not previously received anthracycline therapy (*98*).

3.3. Newer Developmental Agents

If one were to summarize the record of accomplishments of anthracycline analog development up to this point, it is clearly one of unfulfilled promise, with the various "me too" agents showing only marginal clinical differences from their respective parental agents and none clearly demonstrating activity in anthracycline-insensitive or resistant tumors. Notwithstanding these disappointments, it has become increasingly apparent from structure–activity studies that only minor modifications of the anthracycline structure can result not only in inactive agents, but more importantly analogs with in vitro activity, not only against MDR tumor cell lines, but also those expressing MRP and at-MDR phenotypes. It should also be recognized that minor changes in structure can result in differences in the way in which these agents are metabolized and eliminated (*99*). The principal structural modifications have been made on: (1) the daunosamine sugar, whose structural features are implicated by many investigators (*see* Priebe et al. [*100*]) in DNA and cellular binding and intracellular drug transport, and/or (2) substitution at the C-14 position of the chromophore, which affects in vitro binding of drug with topoisomerase II, intracellular drug accumulation, and possibly intracellular drug targets.

Additionally, one cannot overlook the possible importance of the quinone structure in the anthracycline chromophore to the overall biological activity of such agents. Thus, the difference in the pattern of cytotoxicity seen for 5-iminodaunorubicin in the NCI's disease-oriented screen compared with doxorubicin is suggestive of a change in biological activity for this agent. Based on these data, Acton has proposed structure-activity studies using a series of phenazine-di-*N*-oxides as models (*101*); however, this worthwhile work is incomplete at present.

Several thousand analogs have been synthesized to data, and new ones appear with regularity in the scientific literature. As Acton (*101*) noted, "it has always been easier to find active analogues than to choose among them." For the sake of expediency then, we will consider only selected novel analogs that have either reached clinical trials or are in late-stage preclinical development and for which a considerable body of scientific data therefore exists. It is important to note that although these agents

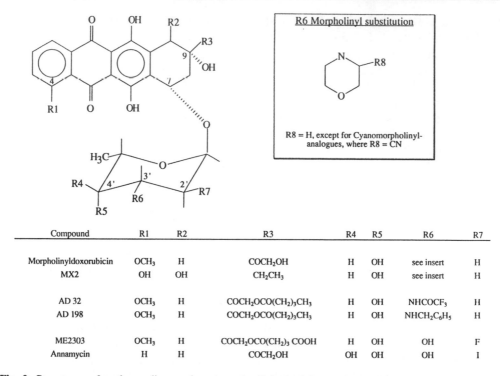

Compound	R1	R2	R3	R4	R5	R6	R7
Morpholinyldoxorubicin	OCH₃	H	COCH₂OH	H	OH	see insert	H
MX2	OH	OH	CH₂CH₃	H	OH	see insert	H
AD 32	OCH₃	H	COCH₂OCO(CH₂)₃CH₃	H	OH	NHCOCF₃	H
AD 198	OCH₃	H	COCH₂OCO(CH₂)₃CH₃	H	OH	NHCH₂C₆H₅	H
ME2303	OCH₃	H	COCH₂OCO(CH₂)₃ COOH	H	OH	OH	F
Annamycin	H	H	COCH₂OH	OH	OH	OH	I

Fig. 2. Structures of anthracycline analogs in early clinical trials or advanced preclinical development.

are representative of the various types of modification that have been investigated, there may be other analogs from each group under active investigation around the world. Thus, the selected agents include: some of the morpholinyl-anthracycline derivatives that appear to possess different nuclear targets and to require metabolic activation for their full biological effect; the lipophilic *N*-alkyl- and *N*-acyl-analogs AD 32 and AD 198, which appear to possess novel mechanistic properties, in part unrelated to a topoisomerase II-directed target; two halogenated, deaminated topoisomerase II-directed analogs ME2303 and Annamycin; and the dual-mechanistic hybrid anthracycline–nitrosourea, AD 312. Chemical structures for all of these agents are to be found in Figs. 2 and 3.

3.3.1. MORPHOLINYL ANTHRACYCLINES: MX2

With the exception of studies with liposomally formulated daunorubicin and doxorubicin, there are currently no clinical trials of systemic anthracycline therapy in the US. However, a number of interesting morpholinyl analogs have been synthesized; some of these are currently undergoing clinical trials in Japan (*102*). This group of agents has arisen, in part, from the initial observations by Acton and colleagues (*103,104*) that cyclo-alkylation of the amino nitrogen on the daunosamine sugar, to reduce the basicity of the nitrogen and avoid P-gp-mediated efflux, dramatically increases antitumor activity (Fig. 2). Subsequently, a large number of analogs have been synthesized to investigate the effects of substitution on the morpholine ring. These efforts have yielded analogs that, in general, are 10–1000 times more potent than doxorubicin, in vitro. Of these, cyanomorpholinyl provided the most notable

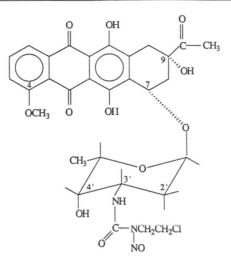

Fig. 3. Structure of the novel hydrid anthracycline-alkylator *N*-(2-chloroethyl)-*N*-nitrosoureidodauno-rubicin (AD 312).

increase in biological activity with no evidence of either cardiotoxicity or crossresistance to doxorubicin (*103,105,106*). Unlike parental doxorubicin, methoxymorpholinyl-, morpholinyl- and cyanomorpholinyldoxorubicin all undergo covalent binding, producing DNA crosslinking in cells with an active metabolism, the last analog yielding cyanide in the process (*107*). This metabolically dependent DNA interaction, for which an intact morpholine ring structure appears critical, is considered the explanation for their greater antitumor activity vs doxorubicin in vivo, relative to in vitro studies (*108–110*). As noted earlier, mechanistic differences are evident between the actions of morpholinyl-doxorubicin and doxorubicin on topoisomerase (Table 2). Whereas doxorubicin produces protein-associated double-strand breaks in DNA, morpholinyl-doxorubicin yields only single-strand breaks (*111*). Subsequently, problems with the stability of the cyanomorpholinyl analog appear to have precluded its further development as a clinical agent. However, morpholine substitution remains an active area of interest; a number of analogs, e.g., MX2 and Ro31-3294, that incorporate this substituent have been investigated and have proven capable of circumventing P-gp resistance, at least in cell-culture systems. MX2 has reached the stage of clinical evaluation.

3′-Deamino-3′-morpholinyl-13-deoxo-10-hydroxycarminomycin (MX2) is presently in clinical trials in Japan against brain tumors, leukemias, lymphomas, and breast cancer. Preclinical data show that MX2, which is more lipophilic than doxorubicin or daunorubicin, has activity against implanted carcinomas and is effective against a doxorubicin-resistant P388 leukemia line in vitro and in vivo (*112*). This differs from the only partial effectiveness reported for the morpholinyldoxorubicin analog against such cells (*113*). Of potential significance, MX2 is orally active against P388 leukemia at serum levels comparable to those produced by iv drug administration; it also has some activity in an intracerebrally implanted L1210 leukemia model (*114*). The major dose-limiting toxicity of MX2 is myelosuppression, comparable to that of doxorubicin (*112*), although lower cardiotoxicity has been observed in a rabbit cardiotoxicity model (*112*). In escalating dose Phase I trials (1.5–54 mg/m², total dose), neutropenia

Table 2
Comparison of the Interactions of Morpholinyl-Anthracyclines
and Doxorubicin with DNA and Mammalian Topoisomerase I and II

Anthracycline	DNA intercalation[a]	DNA crosslinking[b]	DNA cleavage through	
			Topoisomerase I[c]	Topoisomerase II[d]
Doxorubicin	++	–	–	++
Morpholinyldoxorubicin	+	–	+	–
Cyanomorpholinyldoxorubicin	–	+	(+)	–

[a] Drug intercalation was measured by use of a DNA topoisomerase I unwinding assay in the presence of excess enzyme.
[b] DNA crosslinking was measured by incubating the respective drugs with 5′-end-labeled DNA fragments and analyzing the product by agarose gel electrophoresis under denaturing conditions.
[c] Inhibition of DNA topoisomerase I catalytic activity was measured by relaxation of native supercoiled SV40 DNA in the presence of limited amounts of enzyme. The kinetics of the reactions in the presence and absence of test anthracyclines were compared.
[d] Inhibition of DNA topoisomerase II catalytic activity by the various test agents was measured in the presence of excess enzyme by cleavage of 3′-terminus end-labeled (³²P) BanI-HpaII SV40 DNA fragments and subsequent analysis by agarose gel electrophoresis.

For full experimental details, see ref(111).

and thrombocytopenia were evident as the dose-limiting toxicities (*102*); no objective responses were seen.

Despite these encouraging data, questions have been raised regarding the potential therapeutic variability of such drugs as the morpholinyl-anthracyclines, which rely, in part, on metabolic activation by cytochrome P450 enzymes for their full biological activity (*46*). If expression of this family of enzymes is as variable in tumors as it is in normal tissue, such as liver, this would predict potentially yet a further form of (partial) resistance to this type of agent. The full implications of this process for morpholinyl analogs must await clinical evaluation.

3.3.2. *N*-ACYL-ANALOGS: AD 32

A change in the basicity of the daunosamine nitrogen has also been effected by 3'-*N*-acyl substituents. However, simple *N*-acyl substituents on daunorubicin or doxorubicin, e.g., acetate, propionate, and so forth, are easily cleaved enzymatically and, as a consequence, such substituted antracyclines simply serve as prodrugs of the parent antibiotics. As discussed below, however, trifluoroacetylation yields a stable amide bond and results in an agent with remarkably different pharmacologic properties compared with doxorubicin. Various acyl substituents on the 14-carbinol moiety of trifluoroacetylated anthracyclines have also been examined with a view to improving drug lipophilicity and more effective drug cell penetration. One such analog of current clinical interest is *N*-trifluoroacetyladriamycin-14-valerate (AD 32).

AD 32 differs from doxorubicin in having a five-carbon aliphatic ester at the 14-carbinol position and a trifluoroacetyl substitution on the glycosidic amino group. As a result of high lipid solubility, AD 32 rapidly traverses cell membranes, and drug-associated fluorescence accumulates in the cytoplasm, whereas doxorubicin is transported slowly into cells and becomes localized in nuclei and on chromosomes (*115,116*). AD 32 does not intercalate or bind to DNA by any other mechanism (*117*), long considered to be the principal mechanistic basis of cytotoxicity for anthracyclines. Thus, doxorubicin inhibits primarily DNA synthesis, whereas AD 32, despite a failure to complex with DNA, produces rapid inhibition of both DNA and RNA synthesis. Extensive studies have shown unequivocally that AD 32 does not serve as a doxorubicin prodrug. Furthermore, although extensively metabolized, neither can the biological activity of AD 32 be ascribed simply to a biotransformation product. Thus, whereas doxorubicin is a potent intercalator of DNA and an inhibitor of topoisomerase II (Table 3), AD 41 (*N*-trifluoroacetyladriamycin), the principal (in vitro and in vivo) biotransformation product of AD 32, undergoes only a minor degree of DNA intercalation and comparatively low inhibition of topoisomerase II activity (*118*). AD 32 is superior to doxorubicin in a broad range of rodent leukemia and solid tumor models with respect to both antitumor activity and degree of toxicity (*119–121*). In Lewis lung tumor-bearing animals, AD 32 persists in tumor tissue for a longer time than doxorubicin; this selectivity could result in greater exposure of tumor tissue to the drug or its active metabolites (*119*). Based on clinical studies of systemically administered drug conducted at the Dana-Farber Cancer Institute, this drug is well tolerated at doses up to 600 mg/m^2, with leukopenia and thrombocytopenia being the dose-limiting toxicities (*122–125*). Overall the toxicity profile of AD 32 in these earlier clinical studies showed several significant advantages over that of doxorubicin: no cardiotoxicity was observed, even at cumulative dose levels of 16.5 g/m^2; no contact

Table 3

The Effects of 3'-N-Acyl and 3'-N-Alkyl Substitution on the Biological Activity and DNA/Topoisomerase II Interactions of Selected Anthracycline Analogs and Their Principal Biotransformation Products

Anthracycline analog, abbreviation	Activity		DNA intercalation[c]	Topoisomerase II-mediated cleavage[d]
	In vivo[a]	In vitro[b]		
Doxorubicin	+ +	+ + +	+ + +	+ + +
Daunorubicin	+ +	+ + +	+ + +	+ + +
4'-Epi-doxorubicin (Epirubicin)	+ +	+ + +	+ + +	+ + +
3'-N-Acyl substituted analogs				
N-Trifluoroacetyladriamycin-14-valerate (AD 32)	+ + +	+ +	0	0
N-Trifluoroacetyladriamycin (AD 41)	+ + +	+ +	+	+
3'-N-Alkyl substituted analogs				
N-Benzyladriamycin-14-valerate (AD 198)	+ + +	+ +	+ +	0
N-Benzyladriamycin (AD 288)	+	+ +	+ + +	0

[a]In vivo activities (percentage increase in life-span) were compared against P388 cells at the respective optimal drug doses.
[b]In vitro activities (LD$_{50}$ and LD$_{90}$) were compared against CEM and L1210 cells by growth inhibition and clonogenic assays, respectively.
[c]DNA intercalation was assessed by relaxation of Form 1pC15 DNA by topoisomerase I in the presence of various concentrations of the test analogs.
[d]Plasmid DNA in a cell-free system was used to compare drug-induced topoisomerase II-mediated DNA cleavage.

toxicity was evident during inadvertent paravenous extravasation; and less gastrointestinal irritation and alopecia were produced. These initial studies also documented clinical activity against several different tumor types (*124*).

Based on the penetrant qualities of AD 32 and, for an anthracycline-type drug, a remarkable absence of cardio- and contact-toxicity, the potential utility of this drug as an intracavitary agent has been pursued. Initial evaluation of AD 32 administration by topical application was undertaken using the intravesical (ive) route (*125–128*), with a view toward managing superficial bladder carcinoma. Based on these findings, AD 32 progressed to Phase I clinical trials of ive drug instillation in patients with superficial bladder cancer. Clinical pharmacologic monitoring shows comparable negligible systemic drug pharmacology to that observed in the animal model, consistent with a lack of systemic toxicity (*129*). Presently, complete responses have been sustained (mean followup = 2 yr) in 8/32 previously heavily treated patients who presented with recurrent tumor (*130*). Phase II/III studies of AD 32 ive for treatment of BCG-refractory carcinoma *in situ* are currently ongoing. In addition, Phase I studies of ive AD 32 employed in an adjunctive role to prevent reseeding of tumor, immediately following transurethral resection, are now under way with appropriate clinical pharmacology monitoring. Clinical studies with ive AD 32 are in progress as a neoadjuvant approach to the treatment of Stage T_a/T_1 papillary disease. The potential role of ive AD 32 in the treatment of muscle-invasive (Stage T_2) bladder cancer is currently under active consideration.

The potential use of AD 32 as an intraperitoneal (ip) agent against ovarian carcinoma has also been examined in preclinical studies, wherein ip instillation (q 14 d × 3) of AD 32 at concentrations up to 900 mg/m² in rats produced no evidence of inflammatory response, contact toxicity, or peritonitis (*131*), whereas parallel metabolic studies indicated a pharmacokinetic advantage for drug administration by this route (*132*). These data have been confirmed in a Phase I trial of ip AD 32 involving dose escalation up to the maximally tolerated dose of 600 mg/m² (*133*). Normalization of CA-125 antigen levels was evident in 26% of patients, and elimination or control of peritoneal ascites was accomplished in 44% of subjects, brief neutropenia being the dose-limiting toxicity. Additional clinical studies of ip AD 32 are now beginning. Experimental studies have now expanded into other topical applications for AD 32, including intrapleural (*134*), intraprostatic (*135,136*), and more recently, intralesional injection for tumors of the oral cavity and intraventricular administration for brain tumors.

3.3.3. *N*-Alkyl Analogs: **AD 198**

In addition to circumventing P-gp-mediated drug efflux, alkylation at the basic nitrogen site on the anthracycline daunosamine sugar can also modulate the ability of a drug to interact with topoisomerases and to intercalate DNA. A novel anthracycline analog representative of this structural change currently under development is *N*-benzyladriamycin-14-valerate (AD 198), which additionally contains the same lipophilic acyl substituent at the 14-carbinol position as seen in AD 32. Thus, this highly lipophilic adriamycin analog combines superior antitumor activity relative to doxorubicin in several syngeneic tumor models (Table 3) with significantly lower systemic toxicity (*137,138*). Furthermore, AD 198 demonstrates the ability to bypass multiple mechanisms of drug resistance, not only in vitro, but in vivo, as well. For example, against a resistant subline of B16 melanoma totally unresponsive to doxorubicin, AD 198 remains as effective as against the parent sensitive line (*138*). *N*-Benzyladriamycin (AD 288) is the principal biotransformation product formed from AD 198, both in vitro and in vivo, with lower levels of *N*-benzyladriamycinol (AD 298) also being seen. Although AD 288 is more cytotoxic than doxorubicin in vitro, this agent, when given directly, is significantly less effective than AD 198 against P388 and L1210 leukemias in vivo (*137,139*). In vitro differences between AD 198 and doxorubicin include: irreversible G_2/M blockade of the cell cycle (*140*); a weaker binding with isolated purified DNA (*138,141*); production of DNA strand breaks on alkaline elution assays, despite an inability to inhibit isolated mammalian DNA topoisomerase II (*142*); potent membrane lytic activity (*138*); rapid and extensive drug accumulation and high retention in both sensitive and resistant cell lines (*139,143,144*); and lack of crossresistance in MDR phenotypic, as well as "atypical" (topo II-mutant) cell lines (*139,145,146*).

Although the mechanism(s) by which AD 198 exerts its cytotoxicity remains to be fully elucidated, it is clear that the overall effect contains both a nuclear and a cytoplasmic component, the latter occurring as a result of biotransformation. In this regard, a series of studies examining the cellular actions of AD 198 have highlighted the concept that anthracycline metabolites can be distinct from their parental agents both in the mechanism(s) of cytotoxicity and potential cellular resistance. Thus, AD 288, the major biotransformation product of AD 198, localizes in the nucleus an shows comparable DNA intercalation to that of doxorubicin, but is without activity against topoisomerase II, at least in isolated systems (Table 3). By contrast, AD 198, which is also without activity against isolated topoisomerase II, does not enter the nuclei of intact cells, but localizes in the perinuclear region of the cytoplasm in a punctate pattern suggestive of lysosomal/mitochondrial distribution (*147*). Cells expressing either the MDR or at-MDR phenotypes are crossresistant to AD 288. However they are sensitive to AD 198. Mouse macrophage-like J774.2 and P388 AD 198-resistant sublines, produced through selective (AD 198) pressure, independently express the mdr-1b isoform of P-gp as a result of the metabolic conversion of AD 198 to AD 288 under the selective conditions used; modified conditions of high concentration-short duration exposure do not result in P-gp overexpression. J774.2 AD 198-resistant variants show no change in topoisomerase II activity, based on the P4 DNA unwinding assay, an unsurprising result since AD 198 does not appear to interact with this enzyme. Additionally, no increased levels of glutathione-S-transferase activity and no difference in total cytoplasmic AD 198 accumulation are found when compared to parental cells (*148*). Reversal of AD 198 resistance by verapamil in the absence of changes in drug efflux suggests that resistance to this novel lipophilic anthracycline may be related to changes in intracellular drug compartmentalization, possibly into phagosomes that are abundant in macrophages. AD 198 has clearly demonstrated membrane perturbation effects, both in terms of structural integrity and, at minimally cytotoxic doses, in synergizing the cytotoxic effects of nuclear directed drugs, such as doxorubicin (*149*). Whether the effects of this highly lipophilic agent are nonspecific "detergent-like" or have targets within the membrane remains to be established, as does the apparent unique resistance mechanism seen in the mouse macrophage-like cell line.

Thus, AD 198 has proven capable of circumventing the clinically significant forms of drug resistance, and it appears to produce cytotoxicity, in part, through a novel mechanism. Based on its absence of cardiotoxicity, lower systemic toxicity when compared with doxorubicin, superior antitumor activity seen in appropriate models, and its proven ability to circumvent mechanisms of drug resistance, AD 198 is expected soon to enter Phase I clinical trials in the U.S. Recent studies have demonstrated the ability of AD 198 to accumulate and persist at high concentration in rat lung tissue following iv administration (150). Such drug concentrations, in excess of the LD_{90} for AD 198 against a panel of human lung carcinoma cell lines (clonogenic assay; 3-h drug exposure), suggest the potential for lung tumor-directed therapy with this agent.

3.3.4. 3'-DEAMINOANTHRACYCLINES: ME2303 AND ANNAMYCIN

It is now evident from a number of different types of anthracycline analogs that substrate specificity for the P-gp-mediated efflux pump is, in part, dependent on the basicity of the C-3' nitrogen on the daunosamine sugar, but that neither loss of charge at this position nor extreme lipophilicity of the drug molecule alone necessarily circumvents resistance in MDR cells (151). As an alternative to the N-substituted analogs like the morpholinyl-anthracyclines or AD 32 and AD 198, modulation of the basicity at this position has also been accomplished by a number of 3'-OH analogs. In addition, halogens, such as fluorine or iodine at the C-2' position, show electron-withdrawing properties, which assist in stabilizing the glycosidic bond. Two such analogs, having a C-3' hydroxyl substitution and a halogen at the C-2' position, have undergone extensive preclinical/clinical evaluation.

2'-Fluoro-3'-hydroxyldoxorubicin-14-pimelate (ME2303) is one of a series of such substituted analogs (152), in this instance, a pimelate on the C-14 position functions to increase solubility (Fig. 1). ME2303 is superior to doxorubicin in vitro against a panel of resistant human and murine tumor cell lines (153). In vivo, ME2303 is effective by iv and ip administration against P388 leukemia and iv against colon carcinoma, Lewis lung carcinoma, and M5076 melanoma. Partial activity was also claimed in vivo against a doxorubicin-resistant P388 subline (153). Entry of this compound into Phase II clinical trials in Japan has been reported (79), although subsequent literature reports are lacking.

Substantial differences between 3'-deamino-4'-epi-3'-hydroxy-2'-iodo-4-demethoxyadriamycin (Annamycin) and ME2303 include an iodine rather than a fluorine on the C-2' position, epimerization of the C-4' hydroxyl function, and demethoxylation at C-4. These factors provide for increased drug lipophilicity and improved liposomal drug entrapment. Priebe and Perez-Soler have called these two factors, modification of the anthracycline structure to allow both circumvention of P-gp and easy packaging in liposomes for improved drug delivery, the "double advantage" (154). In vitro, liposomal Annamycin (L-Anna) has comparable potency to doxorubicin against sensitive P388, CEM, and KB-3-1 cells, but is more effective than doxorubicin against doxorubicin-resistant sublines (80). Uptake of L-Anna in these lines is less than for the sensitive cells, but is unaffected by inhibitors of P-gp, such as verapamil or cyclosporin A. Anthracycline concentrations in Annamycin-dosed mice bearing B16 melanomas are consistently higher than for doxorubicin-treated animals, especially in tumor and lung (155). Activity of Annamycin in vivo is related to the liposomal formulation used, with small unilamellar vesicles producing greater survival (74–95%) than L-Anna (63–73%) or Annamycin (39–45%) against Lewis lung carcinoma, M5076 reticulosarcoma, and KB-3-1 and KB-V1 human tumor xenografts

(*156*). Based on these data and a positive evaluation in preclinical toxicity studies, liposomal Annamycin has recently entered Phase I clinical trials in the US.

3.3.5. Novel Hybrid Anthracyclines: AD 312

N-(2-Chloroethyl)-*N*-nitrosoureidodaunorubicin (AD 312) combines within the molecule two structural features that are associated with antitumor efficacy, the anthracycline structure, which provides for DNA intercalation and protein-associated DNA strand breaks through an interaction with topoisomerase II, and a nitrosourea alkylating moiety, as in drugs like lomustine (CCNU) and carmustine (BCNU), to inhibit DNA synthesis and repair (*118,157*). Animal studies have confirmed the ability of the AD 312 molecule to distribute into tissues following iv administration (*158*). Glutathione conjugates characteristic of a nitrosourea alkylating agent are evident in rat urine following AD 312 administration (*159*); additionally, the functionality of DNA alkylation by AD 312 has been confirmed by in vitro assay (*157*). The relative lack of toxicity of AD 312 vs doxorubicin is evident in the Bertazzoli mouse model (*160*), wherein AD 312 at 5x the doxorubicin dose produces only minimal evidence of cardiotoxicity compared to the extensive cardiomyopathy seen with doxorubicin (*161*).

AD 312 is active in vitro against sensitive and doxorubicin-resistant P388 cells. In vivo, AD 312 is 100% curative of disease against parental or doxorubicin-resistant P388 leukemia cell lines, with single, multiple, and even following delayed treatment (*157*). AD 312 activity in the P388 doxorubicin-resistant subline, which has reduced levels of topoisomerase II enzyme (*146*), may be partly attributed to the nitrosourea portion of the molecule; the doxorubicin-resistant P388 subline is known to retain sensitivity to alkylating agents (*162*). Additionally, AD 312 shows significant activity against a P388 subline made resistant to BCNU. Significantly, the activity of AD 312 in this model is markedly superior to that of doxorubicin, daunorubicin, or admixtures of daunorubicin and BCNU or CCNU (*163,164*), and is effective at doses that are not associated with significant bone marrow suppression, the latter observation being remarkable for an agent than incorporates two normally potent hematotoxic moieties. Human xenograft studies have revealed AD 312 to possess markedly superior activity against doxorubicin-resistant ovarian (A2780/DOX5) and doxorubicin-insensitive advanced bladder (UCRU-BL13) carcinoma lines (*165*). Against the A549 human lung tumor model, AD 312 shows superior activity (56-> 80 d tumor growth delay) compared to doxorubicin or cisplatin (*165*). Activity against lung tumors is further confirmed in the aggressive FCCL-8 human-derived tumor model, wherein AD 312 produces dramatic tumor regression at all dose levels tested (27–40.8 mg/kg); doxorubicin is without significant effect in this assay (*166*). These finding and the apparent persistence of AD 312 in lung tissue following iv administration (*158*) suggest that AD 312 may have clinical utility against human lung carcinoma, in addition to other drug-refractory tumor types. Based on these data, the novel hydrid drug AD 312 is anticipated to enter clinical trials in the US soon.

4. SUMMARY: WHERE DO WE GO FROM HERE?

Despite the considerable toxicity problems associated with anthracyclines, continued use of such agents as front-line tumor therapy is testimony to their effectiveness relative to other chemotherapeutics. With the passage of time, there has necessarily been a greater understanding of the processes involved in cardiotoxicity, and the use of cardioprotective agents, such as Dezrazoxane, offers the hope that this life-threatening side effect will ultimately be therapeutically controllable. Nevertheless, the emergence of drug-resistant cell populations, through mechanisms that we now recognize as potentially being infinitely more complex than simple overexpression of a P-gp membrane pump, remains as the greatest hurdle for improved anthracycline chemotherapy. All of the various anthracycline analogs outlined above appear, at least in experimental systems, to have potential for improved chemotherapy by their ability to circumvent some experimental resistance mechanisms; their ultimate test will come in the clinical trials where so many earlier aspirations have fallen short. However, the collective knowledge gained from these earlier disappointments, coupled with the many structure–activity studies that have now been conducted and the greater sophistication of current laboratory techniques, predicts a brighter future in anthra-cycline research. As outlined above, our capacity to control both cellular drug trans-port and lethal targets is at hand. Combination of one or more relatively nontoxic anthracyclines with different cellular target sites into a drug "cocktail" and/or for-mulation of drugs in liposomes may ultimately yield a better therapeutic result than our current concepts of anthracycline therapy. Conversely, the potential exists for "dual mechanistic" drugs that either combine two distinct antitumorals into one molecule or are structurally configured such that on biotransformation, they liberate a product with a different mechanism of action and cellular target site. An obvious need for improved anthracycline antitumor drugs remains. In answer to Weiss' ques-tion, "Will we ever find a better doxorubicin?" we believe the answer is yes, but probably not in terms of a major new systemic entity with a wide spectrum of activity, but rather for well-prescribed indications based on clear pharmacologic rationales and appropriate pharmacokinetic support.

REFERENCES

1. Grein A, Spella C, DiMarco A, Canevazzi G. Descrizione e classificazione di un attionamicette (Streptomyces Peucetius sp nova) produltore di un sostanza ad attivite antitumorale; la dauno-micina. *Giorn Microbiol* 1963; 11:109–118.
2. Dubost M, Gauter P, Maral R, et al. Un novel antibiotique a proprietes cytostatiques; la rubi-domycine. *CR Acad Sci Paris* 1963; 257:1813–1815.
3. Pigram WJ, Fuller W, Hamilton LD. Stereochemistry of intercalation: interaction of dauno-mycin with DNA. *Nature New Biol* 1972; 235:17–19.
4. Fogleson PD, Reckord C, Swink S. Doxorubicin inhibits human DNA topoisomerase I. *Cancer Chemother Pharmacol* 1992; 30:123–125.
5. Tewey KM, Rowe TC, Yang L, et al. Adriamycin-induced DNA damage mediated by mam-malian DNA topoisomerase II. *Science* 1984; 226:466–468.
6. Bachur NR, Yu F, Johnson R, et al. Helicase inhibition by anthracycline anticancer agents. *Mol Pharmacol* 1992; 41:993–998.
7. Bachur NR, Gordon SL, Gee MW. Anthracycline antibiotic augmentation of microsomal elec-tron transport and free radical formation. *Mol Pharmacol* 1977; 13:901–910.
8. Murphree SA, Cunningham LS, Hwang KM, Sartorelli AC. Effects of adriamycin on surface properties of sarcoma 180 ascites cells. *Biochem Pharmacol* 1976; 25:1227–1231.
9. Tritton TR. Cell surface actions of Adriamycin. *Pharmacol Ther* 1991; 49:293–309.
10. Koseki Y, Israel M, Sweatman TW, et al. Inhibitory effects of immobilized adriamycin on cell growth and thymidine uptake in human CEM leukemic lymphocytes. *J Cell Pharmacol* 1991; 2:171–178.

11. Ling YH, Priebe W, Perez-Soler R. Apoptosis induced by anthracycline antibiotics in P388 parent and multidrug resistant cells. *Cancer Res* 1993; 53:1583–1589.
12. Jacquillat C, Tanzer J, Boiron M, et al. Rubidomycin: a new agent active in the treatment of acute lymphoblastic leukemia. *Lancet* 1966; 2:27–28.
13. Boiron M, Jacquillat C, Weil M, et al. Daunorubicin in the treatment of acute myelocytic leukemia. *Lancet* 1969; 1:330–333.
14. Wiernik PH, Serpick AA. Randomized clinical trial of daunorubicin and a combination of pre-dnisone, vincristine, 6-mercaptopurine and methotrexate in adult acute non-lymphocytic leukemia. *Cancer Res* 1972; 32:2023–2026.
15. DiMarco A, Gaetani M, Scarpinato B. Adriamycin (NSC-123,127): a new antibiotic with anti-tumor activity. *Cancer Chemother Rep (Part I)* 1969; 53:33–37.
16. DeVita VT, Hellman S, Rosenberg SA, eds. *Cancer. Principles and Practice of Oncology,* 4th ed. Philadelphia: JB Lippincott Company, 1993.
17. Woodcock TM, Allegra JC, Richman SP, et al. Pharmacology and phase I clinical studies of daunorubicin in patients with advanced malignancies. *Semin Oncol* 1984; 11:28–32.
18. Harvey J, Goodman A, McFadden M, et al. A phase I study of daunorubicin in advanced untreatable malignancies. *Semin Oncol* 1984; 11:33–35.
19. Von Hoff DD. Use of daunorubicin in patients with solid tumors. *Semin Oncol* 1984; 11: 23–27.
20. List AF. Multidrug resistance: clinical relevance in acute leukemia. *Oncology* 1993; 7:23–32.
21. Booser DJ, Hortobagyi GN. Anthracycline antibiotics in cancer therapy. *Drugs* 1994; 47: 223–258.
22. Von Hoff DD, Rozencweig M, Leyard M, et al. Daunomycin-induced cardiotoxicity in children and adults. A review of 110 cases. *Am J Med* 1977; 62:200–208.
23. Steinberg JS, Cohen AJ, Wasserman AG, et al. Acute arrhythmogenicity of doxorubicin administration. *Cancer* 1987; 60:1213–1218.
24. Wortman JE, Lucas VS Jr, Schuster E, et al. Sudden death during doxorubicin administration. *Cancer* 1979; 44:1588–1591.
25. Doroshow JH, Locker GY, Myers CE. Enzymatic defenses of the mouse heart against reactive oxygen metabolites; alterations produced by doxorubicin. *J. Clin Invest* 1980; 65:128–135.
26. Myers CE, McGuire WP, Liss RH, et al. Adriamycin: the role of lipid peroxidation in cardiac toxicity and tumour response. *Science* 1977; 197:165–167.
27. Von Hoff DD, Layard MW, Basa P, et al. Risk factors for doxorubicin-induced congestive heart failure. *Ann Intern Med* 1977; 62:200–208.
28. Watts RG. Severe and fatal anthracycline cardiotoxicity at cumulative doses below 400 mg/m²: evidence for enhanced toxicity with multi-agent chemotherapy. *Am J Hematol* 1991; 36:217,218.
29. Lipschultz SE, Colan SD, Gelber R, et al. Late cardiac effects of doxorubicin therapy for acute lymphoblastic leukemia in childhood. *N Engl J Med* 1991; 324:808–815.
30. Lipschultz SE, Lipsitz SR, Mone SM, et al. Female sex and drug dose as risk factors for late cardiotoxic effects of doxorubicin therapy for childhood cancer. *N Engl J Med* 1995; 332: 1738–1743.
31. Gottlieb SL, Edmiston WE Jr, Haywood LJ. Late, late doxorubicin cardiotoxicity. *Chest* 1980; 78:880–882.
32. Freter CE, Lee TC, Billingham ME, et al. Doxorubicin cardiac toxicity manifesting seven years after treatment. Case report and review. *Am J Med* 1986; 80:483–485.
33. Sunnenberg TD, Kramer B. Long-term effects of cancer chemotherapy. *Compr Ther* 1985; 11:58–67.
34. Goorin AM, Chauvenet AR, Perez-Atayde AR, et al. Initial congestive heart failure six to ten years after doxorubicin chemotherapy for childhood cancer. *J. Pediatr* 1990; 116:144–147.
35. Steinherz L, Steinherz P. Delayed cardiac toxicity from anthracycline therapy. *Paediatrician* 1991; 18:49–52.
36. DeValeriola DL. Dose optimization of anthracyclines. *Anticancer Res* 1994; 14:2307–2314.
37. Mitchell RB, Ratain MJ, Vogelzang NJ. Experimental rationale for continuous infusion chemotherapy. In: Lokich JJ, ed. *Cancer Chemotherapy by Infusion,* 2nd ed. Chicago: Precept Press. 1990:3.

38. Bielack SS, Erttmann R, Winkler K, Landbeck G. Doxorubicin: effect of different schedules on toxicity and antitumor efficacy. *Eur J Cancer Clin Oncol* 1989; 25:873–882.
39. Zalupski M, Metch B, Balcerzak S, et al. Phase III comparisons of doxorubicin and dacarbazine given by bolus versus infusion in patients with soft tissue sarcomas: a Southwest Oncology Group Study. *J Natl Cancer Inst* 1991; 83:926–932.
40. Hortobagyi GN, Frye D, Budzar AU, et al. Decreased cardiac toxicity of doxorubicin administered by continuous intravenous infusion in combination chemotherapy for metastatic breast carcinoma. *Cancer* 1989; 63:37–45.
41. Preisler HD, Gessner T, Azarnia N, et al. Relationship between plasma adriamycin levels and the outcome of remission induction therapy for acute non-lymphocytic leukemia. *Cancer Chemother Pharmacol* 1984; 12:125–130.
42. Robert J, Monnier A, Poutignat N, Herait P. A pharmacokinetic and pharmacodynamic study of the new anthracycline pirarubicin in breast cancer patients. *Cancer Chemother Pharmacol* 1991; 29:75–79.
43. Robert J, Illiadis A, Hoerni B, et al. Pharmacokinetics of adriamycin in patients with breast cancer: correlation between pharmacokinetic parameters and clinical short-term response. *Eur J Cancer Clin Oncol* 1982; 18:739–745.
44. Robert J. Use of pharmacokinetic-pharmacodynamic relationships in the development of new anthracyclines. *Cancer Chemother Pharmacol* 1993; 32:99–102.
45. DeValeriola DL, Ross DD, Forrest A, et al. Use of plasma cytotoxic activity to model cytotoxic pharmacodynamics of anticancer drugs. *Cancer Chemother Pharmacol* 1991; 29:133–140.
46. Robert J, Giani L. Pharmacokinetics and metabolism of anthracyclines. *Cancer Surveys* 1993; 17:219–252.
47. Gabizon AA. Liposomal anthracyclines. *Hematol Oncol Clin North Am* 1994; 8:431–450.
48. Huang SK, Mayhew E, Giliani S, et al. Pharmacokinetics and therapeutics of sterically stabilized liposomes in mice bearing C-26 colon carcinoma. *Cancer Res* 1992; 52:6774–6781.
49. Mayhew EG, Lasic DD, Babbar S, et al. Pharmacokinetics and antitumor activity of epirubicin encapsulated in long-circulating liposomes. *Int J Cancer* 1992; 51:302–309.
50. Papahadjopoulos D, Allen TM, Gabizon AA, et al. Sterically stabilized liposomes: Improvements in pharmacokinetics and antitumor therapeutic efficacy. *Proc Natl Acad Sci* 1991; 88: 11,460–11,464.
51. Gabizon AA, Peretz T, Ben-Yosef R, et al. Phase I study of liposome-associated Adriamycin: Preliminary report. *Proc Am Soc Clin Oncol* 1986; 5:43.
52. Gill PS, Espina BM, Muggia F, et al. Phase I/II clinical and pharmacokinetic evaluation of liposomal daunorubicin. *J. Clin Oncol* 1995; 13:996–1003.
53. Gill PS, Wernz J, Scadden DT, et al. A randomized trial of liposomal daunorubicin (DX) vs Adriamycin, bleomycin and vincristine (ABV) in 232 patients with advanced AIDS-related Kaposi's sarcoma. *Proc Am Assoc Cancer Res* 1995; 14:A830.
54. Law TM, Mencel P, Motzer RJ. Phase II trial of liposomal encapsulated doxorubicin in patients with advanced renal cell carcinoma. *Invest New Drugs* 1994; 12:323–325.
55. Speyer JL, Freedberg R. In: Abeloff MD, et al. eds. *Clinical Oncology*. New York: Churchhill Livingstone. 1995:811.
56. Rajagopalan S, Politi PM, Sinha BK, Myers CE. Adriamycin-induced free radical formation in the perfused rat heart: implications for cardiotoxicity. *Cancer Res* 1988; 48:4766–4769.
57. Buss JL, Hasinoff BB. Ferrous iron strongly promotes the ring opening of the hydrolysis intermediates of the antioxidant cardioprotective agent dexrazoxane (ICR-187). *Arch Biochem Biophys* 1995; 317:121–127.
58. Speyer JL, Green MD, Zeleniuch-Jacquotte A, et al. ICRF-187 permits longer treatment with doxorubicin in women with breast cancer. *J Clin Oncol* 1992; 10:117–127.
59. Jelic S, Radulovic S, Neskovic-Konstantinovic Z, et al. Cardioprotection with ICRF-187 (Cardioxane) in patients with advanced breast cancer having cardiac risk factors for doxorubicin cardiotoxicity, treated with the FDC regimen. *Support Cancer Care* 1995; 3:176–182.
60. Kolaric K, Bradamante V, Cervek J, et al. A phase II trial of cardioprotection with Cardioxane (ICRF-187) in patients with advanced breast cancer receiving 5-fluorouracil, doxorubicin and cyclophosphamide. *Oncology* 1995; 52:251–255.
61. Monte E, Sinha BK. Potentiation of doxorubicin cytotoxicity by (+)-1,2-bis (3,5-dioxopipera-

zinyl-1-yl) propane (ICRF-187) in human leukemic HL-60 cells. *Cancer Commun* 1990; 2: 145–149.

62. Sehested M, Jensen PB, Sorensen BS, et al. Antagonistic effects of the cardioprotector (+)-1,2-bis (3,5-dioxopiperazinyl-1-yl) propane (ICRF-187) on DNA breaks and cytotoxicity induced by the topoisomerase II-directed drugs daunorubicin and etoposide (VP-16). *Biochem Pharmacol* 1993; 46:389–393.

63. Abramowicz M, Ed. *Med Lett Drugs Ther* 1995; 37:110,111.

64. Kessel D, Woo ES, Michalska AE, et al. Uptake and retention of daunomycin by mouse leukemic cells as factors in drug response. *Cancer Res* 1968; 28:938–941.

65. Biedler JL, Riehm H. Cellular resistance to actinomycin D in Chinese hamster cells in vitro: cross-resistance, radioautographic and cytogenetic studies. *Cancer Res* 1970; 30:1174–1184.

66. Roninson IB, Chin JE, Choi K, et al. Isolation of human mdr DNA sequences amplified in multidrug-resistant KB carcinoma cells. *Proc Natl Acad Sci USA* 1986; 83:4538–4542.

67. Ueda K, Cardarelli C, Gottesman MM, Pastan I. Expression of a full length cDNA for the human "MDR 1" gene confers resistance to colchicine, doxorubicin, and vinblastine. *Proc Natl Acad Sci USA* 1987; 84:3004–3008.

68. List AF. Multidrug resistance: clinical relevance in acute leukemia. *Oncology* 1993; 7:23–38.

69. Cole SPC, Bhardwaj G, Gerlach JH, et al. Overexpression of a transporter gene in multidrug-resistant human lung cancer cell line. *Science* 1992; 258:1650–1654.

70. Cole SPC, Sparks KE, Fraser K, et al. Pharmacologic characterization of multidrug resistant MRP-transfected human tumor cells. *Cancer Res* 1994; 54:5902–5910.

71. Cole SPC, Downes HF, Slovak ML. Effect of calcium antagonists on the chemosensitivity of two multidrug-resistant human tumor cell lines which do not overexpress P-glycoprotein. *Br J Cancer* 1989; 59:42–46.

72. Barrand MA, Rhodes T, Center MS, Twentyman PR. Chemosensitization and drug accumulation effects of cyclosporin A, PSC-833, and verapamil in human MDR large cell lung cancer cells expressing a 190k membrane protein distinct from P-glycoprotein. *Eur J Cancer* 1993; 29:408–415.

73. Kuss BJ, Deeley RG, Cole SPC, et al. Deletion of gene for multidrug resistance in acute myeloid leukemia with inversion in chromosome 16: prognostic implications. *Lancet* 1994; 343: 1531–1534.

74. Bordow SB, Haber M, Madafiglio J, et al. Expression of the multidrug resistance-associated protein (MRP) gene correlates with amplification and overexpression of the N-myc oncogene in childhood neuroblastoma. *Cancer Res* 1994; 54:5036–5040.

75. Liu LF. DNA topoisomerase poisons as antitumor drugs. *Annu Rev Biochem* 1989; 58:351–375.

76. Osheroff N. Effect of antineoplastic agents on the DNA cleavage/religation reaction of eukaryotic topoisomerase II: inhibition of DNA religation by etoposide. *Biochemistry* 1989; 28: 6157–6160.

77. Beck WT, Danks MK, Wolverton JS, et al. Resistance of mammalian tumor cells to inhibitors of DNA topoisomerase II. In: Liu LF, ed. Topoisomerase-Targeting Drugs. New York: Academic. 1994:145–169.

78. Akimoto H, Bruno NA, Slate DL, et al. Effect of verapamil on doxorubicin cardiotoxicity: altered muscle gene expression in cultured neonatal rat cardiomyocytes. *Cancer Res* 1993; 53: 4658–4664.

79. Weiss RB. The anthracyclines: will we ever find a better doxorubicin? *Semin Oncol* 1992; 19: 670–686.

80. Priebe W. Mechanism of action-governed design of anthracycline antibiotics: "a turn off/turn on" approach. *Current Drug Design* 1995; 1:73–96.

81. Miller AA, Salewski E. Prospects for Pirarubicin. *Med Pediatr Oncol* 1994; 22:261–268.

82. Goldin A, Venditti JM, Geran R. The effectiveness of the anthracycline analogue 4'-epidoxorubicin in the treatment of experimental tumors: a review. *Invest New Drugs* 1985; 3:3–21.

83. Hurteloup P, for the French Epirubicin Study Group: A prospective randomized Phase III trial comparing combination chemotherapy with cyclophosphamide, fluorouracil, and either doxorubicin or epirubicin. *J Clin Oncol* 1988; 6:679–688.

84. Intimi C, for the Italian Multicentre Breast Study with Epirubicin: Phase III randomized study of fluorouracil, epirubicin and cyclophosphamide v. fluorouracil, doxorubicin and cyclophosphamide in advanced breast cancer: An Italian multicentre trial. *J Clin Oncol* 1988; 6:976–982.

85. Weenen H, Van Maanan JMS, De Planque MM, et al. Metabolism of 4' modified analogs of doxorubicin. Unique glucuronidation pathway for 4' epidoxorubicin. *Eur J Cancer Clin Oncol* 1984; 20:919–926.

86. Perez DJ, Harvey VJ, Robinson BA, et al. A randomized comparison of single-agent doxorubicin and epirubicin as first-line cytotoxic therapy in advanced breast cancer. *J Clin Oncol* 1991; 9:2148–2152.

87. Nielsen D, Jensen JB, Dombernowsky P, et al. Epirubicin cardiotoxicity: A study of 135 patients with advanced breast cancer. *J Clin Oncol* 1990; 8:1806–1810.

88. Dardir MD, Ferrans VJ, Mikhael YS, et al. Cardiac morphologic and functional changes induced by epirubicin chemotherapy. *J Clin Oncol* 1989; 7:947–958.

89. Kuffel MJ, Reid JM, Ames MM. Anthracyclines and their C-13 metabolites: growth inhibition and DNA damage following incubation with human tumor cells in culture. *Cancer Chemother Pharmacol* 1992; 30:51–57.

90. Weiss RB. A third anthracycline for acute leukemia. *Contemp Oncol* 1992; 2:30–39.

91. Wiernik PH, Banks PLC, Case DC, et al. Cytarabine plus idarubicin or daunorubicin as induction and consolidation therapy for previously untreated adult patients with acute myeloid leukemia. *Blood* 1992; 79:313–319.

92. Stewart DJ, Grewaal D, Green RM, et al. Bioavailability and pharmacology of oral idarubicin. *Cancer Chemother Pharmacol* 1991; 27:308–314.

93. Lopez M, Contegiacomo A, Vici P, et al. A prospective randomized trial of doxorubicin versus idarubicin in the treatment of advanced breast cancer. *Cancer* 1989; 64:2431–2436.

94. Stuart NSA, Cullen MH, Priestman TJ, et al. A phase II study of oral idarubicin (4-demethoxy-daunorubicin) in advanced breast cancer. *Cancer Chemother Pharmacol* 1988; 21:351–354.

95. Hurteloup P, Armand JP, Schneider M, et al. Phase II trial of idarubicin (4-demethoxydaunorubicin) in advanced breast cancer. *Eur J Cancer Clin Oncol* 1989; 25:423–428.

96. Michieli M, Michelutti A, Damiani D, et al. A comparative analysis of the sensitivity of multidrug resistant (MDR) and non-MDR cells to different anthracycline derivatives. *Leukemia Lymphoma* 1993; 9:255–264.

97. Klumper E, Pieters R, den Boer ML, et al. In vitro anthracycline cross-resistance pattern in childhood acute lymphoblastic leukaemia. *Br J Cancer* 1995; 71:1188–1193.

98. Bastholt L, Dalmark M. Phase II study of idarubicin given orally in the treatment of anthracycline-naive advanced breast cancer patients. *Cancer Treat Rep* 1987; 71:451–454.

99. Han G, Israel M, Seshadri R, Sweatman TW. Metabolism and elimination of N,N-di(n-butyl) adriamycin-14-valerate in the rat. *Cancer Chemother Pharmacol* 1996; 37:472–478.

100. Priebe W, Van NT, Burke TG, Perez-Soler R. Removal of the basic center from doxorubicin partially overcomes multidrug resistance and decreases cardiotoxicity. *Anticancer Drugs* 1993; 4:37–48.

101. Acton EM. Unresolved structure-activity relationships in anthracycline analogue development. In: Priebe W, ed. *Anthracycline Antibiotics. Novel Analogues, Methods of Delivery and Mechanisms of Action.* Washington DC: American Chemical Society. 1995:1–13.

102. Ogawa M, Ariyoshi Y. New anticancer drugs under clinical trials in Japan. *Hematol Oncol Clin North Am* 1994; 8:277–287.

103. Acton EM, Tong GL, Mosher CW, Wolgemuth RL. Intensely potent morpholinyl anthracyclines. *J Med Chem* 1984; 27:638–645.

104. Mosher CW, Wu HY, Fujiwara AN, Acton EM. Enhanced antitumor properties of 3'-(4-morpholinyl) and 3'-(4-methoxy-1-piperidinyl) derivatives of 3'-deamino-daunorubicin. *J Med Chem* 1982; 25:18–24.

105. Sikic BT, Ehsam MS, Harker WG, et al. Dissociation of antitumor potency from the anthracycline cardiotoxicity in a doxorubicin analogue. *Science* 1985; 228:1544–1546.

106. Streeter PG, Johl JS, Gordon GR, Peters JH. Uptake and retention of morpholinyl anthracyclines by adriamycin-sensitive and -resistant P388 cells. *Cancer Chemother Pharmacol* 1986; 16:247–252.

107. Westendorf J, Aydin M, Groth G, et al. Mechanistic aspects of DNA damage by morpholinyl and cyanomorpholinyl anthracyclines. *Cancer Res* 1989; 49:5262–5266.

108. Graham MA, Clugson CK, King LH, et al. Mechanistic studies with methoxymorpholino-doxorubicin: evidence for a novel covalently bound DNA adduct following activation by CYT P450 3A. *Proc Am Assoc Cancer Res* 1992; 33:513.

109. Lau DH, Duran GE, Sikic BI. Characterization of covalent DNA binding of morpholino and cyanomorpholino derivatives of doxorubicin. *J Natl Cancer Inst* 1992; 84:1587–1592.
110. Lau DH, Lewis AD, Sikic BI. Association of DNA cross-linking with potentiation of the morpholino derivative of doxorubicin by human liver microsomes. *J Natl Cancer Inst* 1989; 81: 1034–1038.
111. Wasserman K, Markovits J, Jaxel C, et al. Effects of morpholinyl doxorubicin, doxorubicin, and actinomycin D on mammalian DNA topoisomerases I and II. *Mol Pharmacol* 1990; 38: 38–45.
112. Watanabe M, Komeshima N, Nakajima S, Tsuruo T. MX2, a morpholino anthracycline, as a new antitumor agent against drug-sensitive and multidrug-resistant human and murine tumor cells. *Cancer Res* 1988; 48:6653–6657.
113. Streeter DG, Taylor DL, Acton EM, Peters JH. Comparative cytotoxicities of various morpholinyl anthracyclines. *Cancer Chemother Pharmacol* 1985; 14:160–164.
114. Komeshima N, Tsuruo T., Umezawa H. Antitumor activity of new morpholino anthracyclines. *J Antibiot* 1988; 41: 548–553.
115. Koseki Y, Sweatman TW, Israel M. *N*-Trifluoroacetyladriamycin-14-valerate (AD 32) cellular pharmacology in human bladder tumor cell lines. *Proc Am Assoc Cancer Res* 1992; 33:428.
116. Israel M, Sweatman TW, Seshadri R, Koseki Y. Comparative uptake and retention of Adriamycin and *N*-benzyladriamycin-14-valerate in human CEM leukemia lymphocyte cell cultures. *Cancer Chemother Pharmacol* 1989; 25:177–183.
117. Israel M, Seshadri R, Sweatman TW, et al. Structure and biological activity of *N*-substituted anthracyclines: correlation with DNA interaction. First Conference on DNA Topoisomerases in Cancer Chemotherapy, New York, November 1988.
118. Israel M, Seshadri R, Koseki Y, et al. New anthracycline analogues directed against DNA topoisomerase II. In Tapiero H, Robert J, Lampidis TJ, eds. Interface on Clinical and Laboratory Responses to Anticancer Drugs. Montrouge France: John Libby Eurotext, 1989; 191:39–47.
119. Israel M, Khetarpal VK. Tissue distribution and metabolism of *N*-trifluorocetyladriamycin-14-valerate (AD 32) compared with adriamycin in mice bearing established Lewis Lung carcinoma. Proceedings of the 13th International Congress of Chemotherapy, Vienna, 1983.
120. Israel M, Modest EJ, Frei E III. *N*-Trifluoroacetyladriamycin-14-valerate, an analog with greater experimental antitumor activity and less toxicity than adriamycin. *Cancer Res* 1975; 35:1365–1368.
121. Vecchi A, Cairo M, Mantovani A, et al. Comparative antineoplastic activity of adriamycin and *N*-trifluoroacetyladriamycin-14-valerate. *Cancer Treat Rep* 1978; 62:111–117.
122. Blum RH, Garnick MB, Israel M, et al. An initial clinical evaluation of *N*-trifluoroacetyl-adriamycin-14-valerate (AD 32), an adriamycin analog. *Cancer Treat Rep* 1979; 63:919–923.
123. Blum RH, Garnick MB, Israel M, et al. Preclinical rationale and phase I clinical trial of the adriamycin analog, AD 32. In: Carter SK, Sakurai Y, Umezawa H, eds. *New Drugs in Cancer Chemotherapy, Recent Results in Cancer Research,* vol. 76. New York: Springer-Verlag. 1981: 7–15.
124. Garnick MB, Griffin JD, Sack MJ, et al. Phase II evaluation of N-trifluoroacetyladriamycin-14-valerate (AD 32). In: Muggia FM, Young CW, Carter SK, eds. *Anthracycline Antibiotics in Cancer Therapy.* The Hague: Martinus Nijhoff. 1982:7.
125. Sweatman TW, Payne C, Koseki Y, et al. Drug penetration into dog bladder wall following intravesical (ive) instillation of *N*-trifluoroacetyladriamycin-14-valerate (AD 32). *Proc Am Assoc Cancer Res* 1993; 34:364.
126. Koseki Y, Sweatman TW, Israel M. *N*-Trifluoroacetyladriamycin-14-valerate (AD 32) cellular pharmacology in human bladder tumor cell lines. *Proc Am Assoc Cancer Res* 1992; 33:428.
127. Sweatman TW, Payne C, Patterson L, et al. *N*-Trifluoroacetyladriamycin-14-valerate (AD 32) penetration into human urinary bladder tissue following intravesical instillation. *Proc Am Assoc Cancer Res* 1996; 37:182.
128. Sweatman TW, Parker RF, Israel M. Pharmacologic rationale for intravesical *N*-trifluoroace-tyladriamycin-14-valerate (AD 32): A preclinical study. *Cancer Chemother Pharmacol* 1991; 28:1–6.

129. Sweatman TW, Payne C, Israel M, et al. Clinical pharmacology of intravesical (IVE) *N*-tri-fluoroacetyladriamycin-14-valerate (AD 32). *Proc Am Soc Clin Oncol* 1993; 12:162.

130. Giantonio B, Greenberg R, Bamberger M, et al. A Phase-I trial of AD 32 administered intra-vesically in patients with superficial transitional cell carcinoma of the bladder. *Proc Am Soc Clin Oncol* 1993; 12:251.

131. Israel M, Chengelis CP, Naas DJ, Sweatman TW. Absence of *N*-trifluoroacetyladriamycin-14-valerate (AD 32) toxicity following intraperitoneal (ip) injection in rats. *Proc Am Assoc Cancer Res* 1993; 34:427.

132. Sweatman TW, Payne C, Israel M, et al. Clinical pharmacology of intraperitoneal (ip) *N*-trifluoroacetyladriamycin-14-valerate. *Proc Am Assoc Cancer Res* 1994; 35:245.

133. Markman M, Homesley H, Norberts DA, et al. Phase I trial of intraperitoneal AD 32 in gyne-cologic malignancies. *Gynecol Oncol* 1996; 61:90–93.

134. Devlin S, Sweatman TW. Pharmacology of intrapleural (ipl) *N*-trifluoroacetyladriamycin-14-valerate (AD 32) in the rat. *Proc Am Assoc Cancer Res* 1994; 35:431.

135. Israel M, Bernacki RJ, Kantcr PM. Pharmacologic rationale for intraprostatic AD 32 (*N*-trifluoroacetyladriamycin-14-valerate). *Proc Am Assoc Cancer Res* 1996; 37:372.

136. DiDomenico D, Brown J, Shaw M, et al. Intralesional AD 32 is efficacious in a prostate cancer model. *Proc Am Assoc Cancer Res* 1996; 37:303.

137. Israel M, Seshadri R. *N*-Alkyl and *N*-benzyladriamycin derivatives. US Patent 4,610,977, 1986. US Patent Office, Washington, DC.

138. Israel M, Seshadri R, Koseki Y, et al. Amelioration of adriamycin toxicity through modifica-tion of drug-DNA binding properties. *Cancer Treat Rev* 1987; 14:163.

139. Ganapathi R, Grabowski D, Sweatman TW, et al. *N*-Benzyladriamycin-14-valerate versus pro-gressively doxorubicin-resistant murine tumours: cellular pharmacology and characterization of cross-resistance in vitro and in vivo. *Br J Cancer* 1989; 60:819–826.

140. Traganos F, Israel M, Seshadri R, et al. Effects of new N-alkyl analogues of adriamycin on in vitro survival and cell-cycle progression. *Cancer Res* 1985; 45:6273–6279.

141. Lameh J, Chuang LF, Israel M, Chuang RY. Mechanistic studies on *N*-benzyladriamycin-14-valerate (AD 198), a highly lipophilic alkyl adriamycin analogue. *Anticancer Res* 1988; 8: 689–694.

142. Bodley A, Liu LF, Israel M, et al. DNA topoisomerase II-mediated interaction of doxorubicin and daunorubicin congeners with DNA. *Cancer Res* 1989; 49:5969–5978.

143. Israel M, Sweatman TW, Seshadri R, Koseki Y. Comparative uptake and retention of adria-mycin and *N*-benzyladriamycin-14-valerate in human leukemic lymphocyte cell cultures. *Cancer Chemother Pharmacol* 1989; 25:177–183.

144. Sweatman TW, Israel M, Seshadri R, et al. Cytotoxicity and cellular pharmacology of *N*-benzyl-adriamycin-14-valerate in mechanistically different multidrug-resistant human leukemic cells. *J Cell Pharmacol* 1990; 1:96–102.

145. Krishan A, Sauerteig A, Gordon K, Swinkin C. Flow cytometric monitoring of cellular anthra-cycline accumulation in murine leukemia cells. *Cancer Res* 1986; 46:1768–1773.

146. Maniar N, Krishan A, Israel M, Samy TSA. Anthracycline-induced DNA breaks and resealing in doxorubicin-resistant murine leukemia P388 cells. *Biochem Pharmacol* 1988; 37:1763–1772.

147. Lothstein L, Sweatman TW, Dockter M, Israel M. Resistance of *N*-benzyladriamycin-14-valerate in mouse J774.2 cells: P-glycoprotein expression without reduced *N*-benzyladriamycin-14-valerate accumulation. *Cancer Res* 1992; 52:3409–3417.

148. Lothstein L, Koseki Y, Sweatman TW. P-glycoprotein overexpression in mouse cells does not correlate with resistance to *N*-benzyladriamycin-14-valerate (AD 198). *Anticancer Drugs* 1994; 5:623–633.

149. Koseki Y, Lothstein L, Sweatman TW, Israel M. Absence of P-glycoprotein (P-gp) mechanism for the synergistic effect of *N*-benzyladriamycin-14-valerate (AD 198) on Adriamycin (ADR) cytotoxicity in human ovarian carcinoma cells. *Proc Am Assoc Cancer Res* 1993; 34:367.

150. Koseki Y, Sweatman TW, Israel M. Pharmacologic rationale for lung cancer therapy with *N*-benzyladriamycin-14-valerate (AD 198). *Proc Am Assoc Cancer Res* 1994; 35:411.

151. Lothstein L, Sweatman TW, Priebe W. Study of the effect of charge and lipophilicity on

anthracycline cytotoxicity in multidrug resistant murine J774.2 cells. *Proc Am Assoc Cancer Res* 1994; 35:342.

152. Tsuchiya T, Takagi Y, Umezawa S, et al. Synthesis and antitumor activities of 14-*O*-acyl derivatives of 7-*O*-(2,6-dideoxy-2-fluoro-a-L-talopyranosyl) adriamycin. *J Antibiotic* 1988; 41: 988–991.

153. Tsuruo T, Yusa K, Sudo Y, et al. A fluorine-containing anthracycline (ME2303) as a new antitumor agent against murine and human tumors and their multidrug resistant sublines. *Cancer Res* 1989; 49:5537–5542.

154. Priebe W, Perez-Soler R. Design and tumor targeting of anthracyclines able to overcome multidrug resistance: a double-advantage approach. *Pharmacol Ther* 1993; 60:215–234.

155. Zou Y, Priebe W, Ling YH, Perez-Soler R. Organ distribution and tumor uptake of annamycin, a new anthracycline derivative with high affinity for lipid membranes, entrapped in multilamellar vesicles. *Cancer Chemother Pharmacol* 1993; 32:190–196.

156. Zou Y, Ling YH, Van NT, et al. Antitumor activity of free and liposome-entrapped annamycin, a lipophilic anthracycline antibiotic with non-cross-resistance properties. *Cancer Res* 1994; 54: 1479–1484.

157. Israel M, Seshadri R. Hybrid nitrosoureidoanthracyclines having antitumor activity. U.S. Patent 4,973,675, 1990. US Patent Office, Washington, DC.

158. Pawlik C, Payne C, Lothstein L, et al. Tissue distribution of *N*-(2-[^{14}C]-chloroethyl)-*N*-nitrosoureidodaunorubicin in the rat. *Proc Am Assoc Cancer Res* 1994; 35:431.

159. Sweatman TW, Rodrigues P, Pawlik C, et al. Metabolism and elimination of *N*-(2-[^{14}C]-chloroethyl)-*N*-nitrosoureidodaunorubicin in the rat. *Proc Am Assoc Cancer Res* 1995; 36:364.

160. Bertazzoli C, Bellini O, Magrini U, Tozana M. Quantitative experimental evaluation of adriamycin cardiotoxicity in the mouse. *Cancer Treat Rep* 1979; 63:1877–1883.

161. Israel M, Chengelis CP. Lack of anthracycline-type cardiotoxicity associated with *N*-(2-chloroethyl)nitrosoureidodaunorubicin (AD 312). *Proc Am Assoc Cancer Res* 1994; 35:407.

162. Johnson RK, Chitnis MP, Embrey WM, Gregory EB. In vivo characteristics of resistance and cross resistance of an adriamycin-resistant subline of P388 leukemia. *Cancer Treat Rep* 1978; 62:1535–1547.

163. Israel M, Koseki Y, Seshadri R. Further in vivo antitumor studies with 2-chloroethylnitrosoureidodaunorubicin (AD 312) in murine P388 leukemia systems. *Proc Am Assoc Cancer Res* 1991; 32:2401.

164. Israel M, Koseki Y, Sweatman TW, Seshadri R. DNA topoisomerase II-directed nitrosoureidoanthracyclines: high in vivo antitumor activity with minimal myelosuppression. *J Cancer Res Clin Oncol* 1990; 116:468.

165. Glaves D, Rustum Y, Bernacki RJ, et al. Therapeutic activity of a nitrosourea: anthracycline hybrid (AD 312) against human bladder, lung, and ovarian xenografts. *Proc Am Assoc Cancer Res* 1995; 36:392.

166. Israel M, Krishan A, Wellham LL. Antitumor activity of 2-chloroethylnitrosoureidodaunorubicin (AD 312) in nude mice bearing xenografts of FCC-8 human lung adenocarcinoma. *Proc Am Assoc Cancer Res* 1995; 36:396.

6

Topoisomerase I Inhibitors

Beppino C. Giovanella, PhD

CONTENTS

1. INTRODUCTION

The helical structure of DNA was proposed in 1953 by Watson and Crick (*1*). Twelve years later, Vinograd and collaborators (*2–4*) found that the helix axis can also be coiled in circular DNA. This structure was called supercoiling. This finding was extended to linear DNA by Pettijohn and others (*5–8*). It is now known that practically all DNA in vivo is supercoiled (*9*). Because most of the functions of DNA require untwisting, the importance of the enzymes required for this is self-evident. The first such enzyme identified was called the protein ω (*10*). It is now called topoisomerase I (top1) because in untwisting the supercoiled DNA, it breaks only one of the two strands, whereas topoisomerase II (top2), initially called gyrase, breaks both. Topoisomerase type I enzymes are ubiquitous, having been found in every prokaryotic or eukaryotic cells investigated so far with the exception of sea urchin sperm (*11*).

Eurkaryotic Topo I enzymes show extensive homology among themselves and form a group distinct from the bacterial topoisomerases I (*12*). Topoisomerase I inhibition became an important topic in cancer chemotherapy through the finding that Camptothecin (CAM), an alkaloid of plant origin, is the best known inhibitor of top1 and also a very potent anticancer agent. CAM is contained in a Chinese tree, *Camptotheca acuminata*. During a systemic search for natural anticancer products in plants, an alcoholic extract from such plant demonstrated high activity against L1210 mouse leukemia. Wall, who had supplied the alcoholic extract, proceeded to identify the active constituent of it (*13,14*) and called it Camptothecin. CAM rapidly reached

From: *Cancer Therapeutics: Experimental and Clinical Agents*
Edited by: B. Teicher Humana Press Inc., Totowa, NJ

clinical testing (*15–19*). Unfortunately, in order to render the compound hydrosoluble, the sodium salt of CAM was prepared and used exclusively for iv injection in the clinical trials. Such sodium salt, which is produced by opening the lactone E ring of the CAM molecule, is practically devoided of anticancer activity (*14,20*). Nor surprisingly, the clinical trials resulted in failure and were abandoned. Contemporary with the clinical trials, research demonstrated that CAM inhibited DNA and RNA synthesis, and caused DNA fragmentation in cultured mammalian cells (*21–28*). Sometime afterward, in the late 1980s, the mechanism of action of CAM started to be clarified. Topoisomerase I was identified as the primary target of CAM (*29,30*) and of its derivatives (*31,32*). Top1, in order to act, has first to form a complex with DNA and then rolls along the DNA molecule releasing the supercoiling. At any moment, there is on one side of the top1 a portion of DNA still supercoiled and on the other another portion uncoiled. CAM and derivatives stabilize and prolong this situation (*33*), rendering the cleavable complex (DNA + top1 + CAM) vulnerable to degradation by other nucleases that first produce reversible, and then irreversible, DNA damage (*34–37*). In effect, cells in the S phase are about 1000 times more sensitive to CAM than cells in other phases of the cell cycle (*38*). Working on the premise that CAM and its derivatives are cytotoxic, by stabilizing the DNA–top1 complex and finding higher content of top1 in colon carcinomas than in the normal colon mucosa in 1989, Giovanella et al. (*39*) successfully treated xenografts of human colon cancer in nude mice with two water-insoluble CAM derivatives (9-amino,20[RS]Camptothecin-9AC and 10-11-Methylene-dioxy,20[RS]Camptothecin). These results were rapidly confirmed and extended to other malignancies (*20,40*). It was established that only the S form of these compounds is active. At about the same time, two water-soluble, but close lactone ring CAM derivatives were also developed, CPT-11 (Irinotecan) (*41*) and Hycamptamin (Topotecan) (*42*). Both these drugs were introduced into clinical research (*43,44*), as were the nonidrosoluble CAM and 9AC. Let us examine in detail the characteristics of the four camptothecin drugs that have reached clinical trials.

1. 20(S)-Camptothecin (NSC 94600)—CAM

CAM, the mother compound of this family, is contained in different parts of several plants, *C. acuminata, Mappia Foetida,* and so forth, and it is extracted from them by organic solvents. Chemically, CAM is 4-Ethyl-4-Hydroxy-1H-pyrano-[3′, 4′:6,7]Indolizino[1,2-b]Quinoline-3,14 (4H,12H)-Dione:

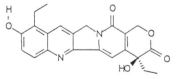

It has a mol wt of 348, and is water-insoluble, and poorly soluble in alcohols and chloroform. It is, however, readily dissolved in sodium hydroxyde with opening of the lactone ring and formation of the sodium salt.

CAM is highly fluorescent and can be detected by fluorescence in nanogram quantities. Several syntheses of CAM have been described (*45–53*), but none of them has been used so far for industrial production. Availability, however, is good because the plants from which it is extracted, first among them *C. acuminata,* grow abundantly and rapidly in tropical and semitropical climates. Extraction is relatively easy and simple, using several solvents. Interest in these compounds was raised first by the finding of antitumor activities in such extracts (54–56), and CAM was the first of them to be identified and isolated (13,14). After the failure of clinical trials owing to the mistaken belief that the sodium salt of CAM possesses the same anticancer activity as the mother compound—whereas it contains only about 10% of the same (14,20)—CAM remained unused for 20 years. After the finding in 1989 of the high antitumor activities of some of its nonwater-soluble derivatives, CAM itself was tested against xenografts of human tumors and found to be very active (20). Extensive toxicological and pharmacological studies in mice, dogs, and pigs determined that this compound is relatively well tolerated with a primary toxicity consisting of inflammatory ileitis totally reversible after treatment cessation (Giovanella et al., unpublished results). Secondary myelosuppression has also been observed under strenuous treatment in dogs. CAM was active when administered im, sc, and orally. It proved largely ineffective when administered iv by bolus injection (Giovanella et al., unpublished results). Because of its intense fluorescence, CAM can be easily detected in biological fluids in nanogram quantities. CAM is excreted mostly through the bile and feces, although a substantial amount is also eliminated in the urine. Plasma levels of CAM have different profiles according to the route of administration. Intramuscular injection supplies the most sustained levels, and oral administration give much shorter profiles. In mice, to maintain the same plasma levels, CAM was administered twice weekly im and daily orally (same dose). Phase I clinical trials of CAM were conducted at the Stehlin Foundation in Houston, Texas (57). Fifty-two patients were enrolled in the study. Thirteen of them had colon cancer, eight breast, seven melanoma, five lung, five prostate, three pancreas, two myeloma, two sarcoma, and one each of liver, kidney, larynx, rectum, cholahgiole cancer, Hodgkin's lymphoma, and non-Hodgkin's lymphoma. All of them had advanced disease refractory to available therapy. The schedule used was daily administration of oral CAM in gelatin capsule for 3 wk followed by 1 wk of rest, 3 wk of treatment, 1 wk of rest, and so on. Initial dose was 0.3 mg/m² escalated following a Fibonacci progression (58–60). Toxicity generally manifested itself around doses of 8–10 mg/m², and consisted mostly of diarrhea (40% of patients) and some episodes of cystitis (17% of patients). Significant drops of leukocyte counts were observed in only two cases, both of whom were heavily pretreated with other chemotherapies. All toxicities were totally reversible. The general policy has been of suspending treatment until normalization of patient condition and then restart of treatment at the lower dose level (toxicity observed at level 10, treatment restarted at level 9). With these precautions, the treatment has been well tolerated. The maximum tolerated dose (MTD) was established to be 8.7 mg/m²/d. Responses have been observed in six patients. One complete response in a non-Hodgkin lymphoma remained in complete remission for 4 mo after discontinuation of CAM treatment, which had been given for 1 yr. The patient died following exploratory celiotomy for diverticulosis. No tumor was present. Two melanoma patients had major regression of multiple skin tumor nodules. Two breast cancer patients had disappearance of liver masses by CAT scan, confirmed in one case by autopsy. One patient with prostate cancer experienced loss of bone pain with fall of rapidly rising PSA from 63 to 29. Three additional patients, one with lung cancer, one with melanoma, and one with breast cancer, exhibited stable disease for more than 6 mo while on the drug. In each case, the disease was in a rapidly escalating phase prior to the treatment. Pharmacokinetics in humans gave the best fit for second-order kinetics. The mean maximum concentration of CAM (total drug) in blood was calculated to be 39 ng/mL. Phase II trials are in progress at the Stehlin Foundation in Houston and at Dana Farber Center in Boston on breast cancer patients.

2. CPT 11 (IRINOTECAN)

CPT 11 is obtained by chemical modification of CAM introducing an ethyl group at the 7-position, then an hydroxyl group at the 10 position (*61,62*), and then binding a piperidinopiperidinocarbonyl group to the hydroxyl group (*62,63*). Chemically, CPT 11 is 7-ethyl-10-[4-(1-piperidino)-1-piperidino]carbonyloxycamptothecin and is water-soluble. Its mol wt is 586.

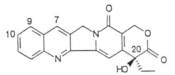

CPT 11 was found to have antitumor activity against murine transplantable tumors (*64,65*) when administered iv, ip, or orally. It also demonstrated activity against xenografts of human tumors (*66,67*). Several Phase I trials have been conducted with iv administration under various schedules in Japan, the US, and Europe (*68–72*). Mostly the drug was administered by 90-min iv infusion. When given once a week, repeated three times (*68*), the maximum tolerated dose (HTD) was 100 mg/m^2/infusion. Daily infusions for 5 d (*69*) had an MTD of 30 mg/m^2/infusion. Gastrointestinal toxicity and leukopenia were the dose-limiting factors. Phase II studies (*73–79*) were conducted on leukemias, lymphomas, cervical cancers, colon cancers, and lung cancer.

As in Phase I studies, gastrointestinal toxicities and myelosuppression were dose-limiting. Twenty to 30% partial responses were observed with some total responses, particularly in non-Hodgkin lymphomas. It is interesting to note that these total responses were observed with prolonged treatment, but not with single-dose schedules (*73*). CPT 11 has been combined with other anticancer agents, particularly cisplatinum (*80,81*) alone, and with granulocyte colony-stimulating factor (*82*). In advanced untreated nonsmall-cell lung cancers, 50% partial responses were observed with these regimens. With the use of the colony-stimulating factor, it was possible to increase the dose of CPT 11 by 33%, and diarrhea became the limiting factors. Cisplatinum was administered on day 1 at 80 mg/m^2. CPT 11 was given (90-min iv infusion) on days 1, 8, and 15 at the dose of 60 mg/m^2 without and 80 mg/m^2 with colony-stimulating factor.

3. TOPOTECAN-SKF104864 (NSC 609699)

Topotecan is prepared by chemical modification of 10 hydroxy CAM, which is a natural product present in small amounts in the tissues of *C. acuminata* and other plants. It is extracted together with CAM and can be separated later. Chemically, Topotecan is 9-dimethylaminomethyl-10-hydroxy-camptothecin and is water-soluble.

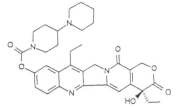

Its mol wt is 421. This compound was found to have anticancer activity in vivo and in vitro (*83–87*) against murine and human tumors.

Shortly afterward, Topotecan entered Phase I clinical trials in the US and in Europe with various schedules iv bolus or infusions of various durations (*88–96*). Dose-limiting toxicity was mostly neutropenia. However, thrombocytopenia was also observed in some continuous infusion regimens (*91–93*). The median MTDs varied depending on the schedule. For 21-d continuous infusion repeated every 4 wk, MTD was 0.53 mg/m²/d. For a 24-h infusion every 3 wk, it was 8.4 mg/m²/d.

Partial responses were observed in patients with nonsmall-cell lung cancer, cancer of the ovary, esophagus, and colon carcinoma (*90–92,97,98*). A complete remission was observed in a patient with nonsmall-cell lung cancer. Another complete remission together with several partial ones were observed in acute leukemias treated with 120-h continuous infusions every 3 wk (*95*). A Phase II trial of nonpretreated metastatic melanomas treated with two 30-min iv infusions at 5-d distance and at the dose of 1.5 mg/m² has given 1 response in 17 treated patients (*99*).

Another Phase II trial in pretreated small-cell lung cancer patients given Topotecan 1.5 mg/m² DX5Q3 for 2 weeks until progression or excessive toxicity results is in progress (*100*). Toxicity so far observed was mostly hematological.

4. 9-AMINO-CAMPTOTHECIN—(NSC 603071);
9-NITRO-CAMPTOTHECIN—(9NC)

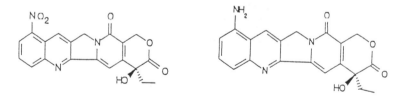

These two derivatives of CAM should be treated as one since the finding by Hinz et al. (*101*) that 9NC is converted in the body of humans and other mammals into 9AC, presumably by reductases that are apparently quite ubiquitous, the same phenomenon having been observed in many tissues (*101,102*). The observation in 1989 (*39*) that 9AC was a potent inhibitor of human colon cancer xenografts was one of the findings that triggered the revival of interest in CAMs as anticancer agents. This compound and 9NC had been synthesized (*103,104*) by nitration of CAM (which produces 9NC and the inactive 12-nitrocamptothecin), separation of 9NC, and reduction of the same to 9AC. Both 9NC and 9AC were found to be very active against L1210 leukemia with the same t/c, 348 (*104*). The amino compound was found to be the most active derivative of CAM in inducing Topo I-mediated cleavage of linear DNA (*32*)—however, 9NC was not tested on this occasion.

After the finding of potent antitumor activity against xenografts by 9AC, several other papers confirmed and extended it, utilizing both in vivo and in vitro systems, and both 9NC and 9AC (*105–111*). Both of these compounds proved to be very potent anticancer agents against a very large spectrum of human tumors. After toxicology studies in mice and dogs, 9AC entered Phase I clinical trials at Dana-Farber Cancer Center in Boston and at the Naval Hospital in Bethesda in 1994, and 9NC in 1995 at the Stehlin Foundation in Houston, TX.

5. PHARMACOLOGY AND PHARMACOKINETICS

Studies with iv injected H^3 generally labeled CAM demonstrated widespread distribution of the drug in the various tissues and organs of the mouse and excretion mostly through bile and feces (*112*). Analytical methods for the determination of CAM and derivatives in biological fluids by HPLC were developed and used to determine the pharmacokinetics of CAMs in the biological fluids of humans and animals (*113–116*). Such methods allow for the determination of the closed and opened lactone forms of CAM and its derivatives at very low concentrations. Using HPLC methods, numerous studies were conducted on the pharmacokinetics of CAMs (*90,92–94,117–126*).

Wide variations have been observed according to route of administration, derivative, and animal species. In humans, terminal half-life, for the closed lactone form, appears to be 30–36 h for oral CPT and iv 9AC, respectively, which are both non-hydrosoluble (our observations; *126*). Hydrosoluble derivatives (CPT 11 and Topotecan) are eliminated more rapidly in the 2–14 h range (*90,94,120,122,123*).

A most imporant finding was that serum albumin binds preferentially to the open lactone form of CAM and its derivatives. This binding alters the equilibrium between the closed and open lactone forms in the serum in favor of the last and because it catalyzes the opening of the lactone ring (*127–129*). Because albumin binds with various avidities to different CAM derivatives, their lactone ring are opened with an efficiency directly proportional to the affinity of albumin for a given derivative. If it is remembered that the opening of the lactone ring completely inactivates these compounds as anticancer agents, the importance of this finding cannot be overemphasized. The same authors found also that albumins of different species are more or less efficient in catalyzing the opening of the lactone ring with the mouse being the less efficient of the species studied and humans having the dubious distinction of being the most effective (*130,131*). Fortunately, it was also found that CAMs bind to lipids and lipoproteins. The lactone ring of CAMs in these complexes remains closed (*130,132–134*).

Data on metabolism of CAMs are scanty, and still not much is known about their excretion, which is accomplished through both urine and bile.

6. RESISTANCE

CAMs, both water-soluble and nonwater-soluble, show little or no crossresistance with other anticancer drugs and appear not to be substrates of the P-glycoprotein multidrug transporter (*135–138*). Only Topotecan seems to be affected by overexpression of the MDR1 resistance gene (*136,139*) and even there, resistance is very low. Cells can become resistant to CAMs, however, both in vitro and in vivo under treatment. Resistant lines contain mutated top1 genes or display a loss of top1 activity more or less pronounced (*140–156*). Interestingly, some of these resistant cells exhibit an increased sensitivity to top2 inhibitors (*157,158*).

7. COMBINATION THERAPY

Combination of Topotecan (*159*) and of CPT 11 (*160*) with cisplatinum has been tried in vitro based on the rationale of interfering with repair of cisplatinum-induced DNA damage (*161*). Clinical trials have been conducted (*80*) and are being run now. It is too soon to draw conclusions.

Attempts to associate CAMs and ionizing radiations have brought very exciting results in vitro and in xenografts (*162–167*). The rationale for such association is that top1 will attach to any fresh break in the DNA. CAMs will block the enzyme–DNA complex, and the irreversible degradation of DNA following will be multiplied by the number of DNA breaks in presence of CAMs. In animal models, doses of ionizing radiations and of 9AC, totally ineffective by themselves, produced total eradication of artificial brain metastases of human lung adenocarcinoma in nude mice (*162,164,176*).

8. CONCLUSIONS

The CAMs have already established themselves as very promising anticancer agents. Other top1 inhibitors have appeared and are under investigation, but it is too soon to evaluate them. Many others will certainly appear in the near future, considering the interest in this type of compound existing now in many laboratories. Although this field is relatively young, the amount of published literature is already considerable. It was obviously already impossible to cover all the papers in existence. For more detailed treatment, consult some recent reviews (*168–175*) where subjects covered in this chapter receive a more comprehensive treatment.

At the present moment, CAMs are undergoing intensive development, and various members of this family of compounds are in clinical trials more or less advanced, and others probably will reach this stage soon.

Summarizing what we know today, we can list the following relatively well-established findings:

1. CAMs can be divided in two categories, water-soluble (Irinotecan, Topotecan, and so on) and water-insoluble (CPT, 9NC, and so forth). The first category is easy to administer, especially iv but appears to have less anticancer activity than the insoluble compound in xenograft models of human tumors.
2. Prolonged administration appears to be more effective than high doses. Scheduling seems to be crucial for these drugs. In our experience, high doses for short periods are totally ineffective. In order to obtain eradication of human cancer xenotransplants in nude mice, sustained treatment for at least 3–4 wk is necessary, no matter what the route of administration.
3. Only the close lactone ring form of CAMs has anticancer activity. Fortunately, such substances are very powerful. In vitro, 10–20 ng/mL will selectively kill tumor cells in 72–96 h, leaving alive nontumor cells. (They stop proliferating, but resume division on removal of the drug.)
4. In the serum, at pH of 7.4 and in the presence of albumin, the lactone ring of CAMs is rapidly open (below pH 7.0, the ring does not open). Every effort is now made to overcome this difficulty, rendered more serious by the finding that human serum albumin is much more effective in catalyzing the opening of the lactone ring than any other albumin tested. Fortunately, it appears that whereas albumin catalyzes the opening of the lactone ring by binding preferentially to the carboxylate form of the CAMs, lipids

and lipoproteins tend to bind to the closed lactone form and to afford a degree of protection to it.

5. Any agent that will cause DNA breaks appears to be a candidate for combination therapy with the CAMs. The most obvious is ionizing radiation, which has already given exciting results in preliminary experiments.

6. Under optimal conditions, against human tumor xenografts, the CAMs have demonstrated an astounding spectrum of activity, proving very effective against all malignant tumors studied. In vitro they have demonstrated a not less astounding degree of selectivity against malignant cells (defined functionally as cells capable of producing a malignant tumor when inoculated into nude mice). CAMs are always cytocidal for tumorigenic cells and cytostatic for nontumorigenic cells at equal doses. Viability of the nontumorigenic cells is preserved at the end of the experiments.

REFERENCES

1. Watson JD, Crick L. A structure for deoxyribose nucleic acid. *Nature* 1953; 171:737,738.
2. Vinograd J, Lebowitz J, Radloff R, Watson R, Laipis P. The twisted circular form of polyoma viral DNA. *Proc Natl Acad Sci* 1965; 53:1104–1111.
3. Vinograd J, Lebowitz J. Physical and topological properties of circular DNA. *J Gen Physiol* 1966; 49:103–125.
4. Vinograd J, Lebowitz J, Watson R. Early and late helix-coil transitions in closed circular DNA: The number of superhelical turns in polyoma DNA. *J Mol Biol* 1968; 33:173–197.
5. Stonington OG, Pettijohn DE. The folded genome of *Escherichia coli* isolated in a protein–DNA–RNA complex. *Proc Natl Acad Sci* 1971; 68:6–9.
6. Worcel A, Burgi E. On the structure of the folded chromosome of *Escherichia coli*. *J Mol Biol* 1972; 72:127–147.
7. Pettijohn DE, Hecht R. RNA molecules bound to the folded bacterial genome stabilize DNA folds and segregate domains of supercoiling. *Cold Spring Harbor Symp Quant Biol* 1974; 38: 31–42.
8. Drlica K, Worcel A. Conformational transitions in the *Escherichia coli* chromosome: Analysis by viscometry and sedimentation. *J Mol Biol* 1975; 98:393–411.
9. Bauer W. Structure and reactions of closed duplex DNA. *Annu Rev Biophys Bioeng* 1978; 7:287–313.
10. Wang JC. Interaction between DNA and an *Escherichia coli* protein ω. *J Mol Biol* 1971; 55:523–533.
11. Poccia DL, Le Vine D, Wang JC. Activity of a DNA topoisomerase (nicking-closing enzyme) during sea urchin development and the cell cycle. *Dev Biol* 1978; 64: 273–283.
12. Hsieh TS. *DNA Topoisomerases in Nucleases,* 2nd ed. Cold Spring Harbor, NY: Cold Spring Harbor Laboratory Press. 1993:209–234.
13. Wall ME, Wani MC, Cook CE, Palmer KH, McPhail AT, Sim GA. Plant antitumor agents. I. The isolation and structure of camptothecin, a novel alkaloidal leukemia and tumor inhibitor from *Camptotheca acuminata*. *J Am Chem Soc* 1966; 88:3888–3890.
14. Wall ME. Alkaloids with antitumor activity. In: Mothes K, Schreiber K, Schutte HR, eds., *International Symposium on Biochemistry and Physiology of the Alkaloids*. Berlin: Academic-Verlag. 1969:77–87.
15. Gottlieb JA, Guarino AM, Call JB, Oliverio VT, Block JB. Preliminary pharmacologic and clinical evaluation of camptothecin sodium (NSC-100880). *Cancer Chemother Rep* 1970; 54: 461–470.
16. Gottlieb JA, Luce JK. Treatment of malignant melanoma with camptothecin (NSC-100880). *Cancer Chemother Rep* 1972; 56:103–105.
17. Moertel CG, Reitemeier RJ, Schutt AJ. A phase II study of camptothecin (NSC-100880) in gastrointestinal cancer. *Proc Am Assoc Cancer Res* 1971; 12:18.
18. Moertel CG, Schutt AJ, Reitemeier RJ, Hahn RG. Phase II study of camptothecin (NSC-100880) in the treatment of advanced gastrointestinal cancer. *Cancer Chemother Rep* 1972; 56: 95.

19. Muggia FM, Creavan PJ, Hansen HH, Cohen MH, Selawry OS. Phase I clinical trial of weekly and daily treatment with camptothecin (NSC-100880): Correlation with preclinical studies. *Cancer Chemother Rep* 1972; 56:515–521.

20. Giovanella BC, Hinz HR, Kozielski AJ, Stehlin JS Jr, Silber R, Potmesil M. Complete growth inhibition of human cancer xenografts in nude mice by treatment with 20-(S)-camptothecin. *Cancer Res* 1991; 51:3052–3055.

21. Bosmann HB. Camptothecin inhibits macromolecular synthesis in mammalian cells but not in isolated mitochondria of *E. coli*. *Biochem Biophys Res Commun* 1970; 41:1412–1420.

22. Horwitz SB, Chang C-K, Grollman AP. Studies on comptothecin. 1. Effects on nucleic acid and protein synthesis. *Mol Pharmacol* 1971; 7:632–644.

23. Horwitz MS, Horwitz SB. Intracellular degradation of HeLa and adenovirus type DNA induced by camptothecin. *Biochem Biophys Res Commun* 1971; 45:723–727.

24. Horwitz SB, Horwitz MS. Effects of camptothecin on the breakage and repair of DNA during the cell cycle. *Cancer Res* 1973; 33:2834–2836.

25. Kessel D. Effects of camptothecin on RNA synthesis in leukemia L1210 cells. *Biochem Biophys Acta* 1971; 246:225–232.

26. Kessel D, Bosmann HB, Lohr K. Camptothecin effects on DNA synthesis on murine leukemia cells. *Biochim Biophys Acta* 1972; 269:210–216.

27. Wu RS, Kumar A, Warner JR. Ribosomal formation is blocked by camptothecin, a reversible inhibitor of RNA synthesis. *Proc Natl Acad Sci USA* 1971; 68:3009–3014.

28. Abelson HT, Penman S. Selective interruption of high molecular weight RNA synthesis in HeLa cells by camptothecin. *Nature (Lond) New Biol* 1972; 237:144–146.

29. Hsiang Y-H, Hertzberg R, Hecht S, Liu LF. Camptothecin induces protein-linked DNA breaks via mammalian DNA topoisomerases I. *J Biol Chem* 1985; 260:14,873–14,878.

30. Hsiang Y-H, Liu LF. Identification of mammalian topoisomerase I as an intracellular target of the antioancer drug camptothecin. *Cancer Res* 1988, 8.1722–1728.

31. Jaxcl C, Kohn KW, Wani MC, Wall ME, Pommeir Y. Structure-activity study of the actions of camptothecin derivatives on mammalian topoisomerase I. Evidence for a specific receptor site and for a relation to antitumor activity. *Cancer Res* 1989; 49:1465–1469.

32. Hsiang Y-H, Liu LF, Wall ME, Wani MC, Kirshenbaum S, Silber R, Potmesil M. DNA topoisomerase I-mediated DNA cleavage and cytotoxicity of camptothecin analogs. *Cancer Res* 1989; 49:4385–4389.

33. Liu LF, DNA topoisomerase poisons as antitumor drugs. *Annu Rev Biochem* 1989; 58:351–375.

34. Avemann K, Knippers R, Koller T, Sogo JM. Camptothecin, a specific inhibitor of type I DNA topoisomerase, induces DNA breakage at replication forks. *Mol Cell Biol* 1988; 8:3026–3034.

35. Holm C, Covey JM, Kerrigan D, Pommier Y. Differential requirement of DNA replication for the cytotoxicity of DNA topoisomerase I and II inhibitors in Chinese hamster DC3F cells. *Cancer Res* 1989; 49:6365–6368.

36. Hsiang Y-H, Lihou MG, Liu LF. Mechanism of cell killing by camptothecin: arrest of replication forks by drug-stabilized topoisomerase 1-DNA cleavable complexes. *Cancer Res* 1989; 49:5077–5082.

37. Ryan AJ, Squires S, Strutt HL, Johnson RT. Camptothecin cytotoxicity in mammalian cells is associated with the induction of persistent double strand breaks in replicating DNA. *Nucleic Acids Res* 1991; 19:3295–3300.

38. Li LH, Fraser TJ, Olin EJ, Bhuyan BK. Action of camptothecin on mammalian cells in culture. *Cancer Res* 1972; 32:2643–2650.

39. Giovanella BC, Stehlin JS, Wall ME, Wani M, Nicholas AW, Liu LF, Silber R, Potmesil M. DNA topoisomerase I-targeted chemotherapy of human colon cancer in xenografts. *Science* 1989; 246:1046–1048.

40. Giovanella BC, Wall ME, Wani MC, Silber R, Stehlin JS, Hochster H, Potmesil M. Efficacy of camptothecin [NSC 94600, CA], 9-amino-camptothecin [NSC 603071, 9-AC] and 10,11-methylenedioxycamptothecin [NSC 606174, 10-11-MDC] in the human cancer xenograft model. *Proc Am Assoc Cancer Res* 1992; 3:432.

41. Kunimoto T, Nitta K, Tanaka T, Uehara N, Baba H, Takeuchi M, Yokokura T, Sawada S, Miyasaka T, Mutai M. Antitumor activity of 7-ethyl-10-[4-(1-piperidino) carbonyloxy-camptothecin, a novel water-soluble derivative of camptothecin against murine tumors. *Cancer Res* 1987; 47:5944–5947.

42. Kingsbury WD, Boehm JC, Jakes DR, Holden KG, Hecht SM, Gallagher G, Caranfa MJ, McCabe FL, Faucette LF, Johnson RK, Hertzberg RP. Synthesis of water-soluble (aminoalkyl) camptothecin analogues; Inhibition of topoisomerase I and antitumor activity. *J Med Chem* 1991; 34:98–107.

43. Negoro S, Fukuoka M, Masuda N, Takada M, Kusunoki Y, Matsui K, Takifuji N, Kudoh S, Niitani H, Taguchi T. Phase I study of weekly intravenous infusion of CPT-11, a new derivative of camptothecin, in the treatment of advanced non-small-cell lung cancer. *J Natl Cancer Inst* 1991; 83:1164–1168.

44. Rowinsky E, Grochow L, Hendricks C, Sartorius S, Ettinger D, McGuire W, Forastiere A, Hurowitz L, Easter V, Donehower R. Phase I and pharmacologic study of topotecan (SK&F 104864): A novel topoisomerase I inhibitor. *Proc Am Soc Clin Oncol* 1991; 10:93.

45. Stork G, Schultz AG. The total synthesis of dl-Camptothecin. *J Am Chem Soc* 1971; 93: 4074–4075.

46. Volkmann R, Danishesky S, Eggler J, Solomon DM. A total synthesis of dl Camptothecin. *J Am Chem Soc* 1971; 93:5576,5577.

47. Winterfeldt E, Korth T, Pike D, Boch M. Biogenetically oriented total synthesis of camptothecin and 7 chlorocamptothecin. *Angew Chem Int Ed Englies* 1972; 11:289,290.

48. Corey EJ, Crouse DN, Anderson JE. A total synthesis of natural 20(S)-camptothecin. *J Org Chem* 1972; 40:2140,2141.

49. Cyril SF, Tang GJ, Morrow J, Rapoport H. A total synthesis of dl-Camptothecin. *J Am Chem* 1975; 97:159–167.

50. Wani MC, Ronman PE, Lindley JT, Wall ME. Plant antitumor agents: 18 Synthesis and biological activity of camptothecin analogues. *J Med Chem* 1980; 23:534–560.

51. Shanghai No 5 and No 1 Pharmaceutical Plant. Shanghai Institute of Pharmaceutical Industrial Research, Shanghai Institute of Materia Medica. The total synthesis dl Camptothecin. *Scientia Sinica (Engl. Ed.)* 1978; 21:27–98.

52. Wani MC, Nicholas W, Wall ME. Plant antitumor agents 28 Resolution of a key tricyclic synthon, 5′(RS)-1,5Dioxo-5′-ethyl-5′-hydroxy-2′H,5′H,6″h-6′-oxopyrana[3′,4-F]6,8-tetrahydro-indolizine: total synthesis and antitumor activity of 20(S)- and 20(R)-camptothecin. *J Med Chem* 1987; 30:2317–2319.

53. Akio E, Hirofumi T, Masamicni S, Hiroaki T. Antitumor agents: Part 2. Asymmetric synthesis of (S) camptothecin. *J Chem Soc Perkin Trans* 1990; 1:27–32.

54. Abbott BJ, Leiter J, Hartwell JL, Perdue RE Jr, Schepartz SA. Screening data from the cancer chemotherapy national service screening laboratory. XXX Plant Extracts. *Cancer Res* 1966; 26 part 2:34–45, 429–470.

55. Perdue RE, Jr, Wall ME, Hartwell JL, Abbott BJ. Comparison of the activity of crude *Camptotheca acuminata* ethanolic extracts against lymphoid leukemia L-1210. *Lloydia* 1968; 31: 229–236.

56. Wall ME, Wani MC. Camptothecin and taxol: discovery to clinic. *Cancer Res* 1995; 55: 753–760.

57. Stehlin JS, Natelson EA, Hinz HR, Giovanella BC, de Ipolyi P, Fehir KM, Trezona TP, Vardeman DM, Harris NJ, Marcee AK, Kozielski AJ, Ruiz-Razura A. Phase I clinical trial and pharmacokinetic results with oral administration of 20(S)-Camptothecin. In: Potmesil M, Pinedo H, eds. *Camptothecins: New Anticancer Agents.* Boca Raton, FL: CRC. 1995:59–65.

58. Goldsmith MA, Slavik M, Carter SK. Quantitative prediction of drug toxicity in humans from toxicology in small and large animals. *Cancer Res* 1975; 35:1354–1364.

59. Lowe Michael C. Large animal toxicological studies of anticancer drugs. In: Hellman K, Carter SK, eds. *Fundamentals of Cancer Chemotherapy.* New York: McGraw-Hill. 1987: 236–247.

60. Carter SK. The Phase I study. In: Hellman K, Carter SK, eds. *Fundamentals of Cancer Chemotherapy.* New York: McGraw-Hill. 1987:285–300.

61. Matsuzono H. Japan Patent; Kokai, 56-158786; 1981.

62. Miyasaka T, Sawada S, Nokata K, Sugino E, Mutai M. US Patent 4604463; 1986.

63. Miyasaka T, Sawada S, Nokata K, Sugino E, Mutai M. Japan Patent, Kowai, 60-17970; 1985.

64. Nitta K, Yokokura T, Sawada S, Takeuchi M, Tanaka T, Uehara N, Baba H, Kunimoto T, Miyasaka T, Mutai M. Antitumor activity of a new derivative of camptothecin. In *Recent Ad-*

vances in Chemotherapy (Proc. 14th Int. Cong. Chemotherapy). Tokyo: University of Tokyo Press. 1985:28–30.

65. Kunimoto T, Nitta K, Tanaka T, Uehara N, Baba H, Takeuchi M, Yokokura T, Sawada S, Miyasaka, T, Muta M. Antitumor activity of 7-ethyl-10[4-(1-Piperidino)-1-Piperidino]carbonyloxy-camptothecin, a novel water-soluble derivative of camptothecin, against murine tumors. *Cancer Res* 1987; 47:5944–5947.

66. Kawato Y, Furuta T, Aonuma M, Yasuoka M, Yokokura T, Matsumoto K. Antitumor activity of a camptothecin derivative, CPT 11 against human tumor xenografts in nude mice. *Cancer Chemother Pharmacol* 1991; 28:192–198.

67. Houghton PJ, Cheshire PJ, Hallman JC, Bissery MC, Mathiew-Boue' A, Houghton JA. Therapeutic efficacy of the topoisomerase I inhibitor 7-ethyl-10-[4[1-Piperidino]-1-Piperidino-carbonyloxy-camptothecin against human tumor xenografts:lack of cross-resistance in vivo in tumors with acquired resistance to the topoisomerase I inhibitor. 9-dimethylaminomethyl-10-hydroxy-camptothecin. *Cancer Res* 1993; 53:2823–2389.

68. Negoro S, Fukuoka M, Masuda N, Takada M, Kasunoki Y, Matsui K, Takifuji N, Kudoh S, Niitani H, Taguchi T. Phase I study of weekly intravenous infusions of CPT 11, a new derivative of camptothecin in the treatment of advanced non-small cell lung cancer. *J Natl Cancer Inst* 1991; 83:1164–1168.

69. Ohe Y, Sasaki Y, Shinkai T, Eguchi K, Tamura T, Kojima A, Kunikane H, Okamoto H, Karato A, Ohmatsu H, Kanzawa F, Saijo N. Phase I study and pharmacokinetics of CPT 11 with 5-day continuous infusion. *J Natl Cancer Inst* 1992; 84:972–974.

70. Clavel M, Mathiew-Boue A, Dumortier A, Chabot GG, Bissery MC, Marty M. Phase I study of CPT-11 administered as a daily infusion for 3 consecutive days. *Proc Am Assoc Cancer Res* 1992; 33:262.

71. Culine S, De Forni M, Extra JM, Chabot GG, Madelaine I, Herait P, Bugat R, Marty M, Mathieu-Boue A. Phase I study of the camptothecin analogue CPT 11 using a weekly schedule. *Proc Am Soc Clin Oncol* 1992; 11:110.

72. Rowinsky E, Grochow L, Ettinger D, Hendricks L, Lubejko B, Sartorius S, Hurowitz L, McGuire W, Rock M, Donehower R. Phase I and pharmacologic study of CPT 11, a semisynthetic topoisomerase I-targeting agent, on a single dose schedule. *Proc Am Soc Clin Oncol* 1992; 11:115.

73. Ohno R, Okada K, Masaoka T, Kuramoto A, Arima T, Yoshida Y, Ariyoshi H, Ichimaru M, Sakai Y, Oguro M, Ito Y, Morishima Y, Yokomaku S, Ota K. An early phase II study of CPT 11: A new derivative of camptothecin for the treatment of leukemia and lymphoma. *J Clin Oncol* 1990; 8:1907–1912.

74. Tsuda H, Takatsuki K, Ohno R, Masaoki T, Okada K, Shirakawa S, Ohashi Y, Oma K, Taguchi T. A late phase II trial of a potent topoisomerase I inhibitor, CPT 11, in malignant lymphoma. *Proc Am Soc Clin Oncol* 1992; 11:1316.

75. Takeuchi S, Dobashi K, Fujimoto S, Tanaka K, Suzuki M, Terashima Y, Hasumi K, Akiya K, Negishi Y, Tamaya T, Tanizawa O, Sugawa T, Umesaka N, Sekiba, K, Aono T, Nakano H, Noda K, Shiota M, Yakushiji M, Sugiyama T, Hashimoto M, Yajima A, Takamizawa H, Sonoda T, Takeda Y, Tomoda Y, Ohta M, Ozaki M, Hirabayashi K, Hiura M, Hate M, Nishigaki K, Taguchi T. A late phase II study of CPT-11 in uterine cervical cancer and ovarian cancer. *Jpn J. Cancer Chemother* 1991; 18:1681–1689.

76. Takeuchi S, Noda K, Yakushiji M. CPT-11 study group on gynecologic malignancy. Late phase II study of CPT-11, topoisomerase I inhibitor, in advanced cervical carcinoma (CC). *Proc Am Soc Clin Oncol* 1992; 22:224 (abstr).

77. Masuda N, Fukuoka M, Kusunoki Y. CPT-11: A new derivative of camptothecin for the treatment of refractory or relapsed small-cell lung cancer. *J Clin Oncol* 1992; 10:1225–1229.

78. Fukuoka M, Niitani H, Suzuki A, Motomiya M, Hasegawa K, Nishiwaki Y, Kuriyama T, Ariyoshi Y, Negoro S, Masuda N, Nakajima S, and Taguchi T. A phase II study of CPT-11, a new derivative of camptothecin, for previously untreated non-small-cell lung cancer. *J Clin Oncol* 1992; 10:16–20.

79. Shimada Y, Yoshino M, Wakui A, Nakao I, Futatasuki K, Sakata Y, Kambe M, Taguchi T, Ogawa N. CPT-11 Gastrointestinal Cancer Study Group. Phase II study of CPT-11, new camptothecin derivative, in metastatic colorectal cancer. *J Clin Oncol* 1993; 11:909–913.

80. Masuda N, Fukuoka M, Takada M, Kusunoki Y, Negoro S, Matsui K, Kudoh S, Takifuji N, Nakagawa K, Kishimoto S. CPT-11 in combination with cisplatin for advanced non-small-cell lung cancer. *J Clin Oncol* 1992; 10:1775–1780.

81. Kudoh S, Kusunoki Y, Matsui K, Nakagawa K, Hirashima T, Tamaoki M, Nitta T, Yana T, Negoro S, Takifuji N, Takada M. Phase I study of irinotecan and cisplatin with granulocyte colony-stimulating factor support for advanced non-small-cell lung cancer. *J Clin Oncol* 1994; 12:90–96.

82. Johnson RK, McCabe FL, Faucette LF, Hertzberg RP, Kingsbury WD, Boehm JC, Caranfa MJ, Holden KG. SKF 104864, a water-soluble analog of camptothecin with broad spectrum activity in preclinical tumor models. *Proc Am Assoc Cancer Res* 1989; 30:623.

83. Tong W, Saltz L, Sirott K, Tookasi F, Cuisoh B. Rapid HPLC assay for topotecan. *Proc Am Assoc Cancer Res* 1991; 32:433.

84. Kingsbury WD, Boehm JC, Jakas DR, Holden KG, Hecht SM, Gallagher GG, Caranfa MJ, McCabe FL, Faucett LF, Johnson RK, Hertzberg RP. Synthesis of water soluble (aminoalkyl) camptothecin analogues: inhibition of topoisomerase I and antitumor activity. *J Med Chem* 1991; 34:98–107.

85. Johnson RK, Herzberg RP, Kingsbury WD, Boehm JC, Caranfa MJ, Faucett LF, McCabe FL, Holden KG. Preclinical profile of SKF104864, a water-soluble analog of camptothecin. Proc. NCI-EORTC 6th Symp. *New Drugs Cancer Ther* 1991:301.

86. Burris HA, Hanauske AR, Johnson RK. Activity of Topotecan, a new topoisomerase I inhibitor, against human tumor colony-forming units *in vitro*. *J Natl Cancer Inst* 1992; 84:1816–1820.

87. Houghton PJ, Cheshire PJ, Myers L, Stewart CF, Synold TW, Houghton JA. Evaluation of 9-dimethylaminomethyl-10-hydroxycamptothecin against xenografts derived from adult and childhood solid tumors. *Cancer Chemother & Pharmacol* 1992; 31:229–239.

88. Recondo G, Abbruzzese J, Newman B, Newman R, Kuhn J, Von Hoff D, Gartiez D, Raber M. A phase I trial of topotecan (TOPO) administered by a 24-hour infusion. *Proc Am Assoc Cancer Res* 1991; 32:206.

89. Wall JG, Burris HA, III, Von Hoff DD, Rodriguez G, Kneuper-Hall R, Shaffer D, O'Rourke T, Brown T, Weiss G, Clark G, McVea S, Brown J, Johnson R, Friedman C, Smith B, Mann WS, Kuhn J. A phase I clinical and pharmacokinetic study of the topoisomerase I inhibitor topotecan (SK&F 104864) given as an intravenous bolus every 21 days. *Anticancer Drugs* 1992; 3:337–345.

90. Rowinsky EK, Grochow LB, Hendricks CB, Ettinger DS, Forastiere AA, Hurowitz LA, McGuire WP, Sartorius SE, Lubejko BG, Kaufmann SH, Donehower RC. Phase I and pharmacologic study of topotecan: A novel topoisomerase I inhibitor. *J Clin Oncol* 1992; 10: 647–656.

91. ten Bokkel Huinink WW, Rodenhuis S, Beijnen J, Dubbelman R, Koier I. Phase I study of the topoisomerase I inhibitor topotecan (SK&F 104864-A). *Proc Am Soc Clin Oncol* 1992; 11:110.

92. Haas NB, LaCreta FP, Walczak J, Hudes GR, Brennan J, Ozols RF, O'Dwyer PJ. Phase I/pharmacokinetic trial of topotecan on a weekly 24-hour infusional schedule. *Proc Am Assoc Cancer Res* 1992; 33:523.

93. Eckardt J, Burris H, Kuhn J, Smith S, Rodriguez G, Weiss G, Smith L, Shaffer D, Johnson R, Von Hoff D. Phase I and pharmacokinetic trial of continuous infusion topotecan in patients with refractory solid tumors. *Proc Am Soc Clin Oncol* 1992; 1:138.

94. Blaney SM, Balis FM, Cole DE, Craig C, Reid JM, Ames MM, Krailo M, Reaman G, Hammond D, Poplack DG. Pediatric phase I trial and pharmacokinetic study of topotecan administered as a 24-hour continuous infusion. *Cancer Res* 1993; 53:1032–1036.

95. Kantarjian HM, Beran M, Ellis A, Zwelling L, O'Brien S, Cazenave L, Koller C, Rios MB, Plunkett W, Keating MJ, Estey EH. Phase I study of topotecan, a new topoisomerase I inhibitor, in patients with refractory or relapsed acute leukemia. *Blood* 1993; 81:146–151.

96. Hochster H, Speyer J, Oratz R, Meyers M, Wernz J, Chachoua A, Raphael B, Lee R, Sorich J, Taubes B, Liebs L, Fry D, Blum R. Topotecan 21 day continuous infusion-Excellent tolerance of a novel schedule. *Proc Am Soc Clin Oncol* 1993; 12:139.

97. Sirott MN, Saltz L, Young C, Tong W, Trochanowski B, Niedzwiecki D, Toomasi F, Kelsen D. Phase I and clinical pharmacologic study of intravenous topotecan. *Proc Am Soc Clin Oncol* 1991; 10:104.

98. Verweij J, Lund B, Beynen J, de Boer M, Koier I, Hansen HH. Clinical studies with topotecan: The EORTC experience, Proc. NCI-EORTC Symp. *New Drugs Cancer Ther* 1992; 7:118 (abstr).

99. Kraut EH, Staubus A, Majernick D, King G, Balcerzak SP. Phase II trial of topotecan in metastatic malignant melanoma. *Proc Am Assoc Cancer Res* 1995; 36:238.

100. Wanders J, Ardizzoni A, Hansen HH, Domernowsky P, Postmus PE, Buitenhuis M, McDonald M, Giacone G, Verweij J. Phase II study of topotecan in refractory and sensitivity small cell lung cancer (SCLC). *Proc Am Assoc Cancer Res* 1995; 36:237.

101. Hinz HR, Harris NJ, Natelson EA, Giovanella BC. Pharmacokinetics of the *in vivo* and *in vitro* conversion of 9-nitro-20(S)-camptothecin to 9-amino-20(S)-camptothecin in humans, dogs and mice. *Cancer Res* 1994; 52:3096–3100.

102. Pantazis P, Harris N, Mendoza J, Giovanella B. Conversion of 9-nitro-camptothecin to 9-aminocamptothecin by human blood cells *in vitro*. *Eur J. Haematol* 1994; 53:246–248.

103. Yakult Honsha CO., Ltd., Japan Patent 59-51288, 1984. Chem. Abstr. 1984, 101, 91319d, 91320x, 91322 2 (9NC and NH).

104. Wani MC, Nicholas AW, Wall ME. Plant antitumor agents, 23 synthesis and antileukemic activity of camptothecin analogues. *J Med Chem* 1986; 29:2358–2363.

105. Potmesil M, Giovanella BC, Wall ME, Liu LF, Silber R, Stehlin JS, Wani MC, Hochster H. Preclinical and clinical development of DNA topoisomerase I inhibitors in the United States. In: Andoh T, Ikeda H, Oguro M, eds. *Molecular Biology of DNA Topoisomerases and Its Application to Chemotherapy.* Nagoya, Japan: CRC. 1993:301–311.

106. Potmesil M, Hinz HR, Marcee A, Vardeman D, Stehlin JS, Wall ME, Wani MC, Silber R, Giovanella BC. Growth inhibition of human cancer metastases in the xenograft model by camptothecin [NSC 94600, CAM], 9-amino-[NSC 603071, 9-AC], and 9-nitrocamptothecin. *Proc Am Asoc Cancer Res* 1992; 33:432.

107. Giovanella BC, Wall ME, Wani MC, Silber R, Stehlin JS, Hochster H, Potmesil M. Efficacy of camptothecin (NSC 94600, CAM], 9-aminocamptothecin [NSC 603071, 9-AC], and 10,11-methylenedioxycamptothecin [NSC 606174, 10-11-MDC] in human cancer xenograft model. *Proc Am Assoc Cancer Res* 1992; 33:432.

108. Pantazis P, Early JA, Kozielski AJ, Mendoza JT, Hinz HR, Giovanella BC. Regression of human breast carcinoma tumors in immunodeficient mice treated with 9-nitrocamptothecin: Differential response of nontumorigenic and tumorigenic human breast cells *in vitro*. *Cancer Res* 1993; 53:1577–1582.

109. Pantazis P, Kozielski AJ, Mendoza JT, Early JA, Hinz HR, Giovanella BC. Camptothecin derivatives induce regression of human ovarian carcinomas grown in nude mice and distinguish between non-tumorigenic and tumorigenic cells *in vitro*. *Int J Cancer* 1993; 53:863–871.

110. Pantazis P, Mendoza JT, Kozielski AJ, Natelson EA, Giovanella BC. 9-nitro-camptothecin delays growth of U-937 leukemia tumors in nude mice and is cytotoxic or cytostatic for human myelomonocytic leukemia lines *in vitro*. *Eur J Haematol* 1993; 50:81–89.

111. Pantazis P, Early JA, Mendoza JT, DeJesus AR, Giovanella BC. Cytotoxic efficacy of 9-nitrocamptothecin in the treatment of human malignant melanoma cells *in vitro*. *Cancer Res* 1994; 54:771–776.

112. Smith PL, Liehr JG, Ahmed AE, Hinz HR, Mendoza J, Kozielski A, Stehlin JS, Giovanella BC. Pharmacokinetics of tritium labeled camptothecin in nude mice. *Proc Am Assoc Cancer Res* 1992; 33:432.

113. Loh JR, Ahmed AE. Determination of camptothecin in biological fluids using reversed-phase high-performance liquid chromatography with fluorescence detection. *J Chromatogr* 1990; 53: 367–376.

114. Beijnen JH, Smith BR, Keijer WJ, Van Gijn R, ten Bokkel Huinink WW, Vlasveld LT, Rodenuhuis S, Underberg WJM. High-performance liquid chromatographic analysis of the new antitumor drug SK&F 104864-A (NSC 609699) in plasma. *J Pharmacol Biomed Anal* 1990; 8:789–794.

115. Supko JG, Malspeis L. A reversed-phase HPLC method for determining camptothecin in plasma with specificity for the intact lactone form of the drug. *J Liquid Chromatogr* 1991; 14: 1779–1803.

116. Supko JG, Malspeis L. Liquid chromatographic analyses of 9-aminocamptothecin in plasma monitored by fluorescence induced upon postcolumn acidification. *J Liquid Chromatogr* 1992; 15:3261–3283.

117. Supko JG, Plowman J, Dykes DJ, Zaharko DS. Relationship between the schedule dependence of 9-amino-20(S)-camptothecin (AC; NSC 603071) antitumor activity in mice and its plasma pharmacokinetics. *Proc Am Assoc Cancer Res* 1992; 33:432.

118. Supko JG, Malspeis L. Pharmacokinetics of the 9-amino and 10,11-methylenedioxy derivatives of camptothecin in mice. *Cancer Res* 1993; 53:3062–3069.

119. Beijnen JH, Rosing H, ten Bokkel Huinink WW, Pinedo HM. High-performance liquid chromatographic analysis of the antitumor drug camptothecin and its lactone ring-opened form in rat plasma. *Cancer Res* 1993; 53:3062–3069.

120. Rowinsky EK, Grochow LB, Ettinger DS, Sartorius SE, Lubjeko BG, Chen T, Rock MK, Donehower RC. Phase I and pharmacological study of the novel topoisomerase I inhibitor 7-ethyl-10[4-(1-piperidino)-1-piperidino]carbonyloxycamptothecin (CPT-11) administered as a ninety-minute infusion every 3 weeks. *Cancer Res* 1994; 54:427–436.

121. Kaneda N, Yokokura T. Nonlinear pharmacokinetics of CPT 11 in rats. *Cancer Res* 1990; 50: 4187–4191.

122. Rothenberg ML, Kuhn JG, Burris HA, Nelson J, Eckhardt JR, Tristan-Morales M, Hilsenbeck SG, Weiss GR, Smith LS, Rodriguez GI, Rock MK, Von Hoff DD. Phase I and pharmacokinetic trial of weekly CPT-11. *J Clin Oncol* 1993; 11:2194–2204.

123. Saltz L, Sirott M, Young C, Tong W, Niedzwiecki D, Tzy-Jyun Y, Tao Y, Trochanowski B, Wright P, Barbosa K, Toomasi F, Kelsen D. Phase I clinical and pharmacology study of topotecan given daily for 5 consecutive days to patients with advanced solid tumors, with attempt at dose intensification using recombinant granulocyte colony-stimulating factor. *J Natl Cancer Inst* 1993; 85:1499–1507.

124. Scott DO, Bindra DS, Stella VJ. Plasma pharmacokinetics of the lactone and carboxylate forms of 20(S)-camptothecin in anesthetized rats. *Pharmacol Res* 1993; 10:1451–1457.

125. de Forni M, Bugat R, Chabot GG, Culine S, Extra J, Couyette A, Madelaine I, Marty ME, Mathiew-Boue A. Phase I and pharmacokinetic study of the camptothecin derivative irinotecan, administered on a weekly schedule in cancer patients. *Cancer Res* 1994; 54:4347–4354.

126. Rubin E, Wood V, Bharti A, Trites D, Lynch C, Hurwitz S, Bartel S, Levy S, Rosowsky A, Toppmeyer D, Kufe D. A phase I and pharmacokinetic study of a new camptothecin derivative, 9-aminocamptothecin. *Clin Cancer Res* 1995; 269:269–276.

127. Burke TG, Mi Z. Preferential binding of the carboxylate form of camptothecin by human serum albumin. *Anal Biochem* 1993; 212:285–287.

128. Burke TG, Mi Z. The structural basis of camptothecin interactions with human serum albumin: Impact on drug stability. *J Med Chem* 1994; 37:40–46.

129. Burke TG, Munshi CB, Mi Z, Jiang Y. The important role of albumin in determining the relative human blood stabilities of the camptothecin anticancer drugs. *J Pharm Sci.* 1995; 84:518,519.

130. Mi Z, Burke TG. Marked interspecies variations concerning interactions of camptothecin with serum albumin. *Biochemistry* 1994; 33:12,540–12,545.

131. Mi Z, Burke TG. Marked interspecies variations concerning interactions of camptothecin analogues with serum albumins. *Proc Am Assoc Cancer Res* 1995; 36:444(2647).

132. Burke TG, Staubus AE, Mishra AK, Malak H. Liposomal stabilization of camptothecin lactone ring. *J Am Chem Soc* 199; 114:8318,8319.

133. Burke TG, Mishra AK, Wan M, Wall ME. Lipid bilayer partitioning and stability of camptothecin drugs. *Biochemistry* 1992; 32:5352–5354.

134. Mi Z, Burke TG. Differential interactions of camptothecin lactone and carboxylate forms with human blood components. *Biochemistry* 1994; 33:10,325–10,336.

135. Tsuruo T, Matsuzaki T, Matsushita M, Saito H, Yokokura T. Antitumor effect of CPT-11, a new derivative of camptothecin, against pleiotropic drug-resistant tumors *in vitro* and *in vivo*. *Cancer Chemother Pharmacol* 1988; 21:71–74.

136. Chen AY, Yu C, Potmesil M, Wall ME, Wani MC, Liu LF. Camptothecin overcomes MDR1-mediated resistance in human KB carcinoma cells. *Cancer Res* 1991; 51:6039–6044.

137. Potmesil M, Giovanella BC, Liu LF, Wall ME, Silber R, Stehlin JS Jr, Hsiang Y-H, Wani MC. Preclinical studies of DNA topoisomerase I-targeted 9-amino and 10,11-methylenedioxy camp-

tothecins. In: Potmesil M, Kohn KW, eds. *DNA Topoisomerases in Cancer*. New York: Oxford University Press. 1991:299.

138. Potmesil M, Giovanella BC, Wall ME, Liu LF, Silber R, Stehlin JS, Wani MC, Hochseer H. Preclinical and clinical development of DNA topoisomerase I inhibitors in the United States. In: Andoh T, Ikeda H, Oguro M, eds. *Molecular Biology of DNA Topoisomerases and Its Application to Chemotherapy*. Nagoya, Japan: CRC. 1993:301–311.

139. Hendricks CB, Rowinsky ER, Grochow LB, Donehower RC, Kaufmann SH. Effect of P-glycoprotein expression on the accumulation and cytotoxicity of topotecan (SK&F 104864), a new camptothecin analogue. *Cancer Res* 1992; 52:2268–2278.

140. Kessel D. Some determinants of camptothecin responsiveness in leukemia L1210 cells. *Cancer Res* 1971; 31:1883–1887.

141. Andoh T, Ishii K, Suzuki Y, Ikegami Y, Kusunki Y, Takemoto Y, Okada K. Characterization of a mammalian mutant with a camptothecin-resistant DNA topoisomerase I. *Proc Natl Acad Sci USA* 1987; 94:5565–5569.

142. Gupta RS, Gupta R, Eng B, Lock RB, Ross WE, Hertzberg RP, Caranfa MJ, Johnson RK. Camptothecin-resistant mutants of Chinese hamster ovary cells containing a resistant form of topoisomerase I. *Cancer Res* 1988; 48:6404–6410.

143. Tan KB, Mattern MR, Eng W-K, McCabe FL, Johnson RK. Nonproductive rearrangement of DNA topoisomerase I and II genes: correlation with resistance to topoisomerase inhibitors. *J Natl Cancer Inst* 1989; 81:1732–1735.

144. Eng WK, McCabe FL, Tan KB, Mattern MR, Hofmann GA, Woessner RD, Hertzberg RP, Johnson RK. Development of stable camptothecin-resistant subline of P388 leukemia with reduced topoisomerase I content. *Mol Pharmacol* 1990; 38:471–480.

145. Kanzawa F, Sugimoto Y, Minato K, Kasahara K, Bungo M, Nakagawa K, Fujiwara Y, Liu LF, Saijo N. Establishment of a camptothecin analogue (CPT-11)-resistant cell line of human non-small cell lung cancer: characterization and mechanism of resistance. *Cancer Res* 1990; 50: 5919–5924.

146. Oguro M, Seki Y, Okada K, Andoh T. Collateral drug sensitivity induced in CPT-11 (a novel derivative of camptothecin)-resistant cell lines. *Biomed & Pharmacother* 1990; 44:209–216.

147. Sugimoto Y, Tsukahara S, Oh-hara T, Isoe T, Tsuruo T. Decreased expression of DNA topoisomerase I in camptothecin-resistant tumor cell lines as determined by a monoclonal antibody. *Cancer Res* 1990; 50:6925–6930.

148. Tamura H-O, Kohichi C, Yamada R, Ikeda T, Koiwa O, Patterson E, Keene JD, Okada K, Kjeldsen E, Nishikawa K, Andoh T. Molecular cloning of a cDNA of a camptothecin-resistant human DNA topoisomerase I and identification of mutation sites. *Nucleic Acids Res* 1991; 19: 69–75.

149. Ishimi Y, Nishizawa M, Andoh T. Characterization of a camptothecin-resistant human DNA topoisomerase I in an *in vitro* system for simian virus 40 DNA replication. *Eur J Biochem* 1992; 202:835–839.

150. Tanizawa A, Pommier Y. Topoisomerase I alterations in a camptothecin-resistant cell line derived from Chinese hamster DC3F cells in culture. *Cancer Res* 1992; 52:1848–1854.

151. Chang J-Y, Dethlefsen LA, Barley LR, Zhou BS, Cheng Y-C. Characterization of camptothecin-resistant Chinese hamster lung cells. *Biochem Pharmacol* 1992; 43:1732–1735.

152. Tanizawa A, Tabuchi A, Bertrand R, Pommier Y. Cloning of Chinese hamster DNA topoisomerase I cDNA and identification of a single-point mutation responsible for camptothecin resistance. *J Biol Chem* 1993; 268:25,463–25,468.

153. Andoh T, Koiwa O, Okada K. Molecular basis of resistance to CPT-11, specific inhibitor of DNA topoisomerase I. In: Miyazaki T, Takaku F, Sakuraba K, eds. *The Mechanisms and New Approach on Drug Resistance of Cancer Cells*. Amsterdam: Elsevier Science Publishers B.U. 1993:95–101.

154. Fujimori A, Harker WG, Hoki Y, Kohlhagen G, Pommier Y. Mutation at the catalytic site of topoisomerase I in a human leukemia cell line resistant to camptothecin. *Proc Am Assoc Cancer Res* 1994; 35:363.

155. Rubin E, Pantazis P, Bharti T, Toppmeyer D, Giovanella BC, Kufe D. Identification of a mutant human topoisomerase I with intact catalytic activity and resistance to 9-nitrocamptothecin. *J Biol Chem* 1994; 269:2433–2439.

156. Pantazia P, Mendoza JT, DeJesus A, Rubin E, Kufe D, Giovanella BC. Partial characterization of human leukemia U-937 cell sublines resistant to 9-nitro-camptothecin. *Eur J Haematol* 1994; 53:135–144.

157. Pantazis P, Mendoza J, DeJesus A, Early J, Shaw M, Giovanella B. Development of resistance to 9-nitro-camptothecin by human leukemia U-937 cells *in vitro* correlates with altered sensitivities to several anticancer drugs. *Anti-Cancer Drugs* 1994; 5:473–479.

158. Pantazis P, Vardeman D, Mendoza J, Early J, Kozielski A, DeJesus A, Giovanella BC. Sensitivity of camptothecin-resistant human leukemia cells and tumors to anticancer drugs with diverse mechanisms of action. *Leuk Res* 1995; 19:45–55.

159. Katz EJ, Vick JS, Kling KM, Andrews PA, Howell SB. Effect of topoisomerase modulators on cisplatin cytotoxicity in human ovarian carcinoma cells. *Eur J Cancer* 1990; 26:724–727.

160. Kano Y, Suzuki K, Akutsu M, Suda K, Inoue Y, Yoshida M, Sakamoto S, Miura Y. Effects of CPT-11 in combination with other anticancer agents in culture. *Int J Cancer* 1992; 50:604–610.

161. Johnson RK, Mattern MR, McCabe FL. Use of topotecan, a topoisomerase I inhibitor, in combination with other anticancer agents to circumvent resistance. Conf. DNA Topoisomerases Ther., 1992, 4th p. 33.

162. Kim JH, Kim SH, Kolozsvary A, Khil MS. Potentiation of radiation response in human carcinoma cells *in vitro* and murine fibrosarcoma *in vivo* by topotecan, an inhibitor of DNA topoisomerase I. *Int J Radiat Oncol Biol Phys* 1992; 22:515–518.

163. Mattern MR, Hofmann GA, McCabe FL, Johnson RK. Synergistic cell killing by ionizing radiation and topoisomerase I inhibitor topotecan (SK&F 104864). *Cancer Res* 1991; 51:5813–5816.

164. Giovanella B, Potmesil M, Wall ME, Stehlin JS, Hinz HR, Vardeman D, Mendoza J. Treatment of human cancer xenografts with camptothecin analogues in combination with cytotoxan or x irradiation. *Proc Am Assoc Cancer Res* 1994; 35:454(2711).

165. Lamond JP, Kirwin R, Wall ME, Boothman DA. Topoisomerase I inhibitors potentiate radiation lethality *in vitro*. *Proc Am Assoc Cancer Res* 1995; 36:605(3599).

166. Tamura K, Tacada M, Masuda N, Fukuoka M. Radiosensitization effect of CPT 11 against human lung tumor xenografts. *Proc Am Assoc Cancer Res* 1995; 605(3599).

167. Giovanella BC, Vardeman DM, Kozieski AK, Stehlin JS, Potmesil M. Enhanced antitumor effectiveness of camptothecin (cpt) and derivatives administered by continuous infusion through scheduling and combination with DNA damaging agents. *Proc Am Assoc Cancer Res* 1995; 36:391(2328).

168. Cozzarelli NR, Wand JC, eds. *DNA Topology and Its Biological Effects*. Cold Spring Harbor, NY: Cold Spring Harbor Laboratory Press, 1990.

169. Li S, Adar KT. *Camptotheca Acuminata Decaisne*. Henry A and Rockwell M. Monographs Stephen F. Austin State University, Nacogdoches, TX 1994.

170. Schneider E, Hsiang Y-H, Liu LF. DNA topoisomerase as anticancer drug targets. In: August T, Anders MW, Murad F, Ikes A, eds. *Advances in Pharmacology,* vol. 21. New York: Academic, 1990:149–183.

171. Andoh T, Ikeda N, Oguro M, eds. *Molecular Biology of DNA Topoisomerases and Its Application to Chemotherapy*. Boca Raton, FL: CRC, 1993.

172. Liu L, ed. *Advances in Pharmacology,* vol. 29A. *DNA Topoisomerases: Biochemistry and Molecular Biology*. San Diego, CA: Academic, 1994.

173. Liu L, ed. *Advances in Pharmacology,* vol. 29B, *DNA Topoisomerases: Topoisomerase-Targeting Drugs*. San Diego, CA: Academic, 1994.

174. Potmesil M, Pinedo H, eds. *Camptothecins: New Anticancer Agents*. Boca Raton, FL: CRC, 1995.

175. Potmesil M. Camptothecins: from bench research to hospital wards. *Cancer Res* 1994; 54:1432–1439.

176. Potmesil M, Vardehar D, Kozielski AI, Mendoza I, Stehlin IS, Giovanella BC. Growth inhibition of human cancer metastases by camptothecins in heavy developed xenograft models. *Cancer Res* 1995; 55:5637–5641.

7

DNA Topoisomerase II Inhibitors

Yves Pommier, MD, PhD

CONTENTS

1. INTRODUCTION

DNA topoisomerases represent a major focus of research not only for cancer chemotherapy, but also for gene regulation, cell cycle, mitosis, and chromosome structure. A number of reviews have been written on the subject (*1–8*).

Several of the most active anticancer drugs, including etoposide (VP-16) and anthracyclines, poison cellular DNA topoisomerases II (top2). The genomic sites of top2 inhibition differ for each class of drug, thereby providing a rationale for the molecular interactions of drugs with top2 ("stacking model") and for the differential activity of top2 inhibitors in the clinic. More recently, another class of top2 inhibitors with a different mechanism of action has been identified. Bis(2,6)-dioxo-piperazines block the catalytic cycle of top2 by preventing the formation of cleavable complexes. This chapter will describe the enzymatic and biological properties of top2 and the peculiarities of each class of inhibitor. Top2 inhibitors will be classified in two groups: top2 poisons, which trap cleavable complexes, and top2 suppressors, which prevent cleavable complexes from forming.

1. DNA TOP2: ENZYMOLOGY AND CELL BIOLOGY

DNA topoisomerases catalyze the unlinking of DNA strands by making transient DNA strand breaks and allowing another DNA to traverse through these breaks. Two types of topoisomerases have been described in mammalian cells, type 1 and type 2 topoisomerases (top1 and top2), and three types in yeast, including topoisomerases III (*3,8–13*). DNA gyrase is the bacterial equivalent of top2. Antibacterial quinolones (nalidixic acid, ciprofloxacin, norfloxacin, and derivatives) are DNA gyrase inhibitors with no or very limited effect on the host human top2. Topoisomerase-mediated DNA breaks correspond to transesterification reactions where a DNA phosphoester bond is transferred to a specific enzyme tyrosine residue.

From: *Cancer Therapeutics: Experimental and Clinical Agents*
Edited by: B. Teicher Humana Press Inc., Totowa, NJ

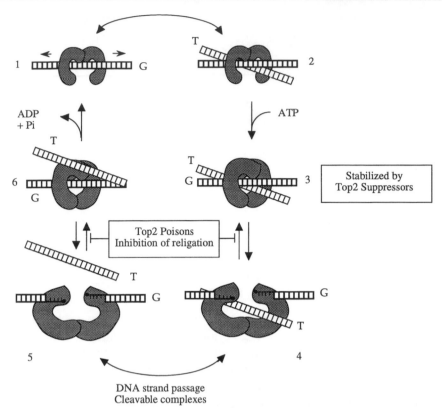

Fig. 1. Top2 catalytic cycle. (1): Noncovalent binding of the top2 dimer to the Gate DNA duplex. (2): DNA recognition and preferential binding to crossovers with G and Transported duplexes. (3): ATP binding promotes the formation of a topological complex on the G duplex; 2-6-dioxopiperazines stabilize this intermediate. (4): DNA cleavage with covalent linking of each top2 monomer to the 5'-DNA terminus of the break on the G duplex (DNA-enzyme transesterification); (5): Poststrand passage cleavable complex; the transported (T) duplex comes out on the other side of the enzyme complex. (6): Religation of the G duplex (DNA–DNA transesterification) followed by ATP hydrolysis and enzyme turnover. Top2 poisons block religation and trap cleavable complexes.

Mammalian DNA top1 and top2 differ in at least two ways. First, top1 relaxes DNA by forming a covalent bond with the 3'-terminus of a DNA single-strand break (for recent review, *see* Gupta et al. [4]), whereas top2 functions as a dimer and forms a double-strand break with each top2 molecule covalently bound to the 5'-terminus of the DNA double-strand break (*see* Fig. 1 and caption). Second, the top1 poisons, camptothecin and its derivatives, do not affect top2 (4,14). Conversely, top2 poisons (etoposides, doxorubicin, amsacrine, and so on) do not trap top1 cleavable complexes with the exception of a few DNA intercalators that trap cleavable complexes of both top1 and top2: actinomycin D (15,16), intoplicine (17), and saintopin (18,19).

Through its ability to open both strands of a DNA duplex (like a Gate; *see* Fig. 1) and to catalyze strand passage (Transport of another duplex through the gate; *see* Fig. 1 [20]), top2 can perform a variety of DNA topoisomerization reactions. Although DNA relaxation is common to top1, conversion of circular DNA to knotted forms, and removal of pre-existing knots are specific to top2. Top2-catalyzed strand passage between independent DNA rings is vital, because it allows decatenation of mitotic and meiotic chromosomes (*see* next paragraph). These biochemical reactions are commonly used to assay topoisomerase activities in vitro: relaxation of supercoiled plasmid DNA in the absence of ATP and Mg^{2+} in the case of top1; and decatenation of kinetoplast DNA (kDNA) and unknotting of P4 DNA in the case of top2 (*12*).

Top1 and top2 can complement each other in yeast, where the absence of one can be compensated by the presence of the other topoisomerase. However, yeast top2 mutants are not viable and die at mitosis, because top2 is essential for chromosome condensation and structure (*3,8–13,21–24*), and for the proper segregation of mitotic (*21–27*) and meiotic (*28,29*) chromosomes. This is because, in addition to its DNA relaxing activity, top2 is essential for the separation of chromatin loops (decatenation of replicated DNA) and condensation of chromosomes, as well as proper segregation of sister chromatids (*25–27,30–34*). The accumulation of top2 at the end of S phase and during G2, and its concentration in the chromosome scaffold are consistent with the enzyme's roles during mitosis. The role of top2 in maintaining the structural integrity of mitotic chromosomes has recently been disputed (*24*). However, a fraction of top2 remains selectively associated with the telophase chromosomes, indicative of an important function during mitosis (*35*). A relationship is possible between top2 and cell-cycle-associated kinases/cyclins, since top2 phosphorylation increases during G2/M (*36*), resulting in enhanced catalytic activity (*see* next paragraph). Both top2α and β proteins are recognized by the monoclonal mitotic phosphoprotein antibody MPM-2 (*37*). The epitope for MPM-2 is conserved for a number of nuclear proteins and is dependent on phosphorylation during or just before M phase. Thus, both top2α and β are probably regulated by mitotic kinase(s). One of the kinases generating immunoreactivity with MPM-2 is MAP kinase (*38*), Today, evidence indicates, however, that top2 phosphorylation during G2/M in yeast is carried out by casein kinase II rather than cdk1-cyclin B (*39,40*).

Phosphorylation at serine/threonines by casein kinase II or protein kinase C enhances top2 catalytic activity (*41,42*), but attenuates the effects of the top2 poisons, etoposide and amsacrine (*43*). Together with the result of Takano et al. (*44*) showing increased phosphorylation in a human KB cell line resistant to etoposide, these observations suggest that top2 phosphorylation is important for determining the enzyme sensitivity to top2 inhibitors. Increased phosphorylation may activate the enzyme catalytic activity while reducing its sensitivity to top2 poisons.

Two top2 isoenzymes have been isolated, top2α and top2β. They differ in their molecular mass (170 dDa for top2α and 180 kDa for top2β), enzymatic properties (*45*), cell-cycle regulation (*46–48*), and cellular distribution (*49,50*). They are encoded by different genes (*45,51–54*). The top2α gene is on chromosome 17q21-22 (*51*), and the top2β gene on chromosome 3p24 (*52,54*). The top2 poison, teniposide (VM-26), and the top2 suppressor, merbarone, have been reported to be three- to eightfold more active on the top2α isoform (*45*). Recently, top2β has been cloned, expressed as a recombinant protein (*55*), and shown to form heterodimers with top2α (Westergaard et al., personal communication).

The top2 catalytic cycle is described in Fig. 1. Top2 dimers first bind reversibly to DNA [step 1 with a preference for DNA crossover regions (step 2)] (*56*). Hence, top2 interaction with DNA is determined both by DNA superstructure (DNA crossovers, bends, and so on) (*56–58*) and local sequence (*59–62*). Although top2 interacts with preferred sequences, its specificity is far less stringent than restriction endonucleases.

This lack of stringency probably allows the enzyme to act at multiple sites of the genome in order to perform its vital functions. On ATP binding, the top2 dimer forms a topological complex with the two DNA duplexes inside the enzyme (step 3) (20,63,64). DNA cleavage (step 4) requires divalent cation (Mg^{2+} in vivo) and corresponds to a nucleophilic attack from the catalytic tyrosine hydroxyl residue (Tyr 804 for human top2 [9]) toward the 5′-side of a DNA phosphodiester bond. This results in the formation of a DNA break associated with the covalent linkage of the 5′-DNA terminus to the catalytic tyrosine (DNA-enzyme transesterification reaction). The other DNA terminus is a 3′-hydroxyl. Each top2 subunit of the homodimer cleaves one strand of the duplex with a stagger of 4 overhanging bases at the 5′-DNA termini (steps 4–5, Fig. 1). The resulting double-strand break opens a gap in the first DNA duplex through which the other duplex can pass (strand passage reaction: steps 4–5). This strand passage reaction is completely dependent on the binding of Mg·ATP, but does not require ATP hydrolysis. Following strand passage, top2 religates the DNA by a reverse transesterification reaction (step 6). In this case, the enzyme catalyzes the nucleophilic attack of the enzyme tyrosine-DNA ester bond by a 3′-DNA hydroxyl terminus. Finally, top2 hydrolyzes ATP and can enter a new catalytic cycle.

Top2 suppressors (bis[2,5]-dioxopiperazines) inhibit the DNA cleavage step (steps 3–4, Fig. 1) by trapping the enzyme in the form of a closed protein clamp (65). Top2 poisons can trap cleavable complexes by inhibiting their religation either before or after DNA strand passage depending on the inhibitor (66,67) (Fig. 1). Formally, the possibility also exists that top2 poisons trap cleavable complexes without a passing DNA duplex inside (not shown in Fig. 1).

2. TOP2 POISONS

Anthracyclines and epipodophyllotoxins (Fig. 2) play key roles in the cancer chemotherapy armamentarium. Formation of cleavable complexes, rather than inhibition of top2 catalytic activity is responsible for activity.

Drug-induced cleavable complexes can be detected in cells as protein-linked DNA breaks by alkaline elution (68,69) and by sodium dodecyl sulfate (SDS)-KCl precipitation assays (70,71) (for review, see 12,72). However, these methods are limited to experimentally growing cells, since they require DNA readiolabeling. There is presently no convenient method to measure DNA cleavage in tumor samples.

Work by Osheroff and coworkers indicates that drugs may act differently in the top2 catalytic cycle (66,73–75). Although etoposide (VP-16) severely inhibits cleavable complex religation and has little effect on strand passage and ATP hydrolysis, genistein and quinolones have little effect on top2-mediated religation, but impair the ability of top2 to carry out its strand passage event and ATP hydrolysis. Amsacrine is unique because it inhibits similarly religation, strand passage, and ATP hydrolysis. These observations strongly suggest that the drugs interact with different top2 protein domains, which is consistent with the finding that some drug-resistant top2 mutant enzymes are not crossresistant to all inhibitors (76–79). Enzyme deletion mutants may prove useful in delineating the top2 domain(s) that interact with the drugs (80), and other cellular proteins involved in the subcellular distribution and phosphorylation of top2 (81,82).

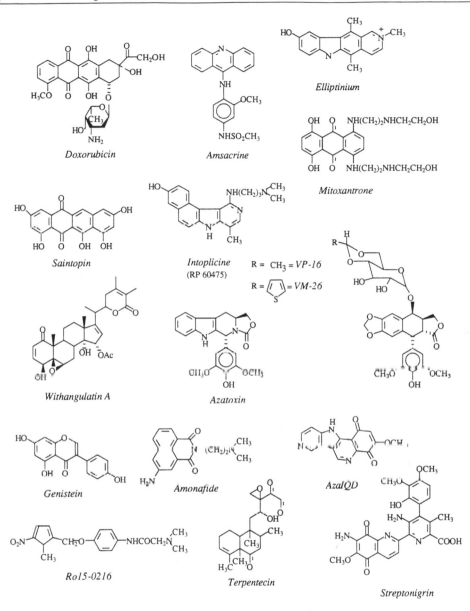

Fig. 2. Chemical structure of top2 poisons.

The molecular interactions of top2 poisons are not known precisely, since the structure of the drug–enzyme–DNA ternary complexes have not been resolved. Drug-induced cleavages do not occur randomly, and each class of inhibitor tends to act at top2 sites with different base sequence preference, either at the 3'- or 5'-terminus of the one of the cleavage sites of the DNA double-strand break (19,83–92). These strong drug-selective preferences for certain bases immediately flanking the cleavage sites suggest that the drugs interact directly with these bases. Top2 inhibitors (whether intercalator or not) have a planar aromatic portion that in some cases mimics a base pair (Fig. 2). Hence, the simplest interpretation is that the drugs stack (intercalate) inside the cleavage sites. Depending on the drug structure, the preferential stacking would take place either at the 3'- or the 5'-terminus with a specific base. This hypothesis implies that topoisomerases first cleave the DNA at many sites, and that the drugs bind specifically to some sites and prevent their religation (*74,75*). The base sequence analyses also imply that stacking at one site is sufficient for the creation of a DNA double-strand break, a view consistent with the concerted action of both enzyme subunits during catalysis (*see* Fig. 1). Recent support for this hypothesis has been provided by Freudenreich and Kreuzer, who showed that an amsacrine derivative alkylates the +1 base of top2 cleavable complexes (*92*). The same type of molecular interaction appears also to account for top1 poisoning by camptothecins (*4,93–95*).

Most clincial antitumor top2 inhibitors are substrates for the P-glycoprotein responsible for the classic multidrug resistance (MDR) phenotype: doxorubicin and analogs, mitoxantrone, anthrapyrazoles, ellipticines, and VP-16 (*96*), and to a lesser extent m-AMSA analogs (*97*). Cells overexpressing the P-glycoprotein are resistant to top2 inhibitors, because the drugs are actively extruded from the cells. In addition, non-*P*-glycoprotein-associated resistance with reduced drug uptake has recently been attributed to overexpression of a 190-kDa protein expressed by the multidrug resistance-associated protein (MRP) gene (*98–102*).

2.1. Demethylepipodophyllotoxins

Extracts from the mayapple or mandrake plant have long been used as a source of folk medicine (*103*). The active principle in this plant, podophyllotoxin, acts as an antimitotic agent that binds to tubulin at a site distinct from that occupied by the vinca alkaloids. A number of semisynthetic derivatives of podophyllotoxin have been made. Two glycosidic derivatives, VM-26 (teniposide) and VP-16 (etoposide) (Fig. 2), are active against a number of human malignancies. Etoposide (VP-16) was introduced in clinical trials in 1971 and approved by the FDA for marketing by Bristol Laboratories under the trade name Vepesid in early 1984. Teniposide (VM-26) has been used in Europe for several years and was approved by the FDA in 1992 for refractory childhood leukemia. More recently, etoposide phosphate has been designed as a prodrug of etoposide in order to obtain a water-soluble compound that could be specifically activated at the tumor sites using antibody–alkaline phosphatase conjugates (*104,105*). In fact, etoposides phosphate (Etopofos®) is almost immediately converted to etoposide in plasma by host endogenous phosphatases, and represents a water-soluble prodrug of etoposide.

The methyl group in *para* of the podophyllotoxin pendant ring is crucial for selectivity toward tubulin, and demethylation at this position is required for top2 poisoning (*106–108*). Demethylepipodophyllotoxins do not bind to DNA significantly in the absence of top2 and can be considered specific top2 poisons. This is in contrast to anthracyclines, which have other cellular targets (*see* below). Top2 cleavable complexes exhibit preference for DNA sites with cytosine at the 3'-DNA terminus opposite to the top2-linked terminus (position -1) (*83*). VP-16 or VM-26 induces similar cleavage patterns (*109,110*), and the cleavage frequency by nucleotide is one of the highest among top2 inhibitors (*61,111*). VM-26 is approximately 10-fold more potent than VP-16 at inducing cleavable complexes both in the presence of purified top2 (*109,110*) and in cells (*107,112*). In cells, cleavable complexes reverse rapidly after drug removal, and consist of a mixture of single- and double-strand breaks (*112,113*).

2.2. Anthracyclines

In contrast to demethylepipodophyllotoxins, anthracyclines (Fig. 2) exert other effects in addition to top2 inhibition: DNA intercalation (*114*) and inhibition of other DNA processing enzymes, such as helicases (*115*), and production of free radicals (*116*) (for recent review, *see 117*). New anthracyclines have also been introduced in the clinics (4-demethoxydaunorubicin [Idarubicin], 4′-epidoxorubicin [Epirubicin]). 4-Demethoxydaunorubicin [Idarubicin] exhibits greater potency against purified top2 than daunorubicin, indicating that removal of the 4-methoxy group yields better top2 inhibitors (*114*). Another approach has been to synthesize analogs with modified sugar to limit the drug recognition by the P-glycoprotein^{MDR}. The amino group on the daunosamine sugar is probably involved in the recognition of the drug by the P-glycoprotein, since the deamino derivative, hydroxyrubicin, is less subject to drug resistance while retaining top2 inhibitory activity (*118*).

The DNA sequence selective inhibition of top2 is common to all anthracyclines (*114, 119*), and the frequency of top2 cleavage per nucleotide is markedly less than in the case of epipodophyllotoxins (*61,120*). Thus, anthracyclines exhibit the highest DNA sequence selectivity among top2 poisons. DNA sequence analyses of the top2-induced cleavage sites indicate a requirement for adenine at the 3′-terminus of one of the two break sites of the top2-induced DNA double-strand break (*85*). In addition, anthracycline-induced cleavable complexes decrease with increasing concentration, probably as a result of DNA intercalation (*114*). Hence, anthracyclines are top2 poisons at low concentrations and suppressors of cleavable complexes at higher concentrations.

The cleavable complexes induced in cells by anthracyclines are also relatively infrequent at a given cytotoxicity level and consist mostly of DNA double-strand breaks. Another difference with the top2 cleavable complexes induced by demethylepipodophyllotoxins and amsacrine is the relatively slow reversibility of the anthracycline-induced top2 cleavable complexes (*121,122*).

2.3. Anthraquinones—Mitoxantrone and Derivatives

Mitoxantrone and derivatives are primarily used in the treatment of breast cancers. They are top2 poisons and DNA intercalators (*123–126*). Hence, they exhibit the dual top2 effects: poisoning at low doses and suppression of cleavable complexes at higher doses. Their pattern of DNA cleavage is unique, although they show similar preference for trapping top2 cleavable complexes with C-1 as in the case of demethylepipodophyllotoxins (*87*). That their top2-induced DNA cleavage patterns are different from those of demethylepipodophyllotoxins implies that other DNA base sequence requirements or structures determine their specificity (*87,126–128*).

MDR cells are usually crossresistant to mitoxantrone, and mitoxantrone can induce P-glycoprotein^{MDR}-mediated (*123,125,129,130*) as well as MRP-mediated (*131*) multidrug resistance. Interestingly, a mitoxantrone-resistant human leukemia HL60 cell line has been shown to exhibit selective alteration of the top2β gene, suggesting that mitoxantrone might preferentially poison top2β (*129,132*).

2.4. Amsacrine

Amsacrine (4′[9-acridinylamino]-methanesulfon-*m*-aniside) (*m*-AMSA) (Fig. 2) was designed and synthesized in 1974 by Cain and Atwell (*133*). It first entered clinical evaluation under National Cancer Institute (NCI) sponsorship in 1976, and its clinical profile is now established. Amsacrine is primarily used in the treatment of hematological malignancies, with emphasis on pediatric and adult acute leukemias, and some activity in lymphomas (*134*). A variety of Phase II trials demonstrated no useful activity against human solid tumors (*135*).

The *m*-AMSA analog, 4-methyl-5-methylcarboxamide (CI-921) (*136,137*), exhibits significantly greater activity against solid tumors both in vitro and in vivo. It has recently entered Phase I and II clinical trials (*138,139*).

m-AMSA is a potent top2 poison; it induces high frequency of top2 cleavable complexes at relatively low concentrations (*121,122*). *m*-AMSA is a relatively weak DNA intercalator (*140*), and the top2 suppressive effect is only observed at high concentrations (generally above 50 μM in the presence of purified top2 and above 100 μM in cells) (*122,141*). These properties turned out to be crucial during the identification of top2 as the target of DNA intercalators, since *m*-AMSA was the first drug used successfully to show top2 poisoning (*142*), and to identify and purify top2 as the nuclear protein forming the protein-linked DNA breaks (*143*). Another interesting feature of *m*-AMSA is that its stereoisomer, *o*-AMSA, which has a methoxygroup in position *ortho* instead of *meta*, is almost inactive as a top2 poison (*122,142*), while being a slightly better DNA intercalator (*140*). This demonstrates a lack of correlation between DNA intercalation and top2 poisoning for acridines (*144*) and probably for most top2 poisons, since the same holds true for anthracyclines (*114*). It has been suggested that the differential anti-top2 activity of *m*-AMSA and *o*-AMSA reflects selective interaction of the *m*-AMSA side chain with the enzyme in the top2–DNA ternary complex (*128,137*).

The frequency of *m*-AMSA-induced top2 cleavable complexes per nucleotide is intermediate between that of anthracyclines and demethylepipodophyllotoxins (*61*). It is comparable to mitoxantrone. The base sequence selectivity of *m*-AMSA-induced top2 cleavable complexes is unique among top2 poisons, since the pattern of cleavage differs from those of other top2 poisons. *m*-AMSA-induced cleavable complexes exhibit preference for an adenine at the 5′-DNA termini of top2 cleavable complexes (*86*). A recent study from Freudenreich and Kreuzer strongly supports the drug stacking model by showing that an *m*-AMSA derivative selectively alkylates the + 1 base of top2 cleavable complexes (*92*).

m-AMSA is less susceptible to P-glycoprotein-mediated MDR than epipodophyllotoxins, anthracyclines, and mitoxantrones (*96,97*). Its cellular uptake and distribution exhibit unique characteristics (*145,146*).

2.5. Ellipticines

Ellipticine is an alkaloid derived from the Apocynaceae family, including *Ochrosia, Bleekeria vitensis,* and *Aspidosperma subincanum* (*103*). Despite its promising preclinical activity, severe toxic effects observed in animal studies hampered the progress of ellipticine toward clinical trials. The semisynthetic derivative, 2-*N*-methyl-9-hydroxy-ellipticinium acetate (NMHE = elliptinium) (Fig. 2), however, exhibited good activity in vivo in various mouse and rat systems, and also lacked hematopoietic toxicity (*147*). Clinical trials of elliptinium were initiated in 1977. Presently, it is used in the treatment of advanced breast cancer in Europe.

Ellipticines are potent DNA intercalators. Hence, top2 cleavable complexes tend to be suppressed at high drug concentrations, and this property, common to all intercalators, was observed early on for ellipticines (*141,148,149*). The DNA sequence selectivity for ellipticines is T-1 (90). In cells, the ellipticine-induced DNA breaks have the unique characteristic to be almost exclusively double-stranded (150,151). A Chinese hamster lung fibroblast cell line made resistant to ellipticine was used first to show that top2 resistance is associated with reduction of top2 cleavable complexes (152,153).

2.6. Other Top2 Poisons

A large number of top2 poisons from diverse chemical families have been identified (amonafide [154–157], flavones, genistein and derivatives [158–160], the nitroimidazole Ro 15-0216 [161], withangulatin [162], streptonigrin [88,89,163], terpenoids [164,165], azatoxins [110,166,167], quinolones [73,168–171], anthraquinones [172], menogaril [173], naphtoquinones [174], the polyaromatic quinone antibiotic UCE6 [175]), and NSC 665517, a compound recently identified from the NCI Anticancer Drug Screen using the COMPARE algorithm (176).

Azatoxin was rationally designed from a pharmacophore analysis of top2 poisons (110,177). It turned out to be a dual inhibitor of tubulin polymerization and of top2 religation without detectable DNA intercalation (110,167). Analogs have recently been made that act only as top2 poisons or tubulin inhibitors (166). Some of the azatoxins with top2 poisoning activity are among the most potent top2 inhibitors without being P-glycoprotein^{MDR} substrates (166,178).

Each class of drug exhibits specific DNA cleavage patterns in the presence of top2. Streptonigrin has the unique property to select top2 cleavable complexes with base preference in the middle of the 4-bp stagger (T + 2 and A + 3) (88,89). Also some, such as terpenoids (164,165) and anthraquinones with alkylating groups (172), produce irreversible cleavable complexes. This last class of compounds might be useful in determining the drug binding sites on top2 (and/or DNA).

3. TOP2 SUPPRESSORS

Inhibition of top2 catalytic activity without trapping of cleavable complexes can also be observed (Fig. 3). This is the case for strong DNA intercalators, such as anthracyclines and ellipticines (120,141,149,179–181). DNA minor groove binders, such as distamycin, have more complex effects with global enhancement of top2 cleavable complexes at low concentrations (< 0.1 μM in purified systems), and DNA sequence-specific redistribution of cleavable complexes at higher concentrations (181).

Hence, three types of dose–response curves can be observed for top2 inhibitors:

1. A monotonal increase of cleavable complexes with drug concentration in the case of weak (or non-) DNA binders (VP-16, VM-26, azatoxins, amsacrine);
2. A bell-shaped curve in the case of anthracyclines, mitoxantrones, ellipticines, and other DNA intercalators; and
3. A monotonal decrease of cleavable complexes in the case of bulky intercalators (ethidium bromide, ditercalinium, aclarubicin) (179,180,189) or non-DNA binders that inhibit the catalytic activity without trapping cleavable complexes (2,6-dioxopiperazines, merbarone, and fostriecin).

Some non-DNA binders can also suppress cleavable complexes and will be described in more details below. They are merbarone (182), bis(dioxopiperazine) derivatives (183,184), suramin (185), and fostriecin, for which contradictory results have been published (186–188) (Fig. 3).

2,6-DIOXOPIPERAZINES

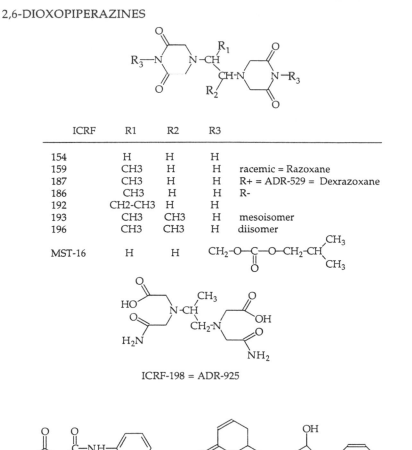

ICRF	R1	R2	R3	
154	H	H	H	
159	CH3	H	H	racemic = Razoxane
187	CH3	H	H	R+ = ADR-529 = Dexrazoxane
186	CH3	H	H	R-
192	CH2-CH3	H	H	
193	CH3	CH3	H	mesoisomer
196	CH3	CH3	H	diisomer
MST-16	H	H	CH₂–O–C–O–CH₂–CH(CH₃)(CH₃)	

ICRF-198 = ADR-925

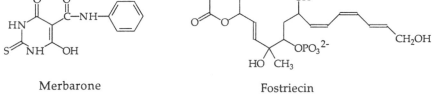

Merbarone   Fostriecin

Fig. 3. Chemical structure of suppressors of top2 cleavable complexes.

3.1. 2,6-Dioxopiperazines

Bis(dioxopiperazines) were originally synthesized as potential intracellular chelating agents, and their biochemical and pharmacological properties, including antitumor activity, were studied extensively well before top2 was identified as their cellular target (*190*). The structures of several 2,6-dioxopiperazines are shown in Fig. 3. ICRF-159 (razoxane) is a racemic mixture, and ICRF-187 (dexrazoxane = ADR529 = NSC 169780) and ICRF-186 (levrazoxane) are its $R+$ and $R-$ stereoisomers, respectively. In 1991, Tanabe and coworkers reported that the ICRF derivatives inhibit top2 catalytic activity without inducing cleavable complexes or binding to DNA (*184*). ICRF-193 was the most potent compound with an IC_{50} around 2 μM, ICRF-154 and ICRF-159 were approximately equipotent with IC_{50}s around 20 μM, and MST-16 was approx 10-fold less potent with an IC_{50} around 300 μM (*184*). The same group also reported that the cellular effects were consistent with inhibition of top2 catalytic activity, since etoposide-induced cleavable complexes were greatly inhibited both in the presence of purified top2 (184) and in cells (183). Drug-treated cells are arrested in G2 and early M phase with fewer condensed and entangled chromosomes and with multilobed nuclei (183). More recent analysis showed that, in the presence ICRF-193, cells traverse many rounds of the cell cycle with their genome replicated, but not segregated, resulting in polyploidization (191). These effects are analogous to those observed in *top2* ts mutants of yeast at nonpermissive temperature (27). 2,6-Dioxopiperazines are presently used to study the cellular functions of top2 (192).

The molecular interactions of ICRF-193 with top2 have been examined, and appear to result from trapping the enzyme in the form of a closed protein clamp as a result of blocking the interconversion between the open- and closed-clamp forms of the enzyme (Fig. 1) (65). Although no cleavable complexes are induced by 2,6-dioxopiperazines, chromosome breakage may be generated as a result of disruption of segregation as in the case of *Saccharomyces cerevisiae top2* mutants (26).

MST-16, a bis(dioxopiperazine) (Fig. 3) derivative developed (193) before knowing its effects on top2 (184), has recently been shown to exhibit significant antitumor activity and selective inhibition of cell proliferation at the G2/M transition (193,194). Clinical trials of orally administered MST-16 in adult T-cell leukemia-lymphoma, which has no standard therapy, showed the drug to be effective (195–197).

ICRF-187 (ADR 529 = dexrazoxane) is very effective in protecting against doxorubicin-induced cardiotoxicity both in animal and clinical studies (198). Anthracyclines produce cumulative, dose-dependent, irreversible cardiomyopathy that can lead to congestive heart failure. Through its semiquinone metabolite, doxorubicin can generate superoxide anion and superhydroxide free radicals with iron as a cofactor. These free radicals cause extensive lipid peroxidation and mitochondrial destruction. Dexrazoxane is hydrolyzed to its active one or two rings-opened (ADR925) metal chelating forms intracellularly in the presence of iron (199. The active ring-opened metabolites displace Fe^{3+} from its complex with doxorubicin, daunorubicin, epirubicin, and idarubicin within minutes (200) to prevent formation of superhydroxide radicals. The protection against anthracyclines effect may also be related to the suppression of anthracycline-induced cleavable complexes by the ring-closed form (ICRF-187, dexrazoxane), an effect that may not be so desirable, because it would also reduce the antitumor activity of the anthracyclines.

3.2. Merbarone

Drake et al. first reported that merbarone (5-[N-phenylcarboxamido]-2-thiobarbituric acid [NSC 336628]) (Fig. 3) (201) inhibits top2 catalytic activity without inducing cleavable complexes (182), and that merbarone exhibited some selectivity for top2α (p170) (45). More recently, Chen and Beck reported that merbarone, like ICRF-193, inhibits chromosome condensation and separation without preventing cells from exiting mitosis. It causes S-phase retardation G2 arrest, and polyploidy in synchronized cultures of HeLa cells (202) and in human leukemic CEM/VM-1 cells (203). Interestingly, the VM-26-resistant cells CEM/VM-1 are not crossresistant to merbarone, indicating that the merbarone and VM-26 interact on different enzyme sites.

Merbarone is in Phase II clinical trials, but so far does not appear active in a variety of solid tumors including renal cell (204), hepatocellular (205), pancreatic (206,207), or gastric (208) carcinomas, or small-cell lung cancer (209).

3.3. Fostriecin

Fostriecin (CI-920) is a phosphate-containing polyene lactone antitumor agent (Fig. 3) isolated from a previously undescribed subspecies of *Streptomyces pulveraceus* cultured from a Brazilian soil sample. Fostriecin is active on a variety of tumor models (*210–212*) and causes an accumulation of cells in the G2 + M phase of the cell cycle (*188,210*).

Fostriecin inhibits the catalytic activity of top2 and the cleavable complexes induced by *m*-AMSA (*188*). As in the case of merbarone, teniposide (VM-26)-resistant cells are not crossresistant to fostriecin (*203*). Recent work by Roberge and coworkers has challenged top2 inhibition as the most relevant cellular effect of fostriecin. Roberge et al. found that fostriecin is 10- to 100-fold more potent against protein phosphatases 1 and 2A, respectively, than against top2 (*213*). They proposed that fostriecin interferes with the mitotic control and induces cycling cells to enter mitosis prematurely. Cells that are in the division cycle by treatment with the DNA replication inhibitor aphidicolin or with the DNA-damaging agents teniposide (VP-16) or camptothecin (*213*) are forced into mitosis by fostriecin. A more recent publication makes an analogy between the cell-cycle effects of fostriecin and another protein phosphatase inhibitor, okadaic acid (*214*). Chromosome condensation induced by fostriecin does not require p34cdc2 kinase activity and histone H1 hyperphosphorylation, but is associated with enhanced histone 2A and H3 phosphorylation (*214*).

4. CONCLUSIONS

DNA topoisomerase poisons are presently a major element of the anticancer armamentarium. Their clinical differences suggest that novel top2 poisons may provide additional progress for cancer chemotherapy. Suppressors top2 cleavable complexes represent another class of drugs with interesting biological, pharmacological, and possibly therapeutic properties.

ACKNOWLEDGMENTS

The author wishes to thank Kurt W. Kohn, Laboratory of Molecular Pharmacology, NCI, for his continuous support and exciting discussions, and Malini Gupta for suggestions on the manuscript.

REFERENCES

1. Wang JC. DNA topoisomerases. *Annu Rev Biochem* 1985; 54:665–697.
2. Wang JC. Recent studies of DNA topoisomerases. *Biochim Biophys Acta* 1987; 909:1–9.
3. Wang JC. DNA topoisomerases: why so many? *J Biol Chem* 1991; 266:6659–6662.
4. Gupta M, Fujimori A, Pommier Y. Eukaryotic DNA topoisomerases I. *Biochim Biophys Acta* 1995; 1262:1–14.
5. Pommier Y, Leteurtre F, Fesen M, Fujimori A, Bertrand R, Solary E, Kohlhagen G, Kohn KW. Cellular determinants of sensitivity and resistance to DNA topoisomerase inhibitors. *Cancer Invest* 1994; 12:530–542.
6. Pommier Y. DNA topoisomerases I and II in cancer chemotherapy: update and perspectives. *Cancer Chemother Pharmacol* 1993; 32:103–108.
7. Watt PM, Hickson ID. Structure and function of type II DNA topoisomerases. *Biochem J* 1994; 303:681–695.

8. Osheroff N, Zechierich EL, Gale KC. Catalytic function of DNA topoisomerase II. *BioEssays* 1991; 13:269–275.

9. Caron PR, Wang JC. DNA topoisomerases as target of therapeutics: a structural overview. In: Andoh T, Ikeda H, Oguro M, eds. *Molecular Biology of DNA Topoisomerases and Its Application to Chemotherapy.* Boca Raton, FL: CRC. 1993:1–18.

10. Champoux J. Mechanistic aspects of type-I topoisomerases. In: Wang JC, Cozarelli NR, eds. DNA topology and its biological effects. Cold Spring Harbor, NY: Cold Spring Harbor Laboratory Press. 1990:217–242.

11. Kohn KW, Pommier Y, Kerrigan D, Markovits J, Covey JM. Topoisomerase II as a target of anticancer drug action in mammalian cells. *NCI Monographs* 1987; 4:61–71.

12. Pommier Y, Kohn KW. Topoisomerase II inhibition by antitumor intercalators and demethyl-epipodophyllotoxins. In: Glazer RI, eds. *Developments in Cancer Chemotherapy.* Boca Raton, FL: CRC. 1989:175–196.

13. Pommier Y, Tanizawa A. Mammalian DNA topoisomerase I and its inhibitors. In: Hickman J, Tritton T, eds. *Cancer Chemotherapy.* Oxford: Blackwell Scientific Publications. 1993: 214–250.

14. Hsiang YH, Hertzberg R, Hecht S, Liu LF. Camptothecin induces protein-linked DNA breaks via mammalian DNA topoisomerase I. *J Biol Chem* 1985; 260:14,873–14,878.

15. Trask DK, Muller MT. Stabilization of type I topoisomerase-DNA covalent complexes by actinomycin D. *Proc Natl Acad Sci USA* 1988; 85:1417–1421.

16. Wasserman K, Markovits J, Jaxel C, Capranico G, Kohn KW, Pommier Y. Effects of morpholinyl doxorubicins, doxorubicin, and actinomycin D on mammalian DNA topoisomerases I and II. *Mol Pharmacol* 1990; 38:38–45.

17. Poddevin B, Riou J-F, Lavelle F, Pommier Y. Dual topoisomerase I and II inhibition by intoplicine (RP-60475) a new antitumor agent in early clinical trials. *Mol Pharmacol* 1993; 44: 767–774.

18. Yamashita Y, Kawada S-Z, Fujii N, Nakano H. Induction of mammalian topoisomerase I and II mediated DNA cleavage by saintopin, a new antitumor agent from fungus. *Biochemistry* 1991; 30:5838–5845.

19. Leteurtre F, Fujimori A, Tanizawa A, Chhabra A, Mazumder A, Kohlhagen G, Nakano H, Pommier Y. Saintopin, a dual inhibitor of DNA topoisomerases I and II, as a probe for drug-enzyme interactions. *J Biol Chem* 1994; 269:28,702–28,707.

20. Roca J, Wang JC. DNA transport by a type II DNA topoisomerase: evidence in favor of a two-gate mechanism. *Cell* 1994; 77:609–616.

21. Adachi Y, Luke M, Laemmli UK. Chromosome assembly in vitro: topoisomerase II is required for condensation. *Cell* 1991; 64:137–148.

22. Earnshaw WC, Heck MM. Localization of topoisomerase II in mitotic chromosomes. *J Cell Biol* 1985; 100:1716–1725.

23. Gasser SM, Laroche T, Falquet J, Boy de la Tour E, Laemmli UK. Metaphase chromosome structure. Involvement of topoisomerase II. *J Mol Biol* 1986; 188:613–629.

24. Hirano T, Mitchison TJ. Topoisomerase II does not play a scaffolding role in the organization of mitotic chromosomes assembled in *Xenopus* egg extracts. *J Cell Biol* 1993; 120:601–612.

25. DiNardo S, Voelkel K, Sternglanz R. DNA topoisomerase II mutant of Saccharomyces cerevisiae: topoisomerase II is required for segregation of daughter molecules at the termination of DNA replication. *Proc Natl Acad Sci USA* 1984; 81:2616–2620.

26. Holm C, Stearns T, Botstein D. DNA topoisomerase II must act at mitosis to prevent nondisjunction and chromosome breakage. *Mol Cell Biol* 1989; 9:159–168.

27. Uemura T, Ohkura H, Adachi Y, Morino K, Shiozaki K, Yanagida M. DNA topoisomerase II is required for condensation and separation of mitotic chromosomes in *S. pombe. Cell* 1987; 50:917–925.

28. Rose D, Holm C. Meiosis-specific arrest revealed in DNA topoisomerase II mutants. *Mol Cell Biol* 1993; 13:3445–3455.

29. Moens PB, Earnshaw WC. Anti-topoisomerase II recognizes meiotic chromosome cores. *Chromosoma* 1990; 98:317–322.

30. Shamu CE, Murray AM. Sister chromatid separation in frog egg extracts requires DNA topoisomerase II activity during anaphase. *J Cell Biol* 1992; 117:921–934.

31. Wood ER, Earnshaw WC. Mitotic chromatin condensation in vitro using somatic cell extracts and nuclei with variable levels of endogenous topoisomerase II. *J Cell Biol* 1990; 111:2839–2850.
32. Newport J. Nuclear reconstitution in vitro: stages of assembly around protein-free DNA. *Cell* 1987; 48:205–217.
33. Newport J, Spann T. Disassembly of the nucleus in the mitotic extracts: membrane vesiculization, lamin disassembly, and chromosome condensation are independent processes. *Cell* 1987; 48:219–230.
34. Downes CS, Mullinger AM, Johnson RT. Inhibitors of DNA topoisomerase II prevent chromatid separation in mammalian cells but do not prevent exit from mitosis. *Proc Natl Acad Sci USA* 1991; 88:8895–8899.
35. Swedlow JR, Sedat JW, Agard DA. Multiple chromosomal populations of topoisomerase II detected in vivo by time-lapse, three-dimensional wide-field microscopy. *Cell* 1993; 73:97–108.
36. Heck MMS, Hittelman WN, Earnshaw WC. In vivo phosphorylation of the 170-kDa form of eukaryotic DNA topoisomerase II. *J Biol Chem* 1989; 264:15,161–15,164.
37. Taagepera S, Rao PN, Drake FH, Gorbsky GJ. DNA topoisomerase II-alpha is the major chromosome protein recognized by the mitotic phosphoprotein antibody MPM-2. *Proc Natl Acad Sci USA* 1993; 90:8407–8411.
38. Kuang J, Ashorn CL. At least two kinases phosphorylate the MPM-2 epitope during *Xenopus oocyte* maturation. *J Cell Biol* 1993; 123:859–868.
39. Cardenas ME, Dang Q, Glover CVC, Gasser SM. Casein kinase II phosphorylates the eukaryote-specific C-terminal domain of topoisomerase II in vivo. *EMBO J* 1992; 11:1785–1796.
40. Bojanowski K, Filhol O, Cochet C, Chambaz EM, Larsen AK. DNA topoisomerase II and casein kinase II associate in a molecular complex that is catalytically active. *J Biol Chem* 1994; 268:22,920–22,926.
41. Ackerman P, Glover CV, Osheroff N. Phosphorylation of DNA topoisomerase II in vivo and in total homogenates of Drosophila Kc cells. The role of casein kinsae II. *J Biol Chem* 1988; 263:12,653–12,660.
42. Corbett AH, Fernald AW, Osheroff N. Protein kinase C modulates the catalytic activity of topoisomerase II by enhancing the rate of ATP hydrolysis: evidence for a common mechanism by regulation by phosphorylation. *J Biol Chem* 1993; 32:2090–2097.
43. De Vore RF, Corbett AH, Osheroff N. Phosphorylation of topoisomerase II by casein kinase II and protein kinase C: effects on enzyme-mediated DNA cleavage/religation and sensitivity to the antineoplastic drugs etoposide and 4'-(9-acridinylamino)methane-sulfon-*m*-anisidide. *Cancer Res* 1992; 52:2156–2161.
44. Takano H, Kohno K, Ono M, Uchida Y, Kuwano M. Increased phosphorylation of DNA topoisomerase II in etoposide-resistant mutants of human KB carcinoma cells. *Cancer Res* 1991; 51:3951–3957.
45. Drake FH, Hofmann GA, Bartus HF, Mattern MR, Crooke ST, Mirabelli CK. Biochemical and pharmacological properties of p170 and p180 forms of topoisomerase II. *Biochemistry* 1989; 28:8154–8160.
46. Tsutsui K, Tsutsui K, Okada S, Watanabe M, Shohmori T, Seki S, Inoue Y. Molecular cloning of partial cDNAs for rat DNA topoisomerase II isoforms and their differential expression in brain development. *J Biol Chem* 1993; 268:19,076–19,083.
47. Woessner RD, Mattern MR, Mirabelli CK, Johnson RK, Drake FH. Proliferation- and cell cycle-dependent differences in expression of the 170 kilodalton and 180 kilodalton forms of topoisomerase II in NIH-3T3 cells. *Cell Growth Differ* 1991; 2:209–214.
48. Capranico G, Tinelli S, Austin CA, Fisher ML, Zunino F. Different patterns of gene expression of topoisomerase II isoforms in differentiated tissues during murine development. *Biochim Biophys Acta* 1992; 1132:43–48.
49. Negri C, Scovassi AI, Braghetti A, Guano F, Astaldi Ricotti GC. DNA topoisomerase II beta: stability and distribution in different animal cells in comparison to DNA topoisomerase I and II alpha. *Exp Cell Res* 1993; 206:128–133.
50. Petrov P, Drake F, Loranger A, Huang W, Hancock R. Localization of DNA topoisomerase II in chinese hamster fibroblasts by confocal and electron microscopy. *Exp Cell Res* 1993; 204:73–81.
51. Tsai-Pflugfelder M, Liu LF, Liu AA, Tewey KM, Whang-Peng J, Knutsen T, Huebner K, Croce CM, Wang JC. Cloning and sequencing of cDNA encoding human DNA topoisomerase

II and localization of the gene to chromosome region 17q21-22. *Proc Natl. Acad Sci USA* 1988; 85:7177–7181.

52. Jenkins JR, Ayton P, Jones T, Davies SL, Simmons DL, Harris AL, Sheer D, Hickson ID. Isolation of cDNA clones encoding the beta isozyme of human DNA topoisomerase II and localisation of the gene to chromosome 3p24. *Nucleic Acids Res* 1992; 20:5587–5592.

53. Patel S, Fisher LM. Novel HeLa topoisomerase II is the II beta isoform: complete coding sequence and homology with other type II topoisomerases. *Br J Cancer* 1993; 67:456–463.

54. Tan KB, Dorman TE, Falls KM, Chung TDY, Mirabelli CK, Crooke ST, Mao J-I. Topoisomerase II-alpha and topoisomerase II-beta genes: characterization and mapping to human chromosomes 17 and 3, respectively. *Cancer Res* 1992; 52:231–234.

55. Austin CA, Marsh KL, Wasserman RA, Willmore E, Sayer PJ, Wang JC, Fisher LM. Expression, domain structure, and enzymatic properties of an active recombinant human DNA topoisomerase II beta. *J Biol Chem* 1995; 270:15,739–15,746.

56. Zechiedrich EL, Osheroff N. Eukaryotic topoisomerases recognize nucleic acid topology by preferentially interacting with DNA crossovers. *EMBO J* 1990; 9:4555–4562.

57. Hsieh C-H, Griffith JD. The terminus of SV40 DNA replication and transcription contains a sharp sequence-directed curve. *Cell* 1988; 52:535–544.

58. Howard MT, Lee MP, Hsieh T-S, Griffith JD. Drosophila topoisomerase II-DNA interactions are affected by DNA structure. *J Mol Biol* 1991; 217:53–62.

59. Sander M, Hsieh TS. Drosophilia topoisomerase II double-strand DNA cleavage: analysis of DNA sequence homology at the cleavage site. *Nucleic Acids Res* 1985; 13:1057–1072.

60. Spitzner JR, Muller MT. A consensus sequence for cleavage by vertebrate DNA topoisomerase I. *Nucleic Acids Res* 1988; 16:5533–5556.

61. Pommier Y, Capranico G, Orr A, Kohn KW. Distribution of topoisomerase II cleavage sites in SV40 DNA and the effects of drugs. *J Mol Biol* 1991; 222:909–924.

62. Pommier Y, Capranico G, Orr A, Kohn KW. Local base sequence preferences for DNA cleavage by mammalian topoisomerase II in the presence of amsacrine and teniposide. *Nucleic Acids Res* 1991; 19:5973–5980.

63. Pommier Y, Kerrigan D, Kohn D. Topological complexes between DNA and topoisomerase II and effects of polyamines. *Biochemistry* 1989; 28:995–1002.

64. Corbett AH, Zechiedrich EL, Osheroff N. A role for the passage helix in the DNA cleavage reaction of eukaryotic topoisomerase II. *J Biol Chem* 1992; 267:683–686.

65. Roca J, Ishida R, Berger JM, Andoh T, Wang JC. Antitumor bisdioxopiperazines inhibit yeast DNA topoisomerase II by trapping the enzyme in the form of a closed protein clamp. *Proc Natl Acad Sci USA* 1994; 91:1781–1785.

66. Corbett AH, Osheroff N. When good enzymes go bad: conversion of topoisomerase II to a cellular toxin by antineoplastic drugs. *Chem Res Toxicol* 1993; 6:585–597.

67. Froelich-Ammon SJ, Osheroff N. Topoisomerase poisons: harnessing the dark side of enzyme mechanism. *J Biol Chem* 1995; 270:21,429–21,432.

68. Kohn KW. Principles and practice of DNA filter elution. *Pharmacol Ther* 1991; 49:55–77.

69. Bertrand R, Pommier Y. Assessment of DNA damage in mammalian cells by DNA filtration methods. In: Studzinski G, Ed. *Cell Growth and Apoptosis: A Practical Approach*. Oxford: IRL, Oxford University Press. 1995:96–117.

70. Trask DK, DiDonato JA, Muller MT. Rapid detection and isolation of covalent DNA/protein complexes: application to topoisomerase I and II. *EMBO J* 1984; 3:671–676.

71. Rowe TC, Chen GL, Hsiang YH, Liu LF. DNA damage by antitumor acridines mediated by mammalian DNA topoisomerase II. *Cancer Res* 1986; 46:2021–2026.

72. Liu LF. DNA topoisomerase poisons as antitumor drugs. *Annu Rev Biochem* 1989; 58:351–375.

73. Robinson MJ, Martin BA, Gootz TD, McGuirk PR, Moynihan M, Sutcliffe JA, Osheroff N. Effects of quinolone derivatives on eukaryotic topoisomerase II. A novel mechanism for enhancement of enzyme mediated DNA cleavage. *J Biol Chem* 1991; 266:14,585–14,592.

74. Robinson MJ, Corbett AH, Osheroff N. Effects of topoisomerase II-targeted drugs on enzyme-mediated DNA cleavage and ATP hydrolysis: evidence for distinct drug interaction domains on topoisomerase II. *Biochemistry* 1993; 32:3638–3643.

75. Robinson MJ, Osheroff N. Effects of antineoplastic drugs on the post-strand passage DNA cleavage/religation equilibrium of topoisomerase II. *Biochemistry* 1991; 30:1807–1813.

76. Zwelling LA, Hinds M, Chan D, Mayes J, Sie KL, Parder E, Silberman L, Radcliffe A, Beran M, Blick M. Characterization of an amsacrine-resistant line of human leukemia cells. *J Biol Chem* 1989; 264:16,411–16,420.

77. Mayes J, Hinds M, Soares L, Altschuler E, Kim P, Zwelling LA. Further characterization of an amsacrine-resistant line of HL-60 human leukemia cells and its topoisomerase II. *Biochem. Pharmacol* 1993; 46:599–607.

78. Huff AC, Ward RE, Kreuzer KN. Mutational alterations of the breakage/resealing subunits of bacteriophage T4 DNA topoisomerase confers resistance to antitumor agent m-AMSA. *Mol Gen Genet* 1990; 221:27–32.

79. Huff AC, Kreuzer KN. Evidence for a common mechanism of action of antitumor and anti-bacterial agents that inhibit type II DNA topoisomerases. *J Biol Chem* 1990; 265:20,496–20,505.

80. Crenshaw DG, Hsieh T-S. Function of the hydrophilic carboxyl terminus of type II DNA topoisomerase from *Drosophila melanogaster. J Biol Chem* 1993; 28:21,328–21,334.

81. Harker WG, Slade DL, Parr RL, Holguin MH. Selective use of an alternative stop codon and polyadenylation signal within intron sequences leads to a truncated topoisomerase IIα messenger RNA and protein in human HL-60 leukemai cells selected for resistance to mitoxantrone. *Cancer Res* 1995; 55:4962–4971.

82. Mirski SEL, Cole SPC. Cytoplasmic localization of a mutant Mr 160,000 topoisomerase II alpha is associated with the loss of putative bipartite nuclear localization signals in a drug-resistant human lung cancer cell line. *Cancer Res* 1995; 55:2129–2134.

83. Pommier Y, Capranico G, Kohn KW. Local DNA sequence requirements for topoisomerase II-induced DNA cleavage produced by amsacrine and teniposide. *Proc Am Assoc Cancer Res* 1991; 32:335.

84. Pommier Y, Kohn KW, Capranico G, Jaxel C. Base sequence selectivity of topoisomerase inhibitors suggests a common model for drug action. In: Andoh T, Ikeda H, Oguro M, eds. *Molecular Biology of DNA Topoisomerase and Its Application to Chemotherapy.* Boca Raton, FL: CRC. 1993:215–227.

85. Capranico G, Kohn KW, Pommier Y. Local sequence requirements for DNA cleavage by mammalian topoisomerase II in the presence of doxorubicin. *Nucleic Acids Res* 1990; 18: 6611–6619.

86. Capranico G, Tinelli S, Zunino F, Kohn KW, Pommier Y. Effects of base mutations on topoisomerase II DNA cleavage stimulated by mAMSA in short DNA oligomers. *Biochemistry* 1993; 32:145–152.

87. Capranico G, De Isabella T, Tinelli S, Bigioni S, Zunino F. Similar sequence specificity of mitoxantrone and VM-26 stimulation of in vitro DNA cleavage by mammalian DNA topoisomerase II. *Biochemistry* 1993; 32:3032–3048.

88. Capranico G, Palumbo M, Tinelli S, Zunino F. Unique sequence specificity by topoisomerase II DNA cleavage stimulation and DNA binding mode of streptonigrin. *J Biol Chem* 1994; 40:25,004–25,009.

89. Leteurtre F, Kohlhagen G, Pommier Y. Streptonigrin-induced topoisomerase II sites exhibit base preference in the middle of the enzyme stagger. *Biochem Biophys Res Commun* 1994; 203:1259–1267.

90. Fosse P, Rene B, Le Bret M, Paoletti C, Saucier J-M. Sequence requirements for mammalian topoisomerase II mediated DNA cleavage stimulated by an ellipticine derivative. *Nucleic Acids Res* 1991; 19:2861–2868.

91. Freudenreich CH, Kreuzer KN. Mutational analysis of a type II topoisomerase cleavage site: distinct requirements for enzyme and inhibitors. *EMBO J* 1993; 12:2085–2097.

92. Freudenreich CH, Kreuzer KN. Localization of an aminoacridine antitumor agent in a type II topoisomerase-DNA complex. *Proc Natl Acad Sci USA* 1994; 91:11,007–11,011.

93. Jaxel C, Capranico G, Kerrigan D, Kohn KW, Pommier Y. Effect of local DNA sequence on topoisomerase I cleavage in the presence or absence of camptothecin. *J Biol Chem* 1991; 266: 20,418–20,423.

94. Tanizawa A, Kohn KW, Pommier Y. Induction of cleavage in topoisomerase I cDNA by topoisomerase I enzymes from calf thymus and wheat germ in the presence and absence of camptothecin. *Nucleic Acids Res* 1993; 21:5157–5166.

95. Pommier Y, Kohlhagen G, Kohn F, Leteurtre F, Wani MC, Wall ME. Interaction of an

alkylating camptothecin derivative with a DNA base at topoisomerase I-DNA cleavage sites. *Proc Natl Acad Sci USA* 1995; 92:8861–8865.

96. Beck WT, Danks MK. Mechanisms of resistance to drugs that inhibit DNA topoisomerases. *Semin Cancer Biol* 1991; 2:235–244.

97. Granzen B, Graves DE, Baguley BC, Danks MK, Beck WT. Structure-activity studies of amsacrine analogs in drug resistant human leukemia cell lines expressing either altered DNA topoisomerase II or P-glycoprotein. *Oncol Res* 1993; 4:489–496.

98. Marquardt D, McCrone S, Center MS. Mechanisms of multidrug resistance in HL60 cells: detection of resistance-associated proteins with antibodies against synthetic peptides that correspond to the deduced sequence of P-glycoprotein. *Cancer Res* 1990; 50:1426–1430.

99. Barrand MA, Heppell-Parton AC, Wright KA, Rabbitts PH, Twentyman PR. A 190-kilodalton protein overexpressed in non-P-glycoprotein-containing multidrug-resistant cells and its relationship to the MRP gene. *J Natl Cancer Inst* 1994; 86:110–117.

100. Cole SP, Bhardwaj G, Gerlach JH, Mackie JE, Grant CE, Almquist KC, Stewart AJ, Kurz EU, Duncan AM, Deeley RG. Overexpression of a transporter gene in a multidrug-resistant human lung cancer cell line (*see* comments). *Science* (*Washington, DC*) 1992; 258:1650–1654.

101. Schneider E, Horton JK, Yang CH, Nakagawa M, Cowan KH. Multidrug resistance-associated protein gene overexpression and reduced drug sensitivity of topoisomerase II in a human breast carcinoma MCF7 cell line selected for etoposide resistance. *Cancer Res* 1994; 54:152–158.

102. Binaschi M, Supino R, Gambetta RA, Giaccone G, Prosperi E, Capranico G, Cataldo I, Zunino F. MRP gene overexpression in a human doxorubicin-resistant SCLC cell line: alterations in cellular pharmacokinetics and in pattern of cross-resistance. *Int J Cancer* 1995; 62:84–89.

103. Cragg G, Suffness M. Metabolism of plant-derived anticancer agents. *Pharmacol Ther* 1988; 37:425–461.

104. Bendixen C, Thomsen B, Alsner J, Westergaard O. Camptothecin-stabilized topoisomerase I-DNA adducts cause premature termination of transcription. *Biochemistry* 1990; 29:5613–5619.

105. Been MD, Burgess RR, Champoux JJ. Nucleotide sequence preference at rat liver and wheat germ type 1 DNA topoisomerase breakage sites in duplex SV40 DNA. *Nucleic Acids Res* 1984; 12:3097–3114.

106. Loike JD, Brewer CF, Sternlicht H, Gensler WJ, Horwitz SB. Structure–activity study of the inhibition of microtubule assembly in vitro by podophyllotoxin and its congeners. *Cancer Res* 1978; 38:2688–2693.

107. Long BH, Musial ST, Brattain MG. Comparison of cytotoxicity and DNA breakage activity of congeners of podophyllotoxin including VP16-213 and VM26: a quantitative structure-activity relationship. *Biochemistry* 1984; 23:1183–1188.

108. Sinha BK, Polita PM, Eliot HM, Kerrigan D, Pommier Y. Structure–activity relations, cytotoxicity and topoisomerase II dependent DNA cleavage induced by pendulum ring analogues of etoposide. *Eur J Cancer* 1990; 26:590–593.

109. Chen GL, Yang L, Rowe TC, Halligan BD, Tewey KM, Liu LF. Nonintercalative antitumor drugs interfere with the breakage-reunion reaction of mammalian DNA topoisomerase II. *J Biol Chem* 1984; 259:13,560–13,566.

110. Leteurtre F, Madalengoitia J, Orr A, Guzi TJ, Lehnert E, Macdonald T, Pommier Y. Rational design and molecular effects of a new topoisomerase II inhibitor, azatoxin. *Cancer Res* 1992; 52:4478–4483.

111. Pommier Y, Orr A, Kohn KW, Riou JF. Differential effects of amsacrine and epipodophyllotoxins on topoisomerase II cleavage in the human c-*myc* proto-oncogene. *Cancer Res* 1992; 52: 3125–3130.

112. Kerrigan D, Pommier Y, Kohn KW. Protein-linked DNA strand breaks produced by etoposide and teniposide in mouse L1210 and human VA-13 and HT-29 cell lines: relationship to cytotoxicity. *NCI Monographs* 1987; 4:117–121.

113. Long BH, Musial ST, Brattain MG. Single- and double-strand DNA breakage and repair in human lung adenocarcinoma cells exposed to etoposide and teniposide. *Cancer Res* 1985; 45: 3106–3112.

114. Capranico G, Zunino F, Kohn KW, Pommier Y. Sequence-selective topoisomerase II inhibition by anthracycline derivatives in SV40 DNA: relationship with DNA affinity and cytotoxicity. *Biochemistry* 1990; 29:562–569.

115. Bachur NR, Johnson R, Yu F, Hickey R, Applegreen N, Malkas L. Antihelicase activity of DNA-binding anticancer agents: relationship to guanosine-cytidine intercalator binding. *Mol Pharmacol* 1993; 44:1064–1069.

116. Zunino F, Capranico G. DNA topoisomerase II as the primary target of anti-tumor anthracyclines. *Anticancer Drug Design* 1990; 5:307–317.

117. Pommier Y. DNA topoisomerases and their inhibition by anthracyclines. In: Priebe W, eds. *Antracycline Antibiotics*. Washington, DC: American Chemical Society. 1995:183–203.

118. Solary E, Ling Y-H, Perez-Soler R, Priebe W, Pommier Y. Hydroxyrubicin, a deaminated derivative of doxorubicin, inhibits mammalian DNA topoisomerase II and partially circumvents multidrug resistance. *Int J Cancer* 1994; 57:1–10.

119. Capranico G, Butelli E, Zunino F. Change of the sequence specificity of daunorubicin-stimulated topoisomerase II DNA cleavage by epimerization of the amino group of the sugar moiety. *Cancer Res* 1995; 55:312–317.

120. Tewey KM, Rowe TC, Yang L, Halligan BD, Liu LF. Adriamycin-induced DNA damage mediated by mammalian DNA topoisomerase II. *Science* 1984; 226:466–468.

121. Zwelling LA, Kerrigan D, Michaels S. Cytotoxicity and DNA strand breaks by 5-iminodaunorubicin in mouse leukemia L1210 cells: comparison with adriamycin and 4′-(9-acridinylamino) methanesulfon-*m*-anisidide. *Cancer Res* 1982; 42:2687–2691.

122. Zwelling LA, Michaels S, Erickson LC, Ungerleider RS, Nichols M, Kohn KW. Protein-associated deoxyribonucleic acid strand breaks in L1210 cells treated with the deoxyribonucleic acid intercalating agents 4′-(9-acridinylamino) methanesulfon-m-anisidide and adriamycin. *Biochemistry* 1981; 20:6553–6563.

123. Capolongo L, Belvedere G, D'Incalci M. DNA damage and cytotoxicity of mitoxantrone and doxorubicin in doxorubicin-sensitive and -resistant human colon carcinoma cells. *Cancer Chemother Pharmacol* 1990; 25:430–434.

124. Neidle S, Jenkins TC. Molecular modeling to study DNA intercalation by antitumor drugs. *Methods Enzymol* 1991; 203:433–458.

125. Smith PJ, Morgan SA, Fox ME, Watson JV. Mitoxantrone-DNA binding and the induction of topoisomerase II associated DNA damage in multi-drug resistant small cell lung cancer cells. *Biochem Pharmacol* 1990; 40:2069–2078.

126. Leteurtre F, Kohlhagen G, Paull KD, Pommier Y. Topoisomerase II inhibition by anthrapyrazoles, DuP 937 & DuP 941 (Losoxanthrone) and cytotoxicity in the NCI cell screen. *J Natl Cancer Inst* 1994; 86:1239–1244.

127. De Isabella P, Capranico G, Palumbo M, Sissi C, Krapcho AP, Zunino F. Sequence selectivity of topoisomerase II DNA cleavage stimulated by mitoxantrone derivatives: relationship to drug DNA binding and cellular effects. *Mol Pharmacol* 1993; 43:715–721.

128. Capranico G, Palumbo M, Tinelli S, Mabilia M, Pozzan A, Zunino F. Conformational drug determinants of the sequence specificity of drug-stimulated topoisomerase II DNA cleavage. *J Mol Biol* 1994; 235:1218–1230.

129. Harker WG, Slade DL, Drake FH, Parr RL. Mitoxantrone resistance in HL-60 leukemia cells: reduced nuclear topoisomerase II catalytic actvity and drug-induced DNA cleavage in association with reduced expression of the topoisomerase IIb isoform. *Biochemistry* 1991; 30: 9953–9961.

130. Kamath N, Grabowski D, Ford J, Kerrigan D, Pommier Y, Ganapathi R. Overexpression of P-glycoprotein and alterations in topoisomerase II in P388 mouse leukemia cells selected in vivo for resistance to mitoxantrone. *Biochem Pharmacol* 1992; 44:937–945.

131. Yang C-HJ, Horton JK, Cowan KH, Schneider E. Cross-resistance to camptothecin analogues in mitoxantrone-resistant human breast carcinoma cell line is not due to DNA topoisomerase I alterations. *Cancer Res* 1995; 55:4004–4009.

132. Harker WG, Slade KL, Parr RL, Feldhoff PW, Sullivan DM, Holguin MH. Alterations in the topoisomerase IIα gene, messenger RNA, and subcellular protein distribution as well as reduced expression of the DNA topoisomerase IIβ enzyme in a mitoxantrone-resistant HL-60 human leukemia cell line. *Cancer Res* 1995; 55:1707–1716.

133. Cain BF, Atwell GJ. The experimental antitumor properties of three congeners of the acridylmethanesulphonanisilide(AMSA)series. *Eur J Cancer* 1974; 10:539–549.

134. Hayat M, Ostronoff M, Gilles G, Zambon E, Baume D, Moran A. Carde P, Droz J, Pico J. Salvage therapy with methyl-gag,high-dose ara-C,m-amsa, and ifosfamide(MAMI) for recur-

rent or refractory lymphoma. *Cancer Invest* 1990; 8:1–5.

135. Louie AC, Issel BF. Amsacrine (AMSA)—a clinical review. *J Clin Oncol* 1985; 3:562–592.

136. Covey JM, Kohn KW, Kerrigan D, Tilchen EJ, Pommier Y. Topoisomerase II-mediated DNA damage produced by 4′-(9-acridinylamino)methanesulfon-m-anisidide and related acridines in L1210 cells and isolated nuclei: relation to cytotoxicity. *Cancer Res* 1988; 48:860–865.

137. Zwelling LA, Mitchell MJ, Satitpunwaycha P, Mayes J, Altschuler E, Hinds M, Baguley BC. Relative activity of structural analogues of amsacrine against human leukemia cell lines containing amsacrine-sensitive or -resistant forms of topoisomerase II: use of computer simulation in new drug development. *Cancer Res* 1992; 52:209–217.

138. Harvey VJ, Hardy JR, Smith S, Grove W, Baguley BC. Phase III study of the amsacrine analogue CI-921(NSC343499) in non-small cell lung cancer. *Eur J Cancer* 1991; 27:1617–1620.

139. Sklarin NT, Wiernik PH, Grove WR, Benson L. A phase II trial of CI-921 in advanced malignancies. *Invest New Drugs* 1992; 10:309–312.

140. Pommier Y. Covey JM, Kerrigan D, Markovits J, Pham R. DNA unwinding and inhibition of mouse leukemia L1210 DNA topoisomerase I by intercalators. *Nucleic Acids Res* 1987; 15: 6713–6731.

141. Pommier Y, Minford JK, Schwartz RE, Zwelling LA, Kohn KW. Effects of the DNA intercalators 4′-(9-acridinylamino)methanesulfon-*m*-anisidide and 2-methyl-9-hydroxyellipticinium on topoisomerase II mediated DNA strand cleavage and strand passage. *Biochemistry* 1985; 24:6410–6416.

142. Nelson EM, Tewey KM, Liu LF. Mechanism of antitumor drug action: poisoning of mammalian DNA topoisomerase II on DNA by 4′-(9-acridinylamino)-methanesulfon-*m*-anisidide. *Proc Natl Acad Sci USA* 1984; 81:1361–1365.

143. Minford J, Pommier Y, Filipski J, Kohn KW, Kerrigan D, Mattern M, Michaels S, Schwartz R, Zwelling LA. Isolation of intercalator-dependent protein-linked DNA strand cleavage activity for cell nuclei and identification as topoisomerase II. *Biochemistry* 1986; 25:9–16.

144. Pommier Y, Covey J, Kerrigan D, Mattes W, Markovits J, Kohn KW. Role of DNA intercalation in the inhibition of purified mouse leukemia (L1210) DNA topoisomerase II by 9-aminoacridines. *Biochem Pharmacol* 1987; 36:3477–3486.

145. Darkin S, Ralph RK. Transport of AMSA drugs into cells. *FEBS Lett* 1985; 190:349–353.

146. Zwelling LA, Kerrigan D, Michaels S, Kohn KW. Cooperative sequestration of m AMSA in L1210 cells. *Biochem Pharmacol* 1982; 31:3269–3277.

147. Paoletti C, Le Pecq JB, Dat Xuong N, Juret P, Garnier H, Amiel JL, Rouessé J. Antitumor activity, pharmacology, and toxicity of ellipticines, ellipticinium and 9-hydroxy-derivatives: preliminary clinical trials of 2-methyl-9-hydroxy-ellipticinium(NSC-264-137). *Recent Res Cancer Res* 1980; 74:107–123.

148. Tewey KM, Chen GL, Nelson EM, Liu LF. Intercalative antitumor drugs interfere with the breakage-reunion reaction of mammalian DNA topoisomerase II. *J Biol Chem* 1984; 259:9182–9187.

149. Pommier Y, Schwartz RE, Zwelling LA, Kohn KW. Effects of DNA intercalating agents on topoisomerase II induced DNA strand cleavage in isolated mammalian cell nuclei. *Biochemistry* 1985; 24:6406–6410.

150. Zwelling LA, Michaels S, Kerrigan D, Pommier Y, Kohn KW. Protein-associated deoxyribonucleic acid strand breaks produced in mouse leukemia L1210 cells by ellipticine and 2-methyl-9-hydroxyellipticinium. *Biochem Pharmacol* 1982; 31:3261–3267.

151. Pommier Y, Schwartz RE, Kohn KW, Zwelling LA. Formation and rejoining of deoxyribonucleic acid double-strand breaks induced in isolated cell nuclei by antineoplastic intercalating agents. *Biochemistry* 1984; 23:3194–3201.

152. Pommier Y, Kerrigan D, Schwartz RE, Swack JA, McCurdy A. Altered DNA topoisomerase II activity in Chinese hamster cells resistant to topoisomerase II inhibitors. *Cancer Res* 1986; 46:3075–3081.

153. Pommier Y, Schwartz RE, Zwelling LA, Kerrigan D, Mattern MR, Charcosset JY, Jacquemin-Sablon A, Kohn KW. Reduced formation of protein-associated DNA strand breaks in Chinese hamster cells resistant to topoisomerase II inhibitors. *Cancer Res* 1986; 46:611–616.

154. Andersson BS, Beran M, Bakic M, Silberman LE, Newman RA, Zwelling LA. *In vitro* toxicity and DNA cleaving capacity of benzisoquinolinedione (nafidimide; NSC 308847) in human leukemia. *Cancer Res* 1987; 47:1040–1044.

155. Hsiang Y-H, Jiang JB, Liu LF. Topoisomerase II-mediated DNA cleavage by amonafide and structural analogs. *Mol Pharmacol* 1989; 36:371–376.

156. Earnshaw WC, Honda BM, Laskey RA, Thomas JO. Assembly of nucleosomes: the reaction involving *X. laevis* nucleoplasmin. *Cell* 1980; 21:373–383.

157. De Isabella P, Zunino F, Capranico G. Base sequence determinants of amonafide stimulation of topoisomerase II DNA cleavage. *Nucleic Acids Res* 1995; 23:223–229.

158. Markovits J, Linassier C, Fosse P, Couprie J, Pierre J, Jacquemin-Sablon A, Saucier J-M, Le Pecq JB, Larsen AK. Inhibitory effects of the tyrosine kinase inhibitor genistein on mammalian DNA topoisomerase II. *Cancer Res* 1989; 49:5111–5117.

159. Austin CA, Patel S, Ono K, Nakane H, Fisher LM. Site-specific DNA cleavage by mammalian DNA topoisomerase II induced by novel flavone and catechin derivatives. *Biochem J* 1992; 282:883–889.

160. Yamashita Y, Kawada S-Z, Nakano H. Induction of mammalian topoisomerase II dependent DNA cleavage by nonintercalative flavonoids, genistein and orobol. *Biochem Pharmacol* 1990; 39:737–744.

161. Sorensen BS, Jensen PS, Andersen AH, Christiansen K, Alsner J, Thomsen B, Westergaard O. Stimulation of topoisomerase II mediated DNA cleavage at specific sequence elements by the 2-nitroimidazole Ro 15-0216. *Biochemistry* 1990; 29:9507–9515.

162. Juang J-K, Huang HW, Chen C-M, Liu HJ. A new compound, withangulatin A, promotes type II DNA topoisomerase-mediated DNA damage. *Biochem Biophys Res Commun* 1989; 159:1128–1134.

163. Yamashita Y, Saitoh Y, Ando K, Takahashi K, Ohno H, Nakano H. Saintopin, a new antitumor antibiotic with topoisomerase II dependent DNA cleavage activity, from Paecilomyces. *J Antibiotics* 1990; 43:1344–1346.

164. Kawada S-Z, Yamashita Y, Fujii N, Nakano H. Induction of heat-stable topoisomerase II-DNA cleavable complex by nonintercalative terpenoides, terpentecin and clerocidin. *Cancer Res* 1991; 51:2922–2925.

165. Kawada S-Z, Yamashita Y, Uosaki Y, Gomi K, Iwasaki T, Takiguchi T, Nakano H. UCT48, a new antitumor antibiotic with topoisomerase II mediated DNA cleavage activity from *streptomyces sp. J Antibiot* 1992; 45:1182–1184.

166. Leteurtre F, Sackett DL, Madalengoitia J, Kohlhagen G, Macdonald T, Hamel E, Paull KD, Pommier Y. Azatoxin derivatives with potent and selective action on topoisomerase II. *Biochem Pharmacol* 1995; 49:1283–1290.

167. Solary E, Leteurtre F, Paull KD, Scudiero D, Hamel E, Pommier Y. Dual inhibition of topoisomerase II and tubulin polymerization by azatoxin, a novel cytotoxic agent. *Biochem Pharmacol* 1993; 45:2449–2456.

168. Yamasahita Y, Ashizawa T, Marimoto M, Hosomi J, Nakano H. Antitumor quinolones with mammalian topoisomerase II mediated DNA cleavage activity. *Cancer Res* 1992; 52:2818–2822.

169. Elsea SH, Osheroff N, Nitiss JL. Cytotoxicity of Quinolones toward eukaryotic cells. *J Biol Chem* 1992; 267:13,150–13,153.

170. Froelich-Ammon SJ, McGuirk PR, Gootz TD, Jefson MR, Osheroff N. Novel 1-8-bridged chiral quinolones with activity against topoisomerase II: stereospecificity of the eukaryotic enzyme. *Antimicrob Agent Chemother* 1993; 37:646–651.

171. Yoshinari T, Mano E, Arakawa H, Kurama M, Iguchi T, Nakagawa S, Tanaka N, Okura A. Stereo(C7)-dependent topoisomerase II inhibition and tumor growth suppression by a new quinolone, BO-2367. *Jpn J Cancer Res* 1993; 84:800–806.

172. Kong XB, Rubin L, Chen LI, Ciszewska G, Watanabe KA, Tong WP, Sirotnak FM, Chou TC. Topoisomerase II-mediated DNA cleavage activity and irreversibility of cleavable complex formation induced by DNA intercalator with alkylating capability. *Mol Pharmacol* 1992; 41:237–244.

173. Ono K, Ikegami Y, Nishizawa M, Andoh T. Menogaril, an anthracycline derivative, inhibits DNA topoisomerase II by stabilizing cleavable complexes. *Jpn J Cancer Res* 1992; 83:1018–1023.

174. Fujii N, Yamashita Y, Arima Y, Nagashima M, Nakano H. Induction of topoisomerase II-mediated DNA cleavage by the plant naphthoquinones plumbagin and shikonin. *Antimicrob Agents Chemother* 1992; 36:2589–2594.

175. Fujii N, Yamashita Y, Chiba S, Uosaki Y, Saitoh Y, Tuji Y, Nakano H. UCE6, a new antitumor antibiotic with topoisomerase I mediated DNA cleavage activity, from actinomycetes

(letter). *J Antibiot* 1993; 46:1173,1174.

176. Gupta M, Abdel-Megeed M, Hoki Y, Kohlhagen G. Paull K, Pommier Y. Eukaryotic DNA topoisomerase mediated DNA cleavage induced by a new inhibitor: NSC 665517. *Mol Pharmacol* 1995; 48:658.

177. Macdonald TL, Lehnert EK, Loper JT, Chow K-C, Ross WE. On the mechanism of interaction of DNA topoisomerase II with chemotherapeutic agents. In: Potmesil M, Kohn KW, eds. *DNA Topoisomerase in Cancer*. New York: Oxford University Press. 1991:199–214.

178. Eymin B, Solary E, Chevillard S, Dubrez L, Goldwasser F, Duchamp O, Genne P, Leteurtre F, Pommier Y. Cellular pharmacology of azatoxins (topoisomerase II and tubulin inhibitors) in P-glycoprotein-positive and negative cell lines. *Int J. Cancer* 1995; 63:268–275.

179. Rowe T, Kupfer G, Ross W. Inhibition of epipodophyllotoxin cytotoxicity by interference with topoisomerase-mediated DNA cleavage. *Biochem Pharmacol* 1985; 34:2483–2487.

180. Markovits J, Pommier Y, Mattern MR, Esnault C, Roques BP, Le Pecq JB, Kohn KW. Effects of the bifunctional antitumor intercalator ditercalinium on DNA in mouse leukemia L1210 cells and DNA topoisomerase II. *Cancer Res* 1986; 46:5821–5826.

181. Fesen M, Pommier Y. Mammalian topoisomerase II activity is modulated by the DNA minor groove binder distamyhcin in simian virus 40 DNA. *J Biol Chem* 1989; 19:11,354–11,359.

182. Drake FH, Hofmann GA, Mong SM, Bartus JO, Hertzberg RP, Johnson RK, Mattern MR, Mirabelli CK. In vitro and intracellular inhibition of topoisomerase II by the antitumor agent merbarone. *Cancer Res* 1989; 49:2578–2583.

183. Ishida R, Miki T, Narita T, Yui R, Sato M, Utsumi KR, Tanabe K, Andoh T. Inhibition of intracellular topoisomerase II by antitumor bis(2,6-dioxopiperazine) derivatives: modes of cell growth inhibition distinct from that of cleavable complex-forming inhibitors. *Cancer Res* 1991; 51:4909–4916.

184. Tanabe K, Ikegami R, Andoh T. Inhibition of topoisomerase II by antitumor agent bis(2,6-dioxopiperazine). *Cancer Res* 1991; 51:4903–4908.

185. Bojanowski K, Lelievre S, Markovits J, Couprie J, Jacquemin-Sablon A, Larsen AK. Suramin is an inhibitor of DNA topoisomerase II in vitro and in chinese hamster fibrosarcoma cells. *Proc Natl Acad Sci USA* 1992; 89:3025–3029.

186. Gedik CM, Collins AR. Comparison of effects of fostriecin, novobiocin, and camptothecin, inhibitors of DNA topoisomerases, on DNA replication and repair in human cells. *Nucleic Acids Res* 1990; 18:1007–1013.

187. Frosina G, Rossi O. Effect of topoisomerase poisoning by antitumor drugs VM 26, fostriecin and camptothecin on DNA repair replication by mammalian cell extracts. *Carcinogenesis* 1992; 13:1371–1377.

188. Boritzki TJ, Wolfard TS, Besserer JA, Jackson RC, Fry DW. Inhibition of type II topoisomerase by fostriecin. *Biochem Pharmacol* 1988; 37:4063–4068.

189. Jensen PB, Jensen PS, Demant EJF, Friche E, Sorensen BS, Sehested M, Wassermann K, Vindelov L, Westergaard O, Hensen HH. Antagonistic effect of aclarubicin on daunorubicin-induced cytotoxicity in human small cell lung cancer cells: relationship to DNA integrity and topoisomerase II. *Cancer Res* 1991; 51:5093–5099.

190. Herman EH, Witiak K, Hellman K, Waravdekar VS. Biological properties of ICRF-159 and related bis(dioxopiperazine) compounds. In: Garattini A, Goldin F, Hawking F, Kopin IJ, eds. *Advances in Pharmacology and Chemotherapy*. New York: Academic. 1982:249–291.

191. Ishida R, Sato M, Narita T, Utsumi KR, Nishimoto T, Morita T, Nagata H, Andoh T. Inhibition of DNA topoisomerase II by ICRF-193 induces polyploidization by uncoupling chromosome dynamics from other cell cycle events. *J Biol Chem* 1994; 26:1341–1351.

192. Takasuga Y, Andoh T, Yamashita J, Yagura T. ICRF-193, an inhibitor of topoisomerase II, demonstrates that DNA replication in sperm nuclei reconstituted in Xenopus egg extracts does not require chromatin decondensation. *Exp Cell Res* 1995; 217:378–384.

193. Narita T, Yaguchi S, Komatsu T, Takase M, Hoshino A, Inaba M, Tsukagoshi S. Antitumor activity of MST-16, a novel derivative of bis(2,6-dioxopiperazine), in murine models. *Cancer Chemother Pharmacol* 1990; 26:193–197.

194. Narita T, Koide Y, Yaguchi S, Kimura S, Izumisawa Y, Takase M, Inaba M, Tsukagoshi S. Antitumor activities and schedule dependence of orally administered MST-16, a novel derivative of bis(2,6-dioxopiperazine). *Cancer Chemother Pharmacol* 1991; 28:235–240.

195. Ohno R, Yamada K, Hirano M, Shirakawa S, Tanaka M, Oguri T, Kodera Y, Mitomo Y, Ikeda Y, Yokomaku S, et al. Phase II study: treatment of non-Hodgkin's lymphoma with an oral antitumor derivative of bis(2,6-dioxopiperazine). *J Natl Cancer Inst* 1992; 84:435–438.

196. Ichihashi T, Kiyoi H, Fukutani H, Kubo K, Yamauchi T, Naoe T, Yamada K, Ohno R. Effective treatment of adult T cell leukemia/lymphoma with a novel oral antitumor agent, MST-16. *Oncology* 1992; 49:333–335.

197. Ohno R, Masaoka T, Shirakawa S, Sakamoto S, Hirano M, Hanada S, Yasunage K, Yokomaku S, Mitomo Y, Nagai K, et al. Treatment of adult T-cell leukemia/lymphoma with MST-16, a new oral antitumor drug and a derivative of bis(2,6-dioxopiperazine). The MST-16 Study Group. *Cancer* 1993; 71:2217–2221.

198. Seifert CF, Nesser ME, Thompson DF. Dexrazoxane in the prevention of doxorubicin-induced cardiotoxicity [published erratum appears in Ann Pharmacother 1994 Dec;28(12):1413]. *Ann Pharmacother* 1994; 28:1063–1072.

199. Buss JL, Hasinoff BB. Ferrous ion strongly promotes the ring opening of the hydrolysis intermediates of the antioxidant cardioprotective agent dexrazoxane (ICRF-187). *Arch Biochem Biophys* 1995; 317:121–127.

200. Buss JL, Hasinoff BB. The one-ring open hydrolysis product intermediates of the cardioprotective agent ICRF-187 (dexrazoxane) displace iron from iron-anthracycline complexes. *Agents Actions* 1993; 40:86–95.

201. Cooney DA, Covey JM, Kang GJ, Dalal M, McMahon JB, Johns DG. Initial mechanistic studies with merbarone (NSC 336628). *Biochem Pharmacol* 1985; 34:3395–3398.

202. Chen M, Beck WT. Differences in inhibition of chromosome separation and G2 arrest by DNA topoisomerase II inhibitors merbarone and VM-26. *Cancer Res* 1995; 55:1509–1515.

203. Chen M, Beck WT. Teniposide-resistant CEM cells, which express mutant DNA topoisomerase IIα, when treated with the non-complex-stabilizing inhibitors of the enzyme, display no cross-resistance and reveal aberrant functions of the mutant enzyme. *Cancer Res* 1993; 53: 5946–5953.

204. Flanigan RC, Saiers JH, Wolf M, Kraut EH, Smith AY, Blumenstein B, Crawford ED. Phase II evaluation of merbarone in renal cell carcinoma. *Invest New Drugs* 1994; 12:147–149.

205. Poplin EA, Tangen CM, Harvey WH, Macdonald JS. Hepatoma/merbarone. A Southwest Oncology Group study. *Invest New Drugs* 1994; 12:337–340.

206. Jones DV, Jr., Ajani JA, Winn RJ, Daugherty KR, Levin B, Krakoff IH. A phase II study of merbarone in patients with adenocarcinoma of the pancreas. *Cancer Invest* 1993; 11:667–669.

207. Kraut EH, Bendetti J, Balcerzak SP, Doroshow JH. Phase II trial of merbarone in soft tissue sarcoma. A Southwest Oncology Group study. *Invest New Drugs* 1992; 10:347–249.

208. Ajani JA, Winn R, Baez L, Pollock T, Maher T, Hallinan-Fueger B, Newman J. Phase II study of merbarone (NSC 336628) in patients with advanced gastric carcinoma. *Cancer Invest* 1994; 12:488–490.

209. Chang AY, Kim K, Glick J, Anderson T, Karp D, Johnson D. Phase II study of taxol, merbarone, and piroxantrone in stage IV non-small-cell lung cancer: The Eastern Cooperative Oncology Group Results (*see* comments). *J Natl Cancer Inst* 1993; 85:388–394.

210. Jackson RC, Fry DW, Boritzki TJ, Roberts BJ, Hook KE, Leopold WR. The biochemical pharmacology of CI-920, a structurally novel antibiotic with antileukemic activity. *Adv Enzyme Regul* 1985; 23:193–215.

211. Scheithauer W, Von Hoff DD, Clark GM, Shillis JL, Elslager EF. In vitro activity of the novel antitumor antibiotic fostriecin (CI-920) in a human tumor cloning assay. *Eur J Cancer Clin Oncol* 1986; 22:921–926.

212. Baguley BC, Calveley SB, Crowe KK, Fray LM, O'Rourke SA, Smith GP. Comparison of the effects of flavone acetic acid, fostriecin, homoharringtonine and tumour necrosis factor alpha on colon 38 tumours in mice. *Eur J Cancer Clin Oncol* 1989; 25:263–269.

213. Roberge M, Tudan C, Hung SM, Harder KW, Jirik FR, Anderson H. Antitumor drug fostriecin inhibits the mitotic entry checkpoint and protein phosphatases 1 and 2A. *Cancer Res* 1994; 54:6115–6121.

214. Guo XW, Th'ng JP, Swank RA, Anderson HJ, Tudan C, Bradbury EM, Roberge M. Chromosome condensation induced by fostriecin does not require p34cdc2 kinase activity and histone H1 hyperphosphorylation, but is associated with enhanced histone H2A and H3 phosphorylation. *EMBO J* 1995; 14:976–985.

8 The Taxoids

Marie-Christine Bissery, PhD and François Lavelle, PhD

CONTENTS

1. INTRODUCTION

Paclitaxel and docetaxel belong to the taxoid family, a new class of antineoplastic drugs. The name taxoids refers to compounds, natural or modified, having a taxane skeleton.

Paclitaxel (Taxol®, NSC 125973) was extracted in the late 1960s from the bark of the Pacific Yew, *Taxus brevifolia*. Because of the scarcity of the drug and the difficulties of formulation, the development was initially slow. Once these problems were solved, development accelerated. Docetaxel (Taxotere®, PR 56976) was obtained by hemisynthesis, using the starting material, 10-deacetyl baccatin III extracted from the needles of the European Yew tree, *Taxus baccata* (Fig. 1). This drug was more readily available because of the renewability of the source, and somewhat more soluble, and thus its development was rapid. Paclitaxel consists of an eight-member taxane ring with a four-member oxetane ring and a side chain at the C-13 position (Fig. 1). Docetaxel differs from paclitaxel in the 10-position on the baccatin ring and in the 3'-position of the lateral chain (Fig. 1).

This chapter will summarize the key steps in the development process of these two new exciting antitumor agents.

2. DISCOVERY

2.1. Paclitaxel

In 1960, a vast screening program for antitumor agents derived from plants was initiated by the Cancer Chemotherapy National Service Center under J. L. Hartwell (*1–3*). In 1962, a US Department of Agriculture botanist, A. S. Barclay, collected 650

From: *Cancer Therapeutics: Experimental and Clinical Agents*
Edited by: B. Teicher Humana Press Inc., Totowa, NJ

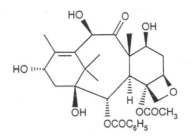

10-Deacetyl Baccatin III

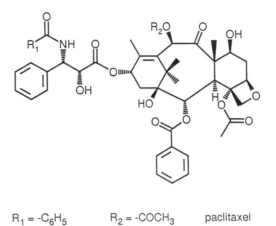

R_1 = -C_6H_5 R_2 = -$COCH_3$ paclitaxel

R_1 = -$OC(CH_3)_3$ R_2 = -H   docetaxel

Fig. 1. Structures of paclitaxel (Taxol®), docetaxel (Taxotere®) and 10-deacetyl-baccatin III.

samples in the West Coast States of the US, including samples of *T. brevifolia*, the Pacific Yew tree. Initial screening of crude extracts showed cytotoxicity toward 9KB cells derived from a nasopharyngeal tumor. M. Wall at Research Triangle Institute was particularly interested in plants with 9KB activity because of his previous experience with *Camptotheca* extracts. This is why he received among other plants, *T. brevifolia*. The isolation procedure of the drug substance was laborious and involved numerous steps (ethanol extraction; partition of the ethanolic residue between water and chloroform; followed by Craig countercurrent distribution), each of them being monitored by an in vivo assay using the rat Walker 256 carcinosarcoma (*2–4*) or/and the P1534 leukemia (*1*). Approximately 0.5 g of paclitaxel could be isolated starting with 12 kg of dried stem and bark (yield 0.004%). The isolation of the pure compound was achieved in 1966 (*1*). In 1971 the structure of paclitaxel was published, and antitumor efficacy was reported in L1210, P388, and P1534 leukemias, and in Walker carcinosarcoma 256 (*5*). However, the activity levels seen against the L1210 and P388 leukemia models were very modest compared to that of other compounds. The only tumor system showing good efficacy, the P1534 leukemia, was not thought to be of predictive value (*1*). Finally, the compound was poorly soluble (i.e., the in vivo evaluation was performed with drug suspension), and supplies were difficult to obtain. Because of this, paclitaxel was not selected for further preclinical development (*1*). Luckily in 1974–1975, extensive in vivo testing was conducted by the National Cancer Institute (NCI), and paclitaxel showed high activity against the murine B16 melanoma model, newly introduced to the NCI screen (*1*). This prompted the NCI to evaluate the compound further. Additional efficacy was noted in colon 26 carcinoma and in MX-1 human breast carcinoma implanted under the renal capsule in nude mice (*6*). However, no efficacy was observed at that time in most of the other models tested, colon 38 adenocarcinoma, Lewis lung carcinoma, CD8F1 mammary, and human xenografts implanted subcutaneously (*6*). Preliminary studies of its mechanism of action indicated that it was a spindle poison that inhibited the cell proliferation at the G2-M phase in the cell cycle and that it blocked mitosis (*7*). The turning point occurred with the demonstration that paclitaxel had a unique mechanism of action by Horwitz. It was established that paclitaxel stabilized microtubules and inhibited depolymerization back to tubulin. This differed from the mechanism of action of other spindle poisons, such as vinca-alkaloids, that bind to tubulin and inhibit its polymerization (*8*). On the basis of the in vivo B16 melanoma efficacy and the uniqueness of mechanism of action, the NCI initiated a very large effort to collect barks and wood to obtain enough material to initiate clinical trials (*1–3*).

Formulation was also an issue, and in 1980, it was reported that toxicology studies would proceed if a satisfactory formulation was developed (*6*). These toxicology and clinical formulation development studies were completed by 1983. Clinical Phase I trials started in 1983. Progress of these trials was hampered by hypersensitivity reactions, which led to the premature closure of some Phase I studies (*9,10*). Since these reactions were observed more commonly with infusions of shorter durations, a decision was made to pursue clinical trials using a 24-h continuous infusion, with premedication to lessen the reactions. The dose-limiting toxicity was neutropenia in seven out of the nine Phase I trial initiated (*1,9,10*).

The final major step in paclitaxel's development was the recognition of its activity against ovarian cancer with responses in approx 30% of patients, many of them having cisplatin or carboplatin refractory disease. These clinical results were reported in 1989 (*11*) (i.e., 6 yr after first clinical entry). Even as evidence of paclitaxel's activity increased, with the report of efficacy in breast and nonsmall-cell lung carcinoma (*12,13*), the clinical development was still prevented by the supply shortage. To address this issue, the NCI sought the assistance of the pharmaceutical industry. A cooperative research and development agreement (CRADA) was awarded to Bristol Myers Squibb in 1991 (*3,9*). In 1992, the company filed a New Drug Application. The Food and Drug Administration approved paclitaxel that same year for the treatment of patients whose ovarian carcinoma had progressed with other chemotherapy (*3,9*) and, in 1994, for metastatic breast cancer.

2.2. Docetaxel

The Institut de Chimie des Substances Naturelles (ICSN) of the Centre National de la Recherche Scientifique and Rhône-Poulenc were interested by the ongoing work on paclitaxel in the US and, in particular, of the newly described mechanism of action of paclitaxel (*8*). The ICSN had expertise in the chemistry and the biochemistry of anti-mitotic compounds, especially vinca-alkaloids, and it was using a test to measure the

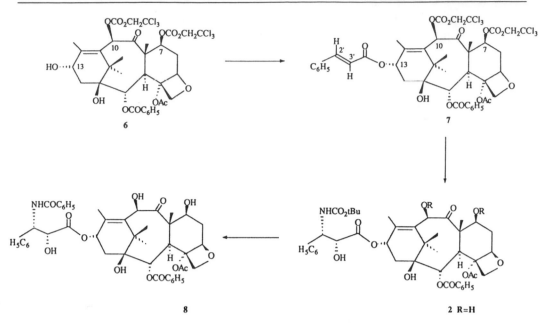

Fig. 2. First hemi-synthesis of docetaxel *2* and 10-deacetyl-paclitaxel *8*.

inhibition of polymerization or depolymerization of tubulin, based on the Shelanski's method (*14*). Finally, the ICSN had a large supply of *T. baccata*, the European species of yew tree that is widely dispersed in France and Europe. Therefore, in 1979, the ICSN decided to undertake research in this area. In 1980, Rhône-Poulenc decided to stop a 20-year period of research on anthracyclines and signed a research agreement concerning taxoids with the ICSN with three main objectives: to explore the chemistry of taxoids, bearing in mind the issue of supply, to build structure–activity relationships, and to select new and patentable antitumor compounds in these series.

From the beginning, P. Potier and colleagues were convinced that semisynthesis was the only realistic approach for preparing paclitaxel and analogs in sufficient quantities for pharmaceutical research and clinical trials. They decided to explore systematically and extensively the different chemical components present in the European yew tree *T. baccata*, in particular in the needles, a renewable source of biological material. The purification of the components present in the needles was monitored by measuring their interactions with tubulin purified from calf brain (*14*). This purification led to the isolation of an abundant precursor of paclitaxel, 10-deacetyl-baccatin III, with a yield of 1 g/kg of fresh needles (*15*) (Fig. 1). This yield was important especially in light of the 150 mg of paclitaxel that could be extracted from 1 kg of dried bark (*16*). It was considered an interesting precursor for hemisynthesis of paclitaxel and other taxoids (*17*). It was 50- to 100-fold less active than paclitaxel in inhibiting microtubules depolymerization (*18*). The closer precursor, baccatin III, was also detected but at much lower concentrations.

2.2.1. First Access to Paclitaxel: Discovery of Docetaxel (Fig. 2)

10-Deacetylbaccatin III, protected at both the C-7 and C-10 positions (compound 6), was converted into the cinnamoyl ester at the C-13 position (compound 7) with a 90% yield. The cinnamic double bond was then oxyminated (*19*), leading to docetaxel (compound 2) and to 10-deacetylpaclitaxel (compound 8) after cleavage of the Boc

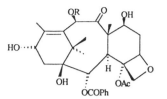

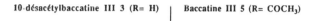

10-désacétylbaccatine III **3** (R= H) | Baccatine III **5** (R= COCH$_3$)

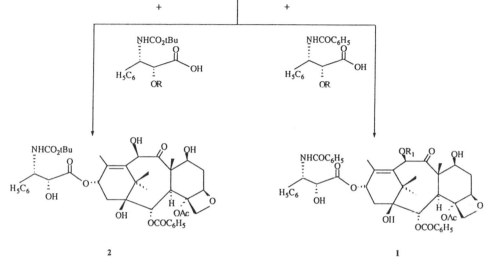

Fig. 3. Convergent synthesis of docetaxel *2* and paclitaxel *1*.

and reacylation (*20*). Paclitaxel was obtained using the same pathway, starting from baccatin III. Similar to all new derivatives of paclitaxel, docetaxel was tested for its interaction with tubulin/microtubules and, surprisingly, was found to be twice more potent than paclitaxel in inhibiting the cold-induced reaction of microtubule depolymerization. At the end of 1985, a small batch of docetaxel was available, and the first demonstration of its in vitro cytotoxicity and in vivo antitumor properties was obtained in the Oncology Department of Rhône-Poulenc, using P388 leukemia. Further in vivo evaluation revealed efficacy against L1210, Lewis lung carcinoma and B16 melanoma (*16,21*).

However, although very successful, this first semisynthetic approach was not applicable at an industrial scale owing to the use of toxic and very expensive reagents, such as osmium tetraoxide.

2.2.2. CONVERGENT SYNTHESIS OF TAXOIDS (FIG. 3)

The convergent synthesis of paclitaxel and docetaxel was performed by direct esterification of 10-deacetyl-baccatin III or baccatin III, with the acids corresponding to the lateral chains present in paclitaxel and docetaxel, respectively. The first asymetric synthesis of the C-13 phenylisoserine chain of paclitaxel was done by Denis and collaborators (*22*). The lateral chain of docetaxel was prepared using benzaldehyde and terbutyl chloroacetate (*23*). Finally, esterification of the acids by baccatin III and 10-deacetyl-baccatin III yielded paclitaxel (*24*) and docetaxel (*23*), respectively. Since these first experiments, the yield of the esterification methods and of the synthesis of the lateral chain have been improved by different teams (*25–28*).

In 1989, the compound was obtained in sufficient amount to initiate extensive pharmacological and toxicological studies and a suitable formulation for iv evaluation was developed. Using the sc B16 melanoma murine model, it was found that iv docetaxel was more active than paclitaxel at an equitoxic dose (*29*).

The compound was also found to be highly active against a large number of murine tumor models, most importantly when treated at an advanced stage (i.e., measurable disease), and schedule studies revealed that the compound was schedule-independent (*29*). Finally, a pharmacokinetic/distribution study in tumor-bearing mice showed that at optimal dosage, the area under the plasma and tumor concentration vs time curves (AUC) were much higher than the AUC required to kill human cancer cell lines in vitro. Toxicology studies were performed according to the NCI guidelines.

Phase I clinical trials were initiated in 1990 in Europe and in the US (*30*). Five different schedules were investigated up front in record time. At the end of the Phase I trials, it was shown that neutropenia was the major dose-limiting toxicity, and responses were reported in different tumor types. Based on considerations, such as dose intensity, toxicity profile, and preclinical data, suggesting absence of schedule dependency, the recommended dose and schedule for Phase II studies were 100 mg/m^2 adminisetred as a 1-h infusion every 3 wk, without prophylactic measures. Broad Phase II testing was initiated in 1992 throughout Europe, North America, and Japan, and a CRADA was signed by the NCI and Rhône-Poulenc Rorer. A broad spectrum of efficacy was reported, including breast, nonsmall-cell lung, and ovarian cancers. A New Drug Application was filed in 1994, and docetaxel has now been approved in more than 30 countries.

3. MECHANISM OF ACTION OF TAXOIDS

3.1. The Cellular Target of Taxoids

Together with actin microfilaments and intermediate filaments, microtubules form the cytoskeleton of eukaryotic cells. The microtubules are involved in a variety of cell functions, including chromosome movement and the regulation of cell shape and motility (*31*). These activities are modulated through associations with several biochemical components, such as guanosine triphosphate (GTP), and a wide range of proteins, the microtubule-associated proteins (MAPs). When a cell begins to divide, interphasic microtubules totally vanish and the mitotic spindle assembles. The depolymerization of mitotic spindle microtubules is essential for specific mitotic events, such as the movement of the chromosomes to the metaphase plate and their correct segregation during anaphase (*32*). Microtubules are long, hollow cylinders assembled from a heterodimeric (α/β) globular protein called tubulin. They consist of 13 aligned protofilaments within which the tubulin subunits interact through longitudinal and lateral bonds (*33*). Not all the tubulin pool assembles into microtubules: a steady state is maintained between assembled tubulin and a concentration of free tubulin called the critical concentration.

3.2. Taxoids Stabilize Microtubules

The polymerization of tubulin purified from mammalian brain usually enhances the turbidity of the solution; thus, the degree of polymerization can be monitored simply by measuring turbidity (*34*). Figure 4 depicts, for example, the effects of doce-

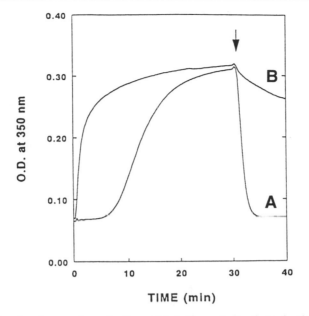

Fig. 4. Effect of docetaxel on polymerization of tubulin and depolymerization of microtubules. Tubulin was polymerized by heating from 3 to 37 °C. Depolymerization of microtubules was obtained by cooling from 37 to 3 °C (arrow). Polymerization or depolymerization was monitored by following the turbidimetry at 350 nm. (A) 10 μM porcine brain tubulin. (B) 10 μM tubulin and 3 μM docetaxel

taxel on the kinetics of tubulin assembly and disassembly. The lag time corresponding to the activation and nucleation of tubulin is notably reduced, and the rate of polymerization is increased (*35*). Finally, microtubules, stabilized by taxoids, do not depolymerize on cold treatment. In fact, paclitaxel and docetaxel analogs are usually evaluated on the basis of the drug concentration that inhibits half of the cold-induced depolymerization. Docetaxel is about twice as efficient as paclitaxel in this respect (*36,37*). The thermodynamic parameters of tubulin assembly are also modified by the taxoids, and the critical concentration is significantly reduced in the presence of paclitaxel (*8*). Docetaxel is twice as efficient as paclitaxel in decreasing the critical concentration of tubulin assembly (*38*).

It should be pointed out that the mechanism of action of the taxoids is unique, since all other known mitotic spindle poisons, in particular, the vinca-alkaloids, shift the tubulin-microtubule equilibrium toward tubulin (*39*) (Fig. 5).

3.3. Characterization of the Interaction Site

Tritiated paclitaxel cosediments with microtubules and dissociates rapidly on the addition of paclitaxel. Thus, a rapid and reversible equilibrium exists between paclitaxel and the microtubules. There is only one high-affinity binding site of paclitaxel per α/β tubulin subunit, indicating that the interaction between microtubules and paclitaxel is specific. The equilibrium dissociation constant was originally found to be 870 n*M* (*40*). Docetaxel competes with paclitaxel for binding to the microtubules, but its equilibrium dissociation constant is two times less, i.e., it has better affinity (*38*). This difference could account for the higher efficiency of docetaxel to promote tubulin polymerization, to stabilize microtubules against cold-induced disassembly, and to

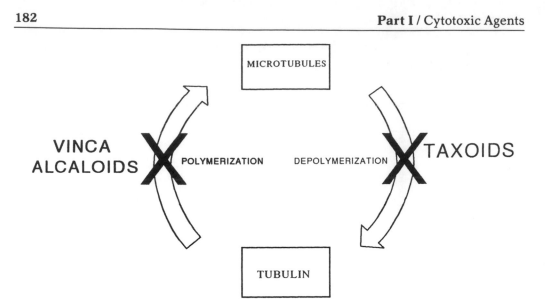

Fig. 5. Mechanism of action of vinca alkaloids and taxoids.

decrease the critical concentration of tubulin assembly. To acquire further insight into the taxoid–microtubule interaction at the molecular level, it is essential to locate the taxoid binding site. So far, it is known that the binding of taxoids is linked to the polymerization process. Furthermore, no binding of taxoids to dimeric tubulin has been detected, indicating that the site is located on assembled tubulin (*38*). This site does not overlap those of other known ligands, such as colchicine, podophyllotoxin, vinblastine, or GTP (*41,42*).

3.4. Models of the Mechanism of Action

Paclitaxel-bound microtubules, the structure of which has been resolved at 3 nm employing X-ray scattering, appear to be constituted of 12 protofilaments instead of the 13 protofilaments usually observed (*43,44*). The solution structure of microtubules induced by docetaxel has been also characterized using the same technique (*45*). The substructures of the microtubule walls are identical in paclitaxel- and docetaxel-induced microtubules; however, the population of docetaxel microtubules has an average of 13 protofilaments like the control microtubules. It is proposed that the chemical substitutions present in docetaxel side chain in its binding site increases slightly the contact angle between adjacent protofilaments. The simple working hypothesis is that taxoids bind between adjacent tubulin molecules, and such a hypothesis is fully compatible with the observed thermodynamic behavior of the taxoid-induced microtubule assembly system (*43*).

4. ANTITUMOR PROPERTIES

4.1. In Vitro Activities

4.1.1. CELLULAR CYTOTOXICITY

Both taxoids have been found extremely potent against a wide variety of murine and human cancer cell lines. Using the COMPARE computer program, it was concluded that docetaxel response profile on 50 human tumor cell lines in the new NCI screening panel, correlated with the data pattern of test agents acting on the tubulin/ microtubule system, the closest compound being paclitaxel (NCI, unpublished results). Several in vitro studies have been done comparing their activities under various experimental conditions (liquid medium, semisolid medium, short- and long-term exposures). The cytotoxicity of paclitaxel and docetaxel at submicromolar concentrations was compared in several murine, P388, SVras, and human tumor cell lines, breast Calc18, colon HCT 116, bladder T24, and nasopharyngeal KB (46). Docetaxel was found to be 1.3- to 12-fold more potent than paclitaxel. The cytotoxic properties of paclitaxel and docetaxel were also compared against nine cell lines established from human ovarian tumors and having intrinsic or acquired resistance to cisplatin. These cell lines were not crossresistant to the taxoids, and docetaxel was found to be active at a twofold lower concentrations than paclitaxel (47).

In addition, the activities of docetaxel and paclitaxel, in a human tumor cloning stem cell assay (starting from fresh human tumor biopsies), were compared at concentrations of taxoids similar to the plasma levels obtained after treatment of patients (48,49). Melanoma, breast, lung, ovarian, and colon tumors cells were significantly inhibited, regardless of the schedule of incubation (1-h exposure or continuous exposure for 14–28 d). Interestingly, 29 samples were found to be more sensitive to docetaxel, whereas 13 were more sensitive to paclitaxel, suggesting partial crossresistance between these two drugs (49). Finally, the in vitro cellular effects of docetaxel and paclitaxel have been recently assessed against a wide range of human normal and tumor samples, including tumor cell lines, primary cultures from tumor biopsies and normal bone marrow samples (50). IC_{50} (50% inhibitory concentrations) values of the two taxoids were in the nanomolar range and docetaxel appeared to be two- to fourfold more cytotoxic than paclitaxel (50).

4.1.2. MECHANISM OF CYTOTOXICITY AND CELLULAR EFFECTS

Uptake and efflux studies were performed on P388 leukemia cells in vitro with radiolabeled docetaxel and paclitaxel. Uptake experiments revealed that a threefold higher intracellular concentration of docetaxel was obtained as compared to paclitaxel, for the same initial extracellular concentration (0.1 μM) (51). Efflux studies revealed that the half-time of efflux of docetaxel from P388 cells was at least three times slower than that of paclitaxel (150 vs 45 min, respectively).

Thus, the higher potency of docetaxel observed in vitro may be explained by the combination of its higher affinity for microtubules, its higher achievable intracellular concentration, and the slower cellular efflux.

Cell-cycle studies revealed that paclitaxel was mainly cytotoxic during mitosis (M phase), as demonstrated by experiments on CHO and A 2780 ovarian tumor cell lines (52). Inhibition of cytokinesis has been observed, but some cells can progress through new cell cycles, leading to the formation of polyploid cells (53,54). Using synchronized HCT116 cells, it was demonstrated that paclitaxel inhibits formation of mitotic spindles in cells without affecting function of preformed spindles and without arresting cells in mitosis (54). Docetaxel has been found to be more active on proliferating than on nonproliferating KB cells (46) and to inhibit mitosis in several cell lines, such as J82 and KB (55). Surprisingly, using synchronized HeLa cells, it has been shown that docetaxel exerts cell killing specifically during the S phase of the cell cycle; no

Table 1
In Vivo Antitumor Activity of Paclitaxel Against Human Tumor Xenografts

sc Human tumor	Highest nontoxic iv dosage mg/kg/dose	Schedule days	Activity[a] rating
A 2780 ovarian	18	7, 9, 11, 13, 15	+ + +
LX-1 lung	24	5, 7, 9, 11, 13	+ + + +
H 2981 lung	24	5, 7, 9, 11, 13	+ +
L 2987 lung	36	14, 16, 18, 20, 22	+ + +
RCA colon	36	4, 6, 8, 10, 12	> + +
HCT-116 colon	36	3, 5, 7, 9, 11	> + + +
A431 vulva	36	3, 5, 7, 9, 11	+ + +

[a] Activity rating: + + + + = highly active (log cell kill > 2.8), + + + = highly active (log cell kill = 2.0 to 2.8), + + = active (log cell kill = 1.3–1.9; T/C ≥ 150% for L1210, + = active (log cell kill = 0.7–1.2 for s.c. tumors, T/C = 125–174% for P388), − = inactive.

cytotoxicity was observed during mitosis, a different situation from what is observed with paclitaxel (56).

Finally, it was found that paclitaxel greatly increases the pool of polymerized tubulin in cells, and new short microtubules free in the cytoplasm were observed (57). In addition, at high concentration, it induced the formation of microtubules bundles (58). Using J82 human bladder and KB 3-1 human carcinoma cells, it was shown that paclitaxel and docetaxel lead to the formation of bundles and asters in a dose- and time-dependent manner (55). Asters were observed in mitotic cells, and bundles were seen in interphase cells. The effects of docetaxel as compared to paclitaxel appeared at a twofold lower concentration (55).

4.2. In Vivo Activity

Paclitaxel and even more docetaxel have been studied in many murine tumor models and human tumor xenografts.

4.2.1. PACLITAXEL

The development of an adequate formulation for paclitaxel led to a re-evaluation of its in vivo antitumor efficacy, using better experimental conditions, i.e., avoiding the previous ip/ip evaluation and administering the drug iv at a site different from the tumor site. The formulation used was 10% Cremophor®, 10% ethanol, 80% NaCl 0.9%. These studies have been recently reviewed, and most of them were performed after initial clinical trials (59,60). Indeed, these studies demonstrated that paclitaxel delivered iv was active against several tumors implanted in distal sites and treated at an early stage: sc Madison 109 murine lung carcinoma and A 431 vulva, A 2780 ovarian, H 2981 and LX-1 lung, and RCA and HCT-116 colon human tumor xenografts implanted under the renal capsule of nude mice (Table 1) (60). When administered sc five times weekly for three consecutive weeks, paclitaxel caused the complete regression of a human breast tumor xenograft, and significantly delayed the growth of endometrial, ovarian, brain, tongue, and lung human tumor xenografts (61). Paclitaxel was also evaluated against ovarian carcinoma xenografts HOC8, HOC18, and HOC22, and was found to have similar efficacy to docetaxel (62).

Table 2
In Vivo Antitumor Activity of Docetaxel Against Human Tumor Xenografts

sc Human tumor	Highest nontoxic iv dosage mg/kg/dose	Schedule days	Activity[a] rating
Calc 18 mammary	32.2	11, 15, 19	+ + +
MX-1 mammary	22	11, 15, 19	+ + + +
LX-1 lung	22	9, 13, 17	+ +
SKMEL-2 melanoma	33	27, 31, 35	+ + + +
CX-1 ovarian	15	12, 16, 20	+ + +
KM20L2 ovarian	33	14, 18, 22	+ +
OVCAR-3	33	3, 7, 11	+ + + +

[a] For activity rating, *see* Table 1.

Further schedule-dependency studies were performed and showed that daily injection for 7 d was the best schedule as opposed to longer spaced administration (*60*).

4.2.2. Docetaxel

The experimental antitumor activity of docetaxel has been evaluated against a panel of 30 tumors of mice and human tumors xenografted in nude mice, representing a variety of tissue types and chemosensitivity patterns. The tumors were grafted in distal sites, and several tumors were treated at advanced and metastatic stages. Dose response was evaluated in all trials to determine accurately the maximum tolerated dose. The formulation used was a 1:1 ethanol polysorbate 80 solution, administered after a 1:10 dilution in glucose 5% in water (*29*). Docetaxel had a broad spectrum of antitumor activity, since 28/30 models responded to this agent (*29,63–65*) (Tables 2 and 3). The experimental antitumor activities of paclitaxel and docetaxel were compared by testing these drugs against B16 melanoma, a tumor sensitive to taxoids using an intermittent schedule, every 2 d × 3. Antitumor activity was expressed by the tumor growth delay (T-C) and by the log cell kill (LCK) of tumor cells obtained at the maximal tolerated dose (MTD) of each drug. According to these criteria, docetaxel was approximately two times more active and potent than paclitaxel (docetaxel: T-C = 12.2 d, LCK = 2.9, MTD = 11.3 mg/kg/d; paclitaxel: T-C = 4.7 d, LCK = 1.1, MTD = 21.7 mg/kg/d) (*29*) (Fig. 6). Among the murine models tested, good activity was observed, with in some cases cures of early stage tumors. However, the most meaningful data were those obtained against advanced stage tumors (i.e., tumors at least 200 mg at start of therapy) where complete tumor regressions could be observed. This occurred with the murine mammary adenocarcinomas 16/C and 13/C, pancreatic ductal carinoma 03, colon 38 adenocarcinoma, and the human xenografts MX-1 mammary and SK-MEL-2 melanoma (*63,64*). Prolonged tumor growth delays were also observed with Calc-18 breast, LX-1 lung, CX-1 colon, head and neck HNX-14C, and HNX-22B xenografts (*64,66*). Since the clinical activity of paclitaxel against ovarian tumors was impressive, five human ovarian xenografts having different sensitivities to the reference drug cisplatin were included in this study. Docetaxel was active against the three tumors sensitive to cisplatin; interestingly, it was also active against OV-Pe, which is resistant to cisplatin (*65*).

Table 3
In Vivo Antitumor Activity of Docetaxel Against Murine Tumors

Tumor	Highest nontoxic iv dosage mg/kg/dose	Schedule days	Activity[a] rating
Solid tumors sc			
Melanoma B16 early	24	3, 5, 7, 9	+ + + +
Pancreas			
PO2	32.2	3, 5, 7	±
PO3 early	20.5	3, 5, 7, 9	+ + + +
PO3 advanced	18.3	22, 24, 26, 28	5/6 CR
Mammary			
MA16/C early	15	3, 5, 7	+ + +
MA16/C advanced	10.8	7, 9, 11	5/5 CR
MA13/C early	14.2	3, 5, 7	+ + + +
MA13/C advanced	15	24, 27, 30	3/5 CR[b]
MA44 early	22	3, 5, 7	±
Colon			
C26 early	5	1–4	+
C38 early	23.5	3, 5, 7	+ + + +
C38 advanced	26.8	14, 16, 18	5/5 CR
C51 early	12.7	3, 5, 7	+ + +
C51 advanced	15.2	10, 12, 14	+ +
Lewis lung early	23.2	3–7	+
Osteosarcoma GOS early	18.6	3–7	+
Hystiocytosarcoma M5076 early	8.6	3–7	–
Leukemias ip			
P388 10⁶ cells	23.2	1–4	+
L1210 10⁵ cells	21.7	1–4	+ +

[a]For activity rating, *see* Table 1.
[b]CR = complete regressions.

Scheduling studies were performed against advanced colon 38 adenocarcinoma. Docetaxel was tested using three different schedules comparing the effect of 2, 3, and 10 administrations over the same duration of treatment. Overall, the administration schedule did not influence markedly the total dosage that can be administered and, thus, the compound was considered schedule-independent for the MTD (*29*).

4.3. Combination Chemotherapy

Since taxoids have clinical activity in ovarian, breast, and lung tumors, most of the experimental studies have been done with drugs active in these diseases: doxorubicin, 5-fluorouracil, cyclophosphamide, cisplatin, and etoposide.

4.3.1. PACLITAXEL

Both in vitro and in vivo studies were performed. The efficacy of combination therapy consisting of paclitaxel plus a topoisomerase II inhibitor, doxorubicin or

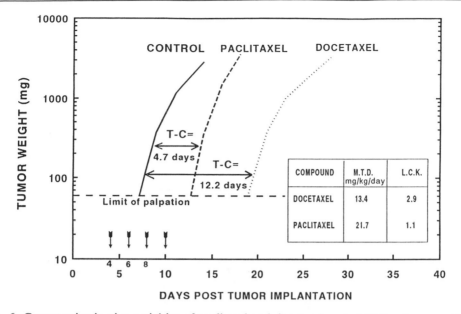

Fig. 6. Comparative in vivo activities of paclitaxel and docetaxel against B16 melanoma. Detailed experimental conditions were described in ref. (*29*). Briefly, B6D2F₁ mice (7 mice/group) were grafted sc on day 0 with 30 mg B16 tumors fragments. Drugs were injected iv on days 4, 6, 8, and 10 at the MTD (21.7 mg/kg/d for paclitaxel; 13.4 mg/kg/d for docetaxel). Tumor growths were measured biweekly. Activity is expressed by the T-C (where T and C are the median time in days necessary for the tumors of the treated group T and the control group C to reach a size of 1 g). Activity is also expressed by the LCK, which quantifies the number of tumor cells killed by the chemotherapy.

etoposide, against various cell lines has been studied in vitro; better results were obtained when cells were first incubated with paclitaxel (*67*). Cisplatin–paclitaxel combination was evaluated using L1210 leukemic cells: maximal effects were observed when cells were incubated for 24 h with paclitaxel, and then treated for 30 min with cisplatin (*68*). Combinations of taxoids and tubulin-interactive agents are of interest because of their complementary mechanism of action. Paclitaxel–estramustine was found to give supra-additive cytotoxic effects on several lines of human prostatic adenocarcinoma. No additive properties were noted when taxoids were combined with vinblastine (*69*).

In vivo combination chemotherapy studies have also been performed with paclitaxel using the M109 tumor model (*60*). The combined agents included cisplatin, etoposide, doxorubicin, cyclophosphamide, methotrexate, pentamethylmelamine, and bleomycin. Taxol-cisplatin and Taxol-bleomycin were the two combinations reported as showing hints of therapeutic synergy (*60*).

In mice grafted with MA16/C mammary adenocarcinoma, the association of doxorubicin-paclitaxel has a synergistic effect, which is observed only when compounds are administered sequentially every 4 d; such a protocol of administration makes this regimen, which is otherwise toxic, acceptable (*70*).

4.3.2. DOCETAXEL

Much of the work has been performed in vivo. Ten two-drug combinations were evaluated in mice bearing sc transplantable tumors (*63, 71,72*). The effects of the optimal docetaxel-based combination were found to be greater than the effect of the best single agent in the case of docetaxel-vinorelbine (against MA16/C), docetaxel-etoposide (against B16 melanoma), docetaxel-cyclophosphamide (against MA13/C), docetaxel-5-fluorouracil (against colon 38), and docetaxel-methotrexate (against P388 leukemia). A similar level of efficacy was obtained in the case of docetaxel-vincristine (against P388) and docetaxel-mitomycin C (against MA13/C), compared to the activity of the best single agent. Good activity was obtained with the docetaxel-vinblastine and docetaxel-doxorubine combinations, both tested against MA13/C. However, their activity was lower than that of docetaxel alone.

In terms of toxicity, the combination toxicity index (CTI, i.e., sum of the fractions of the LD_{50} of each agent used in the combination) ranged from 0.75 for the most toxic combination (docetaxel/cisplatin), indicating complete overlap in dose-limiting toxic effects, to 2 for the least toxic combination docetaxel/vinca alkaloids, indicating that the maximum tolerated dose of each agent could be administered without additional toxicity. All the other combinations had a CTI around 1.2, indicating that approximately 60% of the full dose of each agent can be used in combination without an increase in the overall toxicity (*63, 71, 72*).

Although most of the combinations were evaluated using simultaneous administration, a few studies were performed using different schedules. This factor was found to be important in the case of the docetaxel vincristine combination, where administering the two drugs 24 h apart led to a greater level of host toxicity (*71*).

5. ANIMAL PHARMACOLOGY

Pharmacokinetic data on paclitaxel in animals are scarce because of the lack of a sensitive assay when the drug was being investigated only in the laboratory. None of the bioassays that were developed were suitable for detailed studies. With an assay with a detection limit of 0.1 μM, however, it has been shown that in animals, paclitaxel was almost totally bound to proteins, and had distribution and elimination half-lives of 2.7 and 42 min, respectively, in rabbits (*73*).

In contrast, a sensitive and selective high-performance liquid chromatographic (HPLC) assay for docetaxel was available early in its development (*74*) and was used for studies in animals (*75,76*). In tumor-bearing mice, t1/2α and t1/2β were 7 min and 1.1 h, respectively. The pharmacokinetics were linear. The plasma clearance was 2.2 L/h/kg, and the apparent volume of distribution at steady state 2.2 L/kg. The AUC at doses of 13–62 mg/kg ranged from 4.5 to 29.6 μg/mL/h. Interestingly, the elimination half-life from tumor tissue was more than 20 h, compared to a 2- to 4- h elimination half-life in all other tissues. It was of interest that, at all doses, tumor levels were considerably higher than the IC_{50} values of cytotoxicity in tumor cell cultures, up to 24 h after administration. This long exposure of tumor tissue may be an essential factor to docetaxel activity in human patients, where plasma exposure at therapeutic doses were found later to be in the same range as in the mouse (*77*).

Administration of radiolabeled docetaxel led to a rapid diffusion into all tissues except those of the CNS, with the highest levels seen in liver, bile, intestines, and gastric contents. The plasma protein binding in mice was 76–89%, and the elimination was almost complete at 96 h after administration. In the dog and mouse, the primary route of elimination of radiolabeled docetaxel was hepatic extraction and biliary excretion, whereas urinary excretion was < 10% (*78*). Docetaxel metabolism was found to be similar across species in vivo and in vitro models (*79*). The facts that docetaxel was generally the main circulating compound and that the major metabolites were much less active than docetaxel indicated that parent drug analysis was an appropriate parameter for pharmacokinetic/pharmacodynamic studies of this drug.

6. ANIMAL TOXICOLOGY

Toxicology studies with paclitaxel in rodents were completed by 1982. They were performed with ip drug administration because of the solubility limitation and because of volume constraints. In dogs, the drug was given iv (*1*). The single-dose LD_{10} ip in Sprague-Dawley rats was 138 mg/m², and the LD_{50} was 206 mg/m². For the daily-times-five administration schedule, these doses were 36 and 51 mg/m²/d, respectively, in rats, and 67 and 82 mg/m²/d in CD2F1 mice. The single-dose toxic low (TDL) iv in beagle dogs was 45 mg/m². The major toxic effect in rats and dogs was reversible myelosuppression. In rodents, oligospermia was noted. Gastrointestinal toxicity was most pronounced in the daily-times-five schedule in dogs, and consisted of diarrhea, mucosal ulcerations, and emesis. In dogs, hypotension was also observed, which was believed to be related to histamine released by Cremophor®.

For docetaxel the single-dose LD_{10} in mice was 345 mg/m², and the LD_{50} was 414 mg/m². In dogs, the TDL was 15 mg/m² (*75*). The main toxic effects of docetaxel were reversible myelosuppression and epithelial necrosis in the digestive tract. In mice, cumulative and reversible neurotoxicity was observed. Dogs experienced hypotension, which was thought to be related to the vehicle polysorbate 80. Although there are minor differences, animal toxicology in general appears to be similar for paclitaxel and docetaxel, with similar target organs and more pronounced toxicity with repeated-administration schedules.

The results of the acute toxicity study in dogs served as a basis for the entry dose in humans. Following recommendations of the NCI, one-third of the TDL in dogs was selected as the initial dose level for Phase I clinical trials: 15 mg/m² for paclitaxel and 5 mg/m² for docetaxel.

7. CONCLUSION

New chemical structure, new mechanism of action, coupled with solid preclinical antitumor activity are considered to be key features for the selection of antitumor agents. The taxoids do fit these criteria. Although the discovery process has been very long and tedious, numerous challenges have been overcome. In the case of paclitaxel, a suitable formulation was developed, an adequate supply was ensured, and severe hypersensitivity reactions were diminished. This process took more than 30 years from bark collections to first approval. As a result of the supply difficulties, semisynthetic routes were unveiled, paving the way for the discovery of new compounds. Docetaxel was the first semisynthetic compound in clinical trial and has been developed in record time.

As predicted by their chemical analogies, paclitaxel and docetaxel bear similarities in terms of mechanism of action and experimental antitumor properties in cellular and animal models. These two compounds bind to the same site on microtubules, and consequently, share the same and unique mechanism of action: promotion of tubulin assembly into microtubules resistant to cold-induced depolymerization. However, what seem to be minor chemical differences result in quantitative and qualitative differences. Docetaxel has a twofold increased affinity for binding to microtubules. The population of docetaxel microtubules has an average of 13 protofilaments like normal microtubules, whereas paclitaxel microtubules have an average of 12 protofilaments. Higher intracellular concentration can be achieved and the drug is retained longer owing to a slower efflux from the cells. In addition, whereas paclitaxel is cytotoxic during mitosis, docetaxel exerts its cytotoxic effect during S phase. Docetaxel has been found to be schedule-independent, whereas paclitaxel seems to be schedule-dependent. Finally, crossresistance has not been systematically observed between the two drugs in a tumor cloning assay.

Despite the extraordinary advances obtained during these last few years with the preparation of taxoids by semisynthesis and with the total synthesis of paclitaxel, the chemistry of taxoids is still in its infancy. The first structure–activity relationships for taxoids have been obtained and have revealed key positions both on the lateral chain and on the diterpenoid skeleton. Second-generation compounds could include soluble compounds that are easier to formulate without the use of detergents, such as Cremophor® or polysorbate 80, compounds that are not crossresistant with paclitaxel/docetaxel, and compounds that are better tolerated after acute and/or cumulative administrations.

REFERENCES

1. Suffness M. Taxol: from discovery to therapeutic use. In: Bristol JA ed. *Annual Reports in Medicinal Chemistry*. San Diego, CA: Academic 1993:305–314.
2. Wall ME. Camptothecin and taxol. In: Lednicer D, ed. *Chronicles of Drug Discovery*. Washington DC: American Chemical Society. 1993:327–348.
3. Wall ME, Wani MC. Campthothecin and taxol: discovery to clinic—Thirteenth Bruce F. Cain Memorial Award Lecture. *Cancer Res* 1995; 55:753–760.
4. Wall ME, Wani MC. Recent progress in plant anti-tumor agents. In: 153rd National Meeting of the American Chemical Society, Miami Beach FL, 1967; Paper M-006.
5. Wani MC, Taylor HL, Wall ME, Coggon P, Mc Phail AT. Plant antitumor agents VI. The isolation and structure of taxol, a novel antileukemic and antitumor agent from *Taxus brevifolia*. *J Am Chem Soc* 1971; 93:2325–2327.
6. Douros J, Suffness M. New natural products under development at the National Cancer Institute. Recent results. *Cancer Res* 1981; 76:153–175.
7. Fuchs DA, Johnson RK. Cytologic evidence that taxol, an antineoplastic agent from *Taxus brevifolia*, acts as a mitotic spindle poison. *Cancer Treat Rep* 1978; 62:1219–1222.
8. Schiff PB, Fant J, Horwitz SB. Promotion of microtubule assembly *in vitro* by Taxol. *Nature* 1979; 22:665–667.
9. Pazdur R, Kudelka AP, Kavanagh JJ, Cohen PR, Raber MN. The taxoids: paclitaxel (Taxol®) and docetaxel (Taxotere®). *Cancer Treatment Rev* 1993; 19:351–386.
10. Rowinsky EK, Cazenave LA, Donehower RC. Taxol: A novel investigational antimicrotubule agent. *J Natl Cancer Inst* 1990; 82 (15):1247–1259.
11. McGuire WP, Rowinsky EK, Rosenshein NB, Grumbine FC, Ettinger DS, Armstrong DK, Donehower RC. Taxol: a unique antineoplastic agent with significant activity in advanced ovarian epithelial neoplasms. *Ann Intern Med* 1989; 111:273–279.
12. Holmes FA, Walters RS, Theriault RL, Forman AD, Newton LK, Raber MN, Buzdar AU, Frye DK, Hortobagyi GN. Phase II trial of taxol, an active drug in the treatment of metastatic breast cancer. *J Natl Cancer Inst* 1991: 83:1797–1805.
13. Murphy WK, Fossella FV, Winn RJ, Shin DM, Hynes HE, Gross HM, Davilla E, Leimert JT, Dhingra HM, Raber MN, Krakoff IH, Hong WK. Phase II study of taxol in patients with untreated advanced non-small-cell lung cancer. *J Natl Cancer Inst* 1993; 85:384–388.

14. Shelanski ML, Gaskin F, Cantor CR. Microtubule assembly in the absence of added nucleotides. *Proc Natl Acad Sci USA* 1973; 70:765–769.

15. Senilh V, Blechert S, Colin M, Guénard D, Picot F, Potier P, Varenne P. Mise en évidence de nouveaux analogues du taxol, extraits de *Taxus baccata. J Natural Product* 1984; 47:131.

16. Lavelle F, Guéritte-Voegelein F, Guénard D, Le Taxotere: des aiguilles d'if a la clinique. *Bull Cancer* (Paris) 1993; 80:326–338.

17. Guéritte-Voegelein F, Senilh V, David B, Guénard D, Potier P. Chemical studies of 10-deacetylbaccatin III. Hemisynthesis of taxol derivatives. *Tetrahedron* 1986; 42:4451–4460.

18. Guénard D, Guéritte-Voegelein F, Potier P. Taxol and Taxotere: discovery, chemistry and structure-activity relationships. *Acc Chem Res* 1993; 26:160–167.

19. Herranz E, Biller SA, Sharpless KB. Osmium-catalyzed vicinal oxyamination of olefins by *N*-chloro-*N*-argentocarbamates. *J Am Chem Soc* 1978; 100:3596–3598.

20. Mangatal L, Adeline MT, Guénard D, Guéritte-Voegelein F, Potier P. Application of the vicinal oxyamination reaction with asymmetric induction to the hemisynthesis of taxol and analogues. *Tetrahedron* 1989; 45:4177–4190.

21. Lavelle F, Fizames C, Guéritte-Voegelein F, Guénard D, Potier P. Experimental properties of RP 56976, a Taxol derivative. *Proc Am Assoc Cancer Res* 1989; 30:2254.

22. Denis JN, Greene AE, Serra AA, Luche MJ. An efficient, enantioselective synthesis of the taxol side chain. *J Org Chem* 1986; 51:46–50.

23. Colin M, Guénard D, Guéritte-Voegelein F, Potier P. Preparation of baccatin III derivatives as antitumor agents. Eur. Pat. Appl EP 336841, 89/10/11, FR appl. 884513 (88/04/06).

24. Denis JN, Greene AE, Guénard D, Guéritte-Voegelein F, Mangatal L, Potier P. A highly efficient, practical approach to natural taxol. *J Am Chem Soc* 1988; 110:5917–5919.

25. Commerçon A, Bézard D, Bernard F, Bourzat JD. Improved protection and esterification of a precursor of the Taxotere® and Taxol® side chain. *Tetrahedron Lett* 1992; 33:5185.

26. Holton RA. Eur. Pat. Appl. EP 400,971, 1990. Chem. Abstr. 1991: 114, 164568q.

27. Holton RA. Eur. Pat. Appl. EP 428,376, 1991. Chem. Abstr. 1991: 115, 114817v.

28. Ojima I, Habus I, Zhao M, Georg G, Jayasinghe LR. Efficient and practical asymmetric synthesis of the Taxol C-13 side chain, *N*-Benzoyl-(2R,3S)-3-phenylisoserine, and its analogues via chiral 3-hydroxy-4-aryl-β-lactams through chiral ester enolate-imine cyclocondensation. *J Org Chem* 1991; 56:1681.

29. Bissery MC, Guénard D, Guéritte-Voegelein F, Lavelle F. Experimental antitumor activity of Taxotere (RP 56976, NSC 628503), a taxol analogue. *Cancer Res* 1991; 51:4845–4852.

30. Verweij J, Clavel M, Chevalier B. Paclitaxel (Taxol™) and docetaxel (Taxotere™): Not simply two of a kind. *Ann Oncol* 1994; 5:495–505.

31. Hyams JS, Lloyd CW. in: Harford JB, ed. *Microtubules, Modern Cell Biology Series*, vol. 13. New York: Wiley Liss. 1993:460.

32. Wadsworth P. Mitosis: spindle assembly and chromosome motion. *Current Opinion Cell Biol* 1993; 5:123–128.

33. Beese L, Stubbs G, Cohen C. Microtubule structure at 18 Å resolution. *J Mol Biol* 1987; 194: 257–264.

34. Gaskin F, Cantor CR, Shelanski ML. Turbidimetric studies of the *in vitro* assembly and disassembly of porcine neurotubules. *J Mol Biol* 1974; 89:737–758.

35. Schiff PB, Fant J, Horwitz SB. Promotion of microtubule assembly *in vitro* by taxol. *Nature (Lond.)* 1979; 22:665–667.

36. Ringel I, Horwitz SB. Studies with RP 56976 (Taxotere): a semi-synthetic analog of taxol. *J Natl Cancer Inst* 1991; 83:288–291.

37. Guéritte-Voegelein F, Guénard D, Lavelle F, Le Goff M-T, Mangatal L, Potier P. Relationships between the structure of Taxol analogues and their antimitotic activity. *J Med Chem* 1991; 34:992–998.

38. Diaz JF, Andreu JM. Assembly of purified GDP-tubulin into microtubules induced by RP 56976 and paclitaxel: reversibility, ligand stoichiometry and competition. *Biochemistry* 1993; 32: 2747–2755.

39. Karsenti E. Vers une description du mécanisme d'assemblage du fuseau mitotique a l'échelle moléculaire. *Méd/Sci* 1993; 9:131–139.

40. Parness J., Horwitz SB. Taxol binds to polymerized tubulin in vitro. *J Cell Biol* 1981; 91: 479–487.

41. Schiff PB, Horwitz SB. Taxol assembles tubulin in the absence of exogenous guanosine-5′-triphosphate or microtubule associated proteins. *Biochemistry* 1981; 20:3247–3252.

42. Kumar N. Taxol induced polymerization of purified tubulin. *J Biol Chem* 1981; 256: 10,435–10,441.

43. Diaz JF, Menendez M, Andreu JM. Thermodynamics of ligand-induced assembly of tubulin. *Biochemistry* 1993; 32:10,067–10,077.

44. Andreu JM, Bordas J, Diaz JF, Garcia De Ancos J, Gil R, Medrano FJ, Nogales E, Pantos E, Towns-Andrews E. Low resolution structure of microtubules in solution. *J Mol Biol* 1992; 226:169–184.

45. Andreu JM, Diaz JF, Gil R, De Pereda JM, Garcia De Lacoba M, Peyrot V, Briand C, Towns-Andrews E, Bordas J. Solution structure of microtubules induced by the side chain taxol analogue Taxotere to 3 nm resolution. *J Biol Chem* 1994; 269 no 50:31,785–31,792.

46. Riou JF, Naudin A, Lavelle F. Effects of Taxotere on murine and human tumor cell lines. *Biochem Biophys Res Commun* 1992; 187:164–170.

47. Kelland LR, Abel G. Comparative *in vitro* cytotoxicity of taxol and Taxotere against cisplatin-sensitive and resistant human ovarian carcinoma cell lines. *Cancer Chemother Pharmacol* 1992; 30:444–450.

48. Vogel M, Hilsenbeck SG, Depenbrock H, Danhauser-Riedl S, Block T, Nekarda H, Fellbaum C, Aapro MS, Bissery MC, Rastetter J, Hanauske AR. Preclinical activity of Taxotere (RP 56976, NSC 628503) against freshly explanted clonogenic human tumour cells: comparison with taxol and conventional antineoplastic agents. *Eur J Cancer* 1993; 29A:2009–2014.

49. Hanauske AR, Degen D, Hilsensbeck SG, Bissery MC, Von Hoff DD. Effects of Taxotere and taxol on *in vitro* colony formation of freshly explanted human tumor cells. *Anti-Cancer Drugs* 1992; 3:121–124.

50. Braakhuis BJM, Hill BT, Dietel M, Kelland LR, Aapro MS, Zoli W, Lelieveld P. *In vitro* antiproliferative activity of docetaxel (Taxotere®), paclitaxel (Taxol®) and Cisplatin against human tumors and normal bone marrow cells. *Anticancer Res* 1994; 14:205–208.

51. Riou JF, Petitgenet O, Combeau C and Lavelle F. Cellular uptake and efflux of docetaxel (Taxotere®) and paclitaxel (Taxol®) in P388 cell line. *Proc Am Assoc Cancer Res* 1994; 35:385.

52. Lopes NM, Adams EG, Pitts TW, Bhuyan BK. Cell kill kinetics and cell cycle effects of taxol on human and hamster ovarian cell lines. *Cancer Chemother Pharmacol* 1993; 32:235–242.

53. Roberts JR, Allison DC, Donehower RC, Rowinsky EK. Development of polyploidization in Taxol-resistant human leukemia cells *in vitro*. *Cancer Res* 1990; 50:710–716.

54. Long BH, Fairchild CR. Paclitaxel inhibits progression of mitotic cells to G1 phase by interference with spindle formation without affecting other microtubule functions during anaphase and telophase. *Cancer Res* 1994; 54:4355–4361.

55. Garcia P, Braguer D, Carles G, El Khyari S, Barra Y, De Ines C, Barasoain I, Briand C. Comparative effects of taxol and Taxotere on two different human carcinoma cell lines. *Cancer Chemother Pharmacol* 1994; 34:335–343.

56. Hennequin N, Giocanti N, Favaudon V. S-phase specificity of cell killing by docetaxel (Taxotere) in synchronised HeLa cells. *Br J Cancer* 1995; 71:1194–1198.

57. De Brabander M, Geuens G, Nuydens R, Willebrords R, De Mey J. Taxol induces the assembly of free microtubules in living cells and blocks the organizing capacity of the centrosomes and kinetochores. *Proc Natl Acad Sci USA* 1981; 78:5608–5612.

58. Schiff PB, Horwitz SB. Taxol stabilizes microtubules in mouse fibroblasts cells. *Proc Natl Acad Sci* 1980; 77:1561–1565.

59. Rose WC. Taxol: a review of its preclinical *in vivo* antitumor activity. *Anti-Cancer Drugs* 1992; 3:311–321.

60. Rose WC. Taxol-based combination chemotherapy and other *in vivo* preclinical antitumor studies. *JNCI Monographs* 1993; 15:47–53.

61. Riondel J, Jacrot M, Picot F, Beriel H, Mouriquand C, Potier P. Therapeutic response to taxol of six human tumors xenografted into nude mice. *Cancer Chemother Pharmacol* 1986; 17:137–142.

62. Nicoletti MI, Lucchini V, D'Incalci M, Giavazzi R. Comparison of paclitaxel and docetaxel activity on human ovarian carcinoma xenografts. *Eur J Cancer* 1994; 30A:5:691–696.

63. Bissery MC, Vrignaud P, Lavelle F. Preclinical profile of Docetaxel (Taxotere): Efficacies as a single agent or in combination. *Seminars in Oncology* 1995; 22(Suppl):3–16.
64. Dykes DJ, Bissery MC, Harrison SD, Waud WR. Response of human tumor xenografts in athymic nude mice to docetaxel (RP 56976, Taxotere®). *Invest New Drugs* 1995; 13:1–11.
65. Boven E, Venema-Gaberscek E, Erkelens CAM, Bissery MC, Pinedo HM. Antitumor activity of taxotere (RP 56976, NSC 628503), a new taxol analog, in experimental ovarian cancer. *Ann Oncol* 1993; 4:321–324.
66. Braakhuis BJM, Kegel A, Welters MJP. The growth inhibiting effect of docetaxel (Taxotere®) in head and neck squamous cell carcinoma xenografts. *Cancer Lett* 1994; 81:151–154.
67. Hahn SM, Liebmann JE, Cook J, Fisher J, Goldspiel B, Venzon D, Mitchell JB, Kaufman D. Taxol in combination with doxorubicin or etoposide. *Cancer* 1993; 72:2705–2711.
68. Citardi MJ, Rowinsky EK, Schaefer KL, Donehower RC. Sequence dependent cytotoxicity between cisplatin (C) and the antimicrotubule agents taxol (T) and vincristine (V). *Proc Am Assoc. Cancer Res* 1990; 31:24–31.
69. Speicher LA, Barone L, Tew KD. Combined antimicrotubule activity of estramustine and taxol in human prostatic carcinoma cell lines. *Cancer Res* 1992; 52:4433–4440.
70. Lorusso PM, Demchik LL, Plowman J, Baker L, Corbett TH. Preclinical activity and toxicity of taxol combinations. *Proc Am Assoc Cancer Res* 1993; 34:1794.
71. Bissery MC, Vrignaud P, Bayssas M, Lavelle F. *In vivo* evaluation of Taxotere (RP 56976, NSC 628503) in combination with cisplatin, doxorubicin or vincristine. *Proc Am Assoc Cancer Res* 1992; 33:443.
72. Bissery MC, Vrignaud P, Bayssas M, Lavelle F. Taxotere synergistic combination with cyclophosphamide, etoposide and 5-fluorouracil in mouse tumor models. *Proc Am Assoc Cancer Res* 1993; 34:1782.
73. Hamel E, Lin CM, Johns DG. Tubulin dependent biochemical assay for the antineoplastic agent taxol and application of the drug in serum. *Cancer Treat Rep* 1982; 66:1381–1386.
74. Vergniol JC, Bruno R, Montay G, Frydman A. Determination of Taxotere in human plasma by a semiautomated high-performance liquid chromatographic method. *J Chromatog* 1992; 582:273–278.
75. Bissery MC, Renard A, André S., et al. Preclinical pharmacology and toxicology of Taxotere (RP 56976, NSC 628503). *Ann Oncol* 1992; 3 (suppl 1):121.
76. Bissery MC, Renard A, Montay G, Bayssas M, Lavelle F. Taxotere:Antitumor activity and pharmacokinetics in mice. *Proc Am Assoc Cancer Res* 1991; 32:401.
77. Bruno R, Sanderink GJ. Pharmacokinetics and metabolism of Taxotere™. *Cancer Surveys* 1993; 17:305–313.
78. Marlard M, Gaillard C, Sanderink GJ, Roberts SA, Joannou PP, Facchini V, Chapelle P, Frydman A. Kinetics, distribution, metabolism and excretion of radiolabelled Taxotere® (¹⁴C-RP 56976, docetaxel) in mice and dogs. *Proc Am Assoc Cancer Res* 1993; 34:393.
79. Sanderink GJ, Martinet M, Touzet A, Chapelle P, Frydman A. Docetaxel (Taxotere®), RP 56976) metabolizing enzymes and metabolic drug-drug interactions *in vitro*. *Proc ISSX* 1993; 3:35.

9 Sequence-Selective Groove Binders

Franco Zunino, PhD and Giovanni Capranico, PhD

CONTENTS

1. INTRODUCTION

A large number of agents are known to bind to DNA, interfering with multiple DNA functions in living cells. Their ability to interact with DNA is associated with several biological effects, including antiviral, antibacterial, antiprotozoal, and antitumor activities. Their biological activities are probably related to different effects on cellular targets. From the pharmacological point of view, the most relevant DNA binding agents are antitumor drugs. They exert their cytotoxic effect principally as a consequence of the lack of selectivity by damaging cellular DNA. Cytotoxic and antiproliferative drugs have played and will likely continue to play a major role in cancer chemotherapy.

DNA-interacting cytotoxic agents belong to different chemical classes, and their mode of binding to DNA is quite different depending on the chemical structure and the presence of reactive groups. DNA binding ability is not *per se* a sufficient condition to achieve a significant therapeutic effect. In addition, as a consequence of the lack of selectivity, clinically useful cytotoxic agents often have a low therapeutic index. Indeed, they are expected to cause a large number of DNA lesions not only in tumor, but also in normal cells. However, a certain selectivity toward specific tumor types has been recognized for some agents, as documented by the efficacy of platinum compounds in the treatment of testicular and ovarian cancers. It is conceivable that the different chemosensitivity of tumor cells to cytotoxic agents is related to a different ability of the drug to damage critical genomic sites. However, the genes crucial for a selective effect remain unknown. Most of the known cytotoxic agents have a very limited ability to read sequence information compared to DNA binding proteins.

From: *Cancer Therapeutics: Experimental and Clinical Agents*
Edited by: B. Teicher Humana Press Inc., Totowa, NJ

Molecular pharmacology studies have elucidated several aspects of drug–target interaction and provided a molecular basis for the design of more selective agents.

DNA-interactive drugs include chemically reactive compounds and agents that bind to DNA by noncovalent interactions. The major groups of noncovalently reacting agents are represented by intercalative and nonintercalative drugs. This classification is of course schematic, and there is a large overlap in these groupings. In particular, most known antitumor intercalators contain nonintercalating moieties (e.g., sugars, oligopeptides) able to interact in the helical grooves or along the surface of the phosphate backbone of the double helix. A large number of natural and synthetic DNA-interactive compounds have been described. These small organic ligands (in particular, nonintercalative groove binders) have been extensively used to elucidate aspects of DNA conformation and DNA sequence elements involved in the mechanisms of recognition by regulatory proteins and/or by DNA processing enzymes (1,2). Unfortunately, only a few compounds have proven to be effective antitumor agents. Indeed, DNA interaction can have cellular consequences distinct from cell death. Regardless of the mode of drug–DNA interaction, DNA binding ability is not a sufficient condition for a drug to be an effective antitumor agent. In general, a DNA-interacting agent is endowed with a significant cytotoxic effect when DNA damage (alteration of the nucleic acid structure or persistent inhibition of a critical cellular function) occurs as a consequence of DNA binding. If optimal repair is impossible, persistent lesions may be recognized as an apoptotic stimulus (3).

A number of reviews in the past decade have summarized the DNA binding properties of antitumor agents (4,5). In this chapter, we have focused on the development of antitumor agents for which groove binding ability is a determinant of sequence specificity in induction of DNA damage. Significant research efforts were directed toward elucidating the underlying mechanisms of cytotoxicity of groove binders. In an attempt to interpret the available information on their mode of action and to provide insight into current approaches for the rational development of new effective agents, this chapter will focus on the most representative classes of groove binding agents.

2. MAJOR GROOVE BINDERS

Although the major groove of DNA has greater recognition potential, as predicted on the basis of the number of hydrogen bonds (4), only a few DNA-interacting agents appear to be major-groove-specific. They include bifunctional alkylating agents, methylating agents, and cisplatin (6,7). Typically, such compounds covalently interact with the N-7 position of guanine located in the major groove. In spite of the fact that they apparently do not contain any sequence information, a preferential alkylation by nitrogen mustards occurs at guanines within guanine clusters. This selectivity has been related to the sequence dependence of the electrostatic potential of DNA (8). In fact, guanines surrounded by other guanines are associated with a more negative potential at the N-7 alkylation site than any isolated guanine. A contribution of specific binding interaction of the nonalkylating moieties in influencing selectivity has been proposed (7). Such a possibility may have relevant implications in the development of new agents with increased specificity of DNA binding, as suggested by bis (platinum) compounds, which exhibit a different profile of antitumor activity (9).

Although the sequence specificity of known alkylating (or platinating) agents is not enough to achieve tumor selectivity, the pattern of cell response to these cytotoxic agents is likely to be related to the localization of drug-induced DNA modification within chromatin (*10*) rather than to the variable expression of defense mechanisms. Experimental evidence in resistant cells supports this hypothesis. In tumor cell lines with variable degrees of resistance to cisplatin, no linear relationship has been found between the extent of DNA platination and cytotoxicity (*11*). In the presence of a comparable extent of total platinum-induced DNA-interstrand crosslinks, a marked decrease in formation of these lesions within the ribosomal RNA genes was found in resistant cells (*12*). The finding suggests that differences in the genomic sites of drug-induced lesions could contribute to the resistance phenotype. The molecular aspects of sequence selectivity exhibited by DNA-reactive drugs in DNA covalent modification have been extensively reviewed elsewhere (*5,6*).

3. INTERCALATING AGENTS

DNA intercalators have been extensively studied owing to their efficacy in cancer chemotherapy. The first class of intercalating antitumor agents proven to have clinical antitumor activity is represented by anthracyclines. One of them, doxorubicin, remains one of the most widely used antitumor drugs. The development of anthracyclines is the topic of another chapter of this book. Following identification of the clinical efficacy of anthracyclines, a large number of intercalating agents have been studied in an attempt to find more effective and selective antitumor agents. As already mentioned in Section 1., DNA binding and intercalation are necessary conditions, but not sufficient for optimal antitumor activity (*13*). Indeed, strong intercalators (e.g., ethidium bromide) may have marginal (if any) antitumor activity. It is likely that the mode and site of binding are more critical than the binding affinity. Stabilization of the intercalation complex involves several molecular interactions (*4*). In particular, side chains and bulky groups of the intercalating molecule placed either in the major or minor groove may have a critical role in determining the sequence specificity. Thus, the intercalation site depends not only on the planar drug chromophore, but also on a variety of intrinsic properties (steric and electronic factors) that involve external ligand moieties.

The mechanism of cytotoxic and antitumor activity of intercalating agents is ascribed to their ability to interfere with the function of topoisomerase II (*14*), a nuclear enzyme that regulates DNA topology during multiple metabolic DNA processes (*15*). The agents stabilize an intermediate of the enzyme reaction (the so-called cleavable complex), in which DNA strands are broken and enzyme subunits are covalently linked to DNA. Topoisomerase II inhibitors form a DNA–drug–enzyme ternary complex. A model of drug interaction in the ternary complex has been proposed in which the intercalator is placed at the interface between the topoisomerase II active site and the DNA cleavage site (*14*), thus preventing DNA religation by the enzyme. Studies of anthracycline analogs have not shown precise correlations between a drug's ability to induce DNA cleavage and DNA binding affinity (*13,16,17*). Although drug intercalation may have a role in the mechanism of enzyme inhibition, external interactions involving the sugar residue and the cyclohexene ring, therefore, may be more critical than the strength of intercalation. Relevant to this point is the observation that both these moieties are located in the minor groove (*18*).

Minor groove binders (*see* Section 4. for details on their biochemical and biological activities) have been reported to inhibit the induction of topoisomerase II-mediated DNA damage by *m*-AMSA and etoposide (*19,20*). Although minor groove binding is not a sufficient condition to stimulate enzyme-mediated cleavable complexes (*15*), several antitumor drugs known to be topoisomerase inhibitors have side chains that interact with the minor groove. For example, anthracyclines have a sugar moiety that is located in the minor groove. The presence of a bulky substituent at the 3′-position of doxorubicin (i.e, 3′-morpholinyl derivatives) totally abolishes the drug effect on topoisomerase II. Such derivatives were found to retain their ability to bind to DNA by intercalation (*21*). Available evidence suggests that the amino group at the 3′-position is not required for cytotoxic potency and topoisomerase II-trapping activity (*17*). Thus, the loss of activity of 3′-morpholinyl derivatives on topoisomerase II is not the result of a reduced stabilization of the intercalation complex consequent to loss of an electrostatic interaction of the free protonated amino group in the minor groove. These observations suggest that a bulky substituent at the 3′-position, but not at the 4′-position, is a steric hindrance for formation of the ternary complex and support the hypothesis that the minor groove binding moiety (i.e., amino sugar) is a critical determinant for drug poisoning of topoisomerase II (*17*). The importance of the 3′-substituent (and its orientation in the minor groove) in anthracycline's ability to inhibit topoisomerase II is emphasized by a recent study that indicated that epimerization of the 3′-amino group of the daunorubicin markedly influences the sequence specificity of topoisomerase II-mediated DNA cleavage (*22*). The observation is consistent with a critical role of the 3′-position for specific interaction of daunorubicin-related anthracyclines in the ternary complex. However, it is likely that multiple drug–enzyme interactions contribute to ternary complex stabilization, as suggested by reduced potency of 9-deoxy-doxorubicin in DNA-cleavage stimulation (*16*). Since the latter derivative has DNA binding parameters comparable to those of the parent drug, it is likely that the hydroxyl group at position 9 of the cyclohexene ring is involved in critical interactions with the enzyme. Again, the moiety is located in the minor groove (*18*). In addition to anthracyclines, another classical intercalating antitumor agent, actinomycin D, contains two pentapeptide rings located in the minor groove (*23*), and is a topoisomerase I and II inhibitor (*15,21*).

A peculiar feature of drug-stimulated topoisomerase II DNA cleavage is that the effects of antitumor drugs of different classes are sequence-specific (*24*). The sequence selectivity of different drugs has been rationalized in terms of distinct pharmacophores with similar interaction in the ternary complex. For example, amsacrine and bisantrene were shown to have similar sequence specificity, and also similar drug conformation and electronic properties. It is conceivable that specific interactions involving the drug domain(s) placed externally to the double helix critically influence the drug's ability to form the ternary complex and, hence, the site of DNA cleavage. This interpretation is supported by the effects of streptonigrin on topoisomerase II (*25*). This antitumor agent exhibits unique sequence specificity of topoisomerase II DNA cleavage, since it requires the dinucleotide 5′-TA-3′ from +2 to +3 positions at the DNA cleavage site. Streptonigrin does not intercalate into DNA, but has DNA binding properties resembling those of minor groove binders (*25*).

With few exceptions, known intercalators effective as antitumor agents (e.g., anthracyclines, anthracenediones, actinomycin D, and amsacrines) also have features of external binders, since the intercalation of the planar chromophore is accompanied by groove binding of a part of the molecule. It should be emphasized that the external binding moiety of the drug molecule is a crucial determinant of antitumor efficacy. Other intercalating agents (saintopin, intoplicine, actinomycin D) are dual topoisomerase I and II inhibitors (*15,26–29*), although the structural requirements for topoisomerase I and topoisomerase II are different. Lack of a correlation between activity in stimulation of topoisomerase I DNA cleavage and DNA binding affinity of indolocarbazole derivatives suggests that the mode of binding rather than intercalation is critical for activity (*30*). An interesting feature of intercalator topoisomerase I inhibitors (e.g., 3'-morpholinyl-doxorubicin, actinomycin D) is their preferential inhibition of ribosomal gene transcription (*31*) compared to pure topoisomerase II inhibitors (i.e., doxorubicin). Such a finding suggests a relationship between topoisomerase I inhibition and ribosomal RNA synthesis, and is consistent with an increased cytotoxic potency and a low therapeutic index of these agents.

4. NONCOVALENT DNA MINOR GROOVE BINDERS

Among DNA-interactive drugs, nonintercalating minor groove binders have been most extensively studied for the sequence specificity in DNA binding (*1*). They include agents with broad-spectrum biological activity. Detailed aspects of their biochemical and pharmacological action have been extensively reviewed (*1*) and are not the subject of this chapter. The best studied of these agents are the antiviral antibiotics, distamycin and netropsin, which are known to bind noncovalently to the minor groove with AT preference and to cause widening of the minor groove (*4*). Although incorrectly referred to as antitumor agents, distamycin and noncovalent binders of this group have low cytotoxic potency and negligible antitumor activity. Despite their physical interaction with DNA that causes reversible inhibition of DNA functions, they do not induce a persistent DNA damage, and therefore, they do not have cytotoxic activity. Indeed, among noncovalent minor groove binders, only DNA cleaving agents and topoisomerase I inhibitors show a significant antitumor activity.

Enediyne antibiotics (neocarzinostatin, esperamicin A1, and calicheamicin γ1) are typical examples of cytotoxic drugs with high DNA cleaving ability in the minor groove (*32*). DNA-damaging properties of enediynes have been related to formation of diradical species (*32*). A very potent antitumor antibiotic, C-1027, containing a novel enediyne chromophore has been described (*33*). The compound exhibits high and specific DNA-cleaving ability even in the absence of thiols (*34*). An interesting observation is that in calicheamicin γ1, the sugar residue functions as a minor groove binding element (*35*); such an interaction may be the basis of the site-specific double-strand cleavage (*36*). A similar role has been described for the amino sugar residue of elsamicin A, an agent with a bimodal mechanism of binding (intercalation and minor groove binding) that induces selective DNA cleavage (*37*).

Bleomycin is a well-known glycopeptide antibiotic that exerts cytotoxic activity through oxidative DNA damage. Its binding to DNA involves a partial intercalation of the bithiazole moiety and binding in the minor groove (*38*).

An interesting group of minor groove binding agents is topoisomerase I inhibitors (*39*). In general, drugs that interact with DNA in the minor groove can inhibit the catalytic activity of DNA topoisomerases in a concentration-dependent manner and

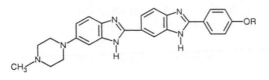

Hoechst 33342, R = OCH₂CH₃

Hoechst 33258, R = OH

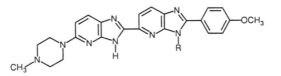

1   R = CH₂ OCH₂CH₃, CH₂O(CH₂)₇CH₃, CH₂CH₂OCH₂CH₃

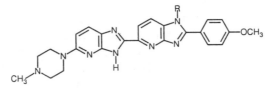

2   R = CH₂ OCH₃, CH₂O(CH₂)₇CH₃,

Fig. 1. Chemical structures of bis-benzimidazoles (Hoechst 33258 and 33342) and N1-alkoxyalkyl derivatives.

interfere with the stabilization of cleavable complexes by topoisomerase-targeted drugs (*40,41*). Thus, these agents act by impeding enzyme action without stabilizing DNA cleavable complexes. Since these compounds apparently inhibit DNA topoisomerase by competing with enzyme binding to DNA, Beerman et al. (*40*) proposed that the action of topoisomerases involves the minor groove. However, a number of minor groove binders (e.g., the bis-benzimidazoles, Hoechst 33342 and 33258 [Fig. 1]) were found to induce DNA cleavage in the presence of purified DNA topoisomerase I (*39*). A peculiar characteristic of single-strand DNA breaks induced by these minor groove binders is the high site specificity. The major cleavage sites have been found in AT rich regions (5'-TCATTTTT-3' with cleavage occurring between T and C), thus suggesting that the T track is a potential binding site of these bis-benzimidazoles, which are indeed highly AT-selective. It has been proposed that this effect could be related to the drug's ability to alter DNA bending, thus preventing ligation of the transiently broken DNA ends (*15*). This interpretation is consistent with the ability of bulgarein to induce topoisomerase I-mediated DNA cleavage and to induce positive DNA super-coils (*42*). The DNA winding produced by low-mol-wt compounds is known only for AT-specific minor groove binders. Topoisomerase I has been involved in the regulation of transcription, since the enzyme is associated with the general transcription factor, TATA box binding protein (TBP) (*43*). The factor has been documented to interact with DNA in the minor groove and share the same sequence preference of minor groove binders (*44*). In addition to a direct effect of minor groove binders as inhibitors of topoisomerase I, the agents are also effective inhibitors of the formation of the DNA/TBP complex (*45*). The structural aspects of minor groove drug–DNA complexes were recently examined by Neidle (*46*), who, on the basis of crystallographic studies, provided a detailed picture of the recognition processes involved. The structural studies emphasized, in addition to electrostatic interactions and hydrogen bonds, the hydrophobic interactions required to maintain the drug in an optimal position within the minor groove.

The pharmacological implications of the specific effects of minor groove binders on topoisomerase I remain to be established. The synthesis and preliminary biological evaluation of minor groove-selective *N*1-alkoxyalkyl-bis-benzimidazoles have been described (*47*) (Fig. 1). A correlation was found between DNA binding and cytotoxic potency. In particular, one of the derivatives with the inward-directed substituent exhibited a 15-fold increased cytotoxic potency compared to Hoechst 33258. Since the compounds may also have inhibitory effects on the catalytic activity of topoisomerases (*41*), the molecular basis of cytotoxicity remains to be defined. Only limited information is available on the cytotoxic and antitumor activity of the bis-benzimidazole derivatives. A selective cytotoxicity of Hoechst 33258 in human melanoma cells has been reported (*48*). The drug effect has been related to inhibition of transcription of specific genes. A plausible explanation for the cell type-specific effects of Hoecst 33258 is that tumor cell lines may differ in drug accessibility of certain AT-rich sequences. The low potency and high toxicity of Hoechst 33258 have precluded clinical evaluation. However, the more lipophylic Hoechst 33342 has been reported to be a potent cytotoxic agent (*49*). Detailed cytotoxicity studies were performed with Hoechst 33342, which exhibits an enhanced membrane permeability compared to the parent compound Hoechst 33258. The pattern of cell response to the former agent was different from that of camptothecin, since it was found less cytotoxic in cell lines expressing multidrug resistance, but only moderately crossresistant in camptothecin-resistant cells, which express a mutant form of topoisomerase I. The aforementioned studies support the potential interest of Hoechst 33342 in cancer chemotherapy.

Other DNA-interacting agents (including mithramycin, chromomycin A3, and nogalamycin) have been reported to stimulate topoisomerase I-mediated DNA cleavage (*15*). Again, such agents are known to bind to the minor groove or to have a moiety located in the minor groove, but with a different sequence specificity (i.e., GC-rich regions) (*50–54*). Although they are well-known cytotoxic agents, only a few have proven useful in clinical therapy. Thus, all DNA binding agents that are known to stimulate topoisomerase I-mediated DNA cleavage have a DNA minor groove binding mode (*15*). The drug interactions with DNA–enzyme in the ternary complex required for an effective stabilization of the cleavage complex have not yet been established. It is likely that minor groove binding is a critical determinant of sequence specificity of these "information-reading" molecules in inducing enzyme-mediated DNA damage.

The DNA sequence-recognizing properties of minor groove binders have suggested their use as carriers for delivering DNA-damaging moieties to specific sequences in DNA. In such approaches (aimed to functionalize minor groove binders), reactive (alkylating/crosslinking) groups or intercalating chromophores have been used. Several minor groove binder–intercalator hybrid molecules (named combilexins) have been developed (*55–57*). An enhanced DNA binding affinity and selectivity, and an interference with DNA topoisomerases at specific DNA sites are the potential advantages of these hybrid molecules. The molecular interactions with DNA and biological activity of a netropsin–acridine hybrid have been described (*57*). The hybrid compound retains its ability to intercalate into DNA, and exhibits lower cytotoxic and antitumor activities than the reference compound *m*-AMSA.

Based on these preliminary observations, other hybrid molecules that combine minor groove ligands and more effective intercalating agents have been synthesized. The most interesting compounds of this category appear to be the distamycin analogs. The DNA binding properties of a series of distamycin–ellipticine hybrid molecules have been extensively studied (*55,56*). One of these agents, Distel (1 +), was found to have a bimodal mechanism of interaction with DNA (i.e., intercalation of the ellepticin chromophore and binding of distamycin in the minor groove), without any apparent sequence specificity (*55*). Molecular modeling studies have suggested that the lack of sequence-selective interaction is related to the lack of a positively charged side chain on the distamycin moiety. Based on these theoretical predictions, a biscationic hybrid, Distel (2 +), has been synthesized to study it interaction with DNA (*56*). The introduction of a second positive charge resulted in a highly sequence-specific, DNA-reading agent. Psoralen (or coumarin) conjugates of minor groove binding AT-selective pyrrole-, or GC-selective imidazole-containing analogs of netropsin have been described (*58*). The linking of psoralen to the AT-selective, pyrrole-containing analogs of netropsin produced a photoactive agent more potent than the corresponding imidazole compound and the 8-methoxy psoralen itself, thus documenting that the minor groove ligand had targeted the photosensitizing agent to cellular DNA. It is noteworthy that in the case of the distamycin–ellipticine hybrid molecule, no direct correlations between DNA binding and cytotoxicity could be found (*55*). The hybrid compound is less cytotoxic than the ellipticine derivative used for conjugation. Such biological effects were interpreted in terms of unfavorable cellular pharmacokinetics of the hybrid compound as a consequence of the hydrophilic nature of distamycin residue. The poor drug uptake may thus represent a relevant limitation in the use of oligopeptide analogs for the development of hybrid antitumor agents.

5. MINOR GROOVE ALKYLATING AGENTS

Mitomycin C is a well-known antitumor antibiotic currently used in clinical cancer chemotherapy. Its cytotoxic action is related to its ability to bind covalently to minor groove DNA, resulting in monofunctional and bifunctional adducts. These processes require reductive activation of the quinone system of the drug and involve exclusively N2 positions of guanines (*59*). A specific DNA sequence recognition by mitomycin C for crosslink formation has been described. A 4-bp sequence preference by the crosslink produced by mitomycin is the result of absolute specificity for CG.

Another example of antitumor agents with minor groove GC sequence selectivity is anthramycin (*6*), which is a member of the pyrrole [1,4]-benzodiazepine group (Fig. 2). In spite of their low molecular weight, anthramycin and tomaymycin have shown a surprising degree of sequence selectivity with preference for adenine flanking the

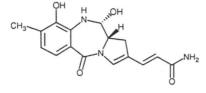

Anthramycin

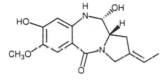

Tomaymycin

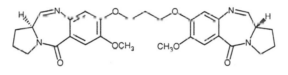

DSB - 120

Fig. 2. Pyrrolo[1,4]benzodiazepine antibiotics (anthramycin and tomaymycin) and dimer of anthramycin (DSB 120).

alkylated guanine (*60*). Crystal structure analysis of a covalent DNA-drug adduct provides insights to understand the molecular basis for sequence specificity in benzodiazepine antibiotics (*61*). This preference is related to a netropsin-like fitting of the acrylamide tail into the minor groove.

In an attempt to find more useful DNA-reading drugs, an interesting development of GC sequence-directed alkylating agents is the synthesis of a C8-linked dimer of anthramycin, with a flexible -0-(CH$_2$)$_3$-0- linker (DSB120) (*62*) (Fig. 2). The dimeric derivative, unlike anthramycin, forms interstrand crosslinks and exhibits a marked cytotoxicity in tumor cell lines. The compound binds to a 6-bp sequence (5´-PuGATCPyr). DNA binding, interstrand crosslinking efficiency, and cytotoxic potency are dependent on the linker chain length, and compounds with even numbers of methylene groups show reduced effectiveness. The observation suggests that, in the design of effective DNA-groove binder alkylators, an optimal size and geometry of the linker are required to ensure that the reactive moiety is in optimal orientation with respect to the target DNA sequence (*63*).

Bifunctional alkylating agents are the first drugs proven to have clinical antitumor efficacy. They are still among the most widely used drugs, with a broad range of activity for the treatment of human tumors. The agents have a limited capacity to read sequence information (*see* Section 2.). In an attempt to increase sequence specificity and

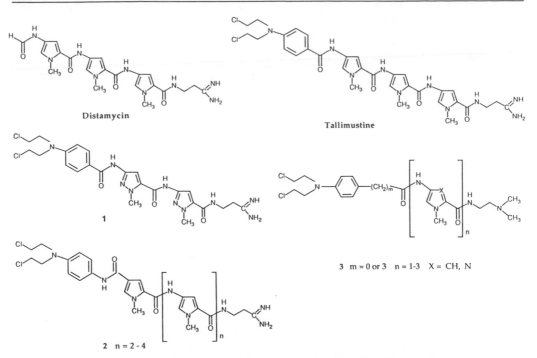

Fig. 3. Minor groove selective alkylating agents related to distamycin A.

to alter the covalent modification of DNA of alkylating/crosslinking agents, several minor groove-directed alkylators have been developed as potential antitumor agents (*64*). In such approaches, the naturally occurring pyrrolic oligopeptides, netropsin and distamycin, or their oligoimidazole analogs were used as a sequence-selective minor groove vectors. One of the most relevant observations in different series of DNA targeted alkylating agents is that the introduction of alkylating functions in minor groove binders results in a substantial increase in cytotoxic potency as compared to the carrier DNA binder itself (*65*). A similar finding was reported for 4-anilino-quinoline-based, minor groove-directed aniline mustards (*66*). Unfortunately, the latter compounds show a negligible in vivo antitumor activity, presumably related to their poor aqueous solubility.

Again, the most studied (and interesting) compounds appear to be the distamycin analogs (Fig. 3). Among recently developed alkylating derivatives of distamycin, a very interesting compound, tallimustine (FCE 24517), has been identified and is being tested in early clinical studies. The derivative was obtained by incorporation of a benzoyl mustard moiety at the N-terminus (*67*). As expected, the compound was found to react covalently with DNA. Whereas distamycin has a low cytotoxic activity and no significant antitumor efficacy, the alkylating derivative exhibits potent cytotoxic activity comparable or superior to that of melphalan, a structurally related alkylating agent (*68*). The compound was not crossresistant with melphalan in a subline of L1210 leukemia selected for resistance to melphalan, but was crossresistant with doxorubicin in a cell line (LoVo/DX) expressing a typical MDR phenotype. Tallimustine exhibits a broad spectrum of antitumor activity against a variety of murine and human solid tumor models, including human melanoma (M14) and small-cell lung carcinoma

(N592). An unexpected finding of in vivo evaluation of tallimustine was a marginal activity against conventional murine leukemia models (P388, L1210). The observation suggests that the pattern of tumor response is not related to the rate of tumor cell proliferation as observed for the conventional alkylating agents and supports a cell-type-specific cytotoxic effect of minor groove alkylators, presumably related to sequence-specific covalent modification of DNA and/or cell type-dependent drug accessibility to critical genes. This interpretation is supported by the toxicity profile observed in a clinical Phase I study of tallimustine (69). Drug treatment causes a highly selective and short-lasting neutropenia, but marginal thrombocytopenia. The pattern of hematological toxicity is peculiar, since treatment was conventional alkylating agents results in both neutropenia and thrombocytopenia.

Distamycin derivatives containing different pyrrole rings have been recently developed (70) (Fig. 3, see compounds 2). Among new compounds, preliminary pre clinical evaluation suggests that MEN 10710, which is a synthetic derivative of distamycin possessing four pyrrole rings in which the bis-(2-chloroethyl)-aminophenyl moiety is linked to the oligopyrrole backbone by the flexible butanamido chain (71), is pharmacologically interesting. The molecular mechanism of DNA interaction, investigated by footprinting experiments and by in vitro DNA interstrand-induced cross-linking, indicated a remarkable difference from tallimustine. Cytotoxic potency was increased by 10- to 50-fold compared to melphalan or tallimustine in human tumor cell lines. In vivo experiments indicated a significant antitumor efficacy against human tumor xenografts, including an ovarian cisplatin-resistant (A2780/DDP) tumor line. In vitro studies also showed a reduced myelotoxicity compared to tallimustine, suggesting a potential degree of selectivity against tumor cells with respect to normal cells.

Since polypyrrole compounds (i.e., distamycin and netropsin) may be susceptible to oxidative breakdown, bispyrazole compounds were prepared as potentially more stable minor groove binding analogs (72) (Fig. 3, compound 1). Although the compounds bind less strongly to DNA and show lower specificity for AT-rich sequences than distamycin, a benzoic acid mustard derivative has a cytotoxic potency comparable to that of the alkylating distamycin analog. A negligible antileukemic activity of the bispyrazole analog was reported in the treatment of P388 murine leukemia. Unfortunately, no solid tumors were used in the preliminary evaluation. Since alkylating derivatives of distamycin exhibit a marginal effectiveness against leukemia systems (68), no definitive conclusions could be drawn on the pharmacological interest of the bispyrazole derivatives.

The increased cytotoxic potency of minor groove binders following incorporation of a reactive moiety is not related to the extent of DNA alkylation. For example, tallimustine is known to alkylate a very limited number of adenines at the N-3 position (73). In spite of the presence of a typical alkylating moiety, tallimustine does not produce detectable covalent links with N-7 guanine, which is the major site of alkylation for conventional bifunctional alkylating agents (6). It appears that the site of alkylation is dependent on the mode of DNA interaction with the polypyrrole chain. This interpretation is supported by a similar mode of action reported for C-1065, the first compound of the minor groove alkylators, that exhibits a somewhat similar sequence recognition (6,64). The sequence selectivity of adenine adduct formation by tallimustine has been recently identified as 5'-TTTTGA-3' (74). A single base modification in the hexamer completely abolishes the adenine alkylation. Such a sequence specificity is unexpected for a low-mol-wt agent and could account for the limited extent of alkylation found in cellular DNA.

Several efforts have been made to modify DNA sequence selectivity of the distamycin/netropsin molecule. Structural modifications have been based on replacement of N-methylpyrrole by an N-methylimidazole to accommodate hydrogen bonding to the 2-amino group of guanine (75). Thus, a novel class of minor groove binding molecules (termed "lexitropsin" to identify information-reading oligopeptides) has been developed. A degree of GC recognition has been found in this series of compounds, but this is associated with a reduction of DNA binding affinity, presumably related to a marked sequence dependence of minor groove width (46). Recently, a GC sequence-specific recognition has been reported for an N-formamido C-terminus-modified lexitropin (76), which represents a new carrier molecule for the development of minor groove alkylators with a different sequence specificity. Alkylating lexitropsins have been used to document groove- and sequence-selective adduct formation by small-mol-wt alkylating agents, thereby providing an insight into the sequence and orientation preferences of the groove binder (77). Imidazole-containing analogs of distamycin were used as vectors for delivery of a variety of alkylating agents to GC-rich sequences (78,79). The most representative compounds of this series are shown in Fig. 3 (scheme 3). In an attempt to identify compounds with GC sequence selectivity and increased efficacy, oligoimidazolecarboxamido analogs of distamycin, wherein the N-terminus contains either a benzyl-mustard or a chloroambucil moiety, were prepared (79). The pattern of DNA alkylation was markedly different from that of other minor groove binder benzoyl mustards, since the former compounds were found to alkylate guanine-N7 in the major groove and to form crosslinks (79). In contrast, benzoyl mustards do not alkylate guanine N-7, but produce highly cytotoxic monoalkylation. Lack of a correlation between the mode of drug binding to DNA (hence the extent of lesions) and cytotoxic potency suggests that comparable cytotoxic potency could be achieved through different mechanisms.

An interesting series of sequence-selective minor groove binders are cyclopropyl-pirroloindole antitumor antibiotics with unique features (64) (Fig. 4). The parent compound of the series is CC-1065, a fermentation product of *Streptomyces zelensis* containing two identical benzopyrrole units and an indolequinone system bearing a reactive cyclopropane ring. CC-1065 binds covalently and noncovalently in the minor groove of AT-rich regions of double-stranded DNA. The covalently bound species results from an alkylation reaction between the cyclopropyl group and N-3 of adenine. A sequence-selective alkylation was observed, with a reactive adenine located inside a 5-bp consensus, i.e., 5'AAAAA and 5'PyNTTA (N = any nucleotide) (80–82). Preclinical studies indicated that CC-1065 is one of the most potent cytotoxic agents ever found, with activity at nanomolar levels (83). However, it was not developed as a clinical candidate because of delayed and irreversible toxicity in preclinical studies (84).

The unique molecular and pharmacological features of CC-1065 led to a marked effort in the chemical modification of parent compound. Among a number of analogs, the first identified as a candidate for clinical development was adozelesin (U-73975) (85). The analog exhibits a similar mechanism of action, with a sequence-selective interaction overlapping at least in part with the parent compound (80). Adozelesin is characterized by a high potency and a promising profile of preclinical activity against murine and human tumor models, but devoided of delayed or irreversible toxicity of the parent compound (64). Phase I studies of adozelesin have been presented using

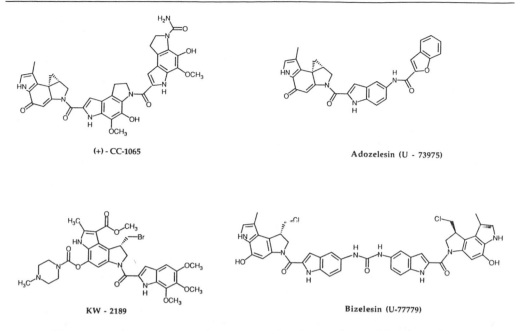

Fig. 4. Chemical structures of CC-1065 and cyclopropyl pyrroleindole analogs.

different iv infusion schedules (85,86). The maximum tolerated dose in a 3-wk schedule of brief iv infusion was 188 μg/m², thus documenting the potency expected on the basis of preclinical studies (85). The dose-limiting toxicity was myelosuppression with thrombocytopenia and leukopenia. The toxicity profile was similar, but not identical to that of other minor groove alkylators (69).

A possible drawback of adozelesin is its pharmacokinetic behavior characterized by a short half-life. In an attempt to modulate the pharmacologic properties, synthetic efforts were directed to the preparation of prodrugs in this series. A very promising compound is carzelesin (U-80244). Although less potent than adozelesin, it possesses a superior efficacy in preclinical evaluation and a more favorable pharmacological behavior (87). As found in other minor groove reactive agents (79), CC-1065 and adozelesin are monoalkylating agents. Based on the observation that clinically useful alkylators are crosslinking agents, cyclopropylpyrrolondole dimers were designed in an attempt to cause DNA damage in a bifunctional manner. Bizelesin (U-77779) emerged from this effort. Bizelesin produces stable interstrand crosslinks with an increased sequence selectivity (81,88). The dimeric bisalkylator derivative inhibits growth of human tumor cells at picomolar levels (89), thus supporting the view that crosslinks are more cytotoxic lesions than monoadducts. On the basis of its potency and good therapeutic index, bizelesin has been chosen for preclinical development (90). A comparative study of DNA binding properties and cytotoxic activity of simplified or extended nonalkylating oligomers of the dihydropyrroloindole ring structure of CC-1065 defined the structural features that contribute to noncovalent DNA minor groove binding, thus identifying the optimal binding unit (91). An interesting observation of the study was a correlation between cytotoxic activity of these oligomers and their molecular size. Although less potent than the alkylating parent compounds, these oligomers were found to be markedly more cytotoxic than other AT-selective, noncovalent minor groove binders (distamycin and netropsin). The finding is consistent with a critical contribution of the noncovalent complex in determining the pharmacological activity of the cyclopropylpyrroloindole drugs.

Duacarmycins are a novel antitumor antibiotic structurally related to CC-1065 (92). Duacarmycin A contains a reactive cyclopropane ring responsible for adenine alkylation at the 3′-end of sequences of three or more consecutive A or T. KW-2189, a synthetic analog of duacarmycin B2, has been selected for development on the basis of its promising pharmacological profile (93). The derivative is considered a prodrug; indeed, although its cytotoxic potency is substantially reduced, it is more effective than the parent compound against experimental tumor models, including drug-resistant human tumors.

On the basis of the mode of interaction with DNA, minor groove binders with alkylating functions should be considered as a novel class of alkylating agents, with a promising preclinical activity. Their clinical efficacy remans to be documented. In contrast to bifunctional alkylating agents (known to interact with N7 or O6 of guanines and cause crosslinks as typlical cytotoxic lesions), minor groove alkylators interact with the N3 of adenines with formation of a mono-adduct. It is likely that this mode of DNA interaction is related to the location of the drug in the minor groove before alkylation (74). In contrast to conventional alkylating agents (which cause selective inhibition of DNA synthesis), no correlation has been found between inhibition of DNA synthesis and cytotoxicity of adozelesin (94) or tallimustine (73). The inhibition of DNA synthesis is a delayed effect that reflects an arrest in G2 phase (73). Although the alkylation of DNA is considered as the primary lesion, the detailed mechanism of the cytotoxic action thus remains to be elucidated. A stimulating hypothesis is that the drug-induced DNA damage (caused by covalent binding) in consensus sequences for the binding of transcription factors may result in persistent impairment of the regulatory mechanisms of transcription of specific genes (7,46). A number of observations support this possibility. For example, distamycin A and its alkylating derivative inhibit the binding of transcription factors that recognize AT-rich consensus sequences in vitro (95). A similar observation has been reported for some synthetic N-methylpiperazine derivatives (Hoechst 33258 and 33342) (48). Minor groove binding drugs are effective inhibitors of formation of the TBP/DNA complex (45). CC-1065, which binds covalently to the DNA, is more effective than the noncovalent binder distamycin A. It is conceivable that the irreversible interaction of the alkylating derivatives may produce a persistent and more effective inhibition of transcription. TFIID, a member of a group of general transcription factors, plays a key role in the initiation step of transcription by RNA polymerase II (44). If the primary mechansim of cell toxicity of minor groove alkylators is related to inhibition of transcription through interference with these regulatory proteins, the mode of actions could not be regarded as tumor cell-specific. Indeed, the cytotoxic potency of these agents is also reflected by their in vivo potency. Thus, the therapeutic index is expected to be a critical pharmacological determinant of the clinical usefulness of the minor groove alkylators.

6. CONCLUSIONS

Most of currently used antitumor agents proven to be clinically effective were discovered through empirical approaches, including random screening of natural and synthetic compounds or systematic chemical maniputations of active agents (i.e., analog development). The identification of their preclinical efficacy led to therapeutic application long before the mechanistic basis of the antitumor effects was understood. Progress in molecular pharmacology of DNA-damaging agents and in molecular biology of tumor cells (oncogene activation, gene regulation, signal transduction) has provided a more rational basis for new drug discovery by exploiting specific macromolecular targets for pharmacological intervention (96).

Groove binding drugs exhibit a striking sequence specificity in DNA interaction and DNA damage (7,46). However, it is evident that the recognition potential of available DNA-interacting agents is not sufficient to provide selective cytotoxicity against tumor cells. Although it appears that DNA lesions produced by DNA-reactive agents are not randomly distributed in the entire genome (10), many of these lesions are probably not required for therapeutic activity. Indeed, cell-specific effects may not be related to the bulk DNA damage (97). Studies performed with tallimustine at the molecular level indicate that a low level of DNA damage sustained at relevant sites of the genome may mediate drug action. Unfortunately, although malignant transformation is known to involve a stepwise accumulation of specific alterations in genes normally regulating growth stimulatory or inhibitory pathways, the critical genes and therefore the DNA sequences most appropriate as useful targets for tumor-specific effects remain to be identified (98). It is possible that efforts directed to the identification of gene-specific sites of DNA damage may provide insight for a better understanding of the molecular/cellular basis of the relative tumor selectivity of available effective antitumor agents. A critical aspect of this molecular pharmacology approach concerns the cellular implications of sequence specificity of drug-induced DNA interaction (and DNA damage) observed in vitro with isolated DNA or oligonucleotide models. Drug interaction is dependent not only on specific sequence, but also on target accessibility and DNA conformation in chromatin. For example, in the presence of the minor groove binder, distamycin A, duocarmycin A induces alkylation of guanine residues that are usually not alkylated by duocarmycin A alone (99). DNA alkylation sites induced by adozelesin and bizelesin in human colon carcinoma cells were mapped in individual genes at the single-nucleotide level (100). The pattern of alkylation induced by these drugs is similar, but not identical to that observed in isolated cell-free DNA. These findings indicated that drug reaction with DNA may be critically influenced by DNA conformation in chromatin.

Among known DNA-interacting compounds, only DNA-damaging drugs have a significant antitumor activity. These agents cause different types of DNA lesions depending on the mode of DNA interactions. It is conceivable that their antitumor efficacy is related to the type of drug-induced lesions and to the persistence of DNA damage. A critical question for the identification of more specific and effective DNA-damaging agents concerns the role played by the sequence specificity and, therefore, the genomic localization of DNA damage. It is conceivable that the cytotoxic and antitumor potency is dependent on the site of drug-induced DNA lesions and the tumor-specific effects of known DNA-kamaging agents are the result of selective DNA damage to critical genes presumably relevant for growth and/or survival (10). Of course, the introduction of a DNA-damaging moiety in more specific DNA-recognizing elements (e.g., oligonucleotides as major groove binders or oligopeptides as minor groove binders) (101) is expected to cause DNA damage at selected genomic sites. However, the exploitation of these highly selective molecules for drug design is still hindered by several chemical and pharmacological problems, including stability of the carriers, poor cellular penetration, and difficulties of synthesis. The available sequence-selective agents can be viewed as structural models for further development of drugs designed to interfere with DNA sites recognized by specific regulatory proteins. The continued development of molecular structural principles in the design process will also provide an increased understanding of the mechanism of tumor inhibition, thus leading to the synthesis of more effective antitumor agents (*46*).

ACKNOWLEDGMENTS

We thank B. Gatto for her critical reading of the manuscript and Laura Zanesi for careful preparation of the manuscript. We gratefully acknowledge grant supports from Associazione Italiana per la Ricerca sul Cancro (Milan), from Progetto Finalizzato ACRO, Consiglio Nazionale delle Ricerche (Rome) and Ministro della Sanita', Italy.

REFERENCES

1. Zimmer C, Wähnert U. Nonintercalating DNA-binding ligands: specificity of the interaction and their use as tools in biophysical, biochemical and biological investigations of the genetic material. *Prog Biophys Mol Biol* 1986; 47:31–112.
2. Hurley LH, Boyd FL. Approaches towards the design of sequence specific drugs for DNA. *Annu Rep Med Chem* 1987; 22:259–268.
3. Smets LA. Programmed cell death (apoptosis) and response to anti-cancer drugs. *Anticancer Drugs* 1994; 5:3–9.
4. Neidle S, Pearl LH, Skelly JV. DNA structure and perturbation by drug binding. *Biochem J* 1987; 243:1–13.
5. Hurley LH. DNA and associated targets for drug design. *J Med Chem* 1989; 32:2027–2033.
6. Warpehoski MA, Hurley LH. Sequence selectivity of DNA covalent modification. *Chem Res Toxicol* 1988; 1:315–333.
7. D'Incalci M, Broggini M, Hartley JA. Sequence and gene-specific drugs. In: Workman P, ed. *New Approaches in Cancer Pharmacology: Drug Design and Development*. Berlin: Springer Verlag, 1992:5–11.
8. Pullman A, Pullman B. Molecular electrostatic potential of the nucleic acids. *Q Rev Biophys* 1981; 14:289–380.
9. Farrell N, Qu Y, Feng L, Van Houten B. Comparison of the chemical reactivity, cytotoxicity, interstrand cross-linking and DNA sequence specificity of bis(platinum) complexes containing monodentate or bidentate coordination spheres with their monomeric analogues. *Biochemistry* 1990; 29:9522–9531.
10. Broggini M, D'Incalci M. Modulation of transcription factor-DNA interactions by anticancer drugs. *Anticancer Drug Design* 1994; 9:373–387.
11. Hamilton TC, Johnson SW, Godwin AK, Bookman MA, O'Dwyer PJ, Hamaguchi K, Jackson K, Ozols RF. Drug resistance in ovarian cancer and potential for its reversal. In: Sharp F, Mason P, Blackett T, Berek J, eds. *Ovarian Cancer 3*. Chapman & Hall Medical, 1994: 203–213.
12. Zhen WP, Link CJ, O'Connor PM. Increased gene-specific repair of cisplatin interstrand cross-links in cisplatin-resistant human ovarian cancer cell lines. *Mol Cell Biol* 1992; 12: 3689–3698.
13. Zunino F, Capranico G. DNA topoisomerase II as the primary target of antitumor anthracyclines. *Anticancer Drug Design* 1990; 5:307–317.
14. Capranico G, Zunino F. DNA topoisomerase-trapping antitumour drugs. *Eur J Cancer* 1992; 28A:2055–2060.
15. Chen AY, Liu LF. DNA topoisomerases: essential enzymes and lethal targets. *Annu Rev Pharmacol Toxicol* 1994; 34:191–218.
16. Capranico G, De Isabella P, Penco S, Tinelli S, Zunino F. Role of DNA breakage in cytotoxicity of doxorubicin, 9-deoxydoxorubicin, and 4-demethyl-6-deoxydoxorubicin in murine leukemia P388 cells. *Cancer Res* 1989; 49:2022–2027.

17. Capranico G, Supino R, Binaschi M, Capolongo L, Grandi M, Suarato A, Zunino F. Influence of structural modifications at the 3' and 4' positions of doxorubicin on the drug ability to trap topoisomerase II and to overcome multidrug resistance. *Mol Pharmacol* 1994; 45: 908–915.

18. Moore MH, Hunter WN, d'Estaintot BL, Kennard O. DNA-drug interactions. The crystal structure of d(CGATCG) complexed with daunomycin. *J Mol Biol* 1989; 206:693–705.

19. Woynarowski JM, Sigmund RD, Beerman TA. DNA minor groove binding agents interfere with topoisomerase II mediated lesions induced by epipodophyllotoxin derivative VM-26 and acridine derivative m-AMSA in nuclei from L1210 cells. *Biochemistry* 1989; 28:3850–3855.

20. Fesen M, Pommier Y. Mammalian topoisomerase II activity is modulated by the DNA minor groove binder distamycin in simian virus 40 DNA. *J Biol Chem* 1989; 264:11,354–11,359.

21. Wassermann K, Markovits J, Jaxel C, Capranico G, Kohn KW, Pommier Y. Effects of morpholinyl doxorubicins, doxorubicin, and actinomycin D on mammalian DNA topoisomerase I and II. *Mol Pharmacol* 1990; 38:38–45.

22. Capranico G, Butelli E, Zunino F. Change of the sequence specificity of daunorubicin-stimulated topoisomerase II DNA cleavage by epimerization of the amino group of the sugar moiety. *Cancer Res* 1995; 55:312–317.

23. Kamitori S, Takusagawa F. Crystal structure of the 2:1 complex between d(GAAGCTTC) and the anticancer drug actinomycin D. *J Mol Biol* 1992; 225:445–456.

24. Capranico G, Palumbo M, Tinelli S, Mabilia M, Pozzan A, Zunino F. Conformational drug determinants of the sequence specificity of drug-stimulated topoisomerase II DNA cleavage. *J Mol Biol* 1994; 235:1218–1230.

25. Caprianico G, Palumbo M, Tinelli S, Zunino F. Unique sequence specificity of topoisomerase II DNA cleavage stimulation and DNA binding mode of streptonigrin. *J Biol Chem* 1994; 269:25,004–25,009.

26. Riou J-F, Fossé P, Nguyen CH, Larsen AK, Bissery M-C, Grondard L, Saucier J-M, Bisagni E, Lavelle F. Intoplicine (RP 60475) and its derivatives, a new class of antitumor agents inhibiting both topoisomerase I and II activities. *Cancer Res* 1993; 53:5987–5993.

27. Trask DK, Muller MT. Stabilization of type I topoisomerase–DNA covalent complexes by actinomycin D. *Proc Natl Acad Sci USA* 1988; 85:1417–1421.

28. Yamashita Y, Kawada SZ, Fujii N, Nakano H. Induction of mammalian DNA topoisomerase I and II mediated DNA cleavage by saintopin, a new antitumor agent from fungus. *Biochemistry* 1991; 30:5838–5845.

29. Riou JF, Helissey P, Grondard L, Giorgi-Renault S. Inhibition of eukaryotic DNA topoisomerase I and II activities by indoloquinolinedione derivatives. *Mol Pharmacol* 1991; 40: 699–706.

30. Yamashita Y, Fujii N, Murakata C, Ashizawa T, Okabe M, Nakano H. Induction of mammalian DNA topoisomerase I mediated DNA cleavage by antitumor indolocarbazole derivatives. *Biochemistry* 1992; 31:12,069–12,075.

31. Wassermann K, Newman RA, Davis FM, Mullins TD, Rose KM. Selective inhibition of human ribosomal gene transcription by the morpholinyl anthracyclines cyanomorpholinyl- and morpholinyldoxorubicin. *Cancer Res* 1988; 48:4101–4106.

32. Nicolaou KC, Smith AL, Yue EW. Chemistry and biology of natural and designed enediynes. *Proc Natl Acad Sci USA* 1993; 90:5881–5888.

33. Sugiura Y, Matsumoto T. Some characteristics of DNA strand scission by macromolecular antitumor antibiotic C-1027 containing a novel enediyne chromophore. *Biochemistry* 1993; 32:5548–5553.

34. Xu YJ, Zhen YS, Goldberg IH. C1027 chromophore, a potent new enediyne antitumor antibiotic, induces sequence-specific double-strand DNA cleavage. *Biochemistry* 1994; 33:5947–5954.

35. Hawley RC, Kiessling LL, Schreiber SL. Model of the interactions of calicheamicin gamma 1 with a DNA fragment from pBR322. *Proc Natl Acad Sci USA* 1989; 86:1105–1109.

36. Zein N, Sinha AM, McGahren WJ, Ellestad GA. Calicheamicin gamma 1I: an antitumor antibiotic that cleaves double-stranded DNA site specifically. *Science* 1988; 240:1198–1201.

37. Uesugi M, Sekida T, Matsuki S, Sugiura Y. Selective DNA cleavage by elsamicin A and switch function of its amino sugar group. *Biochemistry* 1991; 30:6711–6715.

38. Kenani A, Lohez M, Houssin R, Helbecque N, Lemay P, Hénichart JP. Chelating, DNA-binding and DNA-cleaving properties of a bleomycin synthetic model. *Anticancer Drug Design* 1987; 2:47–59.

39. Chen AY, Yu C, Gatto B, Liu LF. DNA minor groove-binding ligands: a different class of mammalian DNA topoisomerase I inhibitors. *Proc Natl Acad Sci USA* 1993; 90:8131–8135.

40. Beerman TA, Woynarowski JM, Sigmund RD, Gawron LS, Rao KE, Lown JW. Netropsin and bis-netropsin analogs as inhibitors of the catalytic activity of mammalian DNA topoisomerase II and topoisomerase cleavable complexes. *Biochim Biophys Acta* 1991; 1090:52–60.

41. Beerman TA, McHugh MM, Sigmund R, Lown JW, Rao KE, Bathini Y. Effects of analogs of the DNA minor groove binder Hoechst 33258 on topoisomerase II and I mediated activities. *Biochim. Biophys Acta* 1992; 1131:53–61.

42. Fujii N, Yamashita Y, Saitoh Y, Nakano H. Induction of mammalian DNA topoisomerase I-mediated DNA cleavage and DNA winding by bulgarein. *J Biol Chem* 1993; 268:13,160–13,165.

43. Merino A, Madden KR, Lane WS, Champoux JJ, Reinberg D. DNA topoisomerase I is involved in both repression and activation of transcription. *Nature* 1993; 365:227–232.

44. Lee DK, Horikoshi M, Roeder RG. Interaction of TFIID in the minor groove of the TATA element. *Cell* 1991; 67:1241–1250.

45. Chiang S-Y, Welch J, Rauscher FJ, Beerman TA. Effects of minor groove binding drugs on the interaction of TATA box binding protein and TFIIA with DNA. *Biochemistry* 1994; 33: 7033–7040.

46. Neidle S. Principles in the design of DNA-interactive molecules. In: Workman P, ed. *New Approaches in Cancer Pharmacology: Drug Design and Development,* vol. II. Heidelberg: Springer Verlag, 1994:9–22.

47. Wang H, Gupta R, Lown JW. Synthesis, DNA binding, sequence preference and biological evaluation of minor groove-selective N1-alkoxyalkyl-bis-benzimidazoles. *Anticancer Drug Design* 1994; 9:153–180.

48. Wong SSC, Sturm RA, Michel J, Zhang X-M, Danoy PAC, McGregor K, Jacobs JJ, Kaushal A, Dong Y, Dunn IS, Parsons PG. Transcriptional regulation of differentiation, selective toxicity and ATGCAAAT binding of bisbenzimidazole derivatives in human melanoma cells. *Biochem Pharmacol* 1994; 47:827–837.

49. Chen AY, Y C, Bodley A, Peng LF, Liu LF. A new mammalian DNA topoisomerase I poison Hoechst 33342: cytotoxicity and drug resistance in human cell cultures. *Cancer Res* 1993; 53: 1332–1337.

50. Kam M, Shafer RH, Berman E. Solution conformation of the antitumor antibiotic chromomycin A3 determined by two-dimensional NMR spectroscopy. *Biochemistry* 1988; 27:3581–3588.

51. Fox KR, Cons BM. Interaction of mithramycin with DNA fragments complexed with nucleosome core particles: comparison with distamycin and echinomycin. *Biochemistry* 1993; 32: 7162–7171.

52. Silva DJ, Goodnow R Jr, Kahne D. The sugars in chromomycin A3 stabilize the $Mg(2+)$-dimer complex. *Biochemistry* 1993; 32:463–471.

53. Gao XL, Mirau P, Patel DJ. Structure refinement of the chromomycin dimer-DNA oligomer complex in solution. *J Mol Biol* 1992; 223:259–279.

54. van Houte LP, van Garderen CJ, Patel DJ. The antitumor drug nogalamycin forms two different intercalation complexes with d(GCGT).d(ACGC). *Biochemistry* 1993; 32:1667–1674.

55. Bailly C, Leclere V, Pommery N, Colson P, Houssier C, Rivalle C, Bisagni E, Hénichart J-P. Binding to DNA, cellular uptake and biological activity of a distamycin-ellipticine hybrid molecule. *Anticancer Drug Design* 1993; 8:145–164.

56. Bailly C, Michaux C, Colson P, Houssier C, Sun J-S, Garestier T, Hélène C, Hénichart J-P, Rivalle C, Bisagni E, Waring MJ. Reaction of a biscationic distamycin-ellipticine hybrid ligand with DNA. Mode and sequence specificity of binding. *Biochemistry* 1994; 33:15,348–15,364.

57. Bailly C, Collyn-D'Hooghe M, Lantoine D, Fournier C, Hecquet B, Fosse P, Saucier J-M, Colson P, Houssier C, Hénichart J-P. Biological activity and molecular interaction of a netropsin-acridine hybrid ligand with chromatin and topoisomerase II. *Biochem Pharmacol* 1992; 43:457–466.

58. Hartley JA, McAdam SR, Das S, Roldan MC, Haskell MK, Lee M. Molecular and cellular pharmacology of novel photoactive psoralen and coumarin conjugates of pyrrole- and imidazole-containing analogues of netropsin. *Anticancer Drug Design* 1994; 9:181–197.

59. Borowy-Borowski H, Lipman R, Tomasz M. Recognition between mitomycin C and specific DNA sequences for cross-link formation. *Biochemistry* 1990; 29:2999–3006.
60. Kizu R, Draves PH, Hurley LH. Correlation of DNA sequence specificity of anthramycin and tomaymycin with reaction kinetics and bending of DNA. *Biochemistry* 1993; 32:8712–8722.
61. Kopka ML, Goodsell DS, Baikalov I, Grzeskowiak K, Cascio D, Dickerson RE. Crystal structure of a covalent DNA-drug adduct: anthramycin bound to C-C-A-A-C-G-T-T-G-G and a molecular explanation of specificity. *Biochemistry* 1994; 33:13,593–13,610.
62. Subhas Bose D, Thompson AS, Ching J, Hartley JA, Berardini MD, Jenkins TC, Neidle S, Hurley LH, Thurston DE. Rational design of a highly efficient non-reversible DNA interstrand cross-linking agent based on the pyrrolobenzodiazepine ring system. *J Am Chem Soc* 1992; 114:4939–4941.
63. Wang JJ, Hill GC, Hurley LH. Template-directed design of a DNA-DNA cross-linker based upon a bis-tomaymycin-duplex adduct. *J Med Chem* 1992; 35:2995–3002.
64. Wierenga W. Sequence-selective DNA-interactive antitumor agents. *Drugs Future* 1991; 16: 741–750.
65. Krowicki K, Balzarini J, De Clercq E, Newman RA, Lown JW. Novel DNA groove binding alkylators: design, synthesis, and biological evaluation. *J Med Chem* 1988; 31:341–345.
66. Gravatt GL, Baguley BC, Wilson WR, Denny WA. DNA-directed alkylating agents. 4. 4-anilinoquinoline-based minor groove directed aniline mustards. *J Med Chem* 1991; 34:1552–1560.
67. Arcamone FM, Animati F, Barbieri B, Configliacchi E, D'Alessio R, Geroni C, Giuliani FC, Lazzari E, Menozzi M, Mongelli N, Penco S, Verini MA. Synthesis, DNA-binding properties, and antitumor activity of novel distamycin derivatives. *J Med Chem* 1989; 32:774–778.
68. Pezzoni G, Grandi M, Biasoli G, Capolongo L, Ballinari D, Giuliani FC, Barbieri B, Pastori A, Pesenti E, Mongelli N, Spreafico F. Biological profile of FCE 24517, a novel benzoyl mustard analogue of distamycin A. *Br J Cancer* 1991; 64:1047–1050.
69. Sessa C, Pagain O, Zurlo MG, de Jong J, Hofmann C, Lassus M, Marrari P, Benedetti MS, Cavalli F. Phase I study of the novel distamycin derivative tallimustine (FCE 24517). *Ann Oncol* 1994; 5:901–907.
70. Animati F, Arcamone F, Bigioni M. DNA sequence selectivity of novel distamycin analogues exhibiting remarkable cytotoxic activity. 8th NCI-EORTC Symposium on New Drugs in Cancer Therapy. Amsterdam, March 15–18, 1994.
71. Bigioni M, Ciucci A, Palma C. Biologicl profile of MEN 10710, a distamycin A derivative possessing antitumor activity and peculiar mode of DNA interaction. 86th Annual Meeting of the American Association for Cancer Research. Toronto, Ontario, Canada, March 18–22, 1995.
72. Lee HH, Boyd M, Gravatt GL, Denny WA. Pyrazole analogues of the bispyrrolocarboxamide anti-tumour antibiotics: synthesis, DNA binding and antitumour properties. *Anticancer Drug Design* 1991; 6:501–517.
73. Broggini M, Erba E, Ponti M, Ballinari D, Geroni C, Spreafico F, D'Incalci M. Selective DNA interaction of the novel distamycin derivative FCE 24517. *Cancer Res* 1991; 51:199–204.
74. Broggini M, Coley H, Mongelli N, Presenti E, Wyatt MD, Hartley JA, D'Incalci M. DNA sequence-specific adenine alkylation by the novel antitumor drug tallimustine (FCE 24517), a benzoyl nitrogen mustard derivative of distamycin. *Nucleic Acids Res.* 1995; 23:81–87.
75. Lown JW. Lexitropsins: rational design of DNA sequence reading agents as novel anti-cancer agents and potential cellular probes. *Anticancer Drug Design* 1988; 3:25–40.
76. Lee M, Preti CS, Vinson E, Wyatt MD, Hartley JA. GC sequence specific recognition by an *N*-formamido, C-terminus-modified and imidazole-containing analogue of netropsin. *J Med Chem* 1994; 37:4073–4075.
77. Zhang Y, Chen F-X, Mehta P, Gold B. Groove- and sequence-selective alkylation of DNA by sulfonate esters tethered to lexitropsins. *Biochemistry* 1993; 32:7954–7965.
78. Lee M, Rhodes AL, Wyatt MD, D'Incalci M, Forrow S, Hartley JA. In vitro cytotoxicity of GC sequence directed alkylating agents related to distamycin. *J Med Chem* 1993; 36:863–870.
79. Lee M, Rhodes AL, Wyatt MD, Forrow S, Harley JA. Design, synthesis, and biological evaluation of DNA sequence and minor groove selective alkylating agents. *Anticancer Drug Design* 1993; 8:173–192.
80. Hurley LH, Warpehoski MA, Lee C-S, McGovren JP, Scahill TA, Kelly RC, Mitchell MA, Wicnienski MA, Gebhard I, Johnson PS, Bradford VS. Sequence specificity of DNA alkylation by the unnatural enantiomer of CC-1065 and its synthetic analogues. *J Am Chem Soc*

1990; 112:4633–4649.

81. Ding Z-M, Hurley LH. DNA interstrand cross-linking, DNA sequence specificity, and induced conformational changes produced by a dimeric analog of (+)-CC-1065. *Anticancer Drug Design* 1991; 6:427–452.

82. Krueger WC, Hatzenbuhler NT, Prairie MD, Shea MH. DNA sequence recognition by the antitumor antibiotic CC-1065 and analogs of CC-1065. *Chem-Biol Interact* 1991; 79:265–286.

83. Wierenga W, Bhuyan BK, Kelly RC, Krueger WC, LI LH, McGovren JP, Swenson DH, Warpehoski MA. Antitumor activity and biochemistry of novel analogs of the antibiotic, CC-1065. *Adv Enzyme Regul* 1986; 25:141–155.

84. McGovren JP, Clarke GL, Pratt EA, DeKoning TF. Preliminary toxicity studies with the DNA-binding antibiotic, CC-1065. *J. Antibiot.* 1984; 37:63–70.

85. Shamdas GJ, Alberts DS, Modiano M, Wiggins C, Power J, Kasunic DA, Elfring GL, Earhart RH. Phase I study of adozelesin (U-73,975) in patients with solid tumors. *Anticancer Drugs* 1994; 5:10–14.

86. Fleming GF, Ratain MJ, O'Brien SM, Schilsky RL, Hoffman PC, Richards JM, Vogelzang NJ, Kasunic DA, Earhart RH. Phase I study of adozelesin administered by 24-hour continuous intravenous infusion. *J Natl Cancer Inst* 1994; 86:368–372.

87. Li LH, DeKoning TF, Kelly RC, Krueger WC, McGovren JP, Padbury GE, Petzold GL, Wallace TL, Ouding RJ, Prairie MD, Gebhard I. Cytotoxicity and antitumor activity of carzelesin, a prodrug cyclopropylpyrroloindole analogue. *Cancer Res* 1992; 52:4904–4913.

88. Lee C-S, Gibson NW. DNA damage and differential cytotoxicity produced in human carcinoma cells by CC-1065 analogues, U-73,975 and U-77,779. *Cancer Res* 1991; 51:6586–6591.

89. Walker DL, Reid JM, Ames MM. Preclinical pharmacology of bizelesin, a potent bifunctional analog of the DNA-binding antibiotic CC-1065. *Cancer Chemother Pharmacol* 1994; 34:317–322.

90. Weiss GR, Burris III HA, Eckardt JR, Fields S, O'Rourke T, Rodriguez GI, Rothenberg ML. New anticancer agents. In: Pinedo HM, Longo DL, Chabner BA, eds. *Cancer Chemotherapy and Biological Response Modifiers Annual 15.* Elsevier Science. 1994:130–151.

91. Boger DL, Invergo BJ, Coleman RS, Zarrinmayeh H, Kitos PA, Collins Thompson S, Leong T, McLaughhlin LW. A demonstration of the intrinsic importance of stabilizing hydrophobic binding and non-covalent van der Waals contacts dominant in the non-covalent CC-1065/B-DNA binding. *Chem-Biol Interact* 1990; 73:29–52.

92. Sugiyama H, Hosoda M, Saito I. Covalent alkylation of DNA with duocarmycin A. Identification of a basic site structure. *Tetrahedron Lett* 1990; 31:7197–7200.

93. Hoshi A, Castaner J. KW-2189. *Drugs Future* 1993; 18:1112,1113.

94. Bhuyan BK, Smith KS, Adams EG, Wallace TL, Vonhoff DD, Li LH. Adozelesin, a potent new alkylating agent. Cell-killing kinetics and cell-cycle effects. *Cancer Chemother Pharmacol* 1992; 30:348.

95. Broggini M, Ponti M, Ottolenghi S, D'Incalci M, Mongelli N, Mantovani R. Distamycins inhibit the binding of OTF-1 and NFE-1 transfactors to their conserved DNA elements. *Nucleic Acids Res* 1989; 17:1051–1059.

96. Zunino F, Capranico G, Pratesi G, Spinelli S. Current approaches to new drug development in cancer chemotherapy. *Farmaco* 1992; 47:1115–1132.

97. Gewirtz DA. Does bulk damage to DNA explain the cytostatic and cytotoxic effects of topoisomerase II inhibitors? *Biochem Pharmacol* 1991; 42:2253–2258.

98. Schwab G, Guroux I, Chavany C, Hélène C, Saison-Behmoaras E. An approach for new anticancer drugs: oncogene-targeted antisense DNA. *Ann Oncol* 1994; 5:S55–S58.

99. Yamamoto K, Sugiyama H, Kawanishi S. Concerted DNA recognition and novel site-specific alkylation by duocarmycin A with distamycin A. *Biochemistry* 1993; 32:1059–1066.

100. Lee CS, Pfeifer GP, Gibson NW. Mapping of DNA alkylation sites induced by adozelesin and bizelesin in human cells by ligation-mediated polymerase chain reaction. *Biochemistry* 1994; 33:6024–6030.

101. Hélène C. Rational design of sequence-specific oncogene inhibitors based on antisense and antigene oligonucleotides. *Eur J Cancer* 1991; 27:1466–1471.

10 Bis-Naphthalimides
Synthesis and Preclinical Evaluation

Cynthia A. Romerdahl, PhD and Miguel F. Braña, PhD

CONTENTS

1. INTRODUCTION

DNA intercalating agents are among the most common anticancer drugs used in the clinical therapy of human tumors. Although some drugs, such as doxorubicin and daunomycin, were originally isolated from natural sources, other compounds are synthetic organic molecules specifically designed as antineoplastic agents. Arcamone has classified these drugs on the basis of DNA interaction into:

1. Compounds that are able to bind covalently to DNA;
2. Agents that cause cleavage of the DNA; and
3. Drugs that bind reversibly to double-helical DNA (*1*).

Our synthetic efforts have focused on this last group, in the hopes that the lack of covalent binding to DNA or DNA nicking would lead to compounds that were less toxic to nontumor tissues. Naphthalimides were synthesized as a new series of potential antitumor compounds in the late 1970s (*2–4*). Since bis-intercalating agents have an even higher binding affinity for DNA (*5*), we later synthesized and evaluated a number of bis-intercalating naphthalimides (designated as bis-naphthalimides) (*6*). In this chapter, we review the origins of this new class of cytotoxic intercalators and summarize the data on the efficacy of these compounds in preclinical models.

2. MONOMERIC NAPHTHALIMIDES

2.1. Synthesis

The naphthalimide series was originally derived by trying to combine structural components of several antitumor compounds into a single molecule (Fig. 1). After

From: *Cancer Therapeutics: Experimental and Clinical Agents*
Edited by: B. Teicher Humana Press Inc., Totowa, NJ

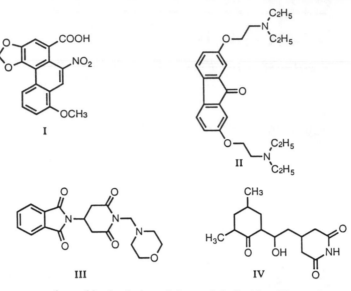

Fig. 1. Cytotoxic compounds used in the design of the naphthalimides. Pictured are aristolochic acid I, tilorone II, CG-603 III, and cycloheximide IV.

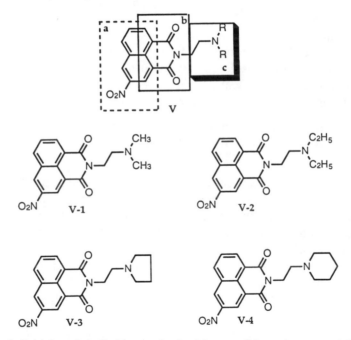

Fig. 2. Initial naphthalimides synthesized for possible antitumor activity.

studying many structures, we selected the following: aristolochic acid 1, a natural product with the intercalating phenanthrene system isolated from different strains of *Aristolochiaceae*; tilorone II, another intercalator that is also an interferon inducer; CG-603 III, a antiproliferative compound; and the protein synthesis inhibitor cyclo-heximide IV. Different moieties were combined into the naphthalimide V system shown in Fig. 2, retaining the β-nitro-naphthalene a of the aristolochic acid, the gluta-

Table 1
Cytotoxic Activity and Acute Toxicity of Selected Naphthalimides

Comp.	IC_{50} μg/mL HeLa Cells	IC_{50} μg/mL KB Cells	LD_{50} mg/kg mouse ip	LD_{50} mg/kg rat ip
V - 1	0.15	0.20	10	6.5
V - 2	2.50	3.50	13	32.5
V - 3	0.30	0.35	12.6	4.5
V - 4	2.0	2.0	40	9.1

rimide rings b that appear in GC-603 and cycloheximide, and the basic chains c present in tilorone and CG-603. The compounds designated as V-1–4 were synthesized and tested for activity using the HeLa and KB cell lines in culture. The data are summarized in Table 1 (3). Two of these derivatives were more active than 6-mercaptopurine, which was used as a reference compound for the cytotoxicity assays. This excellent antitumor activity suggested this was a promising strategy, and a large series of these naphthalimides were then synthesized.

2.2. Biological Activity

The structures and antitumor activities of the naphthalimide derivatives are presented in Table 2. The compounds were compared based on the concentration of drug required to inhibit 50% of the growth of HeLa cells. Growth inhibition was maximal when the side chain was formed by two methylene groups (position Y) and the presence of a basic terminal N group was required at position X (4). The positioning of the substituents in the naphthalic ring seemed optimal at position 5, instead of 4 or 6. These results were subsequently confirmed by other groups (7,8).

Samples from this series were sent to the National Cancer Institute (NCI) for screen- and evaluation (9,10). The activity of these compounds was confirmed by the NCI. One of the series, designated as Amonafide by the WHO (V-10 in Table 2, NSC 308847), was active against the P388 and L1210 leukemia models being used as the primary screen. When Amonafide is given ip 17.5 mg/kg (q 1 d × 5), the increase in life-span is ∼50% over the untreated mice. Amonafide was selected for exploratory clinical development by the NCI. Another active agent from this series, one of the first synthesized (V-1) was designated as Mitonafide (NSC 300288) by the WHO. Mitonafide has in vitro activity against the KB and HeLa cells, as well as in vivo activity against murine and human tumor cell lines (3). The structures of these two compounds are shown in Fig. 3.

Amonafide and Mitonafide bind to double-stranded DNA by intercalation. These drugs stabilize DNA against thermal denaturation, inhibit RNA and DNA synthesis, and initiate DNA cleavage by topoisomerase II, resulting in single-strand breaks (11–14). DNA intercalating agents are known to trap topoisomerase II (15). These compounds appear to hinder the religation step of topoisomerase II action by stabilizing the cleavable complex (16). Mitonafide and Amonafide specifically induce DNA cleavage near nucleotide No. 1830 on pBR322 DNA. It remains unclear, however, if the antitumor effects are due to the alterations of topoisomerase II activity.

In addition to their cytotoxity against tumor cells Amonafide and Mitonafide have other biological activities. Both compounds were active against herpes simplex and

Table 2
Cytotoxic Activity of Naphthalimides V

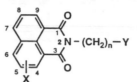

Comp. V	X	Y	n	IC_{50} μM
1	5-NO$_2$	N(CH$_3$)$_2$	2	0.47
2	5-NO$_2$	N(C$_2$H$_5$)$_2$	2	7.00
3	5-NO$_2$	N(CH$_2$)$_4$	2	0.80
4	5-NO$_2$	N(CH$_2$)$_5$	2	5.80
5	5-NO$_2$	N(CH$_2$)$_4$	0	>100
6	5-NO$_2$	N(CH$_2$)$_4$	1	100
7	5-NO$_2$	N(CH$_3$)$_2$	3	3.00
8	5-NO$_2$	N(C$_2$H$_5$)$_2$	3	14.00
9	5-NH$_2$	N(C$_2$H$_5$)$_2$	3	76.00
10	5-NH$_2$	N(CH$_3$)$_2$	2	8.80
11	5-NO$_2$	N(CH$_2$CH$_2$)$_2$O	2	56.00
12	5-NH$_2$	N(CH$_2$CH$_2$)$_2$O	2	30.00
13	5-NO$_2$	(CH$_2$)$_5$NC$_2$H$_5$	0	16.00
14	5-NH$_2$	N(C$_2$H$_5$)$_2$	2	9.60
15	5-NH$_2$	N(CH$_2$)$_4$	2	4.80
16	5-NO$_2$	N(CH$_2$CH$_2$)$_2$NCH$_3$	3	5.20
17	5-NH$_2$	N(CH$_2$CH$_2$)$_2$NCH$_3$	3	28.00
18	5-NH$_2$	N(CH$_2$)$_4$	2	24.00
19	5-Cl	N(CH$_2$CH$_2$)$_2$O	2	>100
20	5-Cl	N(CH$_3$)$_2$	3	6.00
21	5-Cl	N(CH$_2$)$_4$	2	4.50
22	5-Cl	N(CH$_2$)$_5$	2	10.00
23	5-Cl	N(CH$_3$)$_2$	2	2.60
24	5-OH	N(CH$_3$)$_2$	2	10.00
25	5-OH	N(CH$_2$CH$_2$)$_2$O	2	>100
26	5-OH	N(CH$_2$)$_4$	2	11.00
27	5-NO$_2$	N(CH$_3$)$_2$	0	>100
28	5-NO$_2$	N(CH$_3$)$_2$	0	>100
29	5-OCH$_3$	N(CH$_3$)$_2$	2	5.00
30	5-NHCO$_2$C$_2$H$_5$	N(CH$_3$)$_2$	2	28.00
31	5-NHCO$_2$C$_2$H$_5$	N(CH$_2$)$_4$	2	26.00
32	5-OCH$_3$	N(CH$_2$)$_4$	2	2.00
33	5-NHCOCH$_3$	N(CH$_3$)$_2$	2	12.00
34	5-NHCOCH$_3$	N(CH$_2$)$_4$	2	14.00
35	5-NO$_2$	CH(CH$_3$)$_2$	2	>100
36	5-NO$_2$	SH	2	>100
37	H	N(CH$_2$)$_4$	2	11.00
38	H	N(CH$_3$)$_2$	2	3.70
39	5-t-C$_4$H$_9$	N(CH$_3$)$_2$	2	43.00
40	5-NO$_2$	OH	2	>100

Table 2 (Continued)

Comp. V	X	Y	n	IC_{50} μM
41	5-NO$_2$	OCH$_3$	2	>100
42	5-NO$_2$	NH$_2$	2	2.40
43	5-NO$_2$	NHCH$_3$	2	13.00
44	5-NO$_2$	NHCOCH$_3$	2	>100
45	5-NHCO$_2$C$_2$H$_5$	N(C$_2$H$_5$)$_2$	2	26.00
46	5-NHCO$_2$C$_2$H$_5$	N(C$_2$H$_5$)$_2$	3	20.00
47	5-NH$_2$	N(CH$_3$)$_2$	3	16.00
48	5-OH	N(C$_2$H$_5$)$_2$	2	16.00
49	5-NHCOCH$_3$	N(C$_2$H$_5$)$_2$	2	16.00
50	5-NHCOCH$_3$	N(C$_2$H$_5$)$_2$	3	16.00
51	5-NO$_2$	$+$N(CH$_3$)$_3$,I$^-$	2	100
52	6-NO$_2$	N(CH$_3$)$_2$	2	6.30
53	6-NO$_2$	N(CH$_2$)$_4$	2	8.80
54	6-OCH$_3$	N(CH$_2$)$_4$	2	2.30
55	6-OCH$_3$	N(CH$_3$)$_2$	2	5.00
56	6-OCH$_3$	N(C$_2$H$_5$)$_2$	2	12.00
57	6-OCH$_3$	N(CH$_2$)$_5$	2	13.00
58	6-NH$_2$	N(CH$_3$)$_2$	2	3.50
59	6-NH$_2$	N(CH$_2$)$_4$	2	6.00
60	6-NO$_2$	N(C$_2$H$_5$)$_2$	2	16.00
61	6-NO$_2$	N(CH$_2$)$_5$	2	14.00
62	6-Br	N(CH$_3$)$_2$	2	23.00
63	6-Br	N(CH$_2$)$_4$	2	16.00
64	6-Cl	N(CH$_3$)$_2$	2	16.00
65	6-Cl	N(CH$_2$)$_4$	2	21.00
66	6-NH-Bu^n	N(CH$_3$)$_2$	2	11.00
67	6-NH-Bu^n	N(CH$_2$)$_4$	2	10.00
68	6-OH	N-(CH$_3$)$_2$	2	>100
69	6-OH	N(CH$_2$)$_4$	2	>100
70	4-OCH$_3$	N(CH$_3$)$_2$	2	10.00

vaccinia viruses in in vitro assays (*17*). This antiviral activity appears to be specific for DNA viruses, with no activity observed against influenza viruses. Amonafide and Mitonafide were also tested by the NCI in its HIV screen, where the results were negative (data not shown). Mitonafide is an antibiotic with maximum activity against *Bacillus subtilis, Salmonella typi*, and *Shigella dysenteriae (18)*. Amonafide and Mitonafide have also been tested for the ability to kill *Trypanosoma cruzii*, which causes Chagas' disease (*19*). Both compounds were able to kill the parasite in vitro, at concentrations of $10-^7M$. However, in vivo studies with infected mice showed toxicity, so the compounds were not pursued for therapy of Chagas' disease.

2.3. Clinical Evaluation

Both Mitonafide and Amonafide have been tested in clinical trials. Mitonafide was studied in Phase I and II trials using a short administration schedule (1-h infusion every day $\times$ 3–5 d), and it had activity against solid tumors (*20*). However, this dosing

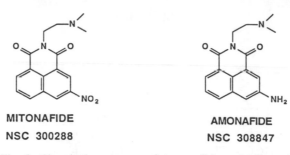

Fig. 3. Chemical structures of Amonafide and Mitonafide.

schedule was associated with central neurotoxicity. When the administration schedule was changed to a 5-d continuous infusion, Mitonafide could safely be administered. Unfortunately, the slow adminstration schedule lacked efficacy in the solid tumors that were tested (non-small cell lung, colorectal, and head and neck cancers) (*21*). Therefore, the clinical development was stopped.

Amonafide has completed several Phase I and II trials. The dose-limiting toxicity appears to be myelosuppression (*22,23*). When given alone, it has limited activity in some solid tumors (*24–26*). When given in combination with cytosine arabinoside, it induced complete remissions in some poor-risk acute leukemias (*27*). Amonafide at a dose of 400 mg/m² was eliminated from plasma with a terminal half-life of 3.5 h (*28*). The peak plasma concentrations were variable and ranged from 2.6 to 9.1 mg/mL. Amonafide undergoes extensive metabolism in vivo, including *N*-acetylation. The rate of acetylation varies owing to genetic differences among patients (*29*). Fast acetylator phenotyping may allow the Amonafide dose to be adjusted for this variability and could be used for future clinical studies.

3. SYNTHESIS OF THE BIS-NAPHTHALIMIDES

Several antibiotics isolated from microorganisms, such as Echinomycin or Luzopeptin, have the ability to intercalate doubly into DNA (*30*). Several groups have attempted to design such bis-intercalators, looking for an improved therapeutic profile. Some new synthetic products have been described, for example, diacridines or ditercalinium (*30*). In the early 1980s, we were interested in improving the activity of naphthalimides by increasing the binding capacity to DNA. Therefore, a new series of bis-intercalating agents was designed using structural features of the lead compounds, Mitonafide and Amonafide. Two of the chromophore units were linked together by bridges containing at least one amine group, because a preliminarily synthesized compound with polymethylenic bridge, V-35, did not showed in vitro activity (*31*). This suggested that the presence of at least an amino group is essential for significant cytotoxic activity, as in the mononaphthalimide series (*4*). We therefore prepared a series of compounds with different substituents in the aromatic system, as well as bridges differing in length and the number of amine groups. The synthesis of these compounds has been described in detail elsewhere (*31,32*). The structures of selected bis-naphthalimides are shown in Table 3. The aromatic substituents were predominantly amino and nitro, since these were the most active in the mononaphthalimide series. In addition, we added the acetylamino substituent, since the main metabolite of Amonafide is the acetyl derivative V-33.

Table 3
Selected Bis-Naphthalimides

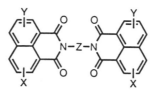

Comp.	X	Y	Z	IC_{50} μM
1	3-NO$_2$	H	(CH$_2$)$_2$-NH-(CH$_2$)$_2$	0.51
2	3-NH$_2$	H	(CH$_2$)$_2$-NH-(CH$_2$)$_2$	30.20
3	3-NH$_2$	6-NO$_2$	(CH$_2$)$_2$-NH-(CH$_2$)$_2$	0.27
4	3-NH$_2$	H	(CH$_2$)$_2$-NCH$_3$-(CH$_2$)$_2$	2.45
5	3-NH$_2$	H	(CH$_2$)$_2$-NH-(CH$_2$)$_3$	0.21
6	3-NH$_2$	H	(CH$_2$)$_2$-NH-(CH$_2$)$_3$	15.50
7	3-NH$_2$	H	(CH$_2$)$_3$-NCH$_3$-(CH$_2$)$_3$	0.07
8	3-NH$_2$	H	(CH$_2$)$_3$-NH-(CH$_2$)$_3$	0.16
9	3-NH$_2$	H	(CH$_2$)$_3$-NH-(CH$_2$)$_3$	4.96
10	3-NH$_2$	6-NO$_2$	(CH$_2$)$_3$-NH-(CH$_2$)$_3$	2.31
11	3-NH$_2$	6-NH$_2$	(CH$_2$)$_3$-NH-(CH$_2$)$_3$	> 100
12	4-NO$_2$	H	(CH$_2$)$_3$-NH-(CH$_2$)$_3$	2.78
13	3-NO$_2$	H	(CH$_2$)$_3$-NCH$_3$-(CH$_2$)$_3$	0.24
14	3-NH$_2$	H	(CH$_2$)$_2$-NCH$_3$-(CH$_2$)$_3$	1.87
15	3-NHCOCH$_3$	H	(CH$_2$)$_3$-NCH$_3$-(CH$_2$)$_3$	7.38
16	3-NO$_2$	6-NO$_2$	(CH$_2$)$_2$-NCH$_3$-(CH$_2$)$_3$	0.77
17	3-NO$_2$	6-NH$_2$	(CH$_2$)$_3$-NCH$_3$-(CH$_2$)$_3$	1.70
18	3-NH$_2$	6-NH$_2$	(CH$_2$)$_2$-NCH$_3$-(CH$_2$)$_3$	> 100
19	3-NO$_2$	H	(CH$_2$)$_3$-NH-C(CH$_3$)$_2$-(CH$_2$)$_2$	0.29
20	3-NO$_2$	H	(CH$_2$)$_3$-NH-(CH$_2$)$_4$	0.19
21	3-NHCOCH$_3$	H	(CH$_2$)$_3$-NH-(CH$_2$)$_4$	> 100
22	3-NO$_2$	H	(CH$_2$)$_2$-C(CH$_3$)$_2$-NH-(CH$_2$)$_4$	0.97
23	3-NH$_2$	H	(CH$_2$)$_3$-NH-(CH$_2$)$_2$-NH-(CH$_2$)$_3$	3.49
24	H	H	(CH$_2$)$_3$-NH-(CH$_2$)$_4$-NH-(CH$_2$)$_3$	2.70
25	3-NH$_2$	H	(CH$_2$)$_3$-NH-(CH$_2$)$_4$-NH-(CH$_2$)$_3$	39.00
26	3-NHCOCH$_3$	H	(CH$_2$)$_3$-NH-(CH$_2$)$_4$-NH-(CH$_2$)$_3$	> 100
27	3-NO$_2$	H	(CH$_2$)$_3$-NH-(CH$_2$)$_4$-NH-(CH$_2$)$_3$	0.72
28	3-NO$_2$	6-NO$_2$	(CH$_2$)$_3$-NH-(CH$_2$)$_4$-NH-(CH$_2$)$_3$	4.00
29	3-NO$_2$	6-NH$_2$	[(CH$_2$)$_2$-C-(CH$_3$)$_2$-NH-(CH$_2$)$_2$]$_2$	4.50
30	3-NO$_2$	H	(H$_2$C)$_3$N⟨piperazine⟩N-(CH$_2$)$_3$	0.23
31	3-NH$_2$	H	(H$_2$C)$_3$N⟨piperazine⟩N-(CH$_2$)$_3$	> 100
32	3-NH$_2$	H	(H$_2$C)$_3$N⟨homopiperazine⟩N-(CH$_2$)$_3$	2.30
33	3-NO$_2$	6-NH$_2$	(CH$_2$)$_3$-NH-(CH$_2$)$_2$-C(CH$_3$)$_2$-NH-CH$_2$-CH$_2$ CH$_2$)$_3$-NH-(CH$_2$)$_2$-C(CH$_3$)$_2$-NH-CH$_2$-CH$_2$	> 100
34	3-NO$_2$	6-NH$_2$	(CH$_2$)$_2$-C(CH$_3$)$_2$-NH-(CH$_2$)$_3$-NH-CH$_2$-CH$_2$ (CH$_2$)$_2$-C(CH$_3$)$_2$-NH-(CH$_2$)$_3$-NH-CH$_2$-CH$_2$	1.77
35	3-NH$_2$	H	(CH$_2$)$_7$	> 100

(continued)

Comp.	X	Y	Z	IC_{50} μM
36	H	H	$(CH_2)_2$-NH-$(CH_2)_2$-NH-$(CH_2)_2$	0.03
37	H	H	$(CH_2)_2$-NH-$(CH_2)_3$-NH-$(CH_2)_2$	0.004
38	H	H	$(CH_2)_2$-NH-$(CH_2)_4$-NH-$(CH_2)_2$ 0.005	
39	H	H		0.002
40	H	H	$CH(CH_3)$-CH_2-NH-$(CH_2)_2$-NH-CH_2-$CH(CH_3)$	0.7
41	H	H	$(CH_2)_2$-NH-$(CH_2)_2$-NH-$(CH_2)_2$-NH-$(CH_2)_2$	0.4
42	H	H	$[(CH_2)_2$-NH-$(CH_2)_2$-NH-$CH_2]_2$	0.6
43	3-NO_2	H	$(CH_2)_2$-NH-$(CH_2)_2$-NH-$(CH_2)_2$	0.002
44	3-NO_2	H	$(CH_2)_2$-NH-$(CH_2)_3$-NH-$(CH_2)_2$	0.0005
45	3-NO_2	H	$(CH_2)_2$-NCH_3-$(CH_2)_3$-NCH_3-$(CH_2)_2$	0.0006
46	3-NO_2	H	$(CH_2)_2$-NCH_3-$(CH_2)_2$-NCH_3-$(CH_2)_2$	0.04
47	4-NO_2	H	$(CH_2)_2$-NH-$(CH_2)_3$-NH-$(CH_2)_2$	0.1
48	3-NH_2	H	$(CH_2)_2$-NH-$(CH_2)_2$-NH-$(CH_2)_2$	0.03
49	3-NH_2	H	$(CH_2)_2$-NH-$(CH_2)_3$-NH-$(CH_2)_2$	0.009
50	3-NH_2	H	$CH(CH_3)$-CH_2-NH-$(CH_2)_2$-NH-(CH_2)-CH-(CH_3)	0.1
51	3-$NHCOCH_3$	H	$(CH_2)_2$-NH-$(CH_2)_2$-NH-$(CH_2)_2$	10
52	3-$NHCOCH_3$	H	$(CH_2)_2$-NH-$(CH_2)_3$-NH-$(CH_2)_2$	3
53	3-$NHCOCH_3$	H	$CH(CH_3)$-CH_2NH-$(CH_2)_2$-$NHCH_2$-$CH(CH_3)$	1
54	3-Br	H	$(CH_2)_2$-NH-$(CH_2)_3$-NH-$(CH_2)_2$	0.008
55	2-OH	H	$(CH_2)_2$-NH-$(CH_2)_3$-NH-$(CH)_2$	0.004
56	4-OH	H	$(CH_2)_2$-NH-$(CH_2)_3$-NH-$(CH_2)_2$	8
57	3-OH	H	$(CH_2)_2$-NH-$(CH_2)_3$-NH-$(CH_2)_2$	0.2

4. ANTITUMOR ACTIVITY

All the compounds were initially evaluated for cytotoxic activity in a standard monolayer cell culture of the HT-29 human colon carcinoma cell line. The IC_{50} values of symmetric and asymmetric bis-naphthalimides are shown in Table 3. In general, bis-naphthalimides have higher cytotoxic activities than the parental compounds, Amonafide and Mitonafide, with some exceptions. Certain aromatic substituents tend to increase cytotoxicity, in the order $CH_3CONH < NH_2 < H < NO_2$ for compounds with the same bridge. These results are consistent with those found for the mononaphthalimides. The length and nature of the bridge also alter the cytotoxicity. Nevertheless, any atempt to obtain accurate quantitative structure–activity relationship studies has failed (32). This suggests the concurrence of different mechanisms of intercalation, which is in agreement with the bis-acridine DNA polyintercalation studies done by Le Pecq and colleagues (33).

Selected bis-naphthalimides were tested for efficacy in animal tumor models. Surprisingly, the most active compound was one that lacked any aromatic substituent (number 37 in Table 3). This compound, designated LU 79553, shows excellent antitumor activity in a number of preclinical models (34). Our initial screen for activity in vivo was to test the compounds at the maximum tolerated dose in the MX-1 model. The MX-1 is a human mammary carcinoma that is xenografted sc into athymic nude mice (35). When LU 79553 is administered to the mice as two cycles of five daily injections, the compound is curative at doses of 20, 25, or 30 mg/kg/d (Fig. 4). This

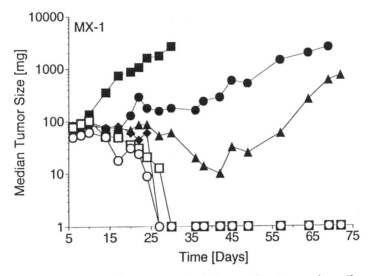

Fig. 4. MX-1 human mammary carcinoma was serially passaged as tumor pieces (3 mm in diameter) implanted sc on day 0. Treatment was initiated on d 6 and consisted of five daily iv injections of LU 79553 (dissolved in sterile water) at 0 (■), 5(●), 10 (▲), 20 (◆), 25 (□), or 30 (○) mg/kg/d. A second cycle was initiated on day 20. Tumors were measured two to three times a week with calipers, and a volume was calculated using the formula $V = (W^2 \times L)/2$. Median tumor size for each treatment group is plotted ($n = 5$).

treatment schedule is also effective when the xenografts are allowed to grow tumor sizes of 1–2 g (*34*). LU 79553 was then tested in a number of different tumor models. The data are summarized in Table 4. Whereas the mononaphthalimide Amonafide has little activity against solid tumor xenografts, LU 79553 treatment has resulted in not only tumor growth inhibition, but tumor regression and tumor-free survivors in several of these models. Based on this dramatic antitumor activity, LU 79553 was selected for clinical development. Phase I clinical trials are currently in progress in Europe and the USA. The absence of a basic terminal nitrogen in the chromophore of LU 79553 may be advantageous, since the nitro substitution on the monomeric compounds appears to be responsible for the CNS toxicity observed in the Mitonafide clinical trials (*20*).

The mechanism of LU 79553's antitumor activity is unknown. The compound intercalates into DNA (M. Waring, in press), as do the monomeric derivatives (*11*). LU 79553 alters the catalytic activity of topoisomerase II in a decatenation assay, but is a much more potent inhibitor than Amonafide (*34*). Although the compound appears to exert its antitumor activity via DNA damage, the critical biochemical target of the bis-naphthalimides remains to be identified.

5. OTHER BIS-NAPHTHALIMIDES

Another series of bis-naphthalimides has been synthesized by investigators at Du Pont Merck (Wilmington, DE) (*36*). The compounds showed a similar spectrum of activity in vitro and in vivo to the bis-naphthalimides described above (*36–39*). The compounds bind to DNA with a high affinity, are active at killing many tumor cell

Table 4
Summary of In Vivo Activity of LU 79553

2 CH$_3$-SO$_3$H

LU 79553

Tumor designation	Tissue type	Activity level[a]
MX-1 early stage	Breast	Curative
MX-1 late stage	Breast	Curative
LX-1	Lung	PR, CR TGD = 42–46 d
LOX	Melanoma	Curative
CX-1	Colon	Some PR TGD = 32–33 d
OVCAR-3	Ovarian	T/C = 198%

[a] PR = partial regressions, CR = complete regressions, TGD = tumor growth delay.

lines in vitro, and some derivatives have impressive activity in preclinical tumor models. One compound, DMP 840, was selected for clinical development. DMP 840 has been evaluated in Phase I studies at several sites (*40–44*). The dose-limiting toxicities are myelosuppression and stomatitis. DMP-840 is currently being studied in Phase II trials.

ACKNOWLEDGMENTS

We thank our many colleagues who have been involved in this research, including T. Barlozzari, P. Bousquet, J. M. Castellano, C. Cocchiaro, D. Conlon, M. D'Autilia, F. Emling, J. George, K. Fitzgerald, R. Kamen, G. Keilhauer, M. Kluge, R. Miller, M. Moran, M.J. Perez de Vega, D. Perron, X. -D. Qian, S. Robinson, E. Schlick, and M. Spigelman.

REFERENCES

1. Arcamone FM, Animati F, Brunella B, Configliacchi E, D'Alessio R, Geroni C, Giuliani FC, Lazzari E, Menozzi M, Mongelli N, Penco S, Verini MA. Synthesis, DNA-binding properties, and antitumor activity of novel dystamycin derivatives. *J Med Chem* 1989; 32:774–778.
2. Braña MF, Castellano JM, Jimenez A, Llombart A, Rabadán FP, Roldán CM, Roldán C, Santos A, Vazquez D. Synthesis, cytostatic activity and mode of action of a new series of imide derivatives of 3-nitro-1,8-naphthalic acid. *Curr Chemother* 1978; 2:1216,1217.
3. Braña MF, Castellano JM, Roldán CM, Santos A, Vazquez D, Jimenez A. Synthesis and mode(s) of action of a new series of imide derivatives of 3-nitro-1,8-naphthalic acid. *Cancer Chemother Pharmacol* 1980; 4:61–66.

4. Braña MF, Sanz AM, Castellano JM, Roldán CM, Roldan C. Synthesis and cytostatic activity of benz[de]isoqinolin-1,3-diones. Structure–activity relationships. *Eur J Med Chem* 1981; 16:207–212.

5. Walkelin LPG, Waring MJ. DNA Intercalating Agents. In: Sammes PG, ed. *Comprehensive Medicinal Chemistry*. Oxford: Pergamon. 1990:702–720.

6. Braña MF, Castellano JM, Morán M, Pérez de Vega MJ, Romerdahl CA, Qian X-D, Bousquet P, Emling F, Schlick E, Keilhauer G. Bis-naphthalimides: a new class of antitumor agents. *Anti-Cancer Drug Design* 1993; 8:257–268.

7. Stevenson KA, Yen S-F, Yang N-C, Bookin DW, Wilson WD. A substituent constant analysis of the interaction of substituted naphthalene monoimides with DNA. *J Med Chem* 1984; 27: 1677–1682.

8. Zee-Cheng RKY, Cheng CC. *N*-(aminoalkyl)imide antineoplastic agents. Synthesis and biological activity. *J Med Chem* 1985; 28:1216–1222.

9. Paull KD, Nasr M, Narayanan VL. Computer assisted structure-activity correlations. *Arzneim-Forsch/Drug Res* 1984; 34:1243–1246.

10. National Cancer Institute. Clinical Brochure, Nafidimide, NSC 308847, November 1984; 6–22.

11. Waring MJ, González A, Jimenez A, Vazquez D. Intercalative binding to DNA of antitumor drugs derived from 3-nitro-1,8-naphthalic acid. *Nucleic Acid Res* 1979; 7:217–230.

12. Andersson BS, Berian M, Bakic M, Silberman LE, Newman RA, Zwelling LA. In vitro toxicity and DNA cleaving capacity of benzisoquinolinedione (nafidimide; NSC-308847) in human leukemia. *Cancer Res* 1986; 47:1040–1044.

13. Nishio A, Uyeki, EM. Induction of DNA strand breaks and chromosome abnormalities by an imide derivative of 3-nitro-1,8-naphthalic acid (mitonafide) in Chinese hamster ovary cells. *J Natl Cancer Inst* 1983; 70:1097–1102.

14. De Isabella P, Zunino F, Capranico G. Base sequence determinants of amonafide stimulation of topoisomerase II DNA cleavage. *Nucleic Acids Res* 1995; 23;223–229.

15. Capranico G, Zunino F. DNA topoisomerase-trapping antitumor drugs. *Eur J Cancer* 1992; 28A:2055–2060.

16. Hsiang Y-H, Jiang JB, Liu LF. Topoisomerase II-mediated DNA cleavage by Amonafide and its structural analogs. *Mol Pharmacol* 1989; 36:371–376.

17. Gancedo APG, Gil C, Vilas P, Pérez S, Paez E, Rodriguez F, Braña MF, Roldán CM. Imide derivatives of 3-nitro-1,8-naphthalic acid: their inhibitory activity against DNA viruses. *Arch Virol* 1982; 74:157–165.

18. Roldán CM, Cubero SJ, Rubio F. Actividad antibiótica del nuevo producto 2-(2-dimetilamino etil)-5-nitrobenzo[d,e]isoquinolein-1,3-diona (Made-4212). *Diag. Biol* 1979; XXVIII:443–446.

19. Osuna A, Castanys C, Mascaró C, Adroher FJ, Braña MF, Roldán CM. In vitro action of three benzo[de]isoquinoline-1,3-dione derivatives against Trypanosoma cruzi. *Rev Inst Med Trop Sao Paulo* 1983; 25:254–258.

20. Llombart M, Poveda A, Forner E, Martos CF, Gaspar C, Muñoz M, Olmos T, Ruiz A, Soriano V, Benavides A, Martín M, Schlick E, Guillem V. Phase I study of Mitonafide in solid tumors. *Invest New Drugs* 1992; 10:177–181.

21. Rosell R, Carles J, Abad A, Ribelles N, Barnadas A, Benavides A, Martín M. Phase I study of Mitonafide in 120 hour continuous infusion in non-small cell lung cancer. *Invest New Drugs* 1992; 10:171–175.

22. Legha SS, Ring S, Raber M, Felder TB, Newman RA, Krakoff IH, Phase I clinical investigation of benzisoquinolinedione. *Cancer Treat Rep* 1987; 71:1165–1169.

23. Saez R,, Craig JB, Kuhn JG, Weiss GR, Koeller J, Phillips J, Havlin K, Harman G, Hardy J, Melink TJ, Sarosy G, VonHoff DD. Phase I investigation of Amondafide. *J Clin Oncol* 1989; 7:1351–1358.

24. Scheithauer W, Kornek G, Haider K, Depisch D. Amonafide in metastatic colorectal carcinoma. *Eur J Cancer* 1990; 26:923–924.

25. Kornek G, Raderer M, Depisch D, Haider K, Fazeny B, Dittrich C, Scheithauer W. Amonafide as first-line chemotherapy for metastatic breast cancer. *Eur J Cancer* 1994; 30A:398–400.

26. Craig J, Crawford E. Phase II trial of amonafide in advanced prostate cancer. *Proc Am Soc Clin Oncol* 1989; 8:147.

27. Allen SL, Budman DR, Fusco D, Kolitz J, Kreis W, Schulman P, Schuster M, DeMarco L,

Marsh J, Haptas K, Fischkoff S. Phase I trial of Amonafide + cytosine arabinoside for poor risk acute leukemias. *Proc Am Assoc Cancer Res* 1994; 35:225.

28. Felder TB, McLean MA, Vestal ML, Lu K, Farquhar D, Legha SS, Shaw R, Newman RA. Pharmacokinetics and metabolism of the antitumor drug Amonafide (NSC-308847) in humans. *Drug Metab Dispos* 1987; 15:773–778.

29. Ratain MJ, Mick R, Berezin F, Janisch L, Schilsky RL, Vogelzang NJ, Lane LB. Phase I study of Amonafide dosing based on acetylator phenotype. *Cancer Res* 1993; 53:2304–2308.

30. Wakelin LPG, Waring MJ. DNA intercalating agents. In: Hansch C, Sammes PG, Taylor JB, eds. *Comprehensive Medicinal Chemistry,* vol. 2. Oxford: Pergamon, 1990:718–721.

31. Braña MF, Castellano JM, Morán M, Pérez de Vega MJ, Romerdahl CR, Qian X-D, Bousquet P, Emling F, Schlick E, Keilhauer G. Bis-naphthalimides: a new class of antitumor agents. *Anti-Cancer Drug Design* 1993; 8:257–268.

32. Braña MF, Castellano JM, Morán M, Perez de Vega MJ, Qian X-D, Romerdahl CA, Keilhauer G. Bis-naphthalimides. 2. Synthesis and biological activity of 5,6-acenaphthalimidoalkyl-1,8-naphthalimidoalkyl amines. *Eur J Med Chem* 1995; 30:235–239.

33. Le Pecq JB, Le Bret M, Barbet J, Roques B. DNA polyintercalating drugs: DNA binding of diacridine derivatives. *Proc Natl Acad Sci USA* 1975; 72:2915–2919.

34. Bousquet PF, Braña MF, Conlon D, Fitzgerald KM, Perron D, Cocchiaro C, Miller R, Moran M, George J, Qian X-D, Keilhauer G, Romerdahl CA. Preclinical evaluation of LU 79553: A novel Bis-naphthalimide with potent antitumor activity. *Cancer Res* 1995; 55:1176–1180.

35. Goldin A, Venditti JM, MacDonald JS, Muggia FM, Henney JE, DeVita JT Jr. Current results of the screening program at the division of cancer treatment, NCI. *Eur J Cancer* 1981; 17: 129–142.

36. Chen SF, Behrens DL, Behrens CH, Czerniak PM, Dexter DL, Dusak BL, Fredericks JR, Gale KC, Gross JL, Jiang JB, Kirshenbaum MR, McRipley RJ, Papp LM, Patten AD, Perrella FW, Seitz SP, Stafford MP, Sun JH, Sun T, Wuonola MA, Von Hoff DD. XB596, a promising bis-naphthalimide anti-cancer agent. *Anticancer Drugs* 1993; 4:447–457.

37. McRipley RJ, Burns-Horwitz PE, Czerniak PM, Diamond RJ, Miller LD, Page RJ, Dexter DL, Chen S-F, Sun J-H, Behrens CH, Seitz SP, Gross JL. Efficacy of DMP-840: a novel bis-naphthalimide cytotoxic agent with human solid tumor xenograft selectivity. *Cancer Res* 1994; 54:159–164.

38. Kirshenbaum MR, Chen S-F, Behrens CH, Papp LM, Stafford MM, Sun J-H, Behrens DL, Fredericks JR, Polkus ST, Sipple P, Patten AD, Dexter D, Seitz SP, Gross JL. (R,R)-2,2′-[1,2-Ethanediylbis [imino(1-methyl-2,1-ethandiyl)]]-bis[5-nitro-1H-benz[de]isoquinoline 1,3-(2H)-dione] dimethanesulfonate (DMP 840), a novel bis-naphthalimide with potent non-selective tumoricidal activity in vitro. *Cancer Res* 1994; 54:2199–2206.

39. Houghton PJ, Cheshire PJ, Hallman JC, Gross JL, McRipley RM, Sun J-H, Behrens CH, Dexter DL, Houghton JA. Evaluation of a novel bis-naphthalimide anticancer agent, DMP 840, against human xenografts derived from adult, juvenile, and pediatric cancers. *Cancer Chemother Pharmacol* 1994:33:265–272.

40. Slichenmyer W, Finizio M, Sartorius S, Rowinsky E, Lai C-M, Grochow L, Pieniaszek H, O'Reilly S, Bunitsky K, Brogdon B, Mabring D, Shifflet C, Donehower R. Phase I and pharmacologic study of DMP 840 as a single infusion every three weeks. *Proc Am Soc Clin Oncol* 1994; 13:142.

41. Cobb P, Burris H, Finizio M, Lai C, Eckardt J, Fields S, Kuhn J, Nelson J, Bunitsky K, Pieniaszek H, Brogdon B, Von Hoff D. Phase I trial and pharmacokinetic study of a new bis-naphthalimide, DMP 840, given daily × 5. *Proc Am Soc Oncol* 1994; 13:159.

42. Maroun J, Stewart D, Goel R, Goss G, Verma S, Yau J, Finizio M, Lai C-M, Bunitsky K, Pieniaszek H, Brodgon B. Phase I Pharmacokinetic study of DMP 840 given in a 3 weekly dosage in a 5 weeks schedule. *Proc Am Soc Clin Oncol* 1994; 13:151.

43. O'Reilly S, Rowinsky EK, Grochow L, Adjei A, Bowling K, Slichenmyer W, Sartorius S, Finizio M, Gray JR, Pieniaszek HJ, Peterman VC, Mabring D, Donehower KC. Phase I and pharmacologic study of DMP 840 as a 24 hour infusion in patients with solid tumors. *Proc Am Soc Clin Oncol* 1995; 14:472.

44. Cobb P. Burris H, Drengler R, Fields S, Smith L, White I, Pieniaszek H, Gray J, Peterman V, Finizio M, Von Hoff D. Phase I trial of DMP 840 given as a 120-hour continuous infusion every 28 days. *Proc Am Soc Clin Oncol* 1995; 14:484.

II NEWER STRATEGIES AND TARGETS

11 The Enediynes

Nina Felice Schor, MD, PhD

Contents

1. INTRODUCTION

In 1965, Ishida et al. (1) reported the identification of an antimicrobial compound isolated from *Streptomyces carzinostaticus*. This compound was given the designation "neocarzinostatin" and was thereafter determined to be an antimitotic agent (2). What followed was a long series of structural and chemical studies of neocarzinostatin, largely spearheaded by Goldberg and his colleagues (reviewed in 3), and culminating in clinical trials in Japan and the US (4–7). The Japanese experience demonstrated difficulty with drug delivery to solid tumors and rapid clearance of the drug from the bloodstream (8). The identification of these limitations led to a series of derivitizations of neocarzinostatin, in an effort to reproduce the demonstrated in vitro efficacy of this drug in an in vivo setting. In addition to lack of efficacy in solid tumors, the American experience was marked by problems with drug toxicity, both of dose-related and idiosyncratic types (4,7), and led to curtailment of preclinical and clinical studies of this drug in this country, and efforts to synthesize and isolate novel enediyne compounds that might not engender these difficulties. This chapter deals with the enediynes as a class. Because of its rich structural and mechanistic history, and because of the reliance of all subsequent developments in this area on prior studies involving this prototypic compound, neocarzinostatin is discussed in detail in each section, followed by a discussion of the compounds, both natural and synthesized, which followed in its wake.

From: *Cancer Therapeutics: Experimental and Clinical Agents*
Edited by: B. Teicher Humana Press Inc., Totowa, NJ

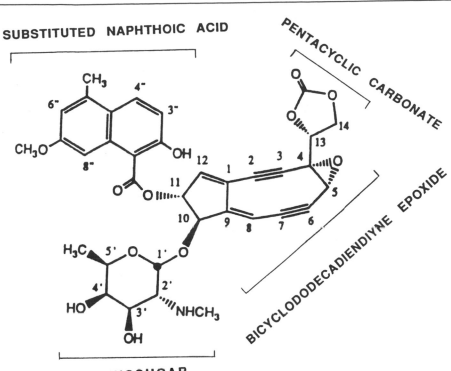

Fig. 1. Structural components of neocarzinostatin chromophore. The molecule consists of four functional components to each of which has been ascribed a role in the cellular activity of the drug.

2. CHEMISTRY AND MECHANISM OF ACTION

Neocarzinostatin consists of a 113-residue protein ($M_r = 11,000$) noncovalently associated with a chromophore of M_r 540 (9–11). The biological activity of the molecule lies primarily in its chromophore (12,13), and it is after this component of neocarzinostatin and other natural enediynes that all of the newer synthesized enediynes have been modeled (14,15). The chromophore consists of four structural subunits: a substituted naphthoic acid, an amino sugar, a pentacyclic carbonate, and a bicyclododecadiendiyne epoxide (16; see Fig. 1). Although the epoxide is the "business end" or "warhead" (17) of the molecule, required for DNA strand cleavage and adduct formation (see this section, below), the other components play important roles in the cytotoxicity of neocarzinostatin. The naphthalene moiety is believed to be important for minor groove binding of the drug; the amino sugar facilitates drug binding to the phosphate backbone of DNA; and the cyclic carbonate appears to mediate traversing of the drug across the cell membrane (16).

Despite the primary importance of the chromophore for the activity of neocarzinostatin, recent studies suggest that the protein does more than just "protect" the chromophore from extracellular inactivation. Modification of the protein moiety can alter cellular uptake of neocarzinostatin chromophore (18), which is believed in large measure to dissociate from the protein en route across the cell membrane (19,20).

The principal mode of action of neocarzinostatin is by the induction of DNA breaks, most of them single-stranded, preferentially at thymidine and adenine residues in AT-rich regions (*11*). The initial interaction of the chromophore with DNA is a two-step process (*21*). First, an external complex is formed between the amino sugar of the drug and the phosphate backbone of the DNA. Next, there is a slow "internalization" of the drug into the minor groove.

Single-strand breaks so predominate in the action of neocarzinostatin that it was originally thought that the occasional double-stranded breaks that arose were the result of close apposition of two randomly placed single-stranded breaks on opposite strands (*12,22*). It has recently become clear, however, that these double-stranded breaks are the result of direct, bistranded cleavage at AGC·GCT sequences (*23–25*).

The reaction of neocarzinostatin with DNA can result in several outcomes: DNA strand breakage, the release of free thymidylic aldehyde, or the formation of adducts between the chromophore and DNA. Both the cleavage of DNA and the liberation of free base aldehydes by neocarzinostatin require oxygen and sulfhydryl reagents. In contrast, the formation of DNA-neocarzinostatin adducts occurs largely under anaerobic conditions (*16*). Furthermore, the requirement of the former reactions for oxygen is independent of that for sulfhydryl groups; that is, in the presence of oxygen, one can observe the formation of spectrophotometrically different products depending on the presence or absence of sulfhydryl reagents (*26*). The kinetics of these reactions suggest that there is sequential reaction with neocarzinostatin of the sulfhydryl reagent followed by the oxygen molecule. The reaction of one sulfhydryl group with the neocarzinostatin chromophore is enough to change its fluorescence spectrum. However, the reaction of the second sulfhydryl reagent molecule with the chromophore requires the prior oxidation of the chromophore molecule (*26*).

Neocarzinostatin has also been found to inhibit *de novo* DNA synthesis (*12*) and to induce mutagenesis, especially at G·C pairs (*27*). However, the roles of these activities in the antineoplastic efficacy of neocarzinostatin are not known.

Since the time of discovery of neocarzinostatin, several other enediynes have been both isolated from natural sources or synthesized *de novo*. All of these compounds have some structural and mechanistic similarity to neocarzinostatin. The first of these to be described was calicheamicin γ^1_1 (*28*). Calicheamicin was isolated from fermentation broths of *Micromonospora echinospora* ssp. calichensis, and, like neocarzinostatin, it binds in the minor groove of DNA and requires oxygen, but not peroxide or superoxide, for its action. Unlike neocarzinostatin, however, calicheamicin consists of a chromophore unassociated with a protein (*28*), and makes sequence-specific double-stranded cuts in DNA (*28,29*). Its particular sequence specificity is apparently partially determined by the carbohydrate domain of this molecule (*30*), although other structural components of the molecule also contribute to this property (*31,32*). Esperamicin A₁ is another enediyne chromophore that makes single-stranded cuts in DNA that differ from those made by neocarzinostatin in their particular base and sequence selectivity. Esperamicin requires thiol, heat, or UV-light activation analogous to that required by neocarzinostatin (*33,34*). Dynemicin A, a hybrid compound containing anthraquinone and enediyne cores, also requires thiol or UV-light activation (*35,36*), but has nicking sequence selectivity that differs from those of esperamicin and calicheamicin. This enediyne is also a natural product, isolated from the fermentation broth of *Micromonospora chersin* (*37*). It induces double-stranded cleavage to the 3'-side of a purine base and staggered by 3 bases on opposite strands. Molecular modeling studies indicate that this cleavage pattern can be predicted from the intercalation position and capacity for enediyne activation of the anthraquinone subunit (38,39). Recently, new natural products with a protein component analogous to aponeocarzinostatin have been described (40–42). One of these, C1027, cleaves duplex DNA to produce single-strand breaks, double-strand breaks, and abasic sites in the absence of thiols (43).

By modeling compounds after dynemicin. A, Nicolaou and colleagues (14) have synthesized a series of "self-triggering" enediynes that do not require sulfydryl compounds for activation. They have made the observation that "pretriggered" enediynes (called stable enediynes) in their series interfere in a competitive fashion with the biological activity of unstable or reactive enediynes, raising the possibility that there is a non-DNA intracellular receptor for the enediynes (15).

3. CELLULAR EFFECTS

There are four principal effects of the enediynes on cells:

1. Mutagenicity;
2. Antimitotic activity associated with cell-cycle arrest;
3. Apoptosis induction; and
4. Differentiation induction.

These effects are not mutually exclusive, and some of them are undoubtedly the result of triggering of endogenous cell-determined responses to antimitosis or to particular mutations (44).

The mutagenicity of enediynes has been shown to be sulfhydryl-dependent and to vary with concentration in parallel with the cytotoxicity of these agents. That is, as the surviving fraction of cells diminishes, so increases the percentage of the remaining cells exhibiting a mutant phenotype. This has been interpreted to mean that the same mechanism, namely DNA cleavage, is responsible for both of these outcomes, and that the quantity of irreparable DNA damage determines whether cell death or mutation is seen in a particular cell or population. In any case, neocarzinostatin is mutagenic in bacteria, yeast, fungi, and mammalian cells (45). Although it had originally been said that cytolysis by neocarzinostatin is dependent only on the concentration of the drug present and not on the drug exposure time, these studies failed to take into account degradation of the chromophore over time at 37°C, and subsequent studies have demonstrated independent exposure time- and concentration-dependent effects (whether cytolysis, mitotic arrest, or differentiation) of this agent (46,47). Hypertonicity of the bathing medium of the cell increases the DNA damage rate and decreases the DNA repair rate in response to neocarzinostatin treatment, but not to DNA crosslinking or intercalating agents (48). The radiosensitivity of tumor cells is enhanced by neocarzinostatin, as is the incidence of "potentially lethal damage" owing to X-irradiation; the degree of enhancement is inversely proportional to the DNA repair capabilities of the particular cell line, even though neocarzinostatin inhibits all repair regardless of the prior capabilities of the line. This almost certainly indicates that neocarzinostatin prohibits repair of residual damage after irradiation, so that the less damage that has been repaired prior to neocarzinostatin addition, the more damaged a cell remains (49,50).

Enediynes act as antimitotic agents by inducing a temporary G2 delay in several cell lines (51,52). Cells remain blocked at G2M for some period of time, demonstrating a decreased mitotic index at 1 h, followed by an "overshoot" at 48 h after drug washout. In neural crest tumor cells, the antimitotic effect is irreversible, perhaps because the G2M block is lengthy enough to trigger an endogenous cellular program for differentiation, and in these cells, the differentiated state is a post mitotic one (19,47,53). Although poly-ADP ribosylation of chromatin protein increases in HeLa cells that undergo G2 delay after neocarzinostatin treatment, inhibitors of this chemical process do not universally inhibit the cell-cycle changes, and the order of potency of the inhibitors that work on both processes is not the same. This implies that these two events are not causally related (51).

Recently, apoptosis induction has been described after enediyne treatment of a variety of cell types (15,54,55). Stable designed enediynes appear to block apoptosis induction by reactive designed enediynes (15), implying that there is a receptor–ligand-like interaction involved in this process. However, this competitive inhibition is not universally seen with natural enediynes, such as calicheamicin (56). Although oligonucleosomal-length cleavage fragments could be produced simply by the direct cleavage of DNA by enediynes in the face of an intact nucleosomal structure, kinetic studies of the cleavage process, and its dependence on protein synthesis and the presence of an endonuclease in at least some cell types make it likely that direct cleavage by the enediynes triggers an endogenous program for cell death (55).

In some neural crest cells treated with enediynes, morphological differentiation results (19,44,53). The precise nature of the differentiation (e.g., whether neuron-like or Schwann cell-like) and the determination of whether a particular cell undergoes apoptosis or differentiation are functions of the endogenous properties of that cell, rather than the concentration or nature of the enediyne with which it is treated (44). Furthermore, even in cases where morphological differentiation along neural lines is apparent, the biochemical accompaniments of this morphological change do not always parallel normal differentiation (57).

Finally, in cell-culture studies, two distinct types of resistance to neocarzinostatin and related enediynes have been described. In one, enediyne resistance is part of a multidrug resistance phenotype, with overexpression of P-glycoprotein, and reversal of the phenomenon with verapamil (58,59). In the other, resistance to neocarzinostatin alone is seen, and is not accompanied by crossresistance to other enediynes or other chemotherapeutic agents. The precise mechanism underlying the latter phenomenon is not known (58).

4. ANTITUMOR EFFECTS OF NEOCARZINOSTATIN: PRECLINICAL AND CLINICAL STUDIES

Since early reports of efficacy of neocarzinostatin against L1210 leukemia in mice (60), this drug has been examined in several of Phase I and Phase II trials for a variety of hematological and solid malignancies. Because pharmacokinetic studies indicated that neocarzinostatin has a short serum half-life, undergoes rapid renal clearance, and is concentrated in the kidney and bladder, Sakamoto et al. (5) undertook a study of newly diagnosed patients with bladder carcinoma confined to the primary organ. Of these 30 patients, each of whom received three or four courses consisting of 1 mg neocarzinostatin iv daily for 7 d followed by a 7-day "rest period," 2 attained complete response, 21 attained partial response, and 6 did not respond to therapy. In all cases, neocarzinostatin treatment was followed by transurethral resection of residual tumor. At followup (12–46 mo), 5 of the 30 patients had recurrences of their tumor. The published recurrence rate for bladder carcinoma with transurethral resection alone is 25–70% within 1 yr and 90% within 2 yr. Toxicity in all patients was reversible and tolerable. The most common problem was myelosuppression, which apparently remitted during the 7-d rest period, and exhibited cumulative severity, which limited the total number of courses of drug that could be given to any patient. Three of the patients treated had transient elevations in SGOT without related symptoms.

These encouraging results led to the undertaking of a Phase II study that included patients with metastatic bladder, prostate, or hepatic carcinoma (4). In contrast to the patients treated for local disease in an organ in which neocarzinostatin is known to attain high concentrations, only 1 of the 35 patients with metastatic disease (a patient with bladder carcinoma) had a partial response to treatment. Myelotoxicity was again the dose-limiting factor in these patients who received iv bolus therapy once daily for 5 d and repeated when their blood cell counts permitted. In addition, two patients sustained dose-limiting toxicity involving pulmonary fibrosis, which responded to steroid treatment and hepatic toxicity, respectively. One patient experienced anaphylaxis during a repeated course of the drug, and was successfully treated with supportive therapy and steroids. Subsequently, 122 patients with disseminated malignant melanoma were randomized to treatment with chlorozotocin, neocarzinostatin, or methyl-CCNU. Although toxicity of neocarzinostatin (thrombocytopenia, leukopenia, and one anaphylactic response) was said to be "tolerable" in this study, the therapeutic response was meager at best. Furthermore, in a Phase II trial of 53 patients with acute leukemia, chronic myelogenous leukemia (CML) in blast crisis, or a variety of solid tumors, only two of the patients with CML responded at all, and both of them relapsed by 6 wk following therapy (7). Thus, although there have been isolated reports since these larger trials of the efficacy of neocarzinostatin as a single, unmodified agent in the therapy of urinary tract malignancies (61), it appears that neocarzinostatin's role may be limited to therapy of tumors in particular sites where high local concentrations of the drug can safely be attained, and as a substrate for the development of more targeted agents and systems for drug delivery. In this regard, Maeda et al. (8) have developed a two-compartment theoretical model of neocarzinostatin as an intra-arterial agent for use in the therapy of malignant gliomas of the central nervous system. They cite the short serum half-life and long CSF half-life of the drug, its several orders of magnitude greater toxicity for glioma cells relative to normal glial elements, and its rapid clearance from the systemic circulation as evidence in favor of this strategy.

5. IMPROVING THE THERAPEUTIC INDEX OF ENEDIYNES

Problems with lack of efficacy in solid tumors, and chromophore-mediated bone marrow and protein-mediated anaphylactoid toxicity of neocarzinostatin have led to several types of attempts at improving the therapeutic index of the enediynes. One early effort to increase the delivery of neocarzinostatin to solid tumors began with the observation that, under angiotensin-induced hypertension, there appeared to be a two-fold increase in neocarzinostatin delivery to tumors with no change in delivery to normal tissues (62). This turned out not to be practical, and more recent efforts in this regard include:

1. Conjugation of neocarzinostatin to a high-mol-wt polymer, which improves its pharmacokinetic properties and decreases the "exposure" of the protein to the immune system;
2. Conjugation of enediynes to monoclonal antibodies (MAb) to target their effects for particular tumor tissues;
3. Targeting of enediynes themselves or their activating (thiol) agents for particular tumor tissues; and
4. Synthesis of novel enediynes, which might have differential delivery to or activity in tumor cells relative to normal cells.

A brief discussion of each of these strategies follows.

The most widely studied modification of neocarzinostatin is the conjugation of this compound to a styrene-maleic acid copolymer (SMANCS; 63–68). SMANCS demonstrates more rapid and more complete internalization by cells than neocarzinostatin (64,65), a finding that probably accounts in part for its improved efficacy against tumor lines. Furthermore, SMANCS appears to be a biologic response modifier, as well. The copolymer appears to elicit increased secretion of interferons γ and β (66), and to increase NK activity, macrophage cytostasis, cytotoxic T-lymphocyte activity, and delayed hypersensitivity to sheep erythrocytes (68,69). Conjugation of neocarzinostatin to a styrene-pyran copolymer perhaps leads to decreased bone marrow toxicity relative to either the native compound or SMANCS. This compound exhibits the same molar cell kill as neocarzinostatin, but has only 70% of the acute toxicity (demonstrated by spleen and bone marrow CFU-C assays) of the native compound, allowing higher doses to be used in the animal models in which it has been tried. It has been suggested that the decrease in toxicity is related to a more tumor-selective pattern of drug delivery, owing to differences between normal and neoplastic vasculature (67). In one study of hepatocellular carcinoma patients who were given intra-arterial SMANCS dissolved in the lipid lymphographic agent ethiodol, radiographic, histologic, and serologic (α-fetoprotein levels) evidence demonstrates promising antitumor activity of this preparation in this particular localized malignancy (70). A method has also been proposed for rescuing patients from the bone marrow toxicity of SMANCS by taking advantage of the more rapid uptake of this compound into tumors relative to normal tissues and by using Tiopronin (N-2-mercaptopropionyl glycine) to inactivate residual SMANCS in the serum (71). Combining local (ip or ia, depending on the tumor model) neocarzinostatin therapy with iv Tiopronin appears to be a promising approach in regionally confined tumors (72,73).

Targeting of tumor tisues for cytotoxic effects by exploiting tumor-specific antigens and MAb made against them has been attempted with conjugates to many cytotoxic agents. The enediynes are no exceptions in this regard. Much of this work has involved the conjugation of neocarzinostatin to the MAb A7. This conjugate demonstrates marked selectivity for tumor relative to normal tissue and, therefore, has a better therapeutic index than neocarzinostatin alone in several tumor models (74). Specific localization of drug has been shown for SC xenografts of colon carcinoma (75,76) and pancreatic carcinoma (77,78). This improvement in therapeutic index is thought to be not only a function of the specific binding of the conjugate to antigens on tumor cells, but also the result of improved serum half-life (both decreased renal clearance and increased stability with a decreased likelihood of dissociation of chromophore from the protein), as well (79). Other promising attempts at antibody conjugation to neocarzinostatin have included thioether linkage to an MAb to astrocytoma cells (80). In addition, several studies have proposed conjugating neocarzinostatin to anti-idiotype antibodies in order to effect specific cytolysis of antisingle-strand DNA targeting or antibody-producing cells in patients with disorders, such as systemic lupus erythematosis (81–83). Recently, a series of calicheamicin analogs have been conjugated to MAb with increased magnitude and specificity of the cytotoxicity for these malignant cells (17). It is particularly interesting that this study demonstrates that the structure–activity relationship obtained for a series of native calicheamicin analogs does not predict the relative activities of the MAb conjugates of these compounds.

Targeting of the toxicity of enediynes has also been attempted using strategies other than antibody conjugation. Taking advantage of the transferrin receptors on leukemia cells, Kohgo and colleagues (84) have improved the tumor cell uptake and in vitro efficacy of neocarzinostatin for K562 cells by conjugating neocarzinostatin to transferrin. The optimal ratio of transferrin to neocarzinostatin in such conjugates is 4.0. Greater proportions of transferrin compromise the DNA cleaving efficacy of the drug; greater proportions of neocarzinostatin compromise the binding of the conjugate to the transferrin receptor. The internalization of the transferrin·4(neocarzinostatin) conjugate proceeds at the same rate as transferrin internalization by these cells (85). Targeting has also been achieved in neuroblastoma cells by sulfhydryl loading of these cells using the neurotransmitter analog 6-mercaptodopamine prior to treatment with neocarzinostatin (86). Since neuroblastoma cells have an active dopamine uptake system, they concentrate 6-mercaptodopamine against a concentration gradient. Most normal cells that actively concentrate dopamine are postmitotic, and so are not readily affected by neocarzinostatin. Neocarzinostatin is therefore selectively activated and effective in neuroblastoma cells, and cytolysis can be effected at much lower concentrations than would ordinarily be required.

Efforts to design or engineer enediynes have led to the production of some that appear to have selectivity for tumor cells relative to normal bone marrow progenitors (14). The mechanism of this selectivity is not clear, but it raises the possibility that such enediynes could be used as therapeutic agents with tolerable toxicity, without the need for conjugation or coupling of these compounds to targeting molecules.

6. CONCLUSIONS

Enediynes have been shown to exhibit antineoplastic activity in a number of tissue-culture and animal models. To the extent that their toxicity is tolerable, they presently have clinical potential in particular localized tumors with pharmacological or anatomical (i.e., site-specific delivery) circumstances that permit attainment of tumoricidal concentrations of these drugs. Harnessing the cytotoxic activity and the known chemical mechanism of these drugs for general clinical use will require improvement of their therapeutic index. Approaches that show promise in this regard include increasing the selectivity of drug delivery and/or drug activation, and selectively rescuing normal tissues from enediyne toxicity.

REFERENCES

1. Ishida N, Miyazaki K, Kumagai K, Rikumaru M. Neocarzinostatin, an antitumor antibioticum of high molecular weight. *J Antibiot* 1965; 18:68–76.
2. Ebina T, Ohtsuki K, Seto M, Ishida N. Specific G_2 block in HeLa-S3 cells by neocarzinostatin. *Eur J Cancer* 1975; 11:155–158.
3. Goldberg IH. Mechanism of neocarzinostatin action: role of DNA microstructure in determination of chemistry of bistranded oxidative damage. *Accounts of Chem Res* 1991; 24:191–196.
4. Natale RB, Yagoda A, Watson RC, Stover DE. Phase II trial of neocarzinostatin in patients with bladder and prostatic cancer. *Cancer* 1980; 45:2836–2842.
5. Sakamoto S, Ogata J, Ikegami K, Maeda H. Chemotherapy for bladder cancer with neocarzinostatin: evaluation of systemic administration. *Eur J Cancer* 1980; 16:103–113.
6. Von Hoff DD, Amato DA, Kaufman JH, Falkson G, Cunningham TJ. Randomized trial of chlorozotocin, neocarzinostatin, or methyl-CCNU in patients with malignant melanoma. *Am J Clin Oncol (CCT)* 1984; 7:135–139.
7. McKelvey EM, Murphy W, Zander A, Bodey GP. Neocarzinostatin: report of a phase II clinical trial. *Cancer Treatment Rep* 1981; 65:699–701.
8. Maeda H, Sano Y, Takeshita J, Iwai Z, Kosaka H, Marubayashi T, Matsukado Y. A pharmacokinetic simulation model for chemotherapy of brain tumor with an antitumor protein antibiotic, neocarzinostatin. *Cancer Chemother Pharmacol* 1981; 5:243–249.
9. Meienhofer J, Maeda H, Glaser CB, Czombos J, Kuromizu K. Primary structure of neocarzinostatin, an antitumor protein. *Science* 1972; 178:875,876.
10. Napier MA, Holmquist B, Strydom DJ, Goldberg IH. Neocarzinostatin: spectral characterization and separation of a non-protein chromophore. *Biochem Biophys Res Commun* 1979; 89:635–642.
11. Dasgupta D, Goldberg IH. Mode of reversible binding of neocarzinostatin chromophore to DNA: base sequence dependency of binding. *Nucleic Acids Res* 1986; 14:1089–1105.
12. Kappen LS, Goldberg IH. Mechanism of the effect of organic solvents and other protein denaturants on neocarzinostatin activity. *Biochemistry* 1979; 18:5647–5653.
13. Kappen LS, Napier MA, Goldberg IH. Roles of chromophore and apo-protein in neocarzinostatin action. *Proc Natl Acad Sci USA* 1980; 77:1970–1974.
14. Nicolaou KC, Dai W-M, Tsay S-C, Estevez VA, Wrasidlo W. Designed enediynes: a new class of DNA-cleaving molecules with potent and selective anticancer activity. *Science* 1992; 256:1172–1178.
15. Nicolaou KC, Stabila P, Esmaeli-Azad B, Wrasidlo W, Hiatt A. Cell-specific regulation of apoptosis by designed enediynes. *Proc Natl Acad Sci USA* 1993; 90:3142–3146.
16. Lee SH, Goldberg IH. Role of epoxide in neocarzinostatin chromophore stability and action. *Mol Pharmacol* 1988; 33:396–401.
17. Hinman LM, Hamann PR, Wallace R, Menendez AT, Durr FE, Upeslacis J. Preparation and characterization of monoclonal antibody conjugates of the calicheamicins: a novel and potent family of antitumor antibiotics. *Cancer Res* 1993; 53:3336–3342.
18. Schonlau F, Kohnlein W, Garnett MC. The acidic groups of the neocarzinostatin protein play an important role in its biological activity. *Mol Pharmacol* 1994; 45:1268–1272.
19. Schor NF. Neocarzinostatin induces neuronal morphology of mouse neuroblastoma in culture. *J Pharmacol Exp Ther* 1989; 249:906–910.
20. Kuroda Y, Sasaki T, Hoshino F. Unusual survival kinetics of neocarzinostatin-treated HeLa cells: its relation to the drug-inactivation. *J Radiat Res* 1991; 32:191–201.
21. Dasgupta D, Auld DS, Goldberg IH. Cryospectrokinetic evidence for the mode of reversible binding of neocarzinostatin chromophore to poly(deoxyadenylic-thymidylic acid). *Biochemistry* 1985; 24:7049–7054.
22. Poon R, Beerman TA, Goldberg IH. Characterization of DNA strand breakage *in vitro* by the antitumor protein neocarzinostatin. *Biochemistry* 1977; 16:486–493.
23. Dedon PC, Goldberg IH. Sequence-specific double-strand breakage of DNA by neocarzinostatin involves different chemical mechanisms within a staggered cleavage site. *J Biol Chem* 1990; 265:14,713–14,716.

24. Meschwitz SM, Schultz RG, Ashley GW, Goldberg IH. Selective abstraction of ²H from C-1' of the C residue in AGC·ICT by the radical center at C-2 of activated neocarzinostatin chromophore: structure of the drug/DNA complex responsible for bistranded lesion formation. *Biochemistry* 1992; 31:9117–9121.

25. McAfee SE, Asley GW. Modulation of neocarzinostatin-mediated DNA double strand damage by activating thiol: deuterium isotope effects. *Nucleic Acids Res* 1992; 20:805–809.

26. Povirk LF, Goldberg IH. Stoichiometric uptake of molecular oxygen and consumption of sulfhydryl groups by neocarzinostatin chromophore bound to DNA. *J Biol Chem* 1983; 258: 11,763–11,767.

27. Povirk LF, Goldberg IH. Detection of neocarzinostatin chromophore-deoxyribose adducts as exonuclease-resistant sites in defined-sequence DNA. *Biochemistry* 1985: 24:4035–4040.

28. Zein N, Sinha AM, McGahren WJ, Ellestad GA. Calicheamicin γ^I_1: an antitumor antibiotic that cleaves double-stranded DNA site specifically. *Science* 1988; 240: 1198–1201.

29. Zein N, Poncin M, Nilakantan R, Ellestad GA. Calicheamicin γ^I_1 and DNA: molecular recognition process responsible for site-specificity. *Science* 1989; 244:697–699.

30. Drak J, Iwasawa N, Danishefsky S, Crothers DM. The carbohydrate domain of calicheamicin γ^I_1 determines its sequence specificity for DNA cleavage. *Proc Natl Acad Sci USA* 1991; 88: 7461–7468.

31. Walker S, Landovitz R, Ding WD, Ellestad GA, Kahne D. Cleavage behavior of calicheamicin γ^I and calicheamicin T. *Proc Natl Acad Sci USA* 1992; 89:4608–4612.

32. Uesugi M, Sugiura Y. New insights into sequence recognition process of esperamicin A_1 and calicheamicin γ^I_1: origin of their selectivities and "induced fit" mechanism. *Biochemistry* 1993; 32:4622–4627.

33. Uesawa Y, Kuwahara J, Sugiura Y. Light-induced DNA cleavage by esperamicin and neocarzinostatin. *Biochem Biophys Res Commun* 1989; 164:903–911.

34. Uesawa Y, Sugiura Y. Heat-induced DNA cleavage by esperamicin antitumor antibiotics. *Biochemistry* 1991; 30:9242–9246.

35. Shiraki T, Sugiura Y. Visible light induced DNA cleavage by the hybrid antitumor antibiotic dynemicin A. *Biochemistry* 1990; 29:9795–9798.

36. Sugiura Y, Arakawa T, Uesugi M, Shiraki T, Ohkuma H, Konishi M. Reductive and nucleophilic activation products of dynemicin A with methyl thioglycolate. A rational mechanism for DNA cleavage of the thiol-activated dynemicin A. *Biochemistry* 1991; 30:2989–2992.

37. Sugiura Y, Shiraki T, Konishi M, Oki T. DNA intercalation and cleavage of an antitumor antibiotic dynemicin that contains anthracycline and enediyne cores. *Proc Natl Acad Sci USA* 1990; 87:3831–3835.

38. Wender PA, Kelly RC, Beckham S, Miller BL. Studies on DNA-cleaving agents: computer modeling analysis of the mechanism of activation and cleavage of dynemicin-oligonucleotide complexes. *Proc Natl Acad Sci USA* 1991; 88:8835–8839.

39. Cardozo MG, Hopfinger AJ, Molecular mechanics and molecular dynamics studies of the intercalation of dynemicin-A with oligonucleotide models of DNA. *Mol Pharmacol* 1991; 40: 1023–1028.

40. Sakata N, S-Tsuchiya K, Moriya Y, Hayashi H, Hori M. Aminopeptidase activity of an antitumor antibiotic, C-1027. *J Antibiot* 1992; 45:113–117.

41. Matsumoto T, Okuno Y, Sugiura Y. Specific interaction between a novel enediyne chromophore and apoprotein in macromolecular antitumor antibiotic C-1027. *Biochem Biophys Res Commun* 1993; 195:659–666.

42. Zein N, Colson KL, Leet JE, Schroeder DR, Solomon W, Doyle TW, Casazza AM. Kedarcidin chromophore: an enediyne that cleaves DNA in a sequence-specific manner. *Proc Natl Acad Sci USA* 1993; 90:2822–2826.

43. Xu Y-J, Zhen Y-S, Goldberg IH. C1027 chromophore, a potent new enediyne antitumor antibiotic, induces sequence-specific double-strand DNA cleavage. *Biochemistry* 1994; 33:5947–5954.

44. Hartsell TL, Schor NF. Neuroblastoma cell type-specific apoptosis and morphological differentiation induced by enediyne agents. *Soc Neurosci Abst* 1994; 20:687.

45. DeGraff WG, Mitchell JB. Glutathione dependence of neocarzinostatin cytotoxicity and mutagenicity in Chinese hamster V-79 cells. *Cancer Res* 1985; 45:4760–4762.

46. Ozawa S, Inaba M. Kinetic analysis of the in vitro cell-killing action of neocarzinostatin. *Cancer Chemother Pharmacol* 1989; 23:279–282.

47. Will P, Guger KA, Schor NF. Effects of neocarzinostatin upon the development of tumors from murine neuroblastoma cells. *Cancer Chemother Pharmacol* 1994; 35:115–120.

48. Terado T, Kimura H, Ikebuchi M, Hill C, Aoyama T. The enhancement of cell lethality and changes in production and repair of DNA damage by hypertonic treatment after exposure to X rays, bleomycin, and neocarzinostatin. *Radiat Res* 1993; 135:189–196.

49. Antoku S, Kura S. Enhancement of radiosensitivity of cultured mammalian cells by neocarzinostatin. I. Inhibition of the repair of sublethal damage. *Int J Radiat Biol* 1990; 58:613–622.

50. Antoku S, Kura S. Enhancement of radiosensitivity of cultured mammalian cells by neocarzinostatin. II. Fixation of potentially lethal damage. *Int J Radiat Biol* 1990; 58:623–632.

51. Iseki S, Mori T. Effect of poly(adenosine diphosphate-ribose) polymerase inhibitors on neocarzinostatin-induced G_2 delay in HeLa-S3 cells. *Cancer Res* 1985; 45:4224–4228.

52. Xu Y-J, Li D-D, Zhen Y-S. Mode of action of C-1027, a new macromolecular antitumor antibiotic with highly potent cytotoxicity, on human hepatoma BEL-7402 cells. *Cancer Chemother Pharmacol* 1990; 27:41–46.

53. Falcione M, Milligan KD, Schwartz MC, Schor NF. Prevention of neocarzinostatin-induced cell death and morphologic change in SK-N-SH human neuroblastoma cells by continuous exposure to nerve growth factor. *Biochem Pharm* 1993; 46:731–738.

54. Hartsell TL, Schor NF. Treatment with neocarzinostatin induces apoptosis in cultured neuroblastoma cells. *Soc Neurosci Abst* 1993; 19:635.

55. Hartsell TL, Yalowich JC, Ritke M, Martinez AJ, Schor NF. Induction of apoptosis in murine and human neuroblastoma cell lines by the enediyne natural product neocarzinostatin. *J Pharmacol Exp Therap* 1995; 275:479–485.

56. Hartsell TL, Hinman LM, Hamann PR, Schor NF. Determinants of the response of neuroblastoma cells to DNA damage: The roles of pretreatment cell morphology and chemical nature of the damage. *J Pharmacol Exp Therap* 1996; 277:1158–1166.

57. Lowengrub JA, Schor NF. Neuronal "differentiation" of murine neuroblastoma cells induced by neocarzinostatin: Neural cell adhesion molecules. *Brain Res* 1993; 613:123–131.

58. Rauscher FJ III, Beerman TA, Baker RM. Characterization of auromomycin-resistant hamster cell mutants that display a multidrug resistance phenotype. *Mol Pharmacol* 1990; 38:198–206.

59. Miyamoto Y, Maeda H. Enhancement of verapamil of neocarzinostatin action on multidrug-resistant Chinese hamster ovary cells: possible release of nonprotein chromophore in cells. *Jpn J Cancer Res* 1991; 82:351–356.

60. Bradner WT, Hutchison DJ. Neocarzinostatin (NSC-69856): An antitumor antibiotic effective against ascitic leukemia L1210 in mice. *Cancer Chemother Rep* 1966; 50:79–84.

61. Satake I, Tari K, Yamamoto M, Nishimura H. Neocarzinostatin-induced complete regression of metastatic renal cell carcinoma. *J Urol* 1985; 133:87–89.

62. Abe I, Hori K, Saito S, Tanda S, Li Y, Suzuki M. Increased intratumor concentration of fluorescein-isothiocyanate-labeled neocarzinostatin in rats under angiotensin-induced hypertension. *Jpn J Cancer Res (Gann)* 1988; 79:874–879.

63. Maeda H, Ueda M, Morinaga T, Matsumoto T. Conjugation of poly(styrene-*co*-maleic acid) derivatives to the antitumor protein of neocarzinostatin: pronounced improvements in pharmacological properties. *J Med Chem* 1985; 28:455–461.

64. Oda T, Maeda H. Binding to and internalization by cultured cells of neocarzinostatin and enhancement of its actions by conjugation with lipophilic styrene-maleic acid copolymer. *Cancer Res* 1987; 47:3206–3211.

65. Oda T, Sato F, Maeda H. Facilitated internalization of neocarzinostatin and its lipophilic polymer conjugate, SMANCS, into cytosol in acidic pH. *JNCI* 1987; 79:1205–1211.

66. Suzuki F, Pollard RB, Maeda H. Stimulation of non-specific resistance to tumors in the mouse using a poly(maleic-acid-styrene)-conjugated neocarzinostatin. *Cancer Immunol Immunother* 1989; 30:97–104.

67. Yamamoto H, Miki T, Oda T, Hirano T, Sera Y, Akagi M, Maeda H. Reduced bone marrow toxicity of neocarzinostatin by conjugation with divinyl ether-maleic acid copolymer. *Eur J Cancer* 1990; 26:253–260.

68. Suzuki F, Matsumoto K, Schmitt DA, Pollard RB, Maeda H. Immunomodulating activities of orally administered SMANCS, a polymer-conjugated derivative of the proteinaceous antibiotic neocarzinostatin, in an oily formulation. *Int J Immunopharmacol* 1993; 15:175–183.

69. Suzuki F, Pollard RB, Uchimura S, Munakata T, Maeda H. Role of natural killer cells and

macrophages in the nonspecific resistance to tumors in mice stimulated with SMANCS, a polymer-conjugated derivative of neocarzinostatin. *Cancer Res* 1990; 50:3897–3904.

70. Konno T, Maeda H, Iwai K, Tashiro S, Maki S, Morinaga T, Mochinaga M, Hiraoka T, Yokoyama I. Effect of arterial administration of high-molecular-weight anticancer agent SMANCS with lipid lymphographic agent on hepatoma: a preliminary report. *Eur J Cancer Clin Oncol* 1983; 19:1053–1065.

71. Oda T, Yamamoto H, Miki T, Maeda H. Differential neutralizing effect on tiopronin on the toxicity of neocarzinostatin and SMANCS: a new rescue cancer chemotherapy. *Jpn J Cancer Res* 1989; 80:394–399.

72. Iwamoto Y, Kuroiwa T, Aoki K, Baba T. "Two-route chemotherapy" using high-dose intra-arterial neocarzinostatin and systemic tiopronin, its antidote, for rat limb tumor. *Cancer Chemother Pharmacol* 1986; 17:247–250.

73. Hasuda K, Kobayashi H, Kuroiwa T, Aoki K, Taniguchi S., Baba T. Efficacy of two-route chemotherapy using intraperitoneal neocarzinostatin and its antidote, intravenous tiopronin, for peritoneally disseminated tumors in mice. *Jpn J Cancer Res* 1989; 80:283–289.

74. Yamaguchi T, Tsurumi H, Kitamura K, Otsuji E, Miyagaki T, Kotani T, Takahashi T. Production, binding and cytotoxicity of human/mouse chimeric monoclonal antibody-neocarzinostatin conjugate. *Jpn J. Cancer Res* 1993; 84:1190–1194.

75. Takashina K-I, Kitamura K, Yamaguchi T, Noguchi A, Noguchi A, Tsurumi H, Takahashi T. Comparative pharmacokinetic properties of murine monoclonal antibody A7 modified with neocarzinostatin, dextran, and polyethylene glycol. *Jpn J. Cancer Res* 1991; 82:1145–1150.

76. Yamaguchi T, Tsurumi H, Kotani T, Yamaoka N, Otsuji E, Kitamura K, Takahashi T. *In vivo* efficacy of neocarzinostatin coupled with Fab human/mouse chimeric monoclonal antibody A7 against human colorectal cancer. *Jpn J. Cancer Res* 1994; 85:167–171.

77. Otsuji E, Yamaguchi T, Yamaoka N, Kitamura K, Yamaguchi N, Takahashi T. Intratumoral administration of neocarzinostatin conjugated to monoclonal antibody A7 in a model of pancreatic cancer. *J Surg Oncol* 1993; 53:215–219.

78. Otsuji E, Yamaguchi T, Yamaoka N, Taniguchi K, Kato M, Kotani T, Kitamura K, Takahashi T. Biodistribution of neocarzinostatin conjugated to chimeric Fab fragments of the monoclonal antibody A7 in nude mice bearing human pancreatic cancer xenografts. *Jpn J. Cancer Res* 1994; 85:530–535.

79. Gottschalk U, Garnett MC, Ward RK, Mailbucher A, Kohnlein W. Increased serum stability and prolonged biological half-life of neocarzinostatin covalently bound to monoclonal antibodies. *J Antibiot* 1991; 44:1148–1153.

80. Kondo S, Nakatsu S, Sakahara H, Kobayashi H, Konishi J, Namba Y. Antitumor activity of an immunoconjugate composed of anti-human astrocytoma monoclonal antibody and neocarzinostatin. *Eur J Cancer* 1993; 29A:420–423.

81. Sasaki T, Muryoi T, Takai O, Tamate E, Ono Y, Koide Y, Ishida N, Yoshinaga K. Selective elimination of anti-DNA antibody-producing cells by antiidiotypic antibody conjugated with neocarzinostatin. *J Clin Invest* 1986; 77:1382–1386.

82. Sasaki T, Tamate E, Muryoi T, Takai O, Yoshingaga K. In vitro manipulation of human anti-DNA antibody production by anti-idiotypic antibodies conjugated with neocarzinostatin. *J Immunol* 1989; 142:1159–1165.

83. Harata N, Sasaki T, Osaki H, Saito T, Shibata S, Muryoi T, Takai O, Yoshinaga K. Therapeutic treatment of New Zealand mouse disease by a limited number of anti-idiotypic antibodies conjugated with neocarzinostatin. *J Clin Invest* 1990; 86:769–776.

84. Kohgo Y, Kondo H, Kato J, Sasaki K, Tsuchima N, Nishisato T, Hirayama M, Fujikawa K, Shintani N, Mogi Y, Niitsu Y. Kinetics of internalization and cytotoxicity of transferrin-neocarzinostatin conjugate in human leukemia cell line, K562. *Jpn J. Cancer Res* 1990; 81:91–99.

85. Sasaki T, Kohgo Y, Kato J, Kondo H, Niitsu Y. Intracellular metabolism and cytotoxicity of transferrin-neocarzinostatin conjugates of differing molar ratios. *Jpn J. Cancer Res* 1993; 84: 191–196.

86. Schor NF. Targeted enhancement of the biological activity of the antineoplastic agent, neocarzinostatin: Studies in murine neuroblastoma cells. *J Clin Invest* 1992; 89:774–781.

12 Matrix Metalloproteinase Inhibitors

William G. Stetler-Stevenson, MD, PhD

Contents

1. EXTRACELLULAR MATRIX DEGRADATION IN CANCER PROGRESSION

1.1. Historical Perspective

The contribution of extracellular matrix turnover to the invasive phenotype of cancer cells has long been recognized. Hippocrates (460–370 BC), who described invading tendrils of tumor tissue and the resulting destruction of bone and soft tissue, ascribed this behavior to an imbalance of the "Four Humors" resulting in a local excess of one of these, which he called "black bile" (*1*). This theory was later extended by Galen (131–203 AD), who proposed that the "black bile" was concentrated in areas of tumor invasion (*2*). Our modern view of the process of cancer invasion and metastasis formation is remarkably similar to these early hypotheses, except that we recognize various lytic enzymes as major components of Hippocrates' "black bile." Furthermore, Hippocrates' concept of a localized imbalance of "Humors" is essentially identical to our current understanding that extracellular matrix degradation and tumor cell migration are dependent on a critical balance between activated proteases and their endogenous inhibitors.

The current view on the role of proteases in cancer metastasis has been refined considerably over the last 20 years. The function of proteases in cancer invasion is now replete with many details, and the role of specific classes of proteases has been defined.

From: *Cancer Therapeutics: Experimental and Clinical Agents*
Edited by: B. Teicher Humana Press Inc., Totowa, NJ

As a result of these studies, several specific proteases have been identified as potential therapeutic targets for novel cancer therapy. Members of the matrix metalloproteinases are one such group. The first members of this family of proteases were the collagenases that were identified through their ability to degrade the collagen triple helix selectivity. However, the role of these proteolytic activities in cancer progression was not appreciated for many years.

In the 1960s and early 1970s, investigators frequently noted the association of a variety of protease activities with invasive tumor cells, including both lysosomal and neutral protease activities (3–9). It had long been recognized that native collagen in fibrillar form was extremely resistant to protease action at neutral pH. Collagenases that selectively degrade these fibrillar collagens within the triple helical domain were initially identified in resorbing tadpole tail and in mammalian tissues showing evidence of collagen breakdown (10,11). In the late 1960s and early 1970s, collagen-degrading activities were reported in association with both epithelial and mesenchymal malignancies. These included basal cell carcinomas of the skin, melanoma, squamous cell carcinomas, soft tissue sarcomas, and breast cancer tissues (12–20). Collagenase activities were also obtained from tumor explants. These collagenases were poorly characterized, and it was difficult to determine if they originated from tumor cells or host response. Furthermore, the correlation between these collagenase activities and the metastatic potential of the tumor was, at best, only broadly demonstrated.

In 1977, Lance Liotta and colleagues used the T241 mouse fibrosarcoma model to demonstrate that tumor cells obtained from the venous effluent of a primary tumor possessed significantly higher basement membrane-degrading and type I collagen matrix-degrading activity when compared to cells of the primary tumor (21). This suggested that metastasizing tumor cells form a distinct subpopulation within the primary tumor and that these cells possessed enhanced invasive potential represented in part by extracellular matrix-degrading protease activity. In that same year, Kuettner and colleagues (22) published a report that described the production of collagenase activity by human osteosarcoma and mammary carcinoma cell lines. This activity was inhibited by a cartilage-derived protein of low molecular weight. Since cartilage is rarely invaded by neoplasms, the authors concluded that the activity of the collagenase and, subsequently, its regulation by the cartilage-derived inhibitor played an important role in tumor cell invasion. These two studies represent a turning point in the view of investigators toward the role of proteases in cancer progression. For the first time, the research focused on degradation of specific components of the extracellular matrix, and this activity was correlated with the aggressive behavior of subpopulations of tumor cells. They are also the first indication that inhibition of collagenase activity might be a useful therapeutic strategy for blocking the spread of tumor cells.

1.2. Basement Membrane as a Barrier to Tumor Invasion

Liotta and colleagues combined the results of these initial experiments with the observation that destruction of basement membranes is often associated with tumor invasion, to formulate a working hypothesis that tumor cells selectively degrade components of the basement membrane (23). Concurrent investigations by other laboratories analyzed the molecular components of the basement membrane and characterized collagen-degrading enzymes from a variety of sources. Type IV collagen was shown to be a major structural component of basement membranes and distinct from the fibrillar collagens previously identified (*24–26*). Specific type IV collagen-degrading activity was first described by Liotta et al. in 1979 (*23*). This activity was derived from the culture media of the T241 metastatic murine fibrosarcoma cell line, and was shown to degrade type IV collagen selectively, generating specific N-terminal 1/4 and C-terminal 3/4 cleavage products. This activity had a molecular mass of approx 65–72 kDa, pH optima around 7.0, and was sensitive to chelating agents suggesting that it was also a neutral metalloproteinase activity. However, the relationship of this type IV collagenase to dermal fibroblast collagenase was not appreciated for several years. Primary sequence information on this interstitial collagenase and on the tumor type IV collagenase would subsequently reveal that these enzymes constituted the first members of a new family of proteases that has become known as the matrix metallo-proteinase (MMP) family (*27,28*). The mammalian interstitial collagenase is recognized as the first member of this family and is often referred to as MMP-1 (*27,28*). The 72-kDa type IV collagenase, first isolated by Liotta, is recognized as the second member and is referred to as MMP-2. Current terminology also refers to this protease as gelatinase A in recognition of the potent gelatinolytic activity that this protease possesses (*27*). Several additional members of this family would also later be identified through their overexpression and association with tumor cells (i.e., transin [rat homolog of human stromelysin-1] [*29*], stromelysin-3 [*30*], and collagenase-3 [*31*]).

Subsequent experiments demonstrated a direct correlation between type IV collagen-degrading activity and metastatic potential of several murine tumor cell lines (*32*). These findings suggested that the basement membrane posed a significant barrier for tumor cell invasion. This concept formed the basis of many studies that attempted to characterize the interaction of tumor cells with the extracellular matrix and formed the basis of the three-step hypothesis of tumor cell interaction with the basement membrane (*33*). This hypothesis defines the invasive phenotype as consisting of three distinct phases: attachment of tumor cells to the basement membrane or extracellular matrix, creation of a proteolytic defect in the basement membrane, and migration of the tumor cells into this defect (*34*). Although initially presented over 10 years ago, this three-step model remains a useful framework for understanding the extracellular matrix–cell interactions that occur during successful cell invasion, whether pathologic or physiologic (*34*). This model highlights tumor cell-mediated extracellular matrix proteolysis as a central feature of tumor invasion and metastasis. It also presents a framework that can be used to test the role of various proteases in cancer invasion.

Subsequent investigations led to the development of in vitro invasion assays, which use either native (*35*) or reconstituted basement membranes (*36,37*). These assays have been useful in demonstrating the requirement of MMP activity during tumor cell invasion. In addition they have also been useful in screening metalloproteinase inhibitors prior to actual in vivo animal testing in either lung colonization or spontaneous metastasis models of tumor progression.

2. THE MMP AND TISSUE INHIBITOR OF METALLOPROTEINASE FAMILIES

2.1. MMPs

Investigation of the biochemistry and molecular biology of chronic diseases, such as arthritis and cancer, has revealed a critical role for extracellular matrix remodeling.

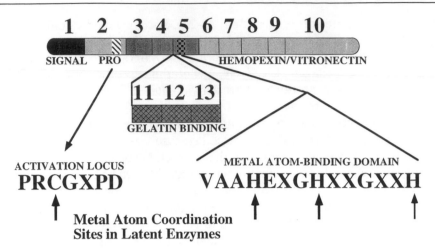

Fig. 1. Domain structure of the matrix metalloproteinases. General structure of a prototypic member of the MMP family is depicted. The exons encoding the full-length protein are represented as 1–10. These include a signal sequence, encoded in exon 1, for extrusion into the endoplasmic reticulum, as well as a prosegment, encoded in exon 2, that contains a highly conserved peptide sequence responsible for the lack of protease activity in the proenzyme. This prosegment contains a unpaired cysteine residue that coordinates the zinc atom of the active site resulting in latency. Exons 4, 5, and 6 encode for the catalytic domain that contains a signature metal atom binding domain that defines this family of proteases. The involvement of these three histidyl residues in zinc atom binding has been confirmed by X-ray diffraction analysis. The gelatinases contain a disruption of the catalytic domain represented by the insertion of three exons immediately upstream of the sequence encoding the metal-atom binding domain. These three exons encode for type II gelatin binding motifs originally observed in fibronectin. The carboxyl region of the MMP family members is the least conserved region. Many members of this protease family show sequence homology to hemopexin and/or vitronectin in this region as illustrated.

These studies also identified several unique matrix-degrading proteases overexpressed in tumor cells that are now known to be members of the MMP family. These are a group of related zinc metallo-endopeptidases with neutral pH optima, which collectively are capable of degrading most, if not all, of the structural components of the extracellular matrix, such as collagens, proteoglycans, and glycoproteins, like fibronectin and laminin (for general review of these enzymes, *see 28,38–40*). These enzymes share a number of common structural domains that identify members of this protease family (Fig. 1). The currently recognized members of the MMP family and their recognized substrates are listed in Table 1. These proteases are subgrouped according to substrate preference (*28,38,39*). The interstitial collagenases, which degrade fibrillar collagens, include fibroblast interstitial collagenase and neutrophil collagenase. The stromelysins have a broad range of substrates, including proteoglycans, glycoproteins, and nonhelical collagens, as well as other latent MMPs resulting in activation. This group includes stromelysin-1, stromelysin-2, and matrilysin. Stromelysin-3 is the newest member of this group and is included primary because of sequence homology, although its substrate specificity is not well defined.

The gelatinase subgroup possesses potent gelatin-degrading activity as well as selective activity against a variety of collagens, such as types IV, V, VII, X, and XI (*28*). This group also degrades other matrix components, such as elastin, fibronectin, and

Table 1
Matrix Metalloproteinase Family Members

Subgroup	E.C. nomenclature/ other designations	MMP number	Molecular species	Substrates
Interstitial collagenases				
	Interstitial collagenase (fibroblast type)	MMP-1	52, 57 kDa	Fibrillar collagens (III > > I)
	PMN collagenase	MMP-8	75 kDa	Fibrillar collagens (I > > III)
	Collagenase-3	MMP-13	54 kDa	Fibrillar collagen
Stromelysins				
	Stromelysin-1	MMP-3	52, 58 kDa	LMN, FBN core protein, other MMP nonhelical collagen
	Stromelysin-2	MMP-10	58 kDa	Same as MMP-3
	Stromelysin-3	MMP-11	29 kDa	α-1-Antitrypsin
	Matrilysin	MMP-7	28 kDa	Similar to MMP-3
Gelatinases				
	Gelatinase-A, 72 kDa type IV collagenase	MMP-2	72 kDa	Gel, col IV, col V FBN, VN, Elastin, col I, cell surface?
	Gelatinase-B, 92 kDa type IV collagenase	MMP-9	92 kDa	Gel, col IV, col V
Other				
	Metalloelastase	MMP-12	53 kDa	Elastin
	Membrane-type MMP	MMP-14	66 kDa	Progelatinase A

vitronectin. Gelatinase A, which is the same as the original 72-kDa type IV collagenase isolated by Liotta and colleagues, as well as gelatinase B, are the current members of this group. Newer members of the MMP family that are less well characterized include macrophage metalloelastase (MMP-12) (*41*) and collagenase-3 (MMP-13) whose expression appears to be selectively associated with human breast cancer (*31*). The newest member of this family contains a transmembrane domain and is referred to as membrane type MMP or MT-MMP (*42*). Some distinguishing features and known substrate specificities of these proteases are briefly outlined in Table 1.

These enzymes are characteristically produced and secreted into the extracellular milieu as proenzymes (*28,38,39*). MT-MMP is the obvious exception to this in that this enzyme is membrane-associated and thus not secreted, but it does appear to be initially produced as a proenzyme. The latency of the proenzyme form of all MMPs is the result of interaction of a highly conserved cysteine of the amino-terminal pro-domain with the zinc atom at the active site (*43*). The cysteine switch hypothesis states that disruption of this interaction results in proenzyme activation. This family of proteases is further defined by the fact that they are selectively inhibited by a group of endogenous inhibitors known as the tissue inhibitors of metalloproteinases or (TIMPs). The balance between the level of activated MMPs and available TIMPs determines the net MMP activity and is therefore a pivotal determinant of extracellular matrix turnover.

TIMP-1	TIMP-2	TIMP-3
28 kDa	21 kDa	24 kDa
Glycosylated	Non-glycosylated	Non-glycosylated
Binds to latent Gel B	Binds to latent Gel A	Binds to ECM
0.9 kb	1.1 and 3.5 kb	4.5 kb
TGF β1: ↑	TGF β1: ↓ ↔	TGF β1: ↑
Xq11	17q25	22q12.1-13.2

Inhibition of all activated MMP's

Fig. 2. Comparison of TIMP family members. The three currently recognized members of the TIMP family are compared and contrasted. Features compared are: molecular mass of the mature protein, glycosylation, unique binding properties, transcript sizes, modulation of gene expression by the action of TGFβ1, and chromosome location of the human gene. Finally, the activity that defines this group of inhibitors is their ability to inhibit all activated members of the MMP family.

2.2. TIMPs

Currently, there are three well-defined members of the TIMP family of inhibitors that share approx 40% homology at the amino acid level (28,40). These are TIMP-1, TIMP-2, and TIMP-3 (Fig. 2). The TIMPs bind with high affinity and 1:1 stoichiometry to active MMPs resulting in the loss of protease activity. All three proteins of this family contain 12 highly conserved cysteine residues. In TIMP-1 and TIMP-2, these cysteine residues have been shown to form disulfide bridges generating six peptide loops and two peptide knots. The exact mechanism of TIMP-mediated inhibition of MMP activity is currently not known.

3. THE ROLE OF MMPs IN CANCER

3.1. From Correlation to Causality

The rapid growth of information on new members of the MMP family has resulted in an explosion of studies on the role of specific MMPs in cancer cell invasion and metastasis formation. Many studies have assessed MMP expression at either the protein or nucleic acid level, and correlated this expression with invasive ability or metastatic potential of the tumor (34). These studies, performed both in vitro and in vivo using a variety of models, consistently demonstrate a direct correlation between the overexpression of MMPs, and increased invasive capacity or metastatic potential of a variety of tumor cell lines.

Similar techniques have been employed to study MMP expression directly in human tumor tissues. A direct correlation between MMP expression and the invasive phenotype of human tumor cells has been observed in lung, prostate, stomach, colon, breast,

Protease / Tumor Type	IC-1 MMP-1	Gel A MMP-2	St-1 MMP-3	Matr MMP-7	Gel B MMP-9	St-2 MMP-10	St-3 MMP-11
Breast		X			X		X
Prostate		X		X	X		
Ovary		X					
Lung	X	X					X
Colo-rectal	X	X		X	X		X
Gastric		X		X			
Thyroid		X					
Liver		X					
Oral (Squamous)	X	X	X	X			
Salivary gland		X					

Fig. 3. Expression of MMPs in human tumor tissues. The results of immunohistochemical and *in situ* hybridization analysis of MMP expression in human tumor tissues are summarized graphically. The results demonstrate the frequent detection of gelatinase A, matrilysin (MMP-7), and gelatinase B in a variety of tumor types. The abbreviations used are IC-1 for interstitial collagenase, Gel A for gelatinase A, St-1 for stromelysin-1, Matr for matrilysin, Gel B for gelatinase B, St-2 for stromelysin-2, and St-3 for stromelysin-3.

ovary, thyroid, and oral squamous cell cancers. Figure 3 summarizes these studies using human tumor tissues. These studies show that many members of the MMP family are overexpressed in human tumor tissue. Although gelatinase A is expressed in all tumor types examined, no single MMP is consistently overexpressed in every single tumor of a given histopathologic classification. This fact probably reflects tumor cell heterogeneity, possible variable MMP expression with tumor progression, as well as differential expression in response to changing extracellular matrices that are encountered during tumor progression.

Three members of the MMP family are overexpressed at a high frequency in many human tumor types. These include stromelysin-3, gelatinase A, and gelatinase B. Stromelysin-3 expression was initially observed in human breast cancer tissues where the level of expression correlated with tumor progression (*30*). More recent studies have demonstrated expression of stromelysin-3 mRNA in a high percentage of primary tumors in the lung (*44*), colon (*45*), squamous cell cancers of the head and neck (*46*), and as basal cell cancers of the skin (*47*). Although stromelysin-3 shows a very strong correlation with the presence of invasive carcinoma, the substrate for this protease remained elusive until recently. This enzyme has now been demonstrated to possess potent degrading activity against a member of the serpin family (**serine p**rotease **in**hibitor), α-1 proteinase inhibitor (*48*). This suggests that MMPs may cooperate with other proteases systems to facilitate matrix turnover.

The specific protease characterized by Liotta as a type IV collagenase of tumor cells is now referred to as gelatinase A. Studies have demonstrated the overexpression of this enzyme in many human tumor tissues, including breast, colon, thyroid, lung, gastric, prostate, and ovarian cancers (*34*). A recent study has demonstrated that expression of pro-MMP-2 in human oral squamous cell carcinomas is associated with an increased frequency of lymph node metastases (49). Those authors suggest that this marker may be useful in evaluating the malignant potential of individual oral squamous cell tumors.

Frequently, the expression of progelatinase A is observed in human tumor tissues prior to the development of frankly invasive carcinoma (i.e., severe dysplasia and/or carcinoma *in situ* (50). This suggests that expression of this proenzyme may be necessary, but is not sufficient for acquisition of the invasive phenotype, and that regulation of progelatinase A activation is a key step during tumor cell invasion.

Recent studies on human tumor cell lines and tumor tissues confirm this hypothesis. Researchers have used the technique of gelatin zymography to assess the contribution of the activated (62-kDa) form of gelatinase A to the invasive phenotype of human breast and nonsmall-cell lung cancer (51–53). These studies demonstrate that although tumors from these tissues may express both progelatinase A and B, only a few tumors expressed small amounts of the activated form of gelatinase B. In contrast, the fraction of total gelatinase A present in the activated (62-kDa) form was consistently elevated in malignant disease and correlated with the tumor grade. Analysis of breast cancer cell lines demonstrates a correlation between the ability to activate progelatinase A with the invasive potential (54). Microdissection of human colorectal tumors and analysis of these microdissected tissues by zymography demonstrate a selective increase in the activated 62-kDa form of gelatinase A in the invasive components of these tumors (55).

These studies highlight the limitations inherent in the measurement of MMP overexpression by both immunohistochemistry and nucleic acid hybridization techniques. A key determinant of invasive behavior is MMP activation. For these enzymes, which are all secreted in the proenzyme form, overproduction of proenzyme and enzyme activity are not equivalent. Future experiments should focus on rigorously correlating tumor stage with levels of active enzyme or direct measurements of enzyme activity. However, the latter is clearly more difficult owing to the presence of endogenous inhibitors.

The correlative evidence presented above clearly suggests that the action of selected MMPs is required during tumor invasion and progression. These correlative data are strongly supported by studies modulating endogenous MMP inhibitors (i.e., TIMPs) to block tumor invasion and metastasis. These studies unequivocally demonstrate a causal role for MMPs in tumor invasion. Numerous studies have correlated low TIMP expression with enhanced invasive and metastatic properties in both murine and human tumor cell lines (56,57). TIMP-1 has been shown to inhibit metastasis in vivo in animal models using B16F10 murine melanoma cells or *ras*-transfected rat embryo fibroblasts (58–60). TIMP-2 transfection and overexpression in *ras*-transfected rat embryo fibroblast resulted in loss of lung colonizing ability following iv injection of these cells, but did not completely block the formation of pulmonary metastases from primary tumors following sc inoculation of tumor cells (58,61). Transfection and overexpression of TIMP-2 have also been shown to inhibit the growth of primary tumors following sc inoculation of *scid* mice with human melanoma cells, but again did not prevent metastasis formation (61). More recently, the ratio of metalloproteinase activity and TIMP-2 has been shown to be a critical determinant in the adhesion and spreading of human melanoma cells (62). Alteration of cell adhesion and spreading in turn alters the ability of tumor cells to migrate and invade. These are cell functions that are essential for the fully competent metastatic phenotype. These experiments using TIMPs have defined the requirement for functional MMP activity during tumor cell invasion. This suggest that targeting the activity of these metalloproteinases may provide a clinically useful mechanism for blocking the local invasion and possibly the metastatic spread of cancer cells.

3.2. Angiogenesis

Endothelial cell invasion during angiogenesis shares a number of functional similarities with invasive tumor cells. This includes crossing a basement membrane connective tissue barrier and the production of MMPs (63,64). The requirement for MMP activity during angiogenesis has been demonstrated in several systems. TIMP-1 blocks basic fibroblast growth factor (bFGF)-induced endothelial cell invasion on human amnion membranes (65). Both TIMP-1 and TIMP-2 block polyamine-stimulated angiogenesis in the chick chorioallantoic membrane assay (66). More recently, Albini and colleagues demonstrated that TIMP-2 can inhibit the angiogenic response induced by Kaposi's sarcoma cell-conditioned media in vivo (67).

Schnaper and colleagues have shown that a critical balance of MMPs and TIMP influences endothelial cell morphogenesis in an in vitro model of angiogenesis (68). In these experiments, the addition of exogenous TIMPs inhibits endothelial tube formation on a reconstituted basement membrane matrix. This effect was also observed following treatment of the endothelial cell cultures with gelatinase A-neutralizing antibodies. Addition of exogenous purified gelatinase A resulted in enhanced tube formation, but this effect was reversed at excess gelatinase A concentrations. As has been observed with tumor cells for both MMPs and other protease systems, excessive protease activity can be detrimental to invasive behavior of endothelial cells (62,69).

Moses et al. have identified a cartilage-derived inhibitor (CDI) of angiogenesis that has collagenase-inhibitory activity and demonstrates amino acid sequence homology to the TIMPs (70). The relationship of this factor to the cartilage-derived collagenase inhibitor originally described by Kuettner and colleagues (22) is not known. CDI has been shown to inhibit endothelial cell migration and proliferation in response to bFGF, a major angiogenic growth factor produced by human tumors. Recent studies have also shown that TIMP-2 can inhibit the bFGF-induced proliferation of human microvascular endothelial cells (71). This effect was not seen with TIMP-1 or synthetic MMP inhibitors, such as Batimastat (vide infra). This identified a unique biological activity of TIMP-2 that is not related to metalloproteinase inhibitory activity. Furthermore, this implies that TIMP-2 may have additional actions that limit neovascularization associated with solid tumor growth and metastasis in vivo.

These findings suggest that the use of either endogenous or synthetic MMP inhibitors to block tumor cell invasion and metastasis may also disrupt the tumor-induced angiogenesis that is required for tumor growth and metastasis. The use of such agents as TIMP-2 may have additional biological activities that could be exploited clinically, i.e., inhibition of bFGF-induced endothelial cell growth.

4. CHANGING RATIONALE
FOR TARGETING MMPs IN HUMAN CANCER

As outlined previously, the MMPs are clearly implicated in the processes of tumor cell invasion and angiogenesis. These processes of tumorigenesis and tumor-induced angiogenesis are interdependent. Elaboration of angiogenic factors and induction of an angiogenic response is a phenotype clearly associated with more aggressive tumors (72,73). In turn, formation of new blood vessels permits the expansion of tumor foci (primary or metastatic) in three dimensions. Following vascularization, tumor foci undergo rapid local expansion and acquire an enhanced metastatic potential that correlates directly with the degree of vascularization of the primary tumor (74–76). Thus, tumor invasion, growth, and metastasis are closely linked to tumor-induced angiogenesis, and both seem to require MMP activity. This suggests that targeting these enzymes in cancer therapy may provide synergistic actions that result in unique therapeutic benefits.

As originally formulated, the strategy of inhibiting MMP activity was directed at preventing metastasis formation. This concept originally met with considerable resistance, because it is well known in the clinic that the majority of cancer patients have metastases at the time of diagnosis of their primary tumor. Thus, the initial presentation of the cancer patient usually occurs at a later stage in the disease when tumor cell invasion and dissemination have already occurred. However, several factors now indicate that inhibition of MMP activity, as therapeutic targets in cancer therapy, may have additional, previously unappreciated therapeutic consequences that are beneficial to the cancer patient. The most compelling of these is the possible use of these agents as cytostatic agents, which would prevent the growth of both primary tumor and metastatic foci. This may be a result of direct action of these agents on the tumor cells or a secondary effect through inhibition of MMP activity required for release of growth factors sequestered in the extracellular matrix or inhibition of tumor-induced angiogenesis required for tumor growth.

The conventional cytotoxic approach to cancer chemotherapy has had limited success in the treatment of advanced solid tumors, and recently the development of new cytotoxic strategies and agents has slowed. This trend, combined with the frequent development of drug resistance to known cytotoxic agents, has led many to explore targets that may lead to the development of a new type of chemotherapy, tumor cell cytostatic agents or "tumoriostatic" agents (Fig. 4). As described previously, endogenous MMP inhibitors, TIMPs, have been shown to inhibit the growth of the primary tumors in experimental models as well as block growth factor stimulation of endothelial cells. Thus, the MMPs are definitely within this class of therapeutic targets that engender cytostatic therapy, as are adhesion molecules, signal transduction pathways, growth factors, and angiogenic responses. The hope is that by the use of selective inhibitors for these targets, one can achieve a halt in tumor progression without significant toxicity. The potential utility of this cytostatic approach to cancer chemotherapy is best exemplified by the recent use of tamoxifen to treat invasive breast cancer (77,78).

Alternatively, the cytostatic strategy could be used as an adjuvant to conventional cytotoxic therapy to prevent regrowth of tumor between cycles of tumor cell killing. One could envisage alternating cycles of cytotoxic and cytostatic therapy. This could prevent tumor regrowth between cycles of cytotoxic agents. Enhancement of cytotoxic therapies that rely on active tumor cell replication might be achieved by initiating cytotoxic therapy immediately prior to release from cytostatic therapy. This could result in improved reduction of tumor burden, which would be amendable to continued cytostatic therapy (see Fig. 4). By limiting the size of the tumor cell population

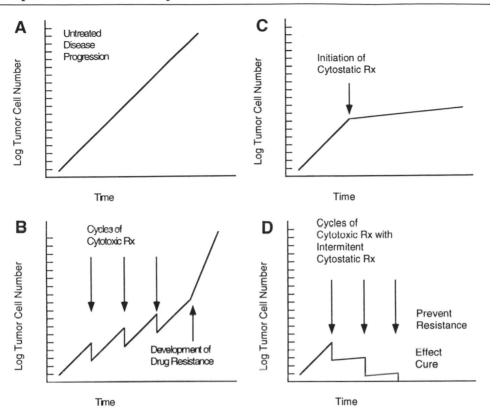

Fig. 4. Cancer therapy paradigms: cytotoxic, cytostatic, and combined therapy. Cancer treatment paradigms are presented in terms of total tumor cell number. (**A**) Untreated cancer. The exponential growth of the early primary is maintained by metastasis formation resulting in exponential increase in tumor burden. (**B**) Cytotoxic therapy. Conventional cytotoxic therapy results in initial reduction of tumor cell burden with eventual regrowth. There is an overall reduction in the rate of tumor cell accumulation, but repeated exposure to cytotoxic agents leads to eventual development of drug resistance and treatment failure. (**C**) Cytostatic therapy. Initiation and continuation of cytostatic therapy with no cytotoxicity prevent further growth of primary tumor and/or metastatic foci. Chronic long-term treatment greatly reduces or eliminates tumor cell accumulation. (**D**) Combined cytotoxic and cytostatic therapy. Administration of cytotoxic agent reduces tumor cell burden, and regrowth is prevented by addition of cytostatic agent. Cytostatic agents are then removed shortly before initiating a second cycle of cytotoxic therapy for further reduction of tumor cell burden. Repeated alternating cycles of cytotoxic and cytostatic therapy could more effectively reduce tumor burden by preventing tumor regrowth between cycles of cytotoxic therapy. Combined therapy may also help prevent development of drug resistance to cytotoxic therapy by limiting the tumor cell population exposed to such agents. The potential clinical utility of combination therapy utilizing an MMP inhibitor and a conventional cytotoxic agent (cyclophosphamide) was recently demonstrated using a murine Lewis lung carcinoma model (*110*).

exposed to the cytotoxic agents, this approach could also help prevent the development of drug resistance. If proven effective at blocking tumor cell spread that is the hallmark of malignant transformation, agents that are well tolerated should also be tested as chemopreventive agents. However, all of these possibilities await the identification of suitable MMP inhibitor(s).

5. INHIBITORS OF MMPs FOR CANCER THERAPY

5.1. Overview

Successful pharmacological targeting of metalloproteinase activity is best exemplified by the development of angiotensin-converting enzyme (ACE) inhibitors to block conversion of angiotensin I to angiotensin II in the treatment of refractory hypertension (*79–81*). This effort led to the identification of Captopril and the prodrug Enalapril, which have become highly successful in the treatment of hypertension and congestive heart failure (*79,81*). This success demonstrates that mechanism-based inhibitors for metalloproteinases can be developed and exploited in the clinical setting. This same strategy has been utilized for the development of MMP inhibitors, since substrate analogs have been modified to target reactive moieties selectively at the active site of MMPs.

5.2. Substrate Analog Inhibitors of MMPs

As mentioned, the most conventional strategy for the development of protease inhibitors has been the substrate analog approach. In this strategy, a peptide analog resembling the native substrate is coupled with either an nonhydrolyzable functionality that replaces the scissile peptide bond or a zinc atom-coordinating or chelating moiety (Fig. 5). This is used as a starting point to synthesize a series of compounds with substitutions at different positions. This strategy designs inhibitors around two regions that interact with the active site of MMPs (*see* Fig. 5). The functionality that interacts with the active site zinc atom is the first region. The second region concerns the design of amino acid side chains on either the amino-terminal (P residues) side or the carboxy-terminal side (P ' residues) of the scissile bond. These residues interact with the active site pocket and thus can give the inhibitor the potential to target a specific MMP. Rational drug design systematically explores the structure–activity relationship of these inhibitors following substitution of various functionalities for the amino acid side chains throughout the parent compound.

This substrate analog approach has been the most widely adopted for the development of MMP inhibitors. In the 1980s, a number of pharmaceutical companies became interested in MMP inhibitors with the specific aim of treating the joint destruction associated with rheumatoid arthritis. These efforts were successful in developing a series of MMP inhibitors. Inhibitors based on a thiol, carboxylic, and phosphinic acid, as well as hydroxamate strategies were developed and explored. The most potent inhibitors are those designed to mimic the carboxy-terminal portion of the substrate and incorporate a hydroxamate moiety attached to the residue at the P_1 ' position (Fig. 5B). The evolution of these efforts has been described elsewhere and is beyond the scope of this chapter (*82–84*). These efforts have resulted in the first generation of MMP inhibitors that are or are about to be tested in phase 1 clinical trials for cancer therapy.

Batimastat, or BB-94 as it had been referred to previously, is a hydroxamic acid analog ([4-{*N*-hydroxyamino}-2*R*-isobutyl-3*S*-{thiophen-2-ylthiomethyl}-succinyl]-L-phenylalanine-*N*-methylamide) with broad-spectrum MMP inhibitory activity, but little activity against other unrelated metalloproteinases (*85*). Batimastat inhibits the metastatic spread of tumor cells in a number of animal models using either murine

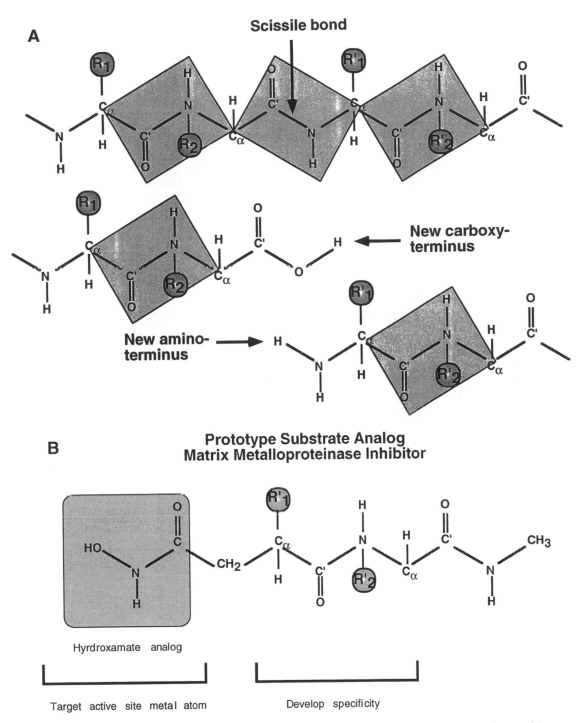

Fig. 5. MMP inhibitor development strategy. (**A**) Structure of the protease substrate. The peptide backbone structure of a protein is illustrated to show the target scissile bond and the nomenclature conventions used to denote amino acid side chains relative to the cleavage site. (**B**) Substrate analog MMP inhibitor. The structural basis for the hydroxamate analog inhibitors currently under development is illustrated. These are derived from the carboxyl side of the putative substrate and include a hydroxamic acid derivative for chelating the active site zinc atom. Potent synthetic MMP inhibitors based on this strategy have been identified, and are in early clinical trials or preclinical development.

B16 melanoma cells, human ovarian cancer cells, or human colon cancer xenografts (53,86). Somewhat unexpectedly, Batismastat also inhibits the growth of the primary tumor, although it is not directly cytotoxic to human tumor cells. Histologic examination of the primary tumor tissues in these experiments suggested that Batimastat treatment resulted in formation of fibrous tissue encapsulation and production of avascular stroma. Inhibition of primary tumor growth has also been observed with other hydroxmate-type, metalloproteinase inhibitors. These include BE16627B (L-N-[N-hydroxy-2-isobutyl-succinyamoyl]-seryl-L-valine), isolated from microbial cultures (87,88), and GM6001 (N-[2R-2-{hydroxamido-carbonymethyl}-4-methylpentanoyl]-L-tryptophan methylamide. The inhibitor BE16627B selectively blocks the in vivo growth of MMP-overproducing human HT1080 fibrosarcoma cells, but does not alter the growth of human colorectal carcinoma cells, HCT116, which secrete only low amounts of MMPs (87). GM6001, also known as Galardin, has been reported to prolong survival in C57/B16 mice with experimental B16/F10 murine melanoma metastases (89).

These findings imply that MMP inhibitors may either alter the angiogenic response required for normal tumor growth and invasion or suppress the proteinase-dependent release of sequestered growth factors from tumor stroma. Taraboletti et al. (90) have shown that Batimastat reduces the growth of experimental hemangiomas by blocking recruitment of normal endothelial cells to these tumors. These effects of Batimastat on endothelial cells suggest that the observed retardation of tumor growth may be owing, at least in part, to alteration of the angiogenic response. Recently, GM 6001 has been shown to inhibit directly the angiogenic response to tumor extract in the rat corneal pocket assay (91).

Batimastat is currently in clinical trials for the treatment of malignant effusions associated with thoracic and peritoneal neoplasms (85). The low solubility and poor oral bioavailability are severe limitations for the formulation and delivery of this compound. However, second-generation compounds with better pharmaceutical properties are currently in preclinical development and should begin clinical trials in the near future. One such compound is BB-2516, also known as Marimastat, which has oral bioavailability, entered phase I clinical trials in the US in mid-1995 (92), and should start early phase II trials by mid-1996.

The substrate analog approach also affords the potential for identifying selective inhibitors for various members of the MMP family based on differences in substrate specificity between these family members. The successful clinical application of an MMP inhibitor may require that it have selective activity and not inhibit other metalloproteinases essential for normal tissue homeostasis. Currently, the need for inhibition of selective subgroups of MMPs or specific members of the MMP family is not clear. The development of selective inhibitors would also provide excellent experimental tools for evaluating the role of various members of the MMP family in both physiologic connective tissue remodeling as well as various pathologic conditions.

Noting the specificity and facility of various MMPs on autoproteolytic processing following activation, Docherty and colleagues at Celltech developed a potent and selective inhibitor for the gelatinases (93). These investigators observed that progelatinase A undergoes rapid autoproteolytic removal of the prodomain to generate an active enzyme species with a tyrosine residue as the new amino-terminus. This group developed inhibitors using tyrosine analogs in the $P_1{'}$ position. This has resulted in the development of the most potent and selective synthetic MMP inhibitor yet characterized. These compounds are again hydroxamate-based inhibitors with tyrosine analogs at the P_1' position and cyclohexyl moiety at the P_2' position (*84,93*). These inhibitors are not yet available for animal testing or clinical trials in cancer patients.

Recent studies have reported the structural characterization of members of the MMP family by X-ray diffraction or nuclear magnetic resonance spectroscopy. These include human fibroblast collagenase, human neutrophil collagenase, stromelysin, and matrilysin (*94–99*). The information represented in these studies will be useful for the development of the next generation of inhibitors that can selectively inhibit individual members of the closely related MMPs.

5.3. Future Directions

Several alternative strategies for inhibition of MMPs also exist and could be exploited for the development of inhibitors. These have received far less attention and support than the substrate analog approach described above. They include inhibitors based on the cysteine switch mechanism in which profragment analogs are targeted to the active site. Other alternatives include TIMP analogs and manipulation of endogenous TIMP production at the tumor site. This last alternative is currently being attempted using a gene therapy approach (Stetler-Stevenson et al., unpublished).

As described previously, all members of the MMP family are secreted in latent form with a profragment that contains a highly conserved sequence responsible for maintenance of latency (*100–102*). This sequence contains a cysteine residue that is thought to coordinate the Zn atom of the active site. This hypothesis is supported by the observation that substitutions in this sequence result in rapid autoactivation of MMPs (*103*). Furthermore, the linear synthetic peptide sequence (MRKPRCGN/VPDV) containing cysteine, but not the conservative substitution of serine for cysteine (MRKPRSGN/VPDV), acts as an inhibitor for gelatinase A (IC_{50}, 8 μM) and stromelysin (IC_{50}, 117 μM) (*101*). This peptide inhibits the MMP-dependent in vitro invasion of tumor cells through a reconstituted basement membrane (*104*). It has also been shown to block neurite outgrowth on reconstituted extracellular matrix, as well as endothelial cell invasion in models of Kaposi's sarcoma (*105,106*).

Recent studies have shown that isocysteine could be substituted for cysteine in these peptides and that other amino acid residues are also essential for inhibitory activity (*107–109*). Introduction of a substituted tyrosine residue at a position located two amino acid residues on the C-terminal side of the cysteine or isocysteine produced a potent inhibitor of stromelysin (IC_{50}, 3 μM). Further exploration of this inhibitor strategy is warranted. Possible combination with other more stable, zinc-chelating strategies could possibly produce a new class of MMP inhibitors.

Little is known about the mechanism through which TIMPs inhibit the MMPs. Structural studies have begun to characterize the domains of the TIMPs that may be involved. Linear peptide analogs of TIMP sequences have had little success in mimicking TIMPs metalloproteinase inhibitory activity. This suggests that the inhibitory action of TIMPs on these proteases is the result of several peptide domains or amino acid side chains that require the correct three-dimensional spatial orientation that is the result of a specific tertiary structure of these proteins. The answer to the mechanism of TIMP action on MMPs will require structural studies on TIMP–MMP complexes.

6. SUMMARY

Malignant tumor cell invasion is now viewed as dysregulated physiologic invasion (*34*). Investigators have started to define the molecular events involved in the process of tumor cell invasion and have found similarities to events involved in angiogenesis, wound healing, and embryonic development. These physiologic invasive processes are strictly regulated both temporally and spatially, and are responsive to negative stimuli that limit these events. Tumor cell invasion and metastasis is also strictly regulated, but is clearly not responsive to negative regulatory signals. In particular, MMP activity is a common denominator for these processes. Regulation of these enzymes is disrupted in tumor cells as evidenced by studies demonstrating transcriptional activation of MMPs and enhanced MMP activation in tumor tissues. Animal models of tumor invasion and metastasis demonstrate that abrogation of MMP activity through the use of synthetic, low/mol/wt, substrate analog inhibitors can effectively block tumor dissemination and also limit primary tumor growth. The suppression of tumor growth has been indirectly linked to suppression of tumor-induced angiogenesis by these MMP inhibitors. This indicates that MMP inhibitors may disrupt a number of key processes involved in cancer progression. The encouraging results of the preclinical testing with these inhibitors, coupled with the strong theoretical basis for this MMP inhibitor approach, lead one to conclude that these inhibitors are a promising new direction in cancer therapy.

ACKNOWLEDGMENTS

The author wishes to thank Mark E. Sobel, Marta L. Corcoran, and David E. Kleiner, Jr., for their critical reading of the manuscript and helpful discussions. The author also thanks Lance Liotta for continued support and encouragement.

REFERENCES

1. Adams F. *The Genuine Works of Hippocrates.* London: Sydeenham Society, 1849.
2. Osler W. *The Evolution of Modern Medicine.* New Haven: Yale University Press, 1921.
3. Koono M, Ushijima K, Hayashi H. Studies on the mechanisms of invasion in cancer. 3. Purification of a neutral protease of rat ascites hepatoma cell associated with production of chemotactic factor for cancer cells. *Int J Cancer* 1974; 13:105–115.
4. Koono M, Katsuya H, Hayashi H. Studies on the mechanisms of invasion in cancer. IV. A factor associated with release of neutral protease of tumor cell. *Int J Cancer* 1974; 13:334–342.
5. Pfleiderer A Jr. Histochemical study of endometrial carcinoma. Systemic investigations of enzymes in infiltrating regions of tumors and interrelations with infiltrated connective tissue. *Am J Obstet Gynecol* 1969; 104:823–828.
6. Sinha B, Goldenberg GJ. The effect of trypsin and neuramidase on the circulation and organ distribution of tumor cells. *Cancer* 1974; 34:1956–1961.
7. Sylven B, Bois-Svenson I. Protein content and enzymatic assays of intersitial fluid from some normal tissues and transplanted mouse tumors. *Cancer Res* 1960; 20:239–248.
8. Sylven B, Bois-Svensson I. On the chemical pathology of interstitial fluid. I. Proteolytic activities in transplanted mouse tumors. *Cancer Res* 1965; 25:458–468.
9. Sylven B. Lysosomal enzyme activity in the interstitial fluid of solid mouse tumour transplants. *Eur J Cancer* 1968; 4:463–474.
10. Nagai Y, Lapiere CM, Gross J. Tadpole collagenase. Preparation and purification. *Biochemistry* 1966; 5:3123–3130.
11. Harris ED, Krane SM. Collagenases. *New Engl J Med* 1974; 291:557–563, 605–609, 652–661.

12. Dresden MH, Hellman SA, Schmidt JD. Collagenolytic enzymes in human neoplasms. *Cancer Res* 1972; 32:993–996.
13. Harris ED Jr., Faulkner CS, Wood S Jr. Collagenase in carcinoma cells. *Biochem Biophys Res Commun* 1972; 48:1247–1253.
14. Carter RL. Metastatic potential of malignant tumours. *Invest Cell Pathol* 1978; 1:275–286.
15. Hashimoto K, Yamanishi Y, Maeyens E. Collagenlytic activities of squamous cell carcinoma of the skin. *Cancer Res* 1973; 33:2790–2801.
16. Robertson DM, Williams DC. *In vitro* evidence of neutral collagenase activity in an invasive mammalian tumour. *Nature* 1969; 221:259,260.
17. Strauch L. The role of Collagenase in tumor invasion. In: Tarin D., ed. *Tissue Interactions in Carcinogenesis*. London: Acedemic. 1972:399–433.
18. Taylor AC, Levy BM, Simpson JW. Collagenlytic activity of sarcoma tissues in culture. *Nature* 1970; 228:366,367.
19. Yamanishi Y, Dabbous MK, Hashimoto K. Effect of Collagenolytic enzymes in basal cell epithelioma of the skin on reconstituted collagen and physical properties and kinetics of the crude enzyme. *Cancer Res* 1972; 32:2551–2560.
20. Yamanishi Y, Maeyens E, Dabbous MK. Collagenlytic activity in malignant melanoma: physiochemical studies. *Cancer Res* 1973; 33:2507–2512.
21. Liotta LA, Kleinerman J, Catanzaro P, Rynbrandt D. Degradation of basement membrane by murine tumor cells. *J Natl Cancer Inst* 1977; 58:1427–1431.
22. Kuettner KE, Soble L, Croxen RL, Marczynska B, Hiti J, Harper E. Tumor cell collagenase and its inhibition by a cartilage-derived protease inhibitor. *Science* 1977; 196:653,654.
23. Liotta LA, Abe S, Robey PG, Martin GR. Preferential digestion of basement membrane collagen by an enzyme derived from a metastatic murine tumor. *Proc Natl Acad Sci USA* 1979; 76:2268–2272.
24. Kleinman HK, McGarvey JL, Liotta LA, Robey PG, Tryggvason K, Matrin GR. Isolation and characterization of type IV porcollagen, laminin and heparan sulfate from the EHS sarcoma. *Biochemistry* 1981; 21:6188–6193.
25. Timpl RA, Dziadek M. Structure, development and molecular pathology of basement membranes. *Int Rev Exp Pathol* 1986; 29:1–112.
26. Yurchenco PD. Assembly of basement membranes. *Ann NY Acad Sci* 1990; 580:195–213.
27. Nagase J, Barrett AJ, Woessner JF. Nomenclature and Glossary of the Matrix Metalloproteinases. *Matrix* 1992; suppl no 1:421,424.
28. Birkedal-Hansen H, Moore WG, Bodden MK, Windsor LJ, Birkedal-Hansen B, DeCarlo A, Engler JA. Matrix metalloproteinases: a review. *Crit Rev Oral Biol Med* 1993; 4:197–250.
29. Matrisian LM, Bowden GT, Krieg P, Fürstenberger G, Briand J-P, Leroy P, Breathnach R. The mRNA coding for the secreted protease transin is expressed more abundantly in malignant than in benign tumors. *Proc Natl Acad Sci* 1986; 83:9413–9417.
30. Bassett P, Bellocq JP, Wolf C, Stoll I, Hutin P, Limacher JM, Podhajcer OL, Chenard MP, Rio MC, Chambon P. A novel metalloproteinase gene specifically expressed in stromal cells of breast carcinoma. *Nature* 1990; 348:699–704.
31. Freije JM, Diez-Itza I, Balbin M, Sanchez LM, Blasco R, Tolivia J, Lopez-Otin C. Molecular cloning and expression of collagenase-3, a novel human matrix metalloproteinase produced by breast carcinomas. *J Biol Chem* 1994; 269:16,766–16,773.
32. Liotta LA, Tryggvason K, Garbisa S, Hart I, Foltz CM, Shafie S. Metastatic potential correlates with enzymatic degradation of basement membrane collagen. *Nature* 1980; 284:67,68.
33. Liotta LA, Rao CN, Barsky SF. Tumor invasion and the extracellular matrix. *Lab Invest* 1983; 49:636–649.
34. Stetler-Stevenson WG, Aznavoorian S, Liotta LA. Tumor cell interactions with the extracellular matrix during invasion and metastasis. *Annu Rev Cell Biol* 1993; 9:541–573.
35. Mignatti P, Robbins E, Rifkin DB. Tumor invasion through the human amnion membrane: requirement for a proteinase cascade. *Cell* 1986; 47:487–498.
36. Hendrix MJ, Gehlsen KR, Wagner HN Jr., Rodney SR, Misiorowski RK, Meyskens FL Jr. In vitro quantification of melanoma tumor cell invasion. *Clin Exp Metastasis* 1985; 3:221–233.
37. Albini A, Iwamoto Y, Kleinman HK, Martin GR, Aaronson SA, Kozlowski JM, McEwan RN. A rapid in vitro assay for quantitating the invasive potential of tumor cells. *Cancer Res* 1987; 47:3239–3245.

38. Matrisian LM. The matrix-degrading metalloproteinases. *BioEssays* 1992; 14:455–462.
39. Kleiner DE Jr., Stetler-Stevenson WG. Structural biochemistry and activation of matrix metalloproteases. *Curr Opinion Cell Biol* 1993; 5:891–897.
40. Ray JM, Stetlerstevenson WG. The role of matrix metalloproteases and their inhibitors in tumor invasion, metastasis and angiogenesis. *Eur Respir J* 1994; 7:2062–2072.
41. Shapiro SD, Kobayashi DK, Ley TJ. Cloning and characterization of a unique elastolytic metalloproteinase produced by human alveolar macrophages. *J Biol Chem* 1993; 268:23,824–23,829.
42. Sato J, Takino T, Okada Y, Cao J, Shinagawa A, Yamamoto E, Seiki M. A matrix metalloproteinase expressed on the surface of invasive tumor cells. *Nature* 1994; 370:61–65.
43. Springman EB, Angleton EL, Birkedalhansen H, Vanwart HE. Multiple modes of activation of latent human fibroblast collagenase—evidence for the role of a cys-73 active-site zinc complex in latency and a cysteine switch mechanism for activation. *Proc Natl Acad Sci* 1990; 87: 364–368.
44. Urbanski SJ, Edwards DR, Maitland A, Leco KJ, Watson A, Kossakowska AE. Expression of metalloproteinases and their inhibitors in primary pulmonary carcinomas. *Br J Cancer* 1992; 66:1188–1194.
45. Urbanski SJ, Edwards DR, Hershfield N, Huchcroft SA, Shaffer E, Sutherland L, Kossakowska AE. Expression pattern of metalloproteinases and their inhibitors changes with the progression of human sporadic colorectal neoplasia. *Diagn Mol Pathol* 1993; 2:81–89.
46. Muller D, Wolf C, Abecassis J, Millon R, Engelmann A, Bronner G, Rouyer N, Rio MC, Eber M, Methlin G, et al. Increased stromelysin 3 gene expression is associated with increased local invasiveness in head and neck squamous cell carcinomas. *Cancer Res* 1993; 53:165–169.
47. Majmudar G, Nelson BR, Jensen TC, Voorhees JJ, Johnson TM. Increased expression of stromelysin-3 in basal cell carcinomas. *Mol Carcinog* 1994; 9:17–23.
48. Pei D, Majmudar G, Weiss SJ. Hydrolytic inactivation of a breast carcinoma cell-derived serpin by human stromelysin-3. *J Biol Chem* 1994; 269:25,849–25,855.
49. Kusukawa J, Sasaguri Y, Shima I, Kameyama T, Morimatsu M. Expression of matrix metalloproteinase-2 related to lymph node metastasis of oral squamous cell carcinoma. A clinicopathologic study. *Am J Clin Pathol* 1993; 99:18–23.
50. Monteagudo C, Merino MJ, San-Juan J, Liotta LA, Stetler-Stevenson WG. Immunohistochemical distribution of type IV collagenase in normal, benign, and malignant breast tissue. *Am J Pathol* 1990; 136:585–592.
51. Brown PD, Bloxidge RE, Stuart NS, Gatter KC, Carmichael J. Association between expression of activated 72-kilodalton gelatinase and tumor spread in non-small-cell lung carcinoma. *J Natl Cancer Inst* 1993; 85: 574–578.
52. Brown PD, Bloxidge RE, Anderson E, Howell A. Expression of activated gelatinase in human invasive breast carcinoma. *Clin Exp Metastasis* 1993; 11:183–189.
53. Davies B, Brown PD, East N, Crimmin MJ, Balkwill FR. A synthetic matrix metalloproteinase inhibitor decreases tumor burden and prolongs survival of mice bearing human ovarian carcinoma xenografts (published erratum appears in *Cancer Res* Aug 1, 1993; 53 [15]:3652). *Cancer Res* 1993; 53:2087–2091.
54. Azzam HS, Arand G, Lippman ME, Thompson EW. Association of MMP-2 activation potential with metastatic progression in human breast cancer cell lines independent of MMP-2 production. *J Natl Cancer Inst* 1993; 85:1758–1764.
55. Emmert-Buck MR, Roth MJ, Zhuang Z, Campo E, Rozhin J, Sloane BF, Liotta LA, Stetler-Stevenson WG. Increased gelatinase A (MMP-2) and cathepsin B activity in invasive tumor regions of human colon cancer samples. *Am J Pathol* 1994; 145:1285–1290.
56. Testa JE. Loss of the metastatic phenotype by a human epidermoid carcinoma cell line, HEp-3, is accompanied by increased expression of tissue inhibitor of metalloproteinase 2. *Cancer Res* 1992; 52:5597–5603.
57. Ponton A, Coulombe B, Skup D. Decreased expression of tissue inhibitor of metalloproteinases in metastatic tumor cells leading to increased levels of collagenase activity. *Cancer Res* 1991; 51:2138–2143.
58. DeClerck YA, Perez N, Shimada H, Boone TC, Langley KE, Taylor SM. Inhibition of invasion and metastasis in cells transfected with an inhibitor of metalloproteinases. *Cancer Res* 1992; 52:701–708.

59. Khokha R, Zimmer MJ, Graham CH, Lala PK, Waterhouse P. Suppression of invasion by inducible expression of tissue inhibitor of metalloproteinase-1 (TIMP-1) in B16-F10 melanoma cells. *J Natl Cancer Inst* 1992; 84:1017–1022.

60. Khokha R. Suppression of the tumorigenic and metastatic abilities of murine B16-F10 melanoma cells in vivo by the overexpression of the tissue inhibitor of the metalloproteinase-1. *J Natl Cancer Inst* 1994; 86:299–304.

61. Montgomery AM, Mueller BM, Reisfeld RA, Taylor SM, DeClerck YA. Effect of tissue inhibitor of the matrix metalloproteinases-2 expression on the growth and spontaneous metastasis of a human melanoma cell line. *Cancer Res* 1994; 54:5467–5473.

62. Ray JM, Stetler-Stevenson WG. Gelatinase-a activity directly modulates melanoma cell-adhesion and spreading. *Embo J* 1995; 14:908–917.

63. Liotta LA, Steeg PS, Stetler-Stevenson WG. Cancer metastasis and angiogenesis: an imbalance of positive and negative regulation. *Cell* 1991; 64:327–336.

64. Braunhut SJ, Moses MA. Retinoids modulate endothelial cell production of matrix-degrading proteases and tissue inhibitors of metalloproteinases (TIMP). *J Biol Chem* 1994; 269: 13,472–13,479.

65. Mignatti P, Tsuboi R, Robbins E, Rifkin DB. In vitro angiogenesis on the human amniotic membrane: requirement for basic fibroblast growth factor-induced proteinases. *J Cell Biol* 1989; 108:671–682.

66. Takigawa M, Nishida Y, Suzuki F, Kishi J, Yamashita K, Hayakawa T. Induction of angiogenesis in chick yolk-sac membrane by polyamines and its inhibition by tissue inhibitors of metalloproteinases (TIMP and TIMP-2). *Biochem Biophys Res Commun* 1990; 171:1264–1271.

67. Albini A, Fontanini G, Masiello L, Tacchetti C, Bigini D, Luzzi P, Noonan DM, Stetler-Stevenson WG. Angiogenic potential in vivo by Kaposi's sarcoma cell-free supernatants and HIV-1 tat product: inhibition of KS-like lesions by tissue inhibitor of metalloproteinase-2. *Aids* 1994; 8:1237–1244.

68. Schnaper HW, Grant DS, Stetler-Stevenson WG, Fridman R, D'Orazi G, Murphy AN, Bird RE, Hoythya M, Fuerst TR, French DL, et al. Type IV collagenase(s) and TIMPs modulate endothelial cell morphogenesis in vitro. *J Cell Physiol* 1993; 156:235–246.

69. Tsuboi R, Rifkin DB. Bimodal relationship between invasion of the amniotic membrane and plasminogen activator activity. *Int J Cncer* 1990; 46:56–60.

70. Moses MA, Sudhalter J, Langer R. Identification of an inhibitor of neovascularization from cartilage. *Science* 1990; 248:1408–1410.

71. Murphy AN, Unsworth EJ, Stetler-Stevenson WG. Tissue inhibitor of metalloproteinases-2 inhibits bFGF-induced human microvascular endothelial cell proliferation. *J Cell Physiol* 1993; 157:351–358.

72. Folkman J. The role of angiogenesis in tumor growth. *Semin Cancer Biol* 1992; 3:65–71.

73. Folkman J, Hanahan D. Switch to the angiogenic phenotype during tumorigenesis. *Princess Takamatsu Symp* 1991; 22:339–347.

74. Weidner N, Semple JP, Welch WR, Folkman J. Tumor angiogenesis and metastasis—correlation in invasive breast carcinoma. *N Engl J Med* 1991; 324:1–8.

75. Weidner N, Folkman J, Pozza F, Bevilacqua P, Allred EN, Moore DH, Meli S, Gasparini G. Tumor angiogenesis: a new significant and independent prognostic indicator in early-stage breast carcinoma (*see* comments). *J Natl Cancer Inst* 1992; 84:1875–1887.

76. Weidner N, Carroll PR, Flax J, Blumenfeld W, Folkman J. Tumor angiogenesis correlates with metastasis in invasive prostate carcinoma. *Am J Pathol* 1993; 143:401–409.

77. Huynh HT, Tetenes E, Wallace L, Pollak M. In vivo inhibition of insulin-like growth factor I gene expression by tamoxifen. *Cancer Res* 1993; 53:1727–1730.

78. Falkson G, Gelman R, Glick J, Falkson CI, Harris J. Reinduction with the same cytostatic treatment in patients with metastatic breast cancer: an Eastern Cooperative Oncology Group study. *J Clin Oncol* 1994; 12:45–49.

79. Abrams WB, Davies RO, Ferguson RK. Overview: the role of angiotensin-converting enzyme inhibitors in cardiovascular therapy. *Fed Proc* 1984; 43:1314–1321.

80. Ashworth RW. Drugs affecting the renin-angiotensin system. *Prog Drug Res* 1982; 26:207–223.

81. Van Zwieten PA, De Jonge A, Timmermans PB. Inhibitors of the angiotensin I converting enzyme as antihypertensive drugs. *Pharm Weekbl (Sci)* 1983; 5:197–204.

82. Vincenti MP, Clark IM, Brinckerhoff CE. Using inhibitors of metalloproteinases to treat arthritis. Easier said than done? *Arthritis Rheum* 1994; 37:1115–1126.
83. Schwartz MA, Van Wart HE. Synthetic inhibitors of bacterial and mammalian interstitial collagenases. *Prog Med Chem* 1992; 29:271–334.
84. Beeley NRA, Ansell PRJ, Docherty AJP. Inhibitors of matrix metalloproteinases (MMPP's). *Curr Opinion Ther Patents* 1994; 4:7–16.
85. Brown PD. Clinical trials of a low molecular weight matrix metalloproteinase inhibitor in cancer. *Ann NY Acad Sci* 1994; 732:217–221.
86. Wang X, Fu X, Brown PD, Crimmin MJ, Hoffman RM. Matrix metalloproteinase inhibitor BB-94 (batimastat) inhibits human colon tumor growth and spread in a patient-like orthotopic model in nude mice. *Cancer Res* 1994; 54:4726–4728.
87. Naito K, Kanbayashi N, Nakajima S, Murai T, Arakawa K, Nishimura S, Okuyama A. Inhibition of growth of human tumor cells in nude mice by a metalloproteinase inhibitor. *Int J Cancer* 1994; 58:730–735.
88. Okuyama A, Naito K, Morishima H, Suda H, Nishimura S, Tanaka N. Inhibition of growth of human tumor cells in nude mice by a metalloproteinase inhibitor. *Ann NY Acad Sci* 1994; 732:408–410.
89. Tressler RJ, Wee J, Summers B, Galardy R. Galardin, a potent metalloproteinase inhibitor, prolongs survival time in a B16-F10 melanoma experimental metastasis model. *Clin Exp Metastasis* 1994; 12:28.
90. Taraboletti G, Garofalo A, Belotti D, Drudis T, Borsotti P, Scanziani E, Brown PD, Giavazzi R. Inhibition of angiogenesis and murine hemangioma growth by Batimastat, a synthetic inhibitor of matrix metalloproteinases. *J Nat Cancer Inst* 1995; 87:293–298.
91. Galardy RE, Grobelny D, Foellmer HG, Fernandez LA. Inhibition of angiogenesis by the matrix metalloprotease inhibitor N-[2R-2-(hydroxamidocarbonymethyl)-4-methylpentanoyl)]-L-tryptoph- an methylamide. *Cancer Res* 1994; 54:4715–4718.
92. Drummond AH, Beckett P, Boone EA, Brown PD, Davis M, Galloway WA, Taupin P, Wood LM, Davidson AH. BB-2516: An orally bioavailable matrix metalloproteinase inhibitor with efficacy in animal cancer models. *Proc Am Assoc Cancer Res* 1995; 36:100
93. Docherty AJP, Cockett MI, Birch ML, Chander S, Willmott N, O'Connell JP, Crabbe T, Mountain A, Morphy JR, Millican TA, Beeley NRA, Murphy G, Hart IR, Stamp G, Mahadevan V. Gelatinase inhibitors for the treatment of cancer. *Clin Exp Metastasis* 1994; 12:12.
94. Spurlino JC, Smallwood AM, Carlton DD, Banks TM, Vavra KJ, Johnson JS, Cook ER, Falvo J, Wahl RC, Pulvino TA, et al. 1.56 A structure of mature truncated human fibroblast collagenase. *Proteins* 1994; 19:98–109.
95. Lovejoy B, Hassell AM, Luther MA, Weigl D, Jordan SR. Crystal structures of recombinant 19-kDa human fibroblast collagenase complexed to itself. *Biochemistry* 1994; 33:8207–8217.
96. Lovejoy B, Cleasby A, Hassell AM, Luther MA, Weigl D, McGeehan G, Lambert MH, Jordan SR. Structural analysis of the catalytic domain of human fibroblast collagenase. *Ann NY Acad Sci* 1994; 732:375–378.
97. Hassell AM, Anderegg RJ, Weigl D, Milburn MV, Burkhart W, Smith GF, Graber P, Wells TN, Luther MA, Jordan SR. Preliminary X-ray diffraction studies of recombinant 19 kDa human fibroblast collagenase. *J Mol Biol* 1994; 236:1410–1412.
98. Bode W, Reinemer P, Huber R, Kleine T, Schnierer S, Tschesche H. The X-ray crystal structure of the catalytic domain of human neutrophil collagenase inhibited by a substrate analogue reveals the essentials for catalysis and specificity. *EMBO J* 1994; 13:1263–1269.
99. Reinemer P, Grams F, Huber R, Kleine T, Schnierer S, Piper M, Tschesche H, Bode W. Structural implications for the role of the N terminus in the "superactivation" of collagenases. A crystallographic study. *FEBS Lett* 1994; 338:227–233.
100. Stetler-Stevenson WG, Krutzsch HC, Wacher MP, Marguiles IMK, Liotta LA. The activation of human type IV Collagenase proenzyme. Sequence identification of the major conversion product following organomercurial activation. *J Biol Chem* 1989; 264:1353–1356.
101. Stetler-Stevenson WG, Talano JA, Gallagher ME, Krutzsch HC, Liotta LA. Inhibition of human type IV collagenase by a highly conserved peptide sequence derived from its prosegment. *Am J Med Sci* 1991; 302:163–170.

102. Van Wart H, Birkedal HH. The cysteine switch: a principle of regulation of metalloproteinase activity with potential applicability to the entire matrix metalloproteinase gene family. *Proc Natl Acad Sci USA* 1990; 87:5578–5582.
103. Sanchez-Lopez R, Nicholson R, Gesnel M-C, Matrisian LM, Breathnach R. Structure–function relationships in the collagenase gene family member transin. *J Biol Chem* 1988; 263: 11,892–11,899.
104. Melchiori A, Albini A, Ray JM, Stetler-Stevenson WG. Inhibition of tumor cell invasion by a highly conserved peptide sequence from the matrix metalloproteinase enzyme prosegment. *Cancer Res* 1992; 52:2353–2356.
105. Benelli R, Adatia R, Ensoli B, Stetler-Stevenson WG, Santi L, Albini A. Inhibition of AIDS-Kaposi's sarcoma cell induced endothelial cell invasion by TIMP-2 and a synthetic peptide from the metalloproteinase propeptide: implications for an anti-angiogenic therapy. *Oncol Res* 1994; 6:251–257.
106. Muir D. Metalloproteinase-dependent neurite outgrowth within a synthetic extracellular matrix is induced by nerve growth factor. *Exp Cell Res* 1994; 210:243–452.
107. Hanglow AC, Lugo A, Walsky R, Finch-Arietta M, Lusch L, Visnick M, Fotouhi N. Peptides based on the conserved predomain sequence of matrix metalloproteinases inhibit human stromelysin and collagenase. *Agents Actions* 1993; 39 spec no:C148–50.
108. Fotouhi N, Lugo A, Visnick M, Lusch L, Walsky R, Coffey JW, Hanglow AC. Potent peptide inhibitors of stromelysin based on the prodomain region of matrix metalloproteinases. *J Biol Chem* 1994; 269:30,227–30,231.
109. Hanglow AC, Lugo A, Walsky R, Visnick M, Coffey JW, Fotouhi N. Inhibition of human stromelysin by peptides based on the N-terminal domain of tissue inhibitor of metalloproteinases-1. *Biochem Biophys Res Commun* 1994; 205:1156–1163.
110. Anderson TC, Shipp MA, Docherty AJP, Teicher BA. Combination therapy including a gelatinase inhibitor and cytotoxic agent reduces local invasion and metastasis of murine Lewis lung carcinoma. *Cancer Res* 1996; 56:715–718.

13 Interferons and Other Cytokines

Jill A. Hendrzak, PhD and Michael J. Brunda, PhD

CONTENTS

INTRODUCTION
INTERFERON α
INTERLEUKIN-2
INTERLEUKIN-12
CONCLUSIONS

1. INTRODUCTION

Cancer therapy with cytokines is a rapidly growing field owing to recent advances in immunology, molecular biology, and cell biology. In normal physiology, cytokines are proteins that regulate cell behavior in a paracrine or autocrine manner. When administered exogenously, these proteins often possess biological activities that make them attractive for cancer therapy. Results of clinical trials to date indicate that cytokines may be used along with other current cancer therapies and may eventually replace some of these.

Interferon alpha (IFN-α) was the first cytokine to be used in clinical trials, and the research experience that was obtained has formed the foundation for the investigation of other cytokines as cancer therapeutics. Preclinical studies with IFN-α have had a substantial impact on its clinical development. Similarly, experimental findings have been critical to the subsequent and more rapid development of another cytokine, interleukin-2 (IL-2). Recent preclinical studies demonstrating the potential of interleukin-12 (IL-12) as an anticancer agent have also led this cytokine to the clinic; however, the clinical data are not yet available. This chapter, not intended to be a comprehensive review of the literature, highlights the important steps in the development of IFN-α, IL-2, and IL-12, the cytokines that currently appear to have the most potential as cancer therapeutics.

2. IFN-α

2.1. Experimental Data

IFNs were discovered more than 30 years ago when Isaacs and Lindenmann demonstrated that cells infected with viruses produced proteins that could induce an antiviral state in uninfected cells (*1*). Extensive research conducted since that time has revealed

From: *Cancer Therapeutics: Experimental and Clinical Agents*
Edited by: B. Teicher Humana Press Inc., Totowa, NJ

263

that there are several different types of IFN proteins and that they have many different effects on cellular functions in addition to their antiviral activity. With the molecular cloning and sequencing of the IFN genes, it has become clear that there are three major types of IFN, α, β, and γ. Although there is only one IFN-β gene and one IFN-γ gene, there are at least 23 different IFN-α genes clustered on chromosome 9, which code for at least 15 functional proteins (2). The recombinant IFN-α proteins have molecular weights of approx 17 kDa. The IFNs, present in small amounts and active under normal physiologic conditions, are produced in much greater amounts following stimulation by an IFN inducer (13). IFN-α is produced primarily by leukocytes, IFN-β is produced by fibroblasts and epithelial cells, and IFN-γ is produced by T-cells and NK cells. The majority of cells in the body possess IFN receptors. IFN-α and IFN-β share components of the same receptor and are known as Type I IFNs, whereas IFN-γ uses a separate receptor and is known as a Type II IFN (2). Several components of the IFN-α receptor have been cloned (4,5), but this receptor complex is not as well characterized as receptors for other cytokines.

Subsequent to its discovery as an antiviral agent, IFN-α has been shown to exert direct effects on cell growth and differentiation. Early studies demonstrating the ability of IFN to inhibit tumor cell growth (6,7) were controversial, because purified IFN was not yet available and impure preparations derived from leukocyte cell cultures, animal tissues, or serum were used. Since then, however, many tumor cell lines have been shown to be sensitive to the growth-inhibitory actions of purified IFN-α in vitro (8). Assays used to measure antiproliferative activity include cellular incorporation of ^{3}H-thymidine, clonogenic assays to measure colony growth in agar (9), and incubation of solid tumor specimens with IFN-α (10). Higher concentrations of IFN-α were often required to achieve the antiproliferative effect, as compared to the antiviral effect, and the result was usually a reversible cytostasis (2).

The in vitro antiproliferative effects of IFN-α in combination with either cytotoxic agents or other cytokines have also been examined. IFN-α has been used in combination with cytotoxic agents, such as doxorubicin, cisplatin, vinblastine, methotrexate, bleomycin, and 5-fluorouracil (5-FU), and synergistic effects on growth inhibition were often observed on a variety of human tumor cell lines or cells from primary tumors (11). The mechanism by which growth is inhibited may involve either modulation of the actions of IFN-α by the cytotoxic drugs or modulation of the action of the cytotoxic drugs by IFN-α (11). Synergistic activity in the inhibition of cell growth can also be obtained when IFN-α is combined with IFN-γ (12,13) or with tumor necrosis factor (TNF) (14,15).

The precise mechanism by which IFN-α inhibits cell growth has been the subject of more recent investigations. IFN-α slows the growth of tumor cells by increasing the length of their cell cycle, particularly at the G_0/G_1 transition phase (2). These cytokinetic effects may occur through the modulation of $2'5'$-oligoadenylate synthetase (a protein translation inhibitor involved in the antiviral activity of IFN-α) or cellular oncogenes, such as c-*myc* and c-*fos* (16–18). In addition, IFN-α can also inhibit the gene for the enzyme ornithine decarboxylase, thus depleting the cell of essential metabolites (19). Basic studies of IFN signaling have identified some of the factors involved in this process (20). Thus, the ability of IFN-α to modulate gene expression may be an important component of its antitumor activity.

In addition to direct effects on tumor growth, IFN-α may also affect tumor growth by indirect mechanisms. Early experiments showed that a mouse L1210 leukemia cell line resistant to the antiproliferative effects of IFN in vitro could be inhibited from growing in vivo by IFN treatment (21,22). It is now known that IFN-α has numerous immunoregulatory activities. IFN-α can induce the differentiation of pre-NK cells (2) as well as stimulate NK activity (23). Furthermore, IFN-α has been shown to enhance antibody-dependent cellular cytotoxicity (ADCC) of both NK cells (24) and neutrophils (25). The cytotoxic function of macrophages is also stimulated by IFN-α (26). In addition, IFN-α can increase the expression of class I major histocompatibility complex (MHC) antigens (27,28) and tumor-specific antigens (29,30) on tumor cells. The increased expression of cell-surface antigens on tumor cells by IFN-α results in more efficient recognition and killing of tumor cells by cytotoxic T-cells and NK cells.

IFN-α also appears to have an indirect effect on tumors by inhibiting angiogenesis, the formation of a blood supply that is critical to the growth of solid tumors. Leukocyte IFN (α/β) was shown to inhibit capillary endothelial cell motility in vitro (31). In another report, the treatment of tumor-bearing mice with IFN-α/β resulted in the early degeneration of the endothelial cells in the vessel of the tumor (32). Studies such as these suggest that the antiangiogenic potential of IFN-α should be further investigated.

Many of the antitumor activities of IFN-α described above have been confirmed in murine tumor models. Using impure preparations of IFN, Gresser and others were the first to show that IFN could inhibit not only the growth of virally induced tumors (33), but also the growth of spontaneous (34) and transplantable (35) tumors. These observations, along with the in vitro data on the antiproliferative effects of IFN-α, led researchers to test the antitumor efficacy of IFN-α against a wide range of tumors, including established sc tumors, murine leukemias, and experimental and spontaneous metastases.

Human tumor xenograft models have been used to investigate the direct effects of human IFN-α on tumor growth, since these mice do not have a competent immune system, and human IFN-α is not active on mouse cells. Often, the response of a particular tumor to IFN-α in vivo is correlated with antiproliferative effects of IFN-α on the tumor cells in vitro. Many types of tumors have responded to IFN-α, including breast, colon, melanoma, and osteosarcoma (36). The results of these studies have shown that the antitumor effect is greater when therapy is initiated soon after tumor injection, repeated doses are more effective than single doses, and tumor stasis is more commonly achieved than tumor regression or cures (36).

Murine tumors growing in syngeneic hosts or transplantable tumor models have been used to examine the indirect antitumor effects of IFN-α. Since human IFN-α is not active on the murine tumors, either murine IFN-α or human IFN-α A/D (a hybrid human IFN-α that has activity on murine cells) has been administered to mice. As with the xenograft model, efficacy of treatment is associated with low tumor load and frequent dosing, and cures are rarely seen (36). In addition, indirect antitumor effects of IFN-α on the immune response have been confirmed. For example, IFN-α A/D-induced inhibition of experimentally induced pulmonary metastases was correlated with enhanced NK cytotoxicity (37). In another report, a variety of effector cells were shown to be involved in the IFN-α/β-induced suppression of Friend erythroleukemia cell (FLC) metastases (38). However, results of studies with animal models have suggested that although indirect effects on the immune system may be involved in mediating the antitumor activity of IFN-α against some tumors, IFN-α appears to exert its major activity primarily through direct effects on tumor growth.

Murine tumor models have also been used to evaluate the antitumor efficacy of IFN-α in combination with cytotoxic drugs or other cytokines. Early observations that IFN could enhance the activity of chemotherapeutic agents in vivo (39,40) have - been extended to human tumor xenografts, in which IFN-α has been found to increase the antitumor activity of cyclophosphamide, doxorubicin, cisplatin, and mitomycin C against various tumor types (41–43). Many studies have addressed the optimal timing for the administration of IFN and cytotoxic agents. Although it was initially thought that the cytotoxic drug should be given first to decrease a large tumor volume so that IFN-α could eradicate the minimum residual disease, recent studies have indicated that the interaction is complex and other types of scheduling may work just as well (11).

The synergy between IFN-α and other cytokines in antitumor efficacy was first demonstrated with the combination of IFN-α and IL-2 using the M5076 reticulum cell sarcoma (44). The synergistic or additive effects of IFN-α used in combination with IL-2 have since been confirmed in many experimental primary sc and metastatic murine tumor models (reviewed in ref. 45). In addition to IL-2, additive or synergistic antitumor activity has also been observed when IFN-α is administered in combination with IFN-γ (46–48), IL-1α (49), or TNF (50). Recent studies have also shown therapeutic efficacy against solid tumors with IFN-α in combination with both a cytokine and a chemotherapeutic agent (51). It should be noted that the combination of cytotoxic drugs or cytokines with IFN-α does not always result in a synergistic or additive effect.

Gene therapy is currently being evaluated in mice as an alternative method to the systemic use of IFN-α. Fibroblasts transfected with the human IFN-α gene secreted human IFN-α and inhibited the growth of chronic myelocytic leukemia in nude mice (52). In addition, metastatic IFN-α/β-resistant FLC (53) or metastatic murine adenocarcinoma cells (54) transfected with a murine IFN-α gene failed to grow in mice and immunized mice to rechallenge with the parental non-IFN-α-secreting tumor cells. Importantly, the IFN-α-producing FLC were also shown to inhibit tumor growth in mice with established metastatic tumors (53). Thus, these results provide a rationale for the use of gene therapy in the clinic.

2.2. Clinical Trials

Information obtained from studying the antitumor efficacy of IFN-α in murine tumor models has been useful in designing clinical trials. In the early clinical trials, natural leukocyte IFN (a mixture of IFNs with only 1% purity) was shown to have antitumor activity against several types of malignancies, including osteosarcoma, lymphoma, and breast cancer (55), and it was believed that IFNs would act on a wide range of tumor types. We now know, using both recombinant and purified natural material, that IFN-α has a more restricted activity, being effective mainly against hematological malignancies. However, the use of IFN-α in the treatment of solid tumors is likely to expand, since it has shown some efficacy and is less toxic than most existing forms of therapy. The effective doses of IFN-α range from 1 million units (MU) to 36 MU/injection and vary with the particular malignancy being treated (56,57). Side effects typically consist of "flu-like" symptoms, such as fever, chills, myalgia, and headache, but may also include gastrointestinal and CNS effects at doses > 18 MU (*16*).

IFN-α has been approved by many health authorities for use in hairy cell leukemia (HCL), a rare B-lymphocyte malignancy, characterized by peripheral blood mononuclear cells that display hair-like protrusions from their cytoplasm. A summary of the largest trials of IFN-α in HCL has shown that long-term treatment with frequent low doses of IFN-α resulted in an overall response rate of 80–90%, with 5% complete remissions (*56*). Responders could be held in remission using prolonged less frequent maintenance doses, and in one study, overall survival rate was 82% (*58*). The antitumor mechanism of IFN-α is mainly owing to direct antiproliferative effects (differentiation, cell-cycle arrest, and/or apoptosis) (*59,60*), but immunomodulatory effects, such as stimulation of NK activity and enhancement of HLA-DR antigens on HCL cells, may add to the activity of IFN-α (*16*).

IFN-α has also shown biological activity in chronic myelogenous leukemia (CML), a progressive myeloproliferative disorder arising from the neoplastic transformation of pluripotent stem cells (*16*). CML is associated with the activation of a cellular oncogene by chromosomal translocation, and a shortened chromosome 22 (the Philadelphia chromosome) is present in hemopoietic cells. Survival prognosis is correlated with a cytogenetic (karyotypic) response. In the largest reported clinical trial, IFN-α treatment resulted in 73% complete hematologic remissions (normalization of peripheral blood counts and disappearance of symptoms) and 19% complete cytogenetic remissions (*61*). It is likely that this antitumor activity was mediated by direct effects of IFN-α on cell growth (*16*). In a recent study, patients were treated first with hydroxyurea and then with IFN-α in combination with ara-C, resulting in a significant increase in the rate of complete cytogenetic remission (*62*). IFN-α may also be effective for the treatment of minimal residual disease following bone marrow transplant (*63*). In addition to CML and HCL, IFN-α has shown some activity against other hematological malignancies, such as multiple myeloma, non-Hodgkin's lymphoma, and cutaneous T-cell lymphoma (*16*).

Although IFN-α activity against solid tumors has been generally disappointing, significant responses have been observed in certain tumors that have been difficult to treat, but are sensitive to immunomodulation, such as malignant melanoma, renal cell carcinoma, and Kaposi's sarcoma. Individuals with malignant melanoma have been treated with IFN-α alone (average response rate 20%) or in combination with cytotoxic drugs, such as cimetidine, decarbazine, cisplatin, and cyclophosphamide (*16*). Thus far, combinations with cytotoxic drugs have not shown increased benefit over IFN-α monotherapy (*16*). Similarly, the combination of IFN-α and IL-2 in Phase I and II trials has been disappointing, with an overall response rate between 0 and 33% (*64*). Recent trials have indicated that IFN-α in combination with both IL-2 and cisplatin may be effective (*65*), but these results must be confirmed. IFN-α therapy is most effective in patients with nonbulky disease limited to cutaneous, soft tissue, or pulmonary sites, or in an adjuvant setting after surgery (*16*).

A review of seven recent studies indicated an overall response rate of 19% for the treatment of renal cell carcinoma with IFN-α (*66*). Combinations of IFN-α with cytotoxic drugs generally did not improve antitumor efficacy; however, a response rate of up to 43% has been observed with IFN-α in combination with vinblastine (*67*). Other drugs that have shown some efficacy in combination with IFN-α are prednisone (*68*) and 5-FU (*69*). IFN-α in combination with IL-2 has given response rates of 0–50%, with a median of 25% (*57*), and has often resulted in severe side effects (*70*). Some recent studies, however, suggest that the combination of IFN-α, IL-2, and 5-FU may prove to be effective (*71*).

IFN-α has demonstrated sufficient efficacy against Kaposi's sarcoma to be approved by the US FDA and other health authorities. Kaposi's sarcoma, a disease of endothelial or spindle-cell origin, has been observed in AIDS patients and other immunosuppressed individuals. Treatment with relatively high doses of IFN-α results in an overall response rate of 30–40%, with better responses in those with higher CD4$^+$ T-cell counts (*72*). The antitumor mechanism of IFN-α is not known, but the activity may be mediated in part by an inhibition of viral replication, with a corresponding increase in CD4$^+$ T-cell numbers (*73*). Also, since Kaposi's sarcoma is an angiogenic disease of endothelial cell origin, IFN-α may exert anti-angiogenic effects. In support of this concept, IFN-α has recently been shown to induce regressions in children with pulmonary hemangioma (*74*). Beneficial effects of IFN-α in combination with AZT has been observed, but were associated with significant toxicity (*75*). In addition to Kaposi's sarcoma and the other solid tumors described above, IFN-α may be effective for localized therapy in bladder and ovarian cancer (*16*).

2.3. Experimental vs Clinical Data

Although there have been limitations, the experimental data on the antitumor effects of IFN-α have been quite useful for the clinical setting. Although IFN-α has clearly demonstrated antitumor efficacy in clinical trials, it is active over a more restricted range of tumor types than what was predicted based on experimental data. This difference cannot be attributed to the use of impure IFN preparations in many experimental studies, since subsequent studies with purified recombinant or natural IFN-α generally confirmed the earlier results. Instead, it may be that antiproliferative effects on tumor cells in vitro were often achieved with higher concentrations of IFN-α than could be used clinically. Owing to the species-restricted activity of IFN-α, animal tumor models failed to predict the toxicity that has been observed in patients given higher doses of IFN-α. Also, some of the antitumor effects of IFN-α observed in animals may have been associated with the use of murine rather than human IFN-α or may have been owing to the increased immunogenicity of some syngeneic tumors.

Some important information has been extrapolated from these experimental data, however. Studies in animal tumor models have indicated that IFN-α may be most effective when it is administered frequently and tumor burden is low. In the clinic, IFN-α is also most effective with frequent dosing, and its usefulness as maintenance therapy for minimal residual disease or as an adjuvant is becoming apparent. Regressions or cures were rarely seen in animals, and the same has been true for humans. The experimental data have also been very useful in elucidating the complex mechanism of the antitumor activity of IFN-α. As in preclinical studies, the clinical data suggest that IFN-α mainly exerts direct effects on tumor cells, but can indirectly affect the immune system as well. Mechanistic studies are important for the identification of novel treatment strategies, and experimental data have already provided some new directions for IFN-α therapy. Clinical studies in which IFN-α is used as an adjuvant, in combination with cytotoxic drugs and/or cytokines, or in gene therapy may result in some very effective treatments for some malignancies.

3. IL-2

3.1. Experimental Data

IL-2 was originally described as a soluble factor, derived from phytohemagglutinin-stimulated human lymphocytes, that could induce the outgrowth of T-cells from bone marrow (76). Subsequent studies have demonstrated that IL-2 is a single-chain glycoprotein of approx 15 kDA (77). Based on its ability to stimulate T-cell proliferation, assays were developed to quantitate its activity (78), and the gene for this cytokine was cloned (79). Although the recombinant protein is nonglycosylated, it retains all of the evaluated biological properties of IL-2.

IL-2 mediates its effect on the immune system by interacting with receptors present on various cell types. The IL-2 receptor (IL-2R) is comprised of three chains, α, β, and γ (80–83). The α chain is a low-affinity receptor for IL-2, the β and γ chains form an intermediate-affinity receptor, but all three chains are necessary for the high-affinity IL-2R (84,85). Signaling results following interaction of IL-2 with either the intermediate- or high-affinity IL-2R (84,85). Ligand–receptor interaction triggers a series of complex biochemical events within cells, which are the focus of much experimental study (84,85), and eventually results in the biological activities associated with IL-2.

In more recent years, it has been demonstrated that IL-2 is produced by the Th1 helper T-cells, a subset of cells that has been implicated in cell-mediated immune responses (86). Consistent with this observation, IL-2 has been shown to be a critical regulator of a variety of biological functions, which have been reviewed in more detail (87,88). With respect to its antitumor potential, one of the most important biological properties of IL-2 is its ability to induce the activation/differentiation of various cell populations that can lyse tumor cells. IL-2 can enhance the generation of murine or human cytotoxic T-lymphocyte (CTL) responses in vitro (89,90), as well as augment responses in animals in vivo (91,92). Likewise, brief exposure of murine or human NK cells in vitro to IL-2 can augment their cytolytic responses (93,94), and increased NK activity has also been demonstrated in animals injected with IL-2 (91,95). Longer-term culture of lymphocytes with IL-2 results in the development of lymphokine-activated killer (LAK) cells (96); LAK cells can kill NK cell-resistant tumor targets and are derived primarily from NK cells (97). Highly specific CTL derived from tumors, tumor-infiltrating lymphocytes (TILs) are also generated by culture of these cells with IL-2 (98). In addition to its effects on lymphocytes, under some conditions, macrophages can also be activated by IL-2, resulting in cells capable of lysing tumor target cells (99). Thus, the cytolytic potential of a diverse set of immune effector cells can be upregulated by IL-2.

IL-2 has also been shown to induce other cytokines, especially IFN-γ (100). In addition to IFN-γ, mRNA, or protein for tumor growth factor-β, TNF-α, lymphotoxin, IL-1, IL-6, IL-5, granulocyte macrophage colony-stimulating factor (GM-CSF), and macrophage colony-stimulating factor (M-CSF) have been demonstrated in IL-2-incubated human peripheral blood mononuclear cells (101). These cytokines may be important in mediating the efficacy of IL-2.

Based on the in vitro and in vivo biological effects of IL-2, substantial interest arose for use of this protein as an antitumor effector molecule. It should be noted that human IL-2, in contrast to IFN-α, is active on both human and mouse cells, thus permitting the use of human IL-2 for studies in rodent animal models. Studies were performed to evaluate the antitumor efficacy of IL-2 as monotherapy in tumor models (*102–106*); positive effects have been observed against experimental and spontaneous pulmonary and hepatic metastases (*102,103,105,106*), in murine leukemia models (*104*), and against established sc tumors (*102,106*). In these models, reduction in the number of metastases (*102,103,105,106*), inhibition of tumor growth (*102,106*), and prolongation of survival were reported (*102,104*). However, in most of these models, treatment with IL-2 was initiated soon after tumor implantation and rarely resulted in long-term cures.

Since many tumor models and experimental conditions have been evaluated, it is difficult to generalize about the optimal utility of IL-2 and its mechanism of action, but a few observations can be made. Although there have been some studies suggesting efficacy at low doses of IL-2 (*105*), the most success has been observed utilizing high doses of IL-2, at or near the maximum tolerated dose of this cytokine (*102,103,106*). At higher doses, IL-2 is quite toxic, and the toxicities in mice (*107*) seem to be similar to those observed in patients. The timing of the initiation of IL-2 therapy seems to play some role in the ability of IL-2 to mediate its antitumor effects. It is more difficult to treat larger, more established sc tumors with IL-2 (G. Truitt, personal communication; M. Brunda, unpublished observations), but this is not necessarily the case with metastases (*102*) or in leukemia (*104*) models.

It is clear that IL-2 does not have a direct antiproliferative effect on tumor cells, but rather mediates its effects through some component of the immune system; however, some of the cytokines induced by IL-2 treatment, for example, IFN-γ or TNF, may directly affect tumor cell proliferation. In various tumor models, the antitumor efficacy of IL-2 is greatly diminished in irradiated mice (*102*) or mice treated with antibodies directed to various immune cell populations (*108*), or in mice concomitantly receiving corticosteroids (*109*). IL-2 treatment induced cytotoxic LAK cells in tumor-bearing mice, and a correlation between the induction of LAK activity and efficacy was observed (*108*). The best effects of IL-2 on metastases were found in the therapy of weakly immunogenic tumors as well as some "nonimmunogenic" tumors, if treatment with IL-2 was initiated on day 3 (*110*). However, initiation of treatment of metastases from nonimmunogenic tumors with IL-2 on day 10 resulted in no therapeutic benefit (*108*). The antitumor effect of IL-2 against poorly responsive tumors, which lack MHC class I, is enhanced following transfection of an MHC class I gene into these tumor cells (*111*), suggesting a role for CD8+ T-cells. Furthermore, an increased lymphocytic infiltrate was evident following histological evaluation of tumors undergoing IL-2-induced regression (*102*), suggesting a possible involvement in the observed tumor inhibition. Whether the immune cells demonstrated in the models inhibit tumor growth through cytolytic mechanisms, cytokine induction, or other mechanisms is not firmly established.

Since IL-2 can induce cytotoxic lymphocyte activity in vitro, a large number of preclinical studies have focused on the use of the combination of IL-2-activated cells and lower levels of systemically administered IL-2 for the therapy of murine metastases. The initial work in this area demonstrated that in several murine pulmonary metastasis models, a substantially greater inhibition of metastases was observed in mice receiving both LAK cells and IL-2 than in mice receiving either component alone (*112–114*). In contrast to the reduced efficacy of IL-2 in irradiated mice, no reduction of the antimetastatic effect of IL-2 plus LAK was seen, most probably reflecting the ability of the transferred LAK cells to mediate the efficacy (*113,115*). One of the main questions associated with this form of therapy is whether the injected LAK cells can selectively migrate to the tumor; accumulation of only small numbers of the injected LAK cells have been found within tumors (*116,117*) and, of possible importance, injected cells were not seen in all metastatic foci (*116*).

Another form of IL-2-adoptive cellular therapy is the use of IL-2 plus TILs (*118*). Therapy with IL-2 plus TILs was found to be up to 100 times more efficacious than IL-2 plus LAK cells in metastatic tumor models; the best synergy was obtained in mice receiving sublethal irradiation or cyclophosphamide treatment, in addition to IL-2 plus TILs (*118–120*). TILs can persist for months in animals, even in the absence of IL-2 therapy (*119,120*).

In animal models, significant effort has also been placed on the therapeutic benefit of IL-2 combined with other antitumor drugs. As discussed earlier, a large amount of data demonstrated substantially increased activity of IL-2 combined with IFN-α (*44,106*); at higher doses of these two cytokines, increased toxicity was also observed (*106*). Combinations with other cytokines, including IFN-γ, TNF, and IL-1, have been evaluated and resulted in modest levels of increased efficacy (*45*). Likewise, combination of IL-2 and cytotoxic drugs has been evaluated in animal models with some improved results (*121,122*).

In addition to the systemic use of IL-2, experimental systems utilizing transfection of tumor cells with the IL-2 gene, resulting in cells secreting IL-2, have also been studied (*123,124*). IL-2-transfected tumor cells do not form tumors and can immunize mice to rechallenge with parental, non-IL-2-secreting tumor cells (*123,124*); variations on this line of research include immunization with tumor cells or tumor antigen and IL-2-secreting fibroblasts (*125*). Antitumor efficacy is dependent on CD8+ T-cells and has been correlated with the induction of CTL (*123–125*). In contrast to the marked effect with IL-2-secreting tumor cells in preimmunizing mice to subsequent tumor challenge, there are few data to support the therapeutic utility of such cells in mice with established tumors.

3.2. Clinical Trials

IL-2 has been clearly demonstrated to have antitumor efficacy in patients with renal cell carcinoma (*126,127*). In the trials used for registration of the drug, 600,000 IU/kg of IL-2 were administered iv every 8 h for 5 d, followed by a second course after 2 wk of rest; dose reduction occurred frequently owing to toxicities (*128*). An objective response rate of 15% (4% complete response, 11% partial response), was observed (*128*); the median duration of response was 23.2 mo (*128*). In other trials utilizing various regimens and high doses of IL-2, the overall response rate in renal cell carcinoma ranged from 0 to 40% with a median response of 20% (*126,127*). Toxicities are quite severe with capillary leak syndrome and hypotension among the major problems (*126,127*). Because of high-dose IL-2 toxicities, a variety of schedules/regimens and combinations have been evaluated in an attempt to maintain efficacy and reduce toxicity (*127*). It does not appear that combinations of IL-2 plus IFN-α (*see* Section 2) or other drugs result in a better response overall (*126,127*), although enhanced efficacy has been reported in some trials. One of the more potentially promising approaches is the use of sc administered IL-2, which in early studies appears to give comparable response rates, but less toxicity (*127*).

IL-2 has been shown to have some activity in several other malignancies. In patients with malignant melanoma, using various regimens/doses, an average response rate of approx 13% (range of 3–60%) was achieved, but at doses often resulting in marked toxicity (*126,127*). Studies evaluating multiple-drug combinations of IL-2, IFN-α, and other chemotherapeutic drugs are in progress and may improve response (*126, 127*). IL-2 has also been tested in a limited number of patients with colorectal, ovarian, bladder, neuroblastoma, non-Hodgkin's lymphoma, and acute myeloid leukemia (*126,127*). Although some responses have been observed, the utility of IL-2 in these malignanies has not been firmly established.

With respect to IL-2 combined with LAK cells, early clinical studies suggested that some efficacy was achievable with this combination (*129*). However, more extensive testing has demonstrated a response rate similar to that obtained with IL-2 alone and with similar toxicities (*126,127*). For example, in a summary of European studies, an overall response rate of 16% (5% CR, 11% PR) was observed in a total of approx 300 renal cell carcinoma patients treated with IL-2 alone or IL-2 plus LAK (*130*). In melanoma patients, although there is no increase in response rate, there is a trend toward longer survival in patients receiving IL-2 plus LAK cells compared to those treated with IL-2 alone (*131*), but additional studies will be needed to confirm this finding. Thus, overall, it appears that there is no significant benefit of IL-2 plus LAK cell therapy compared to treatment with IL-2 alone.

Some of the other experimental approaches developed in animal models are now beginning to be investigated in clinical trials. Early results with IL-2 combined with TILs have also demonstrated some responses, but further testing is required (*132*). Experimental tumor vaccine protocols utilizing IL-2-transfected tumor cells are also in progress.

3.3. Experimental vs Clinical Data

Based on its biological properties and animal experimental data, IL-2 was evaluated in the clinic and shown to have efficacy in some malignancies, in particular renal cell carcinoma. Thus, the experimental data clearly demonstrated the utility of this cytokine for cancer therapy. However, it is also obvious that IL-2 was much more active in murine models than in people. This may reflect the relative immunogenicities of murine vs human tumors, with the murine tumors being more immunogenic. It should be noted that, even in the case of chemotherapeutic drugs, it has been difficult to predict which histologic type of malignancy will respond to therapy by use of animal models. In addition to its potential efficacy, the experimental data have provided a framework for understanding the mechanism(s) mediating the antitumor efficacy observed with IL-2. Thus, IL-2 does not exert its effects on the tumor directly, but rather stimulates the host to mount an immune response through interaction of IL-2 with its receptor on various cell populations. Some useful, but limited information was obtained in animal models for dosing regimen, which began as a starting point for clinical trials.

The marked efficacy of IL-2 combined with cellular therapy, in particular LAK cells, appears not be supported by clinical results to date. However, on closer inspection of these experimental data, cures were rarely obtained in these acute animal models. Furthermore, the large majority of studies utilized metastatic models, which may be "easier" to treat than more established sc tumors. The rather substantial effects seen in animal models may, therefore, translate into marginal effects observed in patients with more chronic disease. Likewise, the success of combination therapy in animal models may translate into only a small incremental effect in patients. However, it should be emphasized that these experimental models have given new directions for therapeutic intervention, which as our knowledge on the use of IL-2 increases, may eventually result in greater benefit to patients. In the future, the use of TILs or IL-2-transfected tumor cells, for example, may result in greater efficacy in some human malignancies.

4. IL-12

In contrast to the relatively long histories of IFNs and IL-2, IL-12 is a more recently discovered cytokine. It has a unique structure, since it is the only characterized interleukin that is composed of two disulfide-bridged subunits, designated p35 and p40 (*133–136*). Full biological activity of this protein is only obtained with the heterodimer and not with the individual subunits alone (*135,136*). Although not fully characterized, the receptor for IL-12 is distinct from the receptor for IL-2 or other cytokines (*137–139*). As with other cytokines, initial studies with recombinant human IL-12 were conducted in various in vitro immunologic assays. A number of the biologic activities of IL-12 (reviewed in *140–143*) are similar to those of IL-2, including enhancement of specific CTL responses, activation of NK/LAK cells, stimulation of T- and NK cell proliferation, and induction of IFN-γ production from both T- and NK cells. However, in addition to activities it shares with IL-2, IL-12 has the unique property of inducing the maturation of the Th1 helper cell population; Th1 cells secrete IL-2 and IFN-γ and promote cell-mediated immune responses. With the availability of recombinant murine IL-12 (rMuIL-12) (*144*), many of these biological effects previously observed in vitro have been confirmed following administration of rMuIL-12 to mice (*145*).

Based on these potent immunomodulatory effects of IL-12, experiments have been performed to evaluate the potential antitumor and antimetastatic effects of IL-12 in murine models. To date, experiments with IL-12 have focused in three areas:

1. Therapeutic effects on sc tumors;
2. Inhibition of experimental and spontaneous metastases; and
3. Tumor cells transfected with the genes for IL-12.

With respect to sc tumors, treatment of tumor-bearing mice with rMuIL-12 can result in tumor growth inhibition, tumor stasis, prolongation of survival, and in some tumor models, regression of established tumors (*146–155*). For example, tumor regression occurs in approx 75% of mice bearing 14-d old Renca renal cell carcinoma tumors that are 1 cm or greater in diameter (*142,146,149,155*); these mice die at 5–7 wk if untreated. Mice whose tumors regressed following treatment with rMuIL-12 rejected subsequent challenge with the same, but not other syngeneic tumors, indicating that tumor-specific immunity had been induced in these animals (*143*). At the effective dose/treatment regiment of IL-12, mild to moderate toxicities (*141;* M. Brunda and T. Anderson, unpublished), primarily leucopenia and elevated hepatic enzymes, were found, demonstrating antitumor efficacy was achievable under conditions that were well tolerated. The antitumor efficacy obtained with IL-12 was superior to treatment with either IFN-α or IL-2 in some models (*153,155;* Brunda et al., unpublished). The mechanism through which IL-12 mediates its antitumor efficacy has not been fully characterized, although IL-12 has no direct antiproliferative effects on tumor cells in vitro (*151*) and is probably immune-mediated, since both T-cells and the induction of IFN-γ are necessary for optimal effects to be seen (*146,151,155*).

Treatment with IL-12 also results in marked antimetastatic effects (*141,146,147, 154*). For example, following iv injection of B16F10 tumor cells, treatment with IL-12 initiated on day 7 resulted in a 75% reduction in the number of pulmonary metastases (*146*). In one experimental metastasis model, treatment with IL-12 gave comparable efficacy, but substantially less toxicity than IL-2 (*147*). Experimental hepatic metastases were also inhibited following treatment with IL-12 (*146*). Similar to its effects in experimental metastasis models, treatment with IL-12 likewise substantially reduced either pulmonary (*154*) or hepatic spontaneous metastases (*141*).

The potential use of IL-12 in tumor vaccines has been demonstrated in a murine model (*150*). When murine fibroblasts secreting biologically active murine IL-12 were mixed with viable BL-6 melanoma cells, a significant delay in tumor growth was observed. Histological evaluation of injection sites demonstrated an increased accumulation of macrophages and a decrease in CD4$^+$ T-cells at sites of IL-12-secreting fibroblasts and tumor cells compared to sites injected with tumor cells alone. Therefore, it appears that IL-12 has the ability to modulate immune responses locally, resulting in increased antitumor efficacy.

Thus, from these preclinical experiments, IL-12 appears to hold promise for the therapy of malignancies in patients. Clinical trials with this cytokine have been initiated, and future studies will determine if the success of IL-12 in animal models will translate into clinical efficacy.

5. CONCLUSIONS

This chapter demonstrates the important role of preclinical studies in the clinical development of cytokines for cancer therapy. Biological activities of a cytokine that are relevant to cancer therapy must first be demonstrated using both in vitro and in vivo assays. Once these effects have been established, the cytokine can be tested in the appropriate animal tumor models. The tumor models are useful in providing the rationale for clinical testing of the cytokine, as well as an initial dose range and treatment schedule to begin clinical trials. Furthermore, the data obtained from these experiments can be used to identify factors that determine a positive response so patient subgroups likely to respond will be identified. However, limitations to these models include the species-specific effects of some cytokines, the immunogenicity of some syngeneic tumors, and the frequent inability of commonly used end points, such as tumor growth inhibition and reduction in metastases, to translate into positive clinical responses. There is a need to refine the animal models used and to evaluate antitumor efficacy in the context of the toxicities induced by the treatment. Nevertheless, the results of these studies provide a starting point for use in the clinic and then continue to influence the direction of clinical testing. Thus, a constant interaction between preclinical and clinical research is essential to realize fully the potential of cytokines in cancer therapy.

In addition, the experience gained from the clinical development of one cytokine can provide some of the directions needed for the development of other cytokines. Almost 30 years passed from the discovery of IFN-α to its approval for clinical use, whereas the time for IL-2 was considerably shorter. Hopefully, the principles learned from the development of these cytokines will lead to the rapid development of IL-12, as well as other cytokines, for the treatment of human malignancies.

REFERENCES

1. Isaacs A, Lindenmann J. Virus interference I. The interferon. *Proc R Soc Lond Ser B* 1957; 147:258–267.
2. Balkwill FR. *Cytokines in Cancer Therapy.* New York: Oxford University Press, 1989.
3. Jahiel RI, Krim M. Interferons: biology, clinical trials, and effects on hematologic neoplasms. In: Chiao JW, ed. *Biological Response Modifiers and Cancer Therapy.* New York: Marcel Dekker. 1988:197–266.
4. Uze G, Lutfalla, Gresser I. Genetic transfer of a functional human interferon α receptor into mouse cells: cloning and expression of its cDNA. *Cell* 1990; 60:225–234.
5. Novick D, Cohen B, Rubinstein M. The human interferon α/β receptor: characterization and molecular cloning. *Cell* 1994; 77:391–400.
6. Paucker K, Cantell K. Henle W. Quantitative studies on viral interference in suspended L cells. III. Effect of interfering viruses and interferon on the growth rate of cells. *Virology* 1962; 17: 324–334.
7. Gresser I. Antitumor effects of interferon. *Adv Cancer Res* 1972; 16:97–140.
8. Taylor-Papadimitriou J, Rozengurt E. Interferons as regulators of cell growth and differentiation. In: Taylor-Papadimitriou J, ed. *Interferons, Their Impact in Biology and Medicine.* Oxford: Oxford Medical Publications. 1985:81–98.
9. Hamburger AW, Salmon SE. Primary bioassay of human tumor stem cells. *Science* 1977; 197: 461–463.
10. Salmon SE, Durie BG, Young L, Liu RM, Trown PW, Stebbing N. Effects of cloned human leukocyte interferons in the human tumor stem cell assay. *J Clin Oncol* 1983; 1:217–225.
11. Wadler S, Schwarz EL. Antineoplastic activity of the combination of interferon and cytotoxic agents against experimental and human malignancies: a review. *Cancer Res* 1990; 50:3473–3486.
12. Denz H. Lechleitner M, Marth Ch, Daxenbichler G, Gastl G, Braunsteiner H. Effect of human recombinant alpha-2 and gamma-interferon on the growth of human cell lines from solid tumors and hematologic malignancies. *J Interferon Res* 1985; 5:147–157.
13. Brunda MJ, Wright RB. Differential antiproliferative effects of combinations of recombinant interferons alpha and gamma on two murine tumor cell lines. *Int J Cancer* 1986; 37:287–291.
14. Kikuchi A, Holan V, Minowada J. Effects of tumor necrosis factor alpha, interferon alpha and interferon gamma on non-lymphoid leukemia cell lines: growth inhibition, differentiation induction and drug sensitivity modulation. *Cancer Immunol Immunother* 1992; 35(4):257–263.
15. Matsubara N, Fuchimoto S, Orita K. Antiproliferative effects of natural human tumor necrosis factor-alpha, interferon-alpha, and interferon-gamma on human pancreatic carcinoma cell lines. *Int J Pancreatol* 1991; 8(3):235–243.
16. Dorr RT. Interferon-α in malignant and viral diseases. *Drugs* 1993; 45(2):177–211.
17. Einhorn S, Showe L, Ostlund L, Juliusson G, Robert KH, Gahrton G, Croce C. Influence of interferon-alpha on the expression of cellular oncogenes in primary chronic lymphocytic leukemia cells. *Oncogene Res* 1988; 3(1):39–49.
18. Hannigan GE, Williams BR. Interferon-alpha activates binding of nuclear factors to a sequence element in the c-fos proto-oncogene 5'-flanking region. *J Interferon Res* 1992; 12(5): 355–361.
19. Baron S. Tyring SK, Fleischmann WR, Coppenhaver DH, Niesel DW, Klimpel GR, Stanton GJ, Hughes TK. The interferons: mechanisms of action and clinical applications. *J Am Med Assoc* 1991; 266:1375–1383.
20. Pelligrini S, Schindler C. Early events in signalling by interferons. *Trends Biochem Sci* 1993; 18:338–342.
21. Gresser I, Brouty-Boye D, Thomas MT, Macieira A. Interferon and cell division. I. Inhibition of the multiplication of mouse leukemia L1210 cells in vitro by interferon preparations. *Proc Natl Acad Sci USA* 1970; 66:1052–1058.
22. Gresser I, Maury C, Brouty-Boye D. Mechanisms of the antitumor effect of interferon in mice. *Nature (Lond)* 1972; 239:167,168.
23. Lee SH, Kelley S, Chiu H, Stebbing N. Stimulation of natural killer cell activity and inhibition of proliferation of various leukemic cells by purified human leukocyte interferon subtypes. *Cancer Res* 1982; 42:1312–1315.
24. Vuist WM, Visseren MJ, Otsen M, Bos K, Vyth-Dreese FA, Figdor CG, Melief CJ, Hekman

A. Enhancement of the antibody-dependent cellular cytotoxicity of human peripheral blood lymphocytes with interleukin-2 and interferon alpha. *Cancer Immunol Immunother* 1993; 36(3):163–170.

25. Hokland P, Berg K. Interferon enhances the antibody-dependent cellular cytotoxicity (ADCC) of human polymorphonuclear lymphocytes. *J Immunol* 1981; 127:1585–1588.

26. Webb DSA, Zur Nedden D, Miller DM, Zoon KC, Gerrard TL. Enhancement of monocyte-mediated tumoricidal activity by multiple interferon-α species. *Cell Immunol* 1989; 124: 158–167.

27. Oberg K. The action of interferon alpha on human carcinoid tumours. *Semin Cancer Biol* 1992; 3(1):35–41.

28. Angus R, Collins CM, Symes MO. The effect of alpha and gamma interferon on cell growth and histocompatibility antigen expression by human renal carcinoma cell in vitro. *Eur J Cancer* 1993; 29A(13):1879–1885.

29. Gaicomini P, Aguzzi A, Pestha S. Modulation by recombinant DNA leukocyte (α) and fibroblast (β) interferons of the expression and shedding of HLA- and tumor-associated antigens by human melanoma cells. *J Immunol* 1984; 133:1649–1655.

30. Greiner JW, Hand PH, Noguchi P, Fisher PB, Pestka S, Schlom J. Enhanced expression of surface tumor associated Ag on human breast and colon tumor cells after recombinant human leukocyte α-interferon treatment. *Cancer Res* 1984; 44:3208–3211.

31. Brouty-Boye D, Zetter BR. Inhibition of cell motility by interferon. *Science* 1980; 208:516–518.

32. Dvorak H, Gresser I. Microvascular injury in pathogenesis of interferon-induced necrosis of subcutaneous tumors in mice. *J Natl Cancer Inst* 1989; 81:497–502.

33. Gresser I, Coppey J, Falcoff E, Fontaine D. Interferon and murine leukemia. I. Inhibitory effects of interferon preparations on development of Friend leukemia in mice. *Proc Soc Exp Biol Med* 1967; 124:84–91.

34. Gresser I, Coppey J, Bourali C. Interferon and murine leukemia. 6. Effect of interferon preparations on lymphoid leukemia of AKR mice. *J Natl Cancer Inst* 1969; 43:1083–1089.

35. Gresser I, Bourali C. Exogenous interferon and inducers of interferon in the treatment of Balb/c mice inoculated with RC_{19} tumor cells. *Nature* 1969; 223:844–845.

36. Thomas H, Balkwill FR. Effects of interferons and other cytokines on tumors in animals: a review. *Pharmacol Ther* 1991; 52:307–330.

37. Brunda MJ, Rosenbaum D, Stern L. Inhibition of experimentally-induced murine metastases by recombinant alpha interferon: correlation between the modulatory effect of interferon treatment on natural killer cell activity and inhibition of metastases. *Int J Cancer* 1984; 34: 421–426.

38. Gresser I, Maury C, Carnaud C, De Maeyer E, Maunroy MT, Belardelli F. Antitumor effects of IFN in mice injected with IFN sensitive and IFN-resistant Friend erythroleukaemia cells. VIII. Role of the immune system in the inhibition of visceral metastases. *Int J Cancer* 1990; 46:468–474.

39. Chirigos MA, Pearson JW. Brief communication: cure of murine leukemia with drug and interferon treatment. *J Natl Cancer Inst* 1973; 51:1367,1368.

40. Gresser I, Maury C, Tovey M. Efficacy of combined interferon cyclophosphamide therapy after diagnosis of lymphoma in AKR mice. *Eur J Cancer* 1978; 14:97–99.

41. Balkwill FR, Moodie EM. Positive interactions between human interferon and cyclophosphamide or Adriamycin in a human tumor model system *Cancer Res* 1984; 44:904–907.

42. Carmichael J, Fergusson RJ, Wolf CR, Balkwill FR, Smyth JF. Augmentation of cytotoxicity of chemotherapy by human α-interferons in human non-small cell lung cancer xenografts. *Cancer Res* 1986; 46:4916–4920.

43. Sklarin NT, Chahinian AP, Feuer EJ, Lahman LA, Szrajer L, Holland JR. Augmentation of activity of cis-diamminedichloroplatinum (II) and mitomycin C by interferon in human malignant mesothelioma xenografts in nude mice. *Cancer Res* 1988; 48:64–67.

44. Brunda MJ, Bellantoni D, Sulich V. In vivo anti-tumor activity of combinations of interferon alpha and interleukin-2 in a murine model. Correlation of efficacy with the induction of cytotoxic cells resembling natural killer cells. *Int J Cancer* 1987; 40:365–371.

45. Brunda MJ. Antitumour activity of interleukin-2 combined with other cytokines. In: Waxman J, Balkwill F, eds. *Interleukin-2*. Oxford: Blackwell Scientific Publications. 1992:106–121.

46. Koren S, Fleischmann WR. Quantitation of *in vivo* potentiation resulting from combined interferon therapy: antitumor effect against B-16 melanoma in mice. *J Interferon Res* 1986; 6: 473–482.

47. Truitt GA, Bontempo JM, Stern LL, Sulich V, Bellantoni D, Trown PW, Brunda MJ. Efficacy and toxicity elicited by recombinant interferons alpha and gamma when administered in combination to tumor-bearing mice. *Biotech Ther* 1989-90; 1(1):1–16.

48. Sayers TJ, Wiltrout TA, McCormick K, Husted C, Wiltrout RH. Antitumor effects of α-interferon and γ-interferon on a murine renal cancer (Renca) *in vitro* and *in vivo*. *Cancer Res* 1990; 50:5414–5420.

49. Brunda MJ, Wright RB, Luistro L, Harbison ML, Anderson TD, McIntyre KW. Enhanced antitumor efficacy in mice by combination treatment with interleukin-1α and interferon-α. *J Immunother* 1994; 15:233–241.

50. Sanada E, Fuchimoto S, Orita, K. Synergistic antiproliferative effect of the combination of natural human tumor necrosis factor-alpha and natural murine interferon-alpha/beta against colon-26 adenocarcinoma hepatic metastases in a murine model. *Acta Med Okayama* 1990; 44(4):217–222.

51. Kedar E, Rutkowski Y, Leshem B. Chemo-immunotherapy of murine solid tumors: enhanced therapeutic effects by interleukin-2 combined with interferon alpha and the role of specific T cells. *Cancer Immunol Immuother* 1992; 35(1):63–68.

52. Ogura H, Tani K, Ozawa K, Nagata S, Asano S, Takaku F. Implantation of genetically manipulated fibroblasts into mice as antitumour alpha-IFN therapy. *Cancer Res* 1990; 50:5102–5106.

53. Ferrantini M, Proietti E, Santodonato L, Gabriele L, Peretti M, Plavec I, Meyer F, Kaido T, Gresser I, Belardelli F. α₁-Interferon gene transfer into metastatic Friend leukemia cells abrogated tumorigenicity in immunocompetent mice: antitumor therapy by means of interferon-producing cells. *Cancer Res* 1993; 53:1107–1112.

54. Ferrantini M, Giovarelli M, Modesti A, Musiani P, Modica A, Venditti M, Peretti E, Lollini P, Nanni P, Forni G, Belardelli F. IFN-α1 gene expression into a metastatic murine adenocarcinoma (TS/A) result in CD8+ T cell-mediated tumor rejection and development of antitumor immunity. *J Immunol* 1994; 153:4604–4615.

55. Came PE. Interferon: its application and future as an antineoplastic agent. In: Ottenbrite RM, Butler GB, eds. *Anticancer and Interferon Agents. Synthesis and Properties*. New York: Marcel Dekker. 1984:301–319.

56. Platanias LC, Golomb HM. Clinical use of interferons: hairy cell, chronic myelogenous and other leukemias. In: Baron S. Coppenhaver DH, Dianzani F, Fleischmann WR, Hughes TK, Klimpel GR, Niesel DW, Stanton GJ, Tyring SK, eds. *Interferon: Principles and Medical Applications*. Galveston: The University of Texas Medical Branch. 1992:487–499.

57. Strander H, Oberg K. Clinical use of interferons: solid tumors. In: Baron S. Coppenhaver DH, Dianzani F, Fleischmann WR, Hughes TK, Klimpel GR, Niesel DW, Stanton GJ, Tyring SK, eds. *Interferon: Principles and Medical Applications*. Galveston: The University of Texas Medical Branch. 1992:533–561.

58. Smith JW, Longo DL, Urba WJ, Clark JW, Watson T, Beveridge J, Conlon K, Sznol M, Creekmore SP, Alvord WG, Lawrence JB, Steis RG. Prolonged, continuous treatment of hairy cell leukemia patients with recombinant interferon-α2a. Blood 1991; 78:1664–1671.

59. Vedantham S, Gamliel H, Golomb HM. Mechanism of interferon action in hairy cell leukemia: a model of effective cancer biotherapy. *Cancer Res* 1992; 52:1056–1066.

60. Gutterman JU. Cytokine therapeutics: lessons from interferon α. *Proc Natl Acad Sci USA* 1994; 91:1198–1205.

61. Talpaz M, Kantarjian H, Kurzrock R, Trujillo JM, Gutterman JU. Interferon-alpha produces sustained cytogenetic responses in chronic myelogenous leukemia. *Ann Intern Med* 1991; 114: 532–538.

62. Arthur CK, Ma DDF. Combined interferon alpha-2a and cytosine arabinoside as first-line treatment for chronic myeloid leukemia. *Acta Haematol* 1992; 89(suppl 1):15–21.

63. Higano CS, Raskind WH, Singer JW. Use of α interferon for the treatment of relapse of chronic myelogenous leukemia in chronic phase after allogeneic bone marrow transplantation. *Blood* 1992; 80:1437–1442.

64. Keilholz U, Scheibenbogen C, MacLachlan D, Jochim A, Bergmann L, Weidmann E, Mitrou

PS, Tilgen W, Hunstein W. Treatment of metastatic melanoma with interferon-α and high dose interleukin-2. In: Bergmann L, Mitrou PS, eds. *Cytokines in Cancer Therapy. Contributions to Oncology.* Basel: Karger. 1994:191–200.

65. Khayat D, Antoine E, Rixe O, Tourani JM, Vuillemin E, Borel C, Benhammouda A, Thill L, Franks C, Auclerc G, et al. Chemoimmunotherapy of metastatic malignant melanoma. The Salpetriere Hospital (SOMPS) experience. *Eur J Cancer* 1993; 29A(S5):S2–S5.

66. Fossa SD. Proc Symp, Progress in the treatment of renal cell carcinoma. Cambridge: Queens College, 1989:12–21.

67. Bergerat JP, Herbrecht R, Dufour P, Jacqmin D, Bollack C, Prevot G, Bailly G, De Garis S, Juraschek F, Oberling F. Combination of recombinant interferon alpha-2a and vinblastine in advanced renal cell cancer. *Cancer* 1988; 62:2320–2324.

68. Fossa SD, Gunderson R, Moe B. Recombinant interferon-alpha combined with prednisone in metastatic renal cell carcinoma. *Cancer* 1990; 65:2451–2454.

69. Sella A, Logothetis J, Fitz K, Dexeus FH, Amato R, Kilbourn R, Wallace S. Phase II study of interferon-α and chemotherapy (5-fluorouracil and mitomycin C) in metastatic renal cell cancer. *J Urol* 1992; 147:573–577.

70. Rosenberg SA, Lotze MT, Yang JC, Linehan WM, Seipp C, Calabro S, Karp SE, Sherry RM, Steinberg S, White DE. Combination therapy with interleukin-2 and alpha-interferon for the treatment of patients with advanced cancer. *J Clin Oncol* 1989; 7:1863,1874.

71. Atzpodien J, Kirchner H, Poliwoda H. Treatment strategies employing chemoimmunotherapy in patients with metastatic renal carcinoma. In: Bergmann L, Mitrou PS, eds. *Cytokines in Cancer Therapy. Contributions to Oncology.* Basel: Karger. 1994:211–217.

72. Evans LM, Itri LM, Campion M, Wyler-Plaut R, Krown SE, Groopman JE, Goldsweig H, Volberding PA, West SB, Mitsuyasu RT, et al. Interferon-alpha-2a in the treatment of acquired immunodeficiency syndrome-related Kaposi's sarcoma. *J Immunother* 1991; 10:39–50.

73. De Wit R, Schattenkerk JKME, Boucher CAB, Bakker PJM, Veenhof KHN, Danner SA. Clinical and virological effects of high-dose recombinant interferon-alpha in disseminated AIDS-related Kaposi's sarcoma. *Lancet* 1988; 2:1214–1217.

74. Folkman J, Shing Y. Minireview: Angiogenesis. *J Biol Chem* 1992; 267:10,931–10,934.

75. Fischl MA. Antiretroviral therapy in combination with interferon for AIDS-related Kaposi's sarcoma. *Am J Med* 1991; 90(suppl 4A):2S–7S.

76. Morgan D, Ruscetti FW, Gallo R. Selective *in vitro* growth of T-lymphocytes from normal bone marrow. *Science* 1976; 193:1007,1008.

77. Welte K, Wang CY, Mertelsmann R, Venuta S, Felman SP, Moore MA. Purification of human interleukin-2 to apparent homogeneity and its molecular heterogeneity. *J Exp Med* 1982; 156: 454–464.

78. Gillis S, Ferm MM, Ou W, Smith KA. T-cell growth factor: Parameters of production and a quantitative microassay for activity. *J Immunol* 1978; 120:2027–2032.

79. Taniguchi T, Matsui H, Fujita T, Fakaoka C, Kashima N, Yoshimoto R, Hamuro J. Structure and expression of a cloned cDNA for human interleukin-2. *Nature* 1983; 302:305–310.

80. Leonard WJ, Depper JM, Crabtree GR, Rudikoff S, Pumphrey J, Robb RJ, Kronke M, Svetlik, PB, Peffer NJ, Waldmann TA, Greene WC. Molecular cloning and expression of cDNAs for the human interleukin-2 receptor. *Nature* 1984; 311:626–631.

81. Nikaido T, Shimizu A, Ishida N, Sabe H, Teshigawara K, Maeda M, Uchiyama T, Yodoi J, Honjo T. Molecular cloning of cDNA encoding human interleukin-2 receptor. *Nature* 1984; 311:631–635.

82. Hatakeyama M, Tsudo M, Minamoto S, Kono T, Doi T, Miyata T, Miyasaka M, Taniguchi T. Interleukin-2 receptor β chain gene: Generation of three receptor forms by cloned human α and β chain cDNAs. *Science* 1989; 244:551–556.

83. Takeshita T, Asao H, Ohtani K, Ishii N, Kumaki S, Tanaka N, Munakata H, Natamura M, Sugamura K. Cloning of the γ chain of the human IL-2 receptor. *Science* 1992; 257:379–382.

84. Smith KA. Lowest dose interleukin-2 immunotherapy. *Blood* 1993; 81:1414–1423.

85. Taniguchi T, Minami Y. The IL-2/IL-2 receptor system: A current overview. *Cell* 1993; 73:5–8.

86. Mosmann TR, Coffman RL. Th1 and Th2 cells: different patterns of lymphokine secretion lead to different functional properties. *Annu Rev Immunol* 1989; 7:145–173.

87. Rees RC. The biological response to interleukin-2. In: Waxman J, Balkwill F, eds. *Interleukin-2.* Oxford: Blackwell Scientific Publications. 1992:47–68.

88. Kintzel PE, Calis KA. Recombinant interleukin-2: a biological response modifier. *Clin Pharm* 1991; 10:110–128.

89. Takai Y, Herrmann S, Greenstein JL, Spitalny GL, Burakoff SJ. Requirement for three distinct lymphocytes for the induction of cytotoxic T lymphocytes from thymocytes. *J Immunol* 1986; 137:3494–3500.

90. Gately MK, Wilson DE, Wong HL. Synergy between recombinant interleukin 2 (rIL 2) and IL 2-depleted lymphokine-containing supernatants in facilitating allogeneic human cytolytic T lymphocyte responses *in vitro*. *J Immunol* 1986; 136:1274–1282.

91. Hefeneider SH, Conlon PJ, Henney CS. Gillis S. *In vivo* interleukin 2 administration augments the generation of alloreactive cytolytic T lymphocytes and resident natural killer cell activity. *J Immunol* 1983; 130:222–227.

92. Rosenberg SA, Grimm EA, McGrogan M, Doyle M, Kawasaki E, Koths K, Mark DF. Biological activity of recombinant human interleukin-2 produced in *Escherichia coli*. *Science* 1984; 223:1412–1415.

93. Henney CS, Kuribayashi K, Kern DE, Gillis S. Interleukin-2 augments natural killer cell activity. *Nature (Lond)* 1981; 291:335–338.

94. Brunda MJ, Tarnowski D, Davatelis V. Interaction of recombinant interferons with recombinant interleukin-2: differential effects on natural killer cell activity and interleukin-2 activated killer cells. *Int J Cancer* 1986; 37:787–793.

95. Talmadge JE, Herberman RB, Chirigos MA, Maluish AE, Schneider MA, Adams JS, Philips H, Thurman GB, Varesio L, Long C, Oldham RK, Wiltrout RH. Hyporesponsiveness to augmentation of murine natural killer cell activity in different anatomical compartments by multiple injections of various immunomodulators including recombinant interferons and interleukin-2. *J Immunol* 1985; 135:2483–2491.

96. Grimm EA, Mazumder A, Zhang HZ, Rosenberg SA. Lymphokine-activated killer cell phenomenon: lysis of natural killer-resistant fresh solid tumor cells by interleukin 2-activated autologous human peripheral blood lymphocytes. *J Exp Med* 1982; 155:1823–1841.

97. Ortaldo JR, Mason AA, Overton R. Lymphokine-activated killer cells. Analysis of progenitors and effectors. *J Exp Med* 1986; 164:1193–1205.

98. Rosenberg SA, Spiess P, Lafreniere R. A new approach to the adoptive immunotherapy of cancer with tumor-infiltrating lymphocytes. *Science* 1986; 233:1318–1321.

99. Espinoza-Delgado I, Bosco MC, Musso T, Gusella GL, Longo DL, Varesio L. Interleukin-2 and human monocyte activation. *J Leuk Biol* 1995; 57:13–19.

100. Farrar WL, Johnson HM, Farrar JJ. Regulation of the production of immune interferon and cytotoxic T lymphocytes by interleukin 2. *J Immunol* 1981; 124:1120–1125.

101. Saraya KA. Interleukin-2 and its place in the cytokine network. In: Waxman J, Balkwill F, eds. *Interleukin-2*. Oxford: Blackwell Scientific Publications. 1992:69–77.

102. Rosenberg SA, Mule JJ, Spiess PJ, Reichert CM, Schwarz SL. Regression of established pulmonary metastases and subcutaneous tumor mediated by the systemic administration of high-dose recombinant interleukin 2. *J Exp Med* 1985; 161:1169–1188.

103. Lafreniere R, Rosenberg SA. Successful immunotherapy of murine experimental hepatic metastases with lymphokine-activated killer cells and recombinant interleukin 2. *Cancer Res* 1985; 45:3735–3741.

104. Thompson JA, Peace DJ, Klarnet JP, Kern DE, Greenberg PD, Cheever MA. Eradication of disseminated murine leukemia by treatment with high-dose interleukin 2. *J Immunol* 1986; 137:3675–3680.

105. Talmadge JE, Philips H, Schindler J. Tribble H, Pennington R. Systematic preclinical study on the therapeutic properties of recombinant human interleukin 2 for the treatment of metastatic disease. *Cancer Res* 1987; 47:5752.

106. Truitt GA, Brunda MJ, Levitt D, Anderson TD, Sherman MI. The therapeutic activity in cancer of IL-2 in combination with other cytokines. *Cancer Surveys* 1989; 8:875–889.

107. Gately MK, Anderson TK, Hayes TJ. Role of asialo-GM$_1$-positive lymphoid cells in mediating the toxic effects of recombinant IL-2 in mice. *J Immunol* 1988; 141:189–200.

108. Mule JJ, Yang JC, Lafreniere RL, Shu S, Rosenberg SA. Identification of cellular mechanisms operational *in vivo* during the regression of established pulmonary metastases by the systemic administration of high-dose recombinant interleukin 2. *J Immunol* 1987; 139:285–294.

109. Papa MZ, Vetto JT, Ettinghausen SE, Mule JJ, Rosenberg SA. Effect of corticosteroid on the

antitumor activity of lymphokine-activated killer cells and interleukin 2 in mice. *Cancer Res* 1986; 46:5618–5623.

110. Papa MZ, Mule JJ, Rosenberg SA. Antitumor efficacy of lymphokine-activated killer cells and recombinant interleukin 2 *in vivo*: Successful immunotherapy of established pulmonary metastases from weakly immunogenic and nonimmunogenic murine tumors of three distinct histological types. *Cancer Res* 1986; 46:4973–4978.

111. Weber JS, Jay G, Tanaka K, Rosenberg SA. Immunotherapy of a murine tumor with interleukin 2. Increased sensitivity after MHC class I gene transfer. *J Exp Med* 1987; 166:1716–1733.

112. Mule JJ, Shu S, Schwarz SL, Rosenberg SA. Adoptive immunotherapy of established pulmonary metastases with LAK cells and recombinant interleukin-2. *Science* 1984; 225:1487–1489.

113. Mule JJ, Shu S, Rosenberg SA. The anti-tumor efficacy of lymphokine-activated killer cells and recombinant interleukin 2 *in vivo*. *J Immunol* 1985; 135:646–652.

114. Lafreniere R, Rosenberg SA. Successful immunotherapy of murine experimental hepatic metastases with lymphokine-activated killer cells and recombinant interleukin 2. *Cancer Res* 1985; 45:3735–3741.

115. Mule JJ, Yan J, Shu S, Rosenberg SA. The anti-tumor efficacy of lymphokine-activated killer cells and recombinant interleukin 2 *in vivo*: Direct correlation between reduction of established metastases and cytolytic activity of lymphokine-activated killer cells. *J Immunol* 1986; 136: 3899–3909.

116. Basse P, Herberman RB, Nannmark U. Johansson BR, Hokland M, Wasserman K, Goldfarb RH. Accumulation of adoptively transferred adherent, lymphokine-activated killer cells in murine metastases. *J Exp Med* 1991; 174:479–488.

117. Futami H, Pilar o AM, Gruys ME, Back TC, Young HA, Wiltrout RH. *In vivo* distribution and cytokine expression by enriched mouse LAK effector cells. *Biotherapy* 1991; 3:219–232.

118. Spiess PJ, Yang JC, Rosenberg SA. In vivo antitumor activity of tumor-infiltrating lymphocytes expanded in recombinant interleukin-2. *J Natl Cancer Inst* 1987; 79:1067–1075.

119. Alexander R, Rosenberg SA. Long term survival of adoptively transferred tumor-infiltrating lymphocytes in mice. *J Immunol* 1990; 145:1615–1620.

120. Alexander RB, Rosenberg SA. Adoptively transferred tumor-infiltrating lymphocytes can cure established metastatic tumor in mice and persist long-term *in vivo* as functional memory T lymphocytes. *J Immunother* 1991; 10:389–397.

121. Salup RR, Back TC, Wiltrout RH. Successful treatment of advanced murine renal cell cancer by bicompartmental adoptive chemoimmunotherapy. *J Immunol* 1987; 138:641–647.

122. Papa MZ, Yang JC, Vetto J, Shiloni E, Eisenthal A, Rosenberg SA. Combined effects of chemotherapy and interleukin 2 in the therapy of mice with advanced pulmonary tumors. *Cancer Res* 1988; 48:122–129.

123. Fearon ER, Pardoll DM, Itaya T, Golumbek P, Levitsky HI, Simons JW, Karasuyama H, Vogelstein B, Frost P. Interleukin-2 production by tumor cells bypasses T helper function in the generation of an antitumor response. *Cell* 1990; 60:397–403.

124. Gansbacher B, Zier K, Daniels B, Cronin K, Bannerji R, Gilboa E. Interleukin 2 gene transfer into tumor cells abrogates tumorigenicity and induces protective immunity. *J Exp Med* 1990; 172:1217–1224.

125. Kim TS, Cohen EP. Interleukin-2-secreting mouse fibroblasts transfected with genomic DNA from murine melanoma cells prolong the survival of mice with melanoma. *Cancer Res* 1994; 54:2531–2535.

126. Whittington R, Faulds D. Interleukin-2. A review of its pharmacological properties and therapeutic use in patients with cancer. *Drugs* 1993; 46:446–514.

127. Bruton JK, Koeller JM. Recombinant interleukin-2. *Pharmacotherapy* 1994; 635–656.

128. Physicians Desk Reference. Proleukin. Medical Economics, Montvale, NJ. 1994:801–804.

129. Rosenberg SA, Lotze MT, Muul LM, Leitman S, Chang AE, Ettinghausen SE, Matory YL, Skibber J, Shiloni E, Vetto JT, Seipp CA, Simpson C, Reichert CM. Observations on the systemic administration of autologous lymphokine activated killer cells and recombinant interleukin-2 to patients with metastatic cancer. *N Eng J Med* 1985; 313:1485–1492.

130. Palmer PA, Vinke J, Evers P, Porreaux C, Oskam R, Roest G, Viems F, Becker L, Loriaux E, Franks GP. Continuous infusion of recombinant interleukin-2 with or without autologous lymphokine activated killer cells for the treatment of advanced renal cell carcinoma. *Eur J Cancer* 1992; 28A:1038–1044.

131. Rosenberg SA, Lotze MT, Yand JC, Topalian SL, Chang AE, Schwartzentruber DJ, Aebersold P, Leitman S, Linehan WM, Seipp CA, White DE, Steinberg SM. Prospective randomized trial of high-dose interleukin-2 alone or in combination with lymphokine-activated killer cells for the treatment of patients with advanced cancer. *J Natl Cancer Inst* 1993; 85:622-632.

132. Rosenberg SA, Packard BS, Aebersold PM, Solomon D, Topalian SL, Toy ST, Simon P, Lotze MT, Yang JC, Seipp CA, Simpson C, Carter C, Bock S, Schwartzentruber D, Wei JP, White DE. Use of tumor-infiltrating lymphocytes and interleukin-2 in the immunotherapy of patients with metastatic melanoma. *N Eng J Med* 1988; 319:1676-1680.

133. Kobayashi M, Fitz L, Ryan M, Hewick RM, Clark SC, Chan S, Loudon R, Sherman F, Perussia B, Trinchieri G. Identification and purification of natural killer cell stimulatory factor (NKSF), a cytokine with multiple biological effects on human lymphocytes. *J Exp Med* 1989; 170:827-845.

134. Stern AS, Podlaski FJ, Hulmes JD, Pan Y-CE, Quinn PM, Wolitzky AG, Familletti PC, Stremio DL, Truitt T, Chizzonite R, Gately MK. Purification to homogencity and partial characterization of cytotoxic lymphocyte maturation factor from human B-lymphoblastoid cells. *Proc Natl Acad Sci USA* 1990; 87:6808-6812.

135. Gubler U, Chua AO, Schoenbaut DS, Dwyer CM, McComas W, Motyka R, Nabavi N, Wolitzky AG, Quinn PM, Familletti PC, Gately MK. Coexpression of two distinct genes is required to generate secreted, bioactive cytoxic lymphocyte maturation factor. *Proc Natl Acad Sci USA* 1991; 88:4143-4147.

136. Wolf SF, Temple PA, Kobayashi M, Young D, Dicig M, Lowe L, Dzialo R, Fitz L, Ferenz C, Hewick RM, Kelleher K, Herrmann SH, Clark SC, Azzoni L, Chan SH, Trinchieri G, Perussia B. Cloning of cDNA for natural killer cell stimulatory factor, a heterodimeric cytokine with multiple biologic effects on T and natural killer cells. *J Immunol* 1991; 146:3074-3081.

137. Chizzonite R, Truitt T, Desai BB, Nunes P, Podlaski FJ, Stern AS, Gately MK. IL-12 receptor. I. Characterization of the receptor on phytohemagglutinin-activated human lymphocytes. *J Immunol* 1992; 148:3117-3124.

138. Desai BB, Quinn PM, Wolitzky AG, Mongini PKA, Chizzonite R, Gately MK. IL-12 receptor. II. Distribution and regulation of receptor expression. *J Immunol* 1992; 148:3125-2132.

139. Chua AO, Chizzonite R, Desai BB, Truitt T, Nunes P, Minetti LJ, Warrier RR, Presky DH, Levine JF, Gately MK, Gubler U. Expression cloning of a human IL-12 receptor component: a new member of the cytokine receptor superfamily with strong homology to gp130. *J Immunol* 1994; 153:128-136.

140. Brunda MJ. Interleukin-12. *J Leukocyte Biol* 1994; 55:280-288.

141. Gately MK, Gubler U, Brunda MJ, Nadeau RR, Anderson TD, Lipman JM, Sarmiento U. Interleukin-12: a cytokine with therapeutic potential in oncology and infectious diseases. *Therapeutic Immunol* 1994; 1:187-196.

142. Brunda MJ, Gately MK. Interleukin-12: potential role in cancer therapy. In: DeVita V, Hellman S, Rosenberg SA, eds. *Important Advances in Oncology 1995*. Philadelphia: JB Lippincott Company. 1995:3-18.

143. Gately MK, Brunda MJ. Interleukin-12: a pivotal regulator of cell-mediated immunity. In: Kurzrock R, Talpaz M. eds. *Cytokines: Interleukins and Their Receptors*. Norwell, MA: Kluwer Academic Publishers. 1995:341-366.

144. Schoenhaut DA, Chua AO, Wolitzky AG, Quinn PM, Dwyer CM, McComas W, Familletti PC, Gately MK, Gubler U. Cloning and expression of murine IL-12. *J Immunol* 1992; 148: 3433-3440.

145. Gately MK, Warrier RR, Honasoge S, Carvajal DM, Faherty DA, Connaughton SE, Anderson TD, Sarmiento U, Hubbard BR, Murphy M. Administration of recombinant IL-12 to normal mice enhances cytolytic lymphocyte activity and induces production of IFN-γ in vivo. *Intl Immunol* 1994; 6:157-167.

146. Brunda MJ, Luistro L, Warrier RR, Wright RB, Hubbard BR, Murphy M, Wolf SF, Gately MF. Antitumor and antimetastatic activity of interleukin-12 against murine tumors. *J Exp Med* 1993; 178:1223-1230.

147. Nastala CL, Edington HD, McKinney TG, Tahara H, Nalesnik M, Brunda MJ, Gately MK, Wolf SF, Schreiber RD, Stewart T, Storkus WJ, Lotze MJ. Recombinant interleukin-12 (IL-12) administration induces tumor regression in association with interferon-gamma production. *J Immunol* 1994; 153:1697-1706.

148. Brunda MJ, Gately MK. Antitumor activity of interleukin-12. *Clin Immunol Immunopath* 1994; 71:253–255.
149. Brunda MJ, Luistro L, Hendrzak JA, Fountoulakis M, Garotta G, Gately MK. Interleukin-12: biology and preclinical studies of a new anti-tumor cytokine. In: Bukowski RM, Finke JH, Klein EA, eds. *The Biology of Renal Cell Carcinoma.* New York: Springer-Verlag, pp. 177–188.
150. Tahara J, Zeh HJ, Storkus WJ III, Pappo I, Watkins SC, Gubler U, Wolf SF, Robbins PD, Lotze MT. Fibroblasts genetically engineered to secrete IL-12 can suppress tumor growth and induce antitumor immunity to murine melanoma in vivo. *Cancer Res* 1994; 54:182–189.
151. Brunda MJ, Luistro L, Hendrzak JA, Fountoulakis M, Garotta G, Gately MK. Role of interferon gamma in mediating the antitumor efficacy of interleukin-12. *J Immunother* 1995; 17:71–77.
152. O'Toole M, Wolf SF, O'Brien C, Hubbard B, Herrmann S. Effect of in vivo IL-12 administration on murine tumor cell growth. *J Immunol* 1993; 150:294A.
153. Stern LL, Tarby CM, Tamborini B, Truitt GA. Preclinical development of IL-12 as an anti-cancer drug: comparison to IL-2. *Proc Am Assoc Cancer Res* 1994; 35:520.
154. Mayor SE, O'Donnell MA, Clinton SK. Interleukin-12 (IL-12) immunotherapy of experimental bladder cancer. *Proc Am Assoc Cancer Res* 1994; 35:474.
155. Hendrzak JA, Luistro L, Gately MK, Garotta G, Brunda MJ. Role of interferon gamma in mediating the antitumor effects of interleukin-12. *Proc Am Assoc Cancer Res* 1994; 35:524.

14 Discovery of TNP-470 and Other Angiogenesis Inhibitors

Donald E. Ingber, MD, PhD

CONTENTS

1. INTRODUCTION

Most types of cancer chemotherapy, either currently available or in development, are cytotoxic in that they are designed to kill rapidly growing tumor cells. Because many normal tissues contain stem cells that also proliferate rapidly (e.g., bone marrow, hair follicles, intestines), these types of agents often cause many side effects, and thus, their clinical effectiveness is limited. For this reason, many in the cancer field have begun to pursue different approaches.

One of the most novel and promising approaches to anticancer therapy does not target the tumor cells directly. Instead, the objective is to inhibit the growth of new capillary blood vessels that feed the growing tumor, a process that is known as tumor "angiogenesis." This chapter will explain the concept behind this approach and review the process of discovery in the field of angiogenesis inhibition. In particular, it will focus on a serendipitous discovery I made 10 years ago while working as a post-doctoral fellow in the laboratory of Judah Folkman. That initial observation led to the development of TNP-470, a potent angiogenesis inhibitor that is now entering Phase II clinical trials. In the process of reviewing these discoveries, preclinical data will be described that, I believe, provide the "proof of principle" for a cancer therapy to be based on angiogenesis inhibition.

Importantly, the chapter that follows is not designed to serve as a thorough introduction to the field or a review of all angiogenesis inhibitors that have been identified. A number of excellent reviews of this type have been published recently (*1–3*). Rather, here I hope to convey the importance of serendipity in the process of cancer drug discovery and the equally important need for a receptive research environment.

From: *Cancer Therapeutics: Experimental and Clinical Agents*
Edited by: B. Teicher Humana Press Inc., Totowa, NJ

2. IN SEARCH OF ANGIOGENESIS INHIBITORS

The search for angiogenesis inhibitors began almost 25 years ago when J. Folkman first suggested that tumors are angiogenesis-dependent (4). This hypothesis was based on results of animal studies and anecdotal observations in human cancer patients, which showed that for tumors to grow larger than approx 1–2 mm^3 in size, they must gain the ability to stimulate ingrowth of new capillaries (5–8). The reason for this is that tumor cells, like all living cells, require a continous supply of oxygen and nutrients in order to grow. In addition, effective blood flow may remove factors that suppress tumor cell death (i.e., apoptosis) (9).

The net result is that tumors generally will not grow significantly in size, and thus, will not be malignant or often clinically detectable if new capillary growth is prevented (5,9–13). A simple example is cutaneous melanoma. Extensive morphometric analysis of histological sections of human melanoma specimens shows that tumors that do not promote angiogenesis tend to remain < 0.76 mm in thickness (these are planar lesions) and exhibit a low incidence of metastasis (14). In contrast, once capillary ingrowth is stimulated, this size restriction is circumvented, and malignancy results. Quantitation of capillary densities in pathological specimens also have been found to be an excellent prognostic indicator in human patients with breast cancer (15).

The proposal that tumors depend on continual neovascularization for their own growth and expansion immediately stimulated a search for a tumor "angiogenesis factor," that is, the soluble mitogen that was thought to be responsible for induction of capillary ingrowth (4,6,16). The concept was simple from a therapeutic perspective: If one could identify this molecule, then specific inhibitors, such as blocking antibodies, could be developed to prevent tumor expansion. Combination of these growth-inhibitory agents with conventional drugs, radiotherapy, and surgical intervention could therefore lead, in theory, to rational management or even cure of this disease.

Great advances have been made in the search for angiogenic factors. Many angiogenic proteins have now been purified, sequenced, and cloned (2,17,18). Some angiogenic factors (e.g., acidic and basic FGFs) are mitogentic for a variety of cell types in addition to capillary cells. In contrast, others appear to be highly specific for endothelium (e.g., VEGF). Other factors (e.g., TGF-B, TNF-α) are not directly mitogenic for endothelial cells, and thus may act indirectly by activating or recruiting other cells, such as macrophages, that in turn release angiogenic mitogens. Alternatively, some angiogenic factors appear to promote angiogenesis directly by stimulating endothelial cell migration and/or capillary tube formation, rather than cell growth *per se* (19).

Importantly, as time went on, it became clear that there was enormous redundancy among angiogenic factors. Many different types of molecules can stimulate capillary growth, and a single tumor can produce more than one angiogenic mitogen (3,17,18, 20). Thus, more recently, emphasis has shifted away from growth factor identification to understanding the molecular basis of capillary growth control.

2.1. Rational Drug Discovery

In the angiogenesis field, as in many other areas of cancer research, the current concept is that a more in depth understanding of the molecular basis of cell and tissue regulation will lead directly to development of new therapeutic agents. In fact, there are many cases where this has been shown to be true. Examples of angiogenesis inhibitors that have been discovered based on a rational approach include: cartilage-derived inhibitor, protamine, platelet factor 4, medroxyprogesterone, proline analogues, retinoids, integrin receptor antagonists, thalidomide, and most recently, angiostatin.

Cartilage-derived inhibitor was first sought after (21,22) and later purified (23) based on the observation that cartilage is a relatively avascular tissue. Interestingly, sharks, which are highly cartilagenous creatures, both contain angiogenesis inhibitory activity in their cartilage and rarely develop solid tumors (24).

Protamine and platelet factor 4 were tested and found to inhibit new capillary growth based on their known high affinity for heparin (25,26). This work followed the discovery that heparin can enhance angiogenic factor activity in vitro (27). At about the same time, Shing and Klagsbrun (again working in Folkman's department) also found that many angiogenic factors can be purified based on their ability to bind heparin (28,29).

The finding that extracellular matrix proteolysis mediates initiation of angiogenesis in vivo (30,31) and endothelial cell migration in vitro (32) led to the testing of known collagenase inhibitors in angiogenesis assays. This approach resulted in the discovery of the antiangiogenic effects of medroxy-progesterone (33). More recently, cartilage-derived inhibitor was found to exhibit anticollagenase activities as well (23). In addition, BB94, a synthetic collagenase antagonist that was initially developed to inhibit tumor growth and metastasis, also has been found to inhibit neovascularization (34). BB94 is currently in Phase I clinical trials.

Proline analogs, retinoids, and other inhibitors of extracellular matrix deposition and processing (e.g., α,α-dipyridyl, β-aminopriopionitrile) were examined because other angiogenesis inhibitors (heparin-angiostatic steroid combinations) were found to induce capillary basement membrane dissolution as part of their action (35). All of these compounds inhibited angiogenesis in the CAM, and their inhibitory effects correlated directly with their ability to suppress collagen deposition in that assay (36).

Soluble antagonists of integrin $\alpha_V\beta_3$ receptors (e.g., blocking antibodies, synthetic RGD peptides) were tested and found to exhibit antiangiogenic activity based on the observation that growing endothelial cells appear to express preferentially this particular extracellular matrix receptor subtype on their surfaces (37,38). Work in my laboratory also had previously shown that extracellular matrix and integrins play a key role in capillary growth control in vitro (39–43) as well as in vivo (35,36).

The discovery of thalidomide's antiangiogenic activity is quite interesting. R. J. D'Amato, an opthalmologist working as a research fellow in Folkman's laboratory, decided that a rational way to identify new angiogenesis inhibitors would be to search the medical literature (using a computer) for existing drugs that exhibit "side effects" that might be expected to be associated with angiogenesis inhibition (e.g., increased rates of spontaneous abortion, large-scale development defects). The discovery of thalidomide's antiangiogenic capabilities resulted (44). Thalidomide has recently entered Phase I clinical trials for treatment of angiogenesis-dependent disease in the eye.

Most recently, angiostatin was discovered based on a search for an endogenous inhibitor in serum that might be responsible for the observed inhibitory influence exerted by large primary tumors on the growth of secondary metastatic lesions (a process that was sometimes referred to as "concomitant immunity" in the past). Although little was known about the mechanism behind this inhibition, Folkman had suspected for many years that it could be due to production of systemic angio-genesis inhibitors that would effectively suppress growth of small tumors at a distance. In this model, tumor expansion would continue at the primary site, because short-lived angiogenic stimulators overcame the inhibitor locally and shifted the balance toward capillary growth at the primary site. However, if clearance of the inhibitors was much slower than that of the angiogenic mitogen, then capillary growth suppres-sion might be expected to dominate systemically. M. O'Reilly, another surgical resident working as a research fellow in Folkman's laboratory, purified a fragment of plamino-gen from serum and urine that has been named "angiostatin" (13). Angiostatin, which appears to be generated or released by primary tumors that suppress the growth of their metastases, effectively prevents the growth of both primary and metastatic lesions when administered to mice and, thus, exhibits all of the properties that Folkman envisioned.

2.2. Discovery by Chance: Angiostatic Steroids

Although the rational approach will likely pay off in the long term, it turns out that other angiogenesis inhibitors were discovered based entirely on chance. A classic example was when S. Taylor, a medical student working in Folkman's laboratory, discovered that heparin and cortisone inhibit angiogenesis (10). She actually made this discovery in the course of trying to optimize a screening assay for angiogenic modulators.

To study angiogenesis, Taylor had been placing tumor extracts on the surface of the chick chorioallantoic membrane (CAM). This embryonic membrane is used as an angiogenesis model, because it is underlined by a continously extending capillary network that grows rapidly from day 6 to day 10 of development (35). In earlier studies, it was shown that application of living tumor cells, tumor extracts, or partially purified angiogenic factor preparations to the surface of the CAM resulted in enhanced angiogenesis, as visualized by increased growth of vessels in a "spoke-wheel" pattern that converged toward the growth stimulus (8,25).

When using this CAM assay, Taylor first added heparin in an attempt to enhance the activity of the tumor-derived angiogenic factors and, thus, increase the sensitivity of the assay (25). Heparin had been previously shown to enhance angiogenic factor-induced capillary cell migration in vitro (27). However, in the assay Taylor used, dust often would fall onto the CAM from the surrounding egg shell causing nonspecific "inflammatory" angiogenesis that complicated the interpretation of her results. In an attempt to suppress this inflammatory activity and increase the signal-to-noise, Taylor and Folkman decided to add cortisone (a potent immune suppressant) to the assay. Surprisingly, they found that not only was this nonspecific background angiogenesis-inhibited, but also both normal embryonic capillary growth and tumor extract-induced angiogenesis were completely prevented as well. In addition, regression of pre-existing capillaries, but not neighboring epithelium, was observed over large regions of the CAM. These studies were extended by Folkman and coworkers to show that com-binations of cortisone and heparin or heparin fragments can inhibit angiogenesis and suppress tumor growth in a variety of animal models (10,45).

Taylor and Folkman's discovery eventually led to the identification and character-ization of an entirely new class of antiangiogenic or "angiostatic" steroids (35, 46–48). These steroids are potent inhibitors of neovascularization when combined with hep-

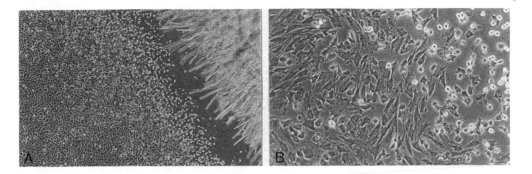

Fig. 1. The fungal contaminant that led to the development of TNP-470. **(A)** A low-magnification phase-contrast view showing the hyphae of the fungal contaminant at the top right of the culture well with the retracting endothelial monolayer below. **(B)** A higher magnification view of the endothelial monolayer near the edge of the fungal colony. A gradient of increased cell rounding can be observed, as one moves from the bottom left to the top right of the view.

arin, yet they have no known glucocorticoid, mineralocorticoid, or sex steroid activities. Importantly, some of these angiostatic steroids occur naturally as "inactive" steroid metabolites in urine (e.g., tetrahydrocortisol). The presence of these endogenous inhibitors may play an important role in maintaining the low cell turnover rate that is characteristic of the normal vascular endothelium (*49*). This work also indirectly led to the search for other angiogenesis inhibitors in urine; the discovery of genistein (*50*) and 2-methoxyestradiol (*51*) soon followed.

3. TNP-470: SERENDIPITY LEADS TO A NEW ANTICANCER DRUG

3.1. Initial Observation

Perhaps one of the best examples of the importance of serendipity in drug discovery in the angiogenesis field is the case of TNP-470 (originally called AGM-1470; *11*). This story is a very personal one since it began with an observation I made while working as a postdoctoral fellow in Folkman's laboratory. In the course of passing standard capillary endothelial cell cultures on November 1, 1985, I discovered fungal contaminants growing in three different wells of the same multiwell culture dish. One of these contaminants I had unfortunately seen many times in the past. Even when small, this type of fungus induced complete cell detachment and death in our endothelial cell cultures. It was a known scourge that would emerge from time to time. My immediate reflex response on seeing this fungus, based on past training and experience, was to immerse the entire culture dish immediately in disinfectant and to place it in line for autoclaving and disposal (the standard approach to contamination in our lab at that time).

However, the fungus in the second well immediately attracted my attention. In contrast to all other fungi I had seen in the past and to the contaminants in the neighboring wells, this fungus did not induce complete cell detachment even though it covered about one-third of a 35-mm well. Instead, this fungus appeared to induce a gradient of cell retraction and rounding in the adjacent endothelial monolayer (Fig. 1). Directly below the fungal colony and along its edge, endothelial cells appeared adherent, but completely spherical, whereas cells only a few diameters away exhibited a normal extended morphology. This morphological change interested me because in other ongoing studies in the laboratory, I had recently found that capillary cells will not grow when stimulated by any angiogenic factor, if cells are induced to round by preventing cell adhesion to extracellular matrix (later published in *35, 39–42*). This basic work was a direct extension of my dissertation research with J Jamieson at Yale, which centered on the importance of cell shape in the control of tissue growth and form (*52–54*). Folkman himself was a pioneer in this area having published an elegant study with A. Moscona (a medical student) in 1978 that was the first to show clearly that cell shape plays a key role in growth control (*55*). In fact, one of the major reasons I chose to carry out my postdoctoral research training in Folkman's laboratory (i.e., rather than complete a clinical residency) was his openness to this novel way of looking at cell growth regulation.

In any case, it was because of my unconventional view of cell growth control that I cultured these fungi. I also cultured the fungus in the third well, which was of similar size, yet it produced only minimal cell detachment or rounding as another control. All three contaminants were cultured in Sabouraud's agar tubes that "happened" to be sitting on a shelf in our mammalian tissue-culture laboratory. Amazingly, it took almost 2 mo before I communicated this finding to Folkman. Basically, I was ambivalent about launching yet another research project given the already overextended state of any postdoctoral fellow. Nevertheless, about 6 wk later in late December of 1985, I could no longer hold back my excitement, and I finally told Folkman of my "discovery." He was extremely enthusiastic and immediately saw the potential importance of this observation. In fact, he was so excited about the finding that he cultured the fungus, collected the medium, and set about testing it for angiogenesis inhibitory activity himself.

The question of whether this fungus might secrete a **soluble** inhibitor was a very important one. About a year before this incident, Folkman had tried to isolate an angiogenesis inhibitor from a fungus that had spontaneously settled on a CAM, apparently inducing capillary regression in that assay. However, that project was a complete failure; if the fungus did produce an angiogenesis inhibitor, it was not secreted in a soluble form that could be detected. The major lesson learned was that isolating a fungus in a mammalian cell tissue-culture laboratory can be a dangerous mistake: rampant contamination (and death) of many endothelial cell cultures resulted. In fact, this fear of contamination was another reason that I questioned whether I should tell Folkman about my discovery. It is also important to point out that the Sabbouraud's agar tubes I used would never have been available in our cell-culture laboratory, if it were not for this prior experience with fungi. Thus, chance played a key role at least twice in the early phase of this discovery process.

Once we cultured the fungus, we confirmed that it indeed secreted a soluble factor that inhibited embryonic angiogenesis in the CAM as well as capillary endothelial cell proliferation in vitro. When the fungus was sent for typing, it was identified as a relatively rare fungus, *Aspergillus fumigatus fresenius*. Conditioned medium from cultures of this fungus also induced cell rounding, and this activity was used as an initial bioassay during subsequent purification of the active molecule.

A third element of chance then came into play. Work in the Folkman laboratory had previously been funded in part by an industrial grant from the Monsanto Company. This grant ended at about this time, and thus, we actively sought funding from a number of different American pharmaceutical companies. When these companies came to review our work, we described our preliminary findings relating to this fungal contaminant. However, there was little interest. At least one of the executives that reviewed our findings very openly stated that he had little interest because he did not see anything "that would be in the clinic within the next six months."

When all seemed to be lost, Folkman received a note from a Dr. Sugino, who had briefly visited the laboratory in the past. It turned out that Sugino now held a high position in a major pharmaceutical company in Japan called Takeda Chemical Industries, Limited. On hearing that Folkman was seeking new funding, Sugino immediately sent a delegation to review our proposal. Rather than send mostly businessman (the approach of the American companies at that time), Takeda sent a delegation that was filled primarily with research scientists. I have two memorable recollections of this meeting: (1) the Takeda scientists were extremely excited about the fungus because microbial analysis and culture were major strengths of their company, and (2) Takeda took a long-term view of the drug discovery process and clearly stated their belief that angiogenesis would represent a major target for therapeutic intervention in the near future. If it were not for Takeda's partnership and incredible talents in the areas of fungal culture, factor purification, and chemical synthesis, TNP-470 would never have been developed.

3.2. Identification of Fumagillin and Analog Development

Immediately after initiating our collaboration with Takeda, we mailed a sample of the fungus that induced a gradient of cell rounding to their scientists. They cultured it in large batches and set out to isolate the putative angiogenesis inhibitory factor. Eventually, they discovered that the active compound that was secreted by the fungus I had isolated was fumagillin, a known antibiotic that had been previously used to treat Amebiasis in humans. Purified fumagillin was shown to inhibit endothelial cell proliferation in vitro, embryonic angiogenesis, and tumor-induced neovascularization in an sc sponge model in mice (52). It also suppressed the growth of a number of mouse tumors. However, its effectiveness was limited because it produced severe weight loss.

For this reason, we then set out to synthesize and test fumagillin analogs that would retain the potent antiangiogenic activity of fumagillin, but lack its toxic side effects. The most potent of these analogs is shown in Fig. 2. It was originally called AGM-1470 (AngioGenesis Modulator-1470). However, Takeda changed its name to TNP-470 (Takeda Neoplastic Product-470) once it entered clinical trials. In this chapter, it will be referred to as TNP-470.

I should note that these studies, which extended over a period of years, were spearheaded by scientists at Takeda, including Katsuichi Sudo, Shoji Kishimoto, Tsuneo Kanamaru, and Takeshi Fugita. Many of the animal studies carried out at our institution were done by Harold Brem, a surgical resident who was working as a research fellow in Folkman's laboratory, along with a number of different surgical residents, technicians, and rotating medical students.

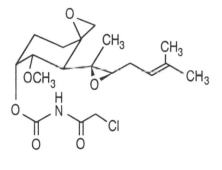

TNP-470

Fig. 2. The structure of the angiogenesis inhibitor, TNP-470 [*O*-(chloroacetyl-carbamoyl)fumagillol].

TNP-470 was found to be a potent inhibitor of endothelial cell proliferation in vitro (half-maximal growth inhibition at approx 100 pg/mL in both human umbilical vein and bovine capillary endothelium; *11*). It also inhibited embryonic and tumor-induced angiogenesis in a variety of models (e.g., CAM, rat and rabbit corneas, sc sponge implants, Matrigel) (*11,56*). Importantly, although TNP-470 prevented cultured endothelial cells from growing when added over a wide range of doses (10 pg to 1 μg/mL), it did not kill these cells. In other words, it produced cytostatic rather than cytotoxic inhibition (*11,57,58*). Furthermore, the same doses that inhibited capillary cell growth had little effect on cultured tumor cells. Nevertheless, TNP-470 effectively suppressed the growth of the same tumor cells when implanted in vivo (*11*). This work has now been extended to include over 30 different solid tumors in mice, rats, rabbits, dogs, and monkeys as well as human tumors in nude mice (*11,57,59–76*; and unpublished data). Almost every solid tumor tested so far has responded well to treatment with this compound, whereas a P388 tumor growing in an ascites (nonsolid) form was found to be relatively resistant (*11*).

Although TNP-470 usually only prevents tumor expansion when used alone, recent studies by B. Teicher (Dana Farber Cancer Institute) have shown that tumor regression can actually be obtained in a high percentage of animals (over 50% in mice bearing Lewis Lung Carcinoma) by combining TNP-470 with standard chemotherapeutic agents, such as cytoxan (*69*). Work at Takeda and in our laboratory also has shown that TNP-470 is a potent inhibitor of tumor metastasis (*59,73*). As expected, angiogenesis inhibition does not inhibit initial implantation of tumor cells; rather, it prevents further tumor expansion at these distant sites. For example, when mice are injected with tumor cells via tail vein and then treated with TNP-470, only small (<1-mm³) lesions are produced in the lungs.

Most importantly, in all of our studies in which mice were injected sc with pure TNP-470 dispersed in saline, we never observed any drug-related toxicities in the range of doses that were necessary to suppress tumor growth. In the thousands of mice tested with this compound, there was no loss of appetite, hair loss, infections, or drug-related deaths. There results were incredibly exciting, to say the least, especially given the history that led to the development of this drug.

3.3. Advantages over Other Anticancer Agents

In summary, based on a serendipitous finding we (the Takeda Scientists, Folkman, Brem, and I) developed a new class of molecules that appear to suppress tumor growth and metastasis by inhibiting angiogenesis. These antiangiogenic compounds are analogs of the fungal product, fumagillin (11). Importantly, this type of angiogenesis inhibitor offers many advantages over curently available anticancer therapies.

The first is low toxicity, which is largely based on the fact that TNP-470 does not kill capillary cells or cells within highly proliferative normal tissues, such as the gut epithelium or lymphoid cells. Rather, it prevents quiescent capillary cells from responding to any mitogenic stimulus. The specificity here comes from the fact that normal capillary cells have extremely low turnover rates, with half-lives on the order of years, whereas cells in tumor capillaries commonly turn over once every few days (49).

A second advantage is that TNP-470 inhibits the growth of both primary and metastatic tumors. Thus, this type of nontoxic compound could be used prophylactically, for example, following resection of a tumor of the breast or colon, which are known to be highly metastatic and, hence, to have a high rate of recurrence. If their low toxicity holds true in humans, then they also may be used in patients with premalignant lesions (e.g., carcinoma in situ of the cervix, patients with high serum PSA levels) or in otherwise healthy people who have a genetically high propensity for tumor development (e.g., as detected by genetic screening methods that are becoming increasingly available).

Another advantage is that the target of this drug, the endothelial cell, is not transformed, and thus, development of drug resistance should be less of a problem than with conventional therapies. In fact, this turns out to be true. Thus far, we have not observed development of drug resistance in any tumors, even when continuously administered in mice for more than 6 mo (Brem et al., unpublished data).

Finally, TNP-470 as well as other angiogenesis inhibitors have been shown to potentiate dramatically the anticancer effects of known chemotherapeutic agents (e.g., cytoxan; 68,69,77). Simultaneous administration of multiple angiogenesis inhibitors also produced additive inhibitory effects (60). Thus, antiangiogenesis agents, such as TNP-470, are perfectly suited to act in concert with other drugs as part of a combined chemotherapeutic regimen.

3.4. Translation from the Lab Bench to the Bedside

Based on these advantages, Phase I clinical trials were initiated with TNP-470 in September 1992 at the National Cancer Institute in patients with Kaposi's sarcoma. More recently, these trials were extended to include adult patients with many different types of solid cancers as well as children with brain tumors.

It should be noted that in the transition to the clinic, an iv route was chosen for the first line of attack. To accomplish this, an entirely new drug formulation had to be developed, which involved adding additional chemicals to TNP-470 to ensure stability and optimize solubility. When this final formulation was administered into beagle dogs by iv bolus injection, toxic effects were observed at high doses in certain organs (e.g., microhemorrhages were visualized in histological specimens of the brain). This toxicity seemed to be partially suppressed by slowing the rate of infusion, and no micro-hemorrhages could be detected when TNP-40 was infused into baboons (unpublished data). Thus, we currently do not know whether this toxicity, although relatively minor compared to conventional cytotoxic agents, relates to the new route or rate of drug administration, the additional chemical components added to the formulation, TNP-470 itself, the animal model being utilized, or combinations of these factors.

In any case, given the relatively minor toxicity observed compared to conventional anticancer agents, TNP-470 quickly moved forward into clinical trials. However, based on the toxicology studies, a slow rate of infusion (over 30 min rather than iv bolus) was incorporated into the clinical protocol. Nevertheless, the take-home message here is that when translating a discovery from the lab bench to the bedside, seemingly small decisions can potentially make an enormous difference. For example, the choice of chemical additives for a new drug formulation usually is not a significant issue for most anticancer agents, which are themselves very toxic. However, this could be a major concern for those interested in developing novel anticancer agents, such as angiogenesis inhibitors, that potentially can suppress tumor growth without significant systemic toxicity.

It is precisely because of concerns such as these that clinical trials involve an initial phase (Phase I), which focuses exclusively on defining dose-limiting toxicities. Animal studies may be useful to identify potential problem areas. However, only results of actual toxicology studies carried out in human patients receiving the final formulation using an appropriate administration route and dose schedule have real meaning in the long term. In the case of TNP-470, the toxicities in Phase I trials have been found to be relatively minor. In fact, this has been a problem in the sense that Phase I trials have extended much longer than is usually required for cytotoxic agents (e.g., the original trial that began in 1992 still continues as of today). Dose-limiting toxicity has only been determined in older male patients with prostate cancer. In these patients, TNP-470 appeared to induce confusion, although this effect reversed when therapy was stopped.

In hindsight, it is interesting that because of our initial toxicology results in beagle dogs, TNP-470 was initially restricted from use in patients with brain cancer, even though there is no effective therapy available for these highly vascular tumors. Given that internal bleeding has not been a problem so far in human testing, Phase I trials in children with brain tumors were recently initiated. Most importantly, Phase II trials also should begin in the near future. However, here again there is a concern. Most oncologists usually only view an anticancer drug as active and useful if they can measure a dramatic and rapid tumor "response," as defined by a measureable shrinkage in tumor size or mass. In contrast, based on our preclinical studies, we expect TNP-470 (and other angiogenesis inhibitors) to produce relatively minor growth suppression (rather than shrinkage) when used alone, especially in the short term. Furthermore, extensive clinical trials in children with hemangioma using another angiogenesis inhibitor, α-interferon, suggest that no clinical effect may be visible for many months, even though complete tumor regression can be obtained by 1 yr in most of these patients (78,79). In fact, this clinical experience with α-interferon provides probably the best indication to date of how antiangiogenesis therapy will need to be administered in the future. Thus, not only must an angiogenesis inhibitor be active, but the clinicians involved in the testing of the drug must also understand that they are dealing with an entirely different type of therapeutic agent and, thus, develop totally new clinical end points. This, of course, may change once angiogenesis inhibitors are tested in combination with conventional chemotherapeutic agents, since dramatic and immediate shrinkage in tumor size should result.

In summary, we must await the publication of results of the ongoing TNP-470 studies and future clinical trials involving drug combinations before we can ascertain the importance of this discovery. There clearly have been many drugs that were promising in early testing and yet only minimally effective when examined in humans. However, I believe that the preclinical results obtained with TNP-470 and other angiogenesis inhibitors, at the very least, provide a glimpse of what an anticancer therapy based on antiangiogenesis might be like in the future.

3.5. Implications for the Future

Probably the most important lesson we have learned from past experience with cancer chemotherapy in human patients is that it is unlikely that there will be a single silver bullet that will cure all cancers. We also know that clinical cures can be obtained with certain types of cancer. However, these dramatic responses almost always require simultaneous administration of multiple drugs. As an example, in treatment of acute lymphocytic leukemia in children, three to four different active agents had to be administered in combination before complete remissions could be produced in almost all patients. However, even then, clinical cures were only obtained in about 15% of these cases. To increase the cure rate to over 75%, as it is today, six to seven different active agents had to be administered in concert. This is likely what a cure of adult human cancer will require in the future. Given our preclinical results with TNP-470, I believe it is likely that one or more angiogenesis inhibitors will be a key part of this type of combined regimen for "cancer management" in the future.

4. CONCLUSIONS

The discoveries in the field of angiogenesis inhibition that I described in this chapter may provide a lesson for those interested in learning how to identify new anticancer drugs. One point was raised repeatedly: the incredible importance of chance and serendipity in the drug discovery process. Contamination of the CAM assay by eggshell dust and of my endothelial culture dish by a fungus are two particular examples of how chance can intervene at a particular time and place. However, these serendipitous events did not occur in a vacuum. No drugs would come from these observations, if the investigators did not have a clear goal in mind and methods on hand to follow up their observations. If the investigators were in a laboratory where rigid focus and strict observance of a preplanned path of inquiry (e.g., as laid out in the specific aims of a government grant proposal) were the rule, these observations also would likely not be made, let alone pursued. In essence, these events would remain no more than cursory observations similar to those made every day in labs around the world, if the research environment was wrong.

In contrast, as you probably can appreciate from my description, the Folkman laboratory of the 1980s (and to this day) was one that was continually open to new ideas and unconventional ways of viewing biological problems, young people (who are not yet tied to convention) were always involved on the front lines, and bioassays that were both novel and highly useful were freely accessible to all. There also was a rare clarity of focus that came directly from Folkman's own vision, and his incredible ability to communicate the excitement and importance of the clinical problem at hand. Finally, gelling all this was sustained financial support from both government (NIH) and industrial sponsors, as well as an active ongoing collaboration with top-notch industrial medicinal chemists and microbiologists. Serendipity without this type of receptive environment would be like a bulb without electricity; the potential for enlightenment would be there, but little light would fall.

In conclusion, if there is any message in this chapter, it is that to best facilitate drug discovery, the scientific and pharmaceutical communities must learn how to develop this type of research incubator in which all of the key elements that are essential for discovery are placed in close proximity in a stable environment. If the final goal is truly translation of basic discoveries directly to the bedside, then ongoing collaborations and paths of communication between academic researchers and industrial scientists also must be established and maintained. Academics have the freedom to change paths at will and to explore serendipitous or counterintuitive results. However, they usually do not understand when to patent a discovery or how to develop a "product" that can be manufactured and distributed worldwide. Industrial scientists, on the other hand, tend to understand the nuts and bolts of true drug development (e.g., toxicology, pharmacokinetics, formulation development, FDA approval, and so forth). Yet, they lack the freedom to change direction at will. The creation of this type of research incubator becomes increasingly more difficult as the funds available to basic researchers and to the biopharmaceutical community become increasingly hard to find. Nevertheless, this is the goal that we must collectively pursue to be sure that new discoveries, both rational and serendipitous, will continue to be made in years to come.

ACKNOWLEDGMENTS

I would like to especially thank Judah Folkman, because essentially none of the discoveries I described would have ever come about without his drive and energy. The work that I described from my laboratory was supported by grants from NIH, American Cancer Society, and Takeda Chemical Industries, Limited. The author is a recipient of a Faculty Research Award from the American Cancer Society.

NOTE ADDED IN PROOF

The first complete tumor regression induced by administration of TNP-470 was recently reported in a woman with metastatic cervical carcinoma (*80*). This patient has now remained free to tumor and toxicity for over a year of continuous therapy with this single angiogenesis inhibitor.

REFERENCES

1. Folkman J, Ingber DE. Inhibition of Angiogenesis. *Semin Cancer Biol* 1992; 3:89–96.
2. Moses MA, Klagsbrun M, Shing Y. The role of growth factors in vascular cell development and differentiation. *Int Rev Cytol* 1995; 161:1–48.
3. Folkman J. Angiogenesis in cancer, vascular, rhematoid and other disease. *Nature Med* 1995; 1:27–30.

4. Folkman J. Tumor angiogenesis: therapeutic implications. *New Engl J Med* 1971; 285:1182–1186.
5. Folkman J. Cole P, Zimmerman S. Tumor behavior in isolated perfused organs: in vitro growth and metastases of biopsy material in rabbit thyroid and canine intestinal segment. *Ann Surg* 1966; 164:491–501.
6. Folkman J, Merler E, Abernathy C, Williams G. Isolation of a tumor factor responsible for angiogenesis. *J Exp Med* 1971; 133:275–288.
7. Gimbrone MA Jr, Leapman SB, Cotran RS, Folkman J. Tumor dormancy in vivo by prevention of neovascularization. *J Exp Med.* 1972; 136:261–276.
8. Knighton D, Ausprunk D, Tapper D, Folkman J. Avascular and vascular phases of tumour growth in the chick embryo. *Br J Cancer* 1977; 35:347–356.
9. Holmgren L, O'Reilly MS, Folkman J. Dormancy of micrometastases: balanced proliferation and apoptosis in the presence of angiogenesis suppression. *Nature Med.* 1995; 1:149–153.
10. Folkman J, Langer R, Linhardt RJ, Haudenchild C, and Tayler S. Angiogenesis inhibition and tumor regression caused by heparin or a heparin fragment in the presence of cortisone. *Science* 1983, 221:719–725.
11. Ingber DE, Fujita T, Kishimoto S, Kanamaru T, Sudo K, Brem H, Folkman J. Synthetic analogues of fumagillin which inhibit angiogenesis and suppress tumour growth. *Nature* 1990; 348: 555–557.
12. Folkman J. What is the evidence that tumors are angiogenesis dependent? *J Natl Cancer Inst* 1990; 82:4–6.
13. O'Reilly MS, Holmgren L, Shing Y, Chen C, Rosenthal RA, Moses M, Lane WS, Cao Y, Sage EH, Folkman J. Angiostatin: a novel angiogenesis inhibitor that mediates the suppression of metastases by a Lewis lung carcinoma. *Cell* 1994; 79:315–328.
14. Srivastava A, Laidler P, Davies RP, Horgan K, Hughes LE. The prognostic significance of tumor vascularity in intermediate-thickness (0.76–4.0 mm thick) skin melanoma. *Am J Pathol* 1988; 133:419–423.
15. Weidner N, Semple JP, Welch WR, Folkman J. Tumor angiogenesis and metastasis-correlation in invasive breast carcinoma. *New Eng J Med* 1991; 324:1–8.
16. Folkman J. The vascularization of tumors. *Sci Am* 1976; 234:58–73.
17. Folkman J, Klagsbrun M. Angiogenic factors. *Science* 1987; 235:442–447.
18. Dvorak HF, Brown LF, Detmar M, Dvorak AM. Vascular permeability factor/vascular endothelial growth factor, microvascular hyperpermeability, and angiogenesis. *Am J Pathol* 1995; 146:1029–1039.
19. Banda MJ, Knighton DR, Hunt TK, Werb Z. Isolation of a nonmitogenic angiogenesis factor from wound fluid. *Proc Natl Acad Sci USA* 1982; 79:7773–7777.
20. Folkman J. The role of angiogenesis in tumor growth. *Semin Cancer Biol* 1992; 3:65–71.
21. Brem H, Folkman J. Inhibition of tumor angiogenesis mediated by cartilage. *J Exp Med* 1975; 141:427–439.
22. Langer R, Conn H, Vacanti J, Haudenschild C, Folkman J. Control of tumor growth in animals by infusion of an angiogenesis inhibitor. *Proc Natl Acad Sci USA* 1980; 77:4331–4335.
23. Moses MA, Sudhalter J, Langer R. Identification of an inhibitor of neovascularization from cartilage. *Science* 1990; 248:1408–1410.
24. Lee A, Langer R. Shark cartilage contains inhibitors of tumor angiogenesis. *Science* 1983; 221: 1185–1187.
25. Taylor S, Folkman J. Protamine is an inhibitor of angiogenesis. *Nature* 1982; 297:307–310.
26. Maione TE, Gray GS, Petro J, Hunt AJ, Donner AL, Bauer SI, Carson HF, Sharpe RJ. Inhibition of angiogenesis by recombinant human platelet factor-4 and related peptides. *Science* 1990; 247:77–79.
27. Azizkhan RG, Azizkhan JC, Zetter BR, Folkman J. Mast cell heparin stimulates migration of capillary endothelial cells in vitro. *J Exp Med* 1980; 152:931–935.
28. Shing Y, Folkman J, Sullivan R, Butterfield C, Murray J, Klagsbrun M. Heparin affinity: purification of a tumor-derived capillary endothelial cell growth factor. *Science* 1984; 223:1296–1299.
29. Klagsbrun M, Shing Y. Heparin affinity of anionic and cationic capillary endothelial cell growth factors: analysis of hypothalamus-derived growth factors and fibroblast growth factors. *Proc Natl Acad Sci USA* 1985; 82:805–809.
30. Ausprunk DH, Folkman J. Migration and proliferation of endothelial cells in preformed and newly formed blood vessels during tumor angiogenesis. *Microvasc Res* 1977; 14:53–65.

31. Berman M, Winthrop S, Ausprunk, Rose J, Langer R, Gage J. Plasminogen activator (uro-kinase) causes vascularization of the cornea. *Invest Ophthalmol Vis Sci* 1982; 22:191–199.
32. Kalebic T, Garbisa S, Glaser B, Liotta LA. Basement membrane collagen degradation by mig-rating endothelial cells. *Science* 1983; 221:281–283.
33. Gross J, Azizkhan RG, Biswas C, Bruns RR, Hsieh DST, Folkman J. Inhibition of tumor growth, vascularization, and collagenolysis in the rabbit cornea by medroxyprogesterone. *Proc Natl Acad Sci USA* 1981; 78:1176–1180.
34. Davies B, Brown PD, East N, Crimmin MJ, Balkwill FR. A synthetic matrix metalloproteinase inhibitor decreases tumor burden and prolongs survival of mice bearing human ovarian car-cinoma xenografts. *Cancer Res* 1993; 53:2087–2091.
35. Ingber DE, Madri JA, Folkman J. A possible mechanism for inhibition of angiogenesis by angiostatic steroids: induction of capillary basement membrane dissolution. *Endocrinology* 1986; 119:1768–1775.
36. Ingber DE, Folkman J. Inhibition of angiogenesis through inhibition of collagen metabolism. *Lab Invest* 1988; 59:44–51.
37. Brooks PC, Clark RA, Cheresh DA. Requirement of vascular integrin alpha v beta 3 for angio-genesis. *Science* 1994; 264:569–571.
38. Brooks PC, Montgomery AM, Rosenfeld M, Reisfeld RA, Hu T, Klier G, Cheresh DA. Integrin alpha v beta 3 antagonists promote tumor regression by inducing apoptosis of angiogenic blood vessels. *Cell* 1994; 79:1157–1164.
39. Ingber DE, Madri JA, Folkman J. Extracellular matrix regulates endothelial growth factor action through modulation of cell and nuclear expansion. *In Vitro Cell Dev Biol* 1987; 23: 387–394.
40. Ingber DE, Folkman J. Mechanochemical switching between growth and differentiation during fibroblast growth factor-stimulated angiogenesis in vitro: role of extracellular matrix. *J Cell Biol* 1989; 109:317–330.
41. Ingber DE. Fibronectin controls capillary endothelial cell growth by modulating cell shape. *Proc Natl Acad Sci USA* 1990; 87:3579–3583.
42. Ingber DE, Prusty D, Frangione J, Cragoe EJ Jr, Lechene C, Schwartz M. Control of in-tracellular pH and growth by fibronectin in capillary endothelial cells. *J Cell Biol* 1990; 110: 1803–1812.
43. Ingber DE. Extracellular matrix as a solid state regulator of angiogenesis: identification of new targets for anti-cancer therapy. *Semin Cancer Biol* 1992; 3:57–63.
44. D'Amato RJ, Loughnan MS, Flynn E, Folkman J. Thalidomide is an inhibitor of angiogenesis. *Proc Natl Acad Sci USA* 1994; 91:4082–4085.
45. Folkman J, Weisz PB, Joullic MM, Li WW, Ewing WR. Control of angiogenesis with synthetic heparin substitutes. *Science* 1989; 243:1490–1493.
46. Crum R, Szabo S, and Folkman J. A new class of steroids inhibits angiogenesis in the presence of heparin or a heparin fragment. *Science* 1985; 230:1375–1378.
47. Folkman J, Ingber DE. Angiostatic steroids: method of discovery and mechanism of action. *Ann Surg* 1987; 206:373,374.
48. Li WW, Casey R, Gonzalez EM, Folkman J. Angiostatic steroids potentiated by sulfated cyclo-dextrins inhibit corneal neovascularization. *Invest Ophthalmol Vis Sci* 1991; 32:2898–2905.
49. Hobson B, Denekamp J. Endothelial proliferation in tumours and normal tissues: continuous labelling studies. *Br J Cancer* 1984; 49:405–413.
50. Fotsis T, Pepper M, Adlercreutz H, Fleischmann G, Hase T, Montesano R, Schweigerer L. Genistein, a dietary-derived inhibitor of in vitro angiogenesis. *Proc Natl Acad Sci USA* 1993; 90:2690–2694.
51. D'Amato RJ, Lin CM, Flynn E, Folkman J, Hamel E. 2-Methoxyestradiol, an endogenous mammalian metabolite, inhibits tubulin polymerization by interacting at the colchicine site. *Proc Natl Acad Sci USA* 1994; 91:3964–3968.
52. Ingber DE, Madri JA, Jamieson JD. Role of basal lamina in the neoplastic disorganization of tissue architecture. *Proc Natl Acad Sci USA* 1981; 78:3901–3905.
53. Ingber DE, Madri JA, Jamieson JD. Basement membrane as a spatial organizer of polarized epithelia: exogenous basement membrane reorients pancreatic epithelial tumor cells in vitro. *Am J Pathol* 1986; 122:129–139.
54. Ingber DE, Jamieson JD. Cells as tensegrity structures: architectural regulation of histodifferen-

tiation by physical forces transduced over basement membrane. In: Andersson LC, Gahmberg CG, Ekblom P, eds. *Gene Expression During Normal and Malignant Differentiation*. Orlando, FL: Academic. 1985:13–32.

55. Folkman J, Moscona A. Role of cell shape in growth control. *Nature* 1978; 273:345–349.
56. Kusaka M, Sudo K, Fujita T, Marui S, Itoh F, Ingber DE, Folkman J. Potent antiangiogenic action of AGM-1470: comparison to the fumagillin parent. *Biochem Biophys Res Commun* 1991; 174:1070–1076.
57. Kusaka M, Sudo K, Matsutani E, Kozai Y, Marui S, Fujita T, Ingber D, Folkman J. Cytostatic inhibition of endothelial cell growth by the angiogenesis inhibitor, TNP-470 (AGM-1470). *Br J Cancer* 1994; 69:212–216.
58. Hori A, Ikeyama S, Sudo K. Suppression of cyclin D1 mRNA expression by the angiogenesis inhibitor TNP-470 (AGM-1470) in vascular endothelial cells. *Biochem Biophys Res Commun* 1994; 204:1067–1073.
59. Brem H, Ingber D, Blood CH, Bradley D, Urioste S, Folkman J. Suppression of tumor metastasis by angiogenesis inhibition. *Surg Forum* 1992; 42:439–441.
60. Brem H, Gresser I, Grosfeld J, Folkman J. The combination of antiangiogenic agents to inhibit primary tumor growth and metastasis. *J Pediatr Surg* 1993; 28:1253–1257.
61. Kamei S, Okada H, Inoue Y, Yoshioka T, Ogawa Y, and Toguchi H. Antitumor effects of angiogenesis inhibitor TNP-470 in rabbits bearing VX-2 carcinoma by arterial administration of microspheres and oil solution. *J Pharmacol Exp Ther* 1993; 264:469–474.
62. Kato T, Sato K, Kakinuma H, Matsuda Y. Enhanced suppression of tumor growth by combination of angiogenesis inhibitor O-(chloroacetyl-carbamoyl)fumagillol (TNP-470) and cytotoxic agents in mice. *Cancer Res* 1994; 54:5143–5147.
63. Morita T, Shinohara N, Tokue A. Antitumour effect of a synthetic analogue of fumagillin on murine renal carcinoma. *Br J Urol* 1994; 74:416–421.
64. Takechi A. Effect of angiogenesis inhibitor TNP-470 on vascular formation in pituitary tumors induced by estrogen in rats. *Neurol Medico-Chirurg* 1994; 34:729–733.
65. Takechi A, Uozumi T, Kawamoto K, Ito A, Kurisu K, Sudo K. Inhibitory effect of TNP-470, a new anti-angiogenic agent, on the estrogen induced rat pituitary tumors. *Anticancer Res* 1994; 14:157–162.
66. Takamiya Y, Brem H, Ojeifo J, Mineta T, Martuza RL. AGM-1470 inhibits the growth of human glioblastoma cells in vitro and in vivo. *Neurosurgery* 1994; 34:869–875.
67. Taki T, Ohnishi T, Arita N, Hiraga S, Saitoh Y, Izumoto S, Mori K, Hayakawa T. Antiproliferative effects of TNP-470 on human malignant glioma in vivo: potent inhibition of tumor angiogenesis. *J Neuro-Oncol* 1994; 19:251–258.
68. Teicher BA, Holden SA, Ara G, Northey D. Response of the FSaII fibrosarcoma to antiangiogenic modulators plus cytotoxic agents. *Anticancer Res* 1993; 13:2101–2106.
69. Teicher BA, Holden SA, Ara G, Sotomayor EA, Huang ZD, Chen YN, Brem H. Potentiation of cytotoxic cancer therapies by TNP-470 alone and with other antiangiogenic agents. *Int J Cancer* 1994; 57:920–925.
70. Toi M, Yamamoto Y, Imazawa T, Takayanagi T, Akutsu K, Tominaga T. Antitumor effect of the angiogenesis inhibitor AGM-1470 and its combination effect with tamoxifen in DMBA induced mammary tumors in rats. *Int J Oncol* 1993; 3:525–528.
71. Yamaoka M, Yamamoto T, Ikeyama S, Sudo K, Fujita T. Angiogenesis inhibitor TNP-470 (AGM-1470) potently inhibits the tumor growth of hormone-independent human breast and prostate carcinoma cell lines. *Cancer Res* 1993; 53:5233–5236.
72. Yamaoka M, Yamamoto T, Masaki T, Ikeyama S, Sudo K, Fujita T. Inhibition of tumor growth and metastasis of rodent tumors by the angiogenesis inhibitor O-(chloroacetyl-carbamoyl)fumagillol (TNP-470; AGM-1470). *Cancer Res* 1993; 53:4262–4267.
73. Yanase T, Tamura M, Fujita K, Kodama S, Tanaka K. Inhibitory effect of angiogenesis inhibitor TNP-470 on tumor growth and metastasis of human cell lines in vitro and in vivo. *Cancer Res* 1993; 53:2566–2570.
74. Yanai S, Okada H, Misaki M, Saito K, Kuge Y, Ogawa Y, Toguchi H. Antitumor activity of a medium-chain triglyceride solution of the angiogenesis inhibitor TNP-470 (AGM-1470) when administered via the hepatic artery to rats bearing Walker 256 carcinosarcoma in the liver. *J Pharmacol Exp Ther* 1994; 271:1267–1273.
75. Yamamoto T, Sudo K, Fujita T. Significant inhibition of endothelial cell growth in tumor

vasculature by an angiogenesis inhibitor, TNP-470 (AGM-1470). *Anticancer Res* 1994; 14:1-3.

76. Tanaka T, Konno H, Matsuda I, Nakamura S, Baba S. Prevention of hepatic metastasis of human colon cancer by angiogenesis inhibitor TNP-470. *Cancer Res* 1995; 55:836-839.

77. Teicher BA, Sotomayor EA, Huang ZD. Antiangiogenic agents potentiate cytotoxic cancer therapies against primary and metastatic disease. *Cancer Res* 1992; 52:6702-6704.

78. White CW, Sondheimer HM, Crouch EC, Wilson H, Fan LL. Treatment of pulmonary hemangiomatosis with recombinant interferon alfa-2a. *New Eng J Med* 1989; 320:1197-1200.

79. Ezekowitz A, Mulliken J, Folkman J. Interferon alpha therapy of haemangiomas in newborns and infants. *Br J Haematol* 1991; 79:67,68.

80. Levy T, Kudelka A, Verschraegen CF, Edwards CL, Freedman RS, Kaplan A, Kieback D, Steger M, Mante R, Gutterman J, Piamsomboon S, Termrungruanglert W, Kavanagh JJ. A Phase I study of TNP-470 administered to patients with advanced squamous cell cancer of the cervix. *Proc Amer Assoc Cancer Res* 1996; 37:166 (Abstract #1140).

15   Antisense Oligonucleotides

Stanley T. Crooke, MD, PhD

CONTENTS

INTRODUCTION
THE ANTISENSE CONCEPT
THE SELECTION OF OPTIMAL RNA RECEPTOR SITES
CHARACTERISTICS OF PHOSPHOROTHIOATE OLIGONUCLEOTIDES
POTENTIAL IN CANCER CHEMOTHERAPY

1. INTRODUCTION

The therapeutic use of oligonucleotides represents a new paradigm for drug discovery. The technology focuses on a class of chemicals, oligonucleotides, that have not been studied as potential drugs before and uses them to intervene in processes that, likewise, have not been studied as sites at which drugs might act. Although the field is still in its infancy, it has generated considerable enthusiasm because of the potential specificity of oligonucleotide drugs and the breadth of potential applications.

The enthusiasm about the technology has been tempered by appropriate reservations concerning the ability of the technology to deliver on its promise. In essence, the questions about the technology reduce to: can oligonucleotide analogs be created that have appropriate properties to be drugs; specifically, what are the pharmocokinetic, pharmacologic, and toxicologic properties of these compounds, and what are the scope and potential of the medicinal chemistry of oligonucleotides? Although much remains to be done, the answers to many of the questions are now available and suggest that the technology may yield important therapeutic advances.

This chapter will focus strictly on the antisense mechanism with particular emphasis on the potential role of this technology in the treatment of cancer.

2. THE ANTISENSE CONCEPT

2.1. History

The antisense concept derives from an understanding of nucleic acid structure and function, and depends on Watson-Crick hybridization (*1*). Thus, arguably, the demonstration that nucleic acid hybridization is feasible (*2*) and the advances in *in situ*

From: *Cancer Therapeutics: Experimental and Clinical Agents*
Edited by: B. Teicher Humana Press Inc., Totowa, NJ

hybridization and diagnostic probe technology (3), lay the most basic elements of the foundation supporting the antisense concept.

However, the first clear enunciation of the concept of exploiting antisense oligonu-cleotides as therapeutic agents was in the work of Zamecnik and Stephenson in 1978 (4). In this publication, these authors reported the synthesis of an oligodeoxyribonu-cleotide 13 nucleotides long that was complementary to a sequence in the respiratory syncitial virus genome. They suggested that this oligonucleotide could be stabilized by 3'- and 5'-terminal modifications, and showed evidence of antiviral activity. More importantly, they discussed possible sites for binding in RNA and mechanisms of action of oligonucleotides.

Though less precisely focused on the therapeutic potential of antisense oligonu-cleotides, the work of Miller and Ts'o and their collaborators during the same period helped establish the foundation for antisense research and re-establish an interest in phosphate backbone modifications as approaches to improve the properties of oligo-nucleotides (5,6). Their focus on methylphosphotriester-modified oligonucleotides as a potential solution to pharmacokinetic limitations of oligonucleotides presaged a good bit of the medicinal chemistry to be performed on oligonucleotides.

Despite the observations of Miller and Ts'o and Zamecnik and colleagues, interest in antisense research was quite limited until the late 1980s, when advances in several areas provided technical solutions to a number of impediments. Since antisense drug design requires an understanding of the sequence of the RNA target, the explosive growth in availability of viral and human genomic sequences provided the informa-tion from which "receptor sequences" could be selected. The development of methods for synthesis of research quantitites of oligonucleotide drugs then supported antisense experiments on both phosphodiester and modified oligonucleotides (7,8). The inception of the third key component (medicinal chemistry) forming the founda-tion of oligonucleotide therapeutics, in fact, was the synthesis in 1969 of phosphoro-thioate poly rI:poly rC as a means of stabilizing the polynucleotide (9). Subsequently, Miller and Ts'o initiated studies on the neutral phosphate analogs, methylphospho-nates (5), and groups at the National Institutes of Health and the Food and Drug Administration and the Worcester Foundation investigated phosphorothioate oligo-nucleotides (10–14). With these advances forming the foundation for oligonucleotide therapeutics and the initial studies suggesting in vitro activities against a number of viral and mammalian targets (12,15–19), interest in oligonucleotide therapeutics in-tensified.

2.2. Strategies to Induce Transcriptional Arrest

An alternative to the inhibition of RNA metabolism and utilization via an anti-sense mechanism is to inhibit transcription by interacting with double-stranded DNA in chromatin. Of the two most obvious binding strategies for oligonucleotides binding to double-stranded nucleic acids, strand invasion and triple-strand formation, triple-stranding strategies, until recently, attracted essentially all of the attention.

Triple helices have been known for polynucleotides since 1957 (20). Triple strands can form via non-Watson-Crick hydrogen bonds between the third strand and purines involved in Watson-Crick hydrogen bonding with the complementary strand of the duplex (for review, see 21). Thus, triple-stranded structures can be formed between a third strand comprised of pyrimidines or purines that interact with a homopurine strand in a homopurine-homopyrimidine strand in a duplex DNA. With the demonstration that homopyrimidine oligonucleotides could indeed form triplex structures (*22–24*), interest in triple-strand approaches to inhibit transcription heightened.

Although there was initially considerable debate about the value of triple-stranding strategies versus antisense approaches (*25*), there was little debate that much work remained to be done to design oligonucleotides that could form triple-stranded structures with duplexes of mixed sequences. Pursuit of several strategies has resulted in significant progress (for review, *see 21*), but resolution of many issues remains to be achieved before triplexing strategies can be used effectively to create pharmacological agents.

Strand invasion, an alternative approach to obstructing transcription by formation of triple strands, has been shown to be feasible if analogs with sufficient affinity can be synthesized. Recently, peptide nucleic acids (PNA) have been shown to have very high affinity and be capable of strand invasion of double-stranded DNA under some conditions (*26*). Again, much remains to be learned about this analog class and other high-affinity analogs before the pharmacological potential of transcriptional arrest via strand invasion is defined.

2.3. Ribozymes and Oligonucleotide-Mediated RNA Cleavage

Ribozymes are RNA molecules that catalyze biochemical reactions (*27*). Ribozymes cleave single-stranded regions of RNA via transesterification of hydrolysis reactions that cleave a phosphodiester bond (*28*). Clearly, a therapeutic oligonucleotide that could specifically bind to and cleave an RNA target should be attractive. Again, however, many technical hurdles must be overcome before modified ribozymes or synthetic oligonucleotides with ribozyme-like activity can be used as drugs.

2.4. Combinatorial Approaches to Oligonucleotide Therapeutics

At least two methods have been published by which oligonucleotides have been identified to interact with cellular proteins by combinatorial methods (*29–31*). The potential advantage of a combinatorial approach is that oligonucleotide-based molecules can be prepared to adopt various structures that support binding to nonnucleic acid targets as well as nucleic acid targets. These can then be screened for potential activities without knowledge about the cause of the disease or the structure of the target.

2.5. The Medicinal Chemistry of Oligonucleotides

Because it was apparent almost immediately that native phosphodiester oligodeoxy- or ribonucleotides are unsatisfactory as drugs because of rapid degradation (*32*), a variety of modifications have been prepared. As previously mentioned, perhaps the most interesting of the initial modifications were the phosphate analogs, the phosphorothioates (*9*) and the methylphosphonates (*5*). Both fully modified oligonucleotides and oligonucleotides "capped" at the 3'- and/or 5'-termini with phosphorothioate or methylphosphonate moieties were tested (*33*). However, studies from many laboratories demonstrated that capped oligonucleotides were relatively rapidly degraded in cells (*34–37*), nor were point modifications with intercalators that enhanced binding to RNA (*38,39*), cholesterol (*40*), or poly-L-lysine (*41,42*) sufficiently active or selective to warrant broad-based exploration.

Since the initial approaches to modifications of oligonucleotides, an enormous range of modifications, including novel bases, sugars, backbones, conjugates, and chimeric oligonucleotides, have been tested (for review, *see 43,44*). Many of these

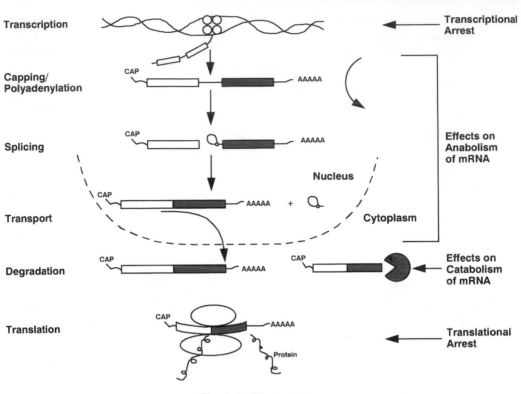

Fig. 1. RNA processing.

modifications have proven to be quite useful and are progressing in testing leading to clinical trials.

2.6. Pharmacological Rationalization of Therapeutic Oligonucleotides

Of central importance to the long-term future of therapeutic oligonucleotides has been the rationalization of oligonucleotides in the context of modern pharmacology (*45*). Progress has been gratifying in that most of the fundamental concerns about oligonucleotides are now answered. These include such issues as questions about the kinetics and characteristics of oligonucleotides binding to RNA targets, proof of activity and mechanism of action in vitro and in vivo, pharmacokinetic and toxicologic properties of oligonucleotides, and the breadth and value of oligonucleotide medicinal chemistry. With six oligonucleotides in clinical trials, numerous demonstrations of potent systemic activities in animals, and clarification of potential toxicities and the therapeutic index of phosphorothioate oligonucleotides, it is reasonable to conclude that substantial progress has been achieved.

2.7. RNA Intermediary Metabolism

Oligonucleotides are designed to modulate the information transfer from the gene to protein—in essence, to alter the intermediary metabolism of RNA. Figure 1 summarizes these processes.

RNA intermediary metabolism is initiated with transcription. The transcription initiation complex contains proteins that recognize specific DNA sequences and locally denature double-stranded DNA, thus allowing a member of the RNA polymerase family to transcribe one strand of the DNA (the antisense strand) into a sense pre-mRNA molecule. Usually during transcription, the 5'-end of the pre-mRNA is capped by adding a methyl-guanosine, and most often by methylation of one or two adjacent sugar residues. This enhances the stability of the pre-mRNA and may play a role in a number of key RNA processing events (46). Between the 5'-cap and the site at which translation is initiated is usually a stretch of nucleotides (5'-untranslated region, 5'-UTR). This area may play a key role in regulating mRNA half-life (47).

Similarly, the 3'-end of the pre-mRNA usually has a stretch of several hundred nucleotides beyond the translation termination signal. This area often plays an important role in determining mRNA half-life. Moreover, posttranscriptionally, most pre-mRNA species are polyadenylated. Polyadenylation stabilizes the RNA, is important in transport of mature mRNA out of the nucleus, and may play important roles in the cytoplasm as well (48,49).

Because eukaryotic genes usually contain intervening sequences (introns), most pre-mRNA species must have these sequences excised and the mature RNA spliced together. Splicing reactions are complex, highly regulated, and involve specific sequences, small-mol-wt RNA species, and numerous proteins. Alternative splicing processes are often used to produce different mature mRNAs and, thus, different proteins. Even though introns are often considered waste, important sequences are conserved, and some introns may play a variety of regulatory roles.

Mature mRNA is exported to the cytoplasm and engages in translation. mRNA half lives vary from a few minutes to many hours, and appears to be highly regulated (47).

Each step shown in the pathway is a composite of numerous steps and is theoretically amenable to intervention with oligonucleotides. For virtually no mRNA is the pathway fully defined; however, available information is insufficient to determine the rate-limiting steps in the intermediary metabolism of any mRNA species (50,51).

2.8. Factors Influencing Antisense Activity

2.8.1. Affinity

The affinity of oligonucleotides for their receptor sequences results from hybridization interactions. The two major contributors to the free energy of binding are hydrogen bonding (usually Watson-Crick base pairing) and base stacking in the double helix that is formed. Affinity is affected by ionic strength. In general, the higher the ionic strength, the higher the affinity of charged oligonucleotides for polynucleotides. As affinity results from hydrogen bond formation between bases and stacking occurs between coplanar bases, affinity increases as the length of the oligonucleotide receptor complex increases. Thus, the affinity per nucleotide unit and the number of hybridizing nucleotide pairs are crucial determinants of overall affinity. Affinity also varies as a function of the sequence in the duplex. Nearest neighbor rules allow the prediction of the free energy binding for DNA–DNA and RNA–RNA hybrids with relatively high precision (52,53). A common misconception is that DNA–RNA duplexes are more stable than DNA–DNA duplexes. In fact, the relative stability of these duplexes varies as a function of the sequence. RNA–RNA duplexes are typically the most stable (S. M. Freier, unpublished results).

As with other drug–receptor interactions, activity requires a minimum level of affinity. For many targets and types of oligonucleotides, the minimum length of an oligonucleotide may be 12–14 nucleotides.

Although theoretical affinities for oligonucleotide–single-strand nucleic acid interactions are very large, in practice, affinity constants are substantially lower. Several factors contribute to the differences between theoretical and realized affinities. Undoubtedly, the most important factor is that RNA can adopt a variety of secondary structures (for review, *see 54*). In addition to secondary structure, RNA can adopt tertiary structures. Tertiary structures result from the interactions of secondary structures in an RNA molecule with other secondary structural elements or single-stranded regions (*55*). A third factor that can potentially reduce the affinity of an oligonucleotide for its RNA receptor is that oligonucleotides can form secondary and tertiary structures themselves. To avoid duplex formation, oligonucleotides that contain self-complementary regions are usually not employed. However, other structures that were not well understood or expected have recently been described. Tetrameric complexes formed by oligonucleotides with multiple guanosines (*29,56–58*) and other base sequences (*59*) can be highly stable, clearly would prevent an antisense interaction, and have a number of biological effects that have confounded interpretation of experiments.

Since RNA and oligonucleotide structures are affected by ionic milieu and nonproductive interactions with proteins and polycations, the in vivo situation is, of course, considerably more complicated. Relatively little is understood about the interplay among all these factors and their effects on the true affinities of oligonucleotides for potential RNA targets.

2.8.2. SPECIFICITY FOR NUCLEIC ACID SEQUENCES

Specificity derives from the selectivity of Watson-Crick or other types of base pairing. The decrease in affinity associated with a mismatched base pair varies as a function of the specific mismatch, the position of the mismatch in a region of complementarity, and the sequence surrounding the mismatch. In a typical interaction between complementary 18-mers, the $\triangle\triangle G_{37}^{\circ}$ or change in Gibbs free energy of binding induced by a single mismatch varies from $+0.2$ to $+4.0$ kcal/mol/modification at 100 mM NaCl. Thus, a single base mismatch could result in a change in affinity of approx 500-fold (*60*). Modifications of oligonucleotides may alter specificity.

At the genomic level, any sequence of 17 residues is expected to occur only once (*61*). Assuming a random distribution of sequences in RNA, any sequence of 13 residues is expected to occur once in the cellular RNA population and, if the nonrandom nature of mammalian RNA sequence is taken into account, an 11-mer oligonucleotide or perhaps smaller could identify and bind to a unique sequence (*62,63*).

To exploit fully the theoretical potential for specificity of an oligonucleotide in a therapeutic context, it is necessary to manipulate the length of the oligonucleotide and its concentration at target. The results of such an exercise have been reported (*64*). In this study, phosphorothioate oligodeoxynucleotides were designed to target the normal or codon 12-point mutation of Ha-*ras* mRNA. Predictions from hybridization experiments suggested that approximately a fivefold specificity for mutant compared to normal Ha-*ras* RNA was possible. By optimizing oligonucleotide length and the extracellular concentration of the oligonucleotide, nearly theoretical specificity was achieved in cells in tissue culture.

Other factors can also be used to enhance specificity. RNA secondary and tertiary structure assures that not all sequences are equally accessible. Design of oligonucleotides to interact with sequences involved in maintenance of RNA structure can theoretically enhance specificity and, if the structure is essential to the stability or function of the RNA, potency. Furthermore, many RNA and DNA sequences interact with proteins, again assuring far more diversity in response to an oligonucleotide and, therefore, greater specificity than might be predicted solely on the basis of differences in nucleic acid sequence.

2.8.3. THERAPEUTIC SPECIFICITY (THERAPEUTIC INDEX)

Clearly, in a therapeutic context, the ability of an oligonucleotide to bind selectively to specific sequences in nucleic acid targets is an important factor in determining its therapeutic index. However, oligonucleotides and analogs can interact with other cellular components, and these interactions can have significant effects on the therapeutic index of oligonucleotides. The factors that determine the significance of nonnucleic interactions of oligonucleotides on the therapeutic index include the affinities for nonnucleic acid sites vs nucleic acids, the numbers of different nonnucleic acid binding sites, the concentrations of each of the binding sites, the biological importance of various binding sites, and kinetic factors. These are, of course, conceptually equivalent to the factors that affect the therapeutic index of drugs of all classes, but very little is understood about these potential interactions.

Chemical classes of oligonucleotides differ in their tendency to interact with various nonnucleic acid targets. For example, phosphorothioates tend to bind to a wide range of proteins with relatively low affinity (36). Nevertheless, detailed in vitro and in vivo toxicological studies have shown that these interactions probably reduce the therapeutic index of phosphorothioates less than perhaps was expected (44,65). We believe that this is owing to the fact that the phosphorothioates bind with very low affinity to a larger number of proteins and their potential toxic effects are consequently "buffered."

2.9. Mechanisms of Action of Antisense Oligonucleotides

The mechanisms by which interactions of oligonucleotides with nucleic acids may induce biological effects are complex and potentially numerous. Furthermore, very little is currently understood about the roles of various mechanisms or the factors that may determine which mechanisms are involved after oligonucleotides bind to their receptor sequences. Consequently, a discussion of mechanisms remains largely theoretical.

2.9.1. OCCUPANCY-ONLY MEDIATED MECHANISMS

Classic competitive antagonists are thought to alter biological activities because they bind to receptors preventing natural agonists from binding and inducing normal biological processes. Binding of oligonucleotides to specific sequences may inhibit the interaction of the RNA or DNA with proteins, other nucleic acids, or other factors required for essential steps in the intermediary metabolism of the RNA or its utilization by the cell.

2.9.1.1. Inhibition of Splicing. A key step in the intermediary metabolism of most mRNA molecules is the excision of introns. These "splicing" reactions are sequence-specific and require the concerted action of spliceosomes. Consequently, oligonucleotides that bind to sequences required for splicing may prevent binding of necessary factors or physically prevent the required cleavage reactions. This then would result in inhibition of the production of the mature mRNA. Although there are several examples of oligonucleotides directed to splice junctions, none of the studies presented data showing inhibition of RNA processing, accumulation of splicing intermediates, or a reduction in mature mRNA, nor are there published data in which the structure of the RNA at the splice junction was probed and the oligonucleotides demonstrated to hybridize to the sequences for which they were designed (*66–69*). Activities have been reported for anti-c-*myc* and antiviral oligonucleotides with phosphodiester, methylphosphonate, and phosphorothioate backbones. Very recently, an oligonucleotide was reported to induce alternative splicing in a cell-free splicing system, and in that system, RNA analyses confirmed the putative mechanism (*70*).

2.9.1.2. Translational Arrest. The mechanism for which the majority of oligonucleotides have been designed is translational arrest by binding to the translation initiation codon. The positioning of the initiation codon within the area of complementarity of the oligonucleotide and the length of oligonucleotide used have varied considerably. Again, unfortunately, only in relatively few studies have the oligonucleotides, in fact, been shown to bind to the sites for which they were designed, and other data that support translation arrest as the mechanism have not been reported.

Target RNA species that have been reported to be inhibited include HIV (*71*), vesicular stomatitis virus (VSV) (*72*), n-*myc* (*73*), and a number of normal cellular genes (*74–77*).

In our laboratories, we have shown that a significant number of targets may be inhibited by binding to translation initiation codons. For example, ISIS 1082 hybridizes to the AUG codon for the UL13 gene of herpes virus types 1 and 2. RNase H studies confirmed that it binds selectively in this area. In vitro protein synthesis studies confirmed that it inhibited the synthesis of the UL13 protein, and studies in HeLa cells showed that it inhibited the growth of herpes type 1 and type 2 with an IC_{50} of 200–400 n*M* by translation arrest (*78*). Similarly, ISIS 1753, a 30-mer phosphorothioate complementary to the translation initiation codon and surrounding sequences of the E2 gene of bovine papilloma virus, was highly effective, and its activity was shown to be owing to translation arrest. ISIS 2105, a 20-mer phosphorothioate complementary to the same region in human papilloma virus, was shown to be a very potent inhibitor. Compounds complementary to the translation initiation codon of the E2 gene were the most potent of the more than 50 compounds studied complementary to various other regions in the RNA (*79*). We have shown inhibition of translation of a number of other mRNA species by compounds designed to bind to the translation codon as well.

In conclusion, translation arrest represents an important mechanism of action for antisense drugs. A number of examples purporting to employ this mechanism have been reported, and recent studies on several compounds have provided data that unambiguously demonstrate that this mechanism can result in potent antisense drugs.

2.9.1.3. Disruption of Necessary RNA Structure. RNA adopts a variety of three-dimensional structures induced by intramolecular hybridization, the most common of which is the stem loop. These structures play crucial roles in a variety of functions. They are used to provide additional stability for RNA and as recognition motifs for a number of proteins, nucleic acids, and ribonucleoproteins that participate in the intermediary metabolism and activities of RNA species. Thus, given the potential general utility of the mechanism, it is surprising that occupancy-based disruption RNA has not been more extensively exploited.

As an example, we designed a series of oligonucleotides that bind to the important stem-loop present in all RNA species in HIV, the TAR element. We synthesized a number of oligonucleotides designed to disrupt TAR, and showed that several indeed did bind to TAR, disrupt the structure, and inhibit TAR-mediated production of a reporter gene (*31*). Furthermore, general rules useful in disrupting stem-loop structures were developed as well (*80*).

Although designed to induce relatively nonspecific cytotoxic effects, two other examples are noteworthy. Oligonucleotides designed to bind to a 17-nucleotide loop in *Xenopus* 28 S RNA required for ribosome stability and protein synthesis inhibited protein synthesis when injected into *Xenopus oocytes* (*81*). Similarly, oligonucleotides designed to bind to highly conserved sequences in 5.8 S RNA inhibited protein synthesis in rabbit reticulocyte and wheat germ systems (*82*).

2.9.2. OCCUPANCY-ACTIVATED DESTABILIZATION

RNA molecules regulate their own metabolism. A number of structural features of RNA are known to influence stability, various processing events, subcellular distribution, and transport. It is likely that, as RNA intermediary metabolism is better understood, many other regulatory features and mechanisms will be identified.

2.9.2.1. 5′-Capping. A key early step in RNA processing is 5′-capping (Fig. 1). This stabilizes pre-mRNA and is important for the stability of mature mRNA. It also is important in binding to the nuclear matrix and transport of mRNA out of the nucleus. Since the structure of the cap is unique and understood, it presents an interesting target.

Several oligonucleotides that bind near the cap site have been shown to be active, presumably by inhibiting the binding of proteins required to cap the RNA. For example, the synthesis of SV40 T-antigen was reported to be most sensitive to an oligonucleotide linked to poly-L-lysine and targeted to the 5′-cap site of RNA (*83*). However, again, in no published study has this putative mechanism been rigorously demonstrated. In fact, in no published study have the oligonucleotides been shown to bind to the sequences for which they were designed.

In studies in our laboratory, we have designed oligonucleotides to bind to 5′-cap structures and reagents to cleave specifically the unique 5′-cap structure (*84*). These studies demonstrated that 5′-cap-targeted oligonucleotides were capable of inhibiting the binding of the translation initiation factor eIF-4α (*85*).

2.9.2.2. Inhibition of 3′-Polyadenylation. In the 3′-untranslated regions of pre-mRNA molecules are sequences that result in the posttranscriptional addition of long (hundreds of nucleotides) tracts of polyadenylate. Polyadenylation stabilizes mRNA and may play other roles in the intermediary metabolism of RNA species. Theoretically, interactions in the 3′-terminal region of pre-mRNA could inhibit polyadenylation and destabilize the RNA species. Although there are a number of oligonucleotides that interact in the 3′-untranslated region and display antisense activities (*86*), to date, no study has reported evidence for alterations in polyadenylation.

2.9.2.3. Other Mechanisms. In addition to 5′-capping and 3′-adenylation, there are clearly other sequences in the 5′- and 3′-untranslated regions of mRNA that affect the stability, localization, and translatability of the molecules. Again, there are a number of antisense drugs that may work by interfering with these processes.

2.9.3. ACTIVATION OF RNASE H

RNase H is an ubiquitous enzyme that degrades the RNA strand of an RNA–DNA duplex. It has been identified in organisms as diverse as viruses and human cells (for review, *see 87*). At least two classes of RNase H have been identified in eukaryotic cells. Multiple enzymes with RNase H activity have been observed in prokaryotics (*87*). Furthermore, there are data that suggest that in eukaryotic cells, there are multiple isozymes.

Although RNase H is involved in DNA replication, it may play other roles in the cells and is found in the cytoplasm as well as the nucleus (*88*). However, the concentration of the enzyme in the nucleus is thought to be greater, and some of the enzyme found in cytoplasmic preparations may be the result of nuclear leakage.

RNase H activity is quite variable. It is absent or minimal in rabbit reticulocytes (*89*), but present in wheat germ extracts (*87*). In HL60 cells, for example, the level of activity in undifferentiated cells is greatest, relatively high in DMSO and vitamin D-differentiated cells, and much lower in PMA-differentiated cells (Hoke, unpublished data).

The precise recognition elements for RNase H are not known. However, it has been shown that oligonucleotides with DNA-like properties as short as tetramers can activate RNase H (*90*). Changes in the sugar influence RNase H activation as sugar modifications that result in RNA-like oligonucleotides, e.g., 2′-fluoro- or 2′-*O*-methyl does not appear to serve as a substrate for RNase H (*91,92*). Alterations in the orientation of the sugar to the base can also affect RNase H activation, since α-oligonucleotides are unable to serve as substrates for RNase H or may require parallel annealing (*93,94*). Additionally, backbone modifications influence the ability of oligonucleotides to activate RNase H. Methylphosphonates do not serve as RNase H substrates (*95,96*). In contrast, phosphorothioates are excellent substrates (*78,97,98;* Hoke, unpublished data). Chimeric oligonucleotides that bind to RNA and activate RNase H have been studied (*99,100*). For example, oligonucleotides comprised of wings of 2′-*O*-methyl sugars and methylphosphonate backbone and a 5-base gap of deoxyoligonucleotides bind to their target RNA and activate RNase H (*99,100*). Furthermore, a single ribonucleotide in a sequence of deoxyribonucleotides was shown to be sufficient to serve as a substrate for RNase H when bound to its complementary deoxyoligonucleotide (*101*).

That it is possible to take advantage of chimeric oligonucleotides designed to activate RNase H and have greater affinity for their RNA receptors and to enhance specificity has also been demonstrated (*102,103*). In a recent study, RNase H-mediated cleavage of target transcript was much more selective when deoxyoligonucleotides comprised of methylphosphonate deoxyoligonucleotide wings and phosphodiester gaps were compared to full phosphodiester oligonucleotides (*103*).

Despite the information about RNase H and the demonstrations that many oligonucleotides may serve as RNase H substrates in lysate and purified enzyme asasys (*104–106*), relatively little is yet known about the role of structural features in RNA targets in activating RNase H and direct proof that RNase H activation is, in fact, the mechanism of action of oligonucleotides in cells.

Recent studies in our laboratories provide additional, although indirect, insights into these questions. ISIS 1939 is a 20-mer phosphorothioate complementary to a sequence in the 3′-untranslated region of ICAM-1 RNA (*86*). It inhibits ICAM-1 production in human umbilical vein endothelial cells, and Northern blots demonstrate that ICAM-1 mRNA is rapidly degraded. A 2'-O-methyl analog of ISIS 1939 displays higher affinity for the RNA than the phosphorothioate, is stable in cells, but inhibits ICAM-1 protein production much less potently than ISIS 1939. It is likely that ISIS 1939 destabilizes the RNA and activates RNase H. In contrast, ISIS 1570, an 18-mer phosphorothioate that is complementary to the translation initiation codon of the ICAM-1 message, inhibited production of the protein, but caused no degradation of the RNA. Thus, two oligonucleotides that are capable of activating RNase H had different effects depending on the site in the mRNA at which they bound (86).

2.9.4. COVALENT MODIFICATION OF THE TARGET NUCLEIC ACID BY THE OLIGONUCLEOTIDE

A large number of oligonucleotides conjugated by alkylating and photoactivable alkylating species have been synthesized and tested for effects on purified nucleic acids and intracellular nucleic acid targets (106–111). The potential disadvantages are obvious: non-specific alkylation may occur in vivo and result in toxicities.

A variety of alkylating agents have been used to modify covalently single-stranded DNA and shown to induce alkylation at sequences predicted by the complementary oligonucleotide to which they were attached (107–111). Similar alkylators have been employed to modify covalently double-stranded DNA after triplex formation (112–115).

Photoactivable crosslinkers and platinates have been coupled to oligonucleotides and shown to crosslink sequence specifically as well. Photoactivable crosslinkers coupled to phosphodiesters, methylphosphonates, and phosphorothioates have been shown to produce sequence-specific crosslinking (116–123). Photoreactive crosslinking has also been demonstrated for double-stranded DNA after triplex formation (124,125).

Preliminary data suggesting that covalent modifications of nucleic acids in cells are feasible and may enhance the potency of oligonucleotides have also been reported. Psoralen-linked methylphosphonate oligonucleotides were reported to be significantly more potent than methylphosphonate oligonucleotides in inhibiting rabbit globin mRNA in rabbit reticulocyte lysate assay (126). Psoralen-linked methylphosphonates were also reported to be more potent in inhibiting herpes simplex virus infection in HeLa cells in tissue culture (67). Additionally, although not producing covalent modification a 9-mer phosphodiester conjugated with an intercalator inhibited mutant Ha-*ras* synthesis in T-24 bladder carcinoma cells (127).

2.9.5. OLIGONUCLEOTIDE-INDUCED CLEAVAGE OF NUCLEIC ACID TARGETS

Another attractive mechanism by which the potency of oligonucleotides might be increased is to synthesize derivatives that cleave their nucleic acid targets directly. Several potential chemical mechanisms are being studied and positive results have been reported.

The mechanism that has been most broadly studied is to conjugate oligonucleotides to chelators of redox-active metals and generate free radicals that can cleave nucleic acids. Dervan and colleagues have developed EDTA-conjugated oligonucleotides that cleave double-stranded DNA sequence specifically after triplex formation (22,128). Dervan and others have also employed EDTA-oligonucleotide conjugates to cleave single-stranded DNA (129,130). It is thought that EDTA-chelated iron generates hydroxyl radicals via a fenton-like reaction that cleaves the DNA. However, the cleavage occurs at several oligonucleotides near the nucleotide at which EDTA is attached rather than with absolute specificity.

In the presence of copper, oligonucleotides conjugated to 2,10 phenanthroline also cleave DNA via a free radical mechanism with some sequence specificity (*131–135*) as do porphyrin-linked oligonucleotides when exposed to light (*136–138*). Porphyrin-linked oligonucleotides, however, oxidize bases and induce crosslinks, as well as cleave the phosphodiester backbone.

To date, no reports have demonstrated selective cleavage of an RNA or enhanced potency of oligonucleotides in cells using oligonucleotides with cleaving moieties that employ these mechanisms. However, it seems likely that studies in progress in a number of laboratories will explore this question shortly.

To date, no reports have demonstrated selective cleavage of an RNA or enhanced potency of oligonucleotides in cells using oligonucleotides with cleaving moieties that employ these mechanisms. However, it seems likely that studies in progress in a number of laboratories will explore this question shortly.

Another mechanism that may be intrinsically more attractive for therapeutic applications, particularly for cleavage of RNA targets, is a mechanism analogous to that used by many ribonucleases, nucleotidyltransferases, phosphotransferases, and ribozymes. Ribozymes are oligoribonucleotides or RNA species capable of cleaving themselves or other RNA molecules (*139*). Furthermore, the Tetrahymena ribozyme has been shown to cleave DNA, but at a slower rate than RNA (*134*). Although several classes of ribozymes have been identified and differ with regard to substrate specificity, the use of internal or external guanosine, and other characteristics, they all employ similar enzymatic mechanisms. Cleavage and ligation involve a Mg^{2+}-dependent transesterification with nucleophilic attack by the 3'-hydroxyl of guanosine (*140*).

Significant progress in achieving a number of key objectives that may result in the therapeutic application of ribozymes has been reported. In addition to studies to understand the basic mechanisms by which ribozymes cleave RNA (*141*), progress in reducing the size of ribozymes and stabilizing them has been reported. A hammerhead ribozyme (*142*) that has been reduced to a minimum length of 22 nucleotides has been shown to cleave RNA (*143*). Most ribonucleotides in several ribozymes have been shown to be nonessential and have been replaced by deoxynucleotides that may stabilize the ribozyme against RNases (*144,145*). Phosphorothioate moieties have been substituted in various positions without loss of activity (*146*). By substituting 2'-fluoro-2'-deoxy uridine for pyrimidines in the conserved region of a hammerhead ribozyme and four phosphorothioate moieties at the 3'-end of the ribozyme, a ribozyme that was as active at the parent ribozyme and stable in undiluted fetal calf serum was reported (*147*). Additionally, a ribozyme containing 2'-fluoro or 2'-amino nucleotides at all pyrimidine positions was reported to be highly active and stable in fetal calf serum (*148*). Other ribozymes containing 2'-modified adenosines and one with 2'-methoxy substituents in a contiguous oligonucleotide have been reported (*149,150*). Thus, it would appear that there is some scope for the application of medicinal chemistry to improve the pharmacokinetic properties of ribozymes.

Although the therapeutic utility of modified synthetic ribozymes is yet to be reported, the progress in this area is gratifying and suggests that this may be a viable approach.

Another approach to the exploitation of ribozyme activities involves the synthesis of oligonucleotides complementary to a target RNA and linked to a sequence that can serve as an external guide sequence for RNase P. RNase P is an enzyme that contains a catalytic RNA (ribozyme) and uses a highly conserved sequence, the external guide sequence, to direct the catalytic RNA to the site of cleavage (*151*). Oligonucleotides incorporating an external guide sequence and expressed by transfection of appropriate plasmids were reported to cause RNase P cleavage of the RNA for chloroamiphenical acetyl transferase (*152*). Thus, it would seem feasible to design stabilized oligonucleotides with external guide sequences that could be employed as drugs.

The notion that a relatively small oligonucleotide could be designed that could interact with and cleave desired sequences as do ribozymes was given impetus by studies that showed activity for ribozymes as short as a 19-mer (*153*) and the demonstration that ribozyme activity can be retained after substitutions, such as phosphorothioates, are introduced (*140*). Consequently, creating oligonucleotides that cleave RNA targets by synthesizing oligonucleotides with appropriate tethers and functionalities positioned to catalyze degradation via acid-base mechanisms (Cook, unpublished data) is an attractive possibility.

2.9.6. CONCLUSIONS

In conclusion, an array of potential postbinding mechanisms has already been identified for oligonucleotides. However, for specific oligonucleotides, insufficient data are available to draw firm conclusions about mechanism, and it is likely that more than one mechanism may play a role in the activity of a given oligonucleotide.

Perhaps more importantly, it is clear that many additional mechanisms are likely to be identified as progress continues. It is important to consider the structure and function of receptor sequences in designing oligonucleotides, and to continue to study potential mechanisms in detail. Clearly, RNase H may play a role in the mechanisms of many oligonucleotides, but equally clearly, it is not critical for the activity of others. In the future, the mechanisms (and resulting efficacy) for which oligonucleotides are designed will probably be optimized for each drug target and chemical class of oligonucleotide.

3. THE SELECTION OF OPTIMAL RNA RECEPTOR SITES

The antisense mechanism begins with the binding of an oligonucleotide to a pre-mRNA or mRNA species via Watson-Crick hybridization. In essence then, antisense oligonucleotides are designed to alter the intermediary metabolism of RNA as described in the previous section. Therefore, at least four factors might influence the receptor sequence that results in the greatest antisense activity: accessibility of receptor sequences to oligonucleotide, RNA structure and the functions of the various structures, terminating mechanism of the oligonucleotide, and chemical properties of the oligonucleotide.

3.1. Factors Influencing Receptor Sequence Accessibility

3.1.1. INTERACTIONS WITH PROTEINS AND OTHER NUCLEIC ACIDS

It is generally accepted that each RNA molecule interacts with multiple proteins at multiple sites, and that there are specialized sequences that interact with selected proteins and other nucleic acids. However, there is relatively little information about the overall accessibility of receptor sites in RNA species or the kinetics of the numerous interactions that must take place between an RNA molecule and other cellular components as the RNA is processed and used. Moreover, there are likely multiple poorly understood cellular processes that affect targeting of antisense drugs that are even yet to be considered. For example, a number of studies have demonstrated that RNA species may be localized to different subcellular compartments. In addition to the obvious compartmentation into nuclear, nucleolar, and cytoplasmic loci, RNA species have been reported to be sorted into a number of different cytoplasmic sites, and this sorting has significant effects on the translation of the mRNA, the half-life, and other properties of the RNA (154,155). Clearly, such events should have a profound influence on the potential effects of antisense drugs. Consequently, the search for optimal sites for antisense interactions has been largely empirical, and at present, meaningful generalizations are not possible. Nevertheless, enough information has been developed to emphasize the complexity of these issues and their effects on antisense drug actions.

3.1.2. THE OPTIMAL ANTISENSE SITE VARIES AS A FUNCTION OF THE RNA SPECIES

To determine whether the pattern of sites that are most sensitive to antisense effects varies depending on the RNA species, it is necessary to study a series of oligonucleotides of the same chemical class that have approximately equivalent theoretical affinities for their target sequences and have equivalent terminating mechanisms against a number of RNA species. We chose to study phosphorothioate oligodeoxynucleotides 20 nucleotides in length against a large number of RNA targets. Each RNA target was "scanned" using one or two concentrations of oligonucleotides targeted to various regions, and then for many oligonucleotides, full-dose response and time-course studies were performed.

Figure 2 shows the effects of phosphorothioate oligonucleotides targeted to different regions in two RNAs, ICAM, and E-selectin. As can be seen, even for oligonucleotides of a single chemical class with equivalent affinities and the ability to terminate RNA activity by serving as substrates for RNase H, enormous variations in potency was observed, depending on the position in the RNA targeted (86,156–158). For example, ISIS 2679 is a potent inhibitor of E-selectin production. Yet ISIS 2687, positioned a few nucleotides from ISIS 2679, is nearly inactive. Similar studies have been performed in our laboratories on many mammalian and viral genes, and the only generalization that is currently supported is that each RNA target (even closely related isotypes) is different. Table 1 represents a qualitative summary of some of our experience. The results are qualitative and represent the "best site" identified after studying multiple oligonucleotides. The number of oligonucleotides studied varies from target to target, as do assay conditions, cell type, and other factors. Consequently, this table and the next are meant to demonstrate the complexity of the problem only, not to provide a definitive statement about the "most active site" in any RNA. Table 2 (Dean et al., unpublished data) summarizes in more detail experience in our laboratories with regard to the activities of phosphorothioate oligodeoxynucleotides active against human and mouse pKC-α. Clearly, although the numbers of oligonucleotides tested are small, it is apparent that all regions may provide active receptor sites, and that mouse and human pKC-α may be different.

3.1.3. THE OPTIMAL ANTISENSE SITE VARIES
AS A FUNCTION OF TERMINATING MECHANISM

To test whether the type of terminating mechanism an oligonucleotide may have influences the sites of optimal antisense activity, we have studied two groups of oligonucleotides, phosphorothioate oligodeoxynucleotides and phosphorothioate oligonucleotides fully modified in the 2'-position as either 2'-fluoro, methoxy, or propoxy. RNase H activation is a terminating mechanism available to the oligodeoxynucleotides. The fully 2'-modified oligonucleotides will not serve as substrates for RNase H. The 2'-fluoro and methoxy oligonucleotides have significantly greater affinity for RNA than the oligodeoxynucleotides. The propoxy oligonucleotides have slightly greater affinities (45,159).

In a study on intercellular adhesion molecule-1 (ICAM-1), a phosphorothioate oligodeoxynucleotide, ISIS 1939, was shown to cause an RNase H-mediated reduction in ICAM-1 RNA. The 2'-methoxy analog is ISIS 1939 caused no reduction in RNA levels and was unable to inhibit ICAM protein synthesis (86). Thus, a position in the untranslated region of ICAM-1 RNA appeared to be sensitive only to an antisense oligonucleotide capable of supporting RNase H-mediated cleavage of the RNA. In contrast, the 2'-methoxy analog of ISIS 1570, a phosphorothioate oligodeoxynucleotide designed to bind to the translation initiation codon of ICAM-1 RNA, was almost as active as the parent molecule (86).

Figure 3 compares the most active receptor sequences in E-selectin RNA for oligodeoxynucleotides and fully modified 2'-propyl analogs (Bennett, unpublished results). There are quite obviously substantial differences in the positions of activity with the non-RNase H-dependent mechanisms displaying somewhat different patterns of activity compared to the oligodeoxynucleotide.

3.1.4. THE OPTIMAL ANTISENSE SITE
MAY VARY AS A FUNCTION OF AFFINITY

Studies in our laboratory have shown that, in a series of compounds that bind to the same receptor sequence and have the same terminating mechanism, potency increases as affinity is enhanced (102). We have also reported that higher-affinity oligonucleotides are required to invade some RNA stem loops (31,55,80,160). It, therefore, is reasonable to speculate that higher-affinity oligonucleotides might be able to bind to receptor sequences unaccessible to lower-affinity compounds, thus producing a different pattern of activities.

One approach to addressing this question is to compare the patterns of activities for higher-affinity RNase H activity "gapmers" to oligodeoxynucleotides. The gapmers display higher affinity and support RNase H. Figure 4 shows the patterns of activities observed when murine VCAM-1 was studied. Some differences were observed (Bennett, unpublished observations). However, given the fact that the propoxy gapmers have only slightly greater affinities for RNA than their parents, relatively small differences were expected and observed. More substantial differences have been observed in patterns of activities for higher-affinity gapmers. For example, in a study of the E-7 mRNA of human papillomavirus, the overall pattern of activity for gapmers was similar to the oligodeoxyoligonucleotides, but a 2'-fluoro gapmer was found that was active in a region not identified by the oligodeoxynucleotides and

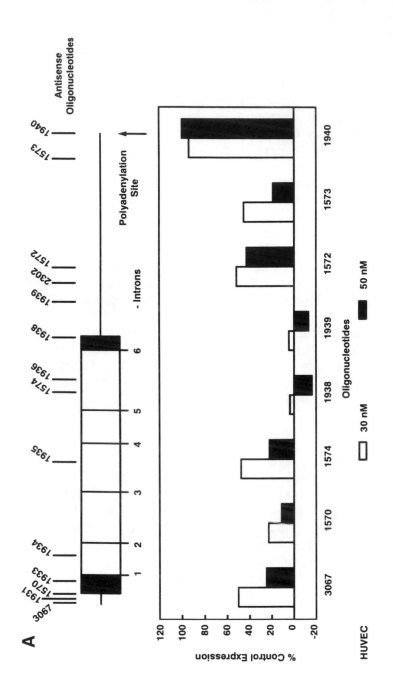

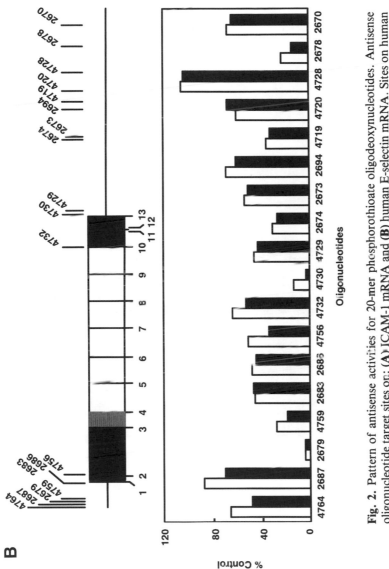

Fig. 2. Pattern of antisense activities for 20-mer phosphorothioate oligodeoxynucleotides. Antisense oligonucleotide target sites on: (**A**) ICAM-1 mRNA and (**B**) human E-selectin mRNA. Sites on human mRNA to which antisense oligonucleotides have been designed to hybridize are shown. Enlarged boxes correspond to translated regions. Activities determined by evaluating protein production as described in Bennett et al. (*158*).

Table 1
Most Active Receptor Sequence[a]

Target	Site	RNA degradation
HSV-UL13	AUG	None
HPV-E2	AUG	Possible
BPV-E2	AUG	—
H-ICAM-1	3'-UTR	Yes
	AUG	No
	5'-cap	No
M-ICAM-1	3'-UTR	Yes
H-ELAM	5'-UTR	No
	3'-UTR	Yes
H-Type II PLA$_2$	3'-UTR	Yes
5-LO	Coding	Yes
HIV	5'-UTR (TAR)	No
HIV-Rev	AUG	Yes
RAS	Coding region	Yes
	AUG	Yes
Influenza	Repetitive sequences	—
PKC-α	5'-UTR	Yes
	3'-UTR	Yes
	AUG	Yes
HCMV major immediate early region	Coding region	Yes
HCV polyprotein	5'-UTR and AUG	Yes

[a]The most active site(s) in each target gene is presented along with comments on whether degradation of the RNA was observed when an oligonucleotide that would form an RNA substrate was studied.

Table 2
Active Sites for Phosphorothioate Oligodeoxynucleotides in Protein Kinase C-α[a]

Target	Oligos tested	Active oligos	% "Hit rate"
Human pKC-α			
5'-UTR	1	1	100
AUG	3	2	66
ORF	6	1	16
3'-UTR	10	2	20
Mouse pKC-α			
5'-UTR	4	2	50
AUG	2	1	50
ORF	1	0	0
3'-UTR	11	5	45

[a]The activities of 23-mer P = S oligonucleotides against different sites on PKC-α in vitro in the presence of cationic lipids as reported by Dean and McKay, 1994. The "activity level" is, of course, somewhat arbitrary since some oligonucleotides are more active than others. However, all assays were conducted similarly, and the minimal activity label observed is biologically significant.

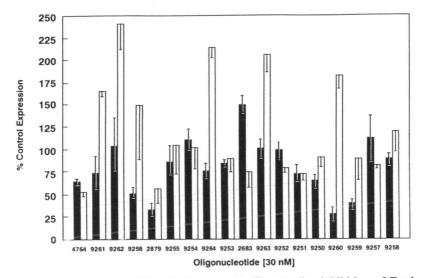

Fig. 3. Comparison of 2´-deoxy (■) with 2´-*O*-propyl (□) P-S oligo inhibition of E-selectin. Most active receptor sequences in E-selectin RNA for oligodeoxynucleotides and fully modified 2´-*O*-propyl analogs. Assays were as described in Bennett et al. (*158*). The positions of the oligonucleotides correspond to location in the RNA 5´- to 3´-ends as shown in the maps in Fig. 2.

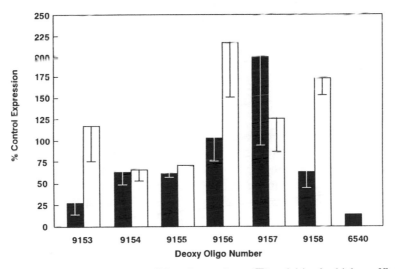

Fig. 4. Comparison of patterns of deoxy (■) and propyl gap (□) activities for higher-affinity RNase H activating gapmers observed when murine VCAM-1 was studied. Assays were as described in Bennett et al. (*158*). The positions of the oligonucleotides correspond to location in the RNA 5´- to 3´-ends in a manner similar to that shown in Fig. 2.

a propoxy gapmer analog of an active oligodeoxynucleotide was inactive (Cowsert, unpublished observations).

Clearly, much more thorough studies are required before firm conclusions about the effect of affinity on the patterns of antisense activities are determined, but it seems likely that affinity will play a major role.

4. CHARACTERISTICS OF
PHOSPHOROTHIOATE OLIGODEOXYNUCLEOTIDES

Of the first-generation oligonucleotide analogs, the class that has resulted in the broadest range of activities and about which the most is known is the phosphorothioate class. Phosphorothioate oligonucleotides were first synthesized in 1969 when a poly rI:poly rC phosphorothioate was synthesized (9). This modification clearly achieves the objective of increased nuclease stability. In this class of oligonucleotides, one of the oxygen atoms in the phosphate group is replaced with a sulfur. The resulting compound is negatively charged as is a phosphodiester, but more resistant to nucleases (161).

4.1. Hybridization

The hybridization of phosphorothioate oligonucleotides to DNA and RNA has been thoroughly characterized (for review, see 43,45,156). The T_m of a phosphorothioate oligonucleotide for RNA is approx 0.5 °C less per nucleotide than for a corresponding phosphodiester oligodeoxynucleotide. This reduction in T_m per nucleotide is virtually independent of the number of phosphorothioate units substituted for phosphodiesters. However, sequence context has some influence as the $\triangle T_m$ can vary from −0.3 to 1.0°C depending on sequence. Compared to RNA:RNA duplex formation, a phosphorothioate oligonucleotide has a T_m approx −2.2°C lower per unit (162). This means that to be effective in vitro, phosphorothioate oligodeoxynucleotides must typically be 17–20 mer in length (64,102) and that invasion of double-stranded regions in RNA is difficult (31,160).

4.2. Interactions with Proteins

Phosphorothioate oligonucleotides bind to proteins. The interactions with proteins can be divided into nonspecific, sequence-specific, and structure-specific binding events, each of which may have different characteristics and effects. Nonspecific binding to a wide variety of proteins has been demonstrated. Exemplary of this type of binding is the interaction of phosphorothioate oligonucleotides with serum albumin. The affinity of such interactions is low. The K_d for albumin is approx 400 μM, thus, in a similar range with aspirin or penicillin (163). Phosphorothioate oligonucleotides can interact with nucleic acid binding protein, such as transcription factors and single-strand nucleic acid binding proteins. However, very little is known about these binding events. Additionally, it has been reported that phosphorothioates bind to an 80-kDa membrane protein that was suggested to be involved in cellular uptake processes (164). However, again, little is known about the affinities, sequence, or structure specificities of these putative interactions.

Phosphorothioates interact with nucleases and DNA polymerases. These compounds are slowly metabolized by both endo- and exonucleases (45) and inhibit these enzymes (165). The inhibition of these enzymes appears to be competitive, and this may account for some early data suggesting that phosphorothioates are almost infinitely stable to nucleases. In these studies, the oligonucleotide-to-enzyme ratio was very high, and thus, the enzyme was inhibited. A phosphodiester oligonucleotide added after degradation of the phosphorothioate plateaued was not degraded. Clearly, such effects could have significant pharmacokinetic consequences.

Phosphorothioates also bind to RNase H when in an RNA–DNA duplex, and the duplex serves as a substrate for RNase H (*166*). At higher concentrations, presumably by binding in a single-strand form to RNase H, phosphorothioates inhibit the enzyme (*166*). Again, the oligonucleotides appear to be competitive antagonists for the DNA–RNA substrate.

Phosphorothioates have been shown to be competitive inhibitors of DNA polymerase α and β with respect to the DNA template, and noncompetitive inhibitors of DNA polymerases γ and δ (*166*). Despite this inhibition, several studies have suggested that phosphorothioates might serve as primers for polymerases and be extended (*165,167,168*). In our laboratories, we have shown extensions of two to three nucleotides only. At present, a full explanation regarding why no longer extensions are observed is not available.

Phosphorothioate oligonucleotides have been reported to be competitive inhibitors for HIV reverse transcriptase (*169*) and inhibit reverse transcriptase-associated RNase H activity (*170*). They have been reported to bind to the cell-surface protein, CD4 (*171*), and to protein kinase C (*172*). Various viral polymerases have also been shown to be inhibited by phosphorothioates (for review, *see 167*). Additionally, we have shown potent, nonsequence-specific inhibition of RNA splicing by phosphorothioates (Hodges & Crooke, unpublished data).

Like other oligonucleotides, phosphorothioates can adopt a variety of structures. As a general rule, self-complementary oligonucleotides are avoided, if possible, to avoid duplex formation between oligonucleotides. However, other structures that are less well understood can also form. For example, oligonucleotides containing runs of guanosines can form tetrameric structures called G-quartets, and these appear to interact with a number of proteins with relatively greater affinity than unstructured oligonucleotides (*173*). ISIS 5320 is exemplary (Fig. 5).

4.3. Nuclease Stability

The principal metabolic pathway for oligonucleotides is cleavage via endo- and exonucleases. Phosphorothioate oligodeoxynucleotides, although quite stable to various nucleases (*32,37,174*), are competitive inhibitors of these same enzymes (*165,166*). Consequently, the stability of phosphorothioate oligonucleotides to nucleases is probably a bit less than initially thought, since high concentrations (that inhibited nucleases) of oligonucleotides were employed in the early studies. Similarly, phosphorothioate oligonucleotides are degraded slowly by cells in tissue culture with a half-life of 12–24 h (*37,165*) and are slowly metabolized in animals (*175*). The pattern of metabolites suggests primarily exonuclease activity with perhaps modest contributions by endonucleases.

4.4. In Vitro Cellular Uptake

Phosphorothioate oligonucleotides are taken up by a wide range of cells in vitro (*176–180*). In fact, very recently, uptake of phosphorothioate oligonucleotides into a prokaryote, *Vibrio parahaemoyticus,* has been reported (*181*). Uptake is time- and temperature-dependent. It is also influenced by cell type, cell-culture conditions, media and sequence, and length of the oligonucleotide (*178*). No obvious correlation between the lineage of cells, whether the cells are transformed or whether the cells are virally infected, and uptake has been identified (*178*), nor are the factors that result in

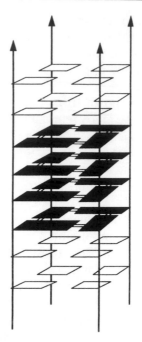

Fig. 5. The structure of ISIS 5320. Tetramer found of $T_sT_sG_sG_sG_sG_sT_sT$.

differences in uptake of different sequences of oligonucleotide understood. Although several studies have suggested that receptor-mediated endocytosis may be a significant mechanism of cellular uptake (*164*), the data are not yet compelling enough to conclude that receptor-mediated endocytosis accounts for a significant portion of the uptake in most cells.

Numerous studies have shown that phosphorothioate oligonucleotides distribute broadly in most cells once taken up (*178,179,182*). Again, however, significant differences in subcellular distribution among various types of cells have been noted.

Cationic lipids have been used to enhance uptake of phosphorothioate oligonucleotides in cells that take up little oligonucleotide in vitro (*183,184*). Again, however, there are substantial variations from cell type to cell type.

4.5. In Vivo Pharmacokinetics

Phosphorothioate oligonucleotides bind to serum albumin and α-2 macroglobulin. The apparent affinity for albumin is quite low (250–400 μM) and comparable to the low-affinity binding observed for a number of drugs, e.g., aspirin, penicillin (*163*). Serum protein binding, therefore, provides a repository for these drugs and prevents rapid renal excretion. Since serum protein binding is saturable, at higher doses, intact oligomer may be found in urine (*168,185*). Studies in our laboratory suggest that in rats, iv doses of 15–20 mg/kg saturate the serum protein binding capacity (Leeds, unpublished data).

Phosphorothioate oligonucleotides are rapidly and extensively absorbed after parenteral administration. For example, in rats, after an id dose 3.6 mg/kg of ¹⁴C-ISIS 2105, a 20-mer phosphorothioate, approx 70% of the dose was absorbed within 4 h, and total systemic bioavailability was in excess of 90% (186). After id injection in humans, absorption of ISIS 2105 was similar to that observed in rats (187).

Distribution of phosphorothioate oligonucleotides from blood after absorption or iv administration is extremely rapid. We have reported distribution half-lives of < 1 h (175,186,187), and similar data have been reported by others (168,185). Blood and plasma clearance is multiexponential with a terminal elimination half-life from 40 to 60 h in all species except humans. In humans, the terminal elimination half-life may be somewhat longer (187).

Phosphorothioates distribute broadly to all peripheral tissues. Liver, kidney, bone marrow, skeletal muscle, and skin accumulate the highest percentage of a dose, but other tissues display small quantitites of drug (175,186). No evidence of significant penetration of the blood–brain barrier has been reported. The rates of incorporation and clearance from tissues vary as a function of the organ studied, with liver accumulating drug most rapidly (20% of a dose within 1–2 h), and other tissues accumulating drug more slowly. Similarly, elimination of drug is more rapid from liver than any other tissue, e.g., terminal half-life from liver: 62 h; from renal medulla: 156 h.

At relatively low doses, clearance of phosphorothioate oligonucleotides is owing primarily to slow metabolism (175,185,186). Metabolism is mediated by exo- and endonucleases that result in shorter oligonucleotides, and ultimately, nucleosides that are degraded by normal metabolic pathways. Although no direct evidence of base excision or modification has been reported, these are theoretical possibilities that may occur. In one study, a larger-mol-wt radioactive material was observed in urine, but was not fully characterized (168). Clearly, the potential for conjugation reactions and extensions of oligonucleotides via these drugs serving as primers for polymerases must be explored in more detail. In a very thorough study, a pair of 20 nucleotide phosphodiester and phosphorothioate oligonucleotides were administered intravenously at a dose of 6 mg/kg to mice. The oligonucleotides were internally labeled with ^{3}H-CH$_3$ by methylation of an internal deoxycytidine residue using HhaI methylase and S-[^{3}H] adenosyl methionine (188). The observations for the phosphorothioate oligonucleotide was entirely consistent with those made in our studies. Additionally, in this paper, autoradiographic analyses showed drug in renal cortical cells (188).

One study of prolonged infusions of a phosphorothioate oligonucleotide to human beings has been reported (189). In this study, five patients with leukemia were given 10-d iv infusions at a dose of 0.05 mg/kg/h. Elimination half-lives reportedly varied from 5.9 to 14.7 d. Urinary recovery of radioactivity was reported to be 30–60% of the total dose, with 30% of the radioactivity being intact drug. Metabolites in urine included both higher- and lower-mol-wt compounds. Obviously, these data differ from observations in other studies. At present, the data are insufficient to determine if the pharmacokinetics of prolonged iv infusions are truly substantially different from the pharmacokinetic behavior of iv bolus injections.

We have also performed oral bioavailability experiments in rodents treated with an H2 antagonist to avoid acid-mediated depurination or precipitation. In these studies, very limited (< 10%) bioavailability was observed.

In summary, pharmacokinetic studies of several phosphorothioates demonstrate that they are well absorbed from parenteral sites, distribute broadly to all peripheral tissues, do not cross the blood–brain barrier, and are eliminated primarily by slow metabolism. In short, once a day or every other day systemic dosing should be feasible. Although the similarities between oligonucleotides of different sequences are far greater than the differences, additional studies are required before determining whether there are subtle effects of sequence on the pharmacokinetic profile of this class of drugs.

4.6. Pharmacological Properties

4.6.1. MOLECULAR PHARMACOLOGY

Antisense oligonucleotides are designed to bind to RNA targets via Watson-Crick hybridization. Since RNA can adopt a variety of secondary structures via Watson-Crick hybridization, one useful way to think of antisense oligonucleotides is as competitive antagonists for self-complementary regions of the target RNA. Obviously, creating oligonucleotides with the highest affinity per nucleotide unit is pharmacologically important, and a comparison of the affinity of the oligonucleotide to a complementary RNA oligonucleotide is the most sensible comparison. In this context, phosphorothioate oligodeoxynucleotides are relatively competitively disadvantaged, since the affinity per nucleotide unit of oligomer is less than RNA ($> -2.0\,°C\ T_m/U$) (190). This results in a requirement of at least 15–17 nucleotides in order to have sufficient affinity to produce biological activity (64).

Phosphorothioate oligonucleotides have also been shown to have effects inconsistent with the antisense mechanism for which they were designed. Some of these effects are owing to sequence- and structure-specific, as well as nonspecific interactions with proteins. These effects are particularly prominent in in vitro tests for antiviral activity since often high concentrations of cells, viruses, and oligonucleotides are coincubated (191,192). Human immune deficiency virus (HIV) is particularly problematic, since many oligonucleotides bind to the gp120 protein and other proteins of the virus (173). In addition to protein interactions, other factors, such as overrepresented sequences of RNA and unusual structures that may be adopted by oligonucleotides, can contribute to unexpected results (173).

Given the variability in cellular uptake of oligonucleotides, the variability in potency as a function of binding site in an RNA target and potential nonantisense activities of oligonucleotides, careful evaluation of dose–response curves and clear demonstration of the antisense mechanism are required before drawing conclusions from in vitro experiments. Nevertheless, numerous well-controlled studies have been reported in which antisense activity was conclusively demonstrated. Since many of these studies have been reviewed previously (43–45,170,193), suffice it to say that antisense effects of phosphorothioate oligodeoxynucleotides against a variety of targets are well documented.

4.6.2. IN VIVO PHARMACOLOGICAL ACTIVITIES

Table 3 summarizes a number of the published reports (abstracts and full publications) demonstrating in vivo activity of oligonucleotides. Local effects have been reported for phosphorothioate and methylphosphonate oligonucleotides. A phosphorothioate oligonucleotide designed to inhibit c-*myb* production and applied locally was shown to inhibit intimal accumulation in the rat carotid artery (194). In this study, a Northern blot showed a significant reduction in c-*myb* RNA in animals treated with the antisense compound, but no effect by a control oligonucleotide. Similar effects were reported for phosphorothioate oligodeoxynucleotides designed to inhibit cylin-dependent kinases (CDC-2 and CDK-2). Again, the antisense oligonucleotide inhibited intimal thickening and cylin-dependent kinase activity, whereas a control

Table 3
Reported Activities of Antisense Drugs in Animals

Target	Animal	Reference
HSV-1	Mouse	67
p120 Oncogene	Mouse	197
c-*myb*	Rat	194
Interleukin 1 receptor	Mouse	201
NF-kB	Mouse	202
CDC-2 and CDK-2	Rat	195
N-*myc*	Mouse	196
Y-Y1 receptors	Rat	198
NMDA-R1 receptor channel	Rat	199
Symptosomal-associated protein 25	Rat	200
NF-kB	Mouse	203
Intercellular adhesion molecule 1	Mouse	213
pKC-α	Mouse	206
BCR-ABL	Mouse	204
c-*myb*	Mouse	205

oligonucleotide had no effect (*195*). Additionally, local administration of a phosphodiester oligonucleotide designed to inhibit N-*myc* resulted in reduction in N-*myc* expression and slower growth to a subcutaneously transplanted human tumor in nude mice (*196*).

Local antitumor effects of phosphorothioate oligodeoxynucleotides have also been reported. An antisense oligonucleotide designed to inhibit the expression of the p120 protein was shown to inhibit the growth of a human tumor transplanted intraperitoneally in nude mice when the compound was administered intraperitoneally (*197*).

Antisense oligonucleotides administered intraventricularly have been reported to induce a variety of effects in the central nervous system. Intraventricular injection of antisense oligonucleotides to neuropeptide-Y-Y1 receptors reduced the density of the receptors and resulted in behavioral signs of anxiety (*198*). Similarly, an antisense oligonucleotide designed to bind to NMDA-R1 receptor channel RNA inhibited the synthesis of these channels and reduced the volume of focal ischemia produced by occlusion of the middle cerebral artery in rats (*199*).

Injection of antisense oligonucleotides to synaptosomal-associated protein-25 into the vitreous body of rat embryos reduced the expression of the protein and inhibited neurite elongation by rat cortical neurons (*200*).

In addition to local and regional effects of antisense oligonucleotides, a growing number of well-controlled studies have demonstrated systemic effects of phosphorothioate oligodeoxynucleotides. Expression of interleukin-1 in mice was inhibited by systemic administration of antisense oligonucleotides (*201*). Oligonucleotides to the NF-kB p65 subunit administered intraperitoneally at 40 mg/kg every 3 d slowed tumor growth in mice transgenic for the human T-cell leukemia viruses (*202*). Similar results with other antisense oligonucleotides were shown in another in vivo tumor model after either prolonged sc infusion or intermittent sc injection (*203*).

Two recent reports further extend the studies of phosphorothioate oligonucleotides as antitumor agents in mice. In one study, phosphorothioate oligonucleotide directed to inhibition of the BCR-ABL oncogene was administered at a dose of 1 mg/d for 9 d iv to immunodeficient mice injected with human leukemic cells. The drug was shown to inhibit the development of leukemic colonies in the mice and to reduce selectively BCR-ABL RNA levels in peripheral blood lymphocytes, spleen, bone marrow, liver, lungs, and brain (*204*). In the second study, a phosphorothioate oligonucleotide antisense to the proto-oncogene *myb*, inhibited the growth of human melanoma in mice. Again, *myb* mRNA levels appeared to be selectively reduced (*205*).

Thus, there is a growing body of evidence suggesting that antisense oligonucleotides (in most cases, phosphorothioate oligodeoxynucleotides) can produce local, regional, and systemic effects at nontoxic doses in vivo. Although proof of mechanism of action is difficult, in most cases, studies with control oligonucleotides demonstrate that the effects are consistent with the proposed antisense mechanism. In the important series of studies by Dean and McKay (*206*), an antisense mechanism and isotype selectivity have been conclusively demonstrated after systemic administration of an antisense oligonucleotide designed to inhibit protein kinase C-α (pKC-α) in mice.

All of these data suggest that phosphorothioate oligodeoxynucleotides may have therapeutic potential.

4.6.3. In Vivo Toxicological Properties

The acute LD_{50} dose in mice of all phosphorothioates tested to date is in excess of 500 mg/kg (Kornbrust, unpublished observations). Although there may be differences among different oligonucleotide sequences and the LD_{50} may be influenced by route of administration, these factors appear to result in minimal variation. Several phosphorothioate oligodeoxynucleotides have been studied for potential fetal toxicities, and to date, no significant adverse effects have been noted (Kornbrust, unpublished observations; *207*).

Although there is no evidence of antigenicity or induction of delayed-type hypersensitivity in animals or humans given multiple doses of phosphorothioate oligonucleotides (*156;* Kornbrust, unpublished observations), multiple doses of these drugs clearly affect the immune system in animals, with rats being the most sensitive species. The manifestations of these toxicities that are observed at lowest doses are increases in spleen weight, production of IgM and IgG, and expansion of B-cell populations in spleens (Kornbrust, unpublished observations; *208*). Although the sequence of the oligonucleotides can affect the dose at which these effects are produced and an antisense sequence designed to inhibit the 65-kDa subunits of NF-kB was reported to be devoid of such effects (*209*), in our experience, all thoroughly tested phosphorothioate oligodeoxynucleotides induced these effects. As a general rule, the doses required to induce these effects have been substantially greater than those demonstrating pharmacologic activity.

In monkeys, several phosphorothioate oligodeoxynucleotides have been shown to cause acute hypotensive events (Kornbrust, unpublished observations; *210*). These effects are transient, if managed appropriately, relatively uncommon, and typically appear to occur in response to the first dose given to an animal. Recent studies suggest that one mechanism responsible for this may be related to complement activation, and that this toxicity can be avoided by giving iv infusions rather than bolus injections. We have evaluated the mechanisms by which phosphorothioate oligonucleotides might induce complement activation and phosphorothioates appear to affect the alternative pathway. In large part, the effects of phosphorothioates are similar to those associated with other polyanions, such as heparin. Complement regulatory factors, such as Factor H and D, appear to be most influenced by these drugs. Based on predictions about studies on animal models, toxicological studies in monkeys, and unpublished studies on systemically administered phosphorothioates currently in the clinic, the therapeutic index relative to this potential toxicity would appear to be likely to be acceptable.

We have also noted prolongation of prothrombin, partial thromboplastin, and bleeding times in monkeys. Again, these effects are plasma concentration-dependent and appear to occur at doses that are sufficient to saturate serum albumin binding sites. The effects on partial thromboplastin time are much more pronounced than those on prothrombin time. The effects appear to be primarily on the extrinsic pathway with clear inhibition of thrombin activity demonstrated. No effects on Factors VIII–XI have been observed. Again, based on predictions from studies in monkeys, the doses likely to produce this toxicity seem substantially greater than the predicted therapeutic doses. Clearly, only carefully controlled clinical trials will define the human toxicities and therapeutic indices of these drugs.

4.6.4. CLINICAL ACTIVITIES

To date, we have studied several hundred patients given multiple doses of three phosphorothioate oligonucleotides and encountered no significant toxicities. Other oligonucleotides are being studied in human beings by other groups, and to date, no significant or dose-related toxicities have been reported.

ISIS 2922, a 20-mer phosphorothioate designed to inhibit cytomegalovirus, has been administered intravitreally to patients with advanced AIDS and advanced drug-resistant CMV retinitis, and showed impressive antiviral activity (*211*).

In this study, three dose groups were studied in patients that had advanced CMV retinitis and had failed ganciclovir and/or foscarnet therapy. The median CD4 count in these patients was 4, so they were extremely immunocompromised. The median time from diagnosis of CMV retinitis was 10 mo. Two patients were treated in the 2-μM dose group and failed. Three of four eyes treated at 4 μM and six of eight eyes at 8 μM responded. The responses were rapid, long-lasting, and substantial. The only adverse event observed was increased inflammation (*212*).

ISIS 2105 is a 20-mer phosphorothioate oligonucleotide designed to inhibit the replication of human papilloma viruses 6 and 11, the viruses responsible for genital warts. Plot ascending-dose multiple-dose studies as primary therapy of genital warts have shown the drug locally and systemically well tolerated after id administration. At doses of 2.5 mg/wart twice weekly and greater, the drug has been associated with resolution of genital warts. In a pivotal placebo-controlled trial of patients treated by surgical removal of the warts and administration of single doses of 0.3 or 1.0 mg/wart ISIS 2105 at the time of surgery, reductions in wart recurrence were observed that were not statistically significant, but suggestive of antiviral activity as a surgical adjuvant.

Development of ISIS 2922 is proceeding with Phase III trials in patients with CMV retinitis. Development of ISIS 2105 is proceeding with a multiple-dose Phase II trial designed to confirm its activity and evaluate its potential utility.

ISIS 2302 is a 20-mer designed to inhibit ICAM (*158,179*). We have completed a single-dose Phase I study in normal volunteers given this drug by 2 h iv infusion at doses up to 2 mg/kg. No significant toxicities were observed.

Table 4
Phosphorothioate Oligonucleotides

Limits
    Pharmacodynamic
        Low affinity per nucleotide unit
        Inhibition of RNase H at high concentrations
    Pharmacokinetic
        Limited bioavailability
        Limited blood–brain barrier penetration
        Dose-dependent pharmacokinetics
    Toxicologic
        Release of cytokines
        Complement-associated effects on blood pressure?
        Clotting effects

4.6.5. CONCLUSIONS

Phosphorothioate oligonucleotides have perhaps outperformed many expectations. They display attractive parenteral pharmacokinetic properties. They have produced potent systemic effects in a number of animal models and, in many experiments, the antisense mechanism has been directly demonstrated as the hoped-for selectivity. Further, these compounds appear to display satisfactory therapeutic indices for many indications.

Nevertheless, phosphorothioates clearly have significant limits (Table 4). Pharmacodynamically, they have relatively low affinity per nucleotide unit. This means that longer oligonucleotides are required for biological activity and that invasion of many RNA structures may not be possible. At higher concentrations, these compounds inhibit RNase H as well. Thus, the higher end of the pharmacologic dose–response curve is lost. Pharmacokinetically, phosphorothioates do not cross the blood–brain barrier, are not significantly orally bioavailable, and may display dose-dependent pharmacokinetics. Toxicologically, clearly the release of cytokines, activation of complement, and interference with clotting will pose dose limits if they are encountered in the clinic.

Since several clinical trials are in progress with phosphorothioates and since others will be initiated shortly, we shall soon have more definitive information about the activities, toxicities, and value of this class of antisense drugs in human beings.

5. POTENTIAL IN CANCER CHEMOTHERAPY

Against a growing number of human tumor xenografts, phosphorothioates and more novel analogs directed to a number of targets have been shown to have potent antitumor effects (for review, *see 44*; Dean, unpublished data; Monia, unpublished data). In a variety of studies, we have observed potent antitumor effects consistent with an antisense mechanisms at doses 2–3 orders of magnitude lower than minimally toxic doses. Furthermore, we have also observed enhanced potency with chimeric analogs (Monia, manuscript in preparation). Thus, it would seem that cautious optimism with regard to the potential of such compounds in the treatment of malignancies is warranted.

A further benefit is the opportunity to use antisense agents to evaluate the roles of specific targets in malignancies.

ACKNOWLEDGMENTS

I am pleased to acknowledge the outstanding assistance in the preparation of this manuscript by Colleen Matzinger. Thanks also to Frank Bennett for his thoughtful review.

REFERENCES

1. Watson JD, Crick FHC. Molecular structure of nucleic acids: A structure for deoxyribose nucleic acid. *Nature* 1953; 171:737.
2. Gillespie D, Spiegelman S. A quantitative assay for DNA-RNA hybrids with DNA immobilized on a membrane. *J Mol Biol* 1965; 12:829–842.
3. Thompson JD, Gillespie D. Current concepts in quantitative molecular hybridization. *Clin Biochem* 1990; 23:261–266.
4. Zamecnik PC, Stephenson ML. Inhibition of Rous sarcoma virus replication and cell transformation by a specific oligodeoxynucleotides. *Proc Natl Acad Sci USA* 1978; 75:280.
5. Ts'o POP, Miller PS, Greene JJ. Nucleic acid analogs with targeted delivery at chemotherapeutic agents. In: Cheng YC, Goz B, Minkoff M, eds. *Development of Target-Oriented Anticancer Drugs*. New York: Raven. 1983:189.
6. Barrett JC, Miller PS, Ts'o POP. Inhibitory effect of complex formation with oligodeoxyribonucleotide ethyl phosphotriesters on transfer ribonucleic acid aminoacylation. *Biochemistry* 1974; 13:4897.
7. Caruthers MH. Gene synthesis machines: DNA chemistry and its uses. *Science* 1985; 230:281.
8. Alvarado-Urbina G, Sathe GM, Liu WC, et al. Automated synthesis of gene fragments. *Science* 1981; 214:270.
9. De Clercq E, Eckstein F, Merigan TC. Interferon induction increased through chemical modification of a synthetic polyribonucleotide. *Science* 1969; 165:1137.
10. Marcus-Sekura CJ, Woerner AM, Shinozuka K, et al. Comparative inhibition of chloramphenicol acetyltransferase gene expression by antisense oligonucleotide analogues having alkyl phosphotriester, methylphosphonate and phosphorothioate linkages. *Nucleic Acids Res* 1987; 15:5749.
11. Matsukura M, Shinozuka K, Zon G, et al. Phosphorothioate analogs of oligodeoxyribonucleotides: inhibitors of replication and cytopathic effects of human immunodeficiency virus. *Proc Natl Acad Sci USA* 1987; 84:7706.
12. Agrawal S, Goodchild J, Civeira MP, et al. Oligodeoxynucleoside phosphoramidates and phosphorothioates as inhibitors of human immunodeficiency virus. *Proc Natl Acad Sci USA* 1988; 85:7079.
13. Goodchild J, Agrawal S, Civeira MP, et al. Inhibition of human immunodeficiency virus replication by antisense oligonucleotides. *Proc Natl Acad Sci USA* 1988; 85:5507.
14. Sarin PS, Agrawal S, Civeira MP. Inhibition of acquired immunodeficiency syndrome virus by oligodeoxynucleotide methylphosphonates. *Proc Natl Acad Sci USA* 1988; 85:7448.
15. Gao W, Stein CA, Cohen JS, et al. Effect of phosphorothioate homo-oligodeoxynucleotides on herpes simplex virus type 2-induced DNA polymerase. *J Biol Chem* 1989; 264:11,521.
16. Smith CC, Aurelian L, Reddy MP, et al. Antiviral effect of an oligo(nucleoside methylphosphonate) complementary to the splice junction of herpes simplex virus type 1 immediate early pre-mRNAs 4 and 5. *Proc Natl Acad Sci USA* 1986; 83:2787.
17. Agris CH, Blake KR, Miller PS, et al. Inhibition of vesicular stomatitis virus protein synthesis and infection by sequence-specific oligodeoxyribonucleoside methylphosphonates. *Biochemistry* 1986; 25:6268.
18. Heikkila R, Schwab G, Wickstrom E, et al. A c-myc antisense oligonucleotide inhibits entry into S phase but not progress from GO to G1. *Nature* 1987; 328:445.

19. Wickstrom EL, Bacon TA, Gonzalez A, et al. Anti-c-myc DNA increases differentiation and decreases colony formation by HL-60 cells *in vitro*. *Cell Dev Biol* 1989; 25:297.

20. Felsenfeld G, Davies DR, Rich A. Formation of a three-stranded polynucleotide molecule. *J Am Chem Soc* 1957; 79:2023.

21. Helene C. Control of gene expression by triplex-helix-forming oligonucleotides. The antigene strategy. In: Crooke ST, Lebleu B, eds. *Antisense Research and Applications*. Boca Raton, FL: CRC. 1993:375.

22. Moser HE, Dervan PB. Sequence-specific cleavage of double helical DNA by triple helix formation. *Science* 1987; 238:645.

23. Le Doan T, Perrouault L, Praseuth D, et al. Sequence-specific recognition, photocrosslinking and cleavage of the DNA double helix by an oligo-[α]-thymidylate covalently linked to an azidoproflavine derivative. *Nucleic Acid Res* 1987; 15:7749.

24. Cooney M, Czernuszewicz G, Postel EH, et al. Site-specific oligonucleotide binding represses transcription of the human c-myc gene *in vitro*. *Science* 1988; 241:456.

25. Mirabelli CK, Crooke ST. Antisense oligonucleotides in the context of modern molecular drug discovery and development. In: Crooke ST, Lebleu B, eds. *Antisense Research and Applications*. Boca Raton, FL: CRC. 1993:7.

26. Nielsen PE, Egholm M, Berg RH, et al. Peptide nucleic acids (PNA): Oligonucleotide analogs with a polyamide backbone. In: Crooke ST, Lebleu B, eds. *Antisense Research and Applications*. Boca Raton, FL: CRC. 1993:363.

27. Cech T. Self-splicing of group 1 introns. *Annu Rev Biochem* 1990; 59:543.

28. Uhlenbeck OC. Using ribozymes to cleave RNAs. In: Crooke ST, Lebleu B, eds. *Antisense Research and Applications*. Boca Raton, FL: CRC. 1993:83.

29. Tuerk C, Gold L. Systematic evolution of ligands by exponential enrichment: RNA ligands to bacteriophage T4 DNA polymerase. *Science* 1990; 249:505.

30. Ellington AD, Szostak JW. In vitro selection of RNA molecules that bind specific ligands. *Nature* 1990; 346:818.

31. Vickers T, Baker BF, Cook PD, et al. Inhibition of HIV-LTR gene expression by oligonucleotides targeted to the TAR element. *Nucleic Acids Res* 1991; 19:3359.

32. Wickstrom E. Oligodeoxynucleotide stability in subcellular extracts and culture media. *J Biochem Biophys Methods* 1986; 13:97.

33. Tidd DM, Warenieus HM. Partial protection on oncogene, antisense oligodeoxynucleotides against serum nuclease degradation using terminal methylphosphonate groups. *Br J Cancer* 1989; 60:343.

34. Dagle JM, Walder JA, Weeks DL. Targeted degradation of mRNA in Xenopus oncytes and embryos directed by modified oligonucleotides: studies of An2 and cylin in embryogenesis. *Nucleic Acids Res* 1990; 18:4751.

35. Dagle JM, Weeks DL, Walder JA. Pathways of degradation and mechanism of action of antisense oligonucleotides in Xenopus laevis embryos. *Antisense Res Dev* 1991; 1:11.

36. Crooke RM. *In vitro* toxicology and pharmacokinetics of antisense oligonucleotides. *Anti-Cancer Drug Design* 1991; 6:609.

37. Hoke GD, Draper K, Freier SM, et al. Effects of phosphorothioate capping on antisense oligonucleotide stability, hybridization and antiviral efficacy versus herpes simplex virus infection. *Nucleic Acids Res* 1991; 19:5743.

38. Asseline U, Delarue M, Lancelot G, et al. Nucleic acid-binding molecules with high affinity and base sequence specificity: intercalating agents covalently linked to oligonucleotides. *Proc Natl Acad Sci USA* 1984; 81:3297.

39. Cazenave C, Stein CA, Loreau N, et al. Comparative inhibition of rabbit globin mRNA translation by modified antisense oligodeoxynucleotides. *Nucleic Acids Res* 1989; 17:4255.

40. Letsinger RL, Zhang G, Sun DK. Cholesteryl-conjugated oligonucleotides: synthesis, properties and activity as inhibitors of replication of human immunodeficiency virus in cell culture. *Proc Natl Acad Sci USA* 1989; 86:6553.

41. Lamaitre M, Bayard B, Lebleu B. Specific antiviral activity of a poly (L-lysine)-conjugated oligodeoxyribonucleotide sequence complementary to vesicular stomatitis virus N protein mRNA initiation site. *Proc Natl Acad Sci USA* 1987; 84:648.

42. Leonetti JP, Rayner B, Lemaitre M, et al. Antiviral activity of conjugates between poly(L-lysine) and synthetic oligodeoxyribonucleotides. *Gene* 1988; 72:323.

43. Crooke ST, Lebleu B, eds. *Antisense Research and Applications.* Boca Raton, FL: CRC, 1993.
44. Crooke ST. Oligonucleotide Therapeutics. In: Wolff ME, ed. *Burger's Medicinal Chemistry and Drug Discovery,* vol. 1, 5th ed. New York: Wiley Interscience. 1995:863.
45. Crooke ST. Therapeutic applications of oligonucleotides. *Annu Rev Pharmacol Toxicol* 1992; 32:329.
46. Mizumoto K, Kaziro Y. Messenger RNA capping enzymes from eukaryotic cells. *Prog Nucleic Acids Res Mol Biol* 1987; 34:1.
47. Ross J. Messenger RNA turnover in eukaryotic cells. *Mol Biol Med* 1988; 5:1.
48. Friedman DI, Imperiale MJ. RNA 3′ end formation in the control of gene expression. *Annu Rev Genet* 1987; 21:453.
49. Manley JL. Polyadenyation of mRNA precursors. *Biochim Biophys Acta* 1988; 950:1.
50. Padgett RA, Grabowski PJ, Konarska MM, et al. Splicing of messenger RNA precursors. *Annu Rev Biochem* 1986; 55:1119.
51. Green MR. Pre-mRNA splicing. *Annu Rev Genet* 1986; 20:671.
52. Breslauer KJ, Frank R, Blocker H. Predicting DNA duplex stability from base sequence. *Proc Natl Acad Sci USA* 1986; 83:3746.
53. Freier SM, Kierzek R, Jaeger J, et al. Improved free-energy parameters for predictions of RNA duplex stability. *Proc Natl Acad Sci USA* 1986; 83:9373.
54. Chastain M, Tinoco I. RNA structure as related to antisense drugs. In: Crooke ST, Lebleu B, eds. *Antisense Research and Applications.* Boca Raton, FL: CRC. 1993:55.
55. Ecker DJ. Strategies for invasion of RNA secondary structure. In: Crooke ST, Lebleu B, eds. *Antisense Research and Applications.* Boca Raton, FL: CRC. 1993:387.
56. Wyatt JR, Vickers TA, Roberson JL, et al. Combinatorially selected guanosine-quartet structure is a potent inhibitor of human immunodeficiency virus envelop-mediated cell fusion. *Proc Natl Acad Sci USA* 1994; 91:1356.
57. Wang KY, McCurdy S, Shea RG, et al. A DNA aptamer which binds to and inhibits thrombin exhibits a new structural motif for DNA. *Biochemistry* 1993; 32:1899.
58. Leroy J-L, Gehring K, Kettani A, et al. Acid multimers of oligodeoxycytidine strands: stoichiometry, base-pair characterization and proton exchange properties. *Biochemistry* 1993; 32:6019.
59. Gehring K, Ley J-L, Gueron M. A tetrameric DNA structure with protonated cytosine-cytosine base pairs. *Nature* 1993; 363:561.
60. Freier SM, Lima WF, Sanghvi YS, et al. Thermodynamics of antisense oligonucleotide hybridization. In: Izant J, Erickson R, eds. *Gene Regulation by Antisense Nucleic Acids.* New York: Raven. 1992:95.
61. Thein SL, Wallace RB. The use of synthetic oligonucleotides as specific hybridization probes in the diagnosis of genetic disorders. In: Davies KE, ed. *Human Genetic Diseases: A Practical Approach.* Oxford: IRL. 1986:33.
62. Helene C, Toulme JJ. Control of gene expression by oligonucleotides covalently linked to intercalating agents and nucleic acid-cleaving reagents. In: Cohen JS, ed. *Oligodeoxynucleotides: Antisense Inhibitors of Gene Expression.* Boca Raton, FL: CRC. 1989:137.
63. Helene C, Toulme JJ. Specific regulation of gene expression by antisense, sense and antigene nucleic acids. *Biochim Biophys Acta* 1990; 1049:99.
64. Monia BP, Johnston JF, Ecker DJ, et al. Selective inhibition of mutant Ha-ras mRNA expression by antisense oligonucleotides. *J Biol Chem* 1992; 267:19,954.
65. Crooke ST. Progress in antisense therapeutics. *Hematol Pathol* 1995; 9:59.
66. McManaway ME, Neckers LM, Loke SL, et al. Tumour-specific inhibition of lymphoma growth by an antisense oligodeoxynucleotide. *Lancet* 1990; 335:808.
67. Kulka M, Smith C, Aurelian L, et al. Site specificity of the inhibitory effects of oligo(nucleoside methylphosphonates) complementary to the acceptor splice junction of herpes simplex virus type 1 immediately early mRNA. *Proc Natl Acad Sci USA* 1989; 86:6868.
68. Zamecnik PC, Goodchild J, Taguchi Y, et al. Inhibition of replication and expression of human T-cell lymphotropic virus type III in cultured cells by exogenous synthetic oligonucleotides complementary to viral RNA. *Proc Natl Acad Sci USA* 1986; 83:4143.
69. Smith CC, Aurelian L, Reddy MP, et al. Antiviral effect of an oligo(nucleoside methylphosphonate) complementary to the splice junction of herpes simplex virus type 1 immediate early pre-mRNAs 4 and 5. *Proc Natl Acad Sci USA* 1985; 83:2787.

70. Dominski Z, Kole R. Restoration of correct splicing in thalassemic pre-mRNA by antisense oligonucleotides. *Proc Natl Acad Sci USA* 1993; 90:8673.

71. Agrawal S, Goodchild J, Civeira MP, et al. Oligodeoxynucleoside phosphoramidites and phosphorothioates as inhibitors of human immunodeficiency virus. *Proc Natl Acad Sci USA* 1988; 85:7079.

72. Lemaitre M, Bayard B, Lebleu B. Specific antiviral activity of a poly(L-lysine)-conjugated oligodeoxyribonucleotide sequence complementary to vesicular stomatitis virus N protein mRNA initiation site. *Biochemistry* 1987; 84:648.

73. Rosolen A, Whitesell L, Olegalo M, et al. Antisense inhibition of single copy N-myc expression results in decreased cell growth without reduction of c-myc protein in a neuroepithelioma cell line. *Cancer Res* 1990; 50:6316.

74. Vasanthakumar G, Ahmed NK. Modulation of drug resistance in a daunorubicin resistant subline with oligonucleotide methylphosphonates. *Cancer Commun* 1989; 1:225.

75. Sburlati AR, Manrow RE, Berger SL. Prothymosin α antisense oligomers inhibit myeloma cell division. *Proc Natl Acad Sci USA* 1991; 88:253.

76. Zheng H, Sahai BM, Kilgannon P, et al. Specific inhibition of cell-surface T-cell receptor expression by antisense oligodeoxynucleotides and its effect on the production of an antigen-specific regulatory T-cell factor. *Proc Natl Acad Sci USA* 1989; 86:3758.

77. Maier JAM, Voulalas P, Roeder D, et al. Extension of the life-span of human endothelial cells by an interleukin-1α antisense oligomer. *Science* 1990; 249:1570.

78. Mirabelli CK, Bennett CF, Anderson K, et al. *In vitro* and *in vivo* pharmacologic activities of antisense oligonucleotides. *Anti-Cancer Drug Design* 1991; 6:647.

79. Cowsert LM, Fox MC, Zon G, et al. In vitro evaluation of phosphorothioate oligonucleotides targeted to the E2 mRNA of papillomavirus: Potential treatment of genital warts. *Antimicrob Agents and Chemotherapy* 1993; 37:171.

80. Ecker DJ, Vickers TA, Bruice TW, et al. Pseudo-half knot formation with RNA. *Science* 1992; 257:958.

81. Saxena SK, Ackerman EJ. Microinjected oligonucleotides complementary to the α-sarcin loop of 28 S RNA abolish protein synthesis in xenopus oocytes. *J Biol Chem* 1990; 265:3263.

82. Walker K, Elela SA, Nazar RN. Inhibition of protein synthesis by anti-5.8 S rNA oligodeoxyribonucleotides. *J Biol Chem* 1990; 265:2428.

83. Westerman P, Gross B, Hoinkis G. Inhibition of expression of SV40 virus large T-antigen by antisense oligodeoxyribonucleotides. *Biomed Biochim Acta* 1989; 48:85.

84. Baker B. Decapitation of a 5' capped oligoribonucleotide by ortho-Phenanthroline:Cu(II). *J Am Chem Soc* 1993; 115:3378.

85. Baker BF, Miraglia L, Hagedorn CH. Modulation of eurkaryotic initiation factor-4E binding to 5' capped oligoribonucleotides by modified antisense oligonucleotides. *J Biol Chem* 1992; 267:11,495.

86. Chiang MY, Chan H, Zounes MA, et al. Antisense oligonucleotides inhibit ICAM-1 expression by two distinct mechanisms. *J Biol Chem* 1991; 266:18,162.

87. Crouch RJ, Dirksen M-L. Ribonucleases H. In: Linn SM, Roberts RJ, eds. *Nucleases.* Cold Spring Harbor, NY: Cold Spring Harbor Laboratory Press. 1985:211.

88. Crum C, Johnson JD, Nelson A, et al. Complementary oligodeoxynucleotide mediated inhibition of tobacco mosaic virus RNA translation *in vitro*. *Nucleic Acids Res* 1988; 16:4569.

89. Haeuptle MT, Frank R, Dobberstein B. Translation arrest by oligodeoxynucleotides complementary to mRNA coding sequences yields polypeptides of predetermined length. *Nucleic Acids Res* 1986; 14:1427.

90. Doris-Keller H. Site specific enzymatic cleavage of RNA. *Nucleic Acid Res* 1979; 7:179.

91. Kawasaki AM, Casper MD, Freier SM, et al. Uniformly modified 2'-deoxy-2'-fluoro phosphorothioate oligonucleotides as nuclease resistant antisense compounds with high affinity and specifity for RNA targets. *J Med Chem* 1993; 36:831.

92. Sproat BS, Lamond AL, Beijer B, et al. Highly efficient chemical synthesis of 2'-O-methyloligoribonucleotides and tetrabiotinylated derivatives; novel probes that are resistant to degradation by RNA or DNA specific nucleases. *Nucleic Acids Res* 1989; 17:3373.

93. Morvan F, Rayner B, Imbach J-L. α-Oligonucleotides: A unique class of modified chimeric nucleic acids. *Anti-Cancer Drug Design* 1991; 6:521.

94. Gagnor C, Rayner B, Leonetti JP, et al. α-DNA IX. Parallel annealing of α-anomeric oligo-doxyribonucleotides to natural mRNA is required for interference in RNaseH mediated hydrolysis and reverse transcription. *Nucleic Acids Res* 1989; 17:5107.

95. Maher JL, III, Wold B, Dervan PG. Inhibition of DNA binding properties by oligonucleotide-directed triple helix formation. *Science* 1989; 245:725.

96. Miller PS. Non-ionic antisense oligonucleotides. In: Cohen JS, ed. *Oligodeoxynucleotides: Antisense Inhibitors of Gene Expression.* Boca Raton, FL: CRC. 1989:79.

97. Stein CA, Cohen JS. Phosphorothiote oligodeoxynucleotide analogues. In: Cohen JS, ed. *Oligodeoxynucleotides: Antisense Inhibitors of Gene Expression.* Boca Raton, FL: CRC. 1989:97.

98. Cazenave C, Stein CA, Loreau N, et al. Comparative inhibition of rabbit globin mRNA translation by modified antisense oligodeoxynucleotides. *Nucleic Acids Res* 1989; 17:4255.

99. Quartin R, Brakel C, Wetmur J. Number and distribution of methylphosphonate linkages in oligodeoxynucleotides affect exo- and endonuclease sensitivity and ability to form RNase H substrates. *Nucleic Acids Res* 1989; 17:7253.

100. Furdon P, Dominski Z, Kole R. RNase H cleavage of RNA hybridized to oligonucleotides containing methylphosphonate, phosphorothioate and phosphodiester bonds. *Nucleic Acids Res* 1989; 17:9193.

101. Eder PS, Walder JA. Ribonuclease H from K562 human erythroleukemia cells. *J Biol Chem* 1991; 206:6472.

102. Monia BP, Lesnik EA, Gonzalez C, et al. Evaluation of 2′ modified oligonucleotides containing 2′-deoxy gaps as antisense inhibitors of gene expression. *J Biol Chem* 1993:268.

103. Giles RV, Tidd DM. Increased specificity for antisense oligodeoxynucleotide targeting of RNA cleavage by RNase H using chimeric methylphosphonodiester structures. *Nucleic Acids Res* 1992; 20:763.

104. Walder RY, Walder JA. Role of RHase H in hybrid-arrested translation by antisense oligonucleotides. *Proc Natl Acad Sci USA* 1988; 85:5011.

105. Minshull J, Hunt T. The use of single-stranded DNA and RNase H to promote quantitative hybrid arrest of translation of mRNA/DNA hybrids in reticulocyte lysate cell-free translations. *Nucleic Acids Res* 1986; 14:6433.

106. Gagnor C, Bertrand J, Thenet S, et al. Alpha-DNA VI: Comparative study of alpha- and beta-anomeric oligodeoxyribonucleotides in hybridization to mRNA and in cell free translation inhibition. *Nucleic Acids Res* 1987; 15:10419.

107. Knorre DG, Vlassov VV, Zarytova VF. Reactive oligonucleotide derivatives and sequence-specific modification of nucleic acids. *Biochimie* 1985; 67:785.

108. Knoore DG, Vlassov VV, Zarytova VF. Oligonucleotides linked to reactive groups. In: Cohen JS, ed. *Oligodeoxynucleotides: Antisense Inhibitors of Gene Expression.* Boca Raton, FL: CRC. 1989:173.

109. Vlassov VV, Zarytova VF, Kutyavin IV, et al. Sequence-specific chemical modification of a hybrid bacteriophage M13 single-stranded DNA by alkylating oligonucleotide derivatives. *FEBS Lett* 1988; 231:352.

110. Summerton J, Bartlett, PA. Sequence-specific crosslinking agents for nucleic acids. Use of 6-bromo-5,5-dimethoxyhexanohydrazide for crosslinking cytidine to guanosine and crosslinking RNA to complementary sequences of DNA. *J Mol Biol* 1978; 122:145.

111. Webb TR, Matteucci MD. Hybridization triggered crosslinking of leoxynucleotides. *Nucleic Acids Res* 1986; 14:7661.

112. Cooney M, Czernuszewicz G, Postel EH, et al. Site-specific oligonucleotide binding represses transcription of the human c-myc gene in vitro. *Science* 1988; 241:456.

113. Moser HE, Dervan PB. Sequence specific cleavage of double helical DNA by triple helix formation. *Science* 1987; 238:650.

114. Le Doan T, Perrouault L, Praseuth D, et al. Sequence-specific recognition, photocrosslinking and cleavage of the DNA double helix by an oligo-[alpha]-thymidylate covalently linked to an azidoproflavine derivative. *Nucleic Acids Res* 1987; 15:7749.

115. Federova OS, Knorre DG, Podust LM, et al. Complementary addressed modification of double-stranded DNA within a ternary complex. *FEBS Lett* 1988; 228:273.

116. Praseuth D, Perrouault L, Le Doan T, et al. Sequence-specific binding and photocrosslinking

of [alpha] and [beta]-oligodeoxynucleotides to the major groove of DNA via triple helix formation. *Proc Natl Acad Sci USA* 1988; 85:1349.

117. Praseuth D, Doan TL, Chassignol M, et al. Sequence-targeted photosensitized reactions in nucleic acids by oligo-α-deoxynucleotides and oligo-β-deoxynucleotides covalently linked to proflavin. *Biochemistry* 1988; 27:3031.

118. Le Doan T, Perrouault L, Chassignol M, et al. Sequence-targeted chemical modifications of nucleic acids by complementary oligonucleotides covalently linked to porphyrins. *Nucleic Acids Res* 1987; 15:8643.

119. Le Doan T, Perrouault L, Thuong NT, et al. Sequence-specific chemical and photochemical reactions on nucleic acids by oligonucleotides linked to porphyrins. *J Inorg Biochem* 1989; 36:274 (abstract).

120. Le Doan T, Praseuth D, Perrouault L, et al. Sequence-targeted photochemical modifications of nucleic acids by complementary oligonucleotides covalently linked to porphyrins. *Bioconj Chem* 1990; 1:108.

121. Lee BL, Blake KR, Miller PS. Interaction of psoralen-derivatized oligodeoxyribonucleoside methylphosphonates with synthetic DNA containing a promoter for T7 RNA polymerase. *Nucleic Acids Res* 1988; 16:10,681.

122. Lee BL, Murakami A, Blake KR, et al. Interaction of psoralen-derivatized oligodeoxyribonucleoside methylphosphonates with single-stranded DNA. *Biochemisty* 1988; 27:3197.

123. Praseuth D, Chassignol M, Takasugi M, et al. Double helices with parallel strands are formed by nuclease-resistant oligo-[alpha]-deoxynucleotides and oligo-[alpha]-deoxynucleotides covalently linked to an intercalating agent with complementary oligo-[beta]-deoxynucleotides. *J Mol Biol* 1987; 196:939.

124. Perrouault L, Asseline U, Rivalle C, et al. Sequence-specific artificial photo-induced endonucleases based on triple-helix forming oligonucleotides. *Nature* 1990; 344:358.

125. Helene C. Artificial control of gene expression by oligonucleotides covalently linked to intercalating agents. *Br J Cancer* 1989; 60:157.

126. Kean JM, Murakami A, Blake KR, et al. Photochemical cross-linking of psoralen-derivatized oligonucleotide methylphosphonates to rabbit globin messenger RNA. *Biochemistry* 1988; 27:9113.

127. Saison-Behmoaras T, Tocque B, Rey I, et al. Short modified oligonucleotides directed against Ha-ras point mutation induce selective cleavage of the mRNA and inhibit T24 cells proliferation. *Embo J* 1991; 10:1111.

128. Dervan PB. Oligonucleotide recognition of double-helical DNA by triple-helix formation. In: Cohen JS, ed. *Oligodeoxynucleotide: Antisense Inhibitors of Gene Expression*. Boca Raton, FL: CRC. 1989;197.

129. Chu BCF, Orgel LE. Nonenzymatic sequence-specific cleavage of single-stranded DNA. *Proc Natl Acad Sci USA* 1985; 82:963.

130. Boutorin AS, Vlassov VV, Kazakov SA, et al. Complementary addressed reagents carrying EDTA-Fe(II) groups for directed cleavage of single-stranded nucleic acids. *FEBS Lett* 1984; 172:43.

131. Francois JC, Saison-Behmoaras T, Chassignol M, et al. Periodic cleavage of poly(dA) by oligothymidylates covalently linked to ^{1,10}-phenanthroline-copper complexes. *Biochemistry* 1988; 27:2272.

132. Francois JC, Saison-Behmoaras T, Barbier C, et al. Sequence-specific recognition and cleavage of duplex DNA via triple helix formation by oligonucleotides covalently linked to a phenanthroline-copper chelate. *Proc Natl Acad Sci USA* 1989; 86:9702.

133. Francois JC, Saison-Behmoaras T, Chassignol M, et al. Sequence-targeted cleavage of single- and double-stranded DNA by oligothymidylates covalently linked to ^{1,10}-phenanthroline. *J Biol Chem* 1989; 264:5891.

134. Sun JS, Francois JC, Lavery R, et al. Sequence-targeted cleavage of nucleic acids by oligo-[α]-thymidylate-phenanthroline conjugates: parallel and anti-parallel double helices are formed with DNA and RNA, respectively. *Biochemistry* 1988; 27:6039.

135. Chen C.-HB, Sigman DS. Nuclease activity of 1,10-phenanthroline-copper: sequence-specific targeting. *Proc Natl Acad Sci USA* 1986; 83:7147.

136. Helene C, Le Doan T, Thuong NT. Sequence-targeted photochemical reactions in single-stranded and double-stranded nucleic acids by oligonucleotide-photosensitizer conjugated. In: Nielson PE, ed. *Photochemical Probes in Biochemistry*. Kluwer Academic Publishers. 1989:219.

137. Helene C, Thuong NT. Oligodeoxynucleotides covalently linked to intercalating agents and to nucleic acid-cleaving reagents. New families of gene regulatory substances. In: Chagas C, Pullman B, eds. *Working Group on Molecular Mechanisms of Carcinogenic and Antitumor Activity*. Vatican City: Pontificaiae Academiae Scientarium Scripta Varia. 1987:205.

138. Helene C, Thuong NT. Control of gene expression by oligonucleotides covalently linked to intercalating agents. *Genome* 1989; 31:413.

139. Cech TR. The chemistry of self-splicing RNA and RNA enzymes. *Science* 1987; 236:1532.

140. McSwiggen JA, Cech TR. Stereochemistry of RNA cleavage by the *tetrahymena* ribozyme and evidence that the chemical step is not rate-limiting. *Science* 1989; 244:679.

141. Uhlenbeck OC. Using ribozymes to cleave RNAs. In: Crooke ST, Lebleu B, eds. *Antisense Research and Applications*. Boca Raton, FL: CRC. 1993:83.

142. Haseloff J, Gerlach WL. Simple RNA enzymes with new and highly specific endoribonuclease activities. *Nature* 1988; 334:585.

143. McCall MJ, Hendry P, Jennings PA. Minimal sequence requirements for ribozyme activity. *Proc Natl Acad Sci* 1992; 89:5710.

144. Chowrira BM, Berzal-Harranz A, Keller CF, et al. Four ribose 2'-hydroxyl groups essential for catalytic function of the hairpin ribozyme. *J Biol Chem* 1993; 268:19,458.

145. Perrouault J-P, Wu T, Cousineau B, et al. Mixed deoxyrib- and ribo-oligonucleotides with catalytic activity. *Nature* 1990; 344:565.

146. Koizumi M, Ohtsuka E. Effects of phosphorothioate and 2-amino groups in hammerhead ribozymes on cleavage rates and Mg^{2+} binding. *Biochemistry* 1991; 30:5145.

147. Heidenreich O, Benseler F, Fahrenholz A, et al. High activity and stability of hammerhead ribozymes containing 2'-modified pyrimidine nucleosides and phosphorothioates *J Biol Chem* 1993; 269:2131.

148. Pieken WA, Olsen DB, Benseler F, et al. Kinetic characterization of ribonuclease-resistant 2'-modified hammerhead ribozymes. *Science* 1991; 253:314.

149. Olsen DB, Benseler F, Aurup H, et al. Study of a hammerhead ribozyme containing 2'-modified adenosine residues. *Biochem* 1991; 30:9735.

150. Goodchild J. Enhancement of ribozyme catalytic activity by a contiguous oligodeoxynucleotide (facilitator) and by 2'-O methylation. *Nucleic Acids Res* 1992; 20:4607.

151. Forster AC, Altman S. External guide sequences for an RNA enzyme. *Science* 1990; 249:783.

152. Yuan Y, Hwang E-S, Altman S. Targeted cleavage of mRNA by human RNase P. *Proc Natl Acad Sci* 1992; 89:8006.

153. Herschlag D, Cech TR. DNA cleavage catalyzed by the ribozyme from *Tetrahymena*. *Nature* 1990; 344:405.

154. Wilhelm JE, Vale RD. RNA on the move: The mRNA localization pathway. *J Cell Biol* 1993; 123:269.

155. Kislauskis EH, Li Z, Singer RH, et al. Isoform-specific 3'-untranslated sequences sort α-cardiac and β-cytoplasmic actin messenger RNAs to different cytoplasmic compartments. *J Cell Biol* 1993; 123:165.

156. Crooke ST. Progress toward oligonucleotide therapeutics: Pharmacodynamic properties. *FASEB J* 1993; 7:533.

157. Bennett CF, Crooke ST. Oligonucleotide-based inhibitors of cytokine expression and function. In: Henderson B, Bodmer M, eds. *Therapeutic Modulation of Cytokines*. Boca Raton, FL: CRC. 1995; in press.

158. Bennett CF, Condon TP, Grimm S, et al. Inhibition of endothelial cell adhesion molecule expression with antisense oligonucleotides. *J Immunol* 1994; 152:3530.

159. Cook PD. Medicinal chemistry strategies for antisense research. In: Crooke ST, Lebleu B, eds. *Antisense Research and Applications*. 1993:149.

160. Lima WF, Monia BP, Ecker DJ, et al. Implication of RNA structure on antisense oligonucleotide hybridization kinetics. *Biochemistry* 1992; 31:12,055.

161. Cohen JS. Phosphorothioate oligodeoxynucleotides. In: Crooke ST, Lebleu B, eds. *Antisense*

Research and Applications. Boca Raton, FL: CRC. 1993:205.

162. Freier SM. Hybridization: Considerations affecting antisense drugs. In: Crooke ST, Lebleu B, eds. *Antisense Research and Applications*. Boca Raton, FL: CRC. 1993:67.

163. Joos RW, Hall WH. Determination of binding constants of serum albumin for penicillin. *J Pharmacol Exp Ther* 1969; 166:113.

164. Loke SL, Stein CA, Zhang XH, et al. Characterization of oligonucleotide transport into living cells. *Proc Natl Acad Sci* 1989; 86:3474.

165. Graham MJ, Cummins L, Cooke ME, et al. *In vitro* metabolism of phosphorothioate antisense oligonucleotides. 1994, submitted.

166. Gao W-Y, Han F-S, Storm C, et al. Phosphorothioate oligonucleotides are inhibitors of human DNA polymerases and RNase H: Implications for antisense technology. *Mol Pharm* 1991; 41:223.

167. Stein CA, Cheng Y-C. Antisense oligonucleotides as therapeutic agents—Is the bullet really magic? *Science* 1993; 261:1004.

168. Agrawal S, Temsamani J, Tang JY. Pharmacokinetics, biodistribution and stability of oligodeoxynucleotide phosphorothioates in mice. *Proc Natl Acad Sci* 1991; 88:7595.

169. Majumdar C, Stein CA, Cohen JS, et al. Stepwise mechanism of HIV reverse transcriptase: primer function of phosphorothioate oligodeoxynucleotide. *Biochem* 1989; 28:1340.

170. Cheng Y-C, Gao W, Han F. Against human immunodeficiency virus and herpes viruses. *Nucleosides & Nucleotides* 1991; 10:155.

171. Stein CA, Neckers LM, Nair BC, et al. Phosphorothioate oligodeoxycytidine interferes with binding of HIV-1 with gp120 to CD4. *J AIDS* 1991; 4:686.

172. Fields AP, Bednarik DP, Hess A, et al. Human immunodeficiency virus induces phosphorylation of its cell surface receptor. *Nature* 1991; 333:278.

173. Wyatt JR, Vickers TA, Roberson JL, et al. Combinatorially selected guanosine-quartet structure is a potent inhibitor of human immunodeficiency virus envelop-mediated cell fusion. *Proc Natl Acad Sci* 1994; 91:1356.

174. Campbell JM, Bacon TA, Wickstrom E. Oligodeoxynucleoside phosphorothioate stability in subcellular extracts, culture media, sera and cerebrospinal fluid. *J Biochem Biophys Methods* 1990; 20:259.

175. Cossum PA, Sasmor H, Dellinger D, et al. Disposition of the ^{14}C-labeled phosphorothioate oligonucleotide ISIS 2105 after intravenous administration to rats. *J Pharmacol Exp Ther* 1993; 267:1181.

176. Crooke RM. *In vitro* toxicology and pharmacokinetics of antisense oligonucleotides. *Anti-Cancer Drug Design* 1991; 6:609.

177. Crooke RM. *In vitro* and *in vivo* toxicology of first generation analogs. In: Crooke ST, Lebleu B, eds. *Antisense Research and Applications*. Boca Raton, FL: CRC. 1993:471.

178. Crooke RM, Graham MJ, Cooke ME, et al. *In vitro* pharmacokinetic analysis of tritiated ISIS 2105 and other phosphorothioate antisense oligonucleotides. Submitted, 1994.

179. Nestle FO, Mitra RS, Bennett CF, et al. Cationic lipid is not required for uptake and selective inhibitory activity of ICAM-1 phosphorothioate antisense oligonucleotides in keratinocytes. *J Invest Dermatol* 1994; 103:569.

180. Neckers LM. Cellular internalization of oligodeoxynucleotides. In: Crooke ST, Lebleu B, eds. *Antisense Research and Applications*. Boca Raton, FL: CRC. 1993:451–460.

181. Chrissey LA, Walz SE, Pazirandeh M, et al. Internalizing of oligodeoxyribonucleotides by *Vibrio parahaemolyticus*. *Antisense Res Dev* 1993; 3:367.

182. Crooke RM. Cellular uptake, distribution and metabolism of phosphorothiote, phosphorodiester and methylphosphonate oligonucleotides. In: Crooke ST, Lebleu B, eds. *Antisense Research and Applications*. Boca Raton, FL: CRC. 1993:427.

183. Bennett CF, Chiang M-Y, Chan H, et al. Cationic lipids enhance cellular uptake and activity of phosphorothioate antisense oligonucleotides. *Mol Pharm* 1992; 41:1023.

184. Bennett CF, Chiang M-Y, Chan H, et al. Use of cationic lipids to enhance the biological activity of antisense oligonucleotides. *J Liposome Res* 1993; 3:85.

185. Iversen P. *In vivo* studies with phosphorothioate oligonucleotides: pharmacokinetic prologue. *Anti-Cancer Drug Design* 1991; 6:531.

186. Cossum PA, Truong L, Owens SR, et al. Pharmacokinetics of a ^{14}C labeled phosphorothioate oligonucleotides, ISIS 2105, after intradermal administration to rats. *J Pharmacol Exp Ther* 1994; 269:89.

187. Crooke ST, Grillone LR, Tendolkar A, et al. A pharmacokinetic evaluation of ^{14}C labeled afovirsen sodium in genital wart patients. *Clin Pharm Ther* 1994; 56:641–646.

188. Sands H, Gorey-Feret LJ, Cocuzza AJ, et al. Biodistribution and metabolism of internally ^{3}H-labeled oligonucleotides. I. Comparison of a phosphodiester and a phosphorothioate. *Mol Pharm* 1994; 45:932.

189. Bayever E, Iversen PL, Bishop MR, et al. Systemic administration of a phosphorothioate oligonucleotide with a sequence complementary to p53 for acute myelogenous leukemia and myelodysplastic syndrome: initial results of a phase 1 trial. *Antisense Res Dev* 1993; 3:383.

190. Cook PD. Medicinal chemistry strategies for antisense research. In: Crooke ST, Lebleu B, eds. *Antisense Research and Applications.* Boca Raton, FL: CRC. 1993:303.

191. Azad RF, Driver VB, Tanaka K, et al. Antiviral activity of a phosphorothioate oligonucleotide complementary to RNA of the human cytomegalovirus major immediate-early region. *Antimicrob Agents and Chemother* 1993; 37:1945.

192. Wagner RW, Matteucci MD, Lewis JG, et al. Antisense gene inhibition by oligonucleotides containing C-5 propyne pyrimidines. *Science* 1993; 260:1510.

193. Nagel KM, Holstad SG, Isenberg KE. Oligonucleotide pharmacotherapy. An antigene stratety. *Pharmacotherapy* 1993; 13:177.

194. Simons M, Edelman ER, DeKeyser J-L, et al. Antisense c-myb oligonucleotides inhibit intimal arterial smooth muscle cell accumulation *in vivo. Nature* 1992; 359:67.

195. Abe J, Zhou W, Taguchi J, et al. Suppression of neointimal smooth muscle cell accumulation *in vivo* by antisense CDC2 and CDK2 oligonucleotides in rat carotid artery. *Biochem Biophys Res Commun* 1994; 198:16.

196. Whitesell L, Rosolen A, Neckers LM. *In vivo* modulation of N-myc expression by continuous perfusion with an antisense oligonucleotide. *Antisense Res Dev* 1991; 1:343.

197. Perkaly L, Saijo Y, Busch RK, et al. Growth inhibition of human tumor cell lines by antisense oligonucleotides designed to inhibit p120 expression. *Anti-Cancer Drug Design* 1993; 8:3.

198. Wahlestedt C, Pich EM, Koob GF, et al. Modulation of anxiety and neuropeptide Y-Y1 receptors by antisense oligodeoxynucleotides. *Science* 1993; 259:528.

199. Wahlestedt C, Golanov E, Yamamotop S, et al. Antisense oligodeoxynucleotides to NMDA-R1 receptor channel protect cortical neurons from excitotoxicity and reduce focal ischaemic infarctions. *Nature* 1993; 363:260.

200. Osen-Sand A, Catsicas M, Staple JK, et al. Inhibition of axonal growth by SNAP-25 antisense oligonucleotides *in vitro* and *in vivo. Nature* 1993; 364:445.

201. Burch RM, Mahan LC. Oligonucleotides antisense to the interleukin 1 receptor mRNA block the effects of interleukin 1 in cultured murine and human fibroblasts and in mice. *J Clin Invest* 1991; 88:1190.

202. Kitajima I, Shinohara T, Bilakovics J, et al. Ablation of transplanted HTLV-1 tax-transformed tumors in mice by antisense inhibition of NF-kB. *Science* 1992; 258:1792.

203. Higgins KA, Perez JR, Coleman TA, et al. Antisense inhibition of the p65 subunit of NF-kB blocks tumorigenicity and causes tumor regression. *Proc Natl Acad Sci* 1993; 90:9901.

204. Skorski T, Nieborowska-Skorska M, Nicolaides NC, et al. Suppression of Ph^1 leukemia cell growth in mice by BCR-ABL antisense oligodeoxynucleotide. *Proc Natl Acad Sci* 1994; 91:4504.

205. Hijiya N, Zhang J, Ratajczak MZ, et al. Biological and therapeutic significance of MYB expression in human melanoma. *Proc Natl Acad Sci* 1994; 91:4499.

206. Dean NM, McKay R. Inhibition of PKC-α expression in mice after systemic administration of phosphorothioate antisense oligonucleotides. *Proc Natl Acad Sci* 1994; 91:11,762–11,766.

207. Guadette MF, Hampikian G, Metelev V, et al. Effect on embryos of injection of phosphorothioate-modified oligonucleotides into pregnant mice. *Antisense Res Dev* 1993; 3:391.

208. Branda RF, Moore AL, Mathews L, et al. Immune stimulation by an antisense oligomer complementary to the *rev* gene of HIV-1. *Biochem Pharmacol* 1993; 45:2037.

209. McIntyre KW, Lombard-Gilooly K, Perez JR, et al. A sense phosphorothioate oligonucleotide directed to the initiation codon of transcription factor NF-kB p65 causes sequence-specific

immune stimulation. *Antisense Res Dev* 1993; 3:309.

210. Cornish KG, Iversen P, Smith L, et al. Cardiovascular effects of a phosphorothioate oligonucleotide with sequence antisense to p53 in the conscious rhesus monkey. *Pharmacol Commun* 1993; 3:239.

211. Crooke ST. Advances in oligonucleotide therapeutics. *1994 Experimental Biology Meeting, American Society for Pharmacology and Experimental Therapeutics,* Anaheim, CA, April 24–28, 1994. Abstract.

212. Palestine AG, Cantrill HL, Luckie AP, et al. Intravitreal treatment of CMV retinitis with an antisense oligonucleotide, ISIS 2922. *Tenth International Conference on AIDS.* Yokohama, Japan, August 7–12, 1994. Abstract.

213. Stepkowski SM, Tu Y, Condon TP, et al. Blocking of heart allograft rejection by intercellular adhesion molecule-1 antisense oligonucleotides alone or in combination with other immunosuppressive modalities. *J Immunol* 1994; 153:5336.

16 Growth Factors and Growth Factor Inhibitors

Edward A. Sausville, MD, PhD and Dan L. Longo, MD

CONTENTS

1. INTRODUCTION

This chapter will outline novel treatment strategies predicated on the modulation of growth factor or cytokine-mediated signal transduction pathways. Several excellent recent monographs have addressed this tissue from the point of view of inhibitors of individual pathway constituents (*1,2*). The current focus will be on defining the pathways potentially relevant to the common neoplasms, followed by a consideration of approaches to modulating processes common to the action of various pathways, with mention of individual agents as they exemplify these strategies. In addition, opportunities for interdigitation of "growth-factor directed" and "traditional" therapeutic agents will be considered.

One view of neoplasia (*3*) is that it is fundamentally a disorder of cellular communication induced by somatic mutations of growth regulatory genes. An extension of this hypothesis is the "autocrine" promotion of neoplasia, first put forth in response to the realization that a prominent aspect of the transformed phenotype in tissue culture or other artificial systems is a reduction in the requirement for exogenous growth factors usually supplied in the form of serum (*4*). Thus, as illustrated in Fig. 1, tumor cells could be viewed as secreting their own "autocrine" factors, or responding to

From: *Cancer Therapeutics: Experimental and Clinical Agents*
Edited by: B. Teicher Humana Press Inc., Totowa, NJ

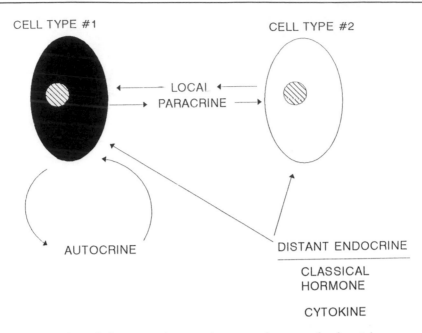

Fig. 1. Growth factors act in autocrine, paracrine, or endocrine styles.

"paracrine" factors secreted by adjacent tumor cells or stroma. The pathways activated by these factors would act in parallel or in addition to the traditional endocrine influences, although with the elucidation of the structures of multiple cytokines, it is clear that the concept of endocrine control of tumor cell growth may have to be altered to include cytokines.

A corollary of this thinking is that manipulation of growth-factor-directed pathways may offer inroads into the therapeusis of neoplasia that actually manipulate neoplastic physiology, rather than "simply" seeking cytotoxicity. From a strategic perspective, an enhanced therapeutic index and more specific targeting of the tumor are the hoped-for consequences, although the tools to begin this endeavor in a clinical sense are only now emerging.

2. SIGNAL TRANSDUCTION PATHWAYS AND MECHANISMS

2.1. Tyrosine Kinase-Linked Signaling

Soon after the elucidation of the structure of Rous sarcoma virus (RSV) genome, it became apparent that neoplastic transformation was caused by a protein kinase activity directed at tyrosine residues detectable in immunoprecipitates using serum from tumor-bearing animals or antibodies raised against the putative v-*src* transforming protein (*5*). Although phosphotyrosine was a relatively minor phosphoamino acid in normal cells, it was possible to demonstrate that RSV-transformed cells had increased levels of phosphotyrosine. The transforming oncogenes of numerous acute transforming viruses were found to have a general structure illustrated in Fig. 2. The SH1(*src* homology) domain refers to the ATP binding region, and two other islands of homology defined the SH2 and SH3 domains represented in the *abl, fps, fgr, yes, lyn, fyn, lck,* and other nonreceptor-linked tyrosine kinases (reviewed in ref. *6*).

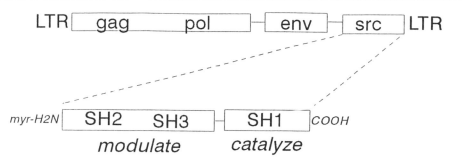

Fig. 2. Overview of non-receptor tyrosine kinase organization. The v-*src* protein arises from the *src* gene present in the RSV genome, downstream of the *gag*, p01, and *env* genes. The SH1 region (*src*-homology) encodes the catalytic domain, and the SH2 and SH3 regions encode regulatory domains.

The importance of these entities to human neoplasia was graphically defined by the demonstration that in certain diseases, pathogenetic alterations of tyrosine kinases could be demonstrated. For example, the Philadelphia chromosome, long known as a cytogenetic marker in chronic myelogenous leukemia (CML) and certain cases of acute lymphoblastic leukemia (ALL), was shown to arise from the translocation of the c-*abl* gene on chromosome 9 into the "breakpoint cluster region" (*bcr*) on chromosome 22 to create a chimeric fusion protein *bcr-abl* with dramatically increased tyrosine kinase activity in comparison to normal c-*abl* (*7–9*). Elevated expression of c-*src* activity was detected in colon carcinomas (*10*), and c-*lck* was aberrantly expressed in certain colon and lung carcinoma cells (*11*). The enzymatic activity of nonreceptor-linked tyrosine kinases can be linked to stimulation of cells by external stimuli. For example, stimulation of T-cells by antigen resulted in increased *lck* activity, and it was possible to demonstrate a physical association between *lck* and the CD4 cell-surface molecule (*12*) that participates in T-cell activation.

Growth factors may be defined as proteins or peptides that stimulate the growth of tissue culture cells in vitro or in organ culture systems. These activities had been defined over the preceding 50 years based primarily on the biologic assay system in which their activity was first manifest (reviewed in *13*). For example, epidermal growth factor (EGF) was first defined as a factor that promoted the development of the neonatal mouse, with potent growth-stimulatory activity for squamous cells. Platelet-derived growth factor (PDGF) was defined as a factor present in platelets that stimulated fibroblast growth. The relation of increased tyrosine kinase activity to growth factor action was strikingly illustrated by the demonstration that the transforming oncogene from the avian erythroblastosis virus consisted of two gene products, one of which, v-*erbB*2, had homology to the EGF-receptor (EGF-R) (*14,15*). A tyrosine kinase activity was clearly encoded by the EGF-R gene, and addition of EGF to cells bearing the EGF-R induced the phosphorylation of numerous intracellular proteins on tyrosine. Subsequent studies revealed this to be a common occurrence after addition of a variety of growth factors and cytokines. Such "growth-factor receptor-linked tyrosine kinases" had common structural features (reviewed in *16*), including an extracellular ligand binding domain, a transmembrane domain, an SH1 domain, and a variety of potential regulatory structural motifs presumed to allow specific signaling. Comparison of sequences of transforming genes from other animal tumors defined the EGF-R as the prototype for a family of growth factor receptors, including c-*erbB*2 (*17*). The clinical importance of the EGF-R family is evident from the frequent elevated expression or amplification of the EGF-R in squamous tumors (*18–20*) or association of adverse prognosis with expression of c-*erbB*2 (*21*).

The most immediate consequence of tyrosine kinase action, altered phosphorylation of proteins in growth factor-stimulated cells, was initially difficult to relate to a specific pathway leading to cellular proliferation, since the phosphorylated molecules included molecules as diverse as cytoskeletal elements and "housekeeping proteins" of uncertain relevance to neoplasia. However, genetic evidence indicated that *ras* oncogene function was required for transformation by oncogenes of the *src* family (*22*), and moreover, it was possible to demonstrate that soon after addition of certain growth factors that acted by tyrosine kinase activation, there was increased activity of the c-*raf* oncogene product (*23*), a serine/threonine kinase. Thus, the concept emerged that there are hierarchical arrangements of protein kinase activities in growth factor-stimulated cells, with growth factor-receptor-linked tyrosine kinases "upstream" of "downstream" serine/threonine kinases.

Three independent approaches were undertaken to define the correct relationships in this signaling pathway. The first was directed at understanding how tyrosine kinases activated their substrates and was based ultimately on the demonstration that transforming oncoproteins existed, such as v-*crk*, which clearly increased the tyrosine phosphate content of transformed cells, but which did not contain an SH1 (phosphoryl-transfer) domain (*24*). By definition, therefore, such a protein could act only by influencing the action of endogenous kinases. However, v-*crk* did contain an SH2-like domain, raising the possibility that SH2 domains could regulate the phosphorylation of substrates for tyrosine kinases. How this might occur was suggested by the demonstration that polyoma middle T-antigen, a tyrosine kinase, could be coimmunoprecipitated with an enzymatic activity, phosphatidylinositol (PI) 3′-kinase, which could also be detected in PDGF- and EGF-stimulated cells. The structure of PI-3′-kinase revealed that it possessed an SH2 domain (*25,26*). This result suggested that SH2 domains could form a physical association with substrates for tyrosine kinases, and indeed, extensive studies have documented that SH2 domains serve as a molecular "docking mechanism" to cause association of phosphotyrosine-containing proteins, including the autophosphorylated growth factor receptors or autophosphorylated tyrosine kinases with the SH2-domain-bearing proteins. In the case of PI-3′-kinase, this association allows a mechanism whereby its activity may be increased after binding to activated signaling molecules (*27*). An analogous mechanism was demonstrated to operate in the case of PDGF-R and EGF-R activation of phospholipase-C-γ (PLC-γ) (*28–30*). The latter finding provided a direct mechanism by which a tyrosine kinase-linked receptor could activate the serine/threonine protein kinase C (PKC), since the product of the activated PLC-γ, diacylglycerol (DAG), is a known endogenous regulator of PKC. The capacity of SH2 domains to subserve an "adapter" function was most dramatically illustrated by the use of a phosphorylated EGF-R as a probe to define proteins that bound phosphorylated tyrosine. This defined a protein *grb2* (which "grabbed" phosphotyrosine) (*31*) with a unique structure consisting of a single SH2 domain flanked by two SH3 domains and no kinase activity. *Grb2* in turn could be demonstrated to be homologous to proteins defined in invertebrate systems as participating in a tyrosine kinase-regulated developmental pathway (*32*), and to form a complex through its SH3 domain with the mammalian homolog of the *son of sevenless* (*Sos*) protein (*33,34*), which was known to regulate *ras* function by causing *ras* proteins to exchange GDP for GTP. Thus, a means for tyrosine kinases to influence *ras* action was demonstrated.

The second approach to define the proper sequence of protein kinase activation after growth factor action was based ultimately on genetic experiments that c-*raf* could be proposed to act "downstream" of *ras*, since "dominant-negative" *ras* mutants did not affect *raf*-transformed systems. This implied a potential interaction between *ras* and *raf*. Such an interaction could be directly demonstrated by high concentrations of cloned and expressed *ras* and *raf* alleles, and ultimately by physical association between *ras* and *raf* in cells (*35,36*). Once *ras* exchanges GDP for GTP, assuming an "activated" conformation, c-*raf* is "recruited" to the membrane, where it undergoes an as yet poorly defined "activation" process, resulting in an increase in the enzymatic activity of c-*raf* (*37,38*).

The final approach that ultimately clarified the downstream effectors of tyrosine kinase action resulted from an examination of the hypothesis that if the "kinase cascade" of growth factor action was correct, then serine/threonine kinase activities should increase following the application of a stimulus of tyrosine kinase activity. Thus, it was possible to demonstrate that after application of EGF, a variety of activities increased, including an activity that phosphorylated a *M*icrotubule *A*ssociated *P*rotein (MAP) kinase and increased its kinase activity for the MAP substrate (*39–41*). This activity was unique in that the MAP kinase could be shown to require both tyrosine and threonine phosphorylation for activity. This allowed the definition of a "dual-specificity" MAP kinase kinase (MAPKK) (*42?*), which was itself regulated by c-*raf* kinase (*43*), thus linking tyrosine kinase action ultimately to the activation of MAP kinase. The significance of this observation is that MAP kinase could be demonstrated to phosphorylate several nuclear proteins, including the *myc* and *jun* oncoproteins, cytoskeletal elements, and transcription factors. Thus, a cell-surface ligand–receptor interaction is linked through a series of direct and indirect steps to the expression of specific genes (*41*).

The current view of tyrosine kinase-mediated signaling is summarized in Fig. 3, where either engagement of a growth factor receptor in quiescent cells or stimulation of a nonreceptor-linked tyrosine kinase through cell-surface molecules with which it forms a noncovalent association leads to stimulation of *ras* activity, which in turn activates c-*raf* and ultimately MAP kinase. The action of the latter protein causes increased transcription of regulatory molecules, which allows either entry into or normal progression through the G1 phase of the cell cycle.

2.2. G-Protein-Linked Signaling

A distinct class of growth factor receptors uses receptors that function not by directly inducing covalent modification of substrate proteins, as is the case with the tyrosine protein kinase-linked receptors, but rather by the elaboration of "second messengers" that allosterically modify the function of effector molecules, including protein kinases and phospholipases. The paradigm for humoral mediators of this class is the β-adrenergic receptor, which activates adenylate cyclase and thereby catalyzes the conversion of ATP to cyclic AMP (cAMP). cAMP in turn binds to regulatory subunits of cAMP-

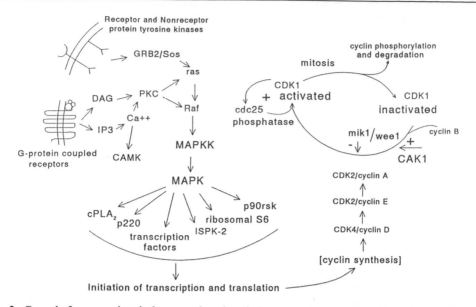

Fig. 3. Growth factor action induces a phosphorylation cascade. Signaling through growth factor receptors leads to activation of *ras* through the adapter molecule grb2 and the GDP release protein *sos*. Activated *ras*, in turn, increases *raf* activity, which then leads to activation of MAP kinase. Transcription "factors" and other signaling pathways are activated, following entry of cells in a path that results in DNA synthesis.

dependent protein kinase (PKA) (*44*). The molecular "switch" that allows ligand-bound receptor to activate adenylate cyclase is a heterotrimeric "G-protein" that consists of a heterotrimer. Ligand-activated receptor (*see* Fig. 4) releases GDP from the $G_s\alpha$ subunit, which then binds GTP, causing the release of $G_s\alpha$ from the $\beta\gamma$ subunits. The $GTP\cdot G_s\alpha$ subunit stimulates adenylate cyclase until the GTP is hydrolyzed, allowing re-formation of the $G_s\alpha\beta\gamma$ heterotrimer, bearing GDP, ready for induction of another catalytic cycle.

The structures of receptors that utilize this general mechanism are all similar in that they have an extracellular domain, seven transmembrane segments, which course in and out of the membrane in a "serpentine" fashion, and an intracellular "loop," which with its carboxyl-terminal portion interacts with G proteins and is the site of receptor-directed regulatory mechanisms, including desensitization and control of receptor internalization controls (reviewed in *45,46*). G proteins exist that, as indicated above, stimulate adenylate cyclase (G_s), inhibit adenylate cyclase (G_i), modulate ion channel activity (G_s and G_o), stimulate phospholipase-$C\beta$ (G_q and G_{16}), and couple photoreceptors to cGMP phosphodiesterase (G_T). Of special relevance to targeting therapeutic measures at the pathways activated by these transducers, G_s is known as the target for cholera toxin, which covalently modifies it to assume a persistently activated state; G_i is the target for pertussis toxin, which causes an inhibitory covalent modification. Note that the heterotrimeric G proteins do have limited homology to the monomeric GTP binding proteins, such as members of the *ras* oncoprotein super-family in the GTP binding domain and in the overall scheme of catalysis, but are distinctive in that the ras alleles in higher eukaryotes have never been shown to regulate

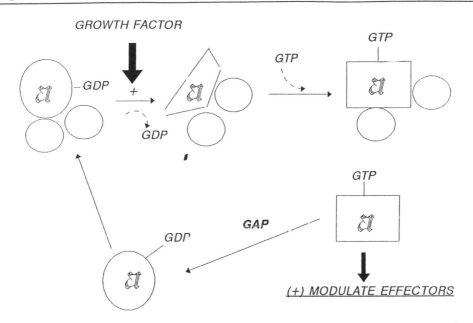

Fig. 4. G protein cycle. The inactive G protein, bearing GDP, is caused to release GDP under the influence of a growth factor or hormone. A transient inactive "empty" subunit exists, but then binds GTP, activating the α subunit to modulate positively effectors, such as adenylate cylase. Hydrolysis of the GTP to GDP under the influence of a GTPase-activating protein (GAP) returns the α subunit to its basal state, bound to G protein β and γ subunits (empty circles).

directly the action of downstream soluble effectors, such as cAMP, but as indicated above, appear to engage in protein–protein interactions in the activated state.

G protein-coupled receptors and their downstream effectors are of potential relevance to a number of human neoplasms. Neuropeptides of the bombesin family, of possible importance in the pathogenesis of lung, breast, and prostate neoplasms, have serpentine receptors (*47*) that activate phospholipase-C (*48*). The consequence of that interaction is elevation of intracellular Ca^{2+} and diacylglycerol, the latter serving in particular to activate PKC. Pituitary tumors have been shown to have "activating" mutations in $G_s\alpha$ (*49*), and in model systems, transfectants from immortalized cell lines bearing heterologous serpentine receptors can apparently cause tumors in a ligand-dependent fashion (*50*). In addition to adrenergic receptors, this class includes receptors for chemotactic cytokines or chemokines (e.g., IL-8, RANTES, IL-10), for f-met-leu-phe, and for autocrine motility factor, which is involved in directed migration of tumor cells (*51*).

2.3. Other Signal Transduction Mechanisms

The tyrosine kinases and the G protein-linked mechanisms account for the transduction mechanisms employed by hundreds of humoral mediators, including growth factors, autocoids, and cytokines. However, in a few specialized instances, other receptor mechanisms have been defined that also have potential therapeutic relevance, although in many cases, aspects of their mechanisms have not been as extensively defined as in the former two receptor types.

2.3.1. A Serine-Kinase-Linked Receptor: Transforming Growth Factor-β (TGF-β)

TGF-β has recently been demonstrated to engage a receptor (receptor II), a constitutively active transmembrane serine/threonine kinase (52), which after binding of TGF-β engages a "receptor I" into a noncovalent complex, allowing propagation by receptor I of a serine/threonine kinase signal to downstream substrates. The definition of those downstream effectors will be of interest to define, since TGF-β is a negative growth regulator of a variety of cell types, perhaps by acting as a negative regulator of cyclin-dependent kinases (53).

2.3.2. Tumor-Necrosis Factor (TNF) Receptors

The TNF family consists of TNF-α (cachectin), TNF-β (lymphotoxin), and lymphotoxin B, which are now recognized as major inflammatory cytokines that may also be paracrine effectors in a variety of tumors. Two distinct receptors (p55 and p75) have been identified (54), and evidence exists that either receptor can activate biologic responses to TNF through a mechanism that involves receptor complexing on the cell surface. TNF-treated cells show activation of PKC, but without increases in Ca^{2+}, suggesting that a phospholipase-C is not responsible. Recently, evidence has been presented that the TNF system can activate a sphingomyelinase (55) with the resulting ceramide acting as a second messenger to activate a ceramide-dependent protein kinase. Also of interest has been the recent recognition that receptors related to TNF, including Fas/APO-1 (CD95), can participate in the activation of an endogenous apoptotic death program important in the physiologic regulation of the immune system, but also with relevance to the therapy of neoplasms, such as gliomas, which express the receptor (56). Other members of this receptor family include CD40, CD30, nerve growth factor receptor, and CD27. These receptors have more limited tissue distribution, but may be manipulable for therapeutic goals.

2.3.3. Interferon Receptors and the JAK-STAT Pathway

The interferons are a diverse family of factors originally recognized by their ability to confer resistance to viral infection through activation of discrete genes in cells bearing receptors specific for each interferon subtype. Recent insights into interferon-induced signal transduction have demonstrated that engagement of either IFN-α or IFN-γ receptors activates so-called Janus kinases (tyrosine kinases with two kinase domains, only one of which is active), which then phosphorylate a p91 molecule, which can then bind another p91, p84, or p113 molecule. The protein complex then undergoes rapid ("STAT") transport to the nucleus, where transcription of IFN-responsive genes occurs (57–60). This recently defined mechanism appears to have relevance not only to the action of the IFNs, but also to IL-6, ciliary neurotrophic factor (CNTF), leukemia inhibitory factor, oncostatin M, IL-2, IL-4, IL-7, IL-9, IL-15, growth hormone prolactin, erythropoietin, and GM-CSF.

2.3.4. Phosphatase Signaling Mechanisms: CD45

CD45 was originally defined as an antigen differentially expressed on a variety of hematopoietic lineages, whose epitope derived from a transmembrane glycoprotein with a complex origin from alternative splicing to yield a family of molecules from 180–220 kDa (61). However, definition of the structure of a protein tyrosine phosphate phosphatase revealed homology, and it rapidly followed that CD45 is itself a transmembrane tyrosine phosphate phosphatase, implying a role in the regulation of signal transduction in hematopoietic cell signaling. Construction of CD45 deletion mutants revealed notable defects in antigen-mediated signaling, implying that the functional outcome of CD45 activity is a positive signal in generation of the immune response (*62*). Although this is of obvious significance to normal T-cell function, since there is a growing list of tyrosine phosphate phosphatases identified by homology cloning (*63*), the formal possibility is that their action similarly may propagate a "positive" signal.

2.3.5. PHOSPHATASE SIGNALING MECHANISMS: CYCLOSPORIN

The immunosuppressants cyclosporin and rapamycin bind to a family of intracellular binding proteins that are peptidyl-prolyl isomerases, perhaps important in protein folding (*64*). However, it also appears that the cyclosporin binding protein complex results in inhibition of the phospho-serine/threonine phosphatase calcineurin, abundant in hematopoietic cells and brain (*65*), which is postulated to regulate transcription factor action. In a way not completely understood, this ultimately results in selective inhibition of signaling in T cells through pathways that normally stimulate cytokine and cytokine receptor gene expression, thus accounting for the observed immunosuppression. However, it is likely that other high-affinity drug binding proteins operate on signals important to cell proliferation, since rapamycin in particular (*66*) can mediate inhibition of tumor cell growth. The direct relationship of this effect to inhibition of a particular phosphatase or to other signaling mechanism action is currently unclear.

2.3.6. GANGLIOSIDE SIGNALING MECHANISMS

Gangliosides are glycosphingolipids containing both hydrophobic ceramide and hydrophilic carbohydrate moieties that include sialic acid residues. Gangliosides are generally represented by the letter G followed by M or D to define whether they contain one or two sialic acid residues, respectively, followed by a number or letter to distinguish monosialic acid and disialic acid members from one another. Gangliosides are present in many cell membranes, but are most abundant in nervous tissue, neural crest, and lymphocytes.

Gangliosides can bind to a number of extracellular proteins, including cholera toxin and diphtheria toxin; however, their physiological ligands are not yet defined. The use of monoclonal antibodies (MAb) to mimic ligand–ganglioside interactions has revealed that gangliosides can initiate a wide variety of intracellular signaling mechanisms (*67*). For example, a subset of T cells expresses the GD3 ganglioside. Antibody to this ganglioside induces tyrosine phosphorylation, nuclear translocation of c-rel, but not NFχB, upregulation of IL-2 receptors and HLA-DR, and secretion of interferon-γ (*68*). In addition, T cells stimulated through GD3 proliferate and develop cytotoxic activity. These effects can be inhibited by cyclosporin, staurosporin, and herbimycin A, implying the involvement of cyclophilin/calcineurin, PKC, and tyrosine kinases in this response. T cells normally require two signals to become activated. No other single stimulus exerts such a wide range of biologic effects on T cells. Similar changes have been noted in tumor cells expressing gangliosides.

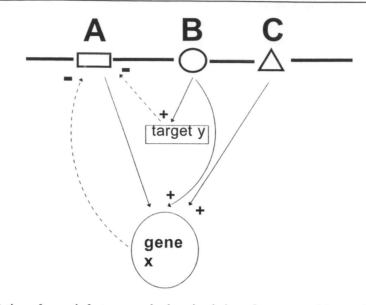

Fig. 5. Regulation of growth factor cascades by stimulation of receptors with negative influence on receptor activation.

3. IMPLICATIONS OF GROWTH FACTOR-DRIVEN CASCADES/NETWORKS

It is apparent that the growth factor-driven signal transduction systems described above do not function independently, but rather act in parallel as well as intersecting arrays. The implications of this arrangement include the possibility that entire pathways may be diminished or augmented in their biologic effect by the action of another pathway at a critical regulatory point in the former pathway. This possibility is illustrated in Fig. 5. Signals propagate from three input receptors and stimulate a particular transcription unit that gives rise to a product that decreases the expression of one of the receptor types. Hence, the result of operation of the signal from ligand A might feedback to decrease response to itself; this is homologous desensitization; however, it is apparent that ligands B and C could also heterologously desensitize the system to the actions of A. In addition, ligand B has a protein-mediated negative regulatory effect on receptor A. This example is not contrived in that, for example, the affinity of EGF-R for EGF is known to be diminished by activated PKC (*67*). The latter could arise from stimulation of EGF-R through PLC-γ, or could arise through activation of G protein kinase-coupled receptors through the action of PLCβ. Another mechanism of receptor desensitization is the modification of the receptor, for example, by phosphorylation, such that its affinity for its ligand is altered or its coupling to its signal transduction mechanism is blocked.

These principles have not been incorporated at all into the design of therapeutically relevant strategies. There has been much focus, as will be shown below, in the design of **specific** antagonists of **specific** targets. Yet it should be clear that narrow therapeutic windows might allow limited biologic effect. What should be pursued are strategies that **decrease** or inappropriately **increase** the activation state of entire pathways in a way that is cell-specific, depending on the array of receptors present.

The most obvious way to effect this goal is to use combinations of growth modulatory large molecules or their antagonists, in conjunction with the small molecules, which although not absolutely specific, may be augmented in their effect or by their action, increase the effect of growth factors or their antagonists acting on their cognate receptors. Such an approach would attempt to capitalize on the pharmacologic tractability of small molecules with the specificity of receptor-mediated processes. Specific types of therapeutic intervention predicated on modulation of growth-factor-related signaling will now be considered.

4. GROWTH FACTORS, ANALOGS, AND ANTAGONISTS

4.1. Suramin

Suramin is a polysulfonated naphthylurea (with a structure that can be viewed as reminiscent of heparan sulfate) that emerged from a screening survey early in the 20th Century to find noncolored analogs of the trypan blue series of antitrypanosomal compounds. Interest in polyanions, such as suramin, as potential antineoplastic agents was renewed following the demonstration that it could reverse simian sarcoma virus transformation (68) and alter the binding of PDGF to its receptor (69). Thus, it was proposed that suramin could antagonize the growth of tumors that depended on autocrine or paracrine mechanisms (70). Antitumor responses in patients have been attributed to suramin in prostate carcinoma, although the exact contribution of suramin to concomitant hormonal manipulation (71), including flutamide withdrawal in that series, remains to be clarified.

An additional difficulty is that the concentration–effect relationship for the inhibition of growth factor binding to receptors is variable with, for example, FGF being somewhat insensitive and FGFs somewhat more sensitive to suramin action. However, it is also clear that the concentrations even where the drug can inhibit the binding of "sensitive" growth factors overlap where effects on a variety of glycosaminoglycan enzymes are also seen, with the consequent risk of anticoagulation.

Nonetheless, it remains formally interesting to consider the development of agents that can specifically bind to growth factors, and suramin is clearly a "lead structure" for this goal with respect to the FGFs in particular. In addition, design of such compounds must take into account the toxicities associated with suramin use, including adrenal injury, neurotoxicity, and susceptibility to infection. Suramin in vivo causes lymphocytopenia and can antagonize IL-2 binding to its receptor (72). It has been incompletely studied in cytokine-driven neoplasms.

4.2. Bombesin-like Peptides

Evidence has been presented that bombesin-like peptides, which in humans include gastrin-releasing peptide and neuromedin-B, function as autocrine growth factors in human small-cell lung carcinoma (73). These peptides function through serpentine receptors (47) coupled to phospholipase-C, with release of Ca^{2+} and phosphatidylinositol turnover (74,75) demonstrable after addition of exogenous peptide. In addition, there is evidence that tumors of diverse histologies, including breast, prostate, and gastrointestinal sites, can respond to peptide addition with similar responses. Since the pharmacophore for this series has been defined and consists of only the C-terminal octapeptide, there has been great interest in developing antagonists (76). SCLC xenografts in athymic mice are susceptible to bombesin antagonists (77). Schally and collaborators have demonstrated antitumor activity in vivo for example, in xenografts of colon, pancreatic, breast, gastric, and CNS origin (*78–80*). Of concern, however, in developing this concept further is the fact that cells have multiple pathways for activation of the Ca^{2+}/phosphatidylinositol signaling pathway (as has been amply demonstrated for SCLC) (*81,82*) and that, therefore, use of alternative receptors for this goal could be accomplished readily in human tumors.

Efforts have also been undertaken to produce antibodies against bombesin peptides, and evidence for some antitumor activity has been observed in SCLC xenografts in athymic mice (*73*). Antibodies to peptides do not localize to tumor masses in vivo in humans and have not been shown to induce responses in a significant fraction of patients. The poor capacity of macromolecules to penetrate tumor masses only heightens the concern that efforts to block Ca^{2+}/PI signaling may elude current therapeutic tools to accomplish this goal by efforts directed at a single-receptor system.

4.3. Somatostatin and Analogs

Lamberts et al. have recently reviewed (*83*) the mechanisms by which somatostatin or its agonists may cause an antitumor effect, including inhibition of the secretion of hormones, such as growth hormone and insulin; direct or indirect inhibition of insulin-like growth factor 1; inhibition of angiogenesis, and a direct antiproliferative effect. The receptors for somatostatin (of which four have been defined) are G protein-coupled receptors that in some systems activate adenylate cyclase. Direct antitumor effects of somatulin have been demonstrated in lung carcinoma xenografts (*84*).

4.4. LHRH Antagonists

In both breast and endometrial carcinoma cells, evidence has been presented that the LHRH antagonist [Ac-D-Nal(2)1,D-Phe(4C1)2,D-Pal(3)3,D-Cit6,D-Ala10]LHRH can inhibit IGF-driven cell proliferation, associated with a decrease in IGF-2 elaboration. A postreceptor mechanism has been proposed (*85,86*), but the nature of the receptor by which the peptide elicits its effect has not been defined.

4.5. Transforming Growth Factor-α

This growth factor is produced by a variety of tumors (e.g., *87,88*) where it signals through the EGF receptor. Efforts to interdict this signaling have included the development of specific antireceptor antibodies (*89,90*) and the synthesis of TGF-α fragments. Most interesting has been the recent observation in model systems (*91,92*) that the combination of an anti-EGF-R antibody plus either cis-platin or doxorubicin appears to increase the likelihood of benefit (*vide intra*). Rieman et al. (*93*) devised a mechanism-based screen of ligand binding to a cell line that overexpresses the receptor, and have examined a series of natural product extracts. One compound series emerged, the methyl pheophorbides, which appear to give evidence not only of blocking the interaction of TGF-α congeners, but also in PDGF and IL-1β assays. In addition, the pheophorbides are related to the protoporphyrins and are dependent on light for efficient action on cells. Although the molecular basis for these effects is not clear, pheophorbides are important as a lead structure for compounds that can "dampen" or eliminate ligand and receptor interaction. Trapidil (*94*) is another compound that, in meningioma cells, inhibits PDGF-R mediated DNA synthesis, yet can also antagonize EGF-driven cell growth in fibroglasts.

4.6 Insulin-like Growth Factor-I (IGF-I)

Convincing evidence by Baserga has recently been summarized (*95*) that IGF-I can function as an important mediator of the transformed state in model systems, and in the maintenance of the transformed phenotype in glioblastoma, breast cancer, small-cell lung cancer, and melanoma cell lines. This system is of interest because in addition to inhibition of IGF-I action by antibodies or potential antagonists, there is a large family of IGF binding proteins (*96,97*) that are coexpressed with IGF-I receptor in, for example, certain breast carcinoma cell lines and, therefore, could represent an alternative strategy to modulating IGF-I action.

4.7. PDGF

The PDGF-R clearly has the potential to transmit an oncogenic signal, since the v-*sis* oncogene product is homologous to the PDGF-β chain. Of interest, evidence has been presented for stimulation of the PDGF-R both at the cell surface and with presentation of the mitogenic signal to the receptor in an intracellular compartment in model systems. Recently, convincing evidence has been presented that an autocrine pathway involving PDGF can drive glioblastoma cell growth (*98*). This result is intriguing because it has been further demonstrated that synthetic peptides can be created that fuse peptide segments from disparate segments of the PDGF molecule to create antagonists of moderate affinity (*99*). Interestingly, these antagonist peptides disrupted receptor dimerization, and although this resulted in clear diminution of receptor autophosphorylation, a decrease in [^{3}H]-thymidine incorporation, which was not restricted to that produced by PDGF, was noted. This finding delineates a potential strategy for the design of antagonists that can affect signals through more than one growth factor system by altering the capacity to dimerize, thus potentially inducing aberrant dimerization.

4.8 Cytokines

Although a comprehensive treatment of this subject would be outside the scope of this chapter, certain cytokine pathways are of clear relevance in considering strategies for clinical exploitation.

The IL2-R consists of the α (T-cell activation antigen; Tac), β, and γ, chains, which together form a heterotrimeric receptor linked to the activation of tyrosine kinase cascades (*100–102*). This receptor system is expressed in a variety of hematopoietic neoplasms (*103*). Current strategies are seeking to target radiolabels or toxins to the IL2-R, either employing antibodies or chimeric fusion proteins (*104–107*) as targeting agents. The latter approach has produced clinical responses in neoplasms bearing the IL2-R (*108–111*). An important feature of the IL2 signaling system is that the γ-chain of the IL2-R is actually shared with the IL4 and IL7 receptors (*112*). A consequence of this is that exposure to IL2 can potentially modulate signaling and mitogenic responses to the other two cytokines. This has been shown to be of functional consequence in cutaneous T-cell lymphoma cells exposed to IL7 (*113*). Of interest to develop are preclinical studies with some of the modulators of protein kinase action to be described below in conjunction with IL2, IL4, or IL7 in neoplasms bearing these receptors.

In multiple myeloma, some evidence exists for an autocrine or paracrine pathway activated by IL6, and although efforts are under way to derive analogous targeting approaches using this cytokine receptor, its expression is more ubiquitous than the IL2 receptor system (*114*), and therefore, the likelihood of a useful therapeutic index is lower. In contrast, the CD30 antigen is a cell-surface molecule with homology to members of the TNF receptor family whose expression is largely restricted to hematopoietic cells, and it is prominently expressed on the Reed-Sternberg cells in Hodgkin's disease. Although it has served as a target for the development of "traditional" toxin or antibody-based targeting strategies, it would be useful to clarify whether TNF-like intracellular signals are elicited by this molecule, since efforts to deregulate their expression could lead to additional therapeutic strategies (*115*).

Cytokine receptors may also be of relevance to the treatment of nonhematopoietic neoplasms. For example, interferon and IL-1 have been clearly demonstrated as potentially useful modulators of the growth of certain gynecologic tumor cells. Recent evidence has been accumulating that IL-1 can inhibit the growth of ovarian carcinoma cells (*116*). IL-1 has also been found to regulate secretion of collagenase, important in mediating invasiveness (*117*) in choriocarcinoma cells. Interferons can also act directly to inhibit the growth of ovarian carcinoma cells (*118*).

5. MODULATION OF CYTOKINE OR GROWTH FACTOR RECEPTOR EXPRESSION

A prominent effect of numerous stimuli for cell activation is an altered display or regulation of cell-surface expression. Examples where this strategy may be of value in developing novel therapeutic strategies include the following cases.

5.1 Interferons

Interferons α and γ can cause marked alterations in apparent expression of EGF-R, perhaps by altering the rate of internalization (*119*). Evidence has been presented for the existence of cell types that, in response to interferons, modulate (*120–122*) expression of the EGF receptor.

5.2. TNF

TNF can act as an autocrine and paracrine (*123*) stimulator of the growth of ovarian carcinoma cells. A striking potential mechanism to consider in explaining these phenomena has recently been demonstrated in pancreatic carcinoma cells, where exposure to TNF caused a decrease in c-*erbB*2 expression, but an increase in EGF-R RNA. The decrease in c-*erbB*2 mRNA was accompanied by decreased protein expression (*124*). Thus, in addition to direct signaling through its own receptor-linked pathways, TNF can clearly influence signaling through these tyrosine kinase linked pathways. The generality of this phenomenon will be of interest to clarify in greater detail.

5.3. Steroids and Retinoids

In breast carcinoma cells, there is considerable evidence that part of the stimulation of growth attributable to estrogens proceeds by activation of growth factor secretion (*125*) with the consequent autocrine or paracrine action of those growth factors on adjacent tumor cells or stroma promoting the growth of the tumor cells. For example, estrogen-treated breast carcinoma cells elaborate TGF-α, FGF, and IGF-like species (*125,126*). Conversely, antiestrogens, such as tamoxifen, droloxifene, and toremifene, can be shown to induce the production of TGF-β, a negative growth regulatory influence (127), as well as to oppose the growth-stimulating effects of IGF-1 (128). Most interesting is the observation that tamoxifen decreases c-erbB2 expression in biopsy specimens from estrogen receptor(-) tumor specimens in patients treated for 3 wk before surgery (129). These results raise the possibility that the antiestrogen can decrease c-erbB2 expression by hormone receptor-linked and hormone receptor-independent mechanisms, although this point has not yet been suggested in studies with cell lines in vitro.

Retinoids are of clear importance in delaying or abrogating the onset of second aerodigestive tract neoplasms in a population at risk; however, the mechanism for this effect is not clear. Recent evidence has been presented that although retinoic acid can enhance EGF-related signaling in normal keratinocytes, human epidermoid carcinoma cells have been described in which retinoids suppress the transcription of the EGF-R through a specific element in the EGF-R promoter that can be related to the activity of the RAR-γ (130). This finding may also have relevance to breast neoplasms, where exposure of mammary carcinoma cells to retinol resulted in a diminished tyrosine phosphorylation of the EGF-R with decreased TGF-α stimulation of the PLC-γ isoform (131). In addition, retinoic acid decreases the estrogen-induced increase in TGF-α secretion by MCF-7 cells (132). Taken together, these molecular mechanisms clearly justify clinical studies of retinoid plus antiestrogen combinations in the treatment or prevention of breast neoplasms.

APL represents an important paradigm for the development of differentiation agents as therapeutic agents, since as a single agent all trans retinoic acid can elicit valuable clinical response. In vitro, HL60 cells or patient-derived APL specimens demonstrate enhanced expression of the GM-CSF receptor after differentiation by the retinoid (133). Whether this is cause or effect has not yet been demonstrated, but modulation of cytokine responsiveness may be a clinically exploitable effect of retinoid exposure (134).

6. MODULATION OF INTRACELLULAR SIGNAL TRANSDUCTION PATHWAYS

6.1. Protein Kinases

Much effort has been expended to design specific antagonists of protein kinases. Yet consideration of Fig. 3 will suggest that a very specific kinase antagonist may be circumvented by the action of additional pathways of cellular activation, or a kinase antagonist directed at a key "final common pathway" kinase, such as PKC, MAP kinase, or the cyclin-dependent kinases, will not have the requisite therapeutic index. The latter consideration is of special relevance, since as discussed by Hunter (135), the catalytic mechanism of all protein kinases studied to date is similar in a way that would suggest descent from a common ancestral gene.

Thus, the design features that should be considered in pursuing protein kinase antagonists for therapeutic development should incorporate not only their ability to function as enzymatic inhibitors, but as deregulators of cellular signal transduction in a way that would achieve the desired end point, which in the case of neoplasia is cell growth inhibition or death. In addition to merely designing "potent" enzymatic inhibitors, one must consider the cellular consequences of that inhibition.

6.2. Tyrosine Protein Kinases

Two general classes of tyrosine protein kinase signaling antagonists are conceivable: those that inhibit the act of phosphoryl transfer, and those that interfere with the protein–protein associations of tyrosine kinase substrates through interruption of SH2 and SH3 domain function. The former are revealed by a decrease in tyrosine phosphates in treated cells and are the class that has received the greatest developmental attention over the past 20 years, whereas the latter are at a very preliminary stage of development, but could afford means of interrupting tyrosine kinase signaling pathways without necessarily affecting the catalytic activity of the kinase. Burke (*136*) and Fry (*137*) have recently reviewed in detail the various chemical classes that have been found to cause tyrosine kinase inhibition. We shall focus here on biological issues pertinent to their development.

6.2.1. INHIBITORS OF PHOSPHORYL TRANSFER

6.2.1.1. Natural Products. Inhibition of *p60src* phosphoryltransfer by flavonoid compounds, such as quercetin, was first described by Graziani et al. (*138*). The structure–activity and kinetic analysis as summarized by ref. (*139*) defines these compounds to be competitive with ATP. Accordingly, there is potential interference with a large number of ATP-requiring enzymatic reactions, and the specificity of this class of compounds can be legitimately questioned. Quercetin is actually a better inhibitor of many serine/threonine kinases in comparison to tyrosine kinases. Genistein, an isoflavone again present in many plants, particularly soy products, shares the general kinetic mechanism, but exhibits greater specificity for tyrosine as compared to serine/threonine kinases (*140*).

Erbstatin (Fig. 6) was isolated from a *Streptomyces* culture filtrate and has a structure clearly relatable to tyrosine. It was found to be a potent inhibitor of the EGF-receptor tyrosine kinase (*141*), as well as the activity of the pp60src in immunoprecipitates from Rous sarcoma virus-infected cells. However, the cellular effects of the agent are less clear. It inhibits the growth of L1210 leukemia cells, and evidence for induction of apoptosis in these cells has recently been presented (*142*). The mechanism of this effect is not clear, but in sea star oocytes, erbstatin can prevent the activation by 1-methyladenine-induced activation of p34cdc2, p44mpk, and ribosomal S6 kinase (*143*). A general criticism of the use of erbstatin and synthetic analogs is that a clear delineation of the responsible mechanism leading to growth inhibition and/or cell death has not been achieved.

Lavendustin was also originally isolated from a *Streptomyces*, and produces inhibition that is of mixed type with respect to both ATP and substrate. The compound is of interest because both amine and nonamineanalogs have demonstrated in one case nanomolar potency vs p56lck. A difficulty with many compounds of this type is exemplified by the recent series (*144,145*) where there is discordance between the compounds' ability to inhibit enzymatic activities as compared to their ability to inhibit cell growth, emphasizing the need to develop this type of inhibitor with a consideration of biologic as well as chemical effects of the drug.

Recently, a novel chemical class of tyrosine kinase antagonist was discovered from marine sponge extracts. Halistanol trisulfdate is a sulfated steroid derivative with micromolar potency for pp60src (*146*). More detailed studies are required to assess the capacity of this class of compound to inhibit cell growth.

A

B

C

D

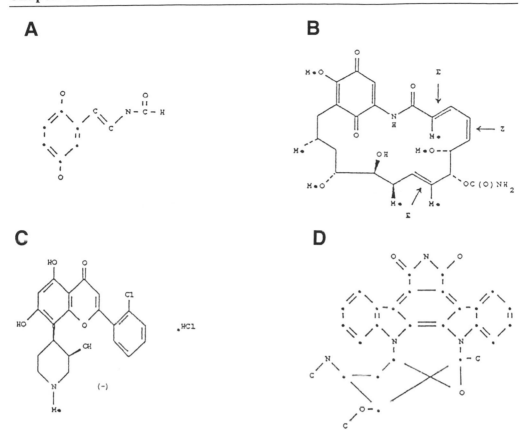

Fig. 6. Structures of protein kinase antagonists. (**A**) Erbstatin (NSC no. 606641). (**B**) Geldanamycin (NSC no. 122750). (**C**) Flavopiridol (NSC no. 649890). (**D**) UNC-01 (NSC no. 638850).

The benzoquinoid ansamycins, including herbimycin A and geldanamycin (Fig. 6), are of interest because recent experiments have suggested novel ways in which interaction of a drug with either its target directly or accessory molecules can lead to apparent modulation of protein kinase activity. The parent compound of the series, herbimycin A, was originally described as an activity isolated from a *Streptomyces* species with activity in a pesticide screening assay (*147*). However, Uehara et al. (*148*) were able to demonstrate that herbimycin caused striking phenotypic reversion of RSV-transformed cells, and pp60^{src} prepared from the cells was inactive in phosphorylating substrate, but the drug added in vitro could not efficiently inhibit the kinase activity of pp60^{src} from untreated cells. This finding suggested to these workers that herbimycin might be acting indirectly to alter the normal cellular function of pp60^{src}. The capacity of herbimycin to reverse many of the protean effects of pp60^{src} in transformed cells (*149*) with relatively few effects on nontransformed cells only heightened interest in the compound, as did documentation of antiangiogenic activity (*150*). However, Uehara et al. (*151*) went on to show that the decreased kinase activity of pp60^{src} was actually accompanied by a decrease in the level of pp60^{src} protein, suggesting that the drug could affect the turnover of the target. This general type of observation has been extended to EGF-R (*152*) and p185$^{c-erbB2}$ (*153*), and thus not simply inhibition of kinase activity *per se*, but a change in the normal dynamics of the target must be considered in assessing activity.

Whitesell et al. (*154*) made a distinction between relatively rapid cytocidal action of herbimycin and geldanamycin in "sensitive" cell types at concentrations below where *src* kinases would be inhibited, again suggesting a cellular target in addition to the kinases alone. Whitesell went on to demonstrate recently (*155*) that the heat-shock protein hsp-90 could form a complex with immobilized geldanamycin, and that soluble benzoquinoid ansamycins inhibited the previously described complex between the *src* kinase and hsp-90. These findings therefore suggest that hsps, pleiotropically involved in a cell's stress response, may also be regarded as the "real" target for the action of the benzoquinoid ansamycins, with indirect effects on apparent tyrosine kinase activity. Although the implications of these findings are continuing to be assessed, it is clear that attempts to develop benzoquinoid ansamycins clinically might profitably consider use of strategies for long exposure to relatively low concentrations, a strategy that has been suggested to cause differentiation of neuroblastoma (*156*) and leukemia cells (*157*). Such a usage may allow function through altered assuration of heat-shock proteins with regulatory kinases.

6.2.1.2. Synthetic Inhibitors of Phosphoryl Transfer. Modeled on the structure of erbstatin, several groups have produced small molecules with the capacity to discriminate between different tyrosine protein kinases. Yaish et al. (*158*) coined the term "tyrphostin" to describe compounds that were modeled on erbstatin and that were designed to inhibit phosphoryl transfer by competing with substrate as opposed to compounds, such as genistein, which were competitive with ATP. A large number of tyrphostins have been synthesized (*159,160*), and as summarized by Levitzki (*161,162*), these compounds can be divided into four structural classes: the malononitriles, the S-arylmalononotriles, the bisubstrate quinoline (where the quinoline portion acts as a pseudo-ATP mimetic), and a series of compounds related to lavendustin. Although the earliest tyrphostins were synthesized with the intention of providing molecules competitive with substrate, actual analysis of the kinetic behavior of tyrphostins suggests that, depending on the particular kinase, there may be mixed inhibition (competitive with respect to both substrate and ATP).

Two immediate problems with this class of compounds is that in many instances, although they have the capacity to discriminate among different tyrosine kinases in in vitro kinase reactions, evidence of activity in living cells in some cases occurs at widely discordant concentrations. Second, clear examples of where these structures actually act in cells to inhibit growth with moderate to good potency, but without reference to inhibition of tyrosine kinases have been demonstrated. For example, the tyrphostin AG 555 is a good inhibitor of topoisomerase I (*163*).

Despite the caveat, therefore, that the mechanism of a tyrphostin in living cells has to be carefully established as relating to the inhibition of a tyrosine kinase, it is possible to show in several systems that cell growth can be blocked through mechanisms that may in some way relate to inhibition of the kinase. For example, Lyall et al. (*164*) showed that tyrphostin-like compounds directed against the EGF receptor could inhibit cell growth in a way that was arguably related to the inhibition of the EGF-R kinase, and could act in athymic mouse xenografts expressing high levels of EGF-R to inhibit tumor growth (*165*). However, the capacity of such compounds to inhibit "outbred" real human tumors in such xenograft systems is less clear.

A number of such tyrphostins that inhibit the p210[bcr-abl] fusion protein have been described (*166*), including those that correlatively inhibit CML cell growth (*167*) or

7. SUMMARY

It is apparent that the immediate future for development of agents that modulate growth factor-mediated signal transduction is bright, with many novel approaches possible predicated on this emerging understanding of cellular pharmacology. However, our understanding remains somewhat primitive, a fact that serves to limit the degree to which our drug development efforts can be said to be clever. An important consequence of our understanding of mechanisms of action of these agents is that the boundary between classical drug development of small molecules and induction of biological responses by antibodies, growth factors, and cytokines is rather blurred by the realization that depending on what growth-promoting influence is paramount, the drug molecules may be expected to have vastly different effects. Thus, development of these agents cannot rely on empiricism, but must incorporate an understanding of the physiology of the intended target in neoplastic as compared to normal tissues if optimal development is to proceed.

REFERENCES

1. Powis G. Signaling pathways as targets for anticancer drug development. *Pharmacol Ther* 1994; 62:57–95.
2. Kerr DJ, Workman P. *New Molecular Targets for Cancer Chemotherapy.* Boca Raton, FL: CRC, 1994.
3. Cantley LC, Auger KR, Carpenter C, Duckworth B, Graziani A, Kapeller R, Soltoff S. Oncogenes and signal transduction. *Cell* 1991; 64:281–302.
4. Sporn MB, Roberts AB. Autocrine secretion—10 years later. *Ann Intern Med* 1992; 117: 408–414.
5. Levinson AD, Oppermann H, Levintow L, Varmus HE, Bishop JM. Evidence that the transforming gene of avian sarcoma virus encodes a protein kinase associated with phosphoprotein. *Cell* 1978; 15:561–572.
6. Bolen JB. Nonreceptor tyrosine protein kinases. *Oncogene* 1993; 8:2025–2031.
7. Witte ON, Kelliher M, Muller AJ, Pendergast AM, Gishizky M, McLaughlin J, Sawyers C, Maru Y, Shah N, Denny C, Rosenberg N. Role of BCR-ABL oncogene in the pathogenesis of Philadelphia chromosome positive leukemias. In: Brugge J, Curran T, Harlow E, McCormick F, eds. *Origins of Human Cancer.* Cold Spring Harbor, NY: Cold Spring Harbor Laboratory Press, 1991:521–526.
8. Shtivelman E, Lifshitz B, Gale RP, Canaani E. Fused transcript of *abl* and *bcr* genes in chronic myelogenous leukaemia. *Nature* 1985; 315:550–554.
9. Lugo TG, Pendergast AM, Muller AJ, Witte ON. Tyrosine kinase activity and transformation potency of *bcr-abl* oncogene products. *Science* 1990; 247:1079–1082.
10. Bolen JB, Veillette A, Schwartz AM, DeSeau V, Rosen N. Activation of pp60^{c-src} protein kinase activity in human colon carcinoma. *Proc Natl Acad Sci USA* 1987; 84:2251–2255.
11. Veillette A, Foss FM, Sausville EA, Bolen JB, Rosen N. Expression of the *lck* tyrosine kinase gene in human colon carcinoma and other non-lymphoid human tumor cell lines. *Oncogene Res* 1987; 1:357–374.
12. Veillette A, Bookman MA, Horak EM, Bolen JB. The CD4 and CD8 T cell surface antigens are associated with the internal membrane tyrosine-protein kinase p56^{lck}. *Cell* 1988; 55:301–308.
13. Sporn M, Roberts A. *Growth Factors: Handbook of Experimental Pharmacology,* vol. 95. Berlin: Springer-Verlag, 1990.
14. Frykberg L, Palmieri S, Beug H, Graf T, Hayman MJ, Vennstrom B. Transforming capacities of avian erythroblastosis virus mutants deleted in the *erbA* or *erbB* oncogenes. *Cell* 1983; 32:227–238.

15. Downward J, Yarden Y, Mayes E, Scrace G, Totty N, Stockwell P, Ullrich A, Schlessinger J, Waterfield MD. Close similarity of epidermal growth factor receptor and v-*erb*B oncogene protein sequences. *Nature* 1984; 307:521–527.

16. Fantl WJ, Johnson DE, Williams LT. Signalling by receptor tyrosine kinases. *Annu Rev Biochem* 1993; 62:453–481.

17. Semba K, Kamata N, Toyoshima K, Yamamoto T. A v-*erb*B-related protooncogene, c-*erb*B-2, is distinct from the c-*erb*B-1/epidermal growth factor-receptor gene and is amplified in a human salivary gland adenocarcinoma. *Proc Natl Acad Sci USA* 1985; 82:6497–6501.

18. Hendler FJ, Ozanne BW. Human squamous cell lung cancers express increased epidermal growth factor receptors. *J Clin Invest* 1984; 74:647–651.

19. Merlino GT, Xu YH, Richert N, Clark AJL, Ishii S, Banks-Schlegel S, Pastan I. Elevated epidermal growth factor receptor gene copy number and expression in a squamous carcinoma cell line. *J Clin Invest* 1985; 75:1077–1079.

20. Yamamoto T, Kamata N, Kawano H, Shimizu S, Kuroki T, Toyoshima K, Rikimaru K, Nomura N, Ishizaki R, Pastan I, Gamou S, Shimizu N. High incidence of amplification of the epidermal growth factor receptor gene in human squamous carcinoma cell lines. *Cancer Res* 1986; 46:414–416.

21. Slamon DJ, Godolphin W, Jones LA, Holt JA, Wong SG, Keith DE, Levin WJ, Stuart SG, Udove J, Ullrich A, Press MF. Studies of the HER-2/*neu* proto-oncogene in human breast and ovarian cancer. *Science* 1989; 244:707–712.

22. Han M, Sternberg PW. *let*-60, a gene that specifies cell fates during *C. elegans* vulval induction, encodes a *ras* protein. *Cell* 1990; 63:921–931.

23. Morrison DK, Kaplan DR, Rapp U, Roberts TM. Signal transduction from membrane to cytoplasm: growth factors and membrane-bound oncogene products increase Raf-1 phosphorylation and associated protein kinase activity. *Proc Natl Acad Sci USA* 1988; 85:8855–8859.

24. Mayer BJ, Hamaguchi M, Hanafusa H. A novel viral oncogene with structural similarity to phospholipase C. *Nature* 1988; 332:272–275.

25. Courtneidge SA, Heber A. An 81 kd protein complexed with middle T antigen and pp60[c-src]: a possible phosphatidylinositol kinase. *Cell* 1987; 50:1031–1037.

26. Otsu M, Hiles I, Gout I, Fry MJ, Ruiz-Larrea F, Panayotou G, Thompson A, Dhand R, Hsuan J, Totty N, Smith AD, Morgan SJ, Courtneidge SA, Parker PJ, Waterfield MD. Characterization of two 85 kd proteins that associate with receptor tyrosine kinases, middle-T/pp60[c-src] complexes, and P13-kinase. *Cell* 1991; 65:91–104.

27. Shoelson SE, Sivaraja M, Williams KP, Hu P, Schlessinger J, Weiss MA. Specific phosphopeptide binding regulates a conformational change in the PI 3-kinase SH2 domain associated with enzyme activation. *EMBO J* 1993; 12:795–802.

28. Margolis B, Rhee SG, Felder S, Mervic M, Lyall R, Levitski A, Ullrich A, Zilberstein A, Schlessinger J. EGF induces tyrosine phosphorylation of phospholipase C-II: a potential mechanism for EGF receptor signaling. *Cell* 1989; 57:1101–1117.

29. Margolis B, Bellot F, Honegger A, Ullrich A, Schlessinger J. Zilberstein A. Tyrosine kinase activity is essential for the association of phospholipase C-γ with the epidermal growth factor receptor. *Mol Cell Biol* 1990; 10:435–441.

30. Margolis B, Li N, Koch A, Mohammadi M, Hurwitz DR, Zilberstein A, Ullrich A, Pawson T, Schlessinger J. The tyrosine-phosphorylated carboxy terminus of the EGF receptor is a binding site for GAP and PLC-γ. *EMBO J* 1990; 9:4375–4380.

31. Lowenstein EJ, Daly RJ, Batzer AG, Li W, Margolis B, Lammers R, Ullrich A, Skolnik EY, Bar-Sagi D, Schlessinger J. The SH2 and SH3 domain-containing protein GRB2 links receptor tyrosine kinases to ras signaling. *Cell* 1992; 70:431–442.

32. Downward J. The GRB2/Sem-5 adaptor protein. *FEBS Lett* 1994; 338:113–117.

33. Egan SE, Giddings BW, Brooks MW, Buday L, Sizeland AM, Weinberg RA. Association of Sos Ras exchange protein with Grb2 is implicated in tyrosine kinase signal transduction and transformation. *Nature* 1993; 363:45–51.

34. Rozakis-Adcock M, Fernley R, Wade J, Pawson T, Bowtell D. The SH2 and SH3 domains of mammalian Grb2 couple the EGF receptor to the Ras activator mSos1. *Nature* 1993; 363:83–85.

35. Warne PH, Viciana PR, Downward J. Direct interaction of Ras and the amino-terminal region of Raf-1 *in vitro*. Activation of serine peptide kinase activity by myelin basic protein kinases *in vitro*. *Nature* 1993; 364:352–355.

36. Zhang XF, Settleman J, Kyriakis JM, Takeuchi-Suzuki E, Elledge SJ, Marshall MS, Bruder JT, Rapp UR, Avruch J. Normal and oncogenic p21^{ras} proteins bind to the amino-terminal regulatory domain of c-Raf-1. *Nature* 1993; 364:308–313.

37. Stokoe D, Macdonald SG, Cadwallader K, Symons M, Hancock JF. Activation of Raf as a result of recruitment to the plasma membrane. *Science* 1994; 264:1463–1467.

38. Wartmann M, Davis RJ. The native structure of the activated Raf protein kinase is a membrane-bound multi-subunit complex. *J Biol Chem* 1994; 269:6695–6701.

39. Ahn NG, Weiel JE, Chan CP, Krebs EG. Identification of multiple epidermal growth factor-stimulated protein serine/threonine kinases from Swiss 3T3 cells. *J Biol Chem* 1990; 265:11,487–11,494.

40. Ahn NG, Krebs EG. Evidence for an epidermal growth factor-stimulated protein kinase cascade in Swiss 3T3 cells. *J Biol Chem* 1990; 265:11,495–11,501.

41. Davis RJ. The mitogen-activated protein kinase signal transduction pathway. *J Biol Chem* 1993; 268:14,553–14,556.

42. Rossomando A, Wu J, Weber MJ, Sturgill TW. The phorbol ester-dependent activator of the mitogen-activated protein kinase p42^{mapk} is a kinase with specificity for the threonine and tyrosine regulatory sites. *Proc Natl Acad Sci USA* 1992; 89:5221–5225.

43. Kyriakis JM, App H, Zhang XF, Banerjee P, Brautigan DL, Rapp UR, Avruch J. Raf-1 activates MAP kinase-kinase. *Nature* 1992; 358:417–421.

44. Taylor SS, Buechler JA, Yonemoto W. cAMP-dependent protein kinase: framework for a diverse family of regulatory enzymes. *Annu Rev Biochem* 1990; 59:971–1005.

45. Strader CD, Fong TM, Tota MR, Underwood D, Dixon RAF. Structure and function of G protein-coupled receptors. *Annu Rev Biochem* 1994; 63:101–132.

46. Allende JE. GTP-mediated macromolecular interactions: the common features of different systems. *FASEB J* 1988; 2:2356–2367.

47. Corjay MH, Dobrzanski DJ, Way JM, Viallet J, Shapira H, Worland P, Sausville EA, Battey JF. Two distinct bombesin receptor subtypes are expressed and functional in human lung carcinoma cells. *J Biol Chem* 1991; 266:18,771–18,779.

48. Sharoni Y, Viallet J, Trepel JB, Sausville EA. Effect of guanine and adenine nucleotides on bombesin-stimulated phospholipase C activity in membranes from Swiss 3T3 and small cell lung carcinoma cells. *Cancer Res* 1990; 50:5257–5262.

49. Landis CA, Masters SB, Spada A, Pace AM, Bourne HR, Vallar L. GTPase inhibiting mutations activate the α chain of G$_s$ and stimulate adenyl cyclase in human pituitary tumours. *Nature* 1989; 340:692–696.

50. Allen LF, Lefkowitz RJ, Caron MG, Cotecchia S. G-protein-coupled receptor genes as protooncogenes: constitutively activating mutation of the α$_{1B}$-adrenergic receptor enhances mitogenesis and tumorigenicity. *Proc Natl Acad Sci USA* 1991; 88:11,354–11,358.

51. Murata J, Lee HY, Clair T, Krutzsch HC, Årestad AA, Sobel ME, Liotta LA, Stracke ML. cDNA cloning of the human tumor motility-stimulating protein, autotaxin, reveals a homology with phosphodiesterase. *J Biol Chem* 1994; 269:30,479–30,484.

52. Wrana JL, Attisano L, Wieser R, Ventura F, Massagué J. Mechanism of activation of the TGF-β receptor. *Nature* 1994; 370:341–347.

53. Koff A, Ohtsuki M, Polyak K, Roberts JM, Massagué J. Negative regulation of G1 in mammalian cells: inhibition of cyclin E-dependent kinase by TGF-β. *Science* 1993; 260:536–539.

54. Heller RA, Krönke M. Tumor necrosis factor receptor-mediated signaling pathways. *J Cell Biol* 1994; 126:5–9.

55. Kolesnick R, Golde DW. The sphingomyelin pathway in tumor necrosis factor and interleukin-1 signaling. *Cell* 1994; 77:325–328.

56. Weller M, Frei K, Groscurth P, Krammer PH, Yonekawa Y, Fontana A. Anti-Fas/APO-1 antibody-mediated apoptosis of cultured human glioma cells. Induction and modulation of sensitivity by cytokines. *J Clin Invest* 1994; 94:954–964.

57. Fu XY, Schindler C, Improta T, Aebersold R, Darnell JE Jr. The proteins of ISGF-3, the interferon α-induced transcriptional activator, define a gene family involved in signal transduction. *Proc Natl Acad Sci USA* 1992; 89:7840–7843.

58. Larner AC, David M, Feldman GM, Igarashi K, Hackett RH, Webb DSA, Sweitzer SM, Petricoin EF III, Finbloom DS. Tyrosine phosphorylation of DNA binding proteins by multiple cytokines. *Science* 1993; 261:1730–1733.

59. Sadowski HB, Shuai K, Darnell JE Jr, Gilman MZ. A common nuclear signal transduction pathway activated by growth factor and cytokine receptors. *Science* 1993; 261:1739–1744.

60. Shuai K, Stark GR, Kerr IM, Darnell JE Jr. A single phosphotyrosine residue of STAT91 required for gene activation by interferon-γ. *Science* 1993; 261:1744–1746.

61. Trowbridge IS. CD45. A prototype for transmembrane protein tyrosine phosphatases. *J Biol Chem* 1991; 266:23,517–23,520.

62. Molina TJ, Kishihara K, Siderovski DP, van Ewijk W, Narendran A, Timms E, Wakeham A, Paige CJ, Hartmann KU, Veillette A, Davidson D, Mak TW. Profound block in thymocyte development in mice lacking p56^{lck}. *Nature* 1992; 357:161–164.

63. Fischer EH, Charbonneau H, Tonks NK. Protein tyrosine phosphatases: a diverse family of intracellular and transmembrane enzymes. *Science* 1991; 253:401–406.

64. Sigal NH, Dumont FJ. Cyclosporin A, FK-506; and rapamycin: pharmacologic probes of lymphocyte signal transduction. *Annu Rev Immunol* 1992; 10:519–560.

65. Clipstone NA, Fiorentino DF, Crabtree GR. Molecular analysis of the interaction of calcineurin with drug-immunophilin complexes. *J Biol Chem* 1994; 269:26,431–26,437.

66. Eng CP, Sehgal SN, Vezina C. Activity of rapamycin (AY-22,989) against transplanted tumors. *J Antibiot (Tokyo)* 1984; 37:1231–1237.

67. Lin CR, Chen WS, Lazar CS, Carpenter CD, Gill GN, Evans RM, Rosenfeld MG. Protein kinase C phosphorylation at Thr 654 of the unoccupied EGF receptor and EGF binding regulate functional receptor loss by independent mechanisms. *Cell* 1986; 44:839–848.

68. Betsholtz C, Johnsson A, Heldin CH, Westermark B. Efficient reversion of simian sarcoma virus-transformation and inhibition of growth factor-induced mitogenesis by suramin. *Proc Natl Acad Sci USA* 1986; 83:6440–6444.

69. Huang SS, Huang JS. Rapid turnover of the platelet-derived growth factor receptor in sis-transformed cells and reversal by suramin. Implications for the mechanism of autocrine transformation. *J Biol Chem* 1988; 263:12,608–12,618.

70. Kopp R, Pfeiffer A. Suramin alters phosphoinositide synthesis and inhibits growth factor receptor binding in HT-29 cells. *Cancer Res* 1990; 50:6490–6496.

71. Myers C, Cooper M, Stein C, LaRocca R, Walther MM, Weiss G, Choyke P, Dawson N, Steinberg S, Uhrich MM, Cassidy J, Kohler DR, Trepel J, Linehan WM. Suramin: a novel growth factor antagonist with activity in hormone-refractory metastatic prostate cancer. *J Clin Oncol* 1992; 10:881–889.

72. Mills GB, Zhang N, May C, Hill M, Chung A. Suramin prevents binding of interleukin 2 to its cell surface receptor: a possible mechanism for immunosuppression. *Cancer Res* 1990; 50: 3036–3042.

73. Cuttitta F, Carney DN, Mulshine J, Moody TW, Fedorko J, Fischler A, Minna JD. Bombesin-like peptides can function as autocrine growth factors in human small-cell lung cancer. *Nature* 1985; 316:823–826.

74. Heikkila R, Trepel JB, Cuttitta F, Neckers LM, Sausville EA. Bombesin-related peptides induce calcium mobilization in a subset of human small cell lung cancer cell lines. *J Biol Chem* 1987; 262:16,456–14,460.

75. Trepel JB, Moyer JD, Heikkila R, Sausville EA. Modulation of bombsin-induced phosphatidylinositol hydrolysis in a small-cell lung-cancer cell line. *Biochem J* 1988; 255:403–410.

76. Jensen RT, Mrozinski JE Jr, Coy DH. Bombesin receptor antagonists: different classes and cellular basis of action. *Recent Results in Cancer Res* 1993; 129:87–113.

77. Thomas F, Arvelo F, Antoine E, Jacrot M, Poupon MF. Antitumoral activity of bombesin analogues on small cell lung cancer xenografts: relationship with bombesin receptor expression. *Cancer Res* 1992; 52:4872–4877.

78. Radulovic S, Miller G, Schally AV. Inhibition of growth of HT-29 human colon cancer xenografts in nude mice by treatment with bombesin/gastrin releasing peptide antagonist (RC-3095). *Cancer Res* 1991; 51:6006–6009.

79. Yano T, Pinski J, Szepeshazi K, Halmos G, Radulovic S, Groot K, Schally AV. Inhibitory effect of bombesin/gastrin-releasing peptide antagonist SB-75 on the growth of MCF-7 MIII human breast cancer xenografts in athymic nude mice. *Cancer* 1994; 73:1229–1238.

80. Qin Y, Ertl T, Cai RZ, Halmos G, Schally AV. Inhibitory effect of bombesin receptor antagonist RC-3095 on the growth of human pancreatic cancer cells in vivo and in vitro. *Cancer Res* 1994; 54:1035–1041.

81. Woll PJ, Rozengurt E. Multiple neuropeptides mobilize calcium in small cell lung cancer: effects of vasopressin, brudykinin, cholecytokinin, galonin and neurostensin. *Biochem Biophys Res Commun* 1989; 164:66–73.

82. Bunn PA, Dienhart DG, Chan D, Puck TT, Tagawa M, Jewett PB, Braunschweiger. Neuropeptide stimulation of calcium flux in human lung cancer cells: delination of alternative pathways. *Proc Natl Acad Sci USA* 1990; 87:2162–2166.

83. Lamberts SWJ, Reubi JC, Krenning EP. The role of somatostatin analogs in the control of tumor growth. *Semin Oncol* 1994; 21:61–64.

84. Bogden AE, Taylor JE, Moreau JP, Coy DH, LePage DJ. Response of human lung tumor xenografts to treatment with a somatostatin analogue (Somatuline). *Cancer Res* 1990; 50: 4360–4365.

85. Hershkovitz E, Marbach M, Bosin E, Levy J, Roberts CT Jr, LeRoith D, Schally AV, Sharoni Y. Luteinizing hormone-releasing hormone antagonists interfere with autocrine and paracrine growth stimulation of MCF-7 mammary cancer cells by insulin-like growth factors. *J Clin Endocrinol Metab* 1993; 77:963–968.

86. Kleinman D, Roberts CT Jr, LeRoith D, Schally AV, Levy J, Sharoni Y. Regulation of endometrial cancer cell growth by insulin-like growth factors and the luteinizing hormone-releasing hormone antagonist SB-75. *Regul Pept* 1993; 20:91–98.

87. Coffey RJ, Goustin AS, Soderquist AM, Shipley GD, Wolfshohl J, Carpenter G, Moses HL. Transforming growth factor α and β expression in human colon cancer lines: implications for an autocrine model. *Cancer Res* 1987; 47:4590–4594.

88. Smith JJ, Derynck R, Korc M. Production of transforming growth factor α in human pancreatic cancer cells: evidence for a superagonist autocrine cycle. *Proc Natl Acad Sci USA* 1987; 84:7567–7570.

89. Masui H, Kawamoto T, Sato JD, Wolf B, Sato G, Mendelsohn J. Growth inhibition of human tumor cells in athymic mice by anti-epidermal growth factor receptor monoclonal antibodies. *Cancer Res* 1984; 44:1002–1007.

90. Ennis BW, Valverius EM, Bates SE, Lippman ME, Bellot F, Kris R, Schlessinger J, Masui H, Goldenberg A, Mendelsohn J, Dickson RB. Anti-epidermal growth factor receptor antibodies inhibit the autocrine-stimulated growth of MDA-468 human breast cancer cells. *Mol Endocrinol* 1989; 3:1830–1838.

91. Fan Z, Baselga J, Masui H, Mendelsohn J. Antitumor effects of anti-epidermal growth factor receptor monoclonal antibodies plus *cis*-diamminedichloroplatinum on well established A431 cell xenografts. *Cancer Res* 1993; 53:4637–4642.

92. Baselga J, Norton L, Masui H, Pandiella A, Coplan K, Miller JH Jr, Mendelsohn J. Antitumor effects of doxorubicin in combination with anti-epidermal growth factor receptor monoclonal antibodies. *J Natl Cancer Inst* 1993; 85:1327–1333.

93. Rieman DJ, Anzano MA, Chan GW, Imburgia TJ, Chan JA, Johnson RK, Greig RG. Antagonism of TGF-α receptor binding and TGF-α induced stimulation of cell proliferation by methyl pheophorbides. *Oncol Res* 1992; 4:193–200.

94. Todo T, Adams EF, Fahlbusch R. Inhibitory effect of trapidil on human meningioma cell proliferation via interruption of autocrine growth stimulation. *J Neurosurg* 1993; 78:463–469.

95. Baserga R. The insulin-like growth factor I receptor: a key to tumor growth? *Cancer Res* 1995; 55:249–252.

96. Figueroa JA, Jackson JG, McGuire WL, Krywicki RF, Yee D. Expression of insulin-like growth factor binding proteins in human breast cancer correlates with estrogen receptor status. *J Cell Biochem* 1993; 52:196–205.

97. Arteaga CL. Interference of the IGF system as a strategy to inhibit breast cancer growth. *Breast Cancer Res Treat* 1992; 22:101–106.

98. Vassbotn FS, Östman A, Langeland N, Holmsen H, Westermark B, Heldin CH, Nistér M. Activated platelet-derived growth factor autocrine pathway drives the transformed phenotype of a human glioblastoma cell line. *J Cell Biochem* 1994; 158:381–389.

99. Engström U, Engström A, Ernlund A, Westermark B, Heldin CH. Identification of a peptide antagonist for platelet-derived growth factor. *J Biol Chem* 1992; 267:16,581–16,587.

100. Nikaido T, Shimizu A, Ishida H, Sabe K, Teshigawara M, Maeda T, Uchiyama J, Yodoi J, Honjo T. Molecular cloning of cDNA encoding human interleukin-2 receptor. *Nature* 1984; 311:631–635.

101. Hatakeyama M, Tsudo M, Minamoto S, Kono T, Doi T, Miyata T, Miyasaka M, Taniguchi T. Interleukin-2 receptor beta chain: generation of three receptor forms by loned alpha and beta chain cDNA's. *Science* 1989; 244:551–556.
102. Takeshita T, Asao H, Ohtani K, Ishii N, Kumaki S, Tanaka N, Munakata H, Nakamura M, Sugamura K. Cloning of the γ chain of the human IL-2 receptor. *Science* 1992; 257:379–382.
103. Strauchen J, Breakstone B. IL-2 receptor expression in human lymphoid lesions. *Am J Pathol* 1987; 126:506–512.
104. Waldmann TA, Goldman C, Top L, Grant A, Burton J, Bamford R, Roessler E, Horak I, Zakorn S, Kaston-Sporks C, White J, England R, Horak E, Martinucci J, Tinubu SA, Mishra B, Junghans R, Dipre M, Carasquillo J, Reynolds J, Gansow O, Nelson D. The interleukin-2 receptor: a target for immunotherapy. *Ann NY Acad Sci* 1993; 685:603–610.
105. Kreitman RJ, Chang CN, Hudson DV, Queen C, Bailon P, Pastan I. Anti-Tac (Fab)-PE40, a recombinant double-chain immunotoxin which kills interleukin-2-receptor-bearing cells and induces complete remission in an in vivo tumor model. *Int J Cancer* 1994; 57:856–864.
106. Williams D, Parker K, Bacha P, Bishai W, Borowski M, Genbauffe F, Strom T, Murphy J. Diphtheria toxin receptor binding domain substitution with interleukin-2: genetic reconstitution and properties of a diphtheria toxin related interleukin-2 fusion protein. *Protein Eng* 1987; 1:493–498.
107. Bacha P, Williams D, Waters C, Murphy J, Strom T. Interleukin-2 receptor mediated action of a diphtheria toxin related interleukin-2 fusion protein. *J Exp Med* 1988; 167:612–622.
108. LeMaistre CF, Meneghetti C, Rosenblum M, Reuben J, Shaw J, Deisseroth A, Woodworth T, Parkinson D. Phase I trial of an interleukin-2 fusion toxin (DAB 486IL2) in hematologic malignancies expressing the IL-2 receptor. *Blood* 1992; 79:2547–2554.
109. LeMaistre CF, Craig F, Meneghetti C, McMullin B, Parker K, Reuben J, Boldt D, Rosenblum M, Woodworth T. Phase I trial of a 90-minute infusion of the fusion toxin DAB(486)IL2 in hematologic cancers. *Cancer Res* 1993; 53:3930–3934.
110. Hesketh P, Caguioa P, Koh H, Dewey H, Facada A, McCaffrey R, Parker K, Nylen P, Woodworth T. Clinical activity of a cytotoxic fusion protein in the treatment of cutaneous T-cell lymphoma. *J Clin Oncol* 1993; 11:1682–1690.
111. Foss FM, Borkowski TA, Gilliom M, Stetler-Stevenson M, Jaffe ES, Figg WD, Tompkins A, Bastian A, Nylen P, Woodworth T, Udey MC, Sausville EA. Chimeric fusion protein toxin DAB486IL-2 in advanced mycosis fungoides and the Sezary syndrome: correlation of activity and interleukin-2 receptor expression in a phase II study. *Blood* 1994; 84:1765–1774.
112. Kondo M, Takeshita T, Ishii N, Nakamura M, Watanabe S, Arai K, Sugamura K. Sharing of the interleukin 2 (IL-2) receptor γ chain between receptors for IL-2 and IL-4. *Science* 1993; 262:1874–1877.
113. Noguchi M, Nakamura Y, Russell SM, Ziegler SF, Tsang M, Cao X, Leonard WJ. Interleukin-2 receptor γ chain: a functional component of the interleukin-7 receptor. *Science* 1993; 262:1877–1880.
114. Foss FM, Koc Y, Stetler-Stevenson MA, Nguyen DT, O'Brien MC, Turner R, Sausville EA. Costimulation of cutaneous T-cell lymphoma cells by interleukin-7 and interleukin-2: potential autocrine or paracrine effectors in the Sézary syndrome. *J Clin Oncol* 1994; 12:326–335.
115. Kishimoto T, Akira S, Taga T. Interleukin-6 and its receptor: a paradigm for cytokines. *Science* 1992; 258:593–597.
116. Falini B, Pileri S, Pizzolo G, Dürkop H, Flenghi L, Stirpe F, Martelli MF, Stein H. CD30 (Ki-1) molecule: a new cytokine receptor of the tumor necrosis factor receptor superfamily as a tool for diagnosis and immunotherapy. *Blood* 1995; 85:1–14.
117. Kilian PL, Kaffka KL, Biondi DA, Lipman JM, Benjamin WR, Feldman D, Campen CA. Antiproliferative effect of interleukin-1 on human ovarian carcinoma cell line (NHI:OVCAR-3). *Cancer Res* 1991; 51:1823–1828.
118. Lewis MP, Sullivan MH, Elder MG. Regulation by interleukin-1 beta of growth and collagenase production by choriocarcinoma cells. *Placenta* 1994; 15:13–20.
119. Powell CB, Manning K, Collins JL. Interferon-alpha (IFN alpha) induces a cytolytic mechanism in ovarian carcinoma cells through a protein kinase C-dependent pathway. *Gynecol Oncol* 1993; 50:208–214.
120. Boente MP, Berchuck A, Rodriguez GC, Davidoff A, Whitaker R, Xu FJ, Marks J, Clarke-Pearson DL, Bast RC Jr. The effect of interferon gamma on epidermal growth factor receptor

expression in normal and malignant ovarian epithelial cells. *Am J Obstet Gynecol* 1992; 167: 1877–1882.

121. Hamburger AW, Pinnamaneni GD. Increased epidermal growth factor receptor gene expression by gamma-interferon in human breast carcinoma cell line. *Br J Cancer* 1991; 4:64–68.

122. Chakravarthy A, Chen LC, Mehta D, Hamburger AW. Modulation of epidermal growth factor receptors by gamma interferon in a breast cancer cell line. *Anticancer Res* 1991; 11:347–351.

123. Wu S, Boyer CM, Whitaker RS, Berchuck A, Wiener JR, Weinberg JB, Bast RC Jr. Tumor necrosis factor alpha as an autocrine and paracrine growth factor for ovarian cancer: monokine induction of tumor cell proliferation and tumor necrosis factor alpha expression. *Cancer Res* 1993; 53:1939–1944.

124. Kalthoff H, Roeder C, Gieseking J, Humburg I, Schmiegel W. Inverse regulation of human ERBB2 and epidermal growth factor receptors by tumor necrosis factor alpha. *Proc Natl Acad Sci USA* 1993; 90:8972–8976.

125. Bates S, McManaway ME, Lippman ME, Dickson RB. Characterization of estrogen responsive transforming activity in human breast cancer cell lines. *Cancer Res* 1986; 46:1707–1713.

126. Dickson RB, McManaway ME, Lippman ME. Estrogen-induced factors of breast cancer cells partially replace estrogen to promote tumor growth. *Science* 1986; 232:1540–1543.

127. Knabbe C, Zugmaier G, Schmahl M, Dietel M, Lippman ME, Dickson RB. Induction of transforming growth factor beta by the antiestrogens droloxifene, tamoxifen, and toremifene in MCF-7 cells. *Am J Clin Oncol* 1991; 14:S15–S20.

128. Kawamura I, Lacey E, Mizota T, Tsujimoto S, Nishigaki F, Manda T, Shimomura K. The effect of droloxifene on the insulin-like growth factor-I stimulated growth of breast cancer cells. *Anticancer Res* 1994; 14:427–431.

129. Le Roy X, Escot C, Brouillet JP, Theillet C, Maudelonde T, Simony-Lafontaine J, Pujol H, Rochefort H. Decrease of c-*erbB*-2 and c-*myc* RNA levels in tamoxifen-treated breast cancer. *Oncogene* 1991; 6:431–437.

130. Zheng ZS, Polakowska R, Johnson A, Goldsmith LA. Transcriptional control of epidermal growth factor receptor by retinoic acid. *Cell Growth Differ* 1992; 3:225–232.

131. Halter SA, Winnier AR, Arteaga CL. Pretreatment with vitamin A inhibits transforming growth factor alpha stimulation of human mammary carcinoma cells. *J Cell Physiol* 1993; 156: 80–87.

132. Fontana JA, Nervi C, Shao ZM, Jetten AM. Retinoid antagonism of estrogen-responsive transforming growth factor alpha and pS2 gene expression in breast carcinoma cells. *Cancer Res* 1992; 52:3938–3945.

133. Hsu HC, Yang K, Kharbanda S, Clinton S, Datta R, Stone RM. All-trans retinoic acid induces monocyte growth factor receptor (c-*fms*) gene expression in HL-60 leukemia cells. *Leukemia* 1993; 7:458–462.

134. de Gentile A, Toubert ME, Dubois C, Krawice I, Schlageter MH, Balitrand N, Castaigne S, Degos L, Rain JD, Najean Y, Chomienne C. Induction of high-affinity GM-CSF receptors during all-trans retinoic acid treatment of acute promyelocytic leukemia. *Leukemia* 1994; 8: 1758–1762.

135. Hunter T. A thousand and one protein kinases. *Cell* 1987; 50:823–829.

136. Burke TR Jr. Protein-tyrosine kinase inhibitors. *Drugs of the Future* 1992; 17:119–131.

137. Fry DW. Protein tyrosine kinases as therapeutic targets in cancer chemotherapy and recent advances in the development of new inhibitors. *Exp Opinion Invest Drugs* 1994; 3:577–595.

138. Graziani Y, Erikson E, Erikson RL. The effect of quercetin on the phosphorylation activity of the Rous sarcoma virus transforming gene product *in vitro* and *in vivo*. *Eur J Biochem* 1983; 135:583–589.

139. Cushman M, Nagarathnam D, Burg DL, Geahlen RL. Synthesis and protein-tyrosine kinase inhibitory activities of flavonoid analogues. *J Med Chem* 1991; 34:798–806.

140. Akiyama T, Ishida J, Nakagawa S, Ogawa H, Watanabe S, Itou N, Shibata M, Fukami Y. Genistein, a specific inhibitor of tyrosine-specific protein kinase. *J Biol Chem* 1987; 262: 5592–5595.

141. Imoto M, Umezawa K, Isshiki K, Kanimoto S, Takeuchi T, Umezawa H. Kinetic studies of tyrosine kinase inhibition by erbstatin. *J Antibiot* 1987; 40:1471–1473.

142. Simizu S, Imoto M, Umezawa K. Induction of apoptosis by erbstatin in mouse leukemia L1210 cells. *Biosci Biotech Biochem* 1994; 58:1549–1552.

143. Daya-Makin M, Pelech SL, Levitzki A, Hudson AT. Erbstatin and tyrphostins block protein-serine kinase activation and meiotic maturation of sea star oocytes. *Biochim Biophys Acta* 1991; 1093:87–94.

144. Smyth MS, Stefanova I, Hartmann F, Horak ID, Osherov N, Levitzki A, Burke TR Jr. Non-amine based analogues of lavendustin A as protein-tyrosine kinase inhibitors. *J Med Chem* 1993; 36:3010–3014.

145. Nussbaumer P, Winiski AP, Cammisuli S, Hiestand P, Weckbecker G, Stütz A. Novel anti-proliferative agents derived from lavendustin A. *J Med Chem* 1994; 37:4079–4084.

146. Slate DL, Lee RH, Rodriguez J, Crews P. The marine natural product, halistanol trisulfate, inhibits pp60^{v-src} protein tyrosine kinase activity. *Biochem Biophys Res Commun* 1994; 203: 260–264.

147. Ōmura S, Iwai Y, Takahashi Y, Sadakane N, Nakagawa A, Ōiwa H, Hasegawa Y, Ikai T. Herbimycin, a new antibiotic produced by a strain of *Streptomyces*. *J Antibiot* 1979; 32:255–261.

148. Uehara Y, Hori M, Takeuchi T, Umezawa H. Phenotypic change from transformed to normal induced by benzoquinonoid ansamycins accompanies inactivation of p60^{src} in rat kidney cells infected with Rous sarcoma virus. *Mol Cell Biol* 1986; 6:2198–2206.

149. Murakami Y, Mizuno S, Hori M, Uehara Y. Reversal of transformed phenotypes by herbimycin A in *src* oncogene expressed rat fibroblasts. *Cancer Res* 1988; 48:1587–1590.

150. Oikawa T, Hirotani K, Shimamura M, Ashino-Fuse H, Iwaguchi T. Powerful antiangiogenic activity of herbimycin A (named angiostatic antibiotic). *J Antibiot* 1989; 42:1202–1204.

151. Uehara Y, Murakami Y, Sugimoto Y, Mizuno S. Mechanism of reversion of Rous sarcoma virus transformation by Herbimycin A: reduction of total phosphotyrosine levels due to reduced kinase activity and increased turnover of p60^{v-src}. *Cancer Res* 1989; 49:780–785.

152. Murakami Y, Mizuno S, Uehara Y. Accelerated degradation of 160 kDa epidermal growth factor (EGF) receptor precursor by the tyrosine kinase inhibitor herbimycin A in the endoplasmic reticulum of A431 human epidermoid carcinoma cells. *Biochem J* 1995; 301:63–68.

153. Miller P, DiOrio C, Moyer M, Schnur RC, Bruskin A, Cullen W, Moyer JD. Depletion of the *erbB*-2 gene product p185 by benzoquinoid ansamycins. *Cancer Res* 1994; 54:2724–2730.

154. Whitesell L, Shifrin SD, Schwab G, Neckers LM. Benzoquinonoid ansamycins possess selective tumoricidal activity unrelated to *src* kinase inhibition. *Cancer Res* 1992; 52:1721–1728.

155. Whitesell L, Mimnaugh EG, De Costa B, Myers CE, Neckers LM. Inhibition of heat shock protein HSP90-pp60^{v-src} heteroprotein complex formation by benzoquinone ansamycins: essential role for stress proteins in oncogenic transformation. *Proc Natl Acad Sci USA* 1994; 91:8324–8328.

156. Preis PN, Saya H, Nádasdi L, Hochhaus G, Levin V, Sadée W. Neuronal cell differentiation of human neuroblastoma cells by retinoic acid plus herbimycin A. *Cancer Res* 1988; 48: 6530–6534.

157. Honma Y, Okabe-Kado J, Hozumi M, Uehara Y, Mizuno S. Induction of erythroid differentiation of K562 human leukemic cells by herbimycin A, an inhibitor of tyrosine kinase activity. *Cancer Res* 1989; 49:331–334.

158. Yaish P, Gazit A, Gilon C, Levitzki A. Blocking of EGF-dependent cell proliferation by EGF receptor kinase inhibitors. *Science* 1988; 242:933–935.

159. Gazit A, Yaish P, Gilon C, Levitzki A. Tyrphostins I: synthesis and biological activity of protein tyrosine kinase inhibitors. *J Med Chem* 1989; 32:2344–2352.

160. Gazit A, Osherov N, Posner I, Yaish P, Poradosu E, Gilon C, Levitzki A. Tyrphostins. Heterocyclic and α-substituted benzylidenemalononitrile tyrphostins as potent inhibitors of EGF receptor and ErbB2/neu tyrosine kinases. *J Med Chem* 1991; 34:1896–1907.

161. Levitzki A. Tyrphostins: tyrosine kinase blockers as novel antiproliferative agents and dissectors of signal transduction. *FASEB J* 1992; 6:3275–3282.

162. Levitzki A, Gazit A. Tyrosine kinase inhibition: an approach to drug development. *Science* 1995; 267:1782–1788.

163. Aflalo E, Iftach S, Segal S, Gazit A, Priel E. Inhibition of topoisomerase I activity by tyrphostin derivatives, protein tyrosine kinase blockers: mechanism of action. *Cancer Res* 1994; 54:5138–5142.

164. Lyall RM, Zilberstein A, Gazit A, Gilon C, Levitzki A, Schlessinger J. Tyrphostins inhibit epidermal growth factor (EGF)-receptor tyrosine kinase activity in living cells and EGF-stimulated cell proliferation. *J Biol Chem* 1989; 264:14,503–14,509.

165. Yoneda T, Lyall RM, Alsina MM, Persons PE, Spada AP, Levitzki A, Zilberstein A, Mundy GR. The antiproliferative effects of tyrosine kinase inhibitors tyrphostins on a human squamous cell carcinoma in vitro and in nude mice. *Cancer Res* 1991; 51:4430–4435.

166. Anafi M, Gazit A, Gilon C, Ben-Neriah Y, Levitzki A. Selective interactions of transforming and normal *abl* proteins with ATP, tyrosine-copolymer substrates, and tyrphostins. *J Biol Chem* 1992; 267:4518–4523.

167. Kaur G, Gazit A, Levitzki A, Stowe E, Cooney DA, Sausville EA. Tyrphostin induced growth inhibition: correlation with effect on p210$^{bcr-abl}$ autokinase activity in K562 chronic myelogenous leukemia. *Anti-Cancer Drugs* 1994; 5:213–222.

168. Anafi M, Gazit A, Zehavi A, Ben-Neriah Y, Levitski A. Tyrphostin-induced inhibition of p210$^{bcr-abl}$ tyrosine kinase activity induces K562 to differentiate. *Blood* 1993; 82:3524–3529.

169. Bryckaert MC, Eldor A, Fontenay M, Gazit A, Osherov N, Gilon C, Levitzki A, Tobelem G. Inhibition of platelet-derived growth factor-induced mitogenesis and tyrosine kinase activity in cultured bone marrow fibroblasts by tyrphostins. *Exp Cell Res* 1992; 199:255–261.

170. Kovalenko M, Gazit A, Böhmer A, Rorsman C, Rönnstrand L, Heldin CH, Waltenberger J, Böhmer FD, Levitzki A. Selective platelet-derived growth factor receptor kinase blockers reverse *sis*-transformation. *Cancer Res* 1994; 54:6106–6114.

171. Fry DW, Kraker AJ, McMichael A, Ambroso LA, Nelson JM, Leopold WR, Connors RW, Bridges AJ. A specific inhibitor of the epidermal growth factor receptor tyrosine kinase. *Science* 1994; 265:1093–5.

172. Songyang Z, Shoelson SE, Chaudhuri M, Gish G, Pawson T, Haser WG, King F, Roberts T, Ratnofsky S, Lechleider RJ, Neel BG, Birge RB, Fajardo JE, Chou MM, Hanafusa H, Schaffhausen B, Cantley LC. SH2 domains recognize specific phosphopeptide sequences. *Cell* 1993; 72:767–778.

173. Waksman G, Kominos D, Robertson SC, Pant N, Baltimore D, Birge RB, Cowburn D, Hanafusa H, Mayer BJ, Overduin M, Resh MD, Rios CB, Silverman L, Kuriyan J. Crystal structure of the phosphotyrosine recognition domain SH2 of v-*src* complexed with tyrosine-phosphorylated peptides. *Nature* 1992; 358:646–653.

174. Burke TR Jr, Smyth MS, Otaka A, Nomizu M, Roller PP, Wolf G, Case R, Shoelson SE. Nonhydrolyzable phosphotyrosyl mimetics for the preparation of phosphatase-resistant SH2 domain inhibitors. *Biochemistry* 1994; 33:6490–6494.

175. Harris W, Hill CH, Lewis EJ, Nixon JS, Wilkinson SE. Protein kinase C inhibitors. *Drugs of the Future* 1993; 18:727–735.

176. Tamaoki T, Nakano H. Potent and specific inhibitors of protein kinase C of microbial origin. *Bio/Technology* 1990; 8:732–735.

177. Ruegg UT, Burgess GM. Staurosporine, K-252 and UCN-01: potent but nonspecific inhibitors of protein kinases. *Trends Pharmacol Sci* 1989; 10:218–220.

178. Seynaeve CM, Kazanietz MG, Blumberg PM, Sausville EA, Worland PJ. Differential inhibition of protein kinase C isozymes by UCN-01, a staurosporine analogue. *Mol Pharmacol* 1994; 45:1207–1214.

179. Seynaeve CM, Stetler-Stevenson M, Sebers S, Kaur G, Sausville EA, Worland PJ. Cell cycle arrest and growth inhibition by the protein kinase antagonist UCN-01 in human breast carcinoma cells. *Cancer Res* 1993; 53:2081–2086.

180. Akinaga S, Gomi K, Morimoto M, Tamaoki T, Okabe M. Antitumor activity of UCN-01, a selective inhibitor of protein kinase C, in murine and human tumor models. *Cancer Res* 1991; 51:4888–4892.

181. Wang Q, Worland PJ, Clark JL, Carlson BA, Sausville EA. Apoptosis in 7-hydroxystaurosporine-treated T lymphoblasts correlates with activation of cyclin-dependent kinases 1 and 2. *Cell Growth Differ* 1995; 6:927–936.

182. Shi L, Nishioka WK, Thing J, Bradburg EM, Litchfield DW, Greenbury AM. Premature p34^{cdc2} activation required for apoptosis. *Science* 1994; 263:1143–1145.

183. Davis PD, Elliott LH, Harris W, Hill CH, Hurst SA, Keech E, Kumar MKH, Lawton G, Nixon JS, Wilkinson SE. Inhibitors of protein kinase C. Substituted bisindolylmaleimides with improved potency and selectivity. *J Med Chem* 1992; 35:994–1001.

184. Bit RA, Davis PD, Elliott LH, Harris W, Hill CH, Keech E, Kumar H, Lawton G, Maw A, Nixon JS, Vesey DR, Wadsworth J, Wilkinson SE. Inhibitors of protein kinase C. Potent and highly selective bisindolylmaleimides by conformational restriction. *J Med Chem* 1993; 36:21–29.

185. Toullec D, Pianetti P, Coste H, Bellevergue P, Grand-Perret T, Ajakane M, Baudet V, Boissin P, Boursier E, Loriolle F, Duhamel L, Charon D, Kirilovsky J. The bisindolylmaleimide GF 109203X is a potent and selective inhibitor of protein kinase C. *J Biol Chem* 1991; 266: 15,771–15,781.
186. Zhang L, Higuchi M, Totpal K, Chaturvedi MM, Aggarwal BB. Staurosporine induces the cell surface expression of both forms of human tumor necrosis factor receptors on myeloid and epithelial cells and modulates ligand-induced cellular response. *J Biol Chem* 1994; 269:10,270–10,279.
187. Sampson LE, Mire-Sluis A, Meager A. Protein kinase C-dependent phosphorylation is involved in resistance to tumour necrosis factor-alpha-induced cytotoxicity in a human monocytoid cell line. *Biochem J* 1993; 292:289–294.
188. Coppock DL, Tansey JB, Nathanson L. 12-*O*-tetradecanoylphorbol-13-acetate induces transient cell cycle arrest in G_1 and G_2 in metastatic melanoma cells: inhibition of phosphorylation of p34^{cdc2}. *Cell Growth Differ* 1992; 1:485–1194.
189. Berkow RL, Kraft AS. Byrostatin, a non-phorbol macrocyclic lactone, activates intact human polymorphonuclear leukocytes and binds to the phorbol ester receptor. *Biochem Biophys Commun* 1985; 131:1109–1116.
190. Kraft AS, Smith JB, Berkow RL. Byrostatin, an activator of the calcium phospholipid-dependent protein kinase, blocks phorbol ester-induced differentiation of human promyelocytic leukemia cells, HL-60. *Proc Natl Acad Sci USA* 1986; 83:1334–1338.
191. Gebbia V, Citarrella P, Miserendino V, Valennza R, Borsellino N. The effects of the macrocytic lactone bryostatin-1 on leukemic cells in vitro. *Tumori* 1992; 78:167–171.
192. Nurse P. Ordering S phase and M phase in the cell cycle. *Cell* 1994; 79:547–550.
193. Sherr CJ. G1 phase progression: cycling on cue. *Cell* 1994; 79:551–555.
194. Vesely J, Havlicek L, Strnad M, Blow J, Donella-Deanna A, Pinna L, Letham DS, Kato J, Detivaud L, Leclerc S, Meijer L. Inhibition of cyclin-dependent kinases by purine analogues. *Eur J Biochem* 1994; 224:771–786.
195. Kitagawa M, Okabe T, Ogino H, Matsumoto H, Suzuki-Takahashi I, Kokubo T, Higashi M, Saitoh S, Taya Y, Yasuda H, Ohba Y, Nishimura S, Tanaka N, Okuyama A, Butyrolactone I. A selective inhibitor of cdk2 and cdc2 kinase. *Oncogene* 1993; 8:2425–2432.
196. Kaur G, Stetler-Stevenson M, Sebers S, Worland P, Sedlacek H, Myers C, Czech J, Naik R, Sausville E. Growth inhibition with reversible cell cycle arrest of carcinoma cells by flavone L86-8275. *J Natl Cancer Inst* 1992; 84:1736–1740.
197. Losiewicz MD, Carlson BA, Kaur G, Sausville EA, Worland PJ. Potent inhibition of Cdc2 kinase activity by the flavonoid L86-8275. *Biochem Biophys Res Commun* 1994; 201:589–595.
198. Worland PJ, Kaur G, Stetler-Stevenson M, Sebers S, Sartor O, Sausville EA. Alteration of the phosphorylation state of p34^{cdc2} kinase by the flavone L86-8275 in breast carcinoma cells. Correlation with decreased H1 kinase activity. *Biochem Pharmacol* 1993; 46:1831–1840.
199. Carlson BA, Sausville EA, Worland PJ. Flavopiridol induced G1-S phase block in MDA-MB-468 breast carcinoma cells with deregulation of CDK2. *Proc Am Assoc Cancer Res* 1995; 36:35.
200. Czech J, Hoffman D, Naik R, Sedlacek HH. Antitumoral activity of flavone L 86-8275. *Int J Oncol* 1995; 6:31–36.
201. Fry MJ. Structure, regulation and function of phosphoinositide 3-kinases. *Biochim Biophys Acta* 1994; 1226:237–268.
202. Escobedo JA, Kaplan DR, Kavanaugh WM, Turck CW, Williams LT. A phosphatidylinositol-3 kinase binds to platelet-derived growth factor receptors through a specific receptor sequency containing phosphotyrosine. *Mol Cell Biol* 1991; 11:1125–1132.
203. Lev S, Givol D, Yarden Y. Interkinase domain of kit contains the binding site for phosphatidylinositol 3′ kinase. *Proc Natl Acad Sci USA* 1992; 89:678–682.
204. Backer JM, Myers MG Jr, Shoelson SE, Chin DJ, Sun XJ, Miralpeix M, Hu P, Margolis B, Skolnik EY, Schlessinger J, White MF. Phosphatidylinositol 3′-kinase is activated by association with IRS-1 during insulin stimulation. *EMBO J* 1992; 11:3469–3479.
205. Raffioni S, Bradshaw RA. Activation of phosphatidylinositol 3-kinase by epidermal growth factor, basis fibroblast growth factor, and nerve growth factor in PC12 pheochromocytoma cells. *Proc Natl Acad Sci USA* 1992; 89:9121–9125.

206. Yamanashi Y, Fukui Y, Wongsasant B, Kinoshita Y, Ichimori Y, Toyoshima K, Yamamoto T. Activation of src-like protein-tyrosine kinase Lyn and its association with phosphatidylinositol 3-kinase upon B-cell antigen receptor-mediated signaling. *Proc Natl Acad Sci USA* 1992; 89: 1118–1122.

207. Gold MR, Chan VW-F, Turck CW, DeFranco AL. Membrane Ig cross-linking regulates phosphatidylinositol 3-kinase in B lymphocytes. *J Immunol* 1992; 148:2012–2022.

208. Thompson PA, Gutkind JS, Robbins KC, Ledbetter JA, Bolen JB. Identification of distinct populations of PI-3 kinase activity following T-cell activation. *Oncogene* 1992; 7:719–725.

209. Prasad KVS, Janssen O, Kapeller R. Raab M, Cantley LC, Rudd CE. Src-homology 3 domain of protein kinase p59^{fyn} mediates binding to phosphatidylinositol 3-kinase in T cells. *Proc Natl Acad Sci USA* 1993; 90:7366–7370.

210. Fantl WJ, Escobedo JA, Martin GA, Turck CW, del Rosario M, McCormick F, Williams LT. Distinct phosphotyrosines on a growth factor receptor bind to specific molecules that mediate different signaling pathways. *Cell* 1992; 69:413–423.

211. Yano H, Nakanishi S, Kimura K, Hanai N, Saitoh Y, Fukui Y, Nonomura Y, Matsuda Y. Inhibition of histamine secretion by wortmannin through the blockade of phosphatidylinositol 3-kinase in RBL-2H3 cells. *J Biol Chem* 1993; 268:25,846–25,856.

212. Powis G, Bonjouklian R, Berggren MM, Gallegos A, Abraham R, Ashendel C, Zalkow L, Matter WF, Dodge J, Grindley G, Vlahos CJ. Wortmannin, a potent a selective inhibitor of phosphatidylinositol-3-kinase. *Cancer Res* 1994; 54:2419–2423.

213. Kiguchi K, Glesne D, Chubb CH, Fujiki H, Huberman E. Differential induction of apoptosis in human breast tumor cells by okadaic acid and related inhibitors of protein phosphatases 1 and 2A. *Cell Growth Differ* 1994; 5:995–1004.

214. Casillas AM, Amaral K, Chegini-Farahani S, Nel AE. Okadaic acid activates p42 mitogen-activated protein kinase (MAP kinase; ERK-2) in B-lymphocytes but inhibits rather than augments cellular proliferation: contrast with phorbol 12-myristate 13-acetate. *Biochem J* 1993; 290:545–550.

215. Roberg M, Tudan C, Hung SMF, Harder KW, Jirik FR, Anderson H. Antitumor drug fostriecin inhibits the mitotic entry checkpoint and protein phosphatases 1 and 2A. *Cancer Res* 1994; 54:6115–6121.

216. Crooke ST, Bennett CF. Mammalian phosphoinositide-specific phospholipase C isoenzymes. *Cell Calcium* 1989; 10:309–323.

217. Merritt JE, Rink TJ. The effects of substance P and carbachol on inositol tris- and tetrakis-phosphate formation and cytosolic free calcium in rat parotid acinar cells. *J Biol Chem* 1987; 262.14,912–14,916.

218. Perrella FW, Chen SF, Behrens DL, Kaltenbach RF III, Seitz SP. Phospholipase C inhibitors: a new class of cytotoxic agents. *J Med Chem* 1994; 37:2232–2237.

219. Kohn EC, Sandeen MA, Liotta LA. In vivo efficacy of a novel inhibitor of selected signal transduction pathways including calcium, arachidonate, and inositol phosphates. *Cancer Res* 1992; 52:3208–3212.

220. Viallet J, Sharoni Y, Frucht H, Jensen RT, Minna JD, Sausville EA. Cholera toxin inhibits signal transduction by several mitogens and the *in vitro* growth of small cell lung cancer. *J Clin Invest* 1990; 86:1904–1912.

221. Bunn PA Jr, Chan D, Stewart J, Gera L, Tolley R, Jewett R, Tagawa M, Alford C, Mochzuki T, Yanaihara N. Effects of neuropeptide analogues on calcium flux and proliferation in lung cancer cell lines. *Cancer Res* 1994; 54:3602–3610.

222. Gordon J, Melamed MD, Ley SC, Hughes-Jones NC. Anti-immunoglobulin inhibits DNA synthesis in Epstein Barr virus-transformed lymphoblastoid cell lines. *Immunology* 1984; 52:79–85.

223. Ashwell JD, Longo DL, Bridges SH. T-cell tumor elimination as a result of T-cell receptor-mediated activation. *Science* 1987; 237:61–64.

224. Beckwith M, Urba WJ, Ferris DK, Freter CE, Kuhns DB, Moratz CM, Longo DL. Anti-IgM-mediated growth inhibition of a human B lymphoma cell line is independent of phosphatidylinositol turnover and protein kinase C activation and involves tyrosine phosphorylation. *J Immunol* 1991; 147:2411–2418.

225. Bridges SH, Kruisbeek AM, Longo DL. Selective in vivo antitumor effects of monoclonal anti-I-A antibody on B cell lymphoma. *J Immunol* 1987; 139:4242–4249.

226. Sussman JJ, Saito T, Shevach EM, Germain RN, Ashwell JD. Thy-1 and Ly-6-mediated lymphokine production and growth inhibition of a T cell hybridoma require coexpression of the T cell antigen receptor complex. *J Immunol* 1988; 140:2520–2526.

227. Funakoshi S, Longo DL, Beckwith M, Conley DK, Tsarfaty G, Tsarfaty I, Armitage RJ, Fanslow WC, Spriggs MK, Murphy WJ. Inhibition of human B-cell lymphoma growth by CD40 stimulation. *Blood* 1994; 83:2787–2789.

228. Aboud-Pirak E, Hurwitz E, Pirak ME, Bellot F, Schlessinger J, Sela M. Efficacy of antibodies to epidermal growth factor receptor against KB carcinoma in vitro and in nude mice. *J Natl Cancer Inst* 1988; 80:1605–1611.

229. Hancock MC, Langton BC, Chan T, Toy P, Monahan JJ, Mischak RP, Shawver LK. A monoclonal antibody against the c-erB-2 protein enhances the cytotoxicity of cis-diamminedichloroplatinum against human breast and ovarian tumor cell lines. *Cancer Res* 1991; 51:4575–4580.

230. Pietras RJ, Fendly BM, Chazin VR, Pegram MD, Howell SB, Slamon DJ. Antibody to HER-2/neu receptor blocks DNA repair after cisplatin in human breast and ovarian cancer cells. *Oncogene* 1994; 9:1829–1838.

231. Kohn KW, Jackman J, O'Connor PM. Cell cycle control and cancer chemotherapy. *J Cell Biochem* 1994; 54:440–452.

17

Immunoconjugates

Walter A. Blättler, DrScNat, Ravi V. J. Chari, PhD, and John M. Lambert, PhD

CONTENTS

1. INTRODUCTION

Successful anticancer drugs must exploit known or unknown, gross or ever so subtle, differences between normal and malignant cells. The development of immunotoxins is one of the first attempts to develop rationally anticancer drugs that are based on known cellular differences associated with cancer cells. Much immunological evidence had accumulated that transformed cells express tumor-specific antigens. However, it was difficult to generate heterosera with well-defined antitumor reactivity. The isolation in 1967 of an agglutinin from wheat germ that identified a tumor-specific determinant on neoplastic cell surfaces (1) marked the first time that a pure molecular species was available for targeting of tumors.

Further probing of cell surfaces with lectins and agglutinins, however, was hampered by the availability of only a small number of lectins with an even smaller number of different binding specificities. This situation changed dramatically with the advent of the monoclonal antibody (MAb) technology (2). The potential for generating a nearly unlimited reservoir of reagents each with its own binding specificity for an antigen was rapidly exploited in creating MAbs that bound to novel tumor cell-specific antigens. Although some naked antibodies were used in clinical tests for the treatment of cancer, many immunologists doubted that the humoral part of the immune system would have sufficient cytotoxic potential to eliminate millions of tumor cells. MAb were, therefore, armed with extraneous cytotoxic effector functions and became delivery vehicles that imparted tumor specificity to otherwise nonselective cytotoxic effector molecules.

From: *Cancer Therapeutics: Experimental and Clinical Agents*
Edited by: B. Teicher Humana Press Inc., Totowa, NJ

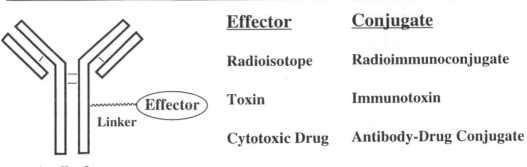

Fig. 1. Schematic representation of immunoconjugates.

The covalent binding of an effector molecule to an MAb yields an immunoconjugate (Fig. 1), which is called an immunotoxin, when the effector molecule is a toxin, an antibody–drug conjugate when cytotoxic drugs are used as effectors, and a radioimmunoconjugate in the case of linked radioisotopes. Common to all three methodologies is their reliance on the tumor-specific binding of their MAb component. Therefore, we shall first discuss the generation of "tumor-specific" MAbs and then describe the development and testing of radioimmunopharmaceuticals, of immunotoxins, and of antibody–drug conjugates.

2. TUMOR-SPECIFIC ANTIBODIES

The ideal MAb for the generation of immunoconjugates would bind to an antigen exclusively present on the surface of tumor cells, and would further be expressed homogeneously on all tumor cells or at least on all tumor stem cells (the latter, however, is difficult to assay). In addition, the antigen should not be shed from cells, should not be present in the serum of patients, and ideally, for practical medical and commercial reasons, should be present on the tumors of all patients with the same type of cancer.

In the infancy of immunotoxin development, several MAb were claimed to be tumor-specific. However, the development and use of more thorough analytical methods, such as analysis with a fluorescence activated cell sorter (FACS), sensitive immunohistochemical staining techniques using large panels of fresh-frozen tissue sections, and modern biochemical and molecular biological techniques, contributed to today's generally accepted view that most antibodies recognize tumor-associated antigens that are expressed only preferentially on tumors. Some antigens may be found on only a limited number of tissues, whereas others are on only one specific tissue type and are, therefore, tissue-specific. In the best case, some tumor-associated antigens may be expressed only during a particular developmental stage of a certain cell type. Some degree of tumor specificity often presents itself by the overexpression of certain surface antigens on transformed cells, such as *erb*B-2/*HER*-2 on breast tumor cells of a subgroup of patients (*3*), or certain carbohydrate antigens on epidermoid carcinomas (*4*). The only surface antigens that are absolutely tumor-specific are the surface immunoglobulin or idiotype present on the cells of B-cell leukemia and lymphomas, and the clonotypic T-cell receptor on T-cell leukemia and lymphoma cells. Not only are these structures tumor-specific, but individualized, patient-specific MAbs have been created (*5*).

To generate MAb with antihuman tumor reactivity, typically mice or rats were immunized with whole cells or cell membrane preparations from tumor cell lines or from tumor biopsies. The spleens of the immunized animals were then used to generate and select antibody-producing hybridomas. However, many MAbs used in immunoconjugates, in particular, antibodies reactive with hematopoietic cells, were originally developed as research tools to differentiate between various normal cell types and were, therefore, generated by injecting animals with normal human cells, such as the various cell types from blood.

MAb that have the potential to be used in anticancer immunoconjugates are conveniently grouped into those that react with hematopoietic tumors and those that bind to antigens on solid tumors. Because of the rapid renewal of hematopoietic cells and the experience of regeneration of blood cells after bone marrow transplantation, tissue-specific antibodies were widely used in immunoconjugates against leukemias and lymphomas. T-cell malignancies were treated, for example, with conjugates binding to the T-cell markers CD5, CD7, or the IL-2 receptor β-chain (CD 25); B-cell malignancies with antibody conjugates against the B-cell differentiation antigens CD19, CD20, and CD22; and analogously, myeloid malignancies with conjugates against the myeloid marker CD33 (6). Most of these antigens are differentiation antigens that are expressed throughout the ontogeny of a particular cell type starting at the earliest lineage restricted stage to ensure that the conjugates were able to treat the yet unidentified clonogenic tumor cells.

It has been much more difficult to identify cell-surface markers useful for immunoconjugates against solid tumors. The principle of tissue specificity is not as easily applied as in the hematopoietic area, except possibly for tumors of nonessential tissues, where the temporary removal of certain cell populations may be tolerated. In the absence of tumor specificity and tissue specificity, the selection of antigens was largely based on their overexpression on tumor cells relative to normal tissues. For lists of possible candidate surface antigens for immunoconjugate targeting, the reader is referred to two comprehensive reviews (7,8).

For the development of highly cytotoxic immunoconjugates that bind to antigens also expressed on some normal tissues, although hopefully at lower levels, it was essential to find animal models for toxicity studies, where similar crossreactivity was observed. Fortunately, many of the antigenic determinants were found to be preserved in nonhuman primates where they were expressed with a similar tissue distribution as in humans. A good example is the data presented for the anti-Le^y antibody in ref. (4).

A problem commonly encountered in solid tumors is the heterogeneous expression of an antigen on cells of a given tumor. Although some cells may express large numbers of an antigen on their surface, other cells in the same biopsy sample, equally having a transformed phenotype, may be antigen-negative. If transformation is a clonogenic event, then these different cell populations may represent differentiation stages that are not necessarily all tumorigenic. Heterogeneous expression of an antigen may, therefore, not necessarily disqualify it from being a target for therapeutic immunoconjugates.

If one surveys the known antigenic cell-surface markers for human solid tumors, (see, e.g., 7,8), one is struck by the paucity of such known markers. Also, when antibodies were generated with different tumor tissues or tumor cell lines, often antibodies to the same antigens were generated. For example, when mice were immunized with the breast tumor line MCF-7, MAb B1 and B3 were obtained that reacted with the Le^y carbohydrate chain (4), and immunization with cell line H3396 derived from a metastatic breast adenocarcinoma yielded antibodies BR64 and BR96, both of which also react with the Le^y carbohydrate chain (9). These results are a reflection of the limitations of the immunological methodology used to identify these antigens. They probably represent the most immunodominant markers recognized by the murine immune system, and only the screening of much larger panels of hybridomas, a work-intensive and time-consuming undertaking, might allow the discovery of further novel antigens with this technology. This realization, far from being discouraging, predicts that we have barely scratched the surface for the discovery of tumor cell-surface markers for therapeutic targeting, and it has spawned the development of several new methodologies. The most promising techniques might be the phage display of the entire murine or human immunological repertoire and its use in the probing of cell surfaces (10), or the searching for interactions on cell surfaces with combinatorial libraries of peptides that carry their genetic information in the form of amplifiable DNA sequences (11).

In most patients treated with murine MAb, a prompt human antimurine antibody (HAMA) response was observed, which led to the development of several "humanization" technologies. Humanization is the attempt to give murine antibodies an appearance that is not recognized as foreign by the human immune system while preserving their specificity and binding avidity.

It was well known that heterosera against xenogeneic immunoglobulins largely reacted with the constant region or Fc portion of the molecule, and the first approach at "humanization" was therefore the genetic construction of chimeric antibodies, comprising the murine variable region and the human constant region of IgG (12). Most chimeric antibodies displayed much reduced immunogenecity, but a response to the murine Fv portion could ultimately be observed. In reshaped or CDR-grafted antibodies, the murine content was further reduced by grafting the murine complementary determining regions (CDRs) or hypervariable region onto a human variable region framework (13). These antibodies were generally found not to be immunogeneic, but it was often difficult to maintain the binding affinity of the parent murine antibodies. Further amino acid changes in the framework region are generally necessary to maintain the original conformations of the CDRs. These changes need to be deduced for each antibody through computer model building, and the ultimate success—preservation of full binding—is often difficult to achieve even with extensive changes that potentially negate the advantage of CDR grafting over chimerization. In the newest approach, called variable domain resurfacing (14), the affinity is maintained by retaining the CDRs and the core of the murine variable region framework. Only the surface residues of the murine variable region framework are replaced by those from a human variable region. A simple algorithm predicts the necessary changes in the framework region, and when this method was applied to two murine antibodies, their affinities were unaffected (14). This approach assumes that the immunogenecity of murine antibody variable regions is determined by the accessible surface residues only, an assumption not yet tested with globulins, but generally accepted for the antigenecity of proteins (15,16).

3. RADIOIMMUNOCONJUGATES

Ever since the appreciation of the cytocidal effects of high doses of radiation, oncologists have attempted to harness the energy of radioactivity to eradicate tumors in patients afflicted with cancer. The goal of radiotherapy is to deliver a sufficiently high dose of radiation locally to the tumor in order to sterilize the tumor without causing lethal damage to the surrounding tissues. Successful killing of all tumor cells requires radiation doses of at least 60 gy to be concentrated at the tumor site, which is at the limit of the dose that can be delivered by external beam radiation while sparing normal tissue. Unfortunately, the wide application of external beam radiotherapy, while improving survival, has rarely resulted in cure. The notion that the ability of oncologists to eradicate tumors could be improved by in vivo administration of a radionuclide was first developed using iodine-131 to treat thyroid carcinomas, which concentrate radioiodine from blood resulting in delivery of local tumoricidal doses of 80–300 gy (*17*).

Radioimmunoconjugate therapy, which exploits the availability of specific antibodies that can localize to tumor cells, has been under investigation for a number of years as one way of improving radiotherapy. The hope of radioimmunoconjugate therapy is that targeting of radioactivity by antibodies could overcome two drawbacks of external beam radiotherapy: (1) specific targeting by radiolabeled antibodies should allow more precise delivery of the radiation dose to the tumor with concomitant sparing of a greater amount of the surrounding normal tissue; and (2) radiolabeled antibody will deliver a radiation dose to small undetected areas of tumor or micrometastases.

Radionuclides that are useful for radioimmunoconjugate therapy must emit particles whose energy can be deposited locally, ideally within a radius that encompasses one or a few cells. Furthermore, such radionuclides should have relatively short half-lives, so that radioactivity incorporated into the patient decays within a reasonable period of time, and in addition, they should be isotopes of elements whose chemistry allows them to be readily conjugated to antibodies. Several radioisotopes that may meet these criteria and that have been used in trials of radioimmunoconjugate therapy are shown in Table 1.

Chemically, the radioisotopes shown in Table 1 comprise two groups, the radiometals and radioactive isotopes of iodine. Iodine (and astatine) is generally conjugated directly to tyrosine residues in antibodies simply by mixing the protein with sodium iodide in the presence of an oxidizing agent, such as Chloramine T or related compounds (*20*). The reaction is extremely rapid, even at 0°C, although one must take care to avoid damage to the antibody by excessive oxidation. Alternatively, radioiodine can be conjugated to antibodies using iodinated compounds that allow labeling without exposing the protein to oxidative conditions, and furthermore, allow the possibility of utilizing iodinated compounds that are not subject to enzymatically catalyzed dehalogenation (*21–23*).

The radioactive metals are conjugated to antibodies by the use of chelating agents that are in turn chemically linked to the protein. Although the early chelates have high stability constants, they are kinetically labile, and in vivo, the radiometal readily exchanges into metal-transport proteins, such as transferrin, thereby losing any target specificity. Once lost from a conjugated chelate, a radiometal, such a yttrium-90, can ultimately be deposited in bone, resulting in prolonged irradiation of bone marrow. Recently, chelating agents that ''cage'' the metal and are far more stable have been developed for diagnostic and therapeutic applications with antibodies (*24,25*). Figure 2 illustrates the structure of two such antibody-conjugated macrocyclic chelators, which are ideal reagents for binding copper-67 and yttrium-90. In vivo studies show that radiometals targeted by antibodies linked to caged chelating agents have greatly

Table 1
Radionuclides with Potential for Radioimmunotherapy[a]

Radioisotope	Half-life	Decay particle	Particle energy, maximum energy, MeV	Path length, mm[b]	Comments
Astatine-211	7.2 h	α	5.9	0.04–0.08	Iodine chemistry
Bismuth-212	1 h	α	6.1	0.04–0.08	
Copper-67	2.4 d	β	0.57	0.6	γ-Emission for imaging
Iodine-125	60.1 d	Auger electron (electron capture)	7.5	0.001–0.02	Requires internalization for cytocidal effect
Iodine-131	8.1 d	β	0.81	0.8	High-energy γ-emission for imaging
Rhenium-186	3.5 d 3.7 d	β	1.1 and 0.93	1.8	γ-Emission for imaging
Rhenium-188	17 h	β	2.1	4.4	γ-Emission for imaging
Yttrium-90	2.5 d	β	2.7	5.3	

[a]Compiled from published data (6,18,19).

[b]The path length is defined as the radius of a sphere within which 90% of the energy emitted by a radionuclide is absorbed (19).

improved tumor localization of the radioactivity, with less deposition into bone and less marrow toxicity (26).

The β-emitters, yttrium-90 and iodine-131, have been the radioisotopes used most extensively in therapeutic studies to date, more because of their ready availability than because they have the most ideal characteristics for therapy (27,28). Iodine-131 is a medium-range β-emitter whose energy is absorbed within one or two cell diameters, whereas the more energetic β-particle of yttrium-90 can penetrate several cell diameters. This is the basis for the theoretical benefit of using radionuclides as the effector killing moiety for antibody-directed therapy, namely that the antigen targeted by the antibody need not be expressed on all of the tumor cells in a tumor mass. Thus, antigen-negative tumor cells may also be killed by the radiation concentrated at the tumor by antigen-positive tumor cells (a "bystander" killing effect). The α-emitters may not share this potential advantage because of the extremely short range of α-particles. However, this property could be an advantage when targeting an antigen expressed homogeneously on all tumor cells and that is internalized by the cells, in that a higher proportion of the energy of the radiation is deposited in the target cell. Unfortunately, the two α-emitters with appropriate chemical properties for conjugation, bismuth-212 (29) and astatine-211 (30), have very short half-lives, which may reduce their effectiveness in vivo (27), and which presents logistical difficulties in their use.

The fate of the antigen/antibody complex on the surface of the tumor cell will influence the best choice of radioisotope or method of linking it to the antibody. Radioiodine is retained better in tumor tissues if it is targeted by an antibody that is not internalized. Otherwise, on internalization, radioimmunoconjugates are enzymatically degraded and dehalogenated with the consequence that the radioactivity

Conjugate Structure **Macrocycle** **Metal Ion**

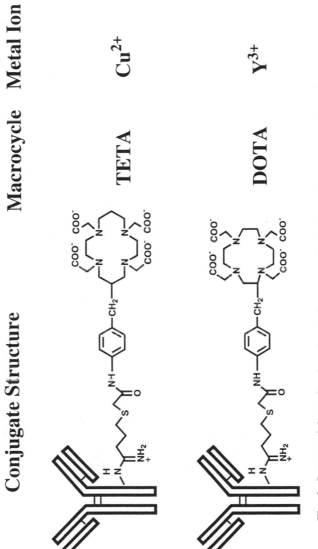

TETA Cu^{2+}

DOTA Y^{3+}

Fig. 2. Structural formula of conjugated macrocyclic chelators for copper and yttrium ions.

rapidly diffuses away and is cleared (*6,18*). Internalizing antibodies are better suited for targeting radiometals, such as yttrium-90 and copper-67, which are retained by the target cells on internalization and eventual degradation of the radioimmunoconjugate (*6*), since cellular proteins are generally good chelators of transition metals. Antibodies that target antigens that readily internalize are necessary for targeting iodine-125 whose decay produces Auger electrons of extremely short path length requiring proximity to the nucleus to elicit cell killing. Iodine-125 is therefore best conjugated via nonmetabolizable adducts (*21–23*).

There has been some debate about what are the most desirable properties for the antibody component of a radioimmunoconjugate, given a high specificity for an antigen selectively expressed on tumor tissue. In contrast to diagnostic uses of radioimmunoconjugates, where the most important parameters are (1) a high ratio of radioisotope delivered to the tumor compared with that delivered to normal tissue and (2) rapid clearance of radioisotope from the blood pool, which otherwise masks the radioactivity concentrated at the tumor (*31*), the most important factor for the radiotherapeutic is the total amount of radioisotope delivered to the tumor and its residence time in the tumor (i.e., dose deposited at the tumor), provided toxicity to normal tissues is tolerated. Although intact IgG penetrates from blood vessels more slowly than Fab or genetically engineered antibody fragments, most studies show that a greater dose of radioactivity is deposited at tumor sites when using radioimmunoconjugates containing intact IgG, suggesting that its slower clearance from blood, and the possibility for bivalent binding to target cells, are the most important parameters for a therapeutic application. Most clinical experience to date has been with mouse IgG in radioimmunoconjugates, which means that the generation of HAMA has been a factor that may limit the ability of patients to receive multiple doses of conjugate. The advent of humanized antibodies may overcome this limitation. Genetic engineering can also be used to make small fragments of humanized antibodies where the single binding domain can have very high affinity, and may, therefore, both penetrate into tumor tissue quickly and be well retained by the tumor, thereby increasing the dose delivered to the tumor.

What is the clinical experience in the evaluation of radioimmunoconjugate therapy in clinical trials? Can a sufficiently high dose of radiation be delivered to tumor in vivo to kill enough tumor cells to effect a therapeutic response? The clinical studies to date can be divided into two general groups, those treating tumors that are particularly radiosensitive, such as lymphomas and leukemias (*6*), and those treating solid tumors (*18*).

Clinical evaluation of radioimmunoconjugate therapy for non-Hodgkin's lymphoma (NHL) has been facilitated by the availability of a variety of B-cell-specific MAb, such as anti-idiotype antibodies, LYM-1 (anti-HLA-DR), anti-B1 (anti-CD20), MB-1 (anti-CD37), and OKB7 (anti-CD21) (*6,32–34*). These antibodies have been coupled to iodine-131 and have been used in cumulative doses of up to 750 mCi/patient. These large doses are well tolerated with the important exception of severe myelosuppression. Even though this severe side effect can be ameliorated by fractionating the dose of radiotherapeutic into multiple smaller doses given over several weeks, it would appear that the best clinical results are obtained in those trials that employ massive myeloablative doses of the radioimmunotherapeutic (*6*). In the studies from the Fred Hutchinson Cancer Center in Seattle, Washington, 16 of 19 patients who were administered therapeutic doses achieved a complete remission (*34*). However, the cost of this therapeutic benefit is that 15 of the patients required an autologous bone marrow transplant (ABMT). These investigators suggest that the only possibility for complete eradication of the tumor is to use massive doses of radioimmunotherapy that are so high as to require bone marrow transplant support. It remains to be determined whether the therapeutic benefit of systemic delivery of massive doses of radiation with ABMT support is superior to other protocols utilizing chemotherapy and total body irradiation (external beam) as ablative regimens for ABMT protocols in the treatment of patients with relapsed lymphoma.

Other leukemias and lymphomas that have been targeted in trials of radioimmunotherapy are acute myelogenous leukemia (AML), T-cell malignancies, and Hodgkin's disease (*6*, and references therein). Iodine-131-labeled anti-CD33 and anti-CD45 antibodies have been used to target AML (*35*), whereas patients with chronic lymphocytic leukemia (CLL) or cutaneous T-cell lymphoma have been treated with anti-CD5 labeled with iodine-131 or yttrium-90, and those with adult T-cell leukemia have been treated with anti-CD25 (IL-2 receptor) conjugated with yttrium-90 (*6*). The most promising responses in these studies were also achieved at dose levels that caused severe myelosuppression as the major side effect (*6*).

In studies where Hodgkin's disease was treated with antiferritin antibodies coupled to yttrium-90 (the tumor cells are rich in ferritin), impressive response rates have been reported (*36*), although again at doses that were also myeloablative so that 17 of 37 patients required ABMT rescue (3 patients died of bone marrow aplasia). The yttrium-90 was conjugated to antibody using diethylenetriamine penta-acetic acid as the chelator, from which yttrium-90 is known to escape in vivo to be taken up by bone, which thus contributes to hematopoietic toxicity (*26*). It may be that the ferritin-rich tumor can also take up the released radiometal by chelation, which may contribute to the therapeutic efficacy of this conjugate.

The clinical experience with the treatment of solid tumors by radioimmunoconjugate therapy has generally been disappointing (*18*). Indeed, if optimal therapeutic effects in relatively radiosensitive neoplasms, such as NHL, can only be achieved at doses of radioimmunoconjugate that are myeloablative, then it is unlikely that therapeutic efficacy in solid tumors can be achieved at doses that are not also myeloablative. Furthermore, the **highest** doses delivered via radioimmunoconjugates are usually estimated to be in the range of 10–20 gy, although it is generally accepted that doses of at least 60 gy are needed to eradicate solid tumors (*27,37*). A Phase II clinical trial of radioimmunotherapy with iodine-131-labeled CC49 antibody in colorectal cancer exemplifies the lack of therapeutic efficacy in the treatment of solid tumors. Despite an antibody of relatively high affinity for the target tumor-associated glycoprotein 72, no tumor responses were observed, and the doses delivered to the tumor were only in the range of 0.2–6.7 gy (*38*). Recent Phase I studies with iodine-131-labeled A33 antibody were similarly disappointing (*39*). A Phase II trial of the CC49 radioimmunoconjugate in metastatic prostate cancer also failed to demonstrate any efficacy with maximal tumor doses estimated in the range of only 2–10 gy (*40*).

One approach to increasing the dose delivered to the tumor, while maintaining the total body dose at tolerable levels, is to treat locally tumors that are confined to particular body cavities. Intralesional radioimmunotherapy of malignant glioma may offer one compartmentalized setting where cytocidal doses of radiation may be delivered to the tumor without significant toxicity to bone marrow, liver, or kidney. Treatment of 17 patients with iodine-131-labeled antitenascin antibodies resulted in 3 partial responses and 3 complete remissions (*41*). Intraperitoneal infusion of yttrium-90-labeled HMFG1 antibody was given to 52 patients with ovarian cancer (*42*). The results were encouraging, with 19 of 21 patients that were regarded as receiving treatment in an adjuvant setting still alive (median followup, 35 mo). However, even in this intra-compartment setting, the authors doubt that the therapeutic effect was due to a cyto-cidal effect of the radiation dose, and suspect that the HMFG1 murine antibody in-duced immunological reactivity against the tumor, an observation also noted by others when treating breast cancer with iodine-131-labeled L6 antibody (*43*).

What are the future prospects for radioimmunotherapy? Several investigators are beginning to think of this modality as a complement to conventional external beam radiotherapy. For example, several patients with AML achieved complete remission when given iodine-131-labeled antibody together with 12 gy of external beam irradia-tion and cytoxan (*6,44*). A similar approach may be appropriate in treatment of certain solid tumors in order to achieve a sterilizing total dose of radiation at the tumor (*45*). The early results in the use of radioimmunotherapy for treating relapsed leukemias and lymphomas have been encouraging, although the therapy is far from optimized and may generally require concomitant ABMT. In particular, the optimal radionu-clide and method of linkage to antibody still need to be defined (*27,28*), and human-ized antibodies need to be tested in the clinic to overcome the limitations on multiple-course therapy imposed by the generation of HAMA (*35*). Nevertheless, even with these improvements, it may be that the long-term prospects for radioimmunotherapy may be confined to treating radiosensitive tumors utilizing myeloablative doses together with bone marrow rescue, or as an adjunct to external beam irradiation, owing to the intrinsic limitations of radiolabeled antibodies to deliver a sterilizing dose of radiation to tumor (*46*). Radioimmunotherapy will likely remain confined to specialized clinical centers with facilities for performing ABMT and for coping with issues, such as radia-tion exposure of medical staff and handling radioactive waste, which are problematic with systemic administration of radioactivity.

4. IMMUNOTOXINS

The limited expression of antigens suitable as targets for immunoconjugates on the surface of tumor cells (in general 10^4–10^5 and very rarely more than 10^6 antigens/cell) coupled with the pharmacodynamics of large molecules, such as γ-immunoglobulins, compelled scientists to search for the most potent cytotoxic agents to be used as effec-tors in immunoconjugates. Known protein toxins from plants, such as ricin, abrin, volkensin, and viscumin, and from bacteria, such as diphtheria toxin and pseudomonas exotoxin A, fit into this category. This spurred research into a better understanding of the mechanism by which these toxins destroy cells, so as to be able to harness their deadly power for the selective killing of tumor cells.

The above-listed toxins kill cells by catalytically inactivating cellular protein synthe-sis. The plant toxins, also called ribosome-inactivating proteins (RIPs) are *N*-glyco-sidases that remove the adenine base of residue 4324 of the 28S ribosomal RNA of the 60S subunit of eukaryotic cells (*47*). The bacterial toxins use NAD$^+$ to ADP-ribosylate elongation factor 2 (*48*). Because the final targets for the toxic action are cytoplasmic, the process of intoxication involves, therefore, at least three functions:

1. A binding function to localize the toxin to a cell surface;
2. A translocation function to transfer the toxin or its catalytic subunit to the cytoplasm, which needs a mechanism to translocate the protein through the lipid bilayer of a membrane, and;
3. An enzymatic function that inactivates the essential cellular process of protein synthesis.

Plant toxins are composed of two protein subunits of approximately equal size, called A-chain and B-chain, that are linked via a disulfide bond. The A-chain contains the enzymatic activity, and the B-chain provides the binding and translocation function. B-chains are lectins with specificity for galactosides and interact tightly with terminal galactose moieties of oligosaccharides found on the surface of eukaryotic cells (49). For ricin, it has been demonstrated that the translocation function is inseparably linked with the binding to galactose residues (50).

Diphtheria toxin (DT) binds to a protein receptor present on human cells and is internalized by endocytosis into acidified vesicles, where it is proteolytically cleaved into disulfide-linked fragments A and B. Cleavage establishes the full enzymatic activity in fragment A and fragment B retains the binding and membrane translocation function (48). (The similarity between the bacterial DT and the plant toxin ricin is remarkable, especially when one considers that ricin is transcribed initially as a single-chain preproricin, where the A and B chains are connected via a 12 amino acid fragment that is proteolytically removed, leaving the disulfide-linked A and B chains.) In pseudomonas exotoxin A (PE), the three functions are located in three molecularly and structurally separated domains of the single-chain protein. The N-terminal domain Ia binds to a protein receptor on human cells, the middle domain II encodes the membrane translocation function, and the C-terminal domain III contains the enzymatic activity. As with DT, only the catalytic domain III reaches the cytosol of the cell after PE is proteolytically cleaved in acidified vesicles following endocytosis (48,51). Interestingly, domain III contains at the C-terminus the amino acid sequence REDLK (ArgGluAspLeuLys) that is required for its cytotoxicity. It may act as an intracellular localization signal, since replacement with the known endoplasmic retention signal KDEL (LysAspGluLys) preserves its toxicity (52).

In all toxins, the binding and enzymatic toxicity functions are physically separated, either into separate subunits or into separate domains. When the first immunotoxins were prepared, the membrane translocation function was little appreciated or understood, and the easily separated toxic subunits ricin A chain or DT fragment A were simply linked to more specific binding moieties, the newly developed MAbs. More elegantly even, it was found that most plants produce single-chain RIPs that have a similar molecular size and the same catalytic function as ricin A chain (53), and immunotoxins could be rapidly produced without fear of contamination by nonspecifically binding B chain. Indeed, it was only the disappointing results with these early immunotoxins—their in vitro cytotoxicities were generally much lower than that of their respective native toxins—that led to the general recognition of the third function of native toxins, the membrane translocation function.

The different structural and functional arrangements found in the above toxins necessitated different approaches for each toxin to eliminate their native, nonselective binding function, while maintaining their membrane translocation and enzymatic activities. For ricin, the binding affinity to its natural cell-surface ligands was lowered by > 1000-fold by covalently linking affinity ligands into the two high-affinity galactose binding sites of its B chain (*54*). This so-called blocked ricin, when incorporated into immunotoxins, killed the antibody target cells with a potency and efficiency similar to native ricin (*55*). Thus, it was concluded that the membrane translocation function in B chain had been preserved. Mechanistic studies demonstrated that the residual low-affinity binding of blocked ricin to galactoside residues, although not interfering with the antibody-directed selectivity and specificity on the cell surface, was necessary for the potency of the immunotoxin (*56*).

The single-chain bacterial toxins PE and DT were cloned, and genetic mutational methods were applied to change their binding characteristics. In PE, where the three domains are each associated with a single function, binding domain Ia was simply deleted to create PE40. When PE40 was then linked chemically to an antibody, the cytotoxicity and specificity of the resulting immunotoxin demonstrated that PE40 contributed the translocation and toxicity function of PE, but not the nonselective binding (*57*). The genetic manipulation not only allowed the removal of the coding region for domain Ia of the PE gene, but allowed its replacement by a gene of another binding protein, therefore creating fusion toxins. Fusion toxins with growth factors, hormones, lymphokines, and single-chain antibodies (Fv) were created (fusion toxins have been reviewed in [*58,59*]), and this chapter only discusses antibody-based toxins, i.e., immunotoxins). Similar genetic approaches have been tried with DT. Indeed, fusion toxins were first created between α-melanocyte-stimulating hormone or interleukin-2 and a truncated form of DT lacking its C-terminal binding domain (*60*). However, the relatively low cytotoxicity of these constructs indicated that efficient membrane penetration was linked to the specific binding of DT to its receptor. Indeed, the most potent specific immunotoxin with DT incorporated the whole toxin with point mutations in the B fragment that lowered the binding activity without affecting the translocation. The promising mutant CRM107 has two point mutations and a 8000-fold lower binding affinity (*61*).

The first immunotoxins evaluated clinically in cancer patients were conjugates of antilymphocyte antibodies linked to ricin A chain. As discussed above, it is the authors' opinion that most of these conjugates lacked adequate cytotoxicity, and not surprisingly, most of these conjugates were not pursued beyond Phase I clinical trials in cancer patients. One lesson learned, however, was that relatively large amounts of foreign proteins—murine IgG and ricin A chain from a plant—could be administered without significant allergic reactions.

The first published report on the clinical use of an immunotoxin that incorporated the translocation domain of a bacterial toxin was the ip administration of OVB3-PE to patients with refractory ovarian cancer (*62*). Dose-limiting toxic encephalopathy, likely owing to crossreactivity of OVB3 with normal human brain tissue, was observed early at the low dose of 5 μg/kg/d × 3 d that was not able to induce any clinical antitumor responses. Intact PE with its binding domain Ia was used, and no PE-directed binding is reported. Conjugation of the antibody via the noncleavable linker might have occurred in the binding domain, and, therefore, diminished its activity. The same authors proceeded then to prepare chemical conjugates or fusion toxins between truncated forms of PE that lacked the binding domain and antibodies or fragments of antibodies. Some of the promising conjugates that might enter clinical evaluation are anti-Tac(Fv)-PE40 for leukemias and transplant rejection, one of the different anti-HER2/*erb*B2-PE40 or anti-HER2/*erb*B2-PE38KDEL conjugates against breast cancer, and B3(Fv)-PE38KDEL against Le^y antigen-positive carcinomas (reviewed in ref. *59*).

The clinical evaluation of conjugates containing mutant whole DT is made more difficult by the immunity of most patients against DT. It was, therefore, proposed to use immunoconjugates with the DT mutant CRM107 for regional therapy at immunologically privileged sites, such as tumors in the central nervous system (*63,64*).

The altered whole ricin toxin, called blocked ricin (bR), was incorporated into three immunoconjugates that were clinically tested. Anti-My9-bR, which binds to CD33 found on cells of myeloid lineage, was used to deplete *ex vivo* AML cells from autologous bone marrow from AML patients (*65,66*). Treatment with Anti-My9-bR eliminated more than 4 logs of leukemic cells, and fewer normal hematopoetic progenitor cells were affected than with a treatment using anti-My9 antibody and complement, leading to a more rapid engraftment (*67*). N901-bR reactive with a neural cell adhesion molecule (NCAM, CD56) uniformly expressed on small-cell lung carcinomas (SCLC) was tested in a Phase I clinical trial on 19 patients with relapsed and/or refractory SCLC at doses ranging from 5 to 40 μg/kg/d given as a continuous infusion over 7 d (*68*). Specific in vivo binding of N901-bR to tumor in the lung, bone marrow, and liver was demonstrated on biopsies. All patients developed human anti-mouse Ig antibodies (HAMA) and antiricin antibodies (HARA). One patient at the maximal tolerated dose (MTD) of 30 μg/kg/d $\times$ 7 d achieved a partial remission. The investigator proposed to use this conjugate when patients are in a state of minimal residual disease (MRD) and plans to initiate a Phase II trial studying patients with SCLC following aggressive induction chemotherapy (*68*).

Anti-B4-bR binds to the B-cell lineage-restricted antigen CD19, which is expressed uniformly on normal and malignant B-cells. The immunoconjugate was first evaluated clinically in a Phase I trial, where 25 patients with refractory B-cell malignancies were treated with daily 1-h infusions on five successive days (*69*). Despite the clinical responses observed—one complete, two partial, and eight mixed or transient responses—it was believed that the chosen schedule of administration was not ideal. The pharmacokinetic results indicated that significant serum levels were only maintained for about 4 h. The same authors undertook, therefore, a second Phase I study, where a 7-d continuous infusion schedule was used to treat 34 patients with NHL, CLL, or acute lymphocytic leukemia (ALL) (*70*). Significant serum levels were now maintained for the duration of drug administration. Two complete responses lasting more than 32 and 15 mo and five partial responses of short duration were reported. Both complete responses were observed in patients with lower tumor burden, which suggested that Anti-B4-bR might be most successfully applied after reduction of the tumor burden by chemotherapy and radiation. Because of the different mechanism of action, Anti-B4-bR would still be capable of eradicating the remaining chemo- and radioresistant tumor cells. This adjuvant immunotoxin therapy was tested in the setting of autologous bone marrow transplantation for NHL patients. After patients had successfully engrafted and were in complete remission, they were treated with the conjugate in the hope of eliminating MRD and to prolong their disease-free survival (*71*). Again, the unique mechanism of killing makes immunotoxins ideal drug candidates for this setting, where the residual tumor cells are often resistant to further chemotherapy.

The above clinical trials evaluate immunotoxins as single agents in different clinical settings. However, as with other anticancer agents, their full potential may ultimately

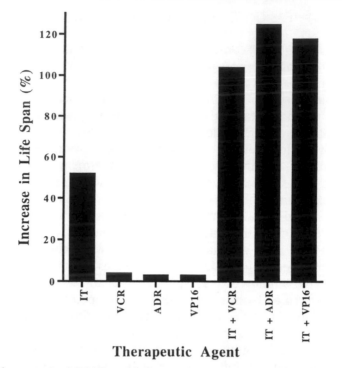

Fig. 3. Synergism between Anti-B4-bR and cytotoxic drugs for the treatment of disseminated mdr-1-expressing Burkitt's lymphoma tumors in SCID mice. Animals bearing 7-d-old tumors administered iv (73) were treated either with Anti-B4-bR alone (IT, 50 μg/kg/d × 5 d) or a chemotherapeutic drug alone at its MTD (VCR, vincristine, 3 × 1 mg/kg qod; ADR, adriamycin, 3 × 3 mg/kg q4d; VP16, etoposide, 3 × 15 mg/kg qod), or with a combination of Anti-B4-bR first (50 μg/kg/d × 5 d on days 7–11) followed by a chemotherapeutic drug (IT + VCR at 3 × 400 μg/kg q5d, on days 12, 17, and 22; IT + ADR at 3 × 3 mg/kg q5d, on d 12, 17, and 22; IT + VP16 at 3 × 15 mg/kg q5d, on days 12, 17, and 22). Untreated control animals died with a mean survival time of 24 d. Chemotherapeutic drugs alone showed no antitumor efficacy against the mdr-1 tumors, since they could not increase the life-span of animals. Immunoconjugate alone increased the life-span by 50%. All three combination treatments increased the life-span by more than 100%, demonstrating a synergistic effect between the immunoconjugate and the chemotherapeutic drugs.

come to fruition in combination treatments with other chemotherapeutic agents. It has already been demonstrated that Anti-B4-bR synergizes with chemotherapeutic agents in the treatment of human disseminated lymphomas in SCID mice (72,73), and more dramatically in the same model for the treatment of disseminated lymphomas expressing the multidrug resistance P-glycoprotein (74) (Fig. 3). These exciting findings have led to the design of several human clinical trials exploring this potential.

Immunotoxins are novel chemotherapeutic agents for the treatment of cancer. However, no drug of this category has yet been approved by health authorities. The most advanced in testing, Anti-B4-bR, is currently undergoing evaluation in a randomized multicenter Phase III trial. The potential of immunotoxins is lodged in their potency, tumor selectivity and, foremost, in their unique killing mechanism. This renders them drug candidates for treatment in disease settings refractory to further standard treatment and for incorporation into multidrug regimens.

5. ANTIBODY–DRUG CONJUGATES

Anticancer drugs in clinical use, such as doxorubicin, methotrexate, and the Vinca alkaloids, have limited selectivity for tumors, and hence, their cytotoxic potency cannot be fully exploited for the destruction of cancer cells. Their high toxicity toward actively proliferating nonmalignant cells, such as cells of the gastrointestinal tract and bone marrow, becomes dose-limiting. The linkage of cytotoxic drugs to MAb binding to specific cell-surface tumor-associated antigens should enhance the selectivity of these drugs by targeted delivery. It was expected that this approach would improve the therapeutic index of these drugs by lowering their systemic toxicity to sensitive normal tissues, while enhancing the local concentration of the cytotoxic agent at the tumor site. Several reports summarize the early development of MAb–drug conjugates (75–79), where, in general, clinically used cytotoxic anticancer drugs, such as daunorubicin, doxorubicin, methotrexate, Vinca alkaloids, mitomycin C, idarubicin, and melphalan, were conjugated to a multitude of murine MAbs. Initially, these drugs were linked directly to antibodies via noncleavable bonds and, in most cases, an average of 4–8 drug molecules were linked/molecule of antibody. Most conjugates lacked cytotoxic potency—they often were less cytotoxic than the free drugs—and attempts were made to improve them by linking to the antibody a larger number of drug molecules via macromolecular carriers, such as dextran, polyglutamic acid, polylysine or human serum albumin. However, the unfavorable pharmacokinetics and pharmacodynamics observed in animals with such conjugates discouraged further development (80).

In the next development phase, the emphasis shifted toward the development of conjugates, where the antibody molecules were linked to drugs via linkers that would be cleaved inside the cell to release active drug. One of the cleavable linkers that has been widely employed is an acid-labile linker that takes advantage of the acidic environment of the endosomes that might be encountered after receptor-mediated endocytosis. Acid-labile linkers based on cis-aconitic acid have been used for the preparation of conjugates of daunorubicin with macromolecular carriers (81), with an antimelanoma antibody (82) and an anti-T-cell antibody (83). Vinblastine and its analogs were linked to antibodies using an acid-labile hydrazide linker (84,85), which was also used for doxorubicin conjugates (86). In an alternative approach, daunorubicin was linked to an antibody via a peptide spacer arm under the premise that free drug would be released from the conjugate by the action of lysosomal peptidases (87).

Evaluation of their in vitro cytotoxicity revealed that these early conjugates were usually less potent than the parent unconjugated drugs, indicating the therapeutic levels of the drugs were not achieved inside target cells. Also, only marginal antigen-specific killing of the target cancer cells in vitro was observed. Typically, a target-specific and an analogous nontargeted conjugate differed in their effective concentrations against a given cell line only by factors of 2–10. Nevertheless, when evaluated in vivo, several of these conjugates showed greater therapeutic efficacy in human tumor xenograft models in immunodeficient mice than the corresponding unconjugated drugs or isotype-matched nonbinding antibody–drug conjugates. For example, it has been recently reported that immunoconjugates prepared with the MAb BR96 and doxorubicin completely cured athymic mice that had been implanted sc with human tumor xenografts (88). This result maybe explained by the high antigen expression ($> 10^6$ antigens/cell for BR96) and the large doses of immunoconjugate administered.

The latter is a common theme in successful treatment of tumor xenografts in animal models.

The preclinical results obtained with antibody–drug conjugates were sufficiently encouraging to warrant evaluation of these agents in humans. An immunoconjugate of methotrexate and the MAb KS1/4, which binds to a 40-kDa glycoprotein antigen that is expressed in human lung, colorectal, pancreatic, and ovarian adenocarcinomas, was evaluated in two different Phase I human clinical trials in nonsmall-cell lung cancer patients (*89,90*). A majority of patients elicited a HAMA response. Immuno-peroxidase staining of carcinoma samples provided evidence of posttreatment localization of the conjugate. However, there were no clinical responses in either study. The same KS1/4 antibody was also linked to vinblastine via either an acid-labile hydrazide linker or an ester link and then evaluated in clinical trials in patients with adenocarcinomas (*91,92*). Again, a majority of the patients elicited a HAMA response, and again, no clinical responses were observed in these studies (*89*). Although conjugates of KS1/4 with methotrexate and vinblastine showed antitumor efficacy in human xenograft tumor models in mice, these results did not translate into clinically useful products and, to the best of our knowledge, human studies with these immunoconjugates have been discontinued. Recently, a human clinical trial has been initiated in colon cancer patients with the MAb BR96 linked to the anti-cancer drug doxorubicin via acid-labile hydrazide bonds (*93*).

Lack of clinical success with these early antibody–drug conjugates suggests that it was not possible to achieve intracellular concentrations of the drug required to kill sufficient numbers of cancer cells. Possible reasons for these outcomes may be:

1. Lack of cytotoxic potency: a majority of commonly used anticancer drugs are only moderately cytotoxic and a large number of drug molecules, too large to be achievable by antibody delivery, have to be internalized to cause cell death;
2. Dearth of antigens on cell surfaces;
3. Inefficient internalization of antigen–antibody complexes; and
4. Inefficient release of the drug from the antibody and often release of a modified, less active form of the drug.

New and very promising antibody–drug conjugates seek to overcome these shortcomings through the use of 100- to 1000-fold more potent cytotoxic drugs and the use of disulfide-containing linkers to ensure rapid release inside target cells. Maytansinoids, CC-1065 analogs, calicheamicin derivatives, and morpholinodoxorubicin were incorporated into new conjugates. Linkage of a highly cytotoxic maytansinoid drug to MAb produced immunoconjugates that exhibited high, antigen-specific cytotoxicity in vitro (*94*). Thus, a disulfide-linked maytansinoid immunoconjugate (C242-May) prepared with the MAb C242, which recognizes the CanAg antigen (*95*) expressed on the surface of human colon cancer cells, kills antigen-positive COLO 205 cells with an IC_{50} value of $1.2 \times 10^{-11}M$, with $> 99.999\%$ of the cells killed at a conjugate concentration of $5 \times 10^{-9}M$. In contrast, the conjugate is at least 600-fold less cytotoxic toward antigen-negative A-375 cells ($IC_{50} = 7.6 \times 10^{-9}M$), demonstrating the antigen specificity of the cytotoxic effect (Fig. 4A). The high antigen-specific cytotoxicity of these conjugates observed in vitro encouraged further evaluation of this conjugate for therapeutic efficacy in vivo in a human tumor xenograft model in SCID mice. Animals were implanted sc with COLO 205 cells, which were allowed to grow for

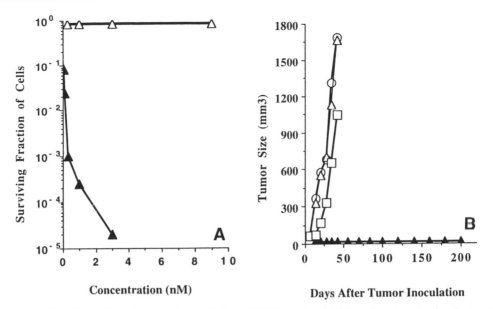

Fig. 4. (A) In vitro cytotoxicity and specificity of C242-maytansinoid conjugate. The in vitro cytotoxicity of C242-maytansinoid conjugate was measured on antigen-positive human colon carcinoma COLO 205 (ATCC CCL 222) cells (closed triangles) and antigen-negative human melanoma A-375 (ATCC CRL 1619) cells (open triangles), using a clonogenic assay. Cells were plated in varying numbers in 96-well plates in 0.2 mL growth media containing varying concentrations of immunoconjugate. The cells were maintained in a humidified atmosphere at 37 °C and 6% CO_2 for 18–21 d. Colonies were then counted, and the plating efficiency and surviving fractions determined. Surviving fractions of cells are plotted as a function of immunoconjugate concentration. **(B)** Antitumor efficacy of C242-May conjugate. The therapeutic efficacy of C242-May was determined in a established human tumor xenograft model in SCID mice that had been implanted sc with COLO 205 colon carcinoma cells. Mice (8–10 animals/group, 4 groups) were inoculated sc with 1×10^7 COLO 205 cells. The tumor was allowed to establish for 7–10 d, and treatment was begun when the average tumor size was between 65 and 100 mm³. One group of mice was left untreated, and a second group was treated iv with C242-May at a maytansinoid dose of 380 μg/kg/d administered every other day for 5 d. The remaining two groups of animals served as negative controls and were treated, using the same schedule, with an equivalent amount of unconjugated C242 antibody (15 mg/kg/d) plus free maytansinoid (380 μg/kg/d), or with the isotype matched yet nonbinding maytansinoid conjugate N901-May (maytansinoid dose 380 μg/kg/d). Tumor size is plotted as a function of time. Control mice: open circles; treated mice: C242-May, closed triangles; C242 + May, open triangles; N901-May, open squares.

7–10 d before treatment started when the tumor size was between 65 and 100 mm³. C242-May, at a maytansinoid dose of 380 μg/kg/d × 5 (conjugate dose 15 mg/kg/d), completely cured all mice of the tumor and animals were disease-free for > 140 d. In contrast, treatment with a mixture of unconjugated maytansinoid and antibody or with the isotype-matched yet nonbinding conjugate N901-May had little effect on the rate of tumor growth when compared with the untreated control mice (Fig. 4B). The results are very encouraging especially in view of the fact that cures with C242-May were also seen at doses (225 μg/kg/d × 5 maytansinoid dose), well below the maximum tolerated dose of the immunoconjugate.

This approach was extended to another potent cytotoxic drug, DC1 (*96*), which is a synthetic analog of the potent natural product CC-1065. An immunoconjugate called

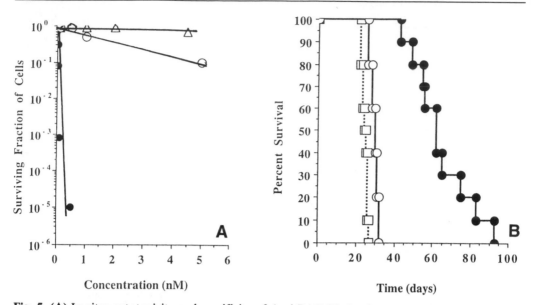

Fig. 5. (A) In vitro cytotoxicity and specificity of Anti-B4-DC1. In vitro cytotoxicity was measured using a growth-back extrapolation assay. Namalwa cells (ATCC CRL 1432) and MOLT-4 cells (ATCC CRL 1582) (4×10^5 cells, 2 mL) were exposed for 24 h to different concentrations of conjugate at 37 °C. Cells were washed, centrifuged, resuspended in fresh growth media, and counted. Cells were then incubated at 37 °C and counted daily using a Coulter counter. Surviving fractions of cells were determined and plotted as a function of conjugate concentration. Namalwa cells: closed circles; Namalwa cells in the presence of $5 \times 10^{-7}M$ unconjugated anti-B4 antibody: open circles; MOLT-4 cells: open triangles. **(B)** Therapeutic efficacy of Anti-B4-DC1. The therapeutic efficacy of Anti-B4-DC1 was determined using an established iv human tumor xenograft survival model in SCID mice. Mice (10 animals/group) were inoculated iv with 4×10^6 Namalwa (Burkitt's lymphoma) cells. Treatment was begun iv after tumor was established (day 7) with either Anti-B4-DC1 (5 mg/kg/d $\times$ 5, corresponding to 82 μg/kg/d DC1 content) or with an equivalent mixture of unconjugated anti-B4 antibody plus free DC1 drug. A control group of animals was left untreated. Control animals: open squares; treated animals: Anti-B4-DC1, closed circles; anti-B4 plus free DC1, open circles.

Anti-B4-DC1 prepared with DC1 and the MAb anti-B4, which recognizes the CD19 antigen found on cells in B-cell malignancies, kills antigen-positive Namalwa cells efficiently with an IC$_{50}$ value of $1.3 \times 10^{-11}M$ after 24 h of exposure to the conjugate. The killing curve is very steep with >99.999% of cells eliminated (surviving fraction of cells $< 1 \times 10^{-5}$) at an immunoconjugate concentration of $5 \times 10^{-10}M$. Again the cytotoxic effect was antigen-specific, since the conjugate was about 400-fold less cytotoxic toward antigen-negative MOLT-4 cells. The addition of a 100-fold excess of unconjugated anti-B4 antibody abolished the cytotoxic effect of anti-B4-DC1 toward antigen-positive Namalwa cells, further demonstrating the antigen specificity of the cytotoxic effect (Fig. 5A). Anti-B4-DC1 also showed significant therapeutic efficacy against an established human tumor survival model in SCID mice (*73*). Mice (10 animals/group) were inoculated intravenously with Namalwa cells (4×10^6 cells/ animal) and iv treatment was begun on day 7, when the tumor had grown to 7×10^7 cells. The group of untreated control mice had a median survival time (MST) of 24 d, whereas the group treated with a mixture of antibody and unconjugated drug showed a slight therapeutic effect with an MST of 30 d. Anti-B4-DC1 (80 μg/kg/d DC1 dose) administered once every day for 5 d showed a pronounced antitumor effect with a 2.6-fold increase in life-span (MST = 62 d) (Fig. 5B).

Similar antitumor efficacy in an animal model was described for an immunoconjugate comprising a hydrazide-linked calicheamicin derivative (97). The preparation and in vitro evaluation of an immunoconjugate with the fourth drug mentioned above, morpholinodoxorubicin, which is about 40-fold more potent than doxorubicin itself, have also been described recently (98).

The new antibody–drug conjugates were built with the experience and insight gained during the last 15 years of immunoconjugate research, and they incorporate features that make them promising improved chemotherapeutic agents whose clinical evaluation is eagerly awaited. All the clinical drugs will include humanized antibodies allowing their use during several cycles of remission induction and consolidation treatment. Whether the size will hamper their efficacy against solid tumors is not at all clear from the preclinical models. However, molecular biological methods allow for the easy production of antibody fragments, such as Fab, F(ab′), and Fv fragments, and it is possible to incorporate them into drug conjugates. Coupled with their smaller size, however, is a much faster clearance rate and often an inability to retain their binding affinity on drug conjugation. Only careful preclinical and clinical evaluation will ultimately allow the determination of the most efficacious type and forms of antibody–drug conjugates.

6. CONCLUSIONS

The use of immunoconjugates for the treatment of cancer, i.e., the selective delivery of cytotoxic agents to tumor cells, seemed to be a simple, straightforward idea whose time had come with the arrival of the MAb technology in 1975. Today, 20 years later, no such agent is yet an approved drug. Every element contributing to the success (antitumor efficacy in patients) of an immunoconjugate had to be newly developed. Specific target antigens had to be discovered, and appropriate effector molecules had to be found and had to be linked via suitable linkers. Killing mechanisms needed to be explored to preserve the potency of toxins. Novel, more potent chemotherapeutic drugs had to be evaluated and had to be modified for covalent linkage to antibodies, and new chelators for radioisotopes had to be synthesized. Pharmacokinetic and pharmacodynamic problems with the large immunoconjugates as well as the patients' immune responses to foreign proteins had to be considered. Today, immunoconjugates are at the stage of evaluation in Phase II and Phase III clinical trials, giving testimony to success in finding solutions to these challenging questions. Important new technologies were also developed, such as the humanization of murine antibodies, the phage display of the antibody repertoire, and combinatorial chemistry, that allowed the identification of novel tumor-selective antibodies at a more rapid pace and their efficient incorporation into effective, nonimmunogenic immunoconjugates. The need for selective anticancer agents has not changed, and immunoconjugate development is positioned well to contribute its part in filling this need.

REFERENCES

1. Burger MM, Goldberg AR. Identification of a tumor specific determinant on neoplastic cell surfaces. *Proc Natl Acad Sci USA* 1967; 57:359–366.

2. Köhler G, Milstein C. Continuous cultures of fused cells secreting antibody of predefined specificity. *Nature* 1975; 256:495–497.

3. Slamon DJ, Clark GM, Wong SG, Levin WJ, Ullrich A, McGuire WL. Human breast cancer: correlation of relapse and survival with amplification of the HER-2/neu oncogene. *Science* 1987; 235:177–182.

4. Pastan I, Lovelace ET, Gallo MG, Rutherford AV, Magnani JL, Willingham MC. Characterization of monoclonal antibodies B1 and B3 that react with mucinous adenocarcinomas. *Cancer Res* 1991; 51:3781–3787.

5. Kwak LW, Campbell MJ, Czerwinski DK, Hart S, Miller RA, Levy R. Induction of immune response in patients with B-cell lymphoma against the surface-immunoglobulin idiotype expressed by their tumors. *N Engl J Med* 1992; 327:1209–1215.

6. Grossbard ML, Press OW, Appelbaum FR, Bernstein ID, Nadler LM. Monoclonal antibody-based therapies of leukemia and lymphoma. *Blood* 1992; 80:863–868.

7. Boyer CM, Lidor Y, Lottich SC, Bast RC Jr. Antigenic cell surface markers in human solid tumors. *Antibody, Immunoconjugates, Radiopharmaceuticals* 1988; 1:105–116.

8. Carroll AM, Greene MI. Tumor cell biology: tumor specific and associated antigens. In: Zalutsky MR, ed. *Antibodies in Radiodiagnostics and Therapy*. Boca Raton, FL: CRC. 1989:13–43.

9. Hellstöm I, Garrigues HJ, Garrigues U, Hellström KE. Highly tumor-reactive internalizing mouse monoclonal antibodies to Le^y-related cell surface antigens. *Cancer Res* 1990; 50:2183–2190.

10. Winter G, Milstein C. Man-made antibodies. *Nature* 1991; 349:293–299.

11. Moos WH, Green GD, Pavia MR. Recent advances in the generation of molecular diversity. In: Bristol JA, ed. *Annual Reports in Medicinal Chemistry*, vol. 28. San Diego, CA: Academic. 1993:315–324.

12. Morrison SL, Johnson MJ, Herzenberg LA, Oi VT. Chimeric human tumor antibody molecules: mouse antigen-binding domains with human constant region domains. *Proc Natl Acad Sci USA* 1984; 81:6851–6855.

13. Reichman L, Clark M, Waldmann H, Winter G. Reshaping human antibodies for therapy. *Nature* 1988; 332:323–327.

14. Roguska MA, Pedersen JT, Keddy CA, Henry AH, Searle SJ, Lambert JM, Goldmacher VS, Blättler WA, Rees AR, Guild BC. Humanization of murine antibodies through variable domain resurfacing. *Proc Natl Acad Sci USA* 1994; 91:969–973.

15. Thornton JM, Edwards MS, Taylor WR, Barlow DJ. Location of "continuous" antigenic determinants in the protruding regions of proteins. *EMBO J* 1986; 5:409–413.

16. Novatny J, Handschumacher M, Haber E, Bruccoleri RE, Carlson WB, Smith DW, Rose GD. Antigenic determinants in protein coincide with surface regions accessible to large probes (antibody domains). *Proc Natl Acad Sci USA* 1986; 83:226–230.

17. Maxon HR, Thomas SR, Hertzberg VS, Kereiakes JG, Chen IW, Sperling MI, Saenger EL. Relation between effective radiation dose and outcome of radioiodine therapy for thyroid cancer. *N Engl J Med* 1983; 309:937–941.

18. Mello AM, Pauwels EKJ, Cleton FJ. Radioimmunotherapy: no news from the newcomer. *J Cancer Res Clin Oncol* 1994; 120:121–130.

19. Simpkin DJ, Mackie TR. EGS4 Monte Carlo determination of the beta dose kernel in water. *Med Phys* 1990; 17:179–186.

20. Fraker PJ, Speck JC. Protein and cell membrane iodinations with a sparingly soluble chloroamide, 1,3,4,5-tetrachloro-3α,6α-diphenyl-glycoluril. *Biochem Biophys Res Commun* 1978; 80:849–857.

21. Ali SA, Warren SD, Richter KY, Badger CC, Eary JF, Press OW, Krohn KA, Bernstein ID, Nelp WB. Improving the tumor retention of radioiodinated antibody: aryl carbohydrate adducts. *Cancer Res* 1990; 50:783s–788s.

22. Zalutsky MR, Narula AS. Radiohalogenation of a monoclonal antibody using an *N*-succinimidyl 2-(tri-*n*-butylstannyl) benzoate intermediate. *Cancer Res* 1988; 48:1446–1450.

23. Ram S, Buchsbaum DJ. Radioiodination of monoclonal antibodies D612 and 17-1A with 3-iodophenylisothiocyanate and their biodistribution in tumor-bearing nude mice. *Cancer* 1994; 73:808–815.

24. Moi MK, DeNardo SJ, Meares CF. Stable bifunctional chelates of metals used in radiotherapy. *Cancer Res* 1990; 50:789s–793s.

25. Kukis DL, Diril H, Grenier DP, DeNardo SJ, DeNardo GL, Salako QA, Meares CF. A comparative study of copper-67 radiolabeling and kinetic stabilities of antibody-macrocycle chelate conjugates. *Cancer* 1994; 73:779–786.

26. DeNardo GL, Kroger LA, DeNardo SJ, Miers LA, Salako Q, Kukis DL, Fand I, Shen S, Renn O, Meares CF. Comparative toxicity studies of yttrium-90 MX-DTPA and 2-IT-BAD conjugated monoclonal antibody (BrE-3). *Cancer* 1994; 73:1012–1022.

27. Rao DV, Howell RW. Time-dose-fractionation in radioimmunotherapy: implications for selecting radionuclides. *J Nucl Med* 1993; 34:1801–1810.

28. Smith A, Alberto R, Blaeuenstein P, Novak-Hofer I, Maecke HR, Schubiger PA. Preclinical evaluation of ⁶⁷Cu-labeled intact and fragmented anti-colon carcinoma monoclonal antibody MAb35. *Cancer Res* 1993; 53:5727–5733.

29. Junghans RP, Dobbs D, Brechbiel MW, Mirzadeh S, Raubitschek AA, Gansow OA, Waldmann TA. Pharmacokinetics and bioactivity of 1,4,7,10-tetra-azacylododecane N,N',N'',N'''-tetraacetic acid (DOTA)-bismuth-conjugated anti-Tac antibody for α-emitter (²¹²Bi) therapy. *Cancer Res* 1993; 53:5683–5689.

30. Larsen RH, Bruland OS, Hoff P, Alstad J, Rofstad EK. Analysis of the therapeutic gain in the treatment of human osteosarcoma microcolonies *in vitro* with ²¹¹At-labelled monoclonal antibody. *Br J Cancer* 1994; 69:1000–1005.

31. Goldenberg DM. New developments in monoclonal antibodies for cancer detection and therapy. *CA Cancer J Clin* 1994; 44:43–64.

32. Kaminski MS, Zasadny KR, Francis IR, Milik AW, Ross CW, Moon SD, Crawford SM, Burgess JM, Petry NA, Butchko GM, Glenn SD, Wahl RL. Radioimmunotherapy of B-cell lymphoma with [¹³¹I]anti-B1 (anti-CD20) antibody. *N Engl J Med* 1993; 329:459–465.

33. Czuczman MS, Straus DJ, Divgi CR, Graham M, Garin-Chesa P, Finn R, Myers J, Old LJ, Larson SM, Scheinberg DA. Phase I dose-escalation trial of iodine-131-labeled monoclonal antibody OKB7 in patients with non-Hodgkin's lymphoma. *J Clin Oncol* 1993; 11:2021–2029.

34. Press OW, Eary JF, Appelbaum FR, Martin PJ, Badger CC, Nelp WB, Glenn S, Butchko G, Fisher D, Porter B, Matthews DC, Fisher LD, Bernstein ID. Radiolabeled-antibody therapy of B-cell lymphoma with autologous bone marrow support. *N Engl J Med* 1993; 329:1219–1224.

35. Caron PC, Schwartz MA, Man Sung Co, Queen C, Finn RD, Graham MC, Divgi CR, Larson SM, Scheinberg DA. Murine and humanized constructs of monoclonal antibody M195 (anti-CD33) for therapy of acute myelogenous leukemia. *Cancer* 1994; 73:1049–1056.

36. Vriesendorp HM, Herpst JM, Germack MA, Klein JL, Leichner PK, Loudenslager DM, Order SE. Phase I-II studies of yttrium-labeled antiferritin treatment for end-stage Hodgkin's disease including radiation therapy: oncology group 87-01. *J Clin Oncol* 1991; 9:918–928.

37. Vaughan ATM, Anderson P, Dykes PW, Chapman CE, Bradwell AR. Limitations to the killing of tumors using radiolabelled antibodies. *Br J Radiol* 1987; 60:567–572.

38. Murray J, Macey DJ, Kasi LP, Rieger P, Cunningham J, Bhadkamkar V, Zhang H-Z, Schlom J, Rosenblum MG, Podoloff DA. Phase II radioimmunotherapy trial with ¹³¹I-CC49 in colorectal cancer. *Cancer* 1994; 73:1057–1066.

39. Welt S, Divgi CR, Kemeny N, Finn RD, Scott AM, Graham M, St Germain J, Richards EC, Larson SM, Oettgen HF, Old LJ. Phase I/II study of iodine 131-labeled monoclonal antibody A33 in patients with advanced colon cancer. *J Clin Oncol* 1994; 12:1561–1571.

40. Meredith RF, Bueschen AJ, Khazaeli MB, Plott WE, Grizzle WE, Wheeler RH, Schlom J, Russell CD, Liu T, LoBuglio AF. Treatment of metastatic prostate carcinoma with radiolabeled antibody CC49. *J Nucl Med* 1994; 35:1017–1022.

41. Riva P, Arista A, Tison V, Sturiale C, Franceschi G, Spinelli A, Riva N, Casi M, Moscatelli G, Frattarelli M. Intralesional radioimmunotherapy of malignant gliomas. *Cancer* 1994; 73:1076–1082.

42. Hird V, Maraveyas A, Snook D, Dhokia B, Soutter WP, Meares C, Stewart JSW, Mason P, Lambert HE, Epenetos AA. Adjacent therapy of ovarian cancer with radioactive monoclonal antibody. *Br J Cancer* 1993; 68:403–406.

43. DeNardo SJ, Mirick GR, Kroger LA, O'Grady LF, Erickson KL, Yuan A, Lamborn KR, Hellström I, Hellström KE, DeNardo GL. The biological window for chimeric L6 radioimmunotherapy. *Cancer* 1994; 73:1023–1032.

44. Applebaum FR, Matthews DC, Eary JF, Badger CC, Kellogg M, Press OW, Martin PJ, Fisher DR, Nelp WB, Thomas ED, Bernstein ID. The use of radiolabeled anti-CD33 antibody to aug-

ment marrow irradiation prior to marrow transplantation for acute myelogenous leukemia. *Transplantation* 1992; 54:829–833.

45. O'Donoghue J. The impact of tumor cell proliferation in radioimmunotherapy. *Cancer* 1994; 73:974–980.

46. Vaughan ATM, Bradwell AR, Dykcs PW, Anderson P. Illusions of tumor killing using radio-labeled antibodies. *Lancet I* 1986:1492,1493.

47. Endo Y. Mechanism of action of ricin and related toxins on the inactivation of eukaryotic ribosomes. In: Frankel AE, ed. *Immunotoxins*. Boston: Kluwer Academic Publishers. 1988:75–89.

48. Collier RJ. Structure–activity relationships in diphtheria toxin and pseudomonas exotoxin A. In: Frankel AE, ed. *Immunotoxins*. Boston: Kluwer Academic Publishers. 1988:25–35.

49. Olsnes S, Sandvig K. How protein toxins enter and kill cells. In: Frankel AE, ed. *Immunotoxins*. Boston: Kluwer Academic Publishers. 1988:39–73.

50. Newton DL, Wales R, Richardson PT, Walbridge S, Saxena SK, Ackerman EJ, Roberts LM, Lord MJ, Youle RJ. Cell surface and intracellular functions for ricin galactose binding. *J Biol Chem* 1992; 267:11,917–11,922.

51. Ogata M, Chaudhary VK, Pastan I, FitzGerald DJ. Processing of pseudomonas exotoxin by a cellular protease results in the generation of a 37,000-Da toxin fragment that is translocated to the cytosol. *J Biol Chem* 1990; 265:20,678–20,685.

52. Chaudhary VK, Jinno Y, FitzGerald D, Pastan I. Pseudomonas exotoxin contains a specific sequence at the carboxyl terminus that is required for cytotoxicity. *Proc Natl Acad Sci USA* 1990; 87:308–312.

53. Barbieri L, Battelli MG, Stirpe F. Ribosome-inactivating proteins from plants. *Biochim Biophys Acta* 1993; 1154:237–282.

54. Lambert JM, McIntyre G, Gauthier MN, Zullo D, Rao V, Steeves RM, Goldmacher VS, Blättler WA. The galactose-binding sites of the cytotoxic lectin ricin can be chemically blocked in high yield with reactive ligands prepared by chemical modification of glycopeptides containing triantennary N-linked oligosaccharides. *Biochemistry* 1991; 30:3234–3247.

55. Lambert JM, Goldmacher VS, Collinson AR, Nadler LM, Blättler WA. An immunotoxin prepared with blocked ricin: a natural plant toxin adapted for therapeutic use. *Cancer Res* 1991; 51:6326–6342.

56. Goldmacher VS, Lambert JM, Blättler WA. The specific cytotoxicity of immunoconjugate containing blocked ricin is dependent on the residual binding capacity of blocked ricin: evidence that the membrane binding and A-chain translocation activities of ricin cannot be separated. *Biochem Biophys Res Commun* 1992; 183:758–766.

57. Pastan I, FitzGerald D. Recombinant toxins for cancer treatment. *Science* 1991; 254:1173–1177.

58. Frankel AE, ed. *Genetically Engineered Toxins*. New York: Marcel Dekker, 1992.

59. Siegall CB. Targeted toxins as anticancer agents. *Cancer (suppl)* 1994; 74:1006–1012.

60. Murphy JR, Lakkis FG, VanderSpek JC, Anderson P. Protein engineering of diphtheria toxin. Development of receptor-specific cytotoxic agents for the treatment of human disease. In: Frankel AE, ed. *Genetically Engineered Toxins*. New York: Marcel Dekker. 1992:365–393.

61. Greenfield L, Johnson VG, Youle RJ. Mutations in diphtheria toxin separate binding from entry and amplify immunotoxin selectivity. *Science* 1987; 238:536–539.

62. Paul LH, Bookman MA, Ozols RF, Young RC, Smith II JW, Longo DL, Gould B, Frankel A, McClay ET, Howell S, Reed E, Willingham MA, FitzGerald DJ, Pastan I. Clinical evaluation of intraperitoneal pseudomonas exotoxin immunoconjugate OVB3-PE in patients with ovarian cancer. *J Clin Oncol* 1991; 12:2095–2103.

63. Johnson VG, Woo C, Wilson D, Zovickian J, Greenfield L, Oldfield EH, Youle R. Improved tumor-specific immunotoxins in the treatment of CNS and ceptomeningeal neoplasia. J Neurosurg 1989; 70:240–248.

64. Lashe DW, Ibercil O, Akbasak A, Youle RJ, Oldfield EH. Efficacy of direct intratumoral therapy with targeted protein toxins for solid human gliomas in nude mice. *J Neurosurg* 1994; 80:520–526.

65. Roy DC, Robertson MJ, Belanger R, Gyger M, Perreault C, Bonny Y, Soiffer R, Epstein C, Ritz J. Engraftment following Anti-My9-bR depleted autologous marrow transplantation for patients with acute myeloid leukemia. *Blood (suppl)* 1992; 80:376a.

66. Roy DC, Griffin JD, Belvin M, Blättler WA, Lambert JM, Ritz J. Anti-My-9-blocked ricin: an immunotoxin for selective targeting of acute myeloid leukemia cells. *Blood* 1991; 77:2404–2412.

67. Robertson MJ, Roy DC, Soiffer R, Belanger R, Gyger M, Perreault C, Anderson K, Freedman A, Nadler LM, Ritz J. More rapid engraftment after infusion of autologous bone marrow treated with Anti-My-9 and complement. *Blood (suppl)* 1993; 82:640a.

68. Lynch TJ, Jr. Immunotoxin therapy of small-cell lung cancer. N901-blocked ricin for relapsed small-cell lung cancer. *Chest* 1993; 103:436s–439s.

69. Grossbard ML, Freedman AS, Ritz J, Coral F, Goldmacher VS, Eliseo L, Spector NK, Lambert JM, Blättler WA, Taylor JA, Nadler LM. Serotherapy of B-cell neoplasms with Anti-B4-blocked ricin: a phase I trial of daily bolus infusion. *Blood* 1992; 79:576–585.

70. Grossbard ML, Lambert JM, Goldmacher VS, Spector NL, Kinsella J, Eliseo L, Coral F, Taylor JA, Blättler WA, Epstein CL, Nadler LM. Anti-B4-blocked ricin: a phase I trial of 7-day continuous infusion in patients with B cell neoplasms. *J Clin Oncol* 1993; 11:726–737.

71. Grossbard ML, Gribben JG, Freedman AS, Lambert JM, Kinsella J, Rabinowe SN, Eliseo L, Taylor JA, Blättler WA, Epstein CL, Nadler LM. Adjuvant immunotoxin therapy with Anti-B4-blocked ricin after autologous bone marrow transplantation for patients with B-cell non-Hodgkin's lymphoma. *Blood* 1993; 81:2263–2271.

72. O'Connor R, Liu C, Ferris CA, Guild BC, Teicher BA, Corvi C, Liu Y, Arceci RJ, Goldmacher VS, Lambert JM, Blättler WA. Anti-B4-blocked recin synergizes with doxorubicin and etoposide on multidrug-resistant and drug-sensitive tumors. *Blood* 1995; 86:4286–4294.

73. Shah SA, Halloran PM, Ferris CA, Levine BA, Bourret LA, Goldmacher VS, Blättler WA. Anti-B4-blocked ricin immunotoxin shows therapeutic efficacy in four different SCID mouse models. *Cancer Res* 1993; 53:1360–1367.

74. Liu C, Lambert JM, Teicher BA, Blättler WA, O'Connor R. Cure of multidrug-resistant human B-cell lymphoma xenografts by combinations of Anti-B4-blocked ricin and chemotherapeutic drugs. *Blood* 1996; 87:3892–3898.

75. Sela M, Hurwitz E. Conjugates of antibodies with cytotoxic drugs. In: Vogel CW, ed. *Immunoconjugates*. New York: Oxford University Press. 1987:189–216.

76. Ghose T, Blair AH, Vaughan K, Kulkarni P. Antibody-directed drug targeting in cancer therapy. In: Goldberg EP, ed. *Targeted Drugs*. New York: John Wiley. 1993:1–22.

77. Rodwell, JD. *Antibody-Mediated Delivery Systems*. New York: Marcel Dekker, 1988.

78. Pietersz GA. The linkage of cytotoxic drugs to monoclonal antibodies for the treatment of cancer. *BioConjugate Chem* 1990; 1:89–95.

79. Garnett MC, Baldwin RW. An improved synthesis of a methotrexate-albumin-791T/36 monoclonal antibody conjugate cytotoxic to human osteogenic sarcoma cell lines. *Cancer Res* 1986; 46:2407–2412.

80. Endo N, Takeda Y, Umemoto N, Kishida K, Watanabe K, Saito M, Kato Y, Hara T. Nature of linkage and mode of action of methotrexate conjugated with antitumor antibodies: implications for future preparation of conjugates. *Cancer Res* 1988; 48:3330–3355.

81. Shen EC, Ryser J-PH. Cis-aconityl spacer between daunomycin and macromolecular carriers: a model of pH sensitive linkage releasing drug from a lysosomotropic conjugate. *Biochem Biophys Res Commun* 1981; 102:1048–1054.

82. Yang HM, Reisfeld RA. Doxorubicin conjugated with a monoclonal antibody directed to a human melanoma-associated proteoglycan suppresses the growth of established tumor xenografts in nude mice. *Proc Natl Acad Sci USA* 1988; 85:1189–1193.

83. Dillman RO, Johnson DE, Shawler DL, Koziol JA. Superiority of an acid-labile daunorubicin-monoclonal antibody immunoconjugate compared to free drug. *Cancer Res* 1988; 48:6097–6102.

84. Laguzza BC, Nichols CL, Briggs SL, Cullinan GJ, Johnson DJ, Starling JJ, Baker AL, Bumol TF, Corvalan JRF. New antitumor monoclonal antibody–vinca conjugate LY203725 and related compounds: design, preparation, and representative in vivo activity. *J Med Chem* 1989; 32:548–555.

85. Apelgren LD, Zimmerman DL, Briggs SL, Bumol TF. Antitumor activity of the monoclonal antibody-Vinca alkaloid immunoconjugate LY203725 (KS1/4-4 desacetylvinblastine-3-carboxhydrazide) in a nude mouse model of ovarian cancer. *Cancer Res* 1990; 50:3540–3544.

86. Greenfield RS, Kaneko T, Daues A, Edson MA, Fitzgerald KA, Olech LJ, Grattan JA, Spitalny

GL, Braslawsky GR. Evaluation in vitro of adriamycin immunoconjugates synthesized using an acid-sensitive hydrazone linker. *Cancer Res* 1990; 50:6600–6607.

87. Trouet A, Masquelier M, Baurain R, de Campenère DD. A covalent linkage between dauno-rubicin and proteins that is stable in serum and reversible by lysosomal hydrolases, as required for a lysosomotropic drug-carrier: *in vitro* and *in vivo* studies. *Proc Natl Acad Sci USA* 1982; 79:626–629.

88. Trail PA, Willner D, Lasch SJ, Henderson AJ, Hofstead S, Casazza AM, Firestone RA, Hellström I, Hellström KE. Cure of xenografted human carcinoma by BR96-doxorubicin immunocon-jugates. *Science* 1993; 261:212–215.

89. Elias DJ, Hirshowitz L, Kline LE, Kroener JF, Dillman RO, Walker LE, Robb JA, Timms RM. Phase I clinical comparative study of monoclonal antibody KS1/4 and KS1/4-methotrexate immunoconjugate in patients with non-small cell lung cancer. *Cancer Res* 1990; 50:4154–4159.

90. Elias DJ, Kline LE, Robbins BA, Johnson HCL, Pekny K, Benz M, Robb JA, Walker LE, Kosty M, Dillman RO. Monoclonal antibody KS1/4-methotrexate immunoconjugate in non-small cell lung carcinoma. *Am J Respir Crit Care Med* 1994; 150:1114–1122.

91. Petersen BF, DeHerdt SV, Schneck DW, Bumol TF. The human immune response to KS1/4-desacetylvinblastine (LY256787) and KS1/4-desacetylvinblastine hydrazide (LY203728) in single and multiple dose clinical studies. *Cancer Res* 1991; 51:2286–2290.

92. Schneck D, Butler F, Dugan W, Littrel D, Dorrbecker S, Petersen B, Browsher R, DeLong A, Zimmerman J. Phase I studies with a murine monoclonal antibody-Vinca conjugate (KS1/4-DAVLB) in patients with adenocarcinoma. *Antibody Immunoconjugate Radiopharmaceuticals* 1989; 2:93–100.

93. Trail PA, Slichenmyer WJ, Birkhofer MJ, Warner G, Knipe J, Willner D, Firestone RA, Sikkema D, Onetto N, Canetta R, Saleh MN, Murray JL, Gilewski TA, Bookman MA, Hellström I, Hellström KE. BR96-doxorubicin immunoconjugate for treatment of patients with carcinoma. *Proc Amer Assoc Cancer Res* 1996; 37:626.

94. Chari RVJ, Martell BA, Gross JL, Cook SB, Shah SA, Blättler WA, McKenzie SJ, Goldmacher VS. Immunoconjugates containing novel maytansinoids: promising anticancer drugs. *Cancer Res* 1992; 52:127–131.

95. Baeckstrom D, Hansson GC, Nilsson O, Johansson C, Gendler SJ, Lindholm L. Purification and characterization of a membrane-bound and secreted mucin-type glycoprotein carrying the carcinoma-associated sialyl-Le[a] epitope on distinct core proteins. *J Biol Chem* 1991; 266:21,537–21,547.

96. Bourret LA, Derr SM, Tadayoni M, Mattocks KM, Shah SA, Liu C, Blättler WA, Goldmacher VS. Enhancement of the selectivity and antitumor efficacy of a CC-1065 analogue through im-munoconjugate formation. *Cancer Res* 1995; 55:4079–4084.

97. Hillman LM, Hamann PR, Wallace R, Menendez AT, Durr FE, Upeslacis J. Preparation and characterization of monoclonal antibody conjugates of the calicheamicins: a novel and potent family of antitumor antibiotics. *Cancer Res* 1993; 53:3336–3342.

98. Mueller BM, Wrasidlo WA, Reisfeld RA. Antibody conjugates with morpholino-doxorubicin and acid-cleavable linkers. *BioConjugate Chem* 1990; 1:325–330.

18

A Case for *ras* Targeted Agents as Antineoplastics

Judith S. Sebolt-Leopold, PhD

CONTENTS

1. INTRODUCTION

Conventional cancer treatment generally employs cytotoxic agents that, by inhibiting DNA replication or mitosis, are most effective against rapidly growing tumors. Clearly we have witnessed successes against various leukemias, lymphomas, and some solid tumors, such as testicular cancer. With some exceptions, there generally exists a close correlation between tumor proliferation rate and sensitivity to cytotoxic drugs (*1*). Therefore, a critical need still exists for the development of agents that will target the more refractory tumors that are distinguished by a low growth fraction, such as colon adenocarcinoma, nonsmall-cell lung cancers, and pancreatic carcinomas. Despite a roughly 40-year search for more efficacious antitumor drugs, very few new agents have shown sufficient broad-spectrum activity for entering mainstream chemotherapy.

During the last decade, our understanding of the molecular basis of neoplasia has been significantly expanded, consequently opening up a number of previously unexplored targets for anticancer drug design. One such target is the *ras* oncogene and its 21-kDa protein product (p21 Ras), which plays a pivotal role in signal transduction pathways involved in growth control and, when mutated, has been linked to transformation. In light of the fact that cancer is a disease of uncontrolled proliferation, *ras* has emerged as an attractive candidate for the design of therapies suppressing its expression or function.

This chapter will describe the normal cellular function of Ras and discuss how *ras* mutations can have dire consequences both with regard to development and subsequent treatment of human malignancies. The rationale behind several diverse strategies for *ras*-directed therapeutic intervention will then be explored along with a review of the progress reported to date.

From: *Cancer Therapeutics: Experimental and Clinical Agents*
Edited by: B. Teicher Humana Press Inc., Totowa, NJ

2. CELLULAR DEPENDENCE ON *ras* FUNCTION

The regulation of normal cell growth involves the interplay of a number of proto-oncogene products that ensure the efficient transmission of extracellular signals to the nucleus. Central to the complex circuitry within the cell are a family of 21-kDa proteins encoded by the *ras* proto-oncogenes, which act as molecular switches by virtue of their guanine nucleotide binding capacity. More than 50 proteins have been identified to date as belonging to the *ras* superfamily and collectively act as signaling molecules for a broad range of cellular functions ranging from cellular proliferation and differentiation to cytoskeleton assembly and vesicular trafficking. The universal importance of Ras proteins is evidenced by their ubiquitous and highly conserved nature among eukaryotic organisms.

Microinjection studies provided perhaps the earliest compelling evidence for the critical role played by Ras in signal transduction. The stimulation of DNA synthesis that normally occurs on the addition of serum to quiescent fibroblasts did not occur when fibroblasts were microinjected with a neutralizing anti-*ras* antibody (2). Conversely, microinjection of oncogenic Ras protein stimulated DNA synthesis in the absence of exogenous growth factors (3). The universal role of Ras in cell growth and differentiation is also supported by microinjection studies showing that anti-Ras antibodies inhibit the neuronal differentiation of PC12 pheochromocytoma cells and block insulin-induced maturation of *Xenopus* oocytes (4,5).

A single base mutation in one of the three mammalian *ras* genes, H(arvey)-, K(irsten)-, and N(euroblastoma)-*ras*, is sufficient to transform cells to malignancy. Although the relevance of *ras* mutations in neoplastic disease has been known for over 20 years, the design of Ras inhibitors has historically been hampered by a lack of clear understanding of the precise role of Ras and its regulatory interactions in signal transduction. This is no longer the case.

Signal transduction begins with an external signal, e.g., a growth factor, hormone, or antigen, binding to its cell-surface receptor. As illustrated in Fig. 1, once the extracellular ligand, e.g., epidermal growth factor (EGF), binds to its receptor, dimerization of the receptor occurs. Intermolecular mechanisms are then responsible for the activation of intrinsic tyrosine kinase activity followed by autophosphorylation of specific tyrosine residues (6).

Subsequent to receptor activation, a number of protein–protein interactions come into play by switching Ras "on" as opposed to its normal state when it is tightly bound to GDP and inactive. One feature shared by these regulatory proteins is that they contain Src-homology domains, responsible for the recognition of specific amino acid sequences containing either phosphotyrosine (SH2) or proline and hydrophobic residues (SH3) (7). The adapter protein Grb-2 contains both SH2 and SH3 domains; Grb-2 first binds to the activated receptor by virtue of its SH2 region and then associates with the Ras activator protein Sos1, the latter event being facilitated by the presence of two SH3 regions within Grb-2 (8). Complex formation between Grb-2 and Sos1 serves to recruit Sos1 into close proximity to Ras, thereby promoting activation of this G protein. Sos1 functions as a guanine nucleotide exchange factor and, on binding to Ras, disrupts its conformation, thereby causing the dissociation of GDP, which leaves the Ras protein free to bind GTP (9,10). In this scenario, Ras must be present at the plasma membrane. Since Ras does not contain a transmembrane domain, membrane

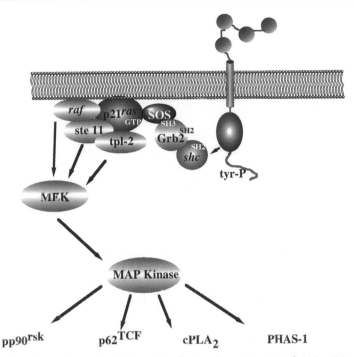

Fig. 1. Key players in the *ras* signaling pathway (*see text* for details).

localization is accomplished by the posttranslational addition of a lipid moiety (farnesyl group) to the carboxyl-terminus of p21, thereby facilitating insertion of the Ras protein into the plasma membrane. This modification will be covered more extensively in Section 4.

Under normal conditions, the cell tightly regulates the proportion of active Ras such that quiescent cells in G_0 generally have < 5% of their total Ras pool in the active state compared to nearly 50% on mitogenic stimulation (*11*). Although Ras, as a G protein, has intrinsic GTPase activity and will eventually hydrolyze bound GTP to GDP and inorganic phosphate, the negative regulatory protein GAP (GTPase-activating protein) acts to accelerate the deactivation of Ras, so that the rate of proliferation is kept under control. GAP was first identified by Trahey and McCormick as an activity that stimulated GTP hydrolysis of microinjected oncogenic Ras in *Xenopus* oocytes (*12*). A dual functionality has been ascribed to GAP, which serves as a downstream target of Ras function in addition to playing the role of negative regulator. Its effector properties were suggested when it was discovered that oncogenic *ras* mutants, despite their unresponsiveness to GAP stimulation, still required interaction with GAP for transforming activity (*13*). GAP, which has a mol wt of 120 kDa, contains two SH2 domains and one SH3 domain at its N-terminus, allowing it to interact with the cellular proteins p62 and p190, a feature that is apparently critical for its signal transducing activity (*14,15*). The cellular functions of p62 and p190 remain unclear, although it is believed that a complex between GAP120 and p190 could serve to couple activated growth factor receptor signals to Ras and Rho/Rac proteins, which are involved in regulation of cytoskeletal actin assembly (*16*). In this manner, cell-cycle progression could be coordinated with cytoskeletal reorganization (*17*).

Once Ras is switched "on," activation of the mitogen-activated protein kinases, i.e., the MAP kinase cascade, is the final series of events leading to transmission of growth signals to the nucleus. The MAP kinases, also referred to as extracellular signal-regulated kinases (ERKs), are serine/threonine kinases. The activity of the first enzyme in this cascade, MAP kinase, depends on a dual specificity kinase capable of phosphorylating both a threonine and a tyrosine residue. Such dual functionality has been ascribed to the c-*raf*-1 proto-oncogene product. Raf, which acts as an MAP kinase kinase, has been found to complex with Ras, only when the latter protein is activated, i.e., in its GTP-bound state (*18*). Recent studies have elegantly shown that if *raf* is genetically manipulated to contain the membrane localization signal of k-Ras conferred by its carboxy-terminus, then it becomes constitutively localized at the plasma membrane and completely bypasses a need for Ras (*19,20*). They conclude that Ras is able to transmit signals downstream by virtue of its ability to recruit Raf to the plasma membrane where a distinct, Ras-independent, Raf activation event occurs. Once Raf is activated, the enzymatic activity of Raf, namely MAP kinase kinase kinase, phosphorylates MEK (MAP kinase kinase), which in turn phosphorylates MAP kinase (ERK). Like Ras, MAP kinase appears to be tightly regulated, becoming activated on phosphorylation and deactivated by various tyrosine phosphatases. The substrates for MAP kinase are diverse; on its own phosphorylation, MAP kinase directs the phosphorylation of transcription factors, including c-*jun* and p62TCF (*21*), and also phosphorylates other kinases, e.g., pp90rsk, promoting their entry into the nucleus to carry out activation of transcription factors (*22*).

The preceding overview highlights only the key interactions of Ras and its many upstream and downstream partners in mitogenic signaling, and points to obvious potential targets for the design of Ras inhibitors. However, it should be kept in mind that the whole picture is considerably more complex, in part because of the existence of multiple Ras partner proteins that sometimes appear to have identical functionality (*see* comprehensive review by Khosravi-Far and Der, ref. *23*). For example, there exist multiple adapter proteins for Ras (Grb-2 and shc) as well as two GAP regulators (p120GAP and neurofibromin-1). Divergent roles for seemingly similar signaling molecules are most likely a reflection of the evolution of the *ras* superfamily, with its large number of structurally homologous, yet functionally unique members. Because of their involvement in distinctly different physiological processes, ensuing crossregulation is likely to occur. For example, the Ras-related protein rap-1 was recently found to compete with Ras for binding to Raf (*24*). Furthermore, p120-GAP is thought to act on all Ras family members. The reader is referred to an excellent review by Boguski and McCormick devoted to the array of proteins identified to date that are known to regulate members of the Ras superfamily (*25*). As we will see in Section 5, the existence of highly homologous proteins within the Ras superfamily is likely to pose special challenges in the design and development of a tumor-specific Ras inhibitor.

3. IMPACT OF *RAS* MUTATIONS IN HUMAN CANCER

ras genes have been intensely studied since 1982, when their ability to induce malignant transformation was first demonstrated (*26*). The critical role played by *ras* mutations in the development of human tumors can be inferred from three separate lines

Table 1
Incidence of *ras* Mutations in Human Malignancies

Tumor	Activated ras gene	Frequency, %[a]
Pancreatic adenocarcinoma	K	75–93
Colon adenocarcinoma	K	40–47
Lung adenocarcinoma	K	22–33
Thyroid carcinoma	H, K, N	53–60
Melanoma	N	8–19
Bladder carcinoma	H	7–17
Hepatocarcinoma	N	0–30
Renal carcinoma	H	7–13
Glioblastoma	—	0
Neuroblastoma	—	0
Prostate	—	5[b]
Ovary	—	0
Cervix	—	0
Sarcoma	—	0
Breast	—	0–8
Lymphoid		
ALL	N	0–18
NHL	—	0
Hodgkins's	N	0–67
Myeloid		
AML	N	11–70
CML	N	0–50

[a]Data represent the range of values reported in individual studies as reported by Bos (*31*).
[b]Data of Gumerlock et al. (*32*).
Abbreviations: ALL (acute lymphocytic leukemia), NHL (non-Hodgkin's lymphoma), AML (acute myelogenous leukemia), CML (chronic myelogenous leukemia).

of evidence. Foremost are the observations made by many groups that oncogenic Ras, but not normal Ras, induces increased cellular proliferation of rodent fibroblasts and also renders them tumorigenic (*27–29*). Second, transgenic mice harboring oncogenic *ras* mutations show an increased incidence of tumor formation (*30*). Finally comes the strong circumstantial evidence from epidemiological studies showing a high frequency of *ras* mutations in a wide variety of tumor types.

In this section, we will see that *ras* mutations occur at a high rate in colon and pancreatic cancers, two tumor types notoriously refractory to standard chemotherapy. Treatment outcome may be further compromised by the ability of oncogenic Ras to enhance a tumor's metastatic potential. Finally, the potential negative impact of *ras* mutations on the outcome of alternative treatment modalities, specifically radiotherapy, will be explored.

3.1. Incidence and Tumor Type

The use of specific recombinant DNA-based assays and the polymerase chain reaction have afforded a ready and accurate means for quantitating the prevalence of *ras* mutations in human tumors. *ras* mutations have been detected in a wide array of human tumors, and are especially prevalent in tumors of the pancreas (90%), colon (50%), and thyroid (50%) (Table 1). These mutations are relatively infrequent in tumors of the breast and prostate. Overall, roughly 30% of all tumors contain an activated *ras* allele. Mutations generally occur in either codon 12, 13, or 61 of one of the three *ras* genes (H-, K-, or N-), most frequently occurring in K-*ras* and least often in H-*ras*.

Evidence in support of a multistep nature of carcinogenesis is compelling and has been most clearly demonstrated for colorectal cancer, where stepwise and cumulative genetic changes are thought to occur *(33)*. Among the early events is hypomethylation of DNA, followed by a mutation in the APC gene and subsequent allelic loss on three different chromosomes. It is thought that these genetic events set the stage for subsequent activating mutations in the *ras* genes.

There is increasing evidence that K-*ras* gene mutations may actually serve as reliable pathogenetic and diagnostic markers of neoplastic disease *(34)*. Mutations in codon 12 of K-*ras* are prevalent in aberrant crypt foci in the colon, which represent lesions that may be preneoplastic *(35)*. Furthermore, mucous cell hyperplasias of the pancreas, which arise in association with chronic pancreatitis, have also been found to harbor K-*ras* mutations with high frequency *(36)*. At the present time, the clinical significance of these findings is unknown. However, should the evidence become compelling for *ras* mutations being confined to neoplastic and preneoplastic tissue, then they may serve as useful markers for earlier diagnosis.

3.2. Role of Oncogenic Ras in Metastasis

The final stage in tumor progression is acquisition by transformed cells of the ability to metastasize, i.e., they invade the bloodstream and lymphatic system, stimulate angiogenesis, and subsequently proliferate in tissues distant to the primary site. When metastatic and nonmetastatic disease has been compared for the incidence of *ras* mutations, a higher frequency has been reported for the invasive tumors *(37,38)*. In view of the selective growth advantage conferred on a cell when Ras activation occurs, one might argue that metastatic potential is an indirect consequence. However, there is compelling evidence suggesting that this is not the case. Expression of oncogenic Ras appears to in effect reprogram the expression of critical genes associated with the metastatic phenotype. Specifically, Ras transformation results in increased expression of key metalloproteinases, i.e., stromelysin and gelatinase, whereas transcription and mRNA levels of TIMP-1 are decreased *(39)*. Along these same lines, expression of the extracellular matrix molecule thrombospondin, which is decreased in metastatic tumors, is also reduced on transfection with viral K-*ras (40)*.

The mechanisms whereby oncogenes, such as *ras*, act to control stromelysin expression are just now beginning to be characterized. Recent work has shown that protein kinase C may play a critical role in PDGF-induced activation of the stromelysin promoter by virtue of a novel palindromic element *(41)*. These data suggest the existence of a bifurcation downstream of *ras*, which leads to stromelysin expression.

3.3. ras Expression and Radiation Resistance

Roughly half of all cancer patients receive radiotherapy at some point during treatment of their disease. Since 30% of all tumors contain oncogenic *ras* mutations, then it stands to reason that a negative impact of activated *ras* on radiosensitivity of tumor cells would be a concern. Sklar first reported in 1988 that increased radiation resistance accompanied Ras transformation *(42)*. Since that time, however, there have been conflicting reports regarding the generality of this phenomenon. Although some researchers have confirmed a correlation between *ras* expression and radioresistance (*43,44*), many groups have reported that *ras* does not confer a change in radiosensitivity (*45–49*). The genetic heterogeneity of the various cell lines studied by these groups may be contributing to the conflicting data, especially in view of the fact that other oncogenes, e.g., *raf* and *myc*, have also been reported to affect radiosensitivity adversely (*50*). Furthermore, simultaneous transformation by two oncogenes, *ras* and *myc*, confers radioresistance to a much greater extent than either oncogene alone (*51*). It has also been suggested that full-length proto-oncogene may influence cellular radiosensitivity in a different manner from that of the activated oncogene (*52*). Data indicating that *ras*-conferred radioresistance is cell-cycle-phase-dependent suggests yet another variable among the various studies (*53*).

4. EMERGENCE OF NEW THERAPEUTIC APPROACHES: RATIONALE AND PROGRESS

4.1. Therapies Targeting ras Expression

Although the concept of repairing a single base mutation by genetic therapy is theoretically appealing, clinically this approach remains in the distance. However, researchers have made excellent progress toward reducing expression of the Ras protein at the translational level as discussed below.

4.1.1. ANTISENSE DNA

One approach that has demonstrated utility in decreasing Ras protein expression involves the use of antisense oligonucleotides complementary to RNA transcripts of the activated *ras* oncogene. Binding of the antisense DNA presumably inhibits expression of mutant *ras* by several mechanisms, including blocking ribosomal translation of the RNA transcript as well as triggering RNase H degradation of the target RNA (*54,55*). Chemical improvements have focused in part on decreasing the general susceptibility of antisense reagents to nuclease degradation. Therefore oligomer analogs containing phosphorothioate linkages in place of the naturally occurring phosphodiester linkage have been employed to increase resistance to nucleases and therefore prolong biological half-life. Oligonucleoside methylphosphonates and phosphoramidates, which are quite hydrophobic and taken up readily by cells, have subsequently been tested with favorable in vitro results reported (*56,57*). Intercalating agents and/or hydrophobic tails have also been employed as linkers to increase affinity for the mRNA target and to promote tumor uptake of the antisense oligomers (*58*).

The short-term nature of the above studies calls into question the degree to which sustained antisense treatment can suppress *ras* expression. Gray and colleagues addressed this issue by treating NIH-3T3 cells transformed with H-*ras* (from the T24 human bladder carcinoma) for 72 h with an appropriate antisense DNA pentadecamer for targeting H-*ras* and then measuring tumorigenicity in athymic nude mice posttreatment (*59*). These investigators were thereby able to demonstrate that tumor growth was significantly reduced for up to 14 d following treatment.

Although these studies demonstrated proof of concept, their clinical significance remained unclear, since treatment of tumor cells with antisense DNA had occurred *ex vivo* prior to inplantation. The critical and logical next step was to address whether antisense DNA reagents could be successfully delivered intact to the tumor site and show efficacy against established tumors without unacceptable toxicity. One approach to delivery, favored over transfection, was to develop a retroviral antisense K-*ras* expression vector; subsequently, this antisense vector was shown to eliminate expression of the mutant Ras protein in human lung cancer cells (*60*). Using an orthotopic human lung cancer model in nude mice, these researchers showed that their antisense K-*ras* retroviral construct, administered by intratracheal instillation on the third day after implantation of the tumor, showed significant activity; 87% of the mice receiving the antisense construct were tumor-free vs only 10% of the control group (*61*).

In general, the concept of antisense DNA therapy to treat mutant *ras*-expressing tumors has shown much promise. The progress of Roth and his colleagues has led to what may be one of the first gene therapy trials for lung cancer (*62*). It remains too early to report clinical results. However, a Phase I trial employing a phosphorothioate oligonucleotide with a sequence complementary to the p53 suppressor gene has been initiated in patients with acute lymphocytic leukemia (AML) or myelodysplastic syndrome; early reports indicate no major toxicity after 10 d of continuous infusion with approx 10–20% of the administered dose recovered in the urine as intact oligonucleotide (*63*).

4.1.2. Ribozymes

The production of catalytic RNA that will specifically cleave within the mutated sequence of mRNA unique to oncogenic *ras* represents another approach for altering Ras protein expression. This approach involves the design of synthetic DNA that encodes hammerhead ribozymes containing thermodynamically stable loop structures to prevent aggregation of ribozymes while also containing the requisite recognition sequence for mutated *ras* mRNA. NIH 3T3 cells have successfully been cotransfected with a plasmid expressing such a ribozyme along with an activated *ras* gene, resulting in abrogation of the transformed phenotype (*64,65*). Furthermore, it has also been reported that transfection of EJ human bladder carcinoma cells with hammerhead ribozyme-encoded DNA results in reduced tumorigenicity in nude mice (*66,67*). These data provide proof of concept that ribozymes can in fact affect Ras protein expression and also support the role of Ras in both tumorigenicity and invasion (*67*). However, it should be kept in mind that the in vivo experiments reported to date with anti-*ras*-directed ribozymes have involved ribozyme-treatment of cells prior to their introduction into animals. Again, as with antisense DNA, successful delivery to the tumor site becomes critical. The exogenous delivery of synthetic ribozymes as well as vector-based approaches to ribozyme therapy are currently being pursued; although great strides have been made chemically to improve catalytic activity and decrease nuclease susceptibility, the major challenge of increasing uptake in order to facilitate localization of RNA remains. It is encouraging in this regard that successful in vivo delivery of ribozymes have been accomplished for noncancer indications (*68*).

4.2. Inhibitors of Ras Function

As we have seen, a single base change mutation is responsible for the conversion of a *ras* proto-oncogene to its activated oncogenic counterpart. Once this molecular switch consequently becomes stuck in the "on" position, uncontrolled proliferation ensues. Because of its complex and critical role in mitogenic signaling, a number of events that involve direct participation of the Ras protein can be envisioned as possibilities for therapeutic intervention.

4.2.1. ANTAGONISTS OF PROTEIN-PROTEIN INTERACTIONS

A review on the subject of the amenability of protein–protein interactions as anticancer targets appears elsewhere (69). With regard to the Ras signaling pathway, one could envision that disruption of the interaction of Ras with either Sos, Raf, or GAP could result in favorable antiproliferative effects. Because technical advances have greatly expedited the synthesis of multiple peptides and also because of the generation of combinatorial peptide libraries, peptidic antagonists of these protein complexes are actively being sought.

Peptide inhibitors that inhibit the interaction of Ras with GAP corresponding to amino acids 19–32 of the Ras protein have been reported (70). These peptide inhibitors should serve as a useful starting point for the design of smaller peptide fragments that will retain activity and not be subject to impermeability and the lability limitations of their predecessors. Inhibitors of Ras/Sos have not yet been reported, but it is noteworthy that peptide inhibitors of Src SH3/SH2 phosphoprotein interactions have recently been reported (71); however, they were found to lack antiproliferative effects, presumably because of poor cell penetration and/or lability of the phosphate group on the tyrosine residue.

Although small molecule inhibitors would be desirable, the likelihood of identifying a specific inhibitor with sufficient affinity may be compromised by virtue of the large surface over which the targeted protein–protein interaction occurs. For instance, the minimal region of Raf required for interaction with Ras appears to be approx 70 amino acids (72). Thus, antagonists of any of the various Ras–protein interactions must be sufficiently large to disrupt Ras binding in a biologically meaningful way, but at the same time be small enough to enter cells readily while not being degraded.

In addition, the existence of multiple SH2 and SH3 domains will most likely make the issue of selectivity a formidable challenge to rational drug design. Encouraging in this regard were the results of a study where *Xenopus* oocytes were microinjected with either a monoclonal antibody (MAb) recognizing the SH3 domain of p120GAP or SH3 domain peptides as short as nine residues; Ras-dependent, but not Ras-independent, maturation of the oocytes was blocked with no adverse effect on GAP activity (73). In general, effective antagonists, whether peptidic or nonpeptidic, should be smaller and demonstrate an improved profile with regard to potency, efficacy, bioavailability, stability, and selectivity compared to the natural ligand (69).

4.2.2. INHIBITORS OF MEMBRANE LOCALIZATION OF RAS

Not only must Ras bind GTP to be active, but it must also be associated with the inner face of the plasma membrane. Initially synthesized as a soluble, cytosolic protein, Ras undergoes a series of posttranslational modifications that provide it with the lipophilicity that is required for membrane association (74,75). To compensate for lack of a transmembrane domain, the Ras protein is prenylated, specifically undergoing addition of a farnesyl group at its carboxy-terminus. All Ras proteins are prenylated by virtue of a common consensus sequence, termed the CAAX motif, at their carboxyl-termini; this CAAX box consists of a cysteine residue (C), followed by two aliphatic amino acids (A), and ending in any one of several amino acids (X). The nature of X

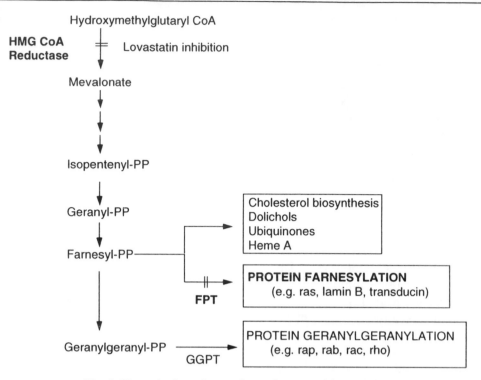

Fig. 2 Biosynthetic pathway of mevalonate and isoprenoids.

determines substrate specificity among the multiple prenylation enzymes. In a series of reactions to be described in more detail below, farnesyl pyrophosphate is enzymatically attached to Ras at the cysteine residue within the CAAX motif, preceding cleavage of the three terminal amino acids followed by methyl esterification of the newly created carboxy-terminal cysteine. Elucidation of the enzymatic events responsible for these chemical modifications of Ras have opened up a number of possibilities for therapeutic intervention.

4.2.2.1. Farnesylation. The cytoplasmic enzyme farnesyl protein transferase (FPT) catalyzes the reaction of farnesyl pyrophosphate, an isoprenoid derived from the mevalonate pathway (Fig. 2), with the CAAX cysteine residue on Ras to form a thioether linkage. FPT, which is ubiquitous among eukaryotic cells, is a heterodimer composed of 48- and 46-kDa subunits. The significant structural homology between mammalian and yeast FPT reveals a high degree of conservation. Three prenylation enzymes have been described. Whereas FPT catalyzes the addition of a 15-carbon farnesyl group, two other prenylation enzymes recognize a 20-carbon isoprenoid substrate and are responsible for protein geranylgeranylation. FPT shares a common subunit, its pyrophosphate binding (α) subunit, with geranylgeranyl protein transferase I (GGPT type 1). The β subunit provides CAAX box specificity; the occurrence of farnesylation as opposed to geranylgeranylation is dictated by the identity of the terminal amino acid in the CAAX motif. Whereas CAAX appears to be invariant for FPT, the geranylgeranylation enzymes recognize CAAL, XXCC, XCXC, and CCXX (*76*).

Table 2
Inhibitors of *ras* Farnesyl Protein Transferase

Inhibitor	IC_{50}, μM	Reference
CAAX analogs		
CVFM and related tetrapeptides	≥ 0.012	79
L-731,735	0.018	80
B581	0.021	81
BZA-2B	0.00085	82
Cys-AMBA-Met	0.15	83
L-739,750	0.018	84
Phenol tripeptides	63–157	85
Biphenyl nonpeptides	0.15	86
FPP analogs		
(α-Hydroxyfarnesyl) phosphonic acid	0.030	87
PD 083176	0.017	88
Farnesylamine	—	89
Natural products		
10'-Desmethoxy-stretonigrin	21	90
Manumycin	5	91
Gliotoxin	1.1	92
Chaetomellic acid A	0.055	87
Zaragozic acid	0.216	87
Pepticinnamin E	0.30	93
Fusidienol	0.30	94
Preussomerin	1.2	95

Interest in FPT as a pharmacological target was initially triggered by the finding that mutants lacking a CAAX motif do not associate with the plasma membrane and furthermore do not transform cells to malignancy (77, 78). This has led to an intensive search in numerous laboratories for potent inhibitors of FPT. A comprehensive list of inhibitors reported to date have been compiled in Table 2 along with their relative potencies against Ras FPT. Reviews appear elsewhere regarding the chemistry of these compounds, as well as further discussion on their potential usefulness as anticancer agents (96–101). I will now focus on six key compounds (structures shown in Fig. 3) to illustrate the progress that has been made in the last five years in achieving cellular activity.

In their initial report describing the identification and purification of FPT, peptides as short as four residues were found by Reiss et al. to act as alternative substrates competing with full-length Ras for farnesylation (79). The tetrapeptide CVFM was found to be a potent inhibitor of FPT (IC_{50} = approx 40 nM) and acted as a true inhibitor since it was not a substrate for farnesylation (102). CVFM and other structurally related tetrapeptides were not serious drug candidates because of inefficient cellular uptake and rapid proteolytic degradation. However, they have served well as first-generation peptide inhibitors of FPT for the design of improved peptidomimetic derivatives of the CAAX motif.

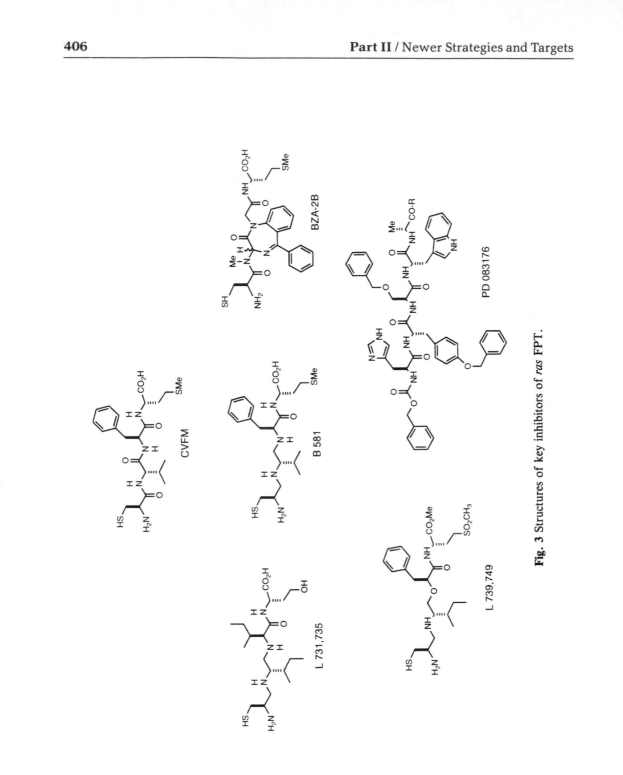

Fig. 3 Structures of key inhibitors of *ras* FPT.

The pseudo-tetrapeptide L 731, 735 (*see* Fig. 3) was designed as a CIIM analog in which the two N-terminal amide bonds were reduced and methionine replaced with homoserine in a successful effort to improve potency (*80*). When the corresponding lactone derivative was synthesized and evaluated, cellular activity could be detected, both with respect to modulation of Ras processing as well as selective inhibition of anchorage-independent growth of *ras*-transformed cells (*80*). Although these synthetic organic inhibitors still lacked sufficient potency to be viable drug candidates, they nevertheless provided evidence that inhibition of FPT can in fact modulate Ras function in whole cells.

B581 represents another CAAX analog that resulted from systematic modification of CVFM by replacement of the amino-terminal amide bonds (*81*). This compound proved to be significantly more stable than CVFM and resulted in cellular modulation of posttranslational processing of prenylated proteins, although at high concentrations (50 μM). Again, limited permeability may have had a detrimental effect on cellular potency. Particularly encouraging was the finding that B581 appeared to be selective for FPT in treated cells; this was reflected in part by a lack of inhibition in the processing of the geranylgeranylated Rap 1A protein (*81,103*).

Replacement of the two aliphatic residues in the CAAX motif with a benzodiazepine-derived mimic of a dipeptide turn led to a subnanomolar inhibitor of FPT (*82*). This compound was designed to allow both the N-terminal cysteine and the C-terminal methionine to coordinate the zinc ion present at the peptide binding site. Cellular activity was observed when the corresponding methyl ester was synthesized, although a 50-fold reduction in enzyme potency accompanied this chemical modification.

A novel compound to emerge from high-volume screening was PD 083176, a protected pentapeptide characterized by the sequence CBZ his-(*O*-benzyl)tyrosine-(*O*-benzyl)serine-tryptophan-D-alanine-NH₂ (*88*). This nonthiol-containing peptide, although highly potent against FPT ($IC_{50} = 20$ nM), proved to be too impermeable for cellular studies. However, if PD 083176 was microinjected into *Xenopus* oocytes, a block in maturation induced by insulin, but not progesterone, was observed, indicating specific inhibition of Ras function. Truncation of PD 083176 has led to a series of modified peptide analogs, e.g. PD 152440, which exhibit a modest reduction in potency against purified FPT relative to PD 083176, but are cell-permeable (*104*). Inhibition of Ras farnasylation was observed when *ras*-transformed cells were treated with concentrations of PD 152440 as low as 1–5 μM.

The first Ras FPT inhibitor reported to have in vivo activity was L-739,750 (*84*). This compound was synthesized in an attempt to decrease the chemical instability of the prodrug of L-731,735 by replacing the nucleophilic nitrogen with an ether oxygen. The absence of systemic toxicity in this study is particularly important as discussed below.

Collectively, evaluation of these six prototype compounds have provided the foundation for an initial determination of the feasibility of developing a Ras FPT inhibitor as a pharmacological agent. First, the studies cited above clearly establish that FPT inhibitors can be designed to enter cells readily and modulate the putative target. Next comes the issue of enzyme specificity, where it is important to show that FPT can be specifically inhibited over other prenylation enzymes. Current dogma dictates that a desirable FPT inhibitory candidate drug should be as selective as possible against FPT relative to GGPT. Since the vast majority of proteins of the Ras superfamily, critical to a wide variety of cellular functions, are prenylated by GGPT, this appears to be a reasonable premise. However, until a successful drug emerges against this target, it remains unclear exactly to what degree FPT prenylation needs to be selectively inhibited. Clearly most of the inhibitors discussed here proved to be highly specific for FPT when tested in vitro against purified enzymes. In some cases, data have begun to emerge at the cellular level supporting the concept that FPT inhibitors can be specific and not result in the concurrent inhibition of processing of geranylgeranylated proteins (*81*).

It is imperative that the toxicity profile of FPT inhibitors also includes an evaluation of their activity against non-Ras-related substrates for farnesylation. Most notably, the structural protein lamin B and proteins involved in visual transduction, i.e., transducin and rhodopsin kinase, are also farnesylated. Therefore, pharmacokinetic parameters, such as whether the inhibitor crosses the blood–brain barrier, may prove important. We still have very little information regarding the relative physiological levels of all of the pertinent substrates for prenylation, nor do we know how their relative substrate affinities compare, what their turnover rates are, and so forth. In the case of irreversible inhibitors, this issue may prove critical. Again, without a clinical precedent directed against this target, we must remain open-minded regarding criteria establishment for advancement of active compounds. Initial indications that administration of an FPT inhibitor to tumor-bearing mice results in efficacy without appreciable systemic toxicity are encouraging (*84*).

Finally, there is the issue of whether FPT inhibitors will selectively target mutant Ras as opposed to endogenous Ras function. It is therefore encouraging that normal fibroblast cells, for instance, continue to grow in monolayer culture at concentrations of BZA-5B that are significantly inhibitory to the growth of *ras*-transformed cells (*82*). The basis for this selectivity, which has been observed for several of the inhibitors reported here, largely remains an enigma.

In addition to specific inhibitors of FPT, some general inhibitors of isoprenylation are actively being investigated for potential clinical utility. Lovastatin, an HMG CoA reductase inhibitor used clinically to lower blood cholesterol levels, has also been reported to inhibit the growth of *ras*-transformed cells in animals (*105*). However, this agent is quite cytotoxic and is 100-fold more potent against cholesterol biosynthesis compared to isoprenylation (*106*). In other studies, phenylacetate, which is the deaminated metabolite of phenylalanine, also appears to be a general inhibitor of protein prenylation (*107*); Phase I testing of phenylactate against glioblastomas has shown early promising signs of activity (*108*). Finally, limonine is a monocyclic monoterpene that along with its metabolites selectivity inhibits the isoprenylation of p21Ras and other 21- to 26-kDa cell-growth-associated proteins (*109*). Preclinical studies have led to current exploration into the feasibility of pursuing limonene as a chemopreventative agent against breast cancer (*110*).

4.2.2.2. Proteolytic Cleavage. On farnesylation, the three terminal amino acids of the CAAX motif are cleaved by proteolytic processing (*111*). Two microsomal enzymes that perform this function have been described; the first is an endoprotease from bovine liver that cleaves a carboxy-terminal tripeptide (*112*), whereas the second enzyme described is a rat brain carboxypeptidase that sequentially removes the terminal amino acids (*113*). Very few inhibitors of these enzymes have been reported. The notable exceptions are farnesyl-CAAX analogs, distinguished by isosteric replacements for the scissile peptide bond, which have significant activity against the endoprotease with K_is as low as 64 nM (*114*). From an anticancer drug standpoint, interest in this target is diminished by the fact that a CAAX mutant of *ras* that did not undergo proteolysis, while compromised in its ability to associate with the plasma membrane, showed a minimal loss in transforming activity (*78*).

4.2.2.3. Methylesterification. Subsequent to proteolytic removal of the three terminal amino acids of the CAAX motif, a protein methyltransferase catalyzes the methyl esterification at the newly terminal cysteine residue (*115,116*). S-farnesyl mercaptopropionic acids have been reported to inhibit weakly methyltransferase with $K_i > 25$ μM. As with the protease, this enzyme modification does not appear to be essential for transforming activity (*78*).

4.2.2.4. Palmitoylation. Farnesylation alone provides Ras proteins with a fairly weak affinity for membrane binding. However, the association of farnesylated Ras with the plasma membrane is enhanced by other structural features of the Ras protein. These may include, in the case of certain K-Ras proteins, a stretch of six lysine residues upstream from the carboxy-terminal CAAX motif; protonation of this polybasic region likely confers a positive charge that provides affinity to the negatively charged phosphate surface of the membrane bilayer (*117*). Cysteine palmitoylation sites may also exist upstream of the CAAX motif, at residues 181 and 184 in the case of H-Ras (*118*). Little is known about the palmitoyl-CoA transferase activity that is responsible for this modification, except that it is associated with an internal membrane compartment (*119*). A potential role for palmitoyl-CoA inhibitors as anticancer drugs does not seem likely based on the studies of Hancock and his colleagues showing that mutant proteins that lack cysteine palmitoylation sites nevertheless retain transforming activity (*117*). Furthermore, most K-Ras proteins, which are most prevalent among human tumors, do not contain sites for palmitoylation.

5. SUMMARY AND FUTURE DIRECTIONS

During the last decade, cytotoxic agents have been de-emphasized in our search for a new generation of anticancer drugs. Certainly it has not been for lack of effort that very few new agents have joined the ranks of the dozen or so drugs from which oncologists have to choose. Conventional chemotherapy has generally exploited the more aggressive growth kinetics exhibited by cancer cells relative to their normal counterparts; we have seen many examples of initially promising drug candidates, often within the DNA intercalator and antimetabolite class, that subsequently fail because tumors become resistant. The tide has therefore shifted toward focusing on the discovery of less toxic compounds designed to exploit fundamental differences between malignant and nonmalignant cells. It is in this context that the *ras* oncogene, expressed in approximately one-third of all human tumors, has become an attractive target for anticancer drug design. Until recently, attempts to discover Ras inhibitors were impeded by a lack of clear understanding of the precise role of Ras in fulfilling its critical obligation to a number of cellular processes, proliferation nonwithstanding. During the last decade, basic research in the signal transduction field has progressed at an astounding rate with Ras emerging from its black box. As a result, the critical Ras interactions that are amenable to therapeutic intervention have been defined, and Ras inhibitors are now being discovered at a rapid rate. In some cases, in vitro studies demonstrating cellular modulation of the putative Ras-directed target have been followed by encouraging reports of in vivo activity, e.g., farnesyl protein transferase inhibitors. We are now faced with many pharmacological questions, previously not germane to the development of cytotoxic agents; the necessary requirements for a signaling antagonist to be worthy of advancement to the clinical testing stage remain to be defined. The next few years are likely to focus on showing that a sufficiently nontoxic Ras inhibitor can target oncogenic *ras* selectively and give a therapeutically meaningful response. If this proves to be the case, Ras inhibitors will likely represent a significant advance in the treatment of many solid tumors for which there is currently no effective treatment.

ACKNOWLEDGMENTS

I would like to thank W. R. Leopold, Gary Bolton, and Alan Saltiel for their assistance with this manuscript. I also wish to express my appreciation to Robert Jackson for introducing me to the challenges of anticancer drug development. I consider myself truly fortunate to have benefited from his mentorship.

REFERENCES

1. Zubrod CG. Chemical control of cancer. *Proc Natl Acad Sci USA* 1972; 69:1042–1047.
2. Stacey DW, DeGudicibus SR, Smith MR. Cellular Ras activity and tumor cell proliferation. *Exp Cell Res* 1987; 171:232.
3. Kung HF, Smith MR, Bekesi E, Stacey DW. Reversal of transformed phenotype by monoclonal antibodies against Ha-Ras p21 proteins. *Exp Cell Res* 1986; 162:363–371.
4. Bar Sagi D, Feramisco JR. Microinjection of the Ras oncogene protein into PC12 cells induces morphological differentiation. *Cell* 1985; 42:841–848.
5. Sadler SE, Maller JL, Gibbs JB. Transforming Ras proteins accelerate hormone-induced maturation and stimulate cyclic AMP phosphodiesterase in *Xenopus* oocytes. *Mol Cell Biol* 1990; 10:1689–1696.
6. Schlessinger J, Ullrich A. Growth factor signaling by receptor tyrosine kinases. *Neuron* 199; 2: 9:383–391.
7. Schlessinger J. SH2/SH3 signaling proteins. *Curr Opinion Genet Dev* 1994; 4:25–30.
8. Lowenstein EJ, Daly RJ, Batzer AG, Li W, Margolis B, Lammers R, Ullrich A, Skolnik EY, Bar-Sagi D, Schlessinger J. The SH2 and SH3 domain-containing protein Grb2 links receptor tyrosine kinases to Ras signalling. *Cell* 1992; 70:431–442.
9. Buday L, Downward J. Epidermal growth factor regulates p21Ras through the formation of a complex of receptor Grb2 adaptor protein, and Sos nucleotide exchange facator. *Cell* 1973: 611–620.
10. Gale NW, Kaplan S, Lowenstein EJ, Schlessinger J, Bar-Sagi D. Grb2 mediates the EGF-dependent activation of guanine nucleotide exchange on Ras. *Nature* 1993; 363:88–92.
11. Osterop AP, Medema RH, v.d.-Zon GC, Bos JL, Moller W, Maassen JA. Epidermal growth factor receptors generate Ras. GTP more efficiently than insulin receptors. *Eur J Biochem* 1993; 212:477–482.
12. Trahey M, McCormick, F. A cytoplasmic protein stimulates normal N-Ras p21 GTPase, but does not affect oncogenic mutants. *Science* 1987; 238:542–554.
13. Cales C, Hancock JF, Marshall CJ, Hall A. The cytoplasmic protein GAP is implicated as the target for regulation by the *ras* gene product. *Nature* 1988; 332:548–551.

14. Wong G, Muller O, Clark R, Conroy L, Moran MF, Polakis P, McCormick F. Molecular cloning and nucleic acid binding properties of the GAP-associated tyrosine phosphoprotein p62. *Cell* 1992; 69:551–558.

15. Settleman J, Narasimhan V, Foster LC, Weinberg RA. Molecular cloning cDNAs encoding the GAP-associated protein p190: implications for a signalling pathway from Ras to the nucleus. *Cell* 1992; 69:539–549.

16. Hall A. Ras-related GTPases and the cytoskeleton. *Mol Biol Cell* 1992; 3:475–479.

17. Pendergast GC, Gibbs JB. Ras regulatory interactions: novel targets for anti-cancer intervention. *BioEssays* 1994; 16:187–191.

18. Moodie SA, Willumsen BM, Weber MJ, Wolfman A. Complexes of Ras-GTP with Raf-1 and mitogen-activated protein kinase kinase. *Science* 1993; 260:1658–1661.

19. Stokoe D, Macdonald SG, Cadwallader K, Symons M, Hancock JF. Activation of Raf as a result of recruitment to the plasma membrane. *Science* 1994; 264:1463–1467.

20. Leevers SJ, Paterson JF, Marshall CJ. Requirement for Ras in Raf activation is overcome by targeting raf to the plasma membrane. *Nature* 1994; 369:411–441.

21. Gille H, Sharrocks AD, Shaw PE. Phosphorylation of transcription factor p62TCF by MAP kinase stimulates ternary complex formation at c-*fos* promoter. *Nature* 1992; 358:414–417.

22. Sturgill TW, Ray LB, Erikson E, Maller JL. Insulin-stimulated MAP-2 kinase phosphorylates and activates ribosomal protein S6 kinase II. *Nature* 1988; 334:715–718.

23. Khosravi-Far R, Der CJ. The Ras signal transduction pathway. *Cancer and Metastasis Rev* 1994; 13:67–89.

24. Cook SJ, Rubinfeld B, Albert A, McCormick F. RapV12 antagonizes Ras-dependent activation of ERK-1 and ERK-2 by LPA and EGF in rat-1 fibroblasts. *EMBO J* 1993; 366:3475–3485.

25. Boguski MS, McCormick F. Proteins regulating Ras and its relatives. *Nature* 1993; 366:43–653.

26. Barbacid M. *Ras* genes. *Ann Rev Biochem* 1987; 56:779–827.

27. Shih C, Padhy LC, Murray M, Weinberg RA. Transforming genes of carcinomas and neuroblastomas introduced into mouse fibroblasts. *Nature* 1981; 290:261–264.

28. Krontiris TG, Cooper GM. Transforming activity of human tumor DNA. *Proc Natl Acad Sci USA* 1981; 78:1181–1184.

29. Wilson DM, Yang D, Dillberger JE, Dietrich SE, Maher VM, McCormick JJ. Malignant transformation of human fibroblasts by a transfected N-*ras* oncogene. *Cancer Res* 1990; 50: 5587–5593.

30. Adams JM, Cory S. Transgenic models of tumor development. *Science* 1991; 254:1161–1167.

31. Bos JL. *Ras* oncogenes in human cancer: a review. *Cancer Res* 1989; 49:4682–4689.

32. Gumerlock P, Poonamallee U, Meyers F. Activated *ras* alleles in human carcinoma of the prostate are rare. *Cancer Res* 1991; 51:1632–1637.

33. Fearon ER, Vogelstein B. A genetic model for colorectal tumorigenesis. *Cell* 1990; 61:759–767.

34. Fearon ER. K-*ras* gene mutation as a pathogenic and diagnostic marker in human cancer. *J Natl Cancer Inst* 1993; 85:1978–1980.

35. Pretlow TP, Brasitus TA, Fulton NC, Cheyer C, Kaplan EL. K-*ras* mutations in putative preneoplastic lesions in human colon. *J Natl Cancer Inst* 1993; 85:2004–2007.

36. Yanagisawa A, Ohtake K, Ohashi K, et al. Frequent c-Ki-*ras* oncogene activation in mucous cell hyperplasias of pancreas suffering from chronic inflammation. *Cancer Res* 1993; 53:953–956.

37. Goretzki PE, Lyons J, Stacy-Phipps S, Rosenau W, Demeure M, Clark OH, McCormick F, Roher HD, Bourne HR. Mutational activation of *ras* and *gsp* oncogenes in differentiated thyroid cancer and their biological implications. *World J Surg* 1992; 16:576–581.

38. Anwar K, Nakakuki K, Naiki H, Inuzuka M. *Ras* gene mutations and HPV infection are common in human laryngeal carcinoma. *Int J Cancer* 1993; 53:22–28.

39. Su ZZ, Austin VN, Zimmer SG, Fisher PB. Defining the critical gene expression changes associated with expression and suppression of the tumorigenic and metastatic phenotype in Ha-*ras*-transformed cloned rat embryo fibroblast cells. *Oncogene* 1993; 8:1211–1219.

40. Zebrenetzky V, Harris CC, Steeg PS, Roberts DD. Expression of the extracellular matrix molecule thrombospondin inversely correlates with malignant progression in melanoma, lung and breast carcinoma cell lines. *Int J Cancer* 1994; 59:191–195.

41. Sanz L, Berra E, Municio MM, Dominguez I, Lozano J, Johansen T, Moscat J. Diaz-Meco MT. Zeta PKC plays a critical role during stromelysin promoter activation by platelet-derived growth factor through a novel palindromic element. *J Biol Chem* 1994; 269:10,044–10,049.

42. Sklar MD. The *ras* oncogenes increase the intrinsic resistance of NIH 3T3 cells to ionizing radiation. *Science* 1988; 239:645–647.

43. Miller AC, Kariko K, Myers CE, Clark EP, Samid D. Increased radioresistance of EJ *ras*-transformed human osteosarcoma cells and its modulation by lovastatin, an inhibitor of p21Ras isoprenylation. *Int J Cancer* 1993; 53:302–307.

44. Hermens AF, Bentvelzen PA. Influence of the H-*ras* oncogene on radiation responses of a rat rhabdomyosarcoma cell line. *Cancer Res* 1992; 52:3073–3082.

45. Grant ML, Bruton RK, Byrd PJ, Gallimore PH, Steele JC, Taylor AM, Grand RJ. Sensitivity to ionising radiation of transformed human cells to mutant *ras* genes. *Oncogene* 1990; 5: 1159–1164.

46. Garden AS, Meyn RE, Weil MM, Lebovitz RM, Lieberman MW. The influence of *ras* oncogene expression on radiation response in the cell. *Int J Radiat Biol* 1992; 307–311.

47. Su LN, Little JB. Transformation and radiosensitivity of human diploid skin fibroblasts transfected with activated *ras* oncogene and SV40 T-antigen. *Int J Radiat Biol* 1992; 62:201–210.

48. Mendonca MS, Boukamp P, Stanbridge EJ, Redpath JL. The radiosensitivity of human keratinocytes: influence of activated c-H-*ras* oncogene expression and tumorigenicity. *Int J Radiat Biol* 1991; 59:1195–1206.

49. Alapetite C, Baroche C, Remvikos Y, Goubin X, Moustacchi E. Studies on the influence of the presence of an activated *ras* oncogene on the in vitro radiosensitivity of human mammary epithelial cells. *Int J Radiat Biol* 1991; 59:385–396.

50. Pirollo KF, Tong YA, Villegas Z, Chen Y, Chang EH. Oncogene-transformed NIH 3T3 cells display radiation resistance indicative of a signal transduction pathway leading to the radiation-resistant phenotype. *Radiat Res* 1993; 135:234–243.

51. McKenna WG, Weiss MC, Endlich B, Ling CC, Bakanauskas VJ, Kelsten ML, Muschel RJ. Synergistic effect of the v-*myc* oncogene with H-*ras* on radioresistance. *Cancer Res* 1990; 50: 97–102.

52. Warenius HM, Browning PG, Britten RA, Peacock JA, Rapp UR. C-*raf*-1 proto-oncogene expression relates to radiosensitivity rather than radioresistance. *Eur J Cancer* 1994; 30A:369–375.

53. Cheong N, Wang Y, Iliakis G. Radioresistance induced in rat embryo cells by transfection with the oncogenes H-*ras* v-*myc* is cell cycle dependent and maximal during S and G2. *Int J Radiat Biol* 1993; 63:623–629.

54. Haeuptle MT, Frank R, Dobberstein B. Translation arrest by oligodeoxynucleotides complementary to mRNA coding sequences yields polypeptides of predetermined length. *Nucleic Acids Res* 1986; 14:1427–1428.

55. Walder RY, Walder JA. Role of RNase H in hybrid-arrested translation by antisense oligonucleotides. *Proc Natl Acad Sci USA* 1988; 85:5011–5015.

56. Chang EH, Miller PS, Cushman C, Devadas K, Pirollo KF, Ts'o PO, Yu ZP. Antisense inhibition of *ras* p21 expression that is sensitive to a point mutation. *Biochemistry* 1991; 30:8283–8286.

57. Chang EH, Miller PS. Ras, an inner membrane transducer of growth stimuli. In: Wilkstrom E, ed. *Prospects for Antisense Nucleic Acid Therapy of Cancer and AIDS.* New York: Wiley-Liss. 1991:115–124.

58. Saison-Behmoaras T, Tocque B, Rey I, Chassignol M, Thuong NT, Helene C. Short modified antisense oligonucleotides directed against Ha-*ras* mutation induce selective cleavage of the mRNA and inhibit T24 cells proliferation. *EMBO J* 1991; 10:1111–1118.

59. Gray GD, Hernandez OM, Hebel D, Root M, Pow-Sang JM, Wickstrom E. Antisense DNA inhibition of tumor growth induced by c-Ha-*ras* oncogene in nude mice. *Cancer Res* 1993; 53: 577–580.

60. Zhang Y, Mukhopadhyay T, Donehower LA, Georges RN, Roth JA. Retroviral vector-mediated transduction of K-*ras* antisense RNA into human lung cancer cells inhibits expression of the malignant phenotype. *Human Gene Therapy* 1993; 4:451–460.

61. Georges RN, Mukhopadhyay T, Zhang Y, Yen N, Roth JA. Prevention of orthotopic human lung cancer growth by intratracheal instillation of a retroviral antisense K-*ras* construct. *Cancer Res* 1993; 53:1743–1746.

62. Drug & Market Development 1994; 4:235.
63. Bayever B, Iversen PL, Bishop MR, Sharp JG, Tewary HK, Arneson MA, Pirrucello SJ, Ruddon RW, Kessinger A, Zon G, Armitage JO. Systemic administration of a phosphorothioate oligonucleotide with a sequence complementary to p53 for acute myelogenous leukemia and myelodysplastic syndrome: initial results of a phase I trial. *Antisense Res Dev* 1993; 3:383–390.
64. Kashani-Sabel M, Funato T, Florenes VA, Fodstad O, Scanlon KJ. Suppression of the neoplastic phenotype in vivo by an anti-*ras* ribozyme. *Cancer Res* 1994; 54:900–920.
65. Koizumi M, Kamiya H, Ohtsuka E. Inhibition of c-Ha-*ras* gene expression by hammerhead ribozymes containing stable C(UUCG)G hairpin loop. *Biol Pharm Bull* 1993; 16:879–883.
66. Tone T, Kashani-Sabet M, Funato T, Shitara T, Yoshida E, Kashfian BI, Horng M, Fodstadt O, Scanlon KJ. Suppression of EJ cells tumorigenicity. *In Vivo* 1993; 7:471–476.
67. Kashini-Sabet M, Funato T, Tone T, Jiao L, Wang W, Yoshida E, Kashfinn BI, Shitara T, Wu AM, Moreno JG, Scanlon KJ, et al. Reversal of the malignant phenotype by an anti-*ras* ribozyme. *Antisense Res Dev* 1992; 2:3–15.
68. Efrat S, Leiser M, Wu YJ, Fusco-DeMane D, Emran OA, Surana M, Jetton TL, Magnuson MA, Weir G, Fleischer N. Ribozyme-mediated attenuation of pancreatic beta-cell glucokinase expression in transgenic mice results in impaired glucose-induced insulin secretion. *Proc Natl Acad Sci USA* 1994; 91:2051–2055.
69. Huber HE, Koblan KS, Heimbrook DC. Protein-protein interactions as therapeutic targets for cancer. *Curr Med Chem* 1994; 1:13–34.
70. Gibbs JB. Pharmacological probes of Ras function. *Sem Cancer Biol* 1992; 3:383–390.
71. Gilmer TG, Rodriguez M, Jordan S, Crosby R, Alligood K, Green M, Kimery M, Wagner C, Kinder D, Charifson P, Hassell AM, Willard D, Luther M, Rusnak D, Sternbach DD, Mehrotra M, Peel M, Shampine L, Davis R, Robbins J, Patel IR, Kassel D, Burkhart W, Moyer M, Bradshaw T, Berman J. Peptide inhibitors of src SH3-SH2-phosphoprotein interactions. *J Biol Chem* 1994; 269:31,711–31,719.
72. Vojtek AB, Hollenberg SM, Cooper JA. Mammalian ras interacts directly with the serine/threonine kinase Raf. *Cell* 1993; 74:205–214.
73. Duchesne M, Schweighoffer F, Parker F, Clerc F, Frobert Y, Thang MN, Tocque B. Identification of the SH3 domain of GAP as an essential sequence for Ras-GAP-mediated signaling. *Science* 1993; 259:525–528.
74. Schafer WR, Kim R, Sterne R, Thorner J, Kim S-H, Rine J. Genetic and pharmacological suppression of oncogenic mutations in RAS genes of yeast and humans. *Science* 1989; 245:379–385.
75. Casey PJ, Solski PA, Der CJ, Buss JE. p21Ras is modified by a farnesyl isoprenoid. *Proc Natl Acad Sci USA* 1989; 86:8323–8327.
76. Gibbs JB. Lipid modifications of proteins in the Ras superfamily. In: Dickey BF, Birnbaumer L, eds. *GTPases in Biology I*. New York: Springer-Verlag. 1993:335–344.
77. Jackson JH, Cochrane CG, Bourne JR, Solski PA, Buss JE, Der CJ. Farnesol modification of Kirsten-*ras* exon 4B protein is essential for transformation. *Proc Natl Acad Sci USA* 1990; 87:3042–3046.
78. Kato K, Cox AD, Hisaka MM, Graham SM, Buss JE, Der CJ. Isoprenoid addition to Ras protein is the critical modification for its membrane association and transforming activity. *Proc Natl Acad Sci USA* 1992; 89:6403–6407.
79. Reiss Y, Goldstein JL, Seabra MC, Casey PJ, Brown MS. Inhibition of purified p21Ras farnesyl: protein transferase by cys-AAX tetrapeptides. *Cell* 1990; 62:81–88.
80. Kohl NE, Mosser SD, deSolms SJ, Giuliani EA, Pompliano DL, Graham SL, Smith RL, Scolnick EM, Oliff A, Gibbs JB. Selective inhibition of Ras-dependent transformation by a farnesyltransferase inhibitor. *Science* 1993; 260:1934–1937.
81. Garcia AM, Rowell C, Ackermann K, Kowalczyk JJ, Lewis MD. Peptidomimetic inhibitors of Ras farnesylation and function in whole cells. *J Biol Chem* 1993; 268:18,415–18,418.
82. James GL, Goldstein JL, Brown MS, Rawson TE, Somers TC, McDowell RS, Crowley CW, Lucas BK, Levinson AD, Marsters JC. Benzodiazepine peptidomimetics: potent inhibitors of Ras farnesylation in animal cells. *Science* 1993; 260:1937–1942.
83. Nigam M, Seong C-M, Qian Y, Hamilton AD, Sebti SM. Potent inhibition of human tumor p21Ras farnesyltransferase by A_1A_2-lacking p21*ras* CA_1A_2X peptidomimetics. *J Biol Chem* 1993; 268:20,695–20,698.

84. Kohl NI, Wilson FR, Mosser SD, Giuliani E, DeSolms SJ, Conner MW, Anthony NJ, Holtz WJ, Gomez RP, Lee T, Smith RL, Graham SL, Hartman GD, Gibbs JB, Oliff A. Protein far-nesyltransferase inhibitors block the growth of Ras-dependent tumors in nude mice. *Proc Natl Acad Sci USA* 1994; 91:9141–9145.

85. Patel DV, Patel MM, Robinson SS, Gordon EM. Phenol based tripeptide inhibitors of Ras farnesyl protein transferase. *Bioorganic Med Chem Lett* 1994; 4:1883–1888.

86. Vogt A, Qian Y, Blaskovich MA, Fossum RD, Hamilton AD, Sebti SM. A non-peptide mimetic of Ras-CAAX:selective inhibition of farnesyltransferase and Ras processing. *J Biol Chem* 1994; 270:660–664.

87. Gibbs JB, Pompliano DL, Mosser SD, Rands E, Lingham RB, Singh SB, Scolnick EM, Kohl NE, Oliff A. Selective inhibition of farnesyl-protein transferase blocks Ras processing in vivo. *J Biol Chem* 1993; 268:7617–7620.

88. Sebolt-Leopold JS, Gowan R, Su T-Z, Leonard D, Sawyer T, Bolton G, Hodges J, Hupe D. Inhibition of Ras farnesyltransferase by a novel class of peptides containing no cysteine or thiol moieties. *Proc Am Assoc Cancer Res* 1994; 35:3535.

89. Kothapalli R, Guthrie N, Chambers AF, Carroll KK. Farnesylamine: an inhibitor of farnesyla-tion and growth of Ras-transformed cells. *Lipids* 1993; 28:969.

90. Liu WC, Barbacid M, Bulgar M, Clark JM, Crosswell AR, Dean L, Doyle TW, Fernandes PB, Huang S, Manne V, Pirnik DM, Wells JS, Meyers E. 10′-Desmethoxystreptonigrin, a novel analog of streptonigrin. *J Antibiotics* 1992; 45:454–457.

91. Hara M, Akasaka K, Akinaga S, Okabe M, Nakano H, Gomez R, Wood D, Uh M, Tamanoi F. Identification of Ras farnesyltransferase inhibitors by microbial screening. *Proc Natl Acad Sci USA* 1993; 90:2281–2285.

92. Van der Pyl D, Inokoshi J, Shiomi K, Yang H, Takeshima H, Omura S. Inhibition of farnesyl-protein transferase by gliotoxin and acetylgliotoxin. *J Antibiotics* 1992; 45:1802–1805.

93. Omura S, Van Der Pyl D, Inokoshi J, Takahashi Y, Takeshima H. Pepticinnamins, new farne-syl-protein transferase inhibitors produced by an actinomycete. *J Antiobiotics* 1993; 46:222–234.

94. Singh SB, Jones ET, Goetz MA, Bills GF, Nallin-Omstead M, Jenkins RG, Lingham RB, Silverman KC, Gibbs JB. Fusidienol: a novel inhibitor of Ras farnesyl-protein transferase from *Fusidium griseum. Tetrahedron Lett* 1994; 35:4693–4696.

95. Singh SB, Zink DL, Liesch JM, Ball RG, Goetz MA, Bolessa EA, Giacobbe RA, Silverman KC, Bills GF, Pelaez F, Cascales C, Gibbs JB, Lingham RB. Preussomerins and deoxypreus-somerins: novel inhibitors of Ras farnesyl-protein transferase. *J Org Chem* 1994; 59:6296–5302.

96. Bolton GL, Sebolt-Leopold JS, Hodges JC. *Ras* oncogene directed approaches in cancer chemotherapy. In: Plattner J, ed. *Annual Reports in Medicinal Chemistry.* New York: Aca-demic. 1994:165–174.

97. Prendergast GC, Gibbs JB. Ras regulatory interactions: novel targets for anticancer interven-tion? *BioEssays* 1994; 16:187–191.

98. Khosravi-Far R, Cox AD, Kato K, Der CJ. Protein prenylation: key to Ras function and cancer intervention? *Cell Growth & Differ* 1992; 3:461–469.

99. Gibbs JB. Ras C-terminal processing enzymes-new drug targets? *Cell* 1991; 65:1–4.

100. Gibbs JB, Oliff A, Kohl NE. Farnesyltransferase inhibitors: Ras research yields a potential cancer therapeutic. *Cell* 1994; 77:175–178.

101. Omura S, Takeshima H. Farnesyl-protein transferase inhibitors. *Drugs of the Future* 1994; 19:751–755.

102. Goldstein JL, Brown MS, Stradley SJ, Reiss Y. Gierasch LM. Nonfarnesylated tetrapeptide inhibitors of protein farnesyltransferase. *J Biol Chem* 1991; 266:15,575–15,578.

103. Cox AD, Garcia AM, Westwick JK, Kowalczyk JJ, Lewis MD, Brenner DA, Der CJ. The CAAX peptidomimetic compound B581 specifically blocks farnesylated, but not geranylgeranylated or myrisylated, oncogenic Ras signaling and transformation. *J Biol Chem* 1994; 269:19,203–19,206.

104. Sebolt-Leopold JS. The therapeutic potential of Ras-targeted protein farnesyltransferase in-hibitors. In: *Emerging Drugs: The Prospect for Improved Medicines.* London: Ashley. 1996: 219–239.

105. Sebti SM, Tkalcevic GT, Jani JP. Lovastatin, a cholesterol biosynthesis inhibitor, inhibits the growth of human H-*ras* oncogene transformed cells in nude mice. *Cancer Commun* 1991; 3: 141–147.

106. Sinensky M, Beck LA, Leonard S, Evans R. Differential inhibitory effects of lovastatin on protein isoprenylation and sterol synthesis. *J Biol Chem* 1990; 265:19,937–19,941.

107. Samid D, Ram Z, Hudgins WR, Shack S, Liu L, Walbridge S, Oldfield EH, Myers CE. Selective activity of phenylacetate against malignant gliomas:resemblance to fetal brain damage in phenylketonuria. *Cancer Res* 1994; 54:891–895.

108. Thibault AM, Cooper MR, Figg WD, Venzon DJ, Oliver Sartor VA, Tompkins AC, Weinberger MS, Headlee DJ, McCall NA, Samid D, Myers CE. A phase I and pharmacokinetic study of intravenous phenylacetate in patients with cancer. *Cancer Res* 1994; 54:1690–1694.

109. Crowell PL, Lin S, Vedejs E, Gould MN. Identification of metabolites of the antitumor agent *d*-limonene capable of inhibiting protein isoprenylation and cell growth. *Cancer Chem Pharmacol* 1992; 31:205–212.

110. Gould MN, Moore CJ, Zhang R, Wang B, Kennen WS, Haag JD. Limonene chemoprevention of mammary carcinoma induction following direct in situ transfer to v-Ha-*ras*. *Cancer Res* 1994; 54:3540–3543.

111. Ashby MN, King DS, Rine J. Endoproteolytic processing of a farnesylated peptide in vitro. *Proc Natl Aci USA* 1992; 89:4613–4617.

112. Ma Y-T, Rando RR. A microsomal endoprotease that specifically cleaves isoprenylated peptides. *Proc Natl Acad Sci USA* 1992; 89:6275–6279.

113. Akopyan TN, Couedel Y, Beaumont A, Foumie-Saluski MC, Roques BP. Cleavage of farnesylated COOH-terminal heptapeptide of mouse N-ras by brain microsomal membranes: evidence for a carboxypeptidase which specifically removes the COOH-terminal methionine. *Biochem Biophys Res Commun* 1991; 187:1336–1339.

114. Ma Y-T, Gilbert, Rando RR. Inhibitors of the isoprenylated protein endopeptidase. *Biochemistry* 1993; 32:2386.

115. Clarke S, Vogel JP, Deschenes RJ, Stock J. Post-translational modification of the H-*ras* oncogene protein: evidence for a third class of protein carboxyl methyltransferase. *Proc Natl Acad Sci USA* 1988; 85:4643–4647.

116. Perez-Sala D, Tan EW, Canada FJ, Rando RR. Methylation and demethylation reactions of guanine nucleotide binding proteins of retinal rod outer segments. *Proc Natl Acad Sci USA* 1991; 88:3043–3046.

117. Hancock JF, Paterson H, Marshall CJ. A polybasic domain or palmitoylation is required in addition to the CAAX motif to localize p21Ras to the plasma membrane. *Cell* 1990; 63:133–139.

118. Hancock JF, Magee AI, Childs JE, Marshall CJ. All Ras proteins are polyisoprenylated but only some are palmitoylated. *Cell* 1989; 57:1167–1177.

119. Gutierrez L, Magee AI. Characterization of an acyltransferase acting on p21N-Ras protein in a cell-free system. *Biochim Biophys Acta* 1991; 1078:147–154.

19

Gene Therapy

Peter I. Schrier, PhD and Susanne Osanto, MD, PhD

1. INTRODUCTION

Cancer is one of the acquired diseases finding its origin in multiple genetic alterations. From studies on several forms of hereditary cancer, we know that part of the alterations are present constitutively in the germ line, leading to a predisposition for getting cancer (*1*). These alterations are heterozygous and affect an allele of one or more tumor suppressor genes, which play a role in controlling cell proliferation and differentiation. Another part of the alterations occurs during life-time as a result of spontaneous mutations in the remaining intact allele, ultimately leading to the formation of the transformed cell. In this development also alterations in proto-oncogenes contribute to the formation of the tumor cell (*2,3*). Sporadic forms of cancer involve similar genetic alterations in tumor suppressor genes and proto-oncogenes, but they usually take much longer to develop. The notion of cancer being a disease anchored in the genes of the cancer cell makes it an attractive target for strategies involving gene therapy.

Gene therapy is commonly defined as "the transfer of new genetic material to cells of an individual with resulting therapeutic benefit to the individual" (*4*). In our view, this definition should be more broadly interpreted, i.e., do not restrict gene therapy only to transfer of new genetic material, but also include manipulation of existing genetic material. This holds true especially for cancer cells in the situation that dominantly activated oncogenes have to be eliminated. In principle, germ line cells as well as somatic cells are targets for genetic alterations. Germ line therapy in humans, however, is for the moment being considered as unethical and not safe, at least as long the experience with the various forms of somatic therapy is limited.

In cancer patients, gene therapy has to be directed to the tumor or, in the case of known hereditary defects, to the (organ) sites were tumor formation is likely to occur.

From: *Cancer Therapeutics: Experimental and Clinical Agents*
Edited by: B. Teicher Humana Press Inc., Totowa, NJ

Strikingly, in the case of cancer, the gene therapy is not confined to the proto-oncogenes or tumor suppressor genes affected. Various other approaches for genetic manipulation allow new forms of cancer therapy, e.g., the transfer of new antigenic determinants into cancer cells, aimed at an enhanced immunogenicity and subsequent destruction by the patient's immune system. These approaches will be first discussed in Section 2. The focus of this chapter, however, will be the implications of somatic gene therapy with regard to interactions of the immune system with neoplastic cells.

2. APPROACHES FOR GENE THERAPY OF CANCER

2.1. Overview

2.1.1. WHY GENE THERAPY?

Since sophisticated tools developed by molecular biologists to modify single genes in individual cells became easily accessible to the field of medical practice, a new area of research opened, aimed at curing diseases by altering human genetic material. This approach has several advantages when compared to conventional drug therapy. First, DNA of the vector carrying the gene can be stably integrated in the host genome, and the subsequent constitutive expression makes the therapy more effective and longer lasting. This will be particularly true for hereditary diseases, where a gene correction is made. Second, vectors can be targeted to certain cells or tissues by making use of tissue-specific promoters regulating the transcription of the transferred genes. Here, one can, for instance, think of altering normal bone marrow stem cells by introducing a multidrug resistance gene to limit myelosuppression of cytostatic drugs in cancer therapy. However, also tumor cells themselves can be modified to produce, for example, enzymes converting prodrugs, or proteins that make the cells more immunogenic. Third, whole cells, modified in vitro to serve as factories of proteins involved in a therapeutic action, can be delivered to patients by adoptive transfer or by surgery. These cells can even be targeted to certain organs or tumors, as in the case of tumor-infiltrating lymphocytes (TIL) homing specifically to the tumor. A number of examples relevant to the treatment of various forms of cancer will be discussed later (cf Section 2.1.3.).

2.1.2. METHODS OF GENE TRANSFER

Various delivery systems suitable for gene therapy have been developed over recent years (Table 1). The most simple one is physical transfer of DNA (or RNA) to cells. This can be achieved in vivo by injection of naked DNA in tumors (5) or by making use of liposome-encapsulated DNA in order to make access of the DNA into tumor cells easier (6). Recently, new techniques using a bombardment of DNA-coated particles into tissues were developed, sometimes referred to as "gene gun" experiments (7). Ex vivo, other techniques are available, including the classical calcium phosphate precipitation method (8), electroporation (9), and lipofection (10). The latter method makes use of liposomes, as in the case of the in vivo situation. The efficiencies of these methods are highly variable and depend on the cells to be transferred. For instance, the calcium phosphate precipitation method works well, with reasonable transfection efficiencies, provided the cells are well dividing in an adherent monolayer. Lipofection can be more efficient, but is more laborious and expensive (10,11). However, in

Table 1
Delivery Systems Used in Gene Therapy

Method	Application in gene therapy		Transient, T, or stable, S, expression
	ex vivo	in vivo	
Physical			
Direct injection of DNA	−	+	T
CaPO₄ precipitation	+	−	S
Lipofection	±	+	T
Transferrinfection	±	+	T
Vector-based			
Retroviruses	+	+	T
Adenovirus	±	+	T
Adeno-associated virus	−	+	S
Herpes virus	±	±	?
Vaccinia virus	±	±	T

+ : major application; ± ; some application; − : minor or no application; S: Stable expression; T: Transient expression; ?: not (yet) known. Data are adapted from ref. *(14)*.

the case that tumors are treated, in fact a 100% efficiency is required, unless a bystander effect is taking place (*see* Section 2.3.1.). The relatively low transfection efficiency makes the physical methods less attractive, because, for instance, selected clones may not express all tumor antigens owing to heterogeneity of the tumor.

Other methods to deliver DNA specifically in dividing cells can be more efficient. One example is the transferrinfection method, which is based on receptor-mediated transfer *(12)*. In this method, DNA is coupled to a transferrin–polylysin conjugate and, thus, results in targeting dividing cells expressing the transferrin receptor. The uptake of the complex can be largely enhanced by including an adenovirus–polylysin conjugate in the complex *(13)*.

Techniques using viral vectors have been widely explored. In the first instance, murine retroviral vectors became the most popular, because of their high efficiency of transduction as a result of high-titered virus stocks *(14)*. These viruses are defective in packaging and can only replicate in a helper cell line harboring the packaging sequences. After infection and reverse transcription to cDNA, the viral genome is integrated in the host genome, and constitutive expression can be obtained for more than a year *(14)*. The gene to be transduced is cloned behind a stong (eukaryotic) promoter, and usually also a selectable marker gene is present allowing selection of transduced cells. The ability of the vector DNA to integrate randomly in the genome, however, can be considered as a potential danger: oncogenes may be activated or tumor suppressor genes inactivated and a new cancer cell may develop. The chance this will happen, however, seems small, since the development of cancer is a multistep process involving multiple alterations in proto-oncogenes as well as in tumor suppressor genes.

One of the major disadvantages of retroviruses is that their integration in the host genome and the subsequent expression of the recombinant gene are limited to dividing cells. This has prompted many investigators to develop viral vectors expressed in nondividing cells. Replicating vectors are preferable, because they usually promote high expression of the recombinant gene (*15*). Examples being explored now are human adenoviruses. They are hardly toxic, and on infection, they accomplish a high gene expression (*16,17*). However, this expression is transient, and more seriously, an immune response against the virus may develop. Adenovirus-associated viruses may be a better choice, because they stably integrate in the genome of the host. The development of these vectors, however, has only recently started (*18*).

2.1.3. SPECIFIC APPROACHES FOR CANCER

Although gene therapy initially had not been designed specifically for cancer, many of its applications have first been tried in cancer patients. Several factors may have contributed to this. First, in the cancer field, there is a large experience with clinical trials, because in many cases, no regular therapy that has been proven successful exists. Second, because of the lack of an alternative, many cancer patients are willing to cooperate in these clinical trials and give their informed consent. Finally, in cancer, the gene therapy is directed to destroying malignant cells, rather than making corrections to improve survival, as is the case for nonneoplastic diseases. This makes the therapy less intrusive for the patient, since, with the exception of corrections made for defects in tumor suppressor genes, no long-term genetic alterations are implemented in the individual.

Several very different concepts, making use of gene therapy in cancer, have been worked out during recent years (Table 2). A distinction can be made between "gene marking" and "gene modification." The former was the first being applied to humans to test the feasibility of gene modification of human cells. TIL from melanomas were transduced with a retroviral vector comprising the neomycin phosphotransferase gene and reinfused into the autologous patients. G418-resistant cells could be recovered from tumor biopsies up to 2 mo after the adoptive transfer (*19*). Later, this technique has been used to assay whether malignant cells were relapsing from purged bone marrow after autologous bone marrow transplantation (BMT). Studies with acute myeloid leukemia (AML) and neuroblastoma patients showed that, in all cases where relapses occurred, the recurrent tumors came from the transplanted bone marrow (*20–22*). This gene marking has also been applied for the labeling of adoptively transferred HIV-specific cytotoxic T-cells (CTL) to patients with non-Hodgkin's lymphoma to prevent HIV infection of healthy donor bone marrow. The transferred CTL were labeled with a resistance gene as well as with the HSV *tk* gene to allow killing off the CTL with ganciclovir in case of unexpected growth (*4*). A similar experiment has been performed with Epstein-Barr virus (EBV)-specific CTL in a patient with post-BMT EBV-related lymphoproliferative disease to allow killing of the EBV-specific CTL (*23*). More examples of the introduction of such a "suicide gene" in tumor cells will be given below (Section 2.3.).

The second group of gene transfer techniques used in cancer consists of those involving gene modification (Table 2). They all aim at the in vivo or in vitro genetic alteration of either normal cells or tumor cells in such a way that the modification will be beneficial for the patient. There are many, conceptually very different, variations possible on this theme. First, one can try to direct the therapy directly to the genes responsible for the oncogenic transformation, and either add deleted genes or replace defect genes. Second, one can try to deliver genes encoding potential therapeutical

Table 2
Approaches of Gene Therapy of Cancer

Form	Example	Goal	Status
Gene marking			
Cell labeling	Labeling TIL cells with a selectable marker	Determine homing	C
	Labeling bone marrow after purging	Determine origin relapse after autologous BMT	C
Cell tracking	Transfer of HSV tk gene in CTL	Killing after adoptive transfer	C
Gene modification			
Addition/replacement	Correct oncogene defect	Kill tumor cell	E
Delivery			
Direct			
Suicide	Transfer of HSV tk gene in tumor cell	Kill tumor cell	C
Intensivation	Transfer of enzymes that activate drugs	Enhance chemotherapy	E
Indirect			
Protection	Transfer of a drug resistance gene	Allow high dose of chemotherapy	E
Immunomodulation	Transfer cytokine gene in tumor cell	Enhance immunogenicity of tumor cell	C

C: Clinically applied in humans.
E: Experimental.

proteins either to tumor cells or normal cells. In the first case, these can be proteins altering the sensitivity of tumor cells to cytostatic drugs (cf Table 2, direct gene therapy). In the second case, these can be proteins protecting normal cells against harmful effects of therapeutical drugs (indirect gene therapy). These forms of gene therapy will be discussed briefly below (Sections 2.2. and 2.3.). Finally, a large number of therapeutical trials making use of gene transfer techniques are focused on the alteration of the immune reactivity of either the tumor cells or the effector cells of the patient. This field of research will be the subject of a separate section (Section 3.).

2.2. Gene Correction

2.2.1. GENES INVOLVED IN CANCER

Genetic defects in proto-oncogenes as well as tumor suppressor genes, in principle, form a good target for gene correction therapy. In recent years, two classes of these tumor-promoting genes have been discerned, the so-called oncogenes and tumor suppressor genes (1). Genetic alterations in the former lead per definition to a "gain of function," and these are genotypically and phenotypically dominant. Such alterations are supposed to be lethal when present in the germ line and are therefore never found as a hereditary property. Alterations in the second type of genes, the tumor suppressor genes, lead to a "loss of function" and may segregate in families as a recessive trait, the lost function being exerted by the nonaffected allele. However, once the intact allele is also affected by sporadic mutation, which probability is considerable during a life-time, cancer will develop. Therefore, in this case, the recessive defect behaves as a dominantly inherited trait.

In the early 1970s, molecular mechanisms of cell transformation were beginning to be unraveled by studies using viruses as transforming agents (24,25). Transforming genes of murine retroviruses, capable of transforming murine cells, were isolated and characterized. Instead of using the viable virus for the induction of transformation, it became feasible to transform cultured cells with purified genes (8). Prominent transforming genes are the oncogenes of acute transforming oncogenic retroviruses, named v-*onc* genes. Well-known examples of retroviral oncogenes are v-*ras* and v-*myc*, encoding proteins involved in signal transduction and transcription, respectively. More than a hundred of these types of genes have been characterized, and all these genes were found to possess cellular counterparts, termed proto-oncogenes or c-*onc* genes. They invariably turned out to play a role in the regulation of cell proliferation and differentiation of normal, noncancerous cells. They mostly mediate the transfer of growth-stimulating signals to the cell nucleus, or are directly involved in the transcription of genes involved in cell proliferation or differentiation.

Several mutated proto-oncogenes were picked up as the transforming genes present in DNA isolates from human tumors, when assayed in an in vitro transformation assay (26). Since only dominantly acting transforming genes could be detected by this assay, our knowledge of tumor suppressor genes emerged largely from cytogenetic and restriction fragment length polymorphism (RFLP) analysis of hereditary forms of cancer. Well-known examples of such tumor suppressor genes are *Rb* and *p53*, the former deleted retinoblastoma, and the latter inactivated by deletion or mutation in numerous forms of human cancer.

2.2.2. CORRECTION OF ONCOGENES

Correcting activated oncogenes by gene therapy is difficult, one of the major problems being that all cells in the tumor have to be hit. Replacing genes by homologous recombination, as performed for germ line cells, seems not to be very effective for this purpose. Also, forcing high expression of the normal products (27) does not seem to be very attractive, since the capacity of the vectors is often limited and, moreover, the alteration in the oncogene is often highly dominant and cannot be simply overruled. Therefore, alternative strategies have been initiated. One of these is making use of antisense constructs, encoding transcripts that counteract expression of the mutated products. Also antisense oligonucleotides have been tried. The feasibility of these methods has been demonstrated for the H-*ras*, c-*myc*, N-*myc*, *bcr-abl*, c-*fos*, and c-*sis* oncogenes (28–33), but for most cases, successful applications in vivo have not been reported. Only for *ras* have the in vitro studies been extended to an in vivo model using human lung cancer cells in nude mice (34). Interestingly, it was recently shown that rat glioma cells could be rendered nontumorigenic in rats by expression of antisense constructs inhibiting insulin-like growth factor (IGF)-1 (35). Strikingly, parental tumor cells at distant sites were also affected, suggesting that inhibition of the growth factor leads to increased expression of immunogenic proteins, raising an immune response also effective against the parental cells (reviewed in *27*). This situation is reminiscent of the effect of transfected cytokine genes in tumor cells on their immune reactivity as will be discussed below.

To counteract oncogene-encoded mRNA effectively in another way, so-called ribozymes have been explored. These RNA molecules offer antisense as well as catalytic properties and allow cleavage of specific RNA sequences. Constructs comprising sequences encoding these ribozymes can be transferred to tumor cells. Effective inhibition of H-*ras* with an activating point mutation at amino acid codon 12 has been shown in melanoma cells, resulting in morphological changes suggestive of a lower degree of malignancy (*27,36*). Similar findings have been reported for the mRNA encoding the tumor-specific *bcr-abl* epitope (*37*).

2.2.3. CORRECTION OF TUMOR SUPPRESSOR GENES

As compared to strategies to counteract activated oncogenes, the introduction of lost or affected tumor suppressor genes into tumor cells seems more attractive and easier to accomplish. An attractive candidate is p53 because:

1. It is affected in numerous forms of human cancer (*38,39*);
2. It is involved in cell-cycle arrest as well as in the induction of apoptosis (*40*); and
3. A number of in vitro studies have shown that (re)introduction of the p53 gene in cancer cells leads to immediate growth arrest (*see 41,42* for review).

Moreover, expression of *p53* in tumor cells has been shown to act synergistically with ionizing radiation or cytostatics in the induction of apoptosis, which makes the combination of gene therapy for *p53* and conventional therapy attractive (*39, 43–46*). Recently, adenoviral vectors comprising the *p53* gene were constructed and shown to be capable of abolishing tumor formation of human tumor cells in nude mice (*45,47*). Another tumor suppressor gene candidate target for therapy is the *Rb* gene, originally discovered in retinoblastoma, but affected in many other forms of human cancer (*48,49*). Furthermore, the product of this gene is involved in cell-cycle regulation, and in fact, its state of phosphorylation controls G1 to S phase transition through its interaction with the nuclear transcription factor E2F (*50,51*). Also, here it has been shown that introduction of an active *Rb* gene may inhibit proliferation of tumor cells (*52*) and vascular proliferative disorders (*53*). Altogether, these experiments show that attractive gene therapy approaches to correct altered oncogene and tumor suppressor gene expression are available and have been proven successful already in experimental tumor models. Their way to the clinic, however, is proceeding slowly, and eventual success in curing cancer patients has to be awaited.

2.3 Drug Delivery

2.3.1. SUICIDE GENES

A large application field in gene therapy does not intend to alter directly genes involved in the origin of cancer as described above, but conducts alterations of either cancer cells or normal cells in such a way that therapy can be improved. The various approaches are summarized in Table 2. A rather spectacular form that is being tested in patients with brain tumors is transfer of the herpes simplex virus thymidine kinase (*tk*) gene into tumor allowing suicide of the cells. The *tk* gene confers sensitivity of human cells to ganciclovir by phosphorylating the drug to a form that is ultimately incorporated in the DNA, leading to inhibition of DNA synthesis and cell death (reviewed in *23*). The ganciclovir can be given to the patient systemically. The *tk* gene can be transferred to the tumor cells in the brain by stereotactic injection either of retrovirus-containing supernatants with a high virus titer or of a murine fibroblast cell line producing a defective retrovirus comprising the *tk* gene (*54,55*). In rat studies, this approach was shown to be extremely effective in destroying the tumor cells macroscopically, as well as microscopically (*56,57*). An important phenomenon observed was that infection of all tumor cells with the virus was not necessary to eradicate the tumor. Apparently, neighboring nontransduced cells were also destroyed, referred to as a "bystander" or "field" effect. This could well be owing to diffusion of toxic products or to disrupture of the tumor vasculature, but another interesting observation was a high invasion of T-lymphocytes and macrophages in *tk* gene-transduced tumors, suggesting that the cells become targets for an enhanced immune reactivity (*58*). The precise mechanism of this is not known, but the effect clearly depended on an intact immune system, because the effect was not seen in nude or irradiated mice (*23,58–60*).

2.3.2. IMPROVEMENT OF DRUG ACTION

Other forms of gene therapy directly targeted to the tumor cells make use of intensification of the action of conventional cytostatic drugs. For example, 5F-uracil (5FU), which has a high systemic toxicity, can be administered in the form of the nontoxic 5F-cytosine when the tumor cells are capable of converting this compound to 5FU. This is possible through transfer of the bacterial enzyme cytosine deaminase (*61*). This transfer can be done by making use of retroviral systems and this type of therapy is therefore named virus-directed enzyme/prodrug therapy (VDEPT) (*62*). Strikingly, also in this case of suicide therapy, an immune component has been shown to be involved in the response, and protective immunity against subsequent challenges with the parental cell line could be gained (*63*). The VDEPT therapy can be made more specific by targeting expression of the enzyme to certain types of tumors by making use of tissue-specific promoters, such as the *CEA* promoter, highly expressed in colon carcinoma, or the *erbB2* or *α-fetoprotein* promoter driving high expression of a transduced gene in hepatocellular and in breast carcinoma, respectively (*62,64*). This approach of enhancing differential transcription is very attractive, since it allows many variations on the theme: various tissues do often express specific genes, and this is reflected in tumors derived from these genes. A prominent example here is the *tyrosinase* gene only expressed in cells of the melanocytic linage. Making use of the *tyrosinase* promotor, genes of choice can be expressed in melanoma (*5,65*).

2.3.3. DIRECTING T-CELLS

Another way to deliver anticancer agents to the tumor site is by making use of specifically homing cells, such as TIL. These can be isolated from surgically removed tumors and transduced with genes encoding, for instance, TNF-α or IFN-γ (*66,67*). After reinfusion in the patient, they home to the tumor and produce locally large amounts of TNF, leading to tumor destruction, in combination with the cytolytic activity of the TIL. One of the problems encountered is the limited production of TNF by the TIL, which can possibly be enhanced by making use of better vectors. Another possibility is to engineer the TNF gene in such a way that a more stable or better secreted protein is produced (*67*). Another problem is that the homing of TIL is not exclusively tumor-specific, causing considerable toxicity of the TIL therapy. To circumvent this problem, one can think of engineering the T-cells in such a way that they express receptors recognizing the tumor cells. Such receptors may be a hybrid of the T-cell receptor with its variable (peptide-recognizing) part replaced by the variable region of a tumor-specific monoclonal antibody (Mab). This approach using the chimeric receptors has been shown to be effective in redirecting cytolytic T-cells to cancer cells (*68–70*).

2.3.4. PROTECTION OF BONE MARROW

In addition to these direct ways to influence gene expression in tumor cells or cells targeted to the tumor, gene modification can be used in a more indirect way, such as to protect bone marrow from being destroyed by conventional chemotherapy. So far, bone marrow stem cell growth factors have been successfully used in combination with high-dose conventional chemotherapy. An alternative strategy may be to protect the bone marrow of the patient by transducing it with genes encoding proteins involved in drug resistance, such as the *mdr-1* gene encoding the P-glycoprotein. This protein functions as a membrane pump to remove toxic compounds out of the cell and is easily induced by a number of different cytostatics rendering tumor cells resistant to further therapy. Animal and human models to explore the feasibility of this system have been reported (*71,72*). Mice reconstituted with *mdr-1*-engineered bone marrow showed less reduction in white blood cell counts than control mice after treatment with taxol. Using this approach, one should keep in mind that *mdr-1* is often also expressed in cancer cells and, therefore, protecting the bone with *mdr-1* makes sense only when the cancer does not express *mdr-1* on treatment. For these reasons, one has sought to modify the P-glycoprotein in such a way that transduced protein can be discerned from endogenous mdr-1 with respect to sensitivity to agents that may reverse its action (*71*). For example, when a Gly185Val mutant is used for transduction bone marrow, verapamil might be used to reverse the resistance of the tumor cells (containing normal mdr-1), because the mutated protein is insensitive to the action of verapamil. In this way, the design of specific mutations altering the properties of mdr-1 may allow very selective action. Another application of *mdr-1* gene transduction is to use it as a selectable marker. For instance, in strategies explained below, where engineered tumor cell vaccines are used, it might be desirable to increase the resistance of the engineered cells as opposed to the parental tumor cells, as to increase exposition of the immune system to these cells, while simultaneously the parental cells are killed off by the used drug. Outgrowth of the engineered tumor cells might be prevented by cotransduction of a suicide gene. In this way, an effective concert action of drug therapy and immune therapy might be obtained. In the next section, we will further elaborate on the use of engineered tumor cell vaccines.

3. THE IMMUNE SYSTEM AS VEHICLE

3.1. Immune Defense Against Cancer Cells

3.1.1. T-CELLS

Over the past few years, exciting new developments in the involvement of the immune system in the defense against neoplastic cells have drawn much attention. Although the results of classical vaccinations with irradiated autologous tumor cells were only of limited success (*73–76*), a new era started when recombinant cytokines, in particular interleukin-2 (IL-2), were introduced in the clinic (*77,78*). These were applied in particular in patients with melanoma and renal cell cancer, which types of cancer had previously been shown to be rather immunogenic, judged on the basis of spontaneous regressions observed (*79–81*). Although the response rates were relatively high, these still did not exceed 40% (*see 82,83* for review). In the earliest studies, lymphokine-activated killer cells (LAK cells) emerging after treatment of peripheral blood lymphocytes (PBL) with IL-2 in vitro were used (*77*). LAK activity is mediated primarily by natural killer (NK) cells and to a lesser extent by MHC-unrestricted T-cells (*84*). LAK cell therapy has been improved by using TIL isolated from fresh tumor specimens rather than the patient's PBL for activation with IL-2 (*78*). In TIL cells, the active effector cells are predominantly T-cells with specific antitumor activity (*85*). In humans, these cells consist of HLA Class II-restricted CD4$^+$ helper T-cells as well as CD8$^+$ MHC Class I-restricted cytotoxic T-cells.

3.1.2. Tumor Antigens

Since MHC antigens are involved in the presentation of altered peptides to reactive T-cells, tumor-reactive T-cells in the TIL cell population interact with tumor-specific peptides bound to the groove of HLA Class I proteins (*86–89*). HLA Class I-restricted T-cell cultures or T-cell clones reacting with the tumor could be established from patients with various forms of human cancer, including melanoma (*90–94*), renal cell carcinoma (*95–98*), ovarian carcinoma (*95–98*), gastric carcinoma (*99*), and pancreatic carcinoma (*100*). Most importantly, specificity of some of the T-cell cultures for allogeneic tumors was found, suggesting that common tumor antigens are involved (*101,102*).

Recently, several tumor antigens recognized by melanoma-specific T-cell clones or T-cell lines have been characterized. These include MAGE-1 and MAGE-3 (*103,104*), Mart-1, also called Melan-A (*105,106*), tyrosinase (*107*), and gp100 (*108,109*). In all these cases, the genes encoding the antigens were not mutated as compared to the genes in normal tissues, indicating that nonmutated self-peptides may serve as CTL target. Tyrosinase is a key enzyme in the melanin synthesis pathway in pigmented cells. The function of the other antigens is not known. With the exception of the testis, MAGE antigens are expressed exclusively in the tumor. This may explain why CTL can be raised against it: inappropriate expression at high density in the tumor cells may elicit an autoimmune reaction. On the contrary, tyrosinase and gp100 are also expressed in normal melanocytes, and here, tumor-specific CTL induction is apparently triggered by bulk expression on tumor cells. The MAGE and Mart antigens are not specific for melanoma, but are also expressed in other tumor types, such as breast carcinoma, neuroblastoma, and lung carcinoma (*110–112*).

3.1.3. Induction of Tumor-Specific CTL

The restriction elements for T-cell recognition of these antigens identified so far were HLA-A*0101, HLA-A*0201, HLA-A*2401, and HLA-Cw*1601 (*105,113–116*). The identification of these targets and the discovery of unique allele-specific peptide binding motifs in the groove of the HLA Class I molecules (*117,118*) made it feasible to determine which peptides in a tumor antigen potentially bind to an HLA Class I allele, and these peptides subsequently could be tested for induction of a T-cell response (*119*). This was done for a number of tumor antigens, such as MAGE-3 and tyrosinase (*120,121*), but also for mutated oncogene products, such as p53 and p21ras (*122,123*). CTL can also be raised against native p53 (*122*), which largely extends the grip of the immune system on tumor cells, because apparently nonmutated proteins present in elevated expression in tumor cells can also serve as a target. Finally, viral proteins in virus-associated human tumors, such as cervical carcinoma, are good targets for T-cells because the viral epitopes are unique and do not resemble cellular proteins (*124,125*). In this latter case, peptide vaccination in an animal model has been shown to be effective in inducing long-term protection of animals against a subsequent challenge with tumor cells (*126*). The power of peptide vaccination for elimination of established tumor, however, has still has to be shown.

An effective method of peptide vaccination may be loading the peptides on professional antigen-presenting cells. In this case, gene technology can play a role because high expression of immunogenic peptides may be reached by transfer of peptide-encoding sequences linked to a signal peptide-encoding sequence, making transport to the endoplasmatic reticulum and assembly into HLA Class I molecules very effective (*127*). Even the HLA Class I expression can be engineered by transfer of individual HLA Class I alleles in cells with an endogenously low HLA Class I expression. Ultimately, this approach may lead to allogeneic vaccination of patients with engineered cells expressing a high density of tumor peptide on the cell surface. Allogenic determinants on these cells are not necessarily a disadvantage, because it has been shown that transfection of syngeneic tumor cells with foreign MHC Class I molecules raises their immunogenicity and may lead to an immune reaction against parental tumor cells owing to the bystander effect (*128–130*). Methods to improve the immunogenicity of tumor cells by genetic engineering as a tool to fight the parental cancer cells will be discussed below.

3.2. Natural Immune Response
Against Human Tumor Is Often Ineffective

Despite the apparent potential of the human immune system to develop a cytotoxic reaction against tumors, an obvious immune reaction seems usually to be absent in patients with cancer. Several reasons may account for this (*see also 131,132* for comprehensive reviews). First, expansion of tumors may be so fast that effector cells are not capable of killing the tumor properly. Second, tumor cells might have escaped an immune response by downmodulation of tumor-specific antigens or MHC Class I antigens in experimental tumors, as well as in humans (*89,133*). For instance, in melanoma, one of the most immune reactive human tumors, downmodulation of particular HLA Class I alleles is a common phenomenon (*134*). Third, suppressor cells consisting mostly of CD4+ T-cells may be activated by tumor cells. This has been clearly shown in animal tumor models (*135*) as well as for human melanomas (*93,136*). Fourth, alterations in the T-cell repertoire leading to aberrant T-cell receptor expression has been found in renal cell carcinomas (*137*). The mechanism leading to this phenomenon is far from clear, but the result is an anergic T-cell population in the tumor. Fifth, the presentation of tumor antigens at the cell surface may be disturbed. This may happen through a defect in genes involved in peptide processing in the cell, required for the generation of peptides and the subsequent assembly of peptide-HLA Class I complexes (*138*). Sixth, local immunosuppressive factors secreted by the tumor, such as transforming growth factor-β (TGF-β) might be involved in the suppression of cytotoxic T-cells (*139,140*). This view is supported by the observation that highly immunogenic tumor cells expressing a transfected TGF-β gene did indeed escape immune surveillance (*141*). Finally, the immunogenicity of spontaneously arising tumors, as human tumors usually are, may be in general too low to elicit a proper immune response (*142*). Altogether, these factors, alone or in combination, may impede recruitment of a proper T-cell helper circuit necessary for proliferation of tumor-specific cytotoxic T-cells. Below, we will discuss several strategies of gene therapy of cancer patients to improve their immune response to the tumor.

3.3. Improving Immunogenicity of Tumor Cells

As mentioned before, naturally occurring tumors, except virally induced ones, have a low immunogenicity. If these tumor cells could be manipulated in such a way that a better response could be evoked by the immune system of the host, vaccination with the manipulated cells could be tested as treatment modality. Recently, attempts to enhance the immunogenicity of murine tumor cells by gene transfer have been remarkably successful. Transfection of allogeneic MHC Class I genes in tumor cells did elicit immune responses directed against the nontransfected tumor cells and could prevent tumor take after immunization (*128,129,143,144*). This situation is reminiscent of immunization of mice with mutated highly immunogenic variants of an originally nonimmunogenic tumor (*145*). The immunized mice became resistant to the mutated tumor cells, as well as to the nonimmunogenic parental tumor. This is probably owing to an adjuvant effect of the mutated antigens on the generation of an immune response against poorly immunogenic (cryptic) antigens present in the mutated tumor cells as well as in the parental tumor. A similar approach was explored by infection of tumor cells with an immunogenic virus, e.g., the Newcastle Disease Virus, or by transfection of a gene encoding an immunogenic viral protein, e.g., hemagglutinin (*146,147*). In all cases, protection was acquired against challenge with the original nonmanipulated tumor cells.

A promising new approach came about with the discovery of so-called accessory molecules, such as B7.1, which plays a role in the physical interaction between antigen-presenting cells and immune effector cells (*148*). This protein represents an essential part of the helper arm of the immune response. Tumor cells are usually devoid of this helper machinery and, therefore, are crippled in their capacity to elicit an onset of an effective immune response. Transfection of the *B7.1* gene in B7.1-negative cells largely stimulates the interaction of effector and target (*149*). This prompted several investigators to see whether transfer of the *B7* gene would make tumor cells more immunogenic. It turned out that, indeed, the introduction of the *B7* gene in nonimmunogenic tumor cells made them less tumorigenic (*150–152*). Moreover, the immune response mounted did protect the animals from a subsequent challenge with the parental cells. Also, long-term memory against the *B7*-engineered as well as the parental cells could be obtained. This approach works particularly well with MHC Class II-negative tumor cells, suggesting that indeed the helper arm of the immune response is restored (*153*). Also in the induction of human tumor-specific CTL in vitro, transfer of the B7 molecule into several human tumor cell lines largely enhances

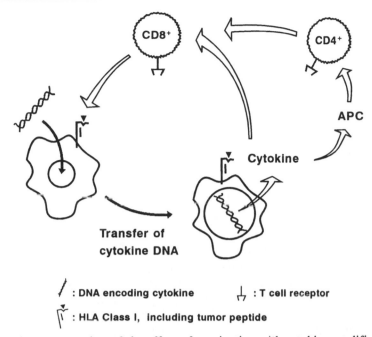

Fig. 1. Schematic representation of the effect of vaccination with cytokine-modified tumor cells. Two alternative routes are depicted: 1. The cytokine in combination with HLA Class I-bound tumor peptide enhances stimulation of CD8 $^+$ T-cells. 2. The cytokine enhances the stimulation of antigen-presenting cells (APC) that present tumor peptide derived from degraded tumor protein to CD4 $^+$ T-cells.

proliferation of tumor-specific CTL in MLTC (*154*). The resulting CTL were not only reactive with the B7-transfected cells, but also with the parental cell line, indicating that B7 is involved in the inductive phase of the immune response.

These experiments clearly show that structural alterations of tumor cells that in some way change their interaction with the immune system may largely improve their immune recognition and enhance the induction of tumor-specific CTL. The most exciting observation is that, in many cases, these CTL recognize not only the modified cells, but also the parental, unaltered, tumor cell. This is also the case when the tumor cells are transduced in order to let them produce cytokines. Since this has been pioneered by many groups over the past few years and has already made its entrance in the cancer clinic, we will discuss this approach in more detail in the next section.

3.4. Enhancing Immunogenicity of Tumor Cells by Cytokine Gene Transfer

3.4.1. CYTOKINES

Very effective protection may be obtained when tumor cells are transfected or transduced with genes encoding growth factors or cytokines. The principle of this approach is schematically represented in Fig. 1. The manifest advantage of this system is the local production and high concentration of immune-modulating factors at the site of the administered tumor cells. Moreover, the side effects of the produced cytokines can be expected to be much lower than on systemic administration. To date, no data have been reported for humans. In animal models, however, promising results have been obtained with the cytokines IL-1 (*155*), IL-2 (*156–161*), IL-4 (*160, 162–164*), IL-6 (*165,166*), IL-7 (*160,167,168*), IL-10 (*155*), IL-12 (*169*), IFN-γ (*160, 170–174*), TNF-α (*66,160, 175–178*), G-CSF (*179*), and GM-CSF (*180,181*). In these cases, at least a significant reduction of tumorigenicity of the cells in syngeneic animals was observed, but in most cases tumor formation was completely abolished. Usually, the reduced tumorigenicity was highly dependent on the amount of cytokine produced: high amounts of cytokine are required for abolishment of tumorigenicity, although bell-shaped dose responses have been reported (*157,182*).

3.4.2. MECHANISM

The mechanism of blocking of tumor growth has not been made unequivocally clear, but definitely depends on the modification made to the tumor cell. The general idea is that the production of the cytokine at the vaccination site attracts immune effector cells, mainly macrophages, neutrophils, NK cells, and CD4+ and CD8+ T-cells. The CD8+ T-cells are ultimately the most important contributors in eliminating the tumor cells, suggesting that one of the main reasons for the effectiveness of the secreted cytokines is the bypassing of the helper arm of the immune system, comprising the antigen presentation through HLA Class II to CD4+ T-cells (Fig. 1). Other effector cells, such as NK cells, may be important too, in particular, in the initial phase of the rejection (*160,183*). It should be stressed, however, that the actual mechanism cannot be generalized, but is largely dependent on the cytokine and on the tumor model used (reviewed in *184,185*). Whatever the actual effectors are, in the above presented view, the cytokine-producing tumor cell interacts directly with the immune system of the host. In an alternative view, however, tumor cells are broken down at the vaccination site, and owing to the local cytokine production of yet intact cells, an effective presentation of tumor antigens is initiated by antigen-presenting cells of the host. This view is substantiated by recent experiments showing that allogeneic cytokine-producing tumor cells are also effective in mounting protective immunity against a subsequent challenge with a syngeneic tumor (*186*). This would actually decimate the necessity of matching for tumor antigen-presenting MHC Class I alleles in vaccination protocols, since the tumor antigens from allogeneic tumor cells would be presented by the autologous antigen-presenting cells and subsequently induce an immune response against the autologous tumor (also *see* Section 4.1.).

Most importantly, in all models studied, animals treated with cytokine gene-engineered tumor cells developed long-term memory against the engineered cells as well as against the parental tumor cells. This effect could not be reached by administration of tumor cells mixed with cytokine or by tumor cells only. In some systems, however, the effect of the cytokine-producing tumor cells could be mimicked by mixing the tumor cells with autologous fibroblasts engineered to produce the cytokine (*186*). In most systems, treatment with live tumor cell vaccines was superior to irradiated cells (*166,187*), stressing that the success of vaccination with engineered tumor cells in human cancer patients may turn out to be limited when the cells are irradiated, as presently required by medical ethical committees.

3.4.3. COMPARISON OF EFFICACY

There is still much discussion about what cytokine is the most effective on transfer in tumor cells in raising an immune response against parental cells. In a series of experiments by various groups, a number of cytokines were compared, and variable results were obtained (*160,166,180,188*). Good choices seem to be IL-2 and GM-CSF, though results are undoubtedly dependent on the tumor model used. Surprisingly, in one study (*187*), the cytokine transfection seemed not to be superior above a mixture of nonmodified tumor cells and *Corynebacterium Parvum* (*C. Parvum*), an adjuvant frequently used in the past as immunostimulator (*189*). The general validity of this observation, however, is hard to evaluate. In particular, for the human situation, vaccination with BCG/tumor cell mixtures was only shown to be effective in rare instances, making a comparison with the animal studies difficult.

Finally, a distantly related, but interesting approach making use of the immunostimulating properties of cytokines is the engineering of immunogenic epitopes that are target for a B-cell response. Constructs harboring sequences encoding tumor-specific idiotypes have been fused to sequences encoding GM-CSF, IL-4, or IL-2, and fusion proteins were synthesized. Such fusion proteins are capable of eliciting significant levels of specific antibodies against the idiotype and can elicit significant antitumor immunity (*190,191*). This strategy is used for the preparation of protein vaccines, but one can speculate that cellular vaccines producing these types of recombinant proteins may be useful too.

In conclusion, vaccination using cytokine transfer techniques seems very promising, although a lot of more research has to be done to fine-tune the experimental conditions. The results so far have encouraged clinicians to initiate clinical studies in patients with melanoma and renal cell carcinoma. In the next section, we will discuss the rationale and outline of these studies.

4. CLINICAL STUDIES

4.1. Rationale

The molecular biology techniques for the modification of tumor cells, discussed in detail before, enable us to explore the new strategies to enhance the immunogenicity of human tumor cells and use these cells for vaccination. Most of the tumor-specific antigens, candidates for such an enhancement in the individual patients, have not yet been identified. The most optimal situation, therefore, is to transfer autologous tumor cells of the patient, either in vivo or *ex vivo*, and let them work as a vaccine. This circumvents the determination of matching for tumor-specific antigens and for the HLA Class I alleles required to present the tumor-specific peptides.

The feasibility and safety of gene therapy with genetically modified cells have been demonstrated by the pioneering work of Rosenberg and coworkers (*19,67,192*). In applying the strategies of cytokine transfection as discussed above, two approaches can be envisioned: (1) transfer of the cytokine genes in vivo locally at the site of the tumor(s), and (2) perform the transfer *ex vivo* on cultured cells and re-administer them to the patient. Both methods have, however, certain disadvantages. Transfer to the tumor *in situ* may be technically difficult, if there is any tumor there. Also, however, the *ex vivo* approach may cause complications. Culturing autologous tumor cells is time-consuming and not always successful. The identification of common tumor antigens presented by either HLA-A*0101 or HLA-A*0201 allows the use of HLA-A*0101 or HLA-A*0201-positive allogeneic cells as a vaccine in melanoma patients harboring these alleles. Approximately 60–70% of white patients will be

HLA-A*0101 and/or HLA-A*0201. Therefore, such a vaccine is expected to be applicable in a considerable number of melanoma patients. Furthermore, the presence of allogeneic HLA Class I or II molecules may be even more advantageous, because it has been shown in animal experiments that foreign MHC genes may induce a similar raise in immunogenicity as obtained with cytokine gene therapy (*see* Section 3.3.). Moreover, as a practical advantage, the allogeneic cells will most likely be rejected by the immune system of the patient, avoiding any risk of tumor recurrences by cells surviving the irradiation. It even may allow vaccination with live tumor cells in patients with a well-functioning immune system, which may be more effective on the basis of the experience with animal vaccination studies (*see* Section 3.4.2.).

Following immunization of patients with genetically modified allogeneic tumor cells that share an HLA Class I allele, the cells may in vivo directly present the shared tumor peptides to HLA Class I-restricted CTL of the patient, provided that the shared HLA Class I allele presents a shared immunodominant peptide. Alternatively, the cells will be degraded and serve as a source of tumor antigens presented by autologous antigen-presenting cells (Fig. 2). These cells will then process and select the appropriate epitopes, which will enter the HLA Class II processing route to stimulate CD4+ T-cells, or even enter the HLA Class I route to induce directly proliferation of CD8+ cytotoxic T-cells (*186*). In this line, one can even think of using a fully allogeneic cell line for vaccination. In this case, a shared tumor antigen is required, and the corresponding tumor peptides can only be presented by the autologous antigen-presenting cells (Fig. 2).

4.2. Trials

A number of clinical trials using gene modification for immune modulatory purposes have been initiated (*193–198*). The studies focused on HLA Class I genes and cytokine genes. The various modes of administration of the ''vaccines'' are:

1. Genes packed in liposomes directly transferred into the tumor *in situ* (*196*);
2. Cytokine-producing fibroblasts admixed with tumor cells (*198*);
3. Autologous tumor cells cultured and transduced with cytokine; and
4. Allogeneic cytokine-transduced or transfected tumor cells (*194,195,197*).

In February 1992, we initiated the first clinical study in which HLA-A*0101 or HLA-A*0201-positive melanoma patients were immunized with an HLA-A*0101, A*0201,B*0801-positive melanoma cell line, transfected with the IL-2 gene. The cell line expresses high levels of HLA Class I. Moreover, the cell line expresses MAGE-1, 2, and 3, tyrosinase, Mart-1, and gp100. The choice of IL-2 was based on the fact that clinical remissions were obtained in patients with metastatic melanoma following IL-2 based treatment regimens. Furthermore, ample evidence exists for the presence of CTL precursors in melanoma patients, and the animal studies testing different cytokines for gene transfer indicated that IL-2 worked well. The IL-2 gene under control of an immediate early cytomegalovirus (CMV) promoter was transfected using the calcium phosphate precipitation technique. This promoter is well expressed in melanoma cells, and the cells produce high amounts of IL-2 up to at least 100 ng IL-2/10^6 cells/24 h. After 100 gy of irradiation, a dose that completely inhibited the proliferation of the cells in vitro, the secretion of biologically active IL-2 on a per-cell basis increased in the first days, decreased thereafter, but after 10 d IL-2 production was

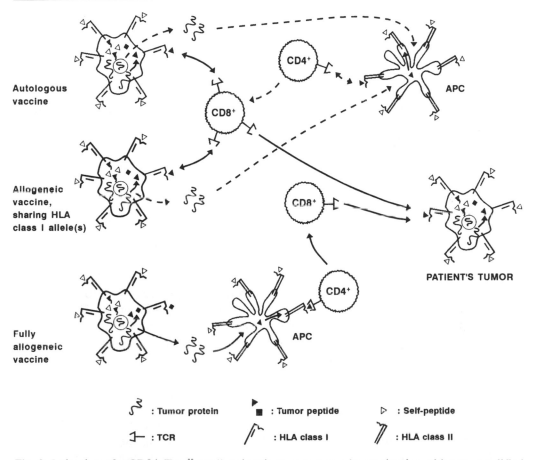

Fig. 2. Induction of a CD8$^+$ T-cell-mediated antitumor response by vaccination with gene-modified tumor cells. Three situations are shown as indicated: 1. autologous tumor cells, 2. allogeneic tumor cells, sharing one or more HLA Class I alleles, or 3. fully allogeneic tumor cells. All vaccination strategies lead to a CD8$^+$-mediated immune response against the patient's own tumor (shown on the right side). Autologous tumor cells or autologous HLA molecules are depicted in gray, and allogeneic tumor cells or allogeneic HLA molecules are depicted in black.

still measurable. The purpose of our study was to evaluate toxicity and antitumor efficacy of weekly subcutaneous injections of the IL-2-secreting irradiated cells. So far, no toxicities have been observed, though we did observe inflammatory reactions at the site of vaccination as well as at the site of distant metastases. Regressions of metastases were observed, but these always represented mixed responses.

Nabel and coworkers (6) reported the enhancement of antitumor immune response by in vivo injection directly in tumors of allogeneic HLA-B7 using DNA–liposome complexes. HLA-B7 protein expression was demonstrated in the tumor cells near the site of injection. No systemic toxicity was observed, whereas a fivefold increase in the frequency of HLA-B7-reactive CTL precursors was demonstrated in one patient following immunization. Furthermore, a distant lung metastasis regressed in one of the five reported patients, suggesting that the allogeneic effects may indeed have enhanced the antitumor immune response.

Altogether these experiments look promising and merit further investigation of gene therapy in cancer patients.

5. EPILOGUE

The present insight into the genetics of cancer development allows an active intervention by means of genetic manipulation. This may be either replacement of affected genes or addition of inactivated or lacking genes. It has been shown that random integration of, for instance, tumor suppressor genes in cancer cells is effectively inhibiting cell-cycle progression. This shows that, in principle, this type of addition therapy can work. Many barriers have to be removed before the delivery of such genes has the power to reach every malignant cell in the body, an absolute requirement for the cure of metastatic cancer. For the moment, however, these techniques can be explored as debulking tools, allowing more effective methods of cancer therapy to be successful. This may, for instance, be triggering the immune system to attack the cancer cell.

The new developments in genetic engineering, in particular the design of new eukaryotic expression vectors, have disclosed an array of possibilities to deliver genes specifically to cancer cells, leaving the surrounding normal cells intact. This has, for instance, led to the clinical use of suicide genes. Another step forward toward precise delivery of genes has been made by invoking the help of the highly selective immune system: on one hand, cytotoxic T-cells have been genetically altered in such a way that they can more effectively interact with the tumor cell; on the other hand, tumor cells have been made immunogenic to enhance the immune system of the host. An intriguing observation has recently been made, i.e., cells harboring suicide genes evoke an immune reaction, leading to a situation that killing by the drug in combination with an immune response may be particularly effective in eradicating the tumor. The gene transfer techniques can be applied to normal cells, too: purged bone marrow of the cancer patient can be engineered is such a way that it becomes resistant to cytostatic drugs, allowing high-dose chemotherapy.

In the clinical setting, the conditions for vaccination will have to be very carefully investigated and evaluated. Based on the animal experiments, the optimal situations for cellular vaccines to be effective were at very low tumor load. Since the clinical trials now performed are all on patients with advanced metastatic disease and probably considerable tumor burden, the outcome may give an underestimated view on the power of the therapy. Therefore, arguments have to be gathered for treating patients with a more favorable prognosis, for instance, in an adjuvant setting. Also, a combination with an adoptive transfer of in vitro expanded tumor-specific CTLs induced by the vaccine might be fruitful. For the moment, however, important data can be gained from the treatment of metastatic patients. First, a careful histological evaluation of biopsies of macroscopic metastases before and after vaccination may give insight into the immune reaction elicited. Second, a minute analysis of tumor-specific CTL in the peripheral blood mononuclease cells (PBMC) of the patients before and after vaccination may reveal whether an increased T-cell reactivity can be induced and toward what antigens these T-cells are directed. On the basis of the outcoming data, further studies can be undertaken to optimize the conditions for this form of gene therapy.

By and large, the search for gene therapy approaches for the treatment of cancer has yielded a number of exciting new developments, with highlights in the "suicide" therapy and immunotherapy. Very powerful new techniques are finding their way to the clinic now. The preliminary clinical data, however, should be evaluated with care and used to allude to new directions for improvement of the present protocols. It is our sincere expectation that the almost indefinite possibilities of the new genetic techniques ultimately will survive in the struggle against cancer.

REFERENCES

1. Bishop JM. Molecular themes in oncogenesis. *Cell* 1991; 64:235–248.
2. Fearon ER, Vogelstein B. A genetic model for colorectal tumorigenesis. *Cell* 1990; 61:759–767.
3. Hunter T. Cooperation between oncogenes. *Cell* 1991; 64:249–270.
4. Morgan RA, Anderson WF. Human gene therapy. *Annu Rev Biochem* 1993; 62:191–217.
5. Hart IR, Vile RG. Targeted therapy for malignant melanoma. *Curr Opinion Oncol* 1994; 6:221–225.
6. Nabel GJ, Nabel EG, Yang ZY, Fox BA, Plautz GE, Gao X, Huang L, Shu S, Gordon D, Chang AE. Direct gene transfer with DNA-liposome complexes in melanoma: expression, biologic activity, and lack of toxicity in humans. *Proc Natl Acad Sci USA* 1993; 90:11,307–11,311.
7. Williams RS, Johnston SA, Riedy M, DeVit MJ, McElligott SG, Sanford JC. Introduction of foreign genes into tissues of living mice by DNA-coated microprojectiles. *Proc Natl Acad Sci USA* 1991; 88:2726–2730.
8. Graham FL, Van der Eb AJ. A new technique for the assay of infectivity of human Adenovirus 5 DNA. *Virology* 1973; 52:456–467.
9. Keating A, Toneguzzo F. Gene transfer by electroporation: a model for gene therapy. *Prog Clin Biol Res* 1990; 333:491–498.
10. Ray J, Gage FH. Gene transfer into established and primary fibroblast cell lines: comparison of transfection methods and promoters. *Biotechniques* 1992; 13:598–603.
11. Jiang CK, Connolly D, Blumenberg M. Comparison of methods for transfection of human epidermal keratinocytes. *J Invest Dermatol* 1991; 97:967–973.
12. Cotten M, Wagner E, Birnstiel ML. Receptor-mediated transport of DNA into eukaryotic cells. *Methods Enzymol* 1993; 217:618–644.
13. Wagner E, Zatloukal K, Cotten M, Kirlappos H, Mechtler K, Curiel DT, Birnstiel ML. Coupling of adenovirus to transferrin-polylysine/DNA complexes greatly enhances receptor-mediated gene delivery and expression of transfected genes. *Proc Natl Acad Sci USA* 1992; 89:6099–6103.
14. Mulligan RC. The basic science of gene therapy. *Science* 1993; 260:926–932.
15. Russell SJ. Replicating vectors for cancer therapy: A question of strategy. *Semin Cancer Biol* 1994; 5:437–443.
16. Haddada H, Ragot T, Cordier L, Duffour MT, Perricaudet M. Adenoviral interleukin-2 gene transfer into P815 tumor cells abrogates tumorigenicity and induces antitumoral immunity in mice. *Hum Gene Ther* 1993; 4:703–711.
17. Kozarsky KF, Wilson JM. Gene therapy: Adenovirus vectors. *Curr Opinion Genet Dev* 1993; 3:499–503.
18. Flotte TR, Afione SA, Conrad C, McGrath SA, Solow R, Oka H, Zeitlin PL, Guggino WB, Carter BJ. Stable in vivo expression of the cystic fibrosis transmembrane conductance regulator with an adeno-associated virus vector. *Proc Natl Acad Sci USA* 1993; 90:10,613–10,617.
19. Rosenberg SA, Aebersold P, Cornetta K, Kasid A, Morgan RA, Moen R, Karson EM, Lotze MT, Yang JC, Topalian SL, Merino MJ, Culver K, Miller AD, Blaese RM, Anderson WF. Gene transfer into humans - Immunotherapy of patients with advanced melanoma, using tumor-infiltrating lymphocytes modified by retroviral gene transduction. *N Engl J Med* 1990; 323:570–578.
20. Rill DR, Buschle M, Foreman NK, Bartholomew C, Moen RC, Santana VM, Ihle JN, Brenner MK. Retrovirus-mediated gene transfer as an approach to analyze neuroblastoma relapse after autologous bone marrow transplantation. *Hum Gene Ther* 1992; 3:129–136.

21. Brenner MK, Rill DR, Moen RC, Krance RA, Mirro J, Jr., Anderson WF, Ihle JN. Gene-marking to trace origin of relapse after autologous bone-marrow transplantation. *Lancet* 1993; 341:85,86.
22. Brenner MK, Rill DR, Heslop HE, Rooney CM, Roberts WM, Li C, Nilson T, Krance RA. Gene marking after bone marrow transplantation. *Eur J Cancer* 1994; 30A:1171–1176.
23. Tiberghien P. Use of suicide genes in gene therapy. *J Leukocyte Biol* 1994; 56:203–209.
24. Bishop JM. Viral oncogenes. *Cell* 1985; 42:23–38.
25. Weinberg RA. The action of oncogenes in the cytoplasm and nucleus. *Science* 1985; 230: 770–776.
26. Land H, Parada LF, Weinberg RA. Tumorigenic conversion of primary embryo fibroblasts requires at least two cooperating oncogenes. *Nature* 1983; 304:596–602.
27. Vile RG. Tumor-specific gene expression. *Semin Cancer Biol* 1994; 5:429–436.
28. Wickstrom EL, Bacon TA, Gonzalez A, Freeman DL, Lyman GH, Wickstrom E. Human promyelocytic leukemia HL-60 cell proliferation and c-myc protein expression are inhibited by an antisense pentadecadeoxynucleotide targeted against c-*myc* mRNA. *Proc Natl Acad Sci USA* 1988; 85:1028–1032.
29. Rosolen A, Whitesell L, Ikegaki N, Kennett RH, Neckers LM. Antisense inhibition of single copy N-*myc* expression results in decreased cell growth without reduction of c-myc protein in a neuroepithelioma cell line. *Cancer Res* 1990; 50:6316–6322.
30. Saison-Behmoaras T, Tocque B, Rey I, Chassignol M, Thuong NT, Helene C. Short modified antisense oligonucleotides directed against Ha-*ras* point mutation induce selective cleavage of the mRNA and inhibit T24 cells proliferation. *EMBO J* 1991; 10:1111–1118.
31. Szczylik C, Skorski T, Nicolaides NC, Manzella L, Malaguarnera L, Venturelli D, Gewirtz AM, Calabretta B. Selective inhibition of leukemia cell proliferation by *bcr-abl* antisense oligodeoxynucleotides. *Science* 1991; 253:562–565.
32. Nitta T, Sato K. Inhibition of c-sis protein synthesis and cell growth with antisense oligonucleotides in human glioma cells. *No Shinkei Geka* 1992; 20:857–863.
33. Robinson-Benion C, Li YX, Holt JT. Gene transplantation: combined antisense inhibition and gene replacement strategies. *Leukemia* 1994; 8:S152–S155.
34. Mukhopadhyay T, Tainsky M, Cavender AC, Roth JA. Specific inhibition of K-*ras* expression and tumorigenicity of lung cancer cells by antisense RNA. *Cancer Res* 1991; 51:1744–1748.
35. Trojan J, Johnson TR, Rudin SD, Ilan J, Tykocinski ML. Treatment and prevention of rat glioblastoma by immunogenic C6 cells expressing antisense insulin-like growth factor I RNA. *Science* 1993; 259:94–97.
36. Ohta Y, Tone T, Shitara T, Funato T, Jiao L, Kashfian BI, Yoshida E, Horng M, Tsai P, Lauterbach K, Kashani-Sabet M, Florenes VA, Fodstad O, Scanlon KJ. H-*ras* ribozyme-mediated alteration of the human melanoma phenotype. *Ann NY Acad Sci* 1994; 716:242–253.
37. Lange W, Cantin EM, Finke J, Dolken G. In vitro and in vivo effects of synthetic ribozymes targeted against bcr/abl mRNA. *Leukemia* 1993; 7:1786–1794.
38. Weinberg RA. Tumor suppressor genes. *Science* 1991; 254:1138–1146.
39. Hall PA, Lane DP. Genetics of growth arrest and cell death: Key determinants of tissue homeostasis. *Eur J Cancer* 1994; 30A:2001–2012.
40. Yonish-Rouach E, Grunwald D, Wilder S, Kimchi A, May E, Lawrence JJ, May P, Oren M. p53-mediated cell death—relationship to cell cycle control. *Mol Cell Biol* 1993; 13:1415–1423.
41. Roemer K, Friedman T. Mechanisms of action of the p53 tumor suppressor and prospects for cancer gene therapy by reconstitution of p53 function. *Ann NY Acad Sci* 1994; 716:265–280.
42. Lane DP. The regulation of p53 function. *Int J Cancer* 1994; 57:623–627.
43. Lotem J, Sachs L. Regulation by bcl-2, c-*myc*, and p53 of susceptibility to induction of apoptosis by heat shock and cancer chemotherapy compounds in differentiation-competent and differentiation-defective myeloid leukemic cells. *Cell Growth Differ* 1993; 4:41–47.
44. Lowe SW, Schmitt EM, Smith SW, Osborne BA, Jacks T. p53 is required for radiation-induced apoptosis in mouse thymocytes. *Nature* 1993; 362:847–849.
45. Clayman GL, Elnaggar AK, Roth JA, Zhang WW, Goepfert H, Taylor DL, Liu TJ. In vivo molecular therapy with p53 adenovirus for microscopic residual head and neck squamous carcinoma. *Cancer Res* 1995; 55:1–6.

46. Oren M. Relationship of p53 to the control of apoptotic cell death. *Semin Cancer Biol* 1994; 5: 221–227.

47. Wills KN, Maneval DC, Menzel P, Harris MP, Sutjipto S, Vaillancourt MT, Huang WM, Johnson DE, Anderson SC, Wen SF, Bookstein R, Shepard HM, Gregory RJ. Development and characterization of recombinant adenoviruses encoding human p53 for gene therapy of cancer. *Hum Gene Ther* 1994; 5:1079–1088.

48. Cobrinik D, Dowdy SF, Hinds PW, Mittnacht S, Weinberg RA. The retinoblastoma protein and the regulation of cell cycling. *Trends Biochem Sci* 1992; 17:312–315.

49. Hollingsworth RE Jr, Hensey CE, Lee WH. Retinoblastoma protein and the cell cycle. *Curr Opinion Genet Dev* 1993; 3:55–62.

50. Cao L, Faha B, Dembski M, Tsai LH, Harlow E, Dyson N. Independent binding of the retinoblastoma protein and p107 to the transcription factor E2F. *Nature* 1992; 355:176–179.

51. Shirodkar S, Ewen M, Decaprio JA, Morgan J, Livingston DM, Chittenden T. The transcription factor E2F interacts with the retinoblastoma product and a p107-Cyclin-A complex in a cell cycle-regulated manner. *Cell* 1992; 68:157–166.

52. Xu HJ, Xu K, Zhou YL, Li J, Benedict WF, Hu SX. Enhanced tumor cell growth suppression by an N-terminal truncated retinoblastoma protein. *Proc Natl Acad Sci USA* 1994; 91: 9837–9841.

53. Chang MW, Barr E, Seltzer J, Jiang YQ, Nabel GJ, Nabel EG, Parmacek MS, Leiden JM. Cytostatic gene therapy for vascular proliferative disorders with a constitutively active form of the retinoblastoma gene product. *Science* 1995; 267:518–522.

54. Oldfield EH, Ram Z, Culver KW, Blaese RM, Devroom HL. Gene therapy for the treatment of brain tumors using intra-tumoral transduction with the thymidine kinase gene and intravenous ganciclovir. *Hum Gene Ther* 1993; 4:39–69.

55. Culver KW, Van Gilder J, Link CJ, Carlstrom T, Buroker T, Yuh W, Koch K, Schabold K, Doornbas S, Wetjen B, et al. Gene therapy for the treatment of malignant brain tumors with in vivo tumor transduction with the herpes simplex thymidine kinase gene/ganciclovir system. *Hum Gene Ther* 1994; 5:343–379.

56. Culver KW, Ram Z, Wallbridge S, Ishii H, Oldfield EH, Blaese RM. In vivo gene transfer with retroviral vector producer cells for treatment of experimental brain tumors. *Science* 1992; 256:1550–1552.

57. Ram Z, Walbridge S, Shawker T, Culver KW, Blaese RM, Oldfield EH, The effect of thymidine kinase transduction and ganciclovir therapy on tumor vasculature and growth of 9L gliomas in rats. *J Neurosurg* 1994; 81:256–260.

58. Caruso M, Panis Y, Gagandeep S, Houssin D, Salzmann JL, Klatzmann D. Regression of established macroscopic liver metastases after in situ transduction of a suicide gene. *Proc Natl Acad Sci USA* 1993; 90:7024–7028.

59. Barba D, Hardin J, Sadelain M, Gage FH. Development of anti-tumor immunity following thymidine kinase-mediated killing of experimental brain tumors. *Proc Natl Acad Sci USA* 1994; 91:4348–4352.

60. Vile RG, Nelson JA, Castleden S, Chong H, Hart IR. Systemic gene therapy of murine melanoma using tissue specific expression of the HSVtk gene involves an immune component. *Cancer Res* 1994; 54:6228–6234.

61. Mullen CA, Kilstrup M, Blaese RM. Transfer of the bacterial gene for cytosine deaminase to mammalian cells confers lethal sensitivity to 5-fluorocytosine: a negative selection system. *Proc Natl Acad Sci USA* 1992; 89:33–37.

62. Huber BE, Richards CA, Austin EA, Virus-directed enzyme/prodrug therapy (VDEPT). Selectively engineering drug sensitivity into tumors. *Ann NY Acad Sci* 1994; 716:104–114.

63. Mullen CA, Coale MM, Lowe R, Blaese RM. Tumors expressing the cytosine deaminase suicide gene can be eliminated in vivo with 5-fluorocytosine and induce protective immunity to wild type tumor. *Cancer Res* 1994; 54:1503–1506.

64. Huber BE, Richards CA, Krenitsky TA. Retroviral-mediated gene therapy for the treatment of hepatocellular carcinoma: an innovative approach for cancer therapy. *Proc Natl Acad Sci USA* 1991; 88:8039–8043.

65. Yasumoto K, Yokoyama K, Shibata K, Tomita Y, Shibahara S. Microphthalmia-associated

transcription factor as a regulator for melanocyte-specific transcription of the human tyrosinase gene. *Mol Cell Biol* 1994; 14:8058–8070.

66. Hwu P, Yannelli JR, Kriegler M, Anderson WF, Perez C, Chiang YWL, Schwarz S, Cowherd R, Delgado C, Mule JJ, et al. Functional and molecular characterization of tumor-infiltrating lymphocytes transduced with tumor necrosis factor-alpha cDNA for the gene therapy of cancer in humans. *J Immunol* 1993; 150:4104–4115.

67. Hwu P, Rosenberg SA. The use of gene-modified tumor-infiltrating lymphocytes for cancer therapy. *Ann NY Acad Sci* 1994; 716:188–197.

68. Eshhar Z, Waks T, Gross G, Schindler DG. Specific activation and targeting of cytotoxic lymphocytes through chimeric single chains consisting of antibody-binding domains and the gamma or zeta subunits of the immunoglobulin and T-cell receptors. *Proc Natl Acad Sci USA* 1993; 90:720–724.

69. Hwu P, Shafer GE, Treisman J, Schindler DG, Gross G, Cowherd R, Rosenberg SA, Eshhar Z. Lysis of ovarian cancer cells by human lymphocytes redirected with a chimeric gene composed of an antibody variable region and the Fc-receptor gamma-chain. *J Exp Med* 1993; 178:361–366.

70. Stancovski I, Schindler DG, Waks T, Yarden Y, Sela M, Eshhar Z. Targeting of T-lymphocytes to *neu/her2*-expressing cells using chimeric single chain Fv receptors. *J Immunol* 1993; 151:6577–6582.

71. Cottesman MM, Germann UA, Aksentijevich I, Sugimoto Y, Cardarelli CO, Pastan I. Gene transfer of drug resistance genes. Implications for cancer therapy. *Ann NY Acad Sci* 1994; 716:26–38.

72. Boesen JJ, Nooter K, Valerio D. Circumvention of chemotherapy-induced myelosuppression by transfer of the *mdr1* gene. *Biotherapy* 1993; 6:291–302.

73. Morton DL. Active immunotherapy against cancer. Present status. *Semin Oncol* 1986; 13: 180–185.

74. McCune CS, O'Donnell RW, Marquis DM, Sahasrabudhe DM. Renal cell carcinoma treated by vaccines for active specific immunotherapy: Correlation of survival with skin testing by autologous tumor cells. *Cancer Immunol Immunother* 1990; 32:62–66.

75. Mitchell MS, Harel W, Kempf RA, Hu E, Kan-Mitchell J, Boswell WD, Dean G, Stevenson L. Active-specific immunotherapy for melanoma. *J Clin Oncol* 1990; 8:856–869.

76. Morton DL, Foshag LJ, Hoon DSB. Prolongation of survival in metastatic melanoma after active specific immunotherapy with a new polyvalent melanoma vaccine. *Ann Surg* 1993; 217:309.

77. Rosenberg SA, Lotze MT, Muul LM, Chang AE, Avis FP, Leitman S, Linehan WM, Robertson CN, Lee RE, Rubin JT, Seipp CA, Simpson CG, White DE. A progress report on the treatment of 157 patients with advanced cancer with lymphokine-activated killer cells and interleukin-2 or high dose interleukin-2 alone. *N Engl J Med* 1987; 316:889.

78. Rosenberg SA, Packard BS, Aebersold PM, Solomon D, Topalian SL, Toy ST, Simon P, Lotze MT, Yang JC, Seipp CA, Simpson C, Carter C, Bock S, Schwarzentruber D, Wei JP, White DE. Use of tumor-infiltrating lymphocytes and interleukin-2 in the immunotherapy of patients with metastatic melanoma. *N Engl J Med* 1988; 319:1676–1680.

79. Cole WH. Spontaneous regression of cancer and the importance of finding its cause. *Natl Cancer Inst Monogr* 1976; 44:5–9.

80. Nathanson A. Spontaneous regression of malignant melanoma: a review of the literature on incidence, clinical features, and possible mechanisms. *Natl Cancer Inst Monogr* 1976; 44: 67–76.

81. Nishimura K, Okada Y, Okada K, Yoshida O, Amitani R, Kubo Y, Ushida S. Spontaneous regression of pulmonary metastasis from renal pelvic cancer. *Urol Int* 1987; 42:461–463.

82. Rosenberg SA. Immunotherapy and gene therapy of cancer. *Cancer Res* 1991; 51:S5074–S5079.

83. Linehan WM, Walther MM, Alexander RB, Rosenberg SA. Adoptive immunotherapy of renal cell carcinoma: studies from the Surgery Branch, National Cancer Institute. *Semin Urol* 1993; 11:41–43.

84. Ortaldo JR, Longo DL. Human natural lymphocyte effector cells: Definition, analysis of activity, and clinical effectiveness. *J Natl Cancer Inst* 1988; 80:999–1010.

85. Topalian SL, Solomon D, Rosenberg SA. Tumor-specific cytolysis by lymphocytes infiltrating human melanomas. *J Immunol* 1989; 142:3714–3725.

86. Bjorkman PJ, Parham P. Structure, function, and diversity of Class I major histocompatibility complex molecules. *Annu Rev Biochem* 1990; 59:253–288.

87. Hoglund P, Ljunggren HG, Kärre K, Jay G. Role of major histocompatibility complex Class I molecules in tumor rejection—new insights from studies with synthetic peptides and transgenic mice. *Immunol Res* 1990; 9:298–313.

88. Browning MJ, Bodmer WF. MHC antigens and cancer-implications for T-cell surveillance. *Curr Opinion Immunol* 1992; 4:613–618.

89. Mellief CJM, Kast WM. Lessons from T-cell responses to virus-induced tumors for cancer eradication in general. *Cancer Surveys* 1992; 13:81–91.

90. Degiovanni G, Lahaye T, Herin M, Hainaut P, Boon T. Antigenic heterogeneity of a human melanoma detected by autologous CTL clones. *Eur J Immunol* 1988; 18:671–676.

91. Anichini A, Mazzocchi A, Fossati G, Parmiani G. Cytotoxic T-lymphocyte clones from peripheral blood and from tumor site detect intratumor heterogeneity of melanoma cells. Analysis of specificity and mechanisms of interaction. *J Immunol* 1989; 142:3692–3701.

92. Wölfel T, Klehmann E, Müller CA, Schütt KH, Meyer zum Büschenfelde KH, Knuth A. Lysis of human melanoma cells by autologous cytolytic T-cell clones. Identification of human histocompatibility leukocyte antigen A2 as a restriction element for three different antigens. *J Exp Med* 1989; 170:797–810.

93. Mukherji B, Chakraborty NG, Sivanandham M. T-cell clones that react against autologous human tumors. *Immunol Rev* 1990; 116:33–62.

94. Knuth A, Wölfel T, Meyer zum Büschenfelde KH. T-cell responses to human malignant tumours *Cancer Surveys* 1992; 13:39–52.

95. Koo AS, Tso CL, Shimabukuro T, Peyret C, Dekernion JB, Belldegrun A. Autologous tumor-specific cytotoxicity of tumor-infiltrating lymphocytes derived from human renal cell carcinoma. *J Immunother* 1991; 10:347–354.

96. Finke JH, Rayman P, Edinger M, Tubbs RR, Stanley J, Klein E, Bukowski R. Characterization of a human renal cell carcinoma specific cytotoxic CD8+ T-cell line. *J Immunother* 1992; 11:1–11.

97. Schendel DJ, Gansbacher B, Oberneder R, Kriegmair M, Hofstetter A, Riethmüller G, Segurado OG. Tumor-specific lysis of human renal cell carcinomas by tumor-infiltrating lymphocytes. I. HLA-A2-restricted recognition of autologous and allogeneic tumor lines. *J Immunol* 1993; 151:4209–4220.

98. Bernhard H, Maeurer MJ, Wölfel T, Karbach J, Schneider J, Storkus W, Huber C, Meyer zum Büschenfelde KH, Knuth A. HLA-A2 restricted cytotoxic T-lymphocytes clones recognize a shared peptide epitope on human renal cancer cells. *Proc Am Assoc Cancer Res* 1994; 35:494.

99. Shimizu Y, Weidmann E, Iwatsuki S, Heberman RB, Whiteside TL. Characterization of human autotumor-reactive T-cell clones obtained from tumor-infiltrating lymphocytes in liver metastasis of gastric carcinoma. *Cancer Res* 1991; 51:6153–6162.

100. Wölfel T, Herr W, Coulie P, Schmitt U, Meyer zum Büschenfilde KH, Knuth A. Lysis of human pancreatic adenocarcinoma cells by autologous HLA- class-I-restricted cytolytic T-lymphocyte (CTL) clones. *Int J Cancer* 1993; 54:636–644.

101. Crowley NJ, Darrow TL, Quinn-Allen MA, Seigler HF. MHC-restricted recognition of autologous melanoma by tumor-specific cytotoxic T-cells—Evidence for restriction by a dominant HLA-A allele. *J Immunol* 1991; 146:1692–1696.

102. Kawakami Y, Zakut R, Topalian SL, Stotter H, Rosenberg SA. Shared human melanoma antigens—recognition by tumor-infiltrating lymphocytes in HLA-A2.1-transfected melanomas. *J Immunol* 1992; 148:638–643.

103. Van der Bruggen P, Traversari C, Chomez P, Lurquin C, De Plaen E, Van den Eynde B, Knuth A, Boon T. A gene encoding an antigen recognized by cytolytic T-lymphocytes on a human melanoma. *Science* 1991; 254:1643–1647.

104. Gaugler B, Van den Eynde B, Van der Bruggen P, Romero P, Gaforio JJ, De Plaen E, Lethe B, Brasseur F, Boon T. Human gene MAGE-3 codes for an antigen recognized on a melanoma by autologous cytolytic T-lymphocytes. *J Exp Med* 1994; 179:921–930.

105. Kawakami Y, Eliyahu S, Delgado CH, Robbins PF, Rivoltini L, Topalian SL, Miki T, Rosenberg SA. Cloning of the gene for a shared human melanoma antigen recognized by autologous T-cells infiltrating into tumor. *Proc Natl Acad Sci USA* 1994; 91:3515–3519.

106. Coulie PG, Brichard V, Van Pel A, Wolfel T, Schneider J, Traversari C, Mattei S, De Plaen E, Lurquin C, Szikora JP, Boon T. A new gene coding for a differentiation antigen recognized by autologous cytolytic lymphocytes on HLA-A2 melanomas. *J Exp Med* 1994; 180:35–42.

107. Brichard V, Van Pel A, Wölfel C, De Plaen E, Lethe B, Coulie P, Boon T. The tyrosinase gene codes for an antigen recognized by autologous cytolytic T-lymphocytes on HLA-A2 melanomas. *J Exp Med* 1993; 178:489–495.

108. Bakker ABH, Schreurs MJW, De Boer AJ, Kawakami Y, Rosenberg SA, Adema GJ, Figdor CG. Melanocyte lineage-specific antigen gp100 is recognized by melanoma-derived tumor infiltrating lymphocytes. *J Exp Med* 1994; 179:1005–1009.

109. Kawakami Y, Eliyahu S, Delgado CH, Robbins PF, Sakaguchi K, Appella E, Yannelli JR, Adema GJ, Miki T, Rosenberg SA. Identification of a human melanoma antigen recognized by tumor-infiltrating lymphocytes associated with in vivo tumor rejection. *Proc Natl Acad Sci USA* 1994; 91:6458–6462.

110. Brasseur F, Marchand M, Van Wijck R, Herin M, Lethe B, Chomez P, Boon T. Human gene MAGE-1, which codes for a tumor rejection antigen, is expressed by some breast tumors. *Int J Cancer* 1992; 52:839–841.

111. Rimoldi D, Romero P, Carrel S. The human melanoma antigen-encoding gene, MAGE-1, is expressed by other tumour cells of neuroectodermal origin such as glioblastomas and neuro-blastomas. *Int J Cancer* 1993; 54:527–528.

112. Weynants P, Lethe B, Brasseur F, Marchand M, Boon T, Expression of Mage genes by non-small-cell lung carcinomas. *Int J Cancer* 1994; 56:826–829.

113. Traversari C, Van der Bruggen P, Leuscher IF, Lurquin C, Chomez P, Van Pel A, De Plaen E, Amarcostesec A, Boon T. A nonapeptide encoded by human gene MAGE-1 is recognized on HLA-A1 by cytolytic T-lymphocytes directed against tumor antigen-MZ2-E. *J Exp Med* 1992; 176:1453–1457.

114. Wölfel T, Van Pel A, Brichard V, Schneider J, Seliger B, Meyer zum Büschenfelde KH, Boon T. Two tyrosinase nonapeptides recognized on HLA-A2 melanomas by autologous cytolytic T-lymphocytes. *Eur J Immunol* 1994; 24:759–764.

115. Robbins PF, El-Gamil M, Kawakami Y, Stevens E, Yannelli JR, Rosenberg SA. Recognition of tyrosinase by tumor-infiltrating lymphocytes from a patient responding to immunotherapy. *Cancer Res* 1994; 54:3124–3126.

116. Van der Bruggen P, Szikora JP, Boel P, Wildmann C, Somville M, Sensi M, Boon T. Autologous cytolytic T-lymphocytes recognize a Mage-1 nonapeptide on melanomas expressing HLA-Cw*1601. *Eur J Immunol* 1994; 24:2134–2140.

117. Falk K, Rötzschke O, Stevanovic S, Jung G, Rammensee HG. Allele-specific motifs revealed by sequencing of self-peptides eluted from MHC molecules. *Nature* 1991; 351:290–296.

118. Hunt DF, Henderson RA, Shabanowitz J, Sakaguchi K, Michel H, Sevilir N, Cox AL, Appella E, Engelhard VH. Characterization of peptides bound to the Class-I MHC molecule HLA-A21.1 by mass spectrometry. *Science* 1992; 255:1261–1263.

119. Nijman HW, Houbiers JGA, Vierboom MPM, Van der Burg SH, Drijfhout JW, Damaro J, Kenemans P, Melief CJM, Kast WM. Identification of peptide sequences that potentially trigger HLA-A2.1-restricted cytotoxic T-lymphocytes. *Eur J Immunol* 1993; 23:1215–1219.

120. Visseren MJW, Van Elsas A, Van der Voort EIH, Ressing ME, Kast WM, Schrier PI, Melief CJM. Cytotoxic T-lymphocytes specific for the tyrosinase autoantigen can be induced from healthy donor blood to lyse melanoma cells. *J Immunol* 1995; 154:3991–3998.

121. Celis E, Tsai V, Crimi C, DeMars R, Wentworth PA, Chesnut RW, Grey HM, Sette A, Serra HM. Induction of anti-tumor cytotoxic T lymphocytes in normal humans using primary cultures and synthetic peptide epitopes. *Proc Natl Acad Sci USA* 1994; 91:2105–2109.

122. Houbiers JGA, Nijman HW, Van der Burg SH, Drijfhout JW, Kenemans P, Van de Velde CJH, Brand A, Momburg F, Kast WM, Melief CJM. In vitro induction of human cytotoxic T-lymphocyte responses against peptides of mutant and wild-type p53. *Eur J Immunol* 1993; 23:2072–2077.

123. Van Elsas A, Nijman HW, Van der Minne CE, Mourer SJ, Kast WM, Melief CJM, Schrier PI. Induction and characterization of cytotoxic T-lymphocytes recognizing mutated p21*ras* peptide presented by HLA-A*0201. *Int J Cancer* 1995; 6:389–396.

124. Stauss HJ, Davies H, Sadovnikova E, Chain B, Horowitz N, Sinclair C. Induction of cytotoxic T-lymphocytes with peptides in vitro—identification of candidate T-cell epitopes in human papilloma virus. *Proc Natl Acad Sci USA* 1992; 89:7871–7875.

125. Kast WM, Brandt RMP, Drijfhout JW, Melief CJM. Human leukocyte antigen-A2.1 restricted candidate cytotoxic T-lymphocyte epitopes of human papillomavirus type-16 E6-protein and E7-protein identified by using the processing-defective human cell line-T2. *J Immunother* 1993; 14:115–120.

126. Feltkamp MCW, Smits HL, Vierboom MPM, Minnaar RP, De Jongh BM, Drijfhout JW, Ter Schegget J, Melief CJM, Kast WM. Vaccination with cytotoxic T-lymphocyte epitope-containing peptide protects against a tumor induced by Human Papillomavirus type-16-transformed cells. *Eur J Immunol* 1993; 23:2242–2249.

127. Minev BR, McFarland BJ, Spiess PJ, Rosenberg SA, Restifo NP. Insertion signal sequence fused to minimal peptides elicits specific CD8+ T-cell responses and prolongs survival of thymoma-bearing mice. *Cancer Res* 1994; 54:4155–4161.

128. Gelber C, Plaksin D, Vadai E, Feldman M, Eisenbach L. Abolishment of metastasis formation by murine tumor cells transfected with "foreign" H-2K genes. *Cancer Res* 1989; 49:2366–2373.

129. Hui KM, Sim TF, Foo TT, Oei AA. Tumor rejection mediated by transfection with allogeneic Class-I histocompatibility gene. *J Immunol* 1989; 143:3835–3843.

130. Ostrand-Rosenberg S, Roby C, Clements VK, Cole GA. Tumor-specific immunity can be enhanced by transfection of tumor cells with syngeneic MHC-Class-II genes or allogeneic MHC-Class-I genes. *Int J Cancer* 1991; 61–68.

131. Greenberg PD. Adoptive T-cell therapy of tumors—mechanisms operative in the recognition and elimination of tumor cells. *Adv Immunol* 1991; 49:281–355.

132. Melief CJM. Tumor eradication by adoptive transfer of cytotoxic T-lymphocytes. *Adv Cancer Res* 58:143–175.

133. Elliott BE, Carlow DA, Rodricks AM, Wade A. Perspectives on the role of MHC antigens in normal and malignant cell development. *Adv Cancer Res* 1989; 53:181–245.

134. Versteeg R, Noordermeer IA, Krüse-Wolters KM, Ruiter DJ, Schrier PI. c-*Myc* downregulates class I HLA expression in human melanomas. *EMBO J* 1988; 7:1023–1029.

135. North RJ, Awwad M, Dunn PL. The immune response to tumors. *Transplant. Proc.* 1989; 21:575–577.

136. Radrizzani M, Benedetti B, Castelli C, Longo A, Ferrara GB, Herlyn M, Parmiani G, Fossati G. Human allogeneic melanoma-reactive T-helper lymphocyte clones—functional analysis of lymphocyte-melanoma interactions. *Int J Cancer* 1991; 49:823–830.

137. Finke JH, Zea AH, Stanley J, Longo DL, Mizoguchi H, Tubbs RR, Wiltrout RH, Oshea JJ, Kudoh S, Klein E, Bukowski RM, Ochoa AC. Loss of T-cell receptor zeta-chain and p56(*lck*) in T-cells infiltrating human renal cell carcinoma. *Cancer Res* 1993; 53:5613–5616.

138. Restifo NP, Esquivel F, Kawakami Y, Yewdell JW, Mule JJ, Rosenberg SA, Bennink JR. Identification of human cancers deficient in antigen processing. *J Exp Med* 1993; 177:265–272.

139. Ranges GE, Figari IS, Espevik T, Palladino MA, Jr. Inhibition of cytotoxic T-cell development by transforming growth factor beta and reversal by recombinant tumor necrosis factor alpha. *J Exp Med* 1987; 166:991–998.

140. Inge TH, Hoover SK, Susskind BM, Barrett SK, Bear HD. Inhibition of tumor-specific cytotoxic T-lymphocyte responses by transforming growth factor-beta 1. *Cancer Res* 1992; 52:1386–1392.

141. Torre-Amione G, Beauchamp RD, Koeppen H, Park BH, Schreiber H, Moses HL, Rowley DA. A highly immunogenic tumor transfected with a murine transforming growth factor type beta 1 cDNA escapes immune surveillance. *Proc Natl Acad Sci USA* 1990; 87:1486–1490.

142. Hewitt HB, Blake ER, Walder AS. *Br J Cancer* 1976; 33:241–259.

143. Isobe K, Hasegawa Y, Iwamoto T, Hasegawa T, Kawashima K, Ding L, Nakashima I. Induction of antitumor immunity in mice by allo-Major Histocompatibility Complex Class-I gene transfectant with strong antigen expression. *J Nat Cancer Inst* 1989; 81:1823–1828.

144. Maio M, Altomonte M, Tatake R, Zeff RA, Ferrone S. Reduction in susceptibility to natural killer cell mediated lysis of human FO-1 melanoma cells after induction of HLA Class-I antigen expression by transfection with β_2m gene. *J Clin Invest* 1991; 88:282–289.

145. Boon T, Van Pel A, De Plaen E. Tum⁻ transplantation antigens, point mutations and antigenic peptides: a model for tumor-specific transplantation antigens. *Cancer Cells* 1989; 1: 25–28.

146. Fearon ER, Itaya T, Hunt B, Vogelstein B, Frost P. Induction in a murine tumor of immunogenic tumor variants by transfection with a foreign gene. *Cancer Res* 1988; 38:2975–2980.

147. Schirrmacher V, Schlag P, Liebrich W, Patel BT, Stoeck M. Specific immunotherapy of colorectal carcinoma with newcastle-disease virus-modified autologous tumor cells prepared from resected liver metastasis. *Ann NY Acad Sci* 1993; 690:364–366.

148. Azuma M, Cayabyab M, Buck D, Phillips JH, Lanier LL. Involvement of CD28 in MHC-unrestricted cytotoxicity mediated by a human natural killer leukemia cell line. *J Immunol* 1992; 149:1115–1123.

149. Hayashi H, Matsubara H, Yokota T, Kuwabara I, Kanno M, Koseki H, Isono K, Asano T, Taniguchi M. Molecular cloning and characterization of the gene encoding mouse melanoma antigen by cDNA library transfection. *J Immunol* 1992; 149:1223–1229.

150. Chen LP, Ashe S, Brady WA, Hellstrom I, Hellstrom KE, Ledbetter JA, Mcgowan P, Linsley PS. Costimulation of antitumor immunity by the B7 counterreceptor for the T-lymphocyte molecules CD28 and CTLA-4. *Cell* 1992; 71:1093–1102.

151. Townsend SE, Allison JP. Tumor rejection after direct costimulation of CD8+ T-cells by B7-transfected melanoma cells. *Science* 1993; 259:368–370.

152. Chen LP, Mcgowan P, Ashe S, Johnston J, Li YW, Hellstrom I, Hellstrom KE. Tumor immunogenicity determines the effect of B7 costimulation on T-cell-mediated tumor immunity. *J Exp Med* 1994; 179:523–532.

153. Baskar S, Ostrand-Rosenberg S, Nabavi N, Nadler LM, Freeman GJ, Glimcher LH. Constitutive expression of B7 restores immunogenicity of tumor cells expressing truncated major histocompatibility complex class-II molecules. *Proc Natl Acad Sci USA* 1993; 90:5687–690.

154. Dohring C, Angman L, Spagnoli G, Lanzavecchia A. T-helper- and accessory-cell-independent cytotoxic responses to human tumor cells transfected with a B7 retroviral vector. *Int J Cancer* 1994; 57:754–759.

155. Douvdevani A, Huleihel M, Zoller M, Segal S, Apte RN. Reduced tumorigenicity of fibrosarcomas which constitutively generate IL-1-alpha either spontaneously or following IL-1-alpha gene transfer. *Int J Cancer* 1992; 51:822–830.

156. Fearon ER, Pardoll DM, Itaya T, Golumbek P, Levitsky HI, Simons JW, Karasuyama H, Vogelstein B, Frost P. Interleukin-2 production by tumor cells bypasses T-helper function in the generation of an antitumor response. *Cell* 1990; 60:397–403.

157. Gansbacher B, Zier K, Daniels B, Cronin K, Bannerji R, Gilboa E. Interleukin-2 gene transfer into tumor cells abrogates tumorigenicity and induces protected immunity. *J Exp Med* 1990; 172:1217–1224.

158. Ley V, Langlade-Demoyen P, Kourilsky P, Larsson-Sciard EL. Interleukin-2-dependent activation of tumor-specific cytotoxic T-lymphocytes in vivo. *Eur J Immunol* 1991; 21:851–854.

159. Connor J, Bannerji R, Saito S, Heston W, Fair W, Gilboa E. Regression of bladder tumors in mice treated with interleukin-2 gene-modified tumor cells. *J Exp Med* 1993; 177:1127–1134.

160. Hock H, Dorsch M, Kunzendorf U, Qin ZH, Diamantstein T, Blankenstein T. Mechanisms of rejection induced by tumor cell-targeted gene transfer of interleukin-2, interleukin-4, interleukin-7, tumor necrosis factor, or interferon-gamma. *Proc Natl Acad Sci USA* 1993; 90: 2774–2778.

161. Porgador A, Gansbacher B, Bannerji R, Tzehoval E, Gilboa E, Feldman M, Eisenbach L. Anti-metastatic vaccination of tumor-bearing mice with IL-2-gene-inserted tumor cells. *Int J Cancer* 1993; 53:471–474.

162. Blankenstein T, Li W, Müller W, Diamantsein T. Retroviral Interleukin-4 gene transfer into a Interleukin-4-dependent cell line results in autocrine growth but not in tumorigenicity. *Eur J Immunol* 1990; 20:935–938.

163. Golumbek PT, Lazenby AJ, Levitsky HI, Jaffee LM, Karasuyama H, Baker M, Pardoll DM. Treatment of established renal cancer by tumor cells engineered to secrete interleukin-4. *Science* 1991; 254:713–716.

164. Tepper RI, Pattengale PK, Leder P. Murine interleukin-4 displays potent anti-tumor activity in vivo. *Cell* 1989; 57:503–512.

165. Mullen CA, Coale MM, Levy AT, Stetler-Stevenson WG, Liotta LA, Brandt S, Blaese RM. Fibrosarcoma cells transduced with the IL-6 gene exhibited reduced tumorigenicity, increased immunogenicity, and decreased metastatic potential. *Cancer Res* 1992; 52:6020–6024.

166. Porgador A, Tzehoval E, Vadai E, Feldman M, Eisenbach L. Immunotherapy via gene therapy - comparison of the effects of tumor cells transduced with the interleukin-2, interleukin-6, or interferon-gamma genes. *J Immunother* 1993; 14:191–201.

167. Hock H, Dorsch M, Diamantstein T, Blankenstein T. Interleukin-7 induces CD4$^+$ T-cell-dependent tumor rejection. *J Exp Med* 1991; 174:1291–1298.

168. Miller AR, McBride WH, Dubinett SM, Dougherty GJ, Thacker JD, Shau HG, Kohn DB, Moen RC, Walker MJ, Chiu R, Schuck BL, Rosenblatt JA, Huang M, Dhanani S, Rhoades K, Economou JS. Transduction of human melanoma cell lines with the human interleukin-7 gene using retroviral-mediated gene transfer - comparison of immunologic properties with interleukin-2. *Blood* 1993; 82:3686–3694.

169. Tahara H, Zeh HJ, Storkus WJ, Pappo I, Watkins SC, Gubler U, Wolf SF, Robbins PD, Lotze MT. Fibroblasts genetically engineered to secrete interleukin-12 can suppress tumor growth and induce antitumor immunity to a murine melanoma in vivo. *Cancer Res* 1994; 54: 182–189.

170. Watanabe Y, Kuribayashi K, Miyatake S, Nishihara K, Nakayama E, Taniyama T, Sakata T. Exogenous expression of mouse interferon-γ cDNA in mouse C1300 neuroblastoma cells results in reduced tumorigenicity by augmented anti-tumor immunity. *Proc Natl Acad Sci USA* 1989; 86:456–9460.

171. Gansbacher B, Bannerji R, Daniels B, Zier K, Cronin K, Gilboa E. Retroviral vector-mediated γ-interferon gene transfer into tumor cells generates potent and long lasting anti-tumor immunity. *Cancer Res* 1990; 50:7820–7825.

172. Restifo NP, Spiess PJ, Karp SE, Mulé JJ, Rosenberg SA. A nonimmunogenic sarcoma transduced with the cDNA for interferon-gamma elicits CD8$^+$ T-cells against the wild-type tumor — correlation with antigen presentation capability. *J Exp Med* 1992; 175:1423–1431.

173. Porgador A, Bannerji R, Watanabe Y, Feldman M, Gilboa E, Eisenbach L. Antimetastatic vaccination of tumor-bearing mice with 2 types of IFN-gamma gene-inserted tumor cells. *J Immunol* 1993; 150:1458–1470.

174. Shiloni E, Karp SE, Custer MC, Shilyansky J, Restifo NP, Rosenberg SA, Mule JJ. Retroviral transduction of interferon-gamma cDNA into a nonimmunogenic murine fibrosarcoma: generation of T-cells in draining lymph nodes capable of treating established parental metastatic tumor. *Cancer Immunol Immunother* 1993; 37:286–292.

175. Blankenstein T, Qin Z, Überla K, Müller W, Rosen H, Volk H-D, Diamantstein T. Tumor suppression after tumor cell-targeted tumor necrosis factor-α gene transfer. *J Exp Med* 1991; 173:1047–1057.

176. Itoh Y, Kohgo Y, Watanabe N, Kanisawa Y, Sakamaki S, Takahashi M, Hirayama Y, Ono H, Himeno T, Niitsu Y. Human tumor-infiltrating lymphocytes transfected with tumor necrosis factor gene could augment cytotoxicity to autologous tumor cells. *Jpn J Cancer Res* 1991; 82: 1203–1206.

177. Hoon DSB, Hayashi Y, Morisaki T, Foshag LJ, Morton DL. Interleukin-4 plus tumor necrosis factor alpha augments the antigenicity of melanoma cells. *Cancer Immunol Immunother* 1993; 37:378–384.

178. Marincola FM, Ettinghausen S, Cohen PA, Cheshire LB, Restifo NP, Mule JJ, Rosenberg SA. Treatment of established lung metastases with tumor-infiltrating lymphocytes derived from a poorly immunogenic tumor engineered to secrete human TNF-alpha. *J Immunol* 1994; 152: 3500–3513.

179. Colombo MP, Ferrara G, Stoppacciaro A, Parenza M, Rodolfo M, Mavilio F, Parmiani G. Granulocyte colony-stimulating factor gene transfer suppresses tumorigenicity of a murine adenocarcinoma in vivo. *J Exp Med* 1991; 173:889–897.

180. Dranoff G, Jaffee EM, Lazenby AJ, Golumbek PT, Levitsky HI, Brose K, Jackson V, Hamada H, Pardoll DM, Mulligan RC. Vaccination with irradiated tumor cells engineered to secrete murine granulocyte-macrophage colony-stimulating factor stimulates potent, specific, and long-lasting anti-tumor immunity. *Proc Natl Acad Sci USA* 1993; 90:3539–3543.

181. Levitsky HI, Lazenby A, Hayashi RJ, Pardoll DM. In vivo priming of two distinct antitumor

effector populations: the role of MHC class I expression. *J Exp Med* 1994; 179:1215–1224.

182. Cavallo F, Giovarelli M, Gulino A, Vacca A, Stoppacciaro A, Modesti A, Forni G. Role of neutrophils and CD4$^+$ T-lymphocytes in the primary and memory response to nonimmunogenic murine mammary adenocarcinoma made immunogenic by IL-2 gene. *J Immunol* 1992; 149:3627–3635.

183. Visseren MJW, Koot M, Van der Voort EIH, Gravestein LA, Schoenmakers HJ, Kast WM, Zijlstra M, Melief CJM. Production of Interleukin-2 by EL4 tumor cells induces natural killer cell- and T-cell-mediated immunity. *J Immunother* 1994; 15:119–128.

184. Gilboa E, Lyerly HK, Vieweg J, Saito S. Immunotherapy of cancer using cytokine gene-modified tumor vaccines. *Semin Cancer Biol* 1994; 5:409–417.

185. Blankenstein T. Increasing tumor immunogenicity by genetic modification. *Eur J Cancer* 1994; 30A:1182–1187.

186. Huang A, Golumbek P, Ahmann DL, Jaffee EM, Pardoll DM, Levitsky HI. Role of bone marrow-derived cells in presenting MHC class I-restricted tumor antigens. *Science* 1994; 264: 961–965.

187. Hock H, Dorsch M, Kunzendorf U, Uberla K, Qin Z, Diamantstein T, Blankenstein T. Vaccinations with tumor cells genetically engineered to produce different cytokines: effectivity not superior to a classical adjuvant. *Cancer Res* 1993; 53:714–716.

188. Vieweg J, Rosenthal FM, Bannerji R, Heston WD, Fair WR, Gansbacher B, Gilboa E. Immunotherapy of prostate cancer in the Dunning rat model: use of cytokine gene modified tumor vaccines. *Cancer Res* 1994; 54:1760–1765.

189. Oettgen HF, Old LJ. The history of cancer immunotherapy. In: De Vita VT, Helman S, Rosenberg SA, eds. *Biologic Therapy of Cancer, Principles and Practice*. Philadelphia: JB Lippincott, 1991:87–119.

190. Tao MH, Levy R. Idiotype/granulocyte-macrophage colony-stimulating factor fusion protein as a vaccine for B-cell lymphoma. *Nature* 1993; 362:755–758.

191. Chen TT, Tao MH, Levy R. Idiotype-cytokine fusion proteins as cancer vaccines. Relative efficacy of IL-2, IL-4, and granulocyte-macrophage colony-stimulating factor. *J Immunol* 1994; 153:4775–4787.

192. Lotze MT, Custer MC, Bolton ES, Wiebke EA, Kawakami Y, Rosenberg SA. Mechanisms of immunologic antitumor therapy: lessons from the laboratory and clinical applications. *Hum Immunol* 1990; 28:198–207.

193. Anonymous. TNF/TIL human gene therapy clinical protocol. *Hum Gene Ther* 1990; 1:441–480.

194. Gansbacher B, Houghton A, Livingston P, Minasian L, Rosenthal F, Gilboa E, Golde D, Oettgen H, Steffens T, Yang SY, Wong G. A pilot study of immunization with HLA-A2 matched allogeneic melanoma cells that secrete interleukin-2 in patients with metastatic melanoma—Memorial Sloan-Kettering Cancer Center. *Hum Gene Ther* 1992; 3:677–690.

195. Gansbacher B, Motzer R, Houghton A, Bander N, Minasian L, Gastl G, Rosenthal F, Gilboa E, Scheinfeld J, Yang SY, Wong G, Golde D, Reuter V, Livingston P, Bosl G, Nanus D, Fair WR. A pilot study of immunization with interleukin-2 secreting allogeneic HLA-A2 matched renal cell carcinoma cells in patients with advanced renal cell carcinoma—Memorial Sloan-Kettering Cancer Center. *Hum Gene Ther* 1992; 3:691–703.

198. Nabel GJ, Chang A, Nabel EG, Plautz G, Fox BA, Huang L, Shu S. Immunotherapy of malignancy by in vivo gene transfer into tumors. *Hum Gene Ther* 1992; 3:339–410.

197. Osanto S, Brouwenstijn N, Vaessen N, Figdor CG, Melief CJM, Schrier PI. Immunization with interleukin-2 transfected melanoma cells—a phase-I-II study in patients with metastatic melanoma. *Hum Gene Ther* 1993; 4:323–330.

198. Lotze MT, Rubin JT, Carty S, Edington H, Ferson P, Landreneau R, Pippin B, Posner M, Rosenfelder D, Watson C, Carlos T, Kirkwood J, Lembersky B, Logan T, Rosenstein M, Rybak ME, Whiteside TL, Elder E, Moen RC, Jacob W, Chen YW, Pinkus RL, Bryant J. Gene therapy of cancer—a pilot study of IL-4-gene-modified fibroblasts admixed with autologous tumor to elicit an immune response. *Hum Gene Ther* 1994; 5:41–55.

Index

POETRY
for Students

Advisors

Erik France: Adjunct Instructor of English, Macomb Community College, Warren, Michigan. B.A. and M.S.L.S. from University of North Carolina, Chapel Hill; Ph.D. from Temple University.

Kate Hamill: Grade 12 English Teacher, Catonsville High School, Catonsville, Maryland.

Joseph McGeary: English Teacher, Germantown Friends School, Philadelphia, Pennsylvania. Ph.D. in English from Duke University.

Timothy Showalter: English Department Chair, Franklin High School, Reisterstown, Maryland. Certified teacher by the Maryland State Department of Education. Member of the National Council of Teachers of English.

Amy Spade Silverman: English Department Chair, Kehillah Jewish High School, Palo Alto, California. Member of National Council of Teachers of English (NCTE), Teachers and Writers, and NCTE Opinion Panel. Exam Reader, Advanced Placement Literature and Composition. Poet, published in *North American Review, Nimrod,* and *Michigan Quarterly Review,* among other publications.

Jody Stefansson: Director of Boswell Library and Study Center and Upper School Learning Specialist, Polytechnic School, Pasadena, California. Board member, Children's Literature Council of Southern California. Member of American Library Association, Association of Independent School Librarians, and Association of Educational Therapists.

Laura Jean Waters: Certified School Library Media Specialist, Wilton High School, Wilton, Connecticut. B.A. from Fordham University; M.A. from Fairfield University.

POETRY
for Students

Presenting Analysis, Context, and Criticism
on Commonly Studied Poetry

VOLUME 33

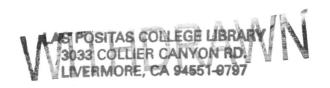
GALE
CENGAGE Learning™

Detroit • New York • San Francisco • New Haven, Conn • Waterville, Maine • London

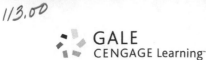
GALE
CENGAGE Learning™

Poetry for Students, Volume 33

Project Editor: Sara Constantakis

Rights Acquisition and Management: Margaret Abendroth, Margaret Chamberlain-Gaston, Sara Crane, Robyn Young

Composition: Evi Abou-El-Seoud

Manufacturing: Drew Kalasky

Imaging: John Watkins

Product Design: Pamela A. E. Galbreath, Jennifer Wahi

Content Conversion: Katrina Coach

Product Manager: Meggin Condino

Gale
27500 Drake Rd.
Farmington Hills, MI, 48331-3535

ISBN-13: 978-1-4144-4181-8
ISBN-10: 1-4144-4181-9

ISSN 1094-7019

This title is also available as an e-book.
ISBN-13: 978-1-4144-4954-8
ISBN-10: 1-4144-4954-2
Contact your Gale, a part of Cengage Learning sales representative for ordering information.

Printed in the United States of America
1 2 3 4 5 6 7 14 13 12 11 10

Table of Contents

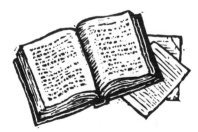

Just a Few Lines on a Page

I have often thought that poets have the easiest job in the world. A poem, after all, is just a few lines on a page, usually not even extending margin to margin—how long would that take to write, about five minutes? Maybe ten at the most, if you wanted it to rhyme or have a repeating meter. Why, I could start in the morning and produce a book of poetry by dinnertime. But we all know that it isn't that easy. Anyone can come up with enough words, but the poet's job is about writing the *right* ones. The right words will change lives, making people see the world somewhat differently than they saw it just a few minutes earlier. The right words can make a reader who relies on the dictionary for meanings take a greater responsibility for his or her own personal understanding. A poem that is put on the page correctly can bear any amount of analysis, probing, defining, explaining, and interrogating, and something about it will still feel new the next time you read it.

It would be fine with me if I could talk about poetry without using the word "magical," because that word is overused these days to imply "a really good time," often with a certain sweetness about it, and a lot of poetry is neither of these. But if you stop and think about magic—whether it brings to mind sorcery, witchcraft, or bunnies pulled from top hats—it always seems to involve stretching reality to produce a result greater than the sum of its parts and pulling unexpected results out of thin air. This book provides ample cases where a few simple words conjure up whole worlds. We do not actually travel to different times and different cultures, but the poems get into our minds, they find what little we know about the places they are talking about, and then they make that little bit blossom into a bouquet of someone else's life. Poets make us think we are following simple, specific events, but then they leave ideas in our heads that cannot be found on the printed page. Abracadabra.

Sometimes when you finish a poem it doesn't feel as if it has left any supernatural effect on you, like it did not have any more to say beyond the actual words that it used. This happens to everybody, but most often to inexperienced readers: regardless of what is often said about young people's infinite capacity to be amazed, you have to understand what usually does happen, and what could have happened instead, if you are going to be moved by what someone has accomplished. In those cases in which you finish a poem with a "So what?" attitude, the information provided in *Poetry for Students* comes in handy. Readers can feel assured that the poems included here actually are potent magic, not just because a few (or a hundred or ten thousand) professors of literature say they are: they're significant because they can withstand close inspection and still amaze the very same people who have just finished taking them apart and seeing how they work. Turn them inside out, and they will still be able to come alive, again and again. *Poetry for Students* gives readers of any age good practice in feeling the ways poems relate to both the reality of the time and place the poet lived in and the reality of our emotions. Practice is just another word for being a student. The information given here helps you understand the way to read poetry; what to look for, what to expect.

With all of this in mind, I really don't think I would actually like to have a poet's job at all. There are too many skills involved, including precision, honesty, taste, courage, linguistics, passion, compassion, and the ability to keep all sorts of people entertained at once. And that is just what they do with one hand, while the other hand pulls some sort of trick that most of us will never fully understand. I can't even pack all that I need for a weekend into one suitcase, so what would be my chances of stuffing so much life into a few lines? With all that *Poetry for Students* tells us about each poem, I am impressed that any poet can finish three or four poems a year. Read the inside stories of these poems, and you won't be able to approach any poem in the same way you did before.

David J. Kelly
College of Lake County

Introduction

Purpose of the Book

The purpose of *Poetry for Students* (*PfS*) is to provide readers with a guide to understanding, enjoying, and studying poems by giving them easy access to information about the work. Part of Gale's "For Students" Literature line, *PfS* is specifically designed to meet the curricular needs of high school and undergraduate college students and their teachers, as well as the interests of general readers and researchers considering specific poems. While each volume contains entries on "classic" poems frequently studied in classrooms, there are also entries containing hard-to-find information on contemporary poems, including works by multicultural, international, and women poets.

The information covered in each entry includes an introduction to the poem and the poem's author; the actual poem text (if possible); a poem summary, to help readers unravel and understand the meaning of the poem; analysis of important themes in the poem; and an explanation of important literary techniques and movements as they are demonstrated in the poem.

In addition to this material, which helps the readers analyze the poem itself, students are also provided with important information on the literary and historical background informing each work. This includes a historical context essay, a box comparing the time or place the poem was written to modern Western culture, a critical overview essay, and excerpts from critical essays on the poem. A unique feature of *PfS* is a specially commissioned critical essay on each poem, targeted toward the student reader.

To further help today's student in studying and enjoying each poem, information on audio recordings and other media adaptations is provided (if available), as well as reading suggestions for works of fiction and nonfiction on similar themes and topics. Classroom aids include ideas for research papers and lists of critical and reference sources that provide additional material on the poem.

Selection Criteria

The titles for each volume of *PfS* are selected by surveying numerous sources on notable literary works and analyzing course curricula for various schools, school districts, and states. Some of the sources surveyed include: high school and undergraduate literature anthologies and textbooks; lists of award-winners, and recommended titles, including the Young Adult Library Services Association (YALSA) list of best books for young adults.

Input solicited from our expert advisory board—consisting of educators and librarians—guides us to maintain a mix of "classic" and contemporary literary works, a mix of challenging and engaging works (including genre titles that are commonly studied) appropriate for different age levels, and a mix of international, multicultural and women authors. These advisors also consult on each volume's entry list, advising on which titles are most studied, most appropriate, and meet the broadest interests across secondary (grades 7–12) curricula and undergraduate literature studies.

How Each Entry Is Organized

Each entry, or chapter, in *PfS* focuses on one poem. Each entry heading lists the full name of the poem, the author's name, and the date of the poem's publication. The following elements are contained in each entry:

Introduction: a brief overview of the poem which provides information about its first appearance, its literary standing, any controversies surrounding the work, and major conflicts or themes within the work.

Author Biography: this section includes basic facts about the poet's life, and focuses on events and times in the author's life that inspired the poem in question.

Poem Text: when permission has been granted, the poem is reprinted, allowing for quick reference when reading the explication of the following section.

Poem Summary: a description of the major events in the poem. Summaries are broken down with subheads that indicate the lines being discussed.

Themes: a thorough overview of how the major topics, themes, and issues are addressed within the poem. Each theme discussed appears in a separate subhead and is easily accessed through the boldface entries in the Subject/Theme Index.

Style: this section addresses important style elements of the poem, such as form, meter, and rhyme scheme; important literary devices used, such as imagery, foreshadowing, and symbolism; and, if applicable, genres to which the work might have belonged, such as Gothicism or Romanticism. Literary terms are explained within the entry, but can also be found in the Glossary.

Historical Context: this section outlines the social, political, and cultural climate in which the author lived and the poem was created. This section may include descriptions of related historical events, pertinent aspects of daily life in the culture, and the artistic and literary sensibilities of the time in which the work was written. If the poem is a historical work, information regarding the time in which the poem is set is also included. Each section is broken down with helpful subheads.

Critical Overview: this section provides background on the critical reputation of the poem, including bannings or any other public controversies surrounding the work. For older works, this section includes a history of how the poem was first received and how perceptions of it may have changed over the years; for more recent poems, direct quotes from early reviews may also be included.

Criticism: an essay commissioned by *PfS* which specifically deals with the poem and is written specifically for the student audience, as well as excerpts from previously published criticism on the work (if available).

Sources: an alphabetical list of critical material quoted in the entry, with full bibliographical information.

Further Reading: an alphabetical list of other critical sources which may prove useful for the student. Includes full bibliographical information and a brief annotation.

In addition, each entry contains the following highlighted sections, set apart from the main text as sidebars:

Media Adaptations: if available, a list of audio recordings as well as any film or television adaptations of the poem, including source information.

Topics for Further Study: a list of potential study questions or research topics dealing with the poem. This section includes questions related to other disciplines the student may be studying, such as American history, world history, science, math, government, business, geography, economics, psychology, etc.

Compare & Contrast: an "at-a-glance" comparison of the cultural and historical differences between the author's time and culture and late twentieth century or early twenty-first century Western culture. This box includes pertinent parallels between the major scientific, political, and cultural movements of the time or place the poem was written, the time or place the poem was set (if a historical work), and modern Western culture. Works written after 1990 may not have this box.

What Do I Read Next?: a list of works that might give a reader points of entry into a classic work (e.g., YA or multicultural titles) and/ or complement the featured poem or serve as a contrast to it. This includes works by the same author and others, works from various genres, YA works, and works from various cultures and eras.

Other Features

PfS includes "Just a Few Lines on a Page," a foreword by David J. Kelly, an adjunct professor of English, College of Lake County, Illinois. This essay provides a straightforward, unpretentious explanation of why poetry should be marveled at and how *Poetry for Students* can help teachers show students how to enrich their own reading experiences.

A Cumulative Author/Title Index lists the authors and titles covered in each volume of the *PfS* series.

A Cumulative Nationality/Ethnicity Index breaks down the authors and titles covered in each volume of the *PfS* series by nationality and ethnicity.

A Subject/Theme Index, specific to each volume, provides easy reference for users who may be studying a particular subject or theme rather than a single work. Significant subjects from events to broad themes are included.

A Cumulative Index of First Lines (beginning in Vol. 10) provides easy reference for users who may be familiar with the first line of a poem but may not remember the actual title.

A Cumulative Index of Last Lines (beginning in Vol. 10) provides easy reference for users who may be familiar with the last line of a poem but may not remember the actual title.

Each entry may include illustrations, including photo of the author and other graphics related to the poem.

Citing Poetry for Students

When writing papers, students who quote directly from any volume of *Poetry for Students* may use the following general forms. These examples are based on MLA style; teachers may request that students adhere to a different style, so the following examples may be adapted as needed.

When citing text from *PfS* that is not attributed to a particular author (i.e., the Themes, Style, Historical Context sections, etc.), the following format should be used in the bibliography section:

> "Angle of Geese." *Poetry for Students*. Ed. Marie Napierkowski and Mary Ruby. Vol. 2. Detroit: Gale, 1998. 8–9.

When quoting the specially commissioned essay from *PfS* (usually the first piece under the "Criticism" subhead), the following format should be used:

> Velie, Alan. Critical Essay on "Angle of Geese." *Poetry for Students*. Ed. Marie Napierkowski and Mary Ruby. Vol. 2. Detroit: Gale, 1998. 7–10.

When quoting a journal or newspaper essay that is reprinted in a volume of *PfS*, the following form may be used:

> Luscher, Robert M. "An Emersonian Context of Dickinson's 'The Soul Selects Her Own Society'." *ESQ: A Journal of American Renaissance* 30.2 (1984): 111–16. Excerpted and reprinted in *Poetry for Students*. Ed. Marie Napierkowski and Mary Ruby. Vol. 1 Detroit: Gale, 1998. 266–69.

When quoting material reprinted from a book that appears in a volume of *PfS*, the following form may be used:

> Mootry, Maria K. "'Tell It Slant': Disguise and Discovery as Revisionist Poetic Discourse in 'The Bean Eaters'." *A Life Distilled: Gwendolyn Brooks, Her Poetry and Fiction*. Ed. Maria K. Mootry and Gary Smith. Urbana: University of Illinois Press, 1987. 177–80, 191. Excerpted and reprinted in *Poetry for Students*. Ed. Marie Napierkowski and Mary Ruby. Vol. 2. Detroit: Gale, 1998. 22–24.

We Welcome Your Suggestions

The editorial staff of *Poetry for Students* welcomes your comments and ideas. Readers who wish to suggest poems to appear in future volumes, or who have other suggestions, are cordially invited to contact the editor. You may contact the editor via E-mail at: **ForStudentsEditors@cengage.com.** Or write to the editor at:

Editor, *Poetry for Students*
Gale
27500 Drake Road
Farmington Hills, MI 48331-3535

Literary Chronology

993: Shmuel ha-Nagid is born in Cordoba, Spain.

1044: Shmuel ha-Nagid's poem "Two Eclipses" is composed.

1056: Smuel ha-Nagid dies in Grenada, Spain.

1572: Ben Jonson is born on or about June 11 in London, England.

1612: Anne Bradstreet is born in Northamptonshire, England.

1616: Ben Jonson's poem "On My First Son" is published in his folio *Epigrams*.

1637: Ben Jonson dies on August 16 in London, England.

1672: Anne Bradstreet dies of tuberculosis on September 16 in Andover, Massachusetts.

1678: Anne Bradstreet's poem "Upon the Burning of Our House, July 10th, 1666" is published in the collection *Several Poems Compiled with Great Variety of Wit and Learning, Full of Delight*.

1770: William Wordsworth is born on April 7 in Cockermouth, Cumberland, England.

1815: William Wordsworth's poem "I Wandered Lonely as a Cloud" is published in the collection *Poems, in Two Volumes*.

1818: Emily Jane Brontë is born on July 30 at Thornton near Bradford, England.

1845: Emily Jane Brontë's poem "The Old Stoic" is published in the Brontë sisters' collection *Poems*, using the pseudonyms Currer, Ellis, and Acton Bell.

1848: Emily Jane Brontë dies of tuberculosis on December 19 at Haworth in Yorkshire, England.

1850: William Wordsworth dies on April 23 at Rydal Mount, Rydal, Westmoreland, England.

1872: Paul Laurence Dunbar is born on June 27 in Dayton, Ohio.

1878: Carl August Sandburg is born on January 6 in Galesburg, Illinois.

1888: T.S. Eliot is born Thomas Stearns Eliot on September 26 in St. Louis, Missouri.

1899: Paul Laurence Dunbar's poem "Sympathy" is published in the collection *Lyrics of the Hearthside*.

1904: Pablo Neruda is born on July 12 in Parral, Chile.

1906: Paul Laurence Dunbar dies of tuberculosis on February 9 in Dayton, Ohio.

1920: Carl Sandburg's poem "Jazz Fantasia" is published in the collection *Smoke and Steel*.

1925: T.S. Eliot's poem "The Hollow Men" is published in *Poems, 1909-1925*.

1928: Maya Angelou is born on April 28 in St. Louis, Missouri.

1932: Sylvia Plath is born on October 27 in Boston, Massachusetts.

1938: Charles Simic is born on May 9 in Belgrade, Yugoslavia.

1942: Pat Mora is born on January 19 in El Paso, Texas.

1943: Carl Sandburg wins the Pulitzer Prize in History for *Abraham Lincoln: The War Years*.

1943: Ellen Bryant Voigt is born on May 9 in Danville, Virginia.

1948: T.S. Eliot receives the Nobel Prize for Literature.

1951: Garrett Kaoru Hongo is born on May 30 in Volcano, Hawaii.

1952: Naomi Shihab Nye is born on March 12 in St. Louis, Missouri.

1953: Carl Sandburg wins the Pulitzer Prize in Poetry for his *Complete Poems*.

1960: Sylvia Plath's poem "Mushrooms" is published in the collection *The Colossus*.

1963: Sylvia Plath commits suicide by gassing herself in an oven on February 11 in London, England.

1965: T.S. Eliot dies on January 4 in London, England.

1967: Carl Sandburg dies of heart failure on July 22 in Flat Rock, North Carolina.

1973: Pablo Neruda dies on September 23 in Santiago, Chile.

1975: Pablo Neruda's poem "Fully Empowered" is published in the collection *Fully Empowered*.

1978: Maya Angelou's poem "Woman Work" is published in the collection *And Still I Rise*.

1980: Charles Simic's poem "Classic Ballroom Dances" is published in the collection *Classic Ballroom Dances*.

1982: Garrett Kaoru Hongo's poem "What For" is published in the collection *Yellow Light*.

1984: Pat Mora's poem "Elena" is published in the collection *Chants*.

1987: Ellen Bryant Voigt's poem "The Lotus Flowers" is published in *The Lotus Flowers*.

1990: Charles Simic wins the Pulitzer Prize in Literature for his collection *The World Doesn't End*.

1994: Naomi Shihab Nye's "Shoulders" is published in the collection *Red Suitcase*.

Acknowledgments

The editors wish to thank the copyright holders of the excerpted criticism included in this volume and the permissions managers of many book and magazine publishing companies for assisting us in securing reproduction rights. We are also grateful to the staffs of the Detroit Public Library, the Library of Congress, the University of Detroit Mercy Library, Wayne State University Purdy/Kresge Library Complex, and the University of Michigan Libraries for making their resources available to us. Following is a list of the copyright holders who have granted us permission to reproduce material in this volume of *PfS*. Every effort has been made to trace copyright, but if omissions have been made, please let us know.

COPYRIGHTED EXCERPTS IN *PfS*, VOLUME 33, WERE REPRODUCED FROM THE FOLLOWING PERIODICALS:

American Book Review, v. 6, January-February, 1984. Copyright © 1984 Writer's Review, Inc. Reproduced by permission.—*Antioch Review*, v. 62, winter, 2004. Copyright © 2004 by the Antioch Review Inc. Reproduced by permission of the Editors.—*Atlantic Online*, November 24, 1999 for "Song and Story" by Steven Cramer. Copyright © 1999 by The Atlantic Monthly Company. All rights reserved. Reproduced by permission of the author.—*Bilingual Review*, v. 21, September-December, 1996. Copyright © 1996 by Bilingual Press/Editorial Bilingüe, Arizona State University, Tempe, AZ. All rights reserved. Reproduced by permission.—*Brontë Studies: The Journal of the Brontë Society*, v. 30, February 5, 2005. Copyright © Bronte Society 2005. Reproduced by permission.—*Canadian Review of American Studies*, v. 34, 2004. © Canadian Review of American Studies 2004. Reprinted by permission of the publisher.—*Centennial Review*, v. 23, summer, 1979; v. 36, spring, 1992. Copyright © 1979, 1992 by *Centennial Review*. Both reproduced by permission.—*Detroit Free Press*, September 10, 2007; March 18, 2009. Copyright © 2007, 2009 Detroit Free Press Inc. Both reproduced by permission of the *Detroit Free Press*.—*Essays in Literature*, v. 21, fall, 1994. Copyright © 1994 by Western Illinois University. Reproduced by permission.—*Explicator*, v. 38, summer, 1980; v. 48, fall, 1989; v. 56, winter, 1998; v. 57, spring, 1999; v. 59, summer, 2001; v. 60, spring, 2002. Copyright © 1980, 1989, 1998, 1999, 2001, 2002 by Helen Dwight Reid Educational Foundation. All reproduced with permission of the Helen Dwight Reid Educational Foundation, published by Heldref Publications, 1319 18th Street, NW, Washington, DC 20036-1802.—*The Journal of Ethnic Studies*, v. 12, winter, 1985. Reproduced by permission.—*MELUS*, v. 27, summer, 2002. Copyright *MELUS: The Society for the Study of Multi-Ethnic Literature of the United States*, 2002. Reproduced by permission.—*Modern Language Quarterly*, v. 3, March, 1942. Copyright © 1992 University of Washington. All rights reserved. Used by permission of the publisher, Duke University Press.—*Nation*, v. 254, January 27, 1992. Copyright © 1992 by *The Nation* Magazine/The Nation Company, Inc. Reproduced by permission.—*New Republic*, v. 214, May 6, 1996. Copyright © 1996 by The New Republic, Inc. Reproduced by permission of *The New Republic*.—*North American Review*, v. 221, March 25, 2009. Copyright © 2009 by the University of Northern Iowa. Reproduced by permission from *The North American Review*.—*Olympian*, February 10, 2008. Copyright © 2008 *The Olympian*. Reproduced by permission.—*Parnassus: Poetry in Review*, v. 25, 2001 for "The Prince and the Paupered: Medieval Hebrew Poetry Meets the Twenty-First Century" by Jay Ladin. Copyright © 2001 Poetry in Review Foundation, NY. Reproduced by permission of the publisher and the author.—*Poets & Writers Magazine*, v. 20, September-October, 1992. Copyright © 1992 Poets & Writers, Inc. Reprinted by permission of the publisher, Poets & Writers, Inc., 90 Broad Street, New York, NY, 10004, www.pw.org.—*South Atlantic Quarterly*, v. 59, 1960. Copyright © 1960 Duke University Press. Copyright renewed 1988 by Duke University Press. All rights reserved. Used by permission of the publisher, Duke University Press.—*Studies in Philology*, v. 75, winter, 1978; v. 86, spring, 1989. Copyright © 1978, 1989 by the University of North Carolina Press. Both used by permission.—*Virginia Quarterly Review*, v. 82, winter, 2006. Copyright 2006, by *The Virginia Quarterly Review*, The University of Virginia. Reproduced by permission of the publisher.—*Washington Report on Middle Eastern Affairs*, v. 25, August 6, 2009. Copyright © 2009 American Educational Trust. All rights reserved. Reproduced by permission.

COPYRIGHTED EXCERPTS IN *PfS*, VOLUME 33, WERE REPRODUCED FROM THE FOLLOWING BOOKS:

Angelou, Maya. From *And Still I Rise*. Random House, 1980. Copyright © 1978 by Maya Angelou. Reproduced by permission of Random House, Inc.—Dunbar, Paul Laurence. From "Sympathy," in *The Collected Poetry of Paul Laurence Dunbar*. Edited by Joanne M. Braxton. University Press of Virginia, 1993. Originally published by Dodd, Mead, and Company, 1913. This edition copyright © 1993 by the Rector and Visitors of the University of Virginia. All rights reserved. Reproduced with permission of the University of Virginia Press.—HaNagid, Shmuel. From *Selected Poems of Shmuel HaNagid*. Translated by Peter Cole from the Hebrew. Princeton University Press, 1996. Copyright © 1996 by Princeton University Press. Reprinted by permission of Princeton University Press.—Hongo, Garrett Kaoru. From *Yellow Light*. Wesleyan University Press, 1982. Copyright © 1982 by Garrett Kaoru Hongo. All rights reserved. Reprinted by permission of Wesleyan University Press.—Nye, Naomi Shihab. From *Red Suitcase*. BOA Editions, 1994. Copyright © 1994 Naomi Shihab Nye. All rights reserved. Reproduced by permission.—Simic, Charles. From "Classic Ballroom Dances," in *Selected Early Poems*. Geroge Braziller, Inc., 1999. Copyright © 1999 by Charles Simic. Reproduced by permission.—Voigt, Ellen Bryant. From "The Lotus Flowers," in *The Made Thing: An Anthology of Contemporary Southern Poetry*. Edited by Leon Stokesbury. University of Arkansas Press, 1999. Copryight © 1987 by Ellen Bryant Voigt. Used by permission of W. W. Norton & Company. Inc.—Wordsworth, William. From "I Wandered Lonely as a Cloud," in *William Wordsworth: The Poems, Volume 1*. Edited by John O. Hayden. Penguin, 1977. Reproduced by permission of Penguin Books, Ltd.

Contributors

Susan K. Andersen: Andersen is a writer and college English teacher. Entry on "Sympathy." Original essay on "Sympathy."

Bryan Aubrey: Aubrey holds a Ph.D. in English. Entries on "Fully Empowered" and "I Wandered Lonely as a Cloud." Original essays on "Fully Empowered" and "I Wandered Lonely as a Cloud."

Jennifer Bussey: Bussey is an independent writer specializing in literature. Entry on "What For." Original essay on "What For."

Catherine Dominic: Dominic is a novelist and a freelance writer and editor. Entries on "Elena" and "Upon the Burning of Our House, July 10th, 1666." Original essays on "Elena" and "Upon the Burning of Our House, July 10th, 1666."

Cynthia Gower: Gower is a novelist, playwright, and freelance writer. Entry on "Jazz Fantasia." Original essay on "Jazz Fantasia."

Diane Andrews Henningfeld: Henningfeld is a professor emerita at Adrian College where she taught literature and writing for many years. She continues to write widely about literature for a variety of educational publishers. Entry on "On My First Son." Original essay on "On My First Son."

Michael J. O'Neal: O'Neal holds a Ph.D. in English literature. Entries on "Classic Ballroom Dances" and "Two Eclipses." Original essays on "Classic Ballroom Dances" and "Two Eclipses."

Claire Robinson: Robinson has an M.A. in English. Entry on "Mushrooms." Original essay on "Mushrooms."

Bradley A. Skeen: Skeen is a classics professor. Entry on "Old Stoic." Original essay on "Old Stoic."

Leah Tieger: Tieger is a freelance writer and editor. Entries on "The Hollow Men" and "The Lotus Flowers." Original essays on "The Hollow Men" and "The Lotus Flowers."

Rebecca Valentine: Valentine is a freelance writer with an emphasis in English literature and history. Entries on "Shoulders" and "Woman Work." Original essays on "Shoulders" and "Woman Work."

Classic Ballroom Dances

CHARLES SIMIC

1980

Charles Simic has come to be regarded as one of America's most important poets—a remarkable achievement given that English is not his native language. "Classic Ballroom Dances" is the title poem in Simic's 1980 collection of poems, *Classic Ballroom Dances*. The collection won the Harriet Monroe Poetry Award and the Poetry Society of America's di Castagnola Award in 1980. Like nearly all of Simic's poems, "Classic Ballroom Dances" is brief, consisting of just sixteen lines, and is written in simple, straightforward language. Its purpose is not to outline a point of view, tell a story, or develop a situation. Rather, its purpose is to evoke an image by drawing a number of implicit comparisons between the people's activities and dancing.

It can be difficult to classify or attach a label to contemporary poets like Simic, including the broader category called Modernism, given that most draw on a wide range of poetic traditions for their inspiration. Nevertheless, many critics see elements of the artistic movement called surrealism in Simic's work. Surrealism was a movement that dominated both literature and the visual arts between World War I and World War II, and that has continued to have an influence on more contemporary poets. The goal of the surrealists was to create startling imagery, often juxtaposing words and phrases in ways that defied reason. The surrealists tried to link conscious and unconscious forms of expression to create a new, fuller reality—what surrealism's

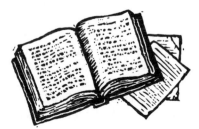

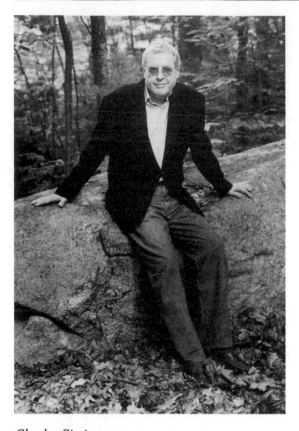

Charles Simic *(© Christopher Felver / Corbis)*

spokesman, French writer André Breton, called a "surreality" in his manifesto of surrealism, published first in 1924, then in a revised version in 1929. (Breton, however, did not coin the word; it was first used by French poet Guillaume Apollinaire in 1917.) Accordingly, the emphasis in surrealist poetry, including that written by Simic, is on the psychological, unconscious thought processes. This surrealist tendency is evident in "Classic Ballroom Dances."

AUTHOR BIOGRAPHY

Simic was born in Belgrade, Yugoslavia, on May 9, 1938. (Yugoslavia, literally "Land of the South Slavs," no longer exists; during most of the twentieth century, the nation called Yugoslavia was an artificial confederation of various ethnic states that have since declared their independence. Belgrade is the capital of Serbia, one of those states.) Simic spent his childhood surviving the horrors of World War II; on numerous occasions he and his

family had to evacuate their home because of bombings. The postwar period was little better. Yugoslavia, like other Eastern European nations, faced economic turmoil as it became a Soviet satellite state ruled by a Communist dictator. Simic's father left for Italy to find work, but when the family tried to leave Yugoslavia to join him, they were stopped by the authorities. Meanwhile, Simic was by all accounts a poor student and was regarded as something of a juvenile delinquent.

The family's fortunes changed in 1954 when they received permission to move to Paris. During his year in Paris, Simic studied English and attended night school. Finally, the family traveled to the United States to join Simic's father, who was working by now for the American company he had worked for before the war. After landing in New York City, the family moved to Chicago, where Simic was enrolled in school. There he encountered teachers who seemed to care about him, and he flourished as a student. During his high school years he became interested in literature, especially poetry. He later quipped, though, that one of his motivations for writing poetry was that at the time it seemed a good way to meet girls.

Simic published his first poems in 1959, and he continued to write poetry while taking night classes and working as an office boy for a Chicago newspaper until he was drafted into the U.S. Army in 1961. Simic destroyed most of these early poems. After finishing his military service in 1963, Simic enrolled at New York University, where he earned his bachelor's degree in 1966. He worked as an editorial assistant for a photography magazine in New York City until 1969. From 1970 to 1973, he taught English at the State University of California at Hayward. Meanwhile, he became a naturalized U.S. citizen in 1971.

Beginning in 1973, Simic taught English literature and creative writing at the University of New Hampshire in Durham, though he has also been a visiting professor at Boston University and Columbia University. He has since retired. A prolific poet, Simic published his first collection, *What the Grass Says*, in 1967. Since then, he has published numerous collections, including *Somewhere among Us a Stone Is Taking Notes* (1969), *Dismantling the Silence* (1971), *White* (1972), *Charon's Cosmology* (1977), *Classic Ballroom Dances* (1980), *Selected Poems, 1963–1983*

(1985), *Unending Blues* (1986), *The World Doesn't End* (1989), *The Book of Gods and Devils* (1990), *Hotel Insomnia* (1992), *Walking the Black Cat: Poems* (1996), *Jackstraws* (2000), and his most recent collection, *Aunt Lettuce, I Want to Peek under Your Skirt* (2005). A collection of sixty of his most popular poems was published in 2008. Simic has also published hundreds of poems in such publications as *New Yorker, Poetry, Nation, Kayak, Atlantic, Esquire, Chicago Review, New Republic, American Poetry Review, Paris Review*, and *Harvard Magazine*. In 1990 Simic received a Pulitzer Prize for his collection *The World Doesn't End*. In addition to writing his own poetry, he has translated the poetry of numerous eastern European writers and has written and published various works of literary criticism. In August 2007, the U.S. Library of Congress appointed Simic as the nation's fifteenth Poet Laureate Consultant in Poetry.

POEM TEXT

Grandmothers who wring the necks
Of chickens; old nuns
With names like Theresa, Marianne,
Who pull schoolboys by the ear;

The intricate steps of pickpockets   5
Working the crowd of the curious
At the scene of an accident; the slow shuffle
Of the evangelist with a sandwich board;

The hesitation of the early-morning customer
Peeking through the window grille   10
Of a pawnshop; the weave of a little kid
Who is walking to school with eyes closed;

And the ancient lovers, cheek to cheek,
On the dance floor of the Union Hall,
Where they also hold charity raffles   15
On rainy Monday nights of an eternal November.

POEM SUMMARY

Title

Unlike many poems, "Classic Ballroom Dances" would make little sense without its title. The title announces the subject matter of the poem, although the poem itself only once uses the word *dance*. The title evokes a number of responses. The word *classic* suggests something traditional, perhaps even old-fashioned, but it also carries numerous other implications:

timelessness, agelessness, stylishness, and elegance, something that will abide and last. This sense of something traditional and enduring from the past is reinforced by the mention not just of dances but of ballroom dances. The reference is to one of the formal, structured dances that were popular in past generations, such as the fox-trot, the jitterbug, the waltz, the polka, and various Latin and South American dances such as the cha-cha and the tango. These dances always involve a partner, and the two partners, who generally maintain physical contact, have to move in synchronization, using precise steps.

The title's reference to dances can be interpreted literally, but the word *dance* can have broader connotations. For instance, a person can *dance around* a topic, meaning to evade it. The word can suggest the social relations between people, who perform a *dance* as they interact with one another. The word suggests movement in time and space. It suggests a rhythm and structure not just on the dance floor but in life. It also suggests that people can engage in stereotypical, predictable movements as they pursue their daily activities.

Stanza 1

"Classic Ballroom Dances" consists of four four-line stanzas. It also comprises a single "sentence," although the sentence is not grammatically complete. The poem is a series of images, each image anchored by a noun modified by various words and phrases. Linking the lines of the first stanza are references to elderly women. Grandmothers are said to wring chickens' necks, perhaps a glancing reference to folk dances such as the chicken dance, a popular rhythm-and-blues dance in the 1950s, or perhaps to a folk dance by the same name in German-speaking countries. Elderly nuns, with stereotypical, old-fashioned names, are then said to yank the ears of schoolboys, the type of discipline that nuns in a former age routinely inflicted on unruly boys. The two images suggest a perverse form of *dancing*: the grandmother is partnered with a chicken as she kills it, presumably to make a meal of it, and the nun is partnered with a schoolboy.

Stanza 2

The second stanza contains images that seem more explicitly related to dancing. Pickpockets are said to engage in *intricate steps*. They move stealthily about a crowd of people who have gathered to gawk at the scene of an accident; the implication is that the attention of the people in the crowd is so riveted on the accident that the pickpocket can easily steal their belongings. The next image employs the word *shuffle* to describe the movement of a preacher who is wearing a sandwich board. This type of advertising tool was commonly used in the past and is still used on occasion today. It consists of two boards hooked together by straps. A person inserts his or her head up through the straps, between the boards, so that one board hangs in front and one hangs in back. In this way a *sandwich* is formed. The boards, then, would be painted with a message. In the case of an evangelist, the message would presumably be of religious beliefs (for example, "Repent" or "The End Is Near"), or perhaps an advertisement for an upcoming revival meeting, an evangelistic gathering intended to promote enthusiasm for faith in a crowd. The evangelist's shuffle is said to be slow, providing an implicit link with the elderly women of the first stanza, who likewise could be presumed to move slowly. Further linkage is provided by the religious references—the nun in stanza 1 and the evangelist in stanza 2.

Stanza 3

Like the first two stanzas, stanza 3 also contains two images. The first invites the reader to imagine a person walking about in the early morning and pausing to look through the barred windows of a pawnshop. The person is described as hesitant, perhaps suggesting that he or she is embarrassed to look at the goods for sale in a pawnshop, which sometimes carries implications of seediness; by reputation, only poor, disreputable people frequent pawnshops. Or perhaps the person is hesitant because he or she longs to own some of the goods for sale but cannot afford them—or perhaps is thinking about raising some money by selling something at the pawnshop. The stanza's second image is a child walking to school with his eyes closed. Again, there are linkages. Reference is made to the child's eyes, just as the customer outside the pawnshop is said to peek inside; further, reference to the child walking to school echoes the earlier reference to the schoolboy whose ear was being pulled by the nun. The child is weaving rather than moving in a straight line, making the nature of the child's movement consistent with the hesitation of the pawnshop customer.

Stanza 4

The fourth stanza makes explicit reference to dancing. Again, as in the previous stanzas, two images are created. The first is of old lovers who dance closely, their cheeks pressed together, on the floor of a union hall. Again there is a reference to advancing age, echoing the images of grandmothers and elderly nuns in stanza 1 and the slow-moving evangelist in stanza 2, and contrasting with the schoolchildren in stanzas 1 and 3. It is unclear—and unimportant—what union hall Simic is referring to. The location is probably generic, referring to any meeting hall used by a local labor union but also used for dances and other events. It is possible that Simic had in mind more specifically a famous nightspot in Brooklyn, New York, call the Union Hall, where bands play and people dance. This type of venue would also be a place where raffles for charity would be held. These raffles are imagined to take place on a rainy weeknight, on Mondays, presumably when people have little else to do after the weekend. They are also imagined to take place during the month of November, but a November that never ends. November, particularly in the northern parts of the United States (Simic wrote the poem while teaching in New Hampshire), is often regarded as the gloomiest, most depressing month of the year. The crisp sunshine and colorful foliage of autumn has ended, trees are barren, the snowfall of winter and the winter holiday season have not started, and the weather is often cloudy, chilly, and rainy.

THEMES

Old Age

"Classic Ballroom Dances" is a poem that does not lend itself readily to thematic analysis. In the first place, the poem consists of just a single sentence, and the sentence is not even grammatically complete. Thus, it never really makes a statement. Rather, the poem consists of a series of images.

Nevertheless, it is possible to discern the glimmerings of a theme. One theme that links the images is that of old age. The first word of the poem is *grandmothers*, followed by a reference to old nuns. Later, the evangelist is said to be shuffling, suggesting the slow, hesitant walk of an elderly man. In the final stanza, reference is made to ancient lovers who are dancing. The

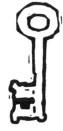

TOPICS FOR FURTHER STUDY

- Write a poem that begins with a three-word title paralleling "Classic Ballroom Dances." Such a title would have two adjectives, then a noun that refers to the subject matter. Examples might include "Ancient Mythic Creatures" or "Cranky Hungry Babies." In your poem, create images that suggest different ways of looking at the topic you have chosen. If your native language is not English, write the poem in your native language and be prepared to translate it for your classmates.

- If you have some knowledge of a foreign language, try writing a similar poem in that language. In a small group discussion, describe for your peers the difficulties you faced in writing poetry in a language that is not your native tongue.

- Conduct research into classic ballroom dances. What are some of the dances? Where did they originate? When were they popular? Find images of people doing these dances on the Internet and create a PowerPoint presentation to introduce classmates to these dances with visuals. Alternatively, find a willing partner and demonstrate some of these dances for your classmates.

- Locate another poem whose subject is dancing. There are numerous possibilities: "Dancer" by Carl Sandburg, "The Harlem Dancer" by Claude McKay, "Indian Dancer" by Sarojini Naidu, "The Baby's Dance" by Ann Taylor, "I cannot dance upon my Toes" by Emily Dickinson, "Sweet Dancer" by William Butler Yeats, "Crazy Jane Grown Old Looks at the Dancers" by William Butler Yeats, "The Dance" by R. S. Thomas, "Dance-Hall Girls" by Robert William Service, "if a living dance upon dead minds" by E. E. Cummings, or "Reasons For Attendance" by Philip Larkin. Write an essay in which you compare the poem you've selected with "Classic Ballroom Dances," focusing on the nature of the imagery the two poets use.

- Surrealism was not confined to literature. Many practitioners of the visual arts used surrealist techniques. Locate a copy of a surrealist painting or sculpture, perhaps in an art book or on the Internet. Display the piece of art to your classmates and explain how the piece you have selected embodies the principles of surrealism, perhaps in much the same way Simic does in "Classic Ballroom Dances."

- Many critics—and Simic himself—note that Simic's poetry is heavily influenced by his early childhood in war-torn Yugoslavia. Investigate the history of Yugoslavia during World War II and the postwar years. Prepare a chart that lists specific events and social/political developments that might have had a profound impact on a boy such as Charles Simic during that time.

- Charles Simic's other passion, besides poetry, is American jazz, which immediately attracted him when he heard it for the first time on the radio when he was living in Paris. Conduct research into the American jazz music of the 1950s. Locate sound recordings of some of this jazz on disc or records. Play some jazz selections that Simic might have listened to as a youth for your classmates. Alternatively, if you play an instrument, perform some jazz selections for your classmates. Explain how you think jazz music might have influenced Simic's poetry.

- In 2007 Simic was appointed the nation's poet laureate by the Library of Congress. Write a brief report on poets laureate of the United States. What does the phrase mean? What other poets have served in this position? What is the history of the poet laureate? What duties does a poet laureate have?

- Use George Ancona's young adult book *Let's Dance* to explore the role of dance in many cultures. Choose a dance and demonstrate it for the class while explaining its purpose in that culture.

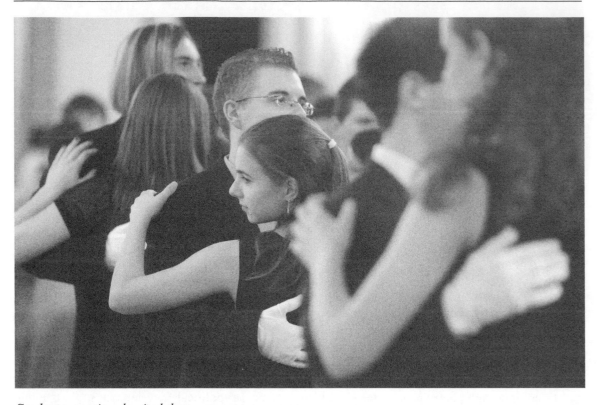

Students practice classical dance (*Michal Cizek | AFP | Getty Image*)

very topic of the poem, classic ballroom dances, suggests something from another age or another generation. These references to age have a counterpoint in the references to schoolchildren; the nun is said to pull schoolboys by their ears, and a small child is said to be walking to school.

Yet Simic never makes an explicit statement about any of these people. The poem simply imagines them engaged in characteristic activities as they go about their lives. The poem ends with an image of sadness, as charity raffles are imagined as taking place on a rainy night in a November that has no end. The reader is left to speculate about the *meaning* of Simic's poem. Perhaps the poem is intended to suggest an eternal cycle of people caught in their routine; the routine of the elderly people has long been established, and that of the schoolchildren is in the process of being formed. Ultimately, though, the poem invites the reader to see such people in a new way and to experience their loneliness and perhaps sorrow as they *dance* their way through their daily existence.

Observation

To state that poets and creative writers in general are astute observers of the human condition is to state the obvious. What is unusual about "Classic Ballroom Dances" is that it is based entirely on observation, with no explicit commentary. Generally, a feature of poetry is the use of simile and metaphor, figures of speech that make comparisons between otherwise unlike objects. "Classic Ballroom Dances" defies this tendency by containing no simile or metaphor. Each of the statements made about the people in the poem or their activities is simply observed and reported, without the implicit commentary of figures of speech. Thus, grandmothers wring the necks of chickens, nuns pull the ears of schoolboys, pickpockets steal from people, an evangelist walks about in a sandwich board, a customer looks into the window of a pawnshop, a child walks to school, and lovers dance. The emphasis is entirely on the person or activity itself, with no comparison to any other thing or activity.

The only expression in the poem that suggests a figure of speech occurs at the very end, where November is said to be eternal. Literally, of course, such a statement is untrue, but figurative the phrase suggests an ongoing depressive state, where gloom and chill seem to last forever. With this one exception, the poem merely presents the results of observation. In this sense, theme and style interact. The style of the poem suggests a theme: that the poet, or anyone, can catch people going about their activities, freeze those activities in time, and allow the activities to speak for themselves, without comment.

That said, however, it must be recognized that the poem taken as a whole is a metaphor. By labeling the poem "Classic Ballroom Dances," Simic makes clear that he sees a metaphorical connection between the activities he reports and dancing. But rather than browbeating the reader with the comparison, the comparison remains implied by the title of the poem. The goal of the poem, then, is to observe and present experience, then invite the reader to see the experience in a new and starling way.

STYLE

Grammar

Normally, readers do not think about traditional grammar when they read poetry. Poetry routinely bends the rules of traditional grammar to create new and interesting verbal effects. Such is the case with Simic's "Classic Ballroom Dances." The poem, consisting of four four-line stanzas, comprises a single sentence, but the *sentence* is incomplete, for it lacks a predicate. (The predicate is the part of a sentence that expresses something about the subject, usually consisting of a verb and an object or objects.) Accordingly, the poem is made up entirely of a sequence of phrases, each anchored by a noun. The noun in the first such phrase is grandmothers, whose activity of wringing chickens' necks is contained in a subordinate clause. (A subordinate clause cannot stand alone, because it depends on the previous phrase for its meaning.) Similarly, the old nuns' activity of pulling the ears of schoolboys is contained in a subordinate clause. In the second stanza, the noun is not the person but the activity. Thus, the anchor noun of the pickpockets is their intricate steps, and that of the evangelist is his slow shuffle. This pattern continues in the third stanza, where the anchor noun of the pawnshop customer is his hesitation, while the anchor noun of the small child walking to school is his weave. In the final stanza, Simic returns to the grammar of the first stanza, with the pair of ancient dancing lovers as his anchor noun. The poem then in a

sense trails off into a description of the place where the ancient lovers are dancing.

The purpose of this kind of grammatical structure is to explicitly avoid making clear, rational statements about the topic at hand. The poem does not have a predicate, meaning that it does not state anything using the conventional grammatical structure of noun plus verb plus modifiers. Rather, it presents the reader with a series of images. The reader is invited to envision the people—grandmothers, nuns, pickpockets, an evangelist, a customer, a little kid, and a pair of ancient lovers—caught in a moment in time doing something that might be regarded as typical of them.

Surrealism

The word *surreal* has entered the everyday vocabulary of English and is often used to mean "odd," "unusual," or "unexpected." Originally, however, it was derived to denote an artistic movement called surrealism. The word joins *realism* to the prefix "sur-," which generally means something like "over" or "above"; thus, the word *surmount* means "to overcome."

Surrealism was an artistic movement that tried to identify and capture a higher psychological reality. It explicitly rejected logic and rationality in favor of artistic forms of expression that emphasized the irrational, illogical movement of the mind as it encountered experience. The movement became popular after World War I. That war, which left millions dead and wounded, came to be regarded as a kind of madness that represented the inevitable outcome of Western rational thought, in particular because war planners used science to find new, more efficient ways to kill: the airplane, mustard gas, the machine gun. Accordingly, during the post-World War I period, many artists and thinkers explored new ways of confronting reality. Many were attracted to the psychological theories of Sigmund Freud, who emphasized the irrational subconscious mind to explain mental disorders (or even to explain the behavior of people who were not mentally disturbed). The result was forms of art that were often puzzling, absurd, startling, and at times unnerving. Readers and art lovers often did not understand them, for the works envisioned experience as chaotic, irrational, and often bizarre.

To label "Classic Ballroom Dances" as a surrealist poem, or Simic as a surrealist poet, is unnecessarily restrictive. Like many contemporary

COMPARE
&
CONTRAST

- **1980:** Another eastern European writer, Cze-slaw Milosz, from Poland, is awarded a major literary prize, in this case the Nobel Prize in Literature. Milosz is regarded as one of the world's most influential poets.

  Today: The 2008 winner of the Nobel Prize in Literature is Frenchman Jean-Marie Gus-tave Le Clézio, who writes novels, essays, short stories, and books for children.

- **1980:** In May, Josip Broz Tito, the Commu-nist dictator of Yugoslavia in the post-World War II period, dies, putting an end to that chapter of Simic's early life.

  Today: Serbia is its own independent nation, one of the last to leave the former Yugosla-via. After terrible violence in the late 1990s, when Serbia, still part of Yugoslavia, sup-ported rebellions in Bosnia and Croatia, as well as incidents of genocide, the country has

been reinstated into the United Nations and the Council of Europe. Incidents of violence continue to occur, such as the arson of the American Embassy in Belgrade in 2008 and outbreaks of bloodshed when the province of Kosovo seceded that same year, contributing to Simic's outspoken opposition to war.

- **1980:** The world political situation is tumul-tuous, with the Iranian Revolution and the consequent seizure of fifty-two American hostages, the invasion of Afghanistan by the Soviet Union, and the subsequent U.S. boycott of the Moscow Olympics.

  Today: America's relationship with Iran con-tinues to be one of hostility and mistrust; the dissolution of the Soviet Union has reduced cold war tensions and allowed new eastern European writers to gain prominence, but the world's hot spot is still the Middle East.

poets, Simic inherited a wide range of poetic tradi-tions that inspired his writing. He differs from the surrealists, for example, in writing poems that are generally regarded as simple—not in the neg-ative sense of "simplistic" but rather in the sense of using ordinary, everyday language rather than the abstruse (or, difficult to understand) language that sometimes characterizes contemporary poetry. Indeed, the source of much of his popularity is that his poems are eminently readable by people who are not themselves poets or literary critics. His poems sometimes contain violence, and often they are marked by sadness, but they also contain humorous elements. It would be more accurate to suggest that Simic's poetry, including "Classic Ballroom Dances," has some of the characteristics of surrealist poetry. In particular, the poem is built around a sequence of images rather than logical statements. This movement from one image to another suggests the movement of the poet's mind as he tries to capture the way in which the stereotypical activities of people resemble the movements of a dance.

HISTORICAL CONTEXT

World War II
One of Charles Simic's major formative experi-ences was World War II. Yugoslavia was invaded by Nazi Germany on April 6, 1941, and surren-dered eleven days later. Thousands of Yugoslav soldiers were taken captive, and much of the country was terrorized by a fascist militia called the Ustaše. However, a strong resistance move-ment developed, led by two groups. One group was the Chetniks, but the most successful resist-ance movement was led by the Communist Yugo-slav Partisans. The Partisans were able to drive the Nazis out of Simic's native Serbia in 1944. Meanwhile, the Red Army of the Soviet Union was making its way westward, leaving Yugoslavia and other eastern and central European countries the scenes of intense fighting and bombing raids. The Simic family was often forced to evacuate their home because of bombing raids. He wit-nessed firsthand the devastation of the war in his hometown of Belgrade.

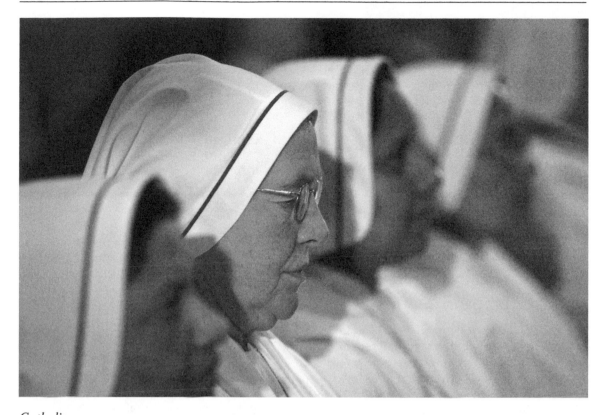

Catholic nuns *(Jonathan Nackstrand / Pool / Getty Images)*

Post-World War II Yugoslavia

As a result of his role as a leader of the Partisans and in the liberation of Yugoslavia from the Nazis, Marshall Josip Tito was an enormously popular figure in the nation. He was head of the nation's provisional government in the years immediately after the war. The Yugoslav people, in a referendum, rejected the monarchy that had ruled the nation before the war. Tito proclaimed the nation a Communist state and ruled with an iron fist until his death in 1980.

The nations of eastern and central Europe were dominated by the Soviet Union. They were Communist states in which the government controlled nearly every aspect of people's lives, and many people lived in fear of running afoul of government authorities. Yugoslavia charted a more independent course, and relations between the nation and the Soviets were often strained. The decade after the war was one of great economic and political turmoil in Yugoslavia, which no doubt motivated the Simic family to leave in 1954 and eventually settle near Chicago. This departure from his native land occurred when Simic was fifteen years old. Most critics

would argue that the turmoil, violence, and bloodshed that Simic witnessed both during the war and in its aftermath affected his view of the world, and therefore had a profound impact on his poetry. Further, his experience as an immigrant gave him the opportunity to meet people from all walks of life in the immigrant community, hearing their distinctive voices and observing their distinctive patterns of behavior.

CRITICAL OVERVIEW

Simic is generally regarded as one of America's most talented and influential poets, as evidenced by his winning of the Pulitzer Prize in Literature and numerous other awards. Nevertheless, the critical reception of his work has sometimes been mixed. Many reviewers of *Classic Ballroom Dances* praised the collection in glowing terms. For example, Robert Hudzik, writing in the *Library Journal*, refers to Simic's "precise surrealistic style" and says that his presentation "changes the way we look at the world and restores our sense of wonder." A reviewer for the *Washington*

Post Book World says that the poems in the collection "move with a grace of understanding and evocation and feeling reminiscent of the movement in the best of Williams' 'simple' poems." "Williams" refers to American poet William Carlos Williams, who was noted for writing poetry in simple language. Anthony Libby, writing for the *New York Times Book Review*, singles out the title poem in the collection as "striking" and "conceptually coherent." Vernon Young, writing in *The Hudson Review*, says of Simic, "Within microcosmic verses which may be impish, sardonic, quasi-realistic or utterly outrageous, he succinctly implies an historical montage, as he does in his poem, 'Classic Ballroom Dances.'" Finally, a *Publishers Weekly* contributor praises the collection for its "carefully chosen words" that have "immediacy and intriguing powers of suggestion."

Other critics, though, were less kind. Libby, while praising the poem "Classic Ballroom Dances," finds that Simic's work as a whole, up to his 1983 collection, *Selected Poems, 1963–1983*, is too reliant on "the customary devices of Surrealism," which "are used with more cleverness than vision." Even less enthusiastic about Simic's poetry is Charles Molesworth, who writes in the *New York Times Book Review* that Simic is "trapped in his own style." He finds the poetry "trifling and even cute," undermined by "false profundity" and "shopworn stylizations."

CRITICISM

Michael J. O'Neal

O'Neal holds a Ph.D. in English literature. In the following essay, he conducts a line-by-line explication of Charles Simic's "Classic Ballroom Dances."

"Classic Ballroom Dances" consists of four four-line unrhymed stanzas. The poem has no strict metrical form. It consists of a single incomplete sentence, using semicolons to link together a series of images that, together, form a gloss (an interlinear explanation, or a description inside the poem's lines) on the poem's title. The title itself is important, for it announces the subject matter of the poem and suggests that the people referred to in the body of the poem are engaged in daily activities that can be compared to dancing. The dances, though, are of a specific type: They are ballroom dances that are said to be

> THE POEM SAYS NOTHING ABOUT THE HISTORY OF THESE PEOPLE, THEIR FUTURES, OR THEIR MOTIVATIONS. IT SIMPLY CAPTURES THEM IN A MOMENT IN TIME DOING A CHARACTERISTIC ACTIVITY."

classic. Ballroom dancing, as opposed to more free-form rock and roll dancing, implies the notion of fixed, predictable steps, suggesting that the people in the poem take part in activities that are likewise fixed and predictable. Further, the dances are classic, suggesting that they have been performed over a long period of time and, as classics, they will likely continue to be performed in the future.

The poem itself begins with a glancing reference to age. The opening reference is to grandmothers who engage in a startling activity: They are said to be wringing chickens' necks. The reader pictures an elderly woman, perhaps one living on a farm, who goes out to the chicken coop to kill a chicken that will be cooked for dinner. One imagines the grandmother chasing the chicken around to catch it, as though the two were engaged in a dance. The next image, still in the first stanza, is again to elderly women, in this case, nuns, who are said to pulling the ears of schoolboys. The reader is invited to imagine a parochial school conducted by aging nuns who routinely use physical punishment as a way of disciplining unruly students, especially boys. Again, the nun and the schoolboy can be thought of as taking part in a kind of dance as the nun jerks him about in order to get him to do something.

In the first stanza, the emphasis in on the person, who is then said to be doing something. In the second stanza, the grammatical structure shifts from the person to the activity itself. The first activity, the intricate steps of a pickpocket, explicitly suggests dancing; people who dance are said to execute the steps of the dance. Again, this "dancer," like the two dancers in the first stanza, has a partner, in this case the crowd of curious onlookers who are so busy gawking at an accident that the pickpocket can

WHAT DO I READ NEXT?

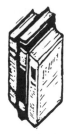

- Denise Roman, who was born in Bucharest, Hungary, is the author of *Maria Dracula* (2003), a novel for younger readers. She adopts surrealist techniques and cites Simic as one of the authors who has influenced her.

- Simic gave an insightful, humorous interview to the *Courtland Review* in August 1998. The interview is available on the review's Web site at http://www.cortlandreview.com/issue four/interview4.htm.

- Simic's commencement speech at Bucknell University on May 18, 2008, available online at http://www.bucknell.edu/x43091.xml, provides insight into his early life and its impact on his poetry.

- Readers interested in "Classic Ballroom Dances" should read the other poems in the 1980 collection by the same name, including such poems as "Ditty" and "December Trees."

- Aimé Césaire is a black poet from Martinique who writes in French, but much of his work has been translated into English and can be found in a 1983 volume, *Aimé Césaire: The Collected Poetry*, translated by Clayton Eshleman and Annette Smith. Cés-

aire's poetry has many characteristics of surrealist poetry.

- Simic himself recommends two eastern European poets whose work is not widely known in the United States: Adam Zagajewski from Poland and Tomaž Šalamun from Slovenia. Zagajewski's work in English includes *Mysticism for Beginners* (1997) and *Canvas* (1991). Šalamun's work in English includes *Feast* (2000), which was edited by Simic, and *The Book for my Brother* (2006).

- Readers interested in surrealism in the visual arts can consult Fiona Bradley's *Surrealism* (1997).

- A wide-ranging collection of surrealist and modernist poetry and drama is collected in Laurence Rainey's *Modernism: An Anthology* (2005).

- Readers who would like to explore the psychological underpinnings of surrealism may consult Sigmund Freud's *The Interpretation of Dreams* (1900). Freud wrote about the relationship between the arts and psychology in *The Psychopathology of Everyday Life* (1901).

---

easily move about and steal their belongings without their noticing.

The second image of the second stanza again throws the focus onto the activity rather than the person. In this case the activity is the shuffle of an evangelist, the word *shuffle* suggesting the kind of dance a couple does to slow music. The person's shuffle is said to be slow, echoing the images of aging from the first stanza. The evangelist is wearing a sandwich board, a "classic" form of advertising regularly used in former generations. The reader is invited to imagine such a person and the message on his sandwich board. Stereotypically, such evangelists would use their sandwich boards to urge people to repent their sins or to otherwise turn to God; alternatively, evangelical preachers would often travel from

town to town conducting tent revivals on the town's outskirts, so the reader might imagine the sandwich board advertising such an event. In either case, the reference to the evangelist provides a linkage with the first stanza and its reference to nuns.

The third stanza continues the pattern of stanza 2 by placing emphasis on the activity rather than the person. The first image of the stanza is that of the hesitation of a customer looking through the window grille of a pawnshop. The word *peeking* suggests a furtive action, as though the customer does not want anyone to notice him looking into the window; the word reinforces the customer's hesitation. The reference to pawnshops carries a number of possible implications. Pawnshops are usually associated with poverty, with being down on one's luck. People pawn goods because they have no other source of money, and people buy goods at a pawnshop generally because they believe they can get them cheaper than they could at other stores. Stolen goods are often pawned for money. Pawnshops carry an implication of seediness, of squalidness. Ultimately, the image of a hesitant customer peeking into a pawnshop window early in the morning conveys a feeling of sadness and loneliness.

The stanza continues with the image of a child walking to school. The child is said to weave, again placing emphasis on the nature of the child's movement. The child weaves because his or her eyes are closed, perhaps because of reluctance to go to school, perhaps because of fear, or perhaps because the child's surroundings are ugly. Alternatively, perhaps the child is simply playing a game by trying to determine whether it is possible to get to school with eyes closed.

The final stanza makes the poem's first explicit reference to dancing. It begins with reference to a pair of old lovers who are dancing, cheeks touching, at a union hall. The age of the lovers provides a link to the aged grandmothers and nuns of the first stanza, and perhaps to the evangelist of stanza 2. The two lovers appear to be engaged in a "classic ballroom dance." Because they are described as ancient, the reader can envision their dance as a shuffle, like that of the evangelist, or as a weave, like that of the child walking to school.

The image of the union hall suggests any one of a thousand such places across the country: nondescript buildings that are used for labor union meetings but are also rented out for dances and other events. One such event might be a charity raffle. But the raffle is not seen in the poem as a source of joy and accomplishment. Rather, it takes place on Monday nights, in the rain. The reader is invited to imagine a dreary weeknight, perhaps in a small town, where people assemble, hoping to win something in the raffle. The event does not take place on the weekend, when people typically engage in fun social activities; rather, on Monday nights the raffle becomes almost an obligation, particularly because of the rain.

Further, these rainy Monday nights all come in a November that is said to be eternal. The implications of November, particularly in the northern stretches of the United States, are of chill, gloom, and dreariness. November lacks the colorful foliage of autumn, and it lacks the charm of winter and the upcoming holiday season. November for many people is a kind of dead month that falls between Halloween and Thanksgiving. It is a month to be endured, to be gotten through. In this poem, however, November is said to be eternal. It never ends, suggesting that the people in the poem are caught in a routine dance that likewise will never end. Thus, the poem trails off on a sad note, leaving readers with an image of people caught in an endless routine—a dance of activity, none of it exciting, inspiring, or joyous. The poem says nothing about the history of these people, their futures, or their motivations. It simply captures them in a moment in time doing a characteristic activity.

Source: Michael O'Neal, Critical Essay on "Classic Ballroom Dances," in *Poetry for Students*, Gale, Cengage Learning, 2010.

Diana Engelmann

In the following essay, Engelmann demonstrates how Simic's poem "Speaking in Tongues" conveys the characteristic duality of exile.

In his essays and interviews, Charles Simic often observes that he thinks of himself primarily as an American poet with profound roots in American literature and culture: the poetry of Whitman, Dickinson, and Roethke, in particular. And to support his case for this "American" lineage, he also points to his interest in contemporary American art, especially that of the New York School; his passion for jazz and blues lyrics from the 1920s and 1930s; and his research in American folklore. While it is true that the experiences of Charles Simic, the "American poet," provide a uniquely cohesive force in his verse, it is also true that the voices of the foreign and of the mother tongue memory still echo in many poems: his childhood memories from Yugoslavia during World War II, before the family emigrated first to Paris and later to Chicago; his reading in European and especially in Serbian folklore and myth; his interest in the French surrealist movement and its specific echo among Serbian poets; his study of modern German and French philosophy; and also his translations of Vasko Popa's poetics.

"I had already begun to wonder," Simic writes, "what kind of poems I would have written had I started writing poetry in Serbian. Are the differences between the two languages on the surface, or is it true what they say about language that each one paints the world in a different way?" (*The Horse Has Six Legs*). We could take Simic's poetry as evidence that language may be permeable and that the structure of one language may shape whatever utterances occur in another. For someone writing in a second language, as Simic has done all along, a poem necessarily evolves out of more than one language and then memory. The result is a "binary vision." This is what it means to be a poet speaking "in tongues": one negotiates languages, the new one and the "other" one that resonates with older memories. These "internal translations" obviously affect pre-verbal silence, the silence where thought begins and then is shaped. The consciousness of an exile, a poet living in a second language and the first's residue, is not a consciousness that rests in memory or history. It is, rather, an "unrest-field," to borrow Vasko Popa's term. And each poem that surfaces from such an unrested consciousness has in it a trace of exile, whether it appears as subject or syntax or tone.

A Simic poem may begin with a corner musician's tune in New York, and then move to the street's end where a gypsy fortuneteller whispers some odd lines resembling old Slavic proverbs, and we suddenly discover that the same street ends in a different country and in a different time. In any Simic landscape—big city, New Hampshire countryside, or the memories of Serbian villages and the war-torn streets of Belgrade—the unexpected patterns of imagery turn back to a place of origin where "the great longing of the visible / to see itself" occurs (*Classic Ballroom Dances*).

In "Pastoral," the speaker arrives at a field that offers peculiar portraits of words and silence:

I came to a field
Where the grass was silence
And flowers
Words

I saw they were both
Of flesh and blood
And that they sense and fear
The wind like a knife

So I sat between the word *obscure*
And the word *gallows*
Took out my small cauldron
And ladle

Whistled to the word *fire*
And she answered me
From her sleep
Spat in the palm of my hand
To catch the stars
Behind my back
And light her way (*Dismantling the Silence*)

The poem moves in cryptic syntax. Surrounded by silence, we experience a sudden turn from the unusual scenery of the field to the stars and the great void above. The sleeping embers of the "word *fire*" send a spark that lands in the speaker's palm, a reminder of his continuing search for signs, for words forgotten and places long gone. Words appear as curious physical representations of their pure linguistic forms facing the speaker. In this strange field, the poet is not in a dialogue with echoes of his past and present self that emerge through the speaker's voice; rather, the voice distances its presence, and searches for the *self* of language. Approaching its essence, the speaker is oddly anonymous, a self without a *self*—a passerby, comfortable in his *self*-imposed exile.

"To be conscious," Simic says, "is to experience distancing" (*The Uncertain Certainty*). The space between the words is the space of longing to engage in a dialogue with the unknown. Here, Simic's path crosses Heidegger's thought on poetizing and metaphor as possibly our only connection to the unknowable. What is inside the unsayable may reach the outside through metaphor, and in that sense poetic language permits discursive thinking to come into being. We can know or perceive any number of things only approximately, and in order to free ourselves from the illusion of knowing, we have to recognize the limitations, the errors, the silences. Just as "flowers" grow through "the grass," "words" materialize through "silence." The reference to "both" may suggest that "grass" and "flowers" in this field are made of "flesh and blood," or that the same may be applied to "silence" and "words." The uncertainty of meaning is intentional because the "field" of translation is unstable. Simic's neo-surrealist image suggests a correlation between Popa's exploration of the "unrest-field" underlying speech and poetry and Heidegger's probing into the essence of language as that which resists thing-for-word interpretation. Every time that the voice in a poem crosses to the silent presence of the past, the poet reveals his exilic desire to recover the mythic space behind the second language and identity, where the self is still untouched by the violence of history and questions of (be)longing.

In "Mother Tongue," native language "travels in a bag," surrounded by other necessary belongings, those few chosen for survival (*Return to a Place Lit by a Glass of Milk*). This poem is one of Simic's most concise presentations of exilic sensibility.

Mother Tongue
Sold by a butcher
Wrapped in newspaper
It travels in a bag
Of the stooped widow
Next to some onions and potatoes

Toward a dark house
Where a cat will
Leap off the stove
Purring
At its entrance.

The setting and the time depicted in the poem are not specified because the suffering and displacement of the lonely widow are too common for the twentieth century. She exists in each decade and at any location: a Warsaw ghetto to a border village somewhere in the Middle East.

Each line contains at least one object essential for the poet's return to a long-gone domestic scene: "newspaper," "widow," "onions and potatoes" "house," "cat," "stove," "entrance." The widow/mother figure has the power to turn the flesh/tongue into the substance of life again and feed the poet's longing. A "butcher" wraps up the "tongue" in newspaper, the most common form of written language. The poet has to unfold pages, dates and years of information covered by the presence of a second language, in order to recapture the sounds and silences of his native speech, the widow's face, the inside of "a dark house," the space of forgetting. The ending word in "Mother Tongue" is " entrance," because the exile's journey does not stop, and the last letter in an alphabet signals the beginning of another.

Simic's poems convey the characteristic duality of exile: they are at once authentic statements of the contemporary American sensibility and vessels of internal translation, offering a passage to what is silent and foreign. Against exile and displaced memory, the quiet voice left behind in "Explorers" responds, "I recognize you. You are all / That has eluded me. / May this be my country."

Source: Diana Engelmann, "*Speaking in Tongues*: Exile and Internal Translation in the Poetry of Charles Simic," in *Antioch Review*, Vol. 62, No. 1, Winter 2004, pp. 44–47.

Ileana A. Orlich
In the following excerpt, Orlich examines Simic's connection to the surrealists.

With *Classic Ballroom Dances* (1980), Charles Simic consolidated his reputation as a major contemporary American poet, whose popularity has steadily increased since the publication of such earlier volumes as *Dismantling the Silence* (1971), *Return to a Place Lit by a Glass of Milk* (1974), *Charon's Cosmology* (1977) and *White* (1970–80). *Classic Ballroom Dances* was selected as a winner of the Poetry Society of America di Castagnola Award and was reviewed in *The New York Times* and *The Yale Review*, where Helen Vendler included Simic in a "Who's Who" gallery of poets worth watching. Simic's recent books include *Unending Blues* (1986), *The World doesn't End* (1989), and *The Book of Gods and Devils* (1990). In 1990 Simic received the Pulitzer Prize for poetry. In more senses than the casual reader of poetry could possibly imagine, Simic's achievements from 1980 to 1990 constitute his progress toward artistic fulfillment—the poet on a roll, conscious of taking extraordinary chances, "spending for vast returns," as Whitman phrased it.

Simic's early poetry was published in *Kayak*, George Hitchcock's small but interesting magazine, whose surrealist experimentations appealed to many poets who, like Simic, were coming of age during and after World War II. Simic found surrealism particularly attractive because it gave him a way of rebelling against the allusive, highly academic, paradoxical poetics of modernism. Surrealism taught him how to rearrange poetic language on a simple, non-connotative basis, in simply-stated metaphors rather than in elaborate conceits, and how to rely on accessible declaratives rather than the detached, ironic use of personae which marked the work of Pound and Eliot. Simic's acknowledgment of the surrealist tendencies in his work is expressed early in 1972 in "Where the Levels Meet: An Interview with Charles Simic."

Source: Ileana A. Orlich, "The Poet on a Roll: Charles Simic's *The Tomb of Stéphane Mallarmé*," in *Centennial Review*, Vol. 36, No. 2, Spring 1992, pp. 413–28.

SOURCES

Breton, André, "Manifesto of Surrealism," 1924, http://www.tcf.ua.edu/Classes/Jbutler/T340/SurManifesto/ManifestoOfSurrealism.htm (accessed September 2, 2009).

Hudzik, Robert, Review of *Classic Ballroom Dances*, in *Library Journal*, Vol. 105, November 1, 1980, p. 2331.

Libby, Anthony, "Gloomy Runes and Loony Spoons," in *New York Times Book Review*, January 12, 1986, p. 17.

Molesworth, Charles, "Fondled Memories," in *New York Times Book Review*, October 12, 1980, p. 36.

Review of *Classic Ballroom Dances*, in *Publishers Weekly*, August 22, 1980, p. 38.

Review of *Classic Ballroom Dances*, in *Washington Post Book World*, November 2, 1980, p. 11

Simic, Charles, "Classic Ballroom Dances," in *Twentieth-Century American Poetry*, edited by Dana Gioia, David Mason, and Meg Schoerke, McGraw Hill, 2004, p. 836.

Young, Vernon, Review of *Classic Ballroom Dances*, in *Hudson Review*, Spring 1981, p. 150.

FURTHER READING

Kolocotroni, Vassiliki, Jane Goldman, and Olga Taxidou, eds., *Modernism: An Anthology of Sources and Documents*, University of Chicago Press, 1999.

> This volume contains primary documents related to modernism in literature and the visual arts; among the topics covered is surrealism. It is not an anthology of literary works but rather an anthology of essays, manifestos, works of criticism, and similar documents that provided the intellectual and aesthetic underpinnings of the Modernist movement.

Passeron, Rene, *The Concise Encyclopedia of Surrealism*, Chartwell Books, 1975.

> This volume provides readers with brief introductions to the artists, movements, works, and styles of surrealist artists in the twentieth century.

Poplawski, Paul, *Encyclopedia of Literary Modernism*, Greenwood Press, 2003.

> The volume, written for readers in grade nine and up, contains several hundred articles on all facets of literary modernism. It includes entries on authors, disciplines, cultures and countries, theories, and movements. It thus provides a wide-ranging examination of the modernist literary culture that Charles Simic inherited.

Solso, Robert L., *The Psychology of Art and the Evolution of the Conscious Brain*, MIT Press, 2003.

> This volume is for readers interested in psychology, particularly neuroscience, and the intersections between psychology and artistic perception. It helps explain how readers see a work of art, and then bring their own histories, experiences, and expectations to bear on their interpretation of the work. The emphasis is on the visual arts, but the theories are equally applicable to works of literature, particularly those written by surrealists, who emphasize the psychology of perception and the unconscious working of the mind.

Elena

PAT MORA

1984

Hispanic American poet Pat Mora, a native Texan, writes about the feelings of struggle and isolation experienced by a Mexican American woman in her poem "Elena." In this free verse poem (a poem that eschews formal structures such as metrical patterns and rhyme schemes), Mora explores the barrier posed by the English language to Mexican immigrants like Elena, the narrator of the poem. English is an obstacle in Elena's ability to understand her children, who have learned to speak English fluently, whereas the Spanish-speaking Elena has not. Mora's descriptive poem evokes sentiments of exclusion, humiliation, and fear, and explores such feelings thematically rather than relating a story or event in a chronological fashion. Mora describes the ways in which Elena attempts to learn English, despite both her husband's disapproval of this decision and her children's exclusion of their mother from their conversations and laughter. In exploring Elena's motivations to learn the language of her adoptive country, Mora demonstrates the subject's urgent sense of need to accomplish her goal, not for her own sake, but for the sake of her children. Despite Elena's missteps and mispronunciations, and her embarrassment regarding her shortcomings, she is depicted by Mora as a brave, loving, and persistent woman.

Mora's "Elena" was first published in the collection *Chants*, originally released in 1984. The second edition was published in 1994 by Arte Publico Press.

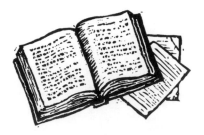

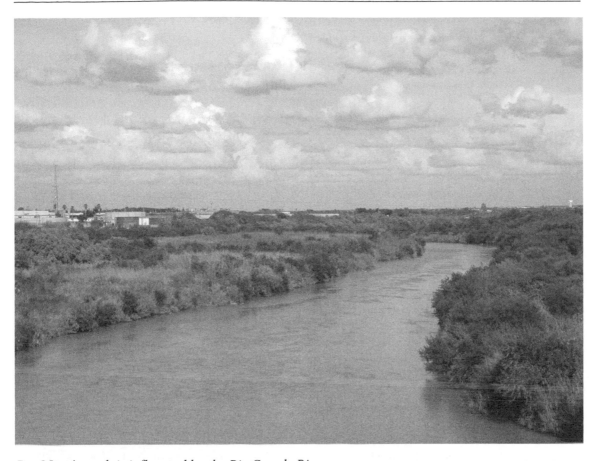

Pat Mora's work is influenced by the Rio Grande River (Image copyright Ricardo Garza, 2009. Used under license from *Shutterstock.com*)

AUTHOR BIOGRAPHY

Born in El Paso, Texas, on January 19, 1942, Mora grew up in the city of her birth and remained in El Paso through her early adulthood. At the age of twenty-one, she married William H. Burnside, Jr. The same year, in 1963, Mora received a bachelor of arts degree in English from Texas Western College. During the next several years Mora worked as a teacher while attending the University of Texas, where she received her master of arts degree in English. While Burnside and Mora were raising their three children, Mora also worked as a part-time teacher of both English and communications at El Paso Community College. She held this position from 1971 through 1978.

After Burnside and Mora divorced in 1981, Mora became an assistant to the vice president of academic affairs at the University of Texas El Paso. At the same time, she judged poetry for the Texas

Institute of Letters and additionally became director of the University Museum at the University of Texas El Paso. While at this institution, Mora also hosted a radio show at the university's radio station from 1983 to 1984. The program concerned the Mexican American perspective on life and society.

In 1984 Mora married anthropologist Vernon Lee Scarborough. After five years together in El Paso, Mora and Scarborough moved to Cincinnati, Ohio. During this year, Mora published her first volume of poetry, *Chants*, a collection containing the poem "Elena." Mora and her husband divide their time between Santa Fe, New Mexico, and Cincinnati, Ohio.

In addition to writing poetry, Mora authors children's books with a multicultural focus. Mora has received awards as both an educator and a writer, including the Harvey L. Johnson Book Award, given by the Southwest Council of Latin American Studies, in 1984, as well as a

Chicano/Hispanic Faculty and Professional Staff Association Award. Additionally, Mora was awarded a National Endowment for the Arts Fellowship in 1994.

POEM SUMMARY

Lines 1–7

Mora's poem "Elena" does not follow any patterns in terms of formal structure and is not divided into stanzas (a stanza is a unit of poetry, or a grouping of lines that divides the poem in the same way that a paragraph divides prose). There are, however, lines that are linked in terms of the subject matter they treat. The poem opens with the narrator of the poem declaring that her native language, Spanish, is insufficient. In the next six lines, Elena recalls her life in Mexico with her children. She remembers listening to her young children and smiling at what they would say. During their time in Mexico, Elena observes, she was able to understand everything her children said. She was empowered by their common language to laugh at the jokes the children told, to delight in the songs they sang. Nothing, not even their secretive childhood plans, was unknown to her. Elena recalls overhearing them plotting to get something from her. In Spanish, she recalls the children convincing each other to ask her for candy. This section of the poem ends abruptly with Elena stating, as emphatically as she asserts in the first line that her Spanish is not enough, that her memories of this special connection with her children through the bond of their language occurred in Mexico, in the past.

Lines 8–11

The tone of "Elena" shifts at the beginning of the eighth line of the poem. Things are different, Elena observes, now that her children are older and enrolled in American schools. Now the children are teenagers who speak fluent English. Elena reveals that the children sit at the table, laughing together, while she stands apart, feeling isolated, unable to understand what they are saying, unable to speak with them in English. Mora's word choice in these lines suggest that Elena feels both incapable of speech and not smart enough to learn what her children have learned. The narrator's shame and embarrassment become as apparent as her sense of exclusion.

Lines 12–20

In the next lines of "Elena," the poet explores Elena's efforts to learn English. Elena reveals that she has bought a book in order to help her learn to speak English. Her husband appears both disapproving and somewhat disinterested. When Elena shows him her book, he frowns and continues to drink his beer. Elena informs the reader that her oldest child attempts to comfort Elena by telling her that the husband does not wish for Elena to become smarter than he is by learning English. Despite this sympathy, Elena admits that at forty, learning the language is challenging. She discusses her embarrassment at not being able to pronounce words properly, and feels that everyone—her children, the grocery store owner, the letter carrier—is laughing at her. Elena confides that she takes her English book into the bathroom with her, where she can practice in private, saying the words that are so strange and difficult for her to enunciate.

Lines 21–22

The final two lines of the poem are succinct expressions of the narrator's fears. Elena insists that she must persist in her efforts, because if she does not keep trying to learn the language her children now speak with ease, she will not be able to hear them when they need her. Much is contained in these two short lines. Mora chooses to express Elena's inability to understand her children's English conversations as deafness. Clearly the family can still speak to one another in Spanish, and so Elena is not truly deaf to her children's needs. Nevertheless, if the children elect to hide something from her, they only need to speak in English. Elena is keenly aware of the fact that being able to comprehend the everyday conversations of her children will enable her to understand their lives and give her the power to advise and guide them, whether or not they directly express a need or ask for help.

THEMES

Language and Languages

Mora's poem "Elena" is concerned with the narrator's native language of Spanish and the English language of her adoptive country, the United States. For Elena, these two languages are symbolic of the conflict between the familiarity of her

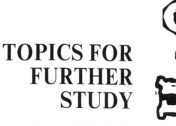

TOPICS FOR FURTHER STUDY

- Mora has written a number of children's picture books, including *The Rainbow Tulip* (1999), *Pablo's Tree* (1994), and *The Desert is My Mother* (1994). Select two or three of Mora's short children's books (choose from those listed here or from others you find in the course of your own research). Read the books and compare them to the poems in the collection that contains "Elena" (*Chants*). The picture books are written for a young audience and the poems are targeted at adults. Despite the differences in the target audience, can you identify similar themes? Does Mora use similar language or imagery to convey those themes? Write a comparative essay in which you discuss Mora's themes, language, style, and imagery, in these different formats. Use examples and quotations from the works to clarify your analysis as needed.

- The history and culture of Mexican Americans is a primary focus in much of Mora's writing. Research Mexican American culture and traditions. Are certain types of traditional foods a part of this culture? What holidays are celebrated? Are certain foods eaten only on special occasions? What type of music is unique to Mexican American culture? Are there religious ceremonies or celebrations particular to this group? What are the subjects and themes of the art and literature of Mexican Americans? Create a presentation for your class on Mexican American culture in which you consider some of these questions. Bring examples of the music, food, artwork, or other items for your class to view or sample.

- Mora's poem "Elena" is focused on a family who has emigrated from Mexico to the United States. Using both print and online resources, research how Mexican citizens become United States citizens. How is legal status attained? Are there immigration quotas (that is, are only certain numbers of people allowed to become U.S. citizens)? What criteria must be met in order to be allowed legal immigrant status? Create a written report, a Power Point presentation, or a Web page in which you discuss your findings. Be sure to cite all of your sources.

- The young-adult novel *White Bread Competition* by Jo Ann Yolanda Hernández, published by Pinata Books in 1997, tells the story of a fourteen-year old Mexican American girl, and the challenges she faces as a member of a minority in her school. The book offers readers of Mora's "Elena" a glimpse of what life might have been like for Elena's children, who are, like the characters in Hernandez's book, teenagers of Mexican descent attending an American school. Read Hernandez's novel, studying the work for ways in which the characters' bilingualism causes conflict at home or in school. Write an essay in which you use both Mora's poem and Hernandez's novel to discuss the ways in which you think speaking both English and Spanish affects the lives of teenage Hispanic American children. What might be the benefits of this bilingualism? How might the ability to speak two languages be perceived as a drawback?

native land and the challenges posed by relocating to a new country. The Spanish language for Elena is comfortable and familiar, the language in which she recalls the early years of her children's lives. It is the language of memory for her. Power over the English language is something Elena's children, now in high school, have achieved. Elena's inability to master the new language is a source of shame, embarrassment, frustration, and fear. Elena can no longer comprehend everything her children say to one another, and she is left out of their jokes. She is uncomfortable with being unable to understand her children's recounting of the day's events. Elena feels excluded because she cannot participate in conversations with her children. Furthermore, the fact that her children have mastered the English language demonstrates the level at which Elena perceives them to be assimilated into their new country.

The negative feelings Mora attributes to Elena convey the narrator's sense of being left behind by her children, who have, through the learning of the English language, become something that she is not; they are truly Americans. Excluded as she is from this transition from immigrant to American, Elena persists in her struggle to learn English. She finds the words difficult to say and is embarrassed when people laugh at her efforts. As frustrated and ashamed as Elena feels, she also understands the power the English language holds for her. Without this mastery, she fears that she will be unable to help her children when they need her. The English language represents Elena's future, while Spanish is the language of her past. Elena struggles to find a way to employ both languages successfully in the present.

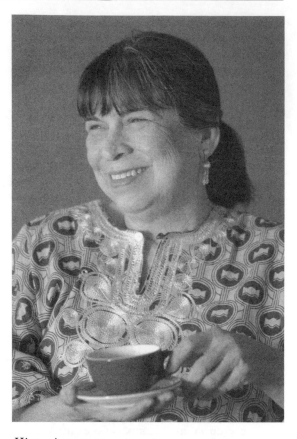

Hispanic woman (Image copyright Elena Ray, 2009. Used under license from Shutterstock.com)

Isolation

The narrator's sense of isolation in the poem "Elena" is a palpable thing, conveyed through Mora's imagery and word choice. The source of Elena's isolation is the English language, as it is spoken fluently by her children but remains a mystery to Elena. From the beginning of the poem, Mora demonstrates the narrator's sense of insufficiency and the feelings of exclusion generated by her inability to master the English language. Her own language, Spanish, is described as not being enough any longer. Before describing Elena's current troubles, Mora depicts a past in which the relationship between Elena and her children is whole, characterized by mutual understanding. Set against this backdrop, Elena's present state of isolation is more clearly understood. Her sense of exclusion is heightened by her knowledge that in the past, her relationship with her children was one in which she felt connected to them. Now, with the children speaking English and her inability to understand their conversations, that feeling of

connection is diminished. Elena fears that this connection may be lost completely.

Mora describes a scene in which the children are seated at the kitchen table, laughing together, while Elena is alone, standing next to the stove, feeling mute and foolish. Elena's physical separation from her children in this image underscores her emotional sense of separation from them. Her isolation intensifies when, as she tries to learn English, her husband frowns upon her efforts, and people, her children included, laugh at the way she mispronounces the English words she struggles so hard to learn. Mora further demonstrates Elena's sense of exclusion when Elena describes how she locks herself away in the bathroom in order to practice her English without a jeering audience. At the end of the poem, Elena's isolation is demonstrated to be a source of intense anxiety for her, as she reveals her fears of not being able to help her children in times of trouble. Without the power of the English language, Elena is set apart from her children, unable to share in the joy and pain of life with them.

STYLE

Free Verse

Mora's "Elena" is a free verse poem. A free verse poem is one in which there is no set structure, rhyme scheme, or the rhythmical pattern known as meter (the pattern of accented and unaccented syllables in formal verse). The poem consists of twenty-two lines that are not divided into stanzas (stanzas are groupings of lines in a poem that divide the poem into sections the way paragraphs divide prose). By writing in free verse, Mora is able to create a poem exploring themes of isolation and the power of language without being fettered to a structure that forces the poem to progress in a formal, linear pattern. Mora moves from the narrator's present thoughts to memories of her past, then back again to the present and the narrator's reflections on her current situation, and finally on to the narrator's expectations regarding her future. The open format of free verse allows the organic development of the poet's themes and the opportunity to develop the character of the narrator.

Persona Poem

As Pat Mora discusses in an interview with Hector A. Torres in the 2007 *Conversations with Contemporary Chicana and Chicano Writers*, "Elena" is what is known as a persona poem. In a persona poem, the poet creates a character and writes in that character's voice from a first-person point of view (in which the character refers to him or herself using "I"). Mora explains that in writing a persona poem, she is able as a poet to delve into the life experiences of individuals quite unlike herself. By using the first-person point of view, Mora creates an intimate portrait of a mother plagued by self-doubt and worry. Not only does Mora use the first person in order to provide a glimpse into Elena's thoughts, she also, in the short span of the poem, gives her character a past, a conflict-laden present existence, and a dream for the future. The personal history Mora ascribes to Elena is one lived in Mexico. While the poet does not reveal why the family left their native land, Elena's memory of her home seems pleasant. The current turmoil Elena experiences in the poem is her sense of being excluded from the lives of her English-speaking children. Driven by the need to be able to participate fully in their lives, Elena struggles to learn English. Mora also reveals that Elena hopes that learning the English language will enable her to be a guiding force in her children's life in the future. Throughout the poem, Elena speaks for herself, in the first person, conveying her fond memories of her children's youth, the current shame she feels, and her hopes and fears. In creating the persona of Elena, Mora strives to present a fully rounded character with a voice of her own.

HISTORICAL CONTEXT

Mexico and the United States in the 1980s

Mora published her poem "Elena" in 1984. During the 1980s, the Mexico that Mora and other Americans observed was a country in transition. Plagued by corruption, abuse of power, and subsequent revolution, the Mexican government began tentatively to regain its footing with the 1982 election of President Miguel de la Madrid. Attempting to remove the heavy influence of the government from Mexico's economy, de la Madrid faced an uphill battle, as Mexico was entering a severe economic recession when he took office. During his presidency, Mexico City was struck by a major earthquake in September 1985. De la Madrid was heavily criticized for the government's sluggish response in rescuing victims and aiding survivors. By the end of his presidency in 1988, de la Madrid was only marginally successful in instituting changes his country's economy.

De la Madrid's presidency overlapped with the presidency of American President Ronald Reagan, who served from 1981 to 1989. Over the years, the two presidents met on several occasions, and the relationship between them and between the two countries was characterized by both political clashes and compromises. In a 1983 meeting between Reagan and de la Madrid, the leaders discussed their mutual efforts to control the flow of illegal drugs from Mexico to the United States, the environmental issues concerning land along the border between the two countries, mutual trade, economic assistance provided by the United States to aid the development of Mexico's agricultural systems, and the political turmoil in Central American countries such as Nicaragua, El Salvador, and Panama. This final topic was perhaps the issue about which the two countries disagreed most. Despite the talk of cooperation in 1983, in 1988 President de la Madrid spoke

COMPARE
&
CONTRAST

- **1980s:** According to U.S. Census Bureau data, over 600,000 people born in Mexico became naturalized United States citizens during the 1980s. (The term naturalized refers to a foreign-born individual being granted legal citizenship.)

  Today: The U.S. Census Bureau reports that from 1990 to 2000, just over 300,000 people born in Mexico became naturalized United States citizens. Since the passage of the North American Free Trade Agreement in 1994, Mexican workers are allowed temporary stays in the United States for seasonal work, making it easier for Mexican citizens to work in the United States and then return home to Mexico, emigrating legally or illegally, and without becoming U.S. citizens.

- **1980s:** The U.S. Census Bureau reports that, as of the 1980 Census, there are 4.9 million foreign-born individuals in the United States who speak Spanish in the home. Forty-three percent of these were born in Mexico. This translates to roughly two million people in the United States who were born in Mexico and who speak Spanish in the home.

  Today: According to the 2000 Census, roughly 8.5 million Mexican-born individuals living in the United States speak Spanish in the home.

- **1980s:** Despite successful bilingual educational programs, which teach native-Spanish speaking children subject areas such as math and science in Spanish, criticism of bilingual programs increases in the 1980s as a parallel movement to make the English language the official language of the United States takes hold.

  Today: Studies in the 1990s and 2000s make the case for continued expansion of bilingual education programs in American schools. Such studies cite, for example, the increased ability to learn a third language by bilingual education students. Other research explores ways of enhancing bilingual programs through increasing knowledge of the students' cultural communities.

- **1980s:** Mexican President Miguel de la Madrid and U.S. President Ronald Reagan meet on several occasions throughout the 1980s to discuss border issues, drug trafficking, environmental issues, and the political conflicts in Central American countries.

  Today: Mexican President Felipe Calderón and U.S. President Barack Obama meet in Mexico City in April 2009 to discuss drug and weapon trafficking between the two countries.

---

out against the interference of the U.S. government in Panamanian affairs. The issue of drug trafficking would also continue to be a source of conflict between the two nations. In 1988, at another meeting between the presidents, de la Madrid defended his nation's effort to curb drug production but criticized the United States for failing to diminish the demand for the illegal substances.

A further issue between the nations during the 1980s was that of immigration of Mexican residents to the United States. In 1986, the

Immigration Reform and Control Act provided legal citizenship to illegal immigrants who lived in the United States as of 1982. In addition to this act, according to George J. Borjas in an introduction to the 2007 *Mexican Immigration to the United States*, border enforcement was enhanced, and employers faced increased fines for employing illegal immigrants. Nevertheless, illegal immigration continued to be prevalent. Borjas cites the sharp decline in income among Mexican citizens during the 1980s as a factor contributing to this increase in immigration.

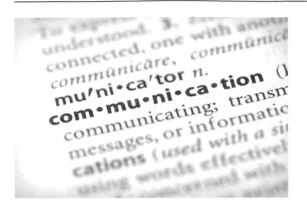

"Communication" in a dictionary (Image copyright
Mark Poprocki, 2009. Used under license from Shutterstock.com)

Hispanic American Poetry in the 1980s

During the late 1960s and throughout much of
the 1970s, the Chicano literary renaissance (a
profusion of literary production by Hispanic
American authors) paralleled the Chicano Movement, a civil rights movement focused on identifying and eliminating discrimination against
Hispanic Americans. The Hispanic American
poetry of the 1980s is built on the foundation of
the earlier renaissance. The poetry of the 1980s
written by Hispanic American poets is diverse,
but it typically reflects a strong sense of cultural
identity and often treats themes related to politics, religion, and family. Additionally, as Virgil
Suarez observes in his 2000 article on Hispanic
literature for *U.S. Society & Values*, Hispanic
American authors are connected by their shared
experience of bilingualism. Being able to think in
two languages creates unique challenges for
expression, Suarez explains. He goes on to discuss the way many Hispanic American writers
incorporate the Spanish language into their
works (written in English).

CRITICAL OVERVIEW

While there is no extensive criticism on Mora's
poem "Elena," several critics discuss her work in
general in introductions to interviews with the
poet. The critics focus on Mora's interest in Mexican and Mexican American culture and heritage
as a driving force in her writing. The passion she
bears for this topic is readily apparent in "Elena"
in its exploration of the frustrations of a Mexican
immigrant learning to speak English. Karin Rosa

Ikas, in her preface to her interview with Mora in
*Chicana Ways: Conversations with Ten Chicana
Writers*, published in 2002, observes that Mora's
writing is largely focused on "the Mexican and
Mexican American cultures and their conservation." In Bruce Allen Dick's 2003 collection of
interviews, *A Poet's Truth: Conversations with
Latino/Latina Poets*, Dick regards Mora as "one
of the best-known Latina writers in the United
States." During the interview, when Dick asks
Mora about her first collection of poetry, *Chants*,
the collection containing "Elena," Mora describes
the work as "the beginning, on paper, for me
to express my fascination with my Mexican
heritage."

Hector A. Torres writes about and interviews Mora in his *Conversations with Contemporary Chicana and Chicano Writers*, published in
2007. Torres introduces his interview with Mora
by discussing the themes prevalent in her poetry,
and by observing the way Mora appears comfortable with her bilingualism, her ability to
speak both Spanish and English fluently. In discussing Mora's collection *Chants*, Torres draws
attention to Mora's examination of the lives and
experiences of Mexican and Mexican American
women, stating that Mora's poetry "traces a
path of identification between indigenous Mexican women and the experiences of modernity
characterizing contemporary Chicanas." Additionally, Torres comments specifically on the
poem "Elena," noting that the poem connects
the title character's desire to learn English with
economic issues, and also that Elena's goal
"hints at Mora's pursuit of her own calling to
write and make a differences in the lives of other
women, Mexicanas and Chicanas alike."

CRITICISM

Catherine Dominic

*Dominic is a novelist and freelance writer and
editor. In the following essay, she demonstrates
the way in which language functions in the poem
"Elena" as a symptom of the larger conflicts Elena
experiences in her relationship with her children.*

Pat Mora's poem "Elena" is a work in which
the narrator expresses her sense of isolation from
her children. Elena pinpoints language as the
source of this growing divide, faulting her Spanish as insufficient, and demonstrating the problems in understanding that the English language

WHAT DO I READ NEXT?

- *House of Houses*, by Pat Mora, was originally published in 1997 and is available in a 2008 edition published by the University of Arizona Press. The work is Mora's memoir, but it is not written in a traditional memoir form. In lyrical prose, Mora gathers all her family members, living and dead, together in one room to talk. The memoir goes on to explore one year in the life of Mora's family.

- *Pat Mora (Who Wrote That?)* by Hal Marcovitz is a biography of Mora geared at a young-adult audience. The book was published by Chelsea House Publishers in 2008 and is part of their larger "Who Wrote That" series of biographies. Marcovitz discusses, among other topics, Mora's youth, her early interest in writing, and her sense of belonging to two cultures, that of Mexico and that of Texas.

- *Parrot in the Oven*, by Victor Martinez, won the 1996 National Book Award for Young People's Fiction. The novel, available through Rayo in a 2004 paperback version, is the coming-of-age story of a Mexican American teenage boy.

- *Cool Salsa: Bilingual Poems on Growing up Latino in the United States*, edited by Lori Carlson, is a collection of poems written in Spanish and in English translation. Some poems utilize both languages; a glossary of Spanish words and terms makes the collection accessible to English-speaking readers. Published by Fawcett in 1995, the collection features the works of well-known and lesser-known poets and treats complex and emotional themes such as the frustrations of being an immigrant, fitting in, and dealing with discrimination, as well as poems simply exploring the ups and downs of everyday life.

- *Ethnicities: Children of Immigrants in America*, edited by Rubén G. Rumbaut and Alejandro Portes, and published by the University of California Press in 2001, is a collection of essays by scholars of immigration studies. The essays focus on the ways in which the children of immigrants from all over the world deal with the process of becoming American.

- *Woman Hollering Creek and Other Stories*, by Sandra Cisneros, is a collection of short fiction about Mexican American women living in Texas in which Cisneros treats themes similar to those explored by Mora: a sense of identification with two cultures, family life, and feelings of isolation. The work was published by Vintage in 1992.

---

generates in her household. Her children speak English well; she does not. Yet underlying the overt conflicts created for the narrator by language is another, more subtle reason for the isolation Elena feels. The poet hints at transitions in Elena's household, transitions that are not confined to the homes of Mexican immigrant families. Elena's children are not only being transformed by their conversion from Spanish speakers to English speakers and by their assimilation to life in America. Elena's children are also growing up. Mora contrasts Elena's memories of her children's youth in Mexico with their teenage life in America; while the contrasts between Mexico and America, between Spanish and English, dominate the poem, the contrast between Elena's children as youngsters and as teenagers is also a central feature of the poem.

In the poem's opening lines, Mora has her narrator Elena recall life in Mexico with her young children. Elena speaks of being able to understand her children, understand their jokes and songs, and their secret conspiring with one another. Yet one may read these lines as imbued

> THE POET HINTS AT TRANSITIONS IN ELENA'S
> HOUSEHOLD, TRANSITIONS THAT ARE NOT
> CONFINED TO THE HOMES OF MEXICAN IMMIGRANT
> FAMILIES. ELENA'S CHILDREN ARE NOT ONLY BEING
> TRANSFORMED BY THEIR CONVERSION FROM
> SPANISH SPEAKERS TO ENGLISH SPEAKERS AND BY
> THEIR ASSIMILATION TO LIFE IN AMERICA. ELENA'S
> CHILDREN ARE ALSO GROWING UP."

with another meaning as well. Not only did Elena understand her children's language when they were young, when they all spoke Spanish with one another, but she was able to understand her children as people. As a mother of youngsters she comprehended the straightforward needs and desires of her children. They wanted to laugh, play, sing, and enjoy some occasional sweets. The lives of the children and the interactions between the children and their mother were uncomplicated when the children were younger. Elena's fondness for this time is captured by Mora through the image of Elena smiling as she listens to her children, and by the affectionate references made about the children in this early part of the poem.

Now, however, Elena finds her home occupied by two American teenagers. There are no sweet references here; the children are no longer little. She speaks of feeling excluded from conversations her children have with one another in English. The imagery of the poem sets her physically apart from the children, underscoring Elena's sense of separation: the children are seated at the kitchen table, and Elena stands by herself, at the stove. While Elena's isolation is intensified by the language differences between herself and her children, one can easily imagine this scene playing out in any American home. The teenagers are speaking to one another in what appears to the listening parent as code. The teens may be using slang terms, or text messaging terms, or they might even be texting one another, laughing at jokes the onlooking mother cannot understand. Whereas earlier in the poem

Elena spoke of being able to understand everything her young children said, suggesting that she truly understood everything about them, now that they are older, Elena feels as if she cannot comprehend her children at all.

Her sense of being disconnected from her children is acutely painful. Mora puts very negative words in Elena's mouth; she speaks of feeling stupid, unable to communicate. Her efforts at learning to speak English generate feelings of embarrassment and shame. If one considers the fact that the children, whose first language is Spanish, are still able to speak Spanish, then the issue of Elena's isolation becomes more apparent, and the intensity of her feelings is more easily understood. Elena and her children are still able to communicate with one another. The children could easily speak Spanish with their mother and in their mother's company. Yet the teenage children choose to make themselves unavailable to their mother by speaking in English instead. It is the fact of this choice that is at least as significant as the language issues at work in the poem. Elena's children, by choosing, like many other teenagers, not to communicate with their mother, by opting to communicate with each other in a way their mother cannot understand, choose to exclude her. The fact that Elena's children make this very deliberate choice is a major part of the sense of isolation that Elena feels. The main conflict in the poem is not simply an internal one within Elena; it is not simply that she cannot understand her children. A major conflict exists between Elena and her children, apart from the conflict Elena has with the English language. Elena's children voluntarily choose not to be understood by their mother. They elect to isolate her. While they attempt to console her when their father disapproves of Elena's efforts to learn English, the children nevertheless intensify their mother's feelings of exclusion by laughing at her when she mispronounces words. Mora skillfully underscores Elena's distance from her children when they are listed along with the grocer and the mailman—familiar strangers—as individuals whose laughter makes her feel embarrassed.

One must not omit from this discussion another cause for Elena's sense of isolation: her husband. Not only does he apparently disapprove of her efforts to learn English, but he also does not seem to be involved in either the life of his wife or the lives of his children. Elena makes no reference to her husband in her reflections on the past in Mexico, when the children were young. Nor does she seem likely to turn to him for support as a parent of teenage children. They do not present a united front in coping with the changes their children are undergoing. Elena stands alone while the husband drinks his beer.

The fear Elena reveals in the poem's last lines is that her children will need help that she will be unable to provide if she does not keep trying. Presumably, Elena is referring to her efforts to learn English, but this is not stated directly. Her desire is to remain a significant presence in the life of her children, to be the person they turn to when help is needed. The husband is notably absent from these lines as well. Elena does not see herself as part of a parenting team, but knows that she, unlike her husband, must not withdraw from her children's lives simply because they have grown older, because they have changed. She insists on trying, despite her fears and embarrassment, despite the fact that her children have made choices to purposefully keep her separated from them. Elena nevertheless endeavors to remain present, to attempt to keep understanding her children. She claims not to want to be deaf to their needs. While her desire to learn English to be able to communicate with them, to hear them in the language in which they choose to speak is an obvious component of her effort to remain a significant part of her children's lives, Elena seeks on a larger scale to remain emotionally connected with her children. Elena must not only overcome the barrier of language, but also the emotional barriers her children have erected in order to keep their mother separate, apart from them.

One final component attributing to Elena's sense of isolation, a factor also related to the issue of language, can be inferred from the poem. Elena does not reveal what has brought her family from Mexico to the United States. Whatever the reasons though, the family is now settled, the children are enrolled in an American high school where they have learned English. From the fact that the children are sitting together in the kitchen, talking and laughing, one can assume that they are relatively happy. Elena has provided opportunities for her children that she apparently did not have; she has given them an American education and the chance to learn English. However, by giving her children such opportunities, Elena has been instrumental in the children's transformation into people who are very different from herself. By exploring this transformation, Mora highlights the irony of parenting. As any mother would, Elena strives to make her children's lives better than her own. In doing so, she isolates herself from them, simply by providing them with the opportunities for experiences she never had. Mora's poem, then, touches on universal themes, despite the specific experiences discussed in "Elena." Within the context of the language conflicts of an immigrant family, Mora examines the isolation a mother creates between herself and her children, and the deliberate exclusion of a mother by her children.

Source: Catherine Dominic, Critical Essay on "Elena," in *Poetry for Students*, Gale, Cengage Learning, 2010.

Diana Huber

In the following interview, Huber speaks with Mora about the importance of reading in general and poetry in particular to young readers.

Bilingual writer Pat Mora is this year's featured writer for the fifth annual Lacey Loves to Read community-wide literacy initiative.

The community is invited to read books by Mora, who will lead writing workshops and speak at a free reception during her Feb. 27–28 visit.

Mora has written more than 30 award-winning children's books that incorporate both English and Spanish. She also has several volumes of poetry for young adults and adults, as well as a memoir that chronicles her experiences of growing up on the Texas-Mexico border.

Mora's upcoming book as a collection of food haiku titled *Yum! ¡Mmm! ¡Que rico!*. She also is working on a compilation of poetry for teenagers.

Mora also is the founder of the family literacy initiative El dia de los ninos / El dia de los libros— Children's Day / Book Day—now housed at the American Library Association. The yearlong commitment of linking all children to books, languages and cultures culminates in celebrations across the country April 30.

She lives in Santa Fe and has three grown children.

Here, Mora tells *The Olympian* about what inspires her writing and why poetry and reading are so important for today's youth.

You decided to become a writer after a career in education and as a university administrator. What prompted this transition?

Growing up, I never saw a writer who was like me. I didn't see a writer who was bilingual. I think young people aspire to be what they see is possible.

I was always a reader, thanks to my mom.... The dream of being a writer came later to me, because I had to work through that notion that it was possible for someone like me to become a writer....

I want young people to understand we often get better at the things we spend a lot of time on. If they spend a lot of time reading and writing, they probably will be better at both, too.

You incorporate Spanish words into many of your stories and poems. Did you intend to write bilingual works from the start?

I grew up in a bilingual home and feel so fortunate.... It's hard to imagine not using both. The comparison I use is the black and white keys on the piano. If you play the piano, you don't want to pass up the black keys.... I want to have that music that I think is part of another language.

Where do you get your inspiration?

Writers are nosy, so we listen and eavesdrop a lot. I'm always looking for a good story. I travel a lot; that gives me the advantage of listening to teachers, librarians and students.

Why is poetry important for young people?

We tend to think something is important when we love it. I love poetry; it is my favorite genre. I love to read it, I love to write it, I love to share it.

On a practical level, I think poetry improves everybody's writing. Poetry demands we delete extra words, and we struggle to find the most vivid example....

I think poetry speaks to us in an interior way. Ideally poetry brings us back in touch with ourselves...not the self that's constantly under stress, but the deeper self. In that way poetry can be incredibly refreshing.

Is poetry going out of style in an age of Internet, MP3 players and video games?

I fear it. My optimistic side wants to believe that books have a particular power that is a magnet to people. But perhaps the more realistic side is that books require quiet time, and if we

> TO BRIDGE THE BORDERS, YOU NEED THE RIGHT COYOTE TO HELP YOU ACROSS. MORA'S COYOTES OR MEDIATORS ARE A STRONG, FEMALE-IDENTIFIED CULTURE AND A BELIEF IN THOSE ASPECTS OF CULTURAL CONSERVATION THAT AFFIRM THE SELF."

don't foster that in our homes and in our schools, it's not a habit that will be easily cultivated, because distractions pull young people away.

What are the challenges of being a Latina writer?

They are many. It's going to be uphill all the way for my generation. Only about 2 percent of children's books published in a year are by or about Latinos, even though Latinos are about 14 percent of the population....

It's so important that we change our definition of what American literature is to reflect the rich diversity of this country.... We want books that make all kinds of children feel at home.

Source: Diana Huber, "Writer Pat Mora Encourages Literacy in Two Languages," in the *Olympian*, February 10, 2008.

Linda C. Fox

In the following review, Fox examines the importance of borders, river cities, and heritage in Mora's poetry.

During a visit to the Fort Wayne Museum of Art in January of 1994 to read from her poetry, Chicana writer Pat Mora remarked that she had grown increasingly aware of the powerful role of water and borders in her life (Mora 1994). At that time Mora was living in Cincinnati, where she had moved in 1989 after many years of residence in El Paso, Texas, one of the principal border towns between the United States and Mexico, with the Rio Grande providing the dividing line. Yet Mora sees Cincinnati as a border city as well, with its river—the Ohio River—serving as separation of the North from the South and its history of crossings from slavery to what was thought to be freedom.

Borders and river cities, then, are paramount in Mora's life experience. This observation will come as no surprise to the reader of her first collection of poetry, *Chants* (Mora 1984), where the imagery of the Texas / Mexico border expresses poignantly the division that Mora feels exists not only between the woman on the other side of the river and herself, but also between parts of her own identity at odds with one another. The burdensome perception by others of her as a cultural misfit, "an American to Mexicans / a Mexican to Americans / a handy token / sliding back and forth / between the fringes of both worlds, / by smiling / by masking the discomfort / of being prejudged / bilaterally," weighs heavily upon Mora as a writer at the border, both geographically and psychologically. Borders can be barriers difficult to overcome, for, as Mora says, "prejudice is in the very air we breathe" (Mora 1992).

Yet it is precisely the tension of this split or pull that leads Mora to forge in time a positive image of who she is. In her first book of essays, *Nepantla: Essays from the Land in the Middle*, Mora reflects often on her world as a border dweller who negotiates constantly the border between the United States and Mexico, between European-American culture and her own Chicana culture. She states: "There probably isn't a week of my life that I don't have at least one experience where I feel that discomfort, the slight frown from someone that wordlessly asks, what is someone like her doing here? But I am in the middle of my life, and well know not only the pain but also the advantage of observing both sides, albeit with my biases, of moving through two, and in fact, multiple spaces, and selecting from both what I want to make part of me, of consciously shaping my space" (Mora 1993, 6). Mora thus emphasizes that the survival skills that she had to learn as a border resident and "translator" of cultures are accompanied by a creative force that frees her to forge a richer, stronger, more integrated self-identity through the choices she makes.

Mora's position as a border dweller has also influenced her poetics. As Leobardo Saravia Quiroz says in his essay "Cultural and Literary Writing on the Border," she is among those writers who "are reclaiming a vision of the border as an internal point of reference for them as individuals and also as writers, though not necessarily the geographical point written about" (Saravia 1989, 66). Mora does begin with geography in *Chants*, but goes well beyond the physical border of the Southwest to portray the socioeconomic, racial, and cultural separations that exist there. For Mora, the Chicana poet compares to the curandera, an indigenous, gentle healer, who learns her craft informally and lives within a strong oral-storytelling culture. Mora recognizes that, like the curandera, she has learned most of her art from hearing and reading others, and she is dedicated to "saving the stories" of her Mexican culture so that the world will appreciate the often unnoticed and devalued aspects of her heritage (Mora 1992). She asks, "How can I be a child of the border and not know with Audre Lorde that in this country 'oppression is as American as apple pie'?" (Mora 1993, 34). A believer in "cultural conservation," a term borrowed from ethnomusicologist Alan Lomax, Mora in her poetry documents, validates, and dignifies her Mexican heritage, a heritage that she ignored as a young woman until one day she awakened to the treasures it held: "Mexico was like a beautiful chest of smooth, dark wood that my mother had in her bedroom," but that was passed by and over until Mora was able to value what it held for her (41).

Mora's feminist beliefs impact her poetics as well. In an interview with Norma Alarcon in 1986, Mora makes clear her bond with women of the past and her hope for those who represent the future: "I am a feminist and totally comfortable with the term. Though I would respect and fight for women's right to choose their political stance in this world, I sometimes have trouble understanding how women cannot see the need for banding together, for some speaking out, for more equity in this world. We have a lot to offer and I feel that I walk on the bones of talented women who were never heard. I am uncomfortable with that and I want change" (Alarcon 1986, 124). Although in the same interview Mora is ambivalent about viewing her writing as feminist, since she wants no message decided on ahead of time as she begins a poem, her focus is on the women who border her, whether they are real (her daughters, her Tia Lobo, her mother, and her mamande) or metaphoric (the desert, "mi madre"). A constant in all three volumes of Mora's poetry, these female figures help her negotiate between the past and the future, and they provide her with lessons in survival and hope, from either side of the geographical or generational border.

Mora recognizes that oppressive traditions need to be rejected, whether they originate in Mexican or Anglo culture. The challenge for Mora is to construct a cultural and feminist identity while straddling what Alvina Quintana calls "two opposing realities that fail to acknowledge her" (Quintana 1991, 76). Gloria Anzaldua, in her now classic *Borderlands / La Frontera*, expresses the need to reject the culturally transmitted paradigms that are harmful to Mexican women while retaining the positive contributions to her self-identity: "Ya no solo [sic] paso toda mi vida botando las costumbres y los valores de mi cultura que me traicionan. Tambien recojo las costumbres que por el tiempo se ran provado [sic] y las costumbres de respeto alas mujeres" (Anzaldua 1987, 15). Anzaldua rejects all imposition of personality on her and fights for the Nahuatl concept of "the freedom to carve and chisel my own face" (22). Mora's words echo Anzaldua's thoughts: "Much as I want us, my daughters, my niece, Chicanas of all ages, to carry the positive aspects of our culture with them for sustenance, I also want us to question and ponder what values and customs we wish to incorporate into our own lives, to continue our individual and collective evolution" (Mora 1993, 53). However, although Mora recognizes along with Anzaldua that such a creature in transition is vulnerable and that there are cures that sting, the psychic unrest that Anzaldua confesses is not characteristic for Mora: "To transform our traditions wisely, we need to know them, be inspired and saddened by them, choose for ourselves what to retain. But we can prize the past together, valuing the positive female and Mexican traditions. We can prize elements of the past as we persist in demanding, and creating, change" (56). Both lived reality and metaphoric construct, Nepantla—and its concomitant image of borders—remains central to Mora's work. Her growing world view gained from travel to other lands and the encounter with other cultures reveals to her borders of many kinds, as an examination of selected poems from the three collections will show.

In *Chants*, some borders are more permeable than others. "The ability to see both sides of the border," as described by Emily Hicks (1991, xxiii), can be seen in Mora's much studied poems dealing with the desert Southwest, where the poetic speaker, a modern "assimilated" Chicana writer, values and is a part of the rituals and traditions that affirm female creativity, strength, and endurance. "Bribe," the initial poem of *Chants*, describes the female connectedness the modern writer feels when, in the search for inspiration, she reenacts the ancient Indian ritual of an offering to the desert. Her ballpoint pen and lined yellowing paper are like the turquoise the Indian women bury as they chant: "Guide my hands, Mother, / to weave singing birds / flowers rocking in the wind, to trap / them on my cloth with a web of thin threads" (Mora 1984).

Kristina Passman points out in her study "Demeter, Kore, and the Birth of the Self" that in Mora's work "the desert world is a place of safety for women, where the worlds of nature and of women are integrated" (Passman 1990, 331). Mother, teacher, and worker of magic, the desert and the females who dwell there serve as a bridge from one generation to another, a border easily traversed. The gentle healing skills of the curandera and of the woman in "Abuelita Magic" who soothes the tears and the cries of her daughter and grandchild with the desert rhythms of a dried chile pod provide an interconnectedness of female nurturance. The abuelita in "Family Ties" who rewards her granddaughter with the pragmatics of white uniforms, not the frills of a hair ornament, and the aging but feisty tia who still savors a full meal at Denny's ("Pushing 100") and a moment of dancing ("Bailando") serve as a source of treasured memories of strong and active Mexican women from a past generation bordering the poet's own.

However, there are characteristics of Chicana life on the border inherited from the Mexican past that Mora rejects as nonaffirming. Mexican women's rigidly prescribed gender roles, especially as they relate to the control of female sexuality, are deconstructed in such poems as "Dream," "Plot," and "Aztec Princess." "Dream" presents the patriarchal value that imposes female virginity at marriage: "Village women say orange blossoms melt on an unclean bride" (Mora 1984). The fear that someone will know that the bride has already acted on her sexual desire is seen as laughable in the light of day (and thus reason), yet frightening at night: "By day I laugh at our Mexican superstitions. / At night they grab me. Draw blood. Like you." The myth of "wild" female sexuality, which must be tightly controlled until marriage, obviously supports the separate spheres for men and women as in "Aztec Princess" where it is the mother, transmitter of male-determined traditions, who insists to a daughter who longs for a fuller life: "Look in the home for happiness." The custom of burying the female umbilical cord in the house is a sign for the female "to nest inside" and symbolizes female confinement against which the young girl rebels by taking the earth, in that no vestige of her cord remains, and carrying it outside to "breathe." In his study "Grandmother Borderland," Patrick Murphy rightly points out that "the girl chooses the outdoors and moonlight against family and domesticity." However, to affirm, as he does, that "Mora sees custom and family as part of the schism between woman and nature, between personal / cultural identity and place" (Murphy 1993, 39–40) is true only with respect to Chicano patriarchal practices, and is not a wholesale rejection of her Mexican heritage of customs and family. In "Plot" it is precisely the mother, herself a victim of the patriarchal view of women as either virgins or whores, who will help her daughter, the next generation, negotiate between her reality and the "proof of virginity" her society requires. She offers the bride-to-be a ring from a Coca Cola can so, by cutting herself, the daughter will be able to prevent the inevitable violence that would result from a lack of a blood stain, whether she is a virgin or not.

If the borders between traditional customs of Mexican / Aztec origin and modern Chicana life are permeable, economic privilege separates social classes and does not permit as easy a crossing. Access to education and to several university posts heightened Mora's awareness of her own privileged position. In her interview with Norma Alarcon in 1986, Mora states: "When I drive to work at the University [of Texas, at El Paso], I see their houses right across the river. So, every day I am aware of the differences between my life and theirs, and of the role of chance in one's life. I could have been born on the other side of the river" (Alarcon 1986, 2). In "Illegal Alien," Socorro, the poetic speaker's Mexican housekeeper, crosses the physical border daily—illegally—to allow her Mexican American senora the freedom to sit "waiting for a poem" (Mora 1984). In "Mexican Maid," skin color is the socioeconomic indicator, and whiteness is desired by the Mexican woman who serves her sunbathing, patronizing Anglo senora. By contrast, in "Illegal Alien" the poet, despite her Mexican heritage, is unable to provide the emotional comfort Socorro needs when,

by revealing the physical violence she endures at the hands of her husband, the housekeeper violates the boundary of social class. The title is ironic, of course, since the poet, with her "cool words" and "plastic bandaid," is the one who is the outsider, the marginalized one, the "alien," at least from the perspective of the human ability to share emotion and to help one another. "Graduation Morning," the story of the relationship between a nurturing Mexican housekeeper and her young Anglo charge, in turn stands in contrast to "Illegal Alien," suggesting that children are more capable of deconstructing the border of economic and class difference: "Though she's small and thin, / black sweater, black scarf, / the boy in the white graduation robe / easily finds her at the back of the cathedral, / finds her amid the swirl of sparkling clothes, / finds her eyes. / Tears slide down her wrinkled cheeks. / Her eyes, luceros, stroke his face." Vicki Ruiz notes the struggle not only for survival but for dignity of many domestic workers in El Paso, one of the most impoverished cities in the United States: "Although frequently victimized, Mexicana domestics are not victims but women who meet each day with integrity and endurance" (Ruiz 1987, 74). Mora recognizes the bravery of these women from the other side of the river who confront oppression daily.

Just as economic privilege in *Chants* distances women of different classes, the clash between English and Spanish is presented as a linguistic border that also separates "them" from "us." Without language there is no communication, and in the United States people of other cultures are silenced when "English only" is the rule. Assimilation can mean deculturation. All too often "linguistic terrorists" in power act to wipe out any trace of other languages in this country for, as Gloria Anzaldua asserts: "Wild tongues can't be tamed, they can only be cut out" (Anzaldua 1987, 54). No wonder, then, that when Mexican families "adapt" to life on this side of the border, they eventually face the dilemma that the "Elena" of Mora's poem has when her own language becomes inadequate in everyday life:

I bought a book to learn English.
My husband frowned, drank more beer.
My oldest said, "Mama, he doesn't want you
to be smarter than he is." I'm forty,
embarrassed at mispronouncing words,
embarrassed at the laughter of my children,
the grocer, the mailman. Sometimes I take

my English book and lock myself in the
   bathroom,
say the thick words softly,
for if I stop trying, I will be deaf
when my children need my help.
(Mora 1984)

Mora has said that "people like Elena are one of the reasons I write" (Mora 1992), that she also writes bilingual children's books peopled with brown faces so that children of Hispanic heritage in this country will learn the value of knowing more than one language as well as see strong cultural role models so rarely present in what they read. Here again, Mora's views coincide with Anzaldua's: "Ethnic identity is twin skin to linguistic identity—I am my language. Until I can take pride in my language, I cannot take pride in myself" (Anzaldua 1987, 59).

In *Borders,* published in 1986, Mora's grounding continues to be Nepantla as she further explores the border concepts between generations, classes, races / ethnicities, and languages seen in *Chants.* The desert appears in fewer poems in this volume, but the rootedness and empowerment that the Southwest symbolizes for Mora in "Desert Women" and "Disguise" are more important here than the real, geographic landscape. Passman points out that "in Borders, Mora develops the theme of the woman 'passing' as an acceptable, assimilated woman, while maintaining her deep sense of connection to the forces that shaped her: her grandmother and the desert" (Passman 1990, 331). It is evident that from the vantage point of the adult lyric speaker the bonds between women of differing generations and retrieved cultural heritage are intertwined. The endurance and strength of "desert women" are underscored in the poem of the same name:

Desert women know
about survival.
Fierce heat and cold
have burned and thickened our skins.
   Like cactus
we've learned to hoard,
to sprout deep roots,
to seem asleep, yet wake
at the scent of softness in the air, to hide
pain and loss by silence,
no branches wail
or whisper our sad songs
safe behind our thorns.

Don't be deceived.
When we bloom, we stun.
(Mora 1986, 80)

Adversity is a toughening influence in the desert, and the apparent passivity of desert women, like that of the cactus, is simply an illusion for, as Mora says, "even in inhospitable places, cactus bears fruit" (Mora 1993, 56).

Just as Southwest women look to the desert as teacher of survival, as nurturer, and as refuge, the speaker's childhood memories in "Disguise" revolve around her grandmother's lap where she curled up after a game of dress-up, a safe haven that allowed her to be "the real me." She likens her present routine as an adult woman who "passes" in a grown-up world to that long-ago pretending to be what is not "the real me," and she dreams of the comfort that special place allowed:

Black heels and a proper gray dress
walk down the hall on a fall afternoon
Grown Up
I stand on tiptoes in there
to smear on make-up every day walk
stilt legs on thin heels, daydream
of shedding this heavy skin, fitting
in a steady lap.
(Mora 1986, 45)

However, the reality is that she must continue to behave as a grown-up whose physical appearance exudes self-confidence despite her desire to shed the outer trappings of adult womanhood.

The class lines initially drawn in *Chants* between senora and maid continue to be divisive and difficult to cross. In "Echoes," feelings of solidarity with the Mexican maid, as before, do not translate into action:

Again and again I hear:
just drop the cups and plates
on the grass. My maid
will pick them up.
Again and again I feel
my silence, the part whirring round me.

I longed to hear this earth
roar, to taste thunder.
to see proper smiles twist
as those black words echoed
in the wind again and again:
just drop...
my maid
just drop...
my maid

Perhaps my desert land waits
to hear me roar, waits to hear

me flash: NO. NO.
Again and again.

In their introduction to *Infinite Divisions,* Rebolledo and Rivero observe that "for middle-class Chicanas, the distinction between mistress and maid is guiltily observed: they are sisters in femaleness above all" (Rebolledo 1993, 112); thus "in the world in that she lives the poetic speaker [of Borders] is not quite at home; there is always a pea under the mattress, a cactus thorn in the flesh" (32). In this case the discomfort comes from the speaker's awareness of the inequity with which she and the Mexican maid are treated because of class difference.

Some of the previous context of separation caused by the language border also continues in *Borders,* yet there are even deeper connections made between language and discrimination, between the linguistic border and its intersections with racial / ethnic ones. Now the focus is not only the Spanish language, which is not valued in the United States, but the denigration of the culture itself. Even though the speaker of "Bilinqual Christmas" and "Now and Then, America" has "made it" into the boardrooms and corporate offices, she is "different" (read Mexican American) and feels patronized, marginalized, and tokenized in a society that pays lip service to diversity by "adding a dash of color / to conferences and corporate parties / one per panel or office / slight south-of-the-border seasoning," but outside the corporate Christmas party office has, instead of "twinkling lights," "search lights / seeking illegal aliens / outside our thick windows" (Mora 1986, 21). In the second poem, "Now and Then, America," the speaker rejects the sterile conformity of the model for success in the United States that does not allow her, despite her socioeconomic class, her authenticity, her mezcla. The lyric voice pleads for true acceptance, not only of her American side, but of her Mexican side as well:

> Who wants to rot
> as she marches through life
> in a pin-striped suit
> neck chained in a soft, silk bow
> in step, in style, insane.
> Let me in
> to board rooms wearing hot colors,
> my hair long and free,
> maybe speaking Spanish.
> Risk my difference, my surprises,
> Grant me a little life, America. (33)

The value placed on the Mexican side, with its liveliness and animated display of emotions, is evident in "Sonrisas," which uses the imagery of "two rooms" to indicate the crossroads that characterize the poetic persona's life:

> I live in a doorway
> between two rooms, I hear
> quiet clicks, cups of black
> coffee, click, click like facts
> budgets, tenure, curriculum,
> from careful women in crisp beige
> suits, quick beige smiles
> that seldom sneak into their eyes.
>
> I peek
> in the other room senoras
> in faded dresses stir sweet
> milk coffee, laughter whirls
> with steam from fresh tamales
> sh, sh, mucho ruido,
> they scold one another,
> press their lips,
> trap smiles
> in their dark Mexican eyes. (20)

The guarded demeanor and conformist dress of the academic community contrast sharply with the casual, "sweet" vivaciousness of the Mexican womanculture, in both of which Mora is capable of participating but between which she feels torn.

This awareness of her border identity informs Mora's casting of two new images in this second volume: the border between mother and children and the border between men and women. Although we cannot assume that in every poem the lyric speaker's experience is that of the poet, it is important to note that in the period that the poetry of *Borders* was being written, Mora was a divorced mother with three children, and her life experiences at that time almost surely shaped the poetic presentation of these boundaries.

As any mother knows, the border between mother and child is a delicate one; it can be bridged but is made ever more difficult because of outside pressures. The mother is the guardian of her young children's safety, both physical and emotional, and despite the fact that the nurturing mother would like to spare her children pain, it is often not possible. The mother in "Same Song" is sensitive to her adolescent children's feelings of dissatisfaction and self-criticism when they look into the mirror, because she knows that in a world that provides images of a perfection impossible to achieve, her twelve-year-old daughter will never be fair-skinned enough and her sixteen-year-old son will never have the perfect body he desires. A visit to the hospital in "Waiting Room: Orthopedic Surgery" reveals just how fragile the human body is:

> Usually I believe my children
> charmed, armed with rubber
> bones and flesh beneath
> their sweet, soft skin.
> Here
> canes, casts, wheelchairs,
> bound feet tell loud tales . . .
>
> . . . we are fragile
> we bleed and break. (42)

Even before a mother's work of raising her offspring is completed, in a rare moment it is possible to gain a glimpse into the relationship between her and her child when the mother will have grown older and the child will be an adult. Whereas now she is the nurturer, it will then be her child who, in reversed roles, becomes the source of encouragement. "Goblin" describes this flash of the future when, in encountering a storm after leaving the movie house, "You pulled my hand gently / jumping puddles, tugging / 'You can make it. Jump' / My eleven-year-old mothering me" (43). Certainly the mother-child border can be a separator, as in "The Heaviest Word in Town"—which is "NO"—but Mora as mother of teenagers, who are at an age marked by particularly difficult passages for both mothers and children to negotiate, is taken back in "Oral History" to the protected feeling of years past when her Tia Lobo would tell her and her siblings stories that linked their past and future, her four lobitos "who even now curl around the memory / of you and rest peacefully / in your warmth" (50). Mora surely realizes that the legacy of the stories of their ancestry will live on long after she, her children's mother, is not here anymore. Thus, "saving the stories" through generations is a task that allows mediation not only between mother and child, but also between her Americanized children and their Mexican roots.

The border between men and women is even less easily crossed, especially when there have been repeated failures of communication and authenticity of self is at stake. The color-separated symbols of male and female placed in opposition on the cover of the book and the positioning of the title poem as the first the reader encounters clearly signal the importance of this particular border.

Mora quotes researcher Carol Gilligan with respect to the difference in men's and women's language: "My research suggests that men and women may speak different languages that they assume are the same" (9). "The side-by-side translations / were the easy ones," says the poetic persona, acknowledging the fact that sexual liaisons and pillowtalk are facile but that really hearing the other in a relationship is much harder to achieve:

> So who can hear
> the words we speak
> you and I, like but unlike,
> and translate us to us
> side by side? (10)

When women are defined primarily as objects for sexual gratification or when motherhood and the accompanying self-sacrifice and nurturing of others become cultural imperatives, expressions of doubt in female self-worth become common, such as in "Diagnosis" when the senora facing a hysterectomy expresses her fear—"No sere mujer, doctor"—to the Anglo who will remove what he calls "a useless uterus" (25). In "Out of Business" the female is the "doctor" and men are her "patients"; she serves their emotional needs by squeezing out the pus from their infected wounds, only to never get repaid or have them reciprocate. The title refers to the statement that leads off the poem: "First Aid Station Closed. Newly Divorced Men Don't Stop By My Door" (61). Vulnerable after divorce, the poet in "Internal Battle" describes the challenge to reconcile the craving for independence with the need for a man in a relationship where she can "gaze at our shadows distinct / yet linked by choice" (55). Bridging this chasm places strength and softness in opposition, yet both are needed for the poetic female persona to reestablish faith in a man. Annihilation of self is a danger as she becomes absorbed in another relationship, and she declares hatred of her softness that allows her, like her cat, to "be bruised again" (57). Her fear of disappearing is countered by a firm grip in "Woman Mysteriously Disappears":

> That's what
> the headline
> would say
> but I'm too clever.
> I grip
> bridge rails
> when inviting rivers
> call me

far down
below
tempting me to dare.
When I'm with you
I secretly
grip furniture
and door handles.
I never stare
into your eyes
for long. (56)

In societies and cultures where male dominance is standard, the female in a heterosexual love relationship may well risk denial, even annihilation, of her very identity. The differences between male and female make revealing one's true self a frightening step ("My Mask"), but ultimately the poet finds the union "by choice" that will allow her to be who she is. Mora's poem "Marriage II" is undoubtedly autobiographical, since the two who unite to "dig together" for the songs of the past and the blooms of the present are archaeologist and poet, in the poem and in real life.

If gender politics and family politics are the prevalent borders in her second volume, in Mora's third collection of poetry, *Communion*, published in 1991, the primary emphasis is on geopolitics. Mora extends her "border feminism"—a term Saldivar Hull uses in her essay "Feminism on the Border" (Saldivar Hull 1991, 211)—as she writes of situations she encounters in her travels. Since 1986, the year in that a Kellogg Scholar grant enabled her to study cultural conservation issues, Mora has traveled to many foreign lands, an experience she considers one of her great teachers (Mora 1993, 153): "It is in my trips out of this country that I best see our weaknesses and our strengths" (159). Although the borders presented in *Chants* and *Borders* are still present in this volume (desert / modern woman in "Desert Pilgrimage"; class difference in "The Other Woman"; American / Mexican culture in "Foreign Spooks"; language in "A Voice"; mother and child in "Teenagers;" men and women in "Probing"; a rejection of violence toward women in "Perfume" and "Emergency Room"), a concern for a broader community (and hence the title, *Communion*) is the salient theme of this collection. Mora says, "Ultimately my community is not only my ethnic community but also all the like-minded souls seeking a more equitable world" (147), and the poet searches on her travels for those who practice the same rites, for those who profess the same faith in creating a better world, as she does.

Communion signifies an act of sharing, of seeing the commonalities, of transcending—not denying—the differences that separate us. Writing from the border(s) has not been a confining experience for Mora, for she is able to deconstruct geopolitical markers thanks to her border dweller's identity; she knows that borders can be crossed in at least two directions. At the same time her feminist solidarity allows her to understand other women's lives, across country and custom and class and ethnicity. Thus, such poems as "Veiled" and "Too Many Eyes" question the silence and gravity of Pakistani women in the face of customs that silence and confine them. In "Veiled," the subversive poetic "we" stealthily takes all the burqas to the river to free the trapped emotions they contain, and wonders:

will the water loosen
laughter trapped inside those threads
will light songs rise
and swirl with the morning mist

or will sighs rise,
heavy, dark like storm clouds?
(Mora 1991, 34)

"Too Many Eyes" captures the clash of customs Mora experienced in Pakistan, where she was stared at constantly, a visitor in a culture that covers women and makes them nearly invisible:

Horseflies, those eyes
nipped at my unveiled skin
day after day wearied me
until I, a vain woman,
avoided mirrors and make-up,
pulled my hair back
with one quick twist,
hid in my wrinkled clothes. (36)

Although American women and Mexican women don't veil themselves physically, Mora is aware that life on the border of any patriarchal culture reveals a shared female experience of suppression. Enforced domesticity and public invisibility of women are common characteristics for women who live in such cultures, and when Mora read her border poems in a "safe," private setting in Pakistan, the women said to her: "You are just like us" (Mora 1993, 97).

Even in revolutionary Cuba, where Mora witnessed improved access to health care for all, streets safe even late at night, and artists happily engaged in their work, observation of the female rituals of life makes Mora question in "The Mystery" the omnipresent smile on women's faces as they work hard, live poor, and follow orders in a society where they are destined to produce cookie-cutter soldiers: "They smile when their children march / by in uniform, all in step, all smiling" (Mora 1991,41).

Children and mothers or grandmothers become the special focus in *Communion* as Mora examines the border between the haves and have-nots. Whether the setting is Peru, Mexico, or the Dominican Republic, the harshness of the struggle for sheer survival is documented by the eyes of children. The disenfranchised little gift in "Fences" who daily touches what she will never own is contrasted with the turistas' easy-flowing wealth:

> Mouths full of laughter,
> the turistas come to the tall hotel
> with suitcases full of dollars.
>
> Once my little sister
> ran barefoot across the hot sand
> for a taste.
>
> My mother roared like the ocean,
> "No. No. It's their beach.
> It's their beach." (50)

Often we look away so as to avoid really seeing poverty's painful injustices, unprepared, as in "Picturesque: San Cristobal de las Casas" to bear witness to the exhaustion that being poor exacts: "But no one told me about the bare feet. / No one told me about the weaver's chair, a rock. / No one told me about the wood bundles bending / women's backs. No one told me about the children / who know how to open their smiles / as they open their dry palms" (57). Just as often, as in "Peruvian Child," we as privileged tourists take snapshots that commodify the subject for "picturesque" consumption:

> We wanted, as usual, to hold a picture
> of the child in a white border, not to hold her
> mud-crusted hands or feet or face,
> not to hold her, the child in our arms. (60)

Mora asks, Whose beach is it, anyway? Why must we look away when we confront inequities in this world? How can we cross the borders that divide us as human beings? How can we reach communion with other peoples and make space for future generations to live in a healthier world?

The answers to Mora's questions go back to lessons learned in Nepantla. If, as Renato Rosaldo says, Anzaldua's *Borderlands / La Frontera* "celebrates the potential of borders in opening new forms of human understanding" (Rosaldo 1989, 216), so too the poetic work of

Pat Mora offers solutions. To bridge the borders, you need the right coyote to help you across. Mora's coyotes or mediators are a strong, female-identified culture and a belief in those aspects of cultural conservation that affirm the self. In "Cissy in a Bonnet," a poem about Mora's daughter's bonnet, which the small child called her brain, worn backward at age four and still carried by Mora wherever she moves, the mother-poet suggests that an integrated self-identity is only fully realized when one is able to look not only ahead but behind:

> Maybe part of the journey is always backwards,
> the careful brushing away of the layers,
> personal archaeology, uncovering forgotten,
> broken pieces, sifting even in our dreams
> until we fit the jagged edges into round wholes
> we cherish privately; and occasionally we
> break the code, with our fingers read our early
> symbols, reunite with the rare spirits we house.
> (Mora 1991, 81)

Mora, like the new mestiza of whom Anzaldua speaks, transcends her duality so she is "on both shores at once" (Anzaldua 1987, 78). Mora calls herself "a compact hybrid, the flor de noche buena" (Mora 1992), that grew wild in Mexico but then became domesticated as the poinsettia in this country. Hybrids are bred to retain the strongest characteristics of at least two strains, and strength is the key. Mora believes, in the empowering words of her poem "The Young for Juana," that "my hands are strong, and from within I rule" (Mora 1991, 78). Pat Mora's ability to negotiate borders is a powerfully positive tool in working for justice in an imperfect world.

Source: Linda C. Fox, "From Chants to Borders to Communion: Pat Mora's Poetic Journey to Nepantla," in *Bilingual Review*, Vol. 21, No. 3, September–December 1996, pp. 219–31.

SOURCES

Borjas, George J., ed., Introduction to *Mexican Immigration to the United States*, University of Chicago Press, 2007, pp. 1–12.

Camp, Roderic Ai, "The Time of the Technocrats and Deconstruction of the Revolution," in *The Oxford History of Mexico*, Oxford University Press, 2000, pp. 609–36.

"De La Madrid Indirectly Hits U.S. Intervention in Panama's Affairs," in *Los Angeles Times*, March 27, 1988, http://articles.latimes.com/1988-03-27/news/mn-431_1_de-la-madrid, (accessed on August 1, 2009).

Dick, Bruce Allen, "Pat Mora," in *A Poet's Truth: Conversations with Latino/Latina Poets*, University of Arizona Press, 2003, pp. 93–106.

Escamilla, Kathleen, "A Brief History of Bilingual Education in Spanish," *ERIC Digest, Education Research Information Center*, March, 1989, http://www.eric.ed .gov/ERICWebPortal/Home.portal?_nfpb = true&ERICExt Search_SearchValue_0 = ED308055&searchtype = keyword &ERICExtSearch_SearchType_0 = kw&_pageLabel = Record Details&objectId = 0900019b8010cdc5&accno = ED308055&_ nfls = false (accessed August 1, 2009).

Gerstenzang, Jame, and Dan Williams, "De la Madrid Lectures Reagan on Drug Effort—Defends Mexico's Fight to Halt Cultivation and Smuggling, Says U.S. Fails to Curb Consumption," in *Los Angeles Times*, February 14, 1988, http://articles.latimes.com/1988-02-14/news/mn-42660_1_de-la-madrid (accessed August 1, 2009).

Ikas, Karin Rosa, "Pat Mora: Poet, Writer, Educator," in *Chicana Ways: Conversations with Ten Chicana Writers*, University of Nevada Press, 2002, pp. 127–52.

Lipski, John M., "The Importance of Spanish in the United States," in *Varieties of Spanish in the United States*, Georgetown University Press, 2008, pp. 1–13.

Moll, Luis C., "Bilingual Classroom Studies and Community Analysis: Some Recent Trends," in *Educational Researcher*, Vol. 21, No. 2, 1992, pp. 20–24.

Mora, Pat, "Elena," in *Chants*, 1984, reprint ed., Arte Publico Press, 1994, p. 58.

Nicholas, Peter, and Tracy Wilkinson, "Obama Pledges Help in Mexico's War on Drug Lords, with an Exception," in *Los Angeles Times*, April 17, 2009, http://www. latimes.com/news/nationworld/world/la-fg-obama-mexico17-2009apr17,0,7867926.story (accessed on August 1, 2009).

"North American Free Trade Agreement," in *United States Department of Agriculture Foreign Agriculture Service*, http://www.fas.usda.gov/itp/Policy/nafta/nafta. asp (accessed August 1, 2009).

Sanz, Cristina, "Bilingual Education Enhances Third Language Acquisition: Evidence from Catalonia," in *Applied Psycholinguistics*, Vol. 21, No. 1, 2000, pp. 23–44.

Suarez, Virgil, "Hispanic American Literature: Divergence and Commonality," in *U.S. Society & Values*, February 2000, pp. 32–37.

Torres, Hector A., Introduction to *Conversations with Contemporary Chicana and Chicano Writers*, University of New Mexico Press, 2007, pp. 1–32.

———, and Pat Mora, "Pat Mora: I was Always at Home in Language," in *Conversations with Contemporary Chicana and Chicano Writers*, University of New Mexico Press, 2007, pp. 244–74.

"United States Foreign-Born Population," in *U.S. Census Bureau*, http://www.census.gov/population/www/ socdemo/foreign/STP-159-2000tl.html (accessed on August 1, 2009).

FURTHER READING

Casanova, Rosa, and Adriana Konzevik, *Mexico: A Photographic History*, Editorial RM, 2007.
> In this work, written and edited by Casanova and Konzevik, the holdings of Mexico's Fototeca Nacional, or national photographic archives, are reproduced, offering a glimpse of Mexico's history over the past 130 years. The photos catalogue the social and political changes in the nation's history, as well as provide an overview of the artistic and cultural developments that have occurred in Mexico.

García, Cristina, ed., *Bordering Fires: The Vintage Book of Contemporary Mexican and Chicano/a Literature*, Vintage, 2006.
> García introduces this collection of essays, stories, and poetry by Hispanic American writers. The collection is organized chronologically by the various movements in Hispanic American literature.

Hakuta, Kenji, *The Mirror of Language: The Debate on Bilingualism*, Basic Books, 1986.
> Hakuta explores the issue of bilingualism and bilingual education, discussing in particular the differences in the ways children and adults learn a second language. Hakuta also studies the educational and intellectual value of the acquisition of a second language.

Worth, Richard, *Mexican Immigrants (Immigration to the United States)*, edited by Robert Asher, Facts On File, 2004.
> Worth provides a brief history of Mexican immigration to the United States. The work is targeted at a young adult audience.

Fully Empowered

PABLO NERUDA

1962

"Fully Empowered" is a poem by Pablo Neruda, who is considered to be one of the greatest twentieth-century poets. The poem was first published in Spanish in 1962 in the volume of the same title, *Plenos poderes*, which was translated into English as *Fully Empowered* by Alastair Reid in 1975. This book was reprinted in 2001 with an introduction by Reid. Both editions are bilingual, with the Spanish text appearing alongside the English translation. The poem can also be found in *The Poetry of Pablo Neruda*, edited and with an introduction by Ilan Stavans, published by Farrar, Straus, and Giroux in 2003. Another translation of the poem, titled "Full Powers," can be found in the collection of Neruda's poems *Five Decades: Poems, 1925–1970*, translated by Ben Belitt and published by Grove Press in 1994.

Neruda wrote "Fully Empowered" quite late in his long poetic career. It is a personal, highly symbolic poem that employs images that recur many times in Neruda's poetry. It might be understood to refer to the poet's creative process and his role as a poet. With its richness of imagery and the affirmative joy of its theme, "Fully Empowered" is an intriguing introduction to Neruda's work.

AUTHOR BIOGRAPHY

One of Latin America's greatest poets, Neruda was born Neftalí Ricardo Reyes Basoalto in Parral, Chile, on July 12, 1904. His mother died

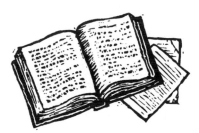

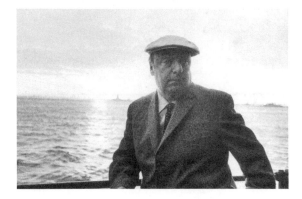

Pablo Neruda *(Sam Falk | Hulton Archive | Getty Images)*

when he was an infant, and in 1906 he moved with his father to Temuco in southern Chile. At school he was encouraged in his early literary efforts by the poet Gabriela Mistral, who recognized his talent. By the time he graduated from high school he had already published poetry in local newspapers and magazines, and while still in his teens he adopted the name Pablo Neruda. Soon after moving to Santiago, Chile, in 1921 to study French, he published the volume that established his poetic fame—*Veinte poemas de amor y una canción desesperada* (1924), translated by W. S. Merwin as *Twenty Love Poems and a Song of Despair* (1969).

In 1927, Neruda traveled to Rangoon, Burma, where he had been appointed Chilean consul. It was the custom in Chile to appoint poets to diplomatic positions abroad. Neruda took the opportunity to travel extensively in the Far East. He also wrote one of his most highly praised poetry books, *Residencia en la tierra*, which was published in two parts in 1933 and 1935. It established his international reputation and was published in English as *Residence on Earth and Other Poems* in 1946. Neruda added a third volume, *Tercera residencia*, in 1947.

In 1934, Neruda was sent to Spain as Chilean consul. However, he was relieved of his post after the Spanish Civil War broke out in 1936 because he wrote a poem in support of the Republican cause against the Fascists. He moved to Paris, where he continued to support the Republicans by founding political and cultural organizations.

In 1943, Neruda joined the Communist Party and was elected to the Senate in 1946. But when President González Videla broke with his former communist allies in 1947, Neruda protested against censorship. He was expelled from the Senate and a warrant was issued for his arrest, but he went into hiding and then fled to Argentina.

One of Neruda's most important poems, an epic celebration of the history and the people of the American continent, *Canto general*, was published in 1950; excerpts translated by Ben Belitt as *Poems from the Canto General* were published in 1968. In the early 1950s, Neruda traveled to Italy and France. He met a Chilean woman, Matilde Urrutia, who on his return to Chile in 1952 became his second wife.

Neruda's *Odas elementales* (1954; *Elementary Odes*, 1961) made poetry subjects out of everyday objects and became some of his most popular poems. Later in the 1950s and continuing for the remainder of his career, Neruda's poetry grew less political and more personal. Notable publications include *Estravagario* (1958; translated by Alastair Reid as *Extravagaria*, 1972); *Plenos poderes* (1962; translated by Reid as *Fully Empowered*, 1975); and *Memorial de Isla Negra* (1964; translated by Reid as *Isla Negra: A Notebook*, 1981).

In 1970, Neruda was the Communist Party candidate for the presidency of Chile, but he withdrew in order to support the socialist candidate, Salvador Allende, a personal friend. After Allende's victory in 1970, Neruda was appointed Chile's ambassador to France. The following year he was awarded the Nobel Prize for Literature.

Neruda died of cancer on September 23, 1973, in Santiago, twelve days after Allende was assassinated in a right-wing coup that toppled Chile's socialist government.

POEM SUMMARY

Stanza 1

"Fully Empowered" is a poem about how the poet writes, how he mines the material for his work. It is also a celebration of the entire range of his life as a human being. The poem must be understood metaphorically, since there is no literal meaning to many of the phrases he uses. In the first stanza, the poet says that he writes outside in the sunshine, in the crowded street. Perhaps he means by this that he writes about matters that everyone can see and participate in, as part of a human community. Varying the metaphor, he continues that he writes when the tide is in, suggesting a seaside location, but again this should not be understood literally. He likely means that he writes when the tide of creativity flows in him. These are all places, he states at the end of line 2, where he can write well. He then uses a musical metaphor, but he is talking about writing and self-expression. In line 3, he identifies something that puts a brake on his creativity, and he calls it night. It stops his work for a while but then he learns how to use the night, perhaps as material for his poetry.

Stanza 2

In stanza 2, the poet continues to write of his own creativity in highly metaphoric language. In line 6 and 7, he writes of the night coming while his eyes focus on something that can be clearly seen and measured, perhaps as material for poetry. In line 8, continuing to explore his creative process, he may be referring to a twenty-four-hour period from one sunrise to the next, including all the hours of darkness. During this time, he is creating the means of understanding so that he can unlock his own creativity. In the twilight, he explores. By this he may be referring metaphorically to things that are not obvious or not clearly seen or understood. He keeps exploring until the sea fills everything. The sea may be a metaphor for truth and knowledge that can bring the light of understanding to all the dark places, the areas of the mind and heart that were formerly empty or unknown.

Stanza 3

The poet writes in stanza 3 of how he loves the process of poetic creativity he has metaphorically described in the previous two stanzas. He mines all aspects of the psyche, from light to dark, and goes back and forth between them. He is not concerned about death; he embraces life and death, it does not matter which.

Stanza 4

In stanza 4, the poet reflects on how he came to have what he feels are his obligations, perhaps to the earth. He questions from whom or what he may have inherited these obligations. Was it from his parents, he wonders, or from some other, nonhuman source, the mountains, perhaps?

Stanza 5

The poet maintains his thought from the previous stanza but does not try to reach any conclusions. The first line continues to explore metaphorically his sense of obligation to life itself, which spreads out in all directions from the central core of his life. All he knows or cares to know is that he continues to live and do what he does simply because that is what he does. His activity is its own reward and justification.

Stanza 6

Stanza 6 continues to emphasize that there is something about his life and his psychic processes that is beyond any explanation that he could give. He digs deep into his own being with closed eyes and finds two contrary forces pulling at him. One pulls him toward death, while the other seems to celebrate life and does so in order that the poet might celebrate, too.

Stanza 7

In this final stanza, the poet reaches an ambiguous conclusion from everything he has said up to this point. He says that he is formed out of something that is not life. He may perhaps be referring to an inner silence or nothingness that is life in its unmanifest form, but he does not say this explicitly. He leaves it to the reader to understand. He continues with a metaphor about the sea. Just as the waves of a sea break against a reef and pull back stones from it as they ebb, so he, too, is a part of death. Something pulls at him too, and it is death, but paradoxically death is what opens him up to life. He continues to express this paradox in the final line, which returns to the images with which the poem began, of day and night, light and dark. The being of the poet inhabits both these realms, which suggests the "fully empowered" state of being referenced in the title.

THEMES

Creativity

As the very first line makes clear, "Fully Empowered" is a poem about writing. It is about the creative process as experienced by the poet. The poem is entirely metaphorical and might give rise to a number of interpretations. The main thrust of meaning, however, seems relatively clear. Although the poet does not explicitly name them, he identifies two regions of the psyche

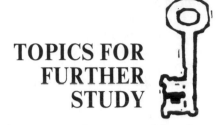

TOPICS FOR FURTHER STUDY

- Sit out in nature, perhaps near a lake, river, or sea, and write a poem in which you use imagery drawn from what you are observing and experiencing in the natural world. How does the scene make you feel? What do your senses observe?

- Find another poem by Neruda that you like and compare it with "Fully Empowered." Give an oral presentation in which you read both poems aloud and comment on their similarities and differences.

- What is the purpose of poetry? Does it fulfill a useful function in society? What might that function be? Read the lecture Neruda gave when he accepted the Nobel Prize for Literature (http://nobelprize.org/nobel_prizes/literature/laureates/1971/neruda-lecture-e.html) for ideas on the topic. Consider the issues Neruda raises in his speech and then give a class presentation, showing your main points using PowerPoint or a similar program.

- Consult Joseph Roman's biography, *Pablo Neruda*, written for young adult readers and published in 1992 by Chelsea House in their Hispanics of Achievement series. Using material from this book, write an essay on Neruda in which you explore how and why he supported the Communist Party. What did he think that communism or socialism might achieve in Chile?

that might be called day and night. The day aspect seems to refer to everything that is clearly visible, since the metaphor used is that of the sun. There is also a social element to this day element; it is that part of the poet that engages with other people. In the first stanza, the poet seems very comfortable with that side of the psyche; his work flows out easily. He is happy and untroubled.

The other half of the psyche is first mentioned in line 3 of the first stanza. The overall metaphor is that of night. This is not so comfortable or easy

for the poet. Night seems to slow down his creativity at first, but he learns how to understand the darkness and use it to yield more knowledge and understanding of life, which, of course, will then be expressed in his poetry. What does he mean by this metaphor of night? He may be referring to those aspects of life that are harder to understand and harder to deal with. They may be less obvious than the "daylight" part of the psyche, but they may hold deeper truths. The poet needs to dig down into the deeper parts of his psyche to access them. When he does this, it makes his work more complete, more satisfying. He understands, or seeks to understand, the totality of his being. He is not content with knowing only isolated parts; he wants a full knowledge of himself, and this will empower him, as the title suggests.

In learning how to access, in the process of poetic creativity, all aspects of the psyche, the poet states in stanzas 4 and 5 that he is aware of how his being is connected to so much on earth, both human and nonhuman. His own self extends in so many directions, and it all becomes material for poetry. In stanza 4, he speculates about this connection, wondering where it comes from, but in the next stanza he shows no desire for intellectual understanding. He is content just to live, without seeking rational explanations for why he thinks or feels the way he does. This is the secret, he suggests in stanza 6, to his creativity. It is an intuitive process that cannot be explained rationally. When he turns his attention within, cutting off the world of sense perception, he somehow manages to access two contrary forces, the impulse to life and the impulse to death. He creates poetry out of this understanding of the whole range of life.

A Celebration of Life

"Fully Empowered" explores poetic creativity yet it is also a celebration of life, the poet's life in particular but only as it represents something universal. Indeed, in this poem it is hard to separate poetry from life. As the poet seeks understanding of his life, he gives out, in his poetry, the wisdom he has gained. Life and poetry are no more than two names for the same phenomenon. As a poet, Neruda writes of life as he lives and knows it. The more knowledge and understanding he has, the more "fully empowered" he feels. It is a process of coming into himself in all his fullness. He celebrates his life in all its manifold aspects, some knowable, some not. There are no regrets in this poem, no complaints, only acceptance and the impulse to explore and to know, to access the deepest stream

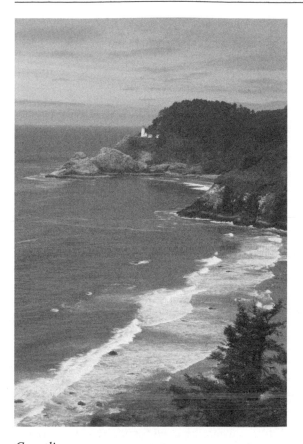

Coastline *(Image copyright Jeff Shanes, 2009. Used under license from Shutterstock.com)*

of life as it manifests in the poet's own being. He aspires to know and embrace everything, leaving nothing out, but this is not a restless search for knowledge. It is ripe with the glow of an achieved state of being that is always fluctuating, never static, and never ceasing to nourish the poet's inner life. This life consists of a coexistence of opposites that the poet explains with the use of various metaphors. Two of these opposites are life and death. He celebrates life whilst always possessing an awareness of death, from which life is inseparable. Death, for example, is mentioned in stanzas 3, 6, and 7, but it does not impinge on the poet's celebration of the totality of existence. On the contrary, death is essential for life.

STYLE

Paradox

One of the main elements in "Fully Empowered" is the coexistence of opposites. Experiencing or being aware of opposing elements (light and dark, life and death, for example) is part of the poet's search for a complete experience of life. This culminates in the occurrence of what is called a paradox. In *A Glossary of Literary Terms*, M. H. Abrams defines paradox as "a statement which seems on its face to be self-contradictory or absurd, yet turns out to make good sense." The paradoxes in the poem occur twice in the final stanza. The poet finds that his awareness of death actually shows him life; and then in the final line he states that although it is daylight, he walks in shade. What he means, perhaps, is that he has learned to live at a deeper level than that of the surface, conscious mind. He has mined the depths of the psyche, so even when he is living out his day-to-day activities, he is in fact functioning from another source, perhaps closer to the heart of life, but described in terms that echo the nighttime he evoked earlier in the poem.

Imagery

This poem is made up of images rather than statements that can be understood in a literal way. Image in its most basic sense means something that can be pictured by the reader. One such image is that of the sun, which also functions as a symbol. A literary symbol, according to Abrams, is "a word or phrase that signifies an object or event which in turn signifies something, or has a range of reference, beyond itself." The sun image perhaps suggests a certain clear-headed consciousness the poet possesses at certain times. This image occurs in stanzas 1 and 2 and is implied in the last line of the final stanza. Another image is that of the sea, which occurs in stanzas 1, 2, 5, and 7, as well as being implied in the water imagery of stanza 6. This imagery symbolizes a certain quality of the poet's consciousness. It may imply his receptiveness to the deeper levels of his mind, the flow of creativity that he is able to access. However, in the final stanza, the meaning of the sea image appears to change. This is an example of a simile, in which two different things are compared in a way that brings out the similarities between them and is often recognized by the occurrence, as in line 27, of the word *as*. The image of the waves of the sea eroding the reef is compared (starting in line 30) to death, which suggests that the sea is life itself eventually wearing down the physical body (the implied equivalent of the reef referred to in line 27).

Night, and associated images of darkness, form another set of images in this poem. Like the sun image, night and darkness may be understood as symbols for states of mind or consciousness. Other images include keys, intended to signify the fact that the poet can unlock the mysteries of life, and stone, which is used in connection with death, meaning it lacks the dynamic quality of sea and life.

In a broader sense, imagery may refer not only to visual images but to all sense perceptions. For example, the speaker repeatedly (stanzas 1, 5, and 6) presents himself as singing, which is an auditory image. Perhaps by this reference to singing he implies that the writing of poetry might be understood as a kind of celebration or song of life.

Persona

The first-person speaker in a lyric poem is referred to as the persona. Persona is from a Latin word meaning mask. Persona refers to the way the poet chooses to present the speaker of the poem. The persona is not to be confused with the author of the poem, although in many lyric poems the two are close, if not identical. In this poem, the persona is, like Neruda, a poet, as the first line states. The persona also presents himself in a number of other guises—as traveler (line 12), although he describes neither a starting point nor a destination because he journeys within the psyche; as a locksmith (lines 8–9) who makes keys and seeks locks to unlock; and throughout the poem as an explorer who absorbs in himself the mysteries of life.

HISTORICAL CONTEXT

Latin American Poets of the Mid-Twentieth Century

While Neruda was the preeminent Latin American poet of his day, there were other poets of distinction during this period. Chilean poet Vicente Huidobro (1893–1948) was well known in his own country and abroad. Huidobro lived in Europe during the 1920s, and it was partly through him that the European movement known as modernism became a force in Latin American poetry, although as D. P. Gallagher points out in *Modern Latin American Literature*, Latin American poets also had the confidence to discard European influences when they chose to.

"It was their own experience, their own sensibility, and their own vision that were ultimately to matter," wrote Gallagher. There was no love lost between Huidobro and Neruda, however. Huidobro appears to have resented the fame of the younger poet and sent Neruda anonymous letters attacking him. This is reported by Neruda in his *Memoirs*, in which he describes Huidobro as "typical of a long line of incurable egocentrics," but also acknowledges that Huidobro was an "extraordinarily gifted poet."

Another noted Chilean poet was Gabriela Mistral (1889–1957), who was one of Neruda's early mentors and later became his close friend. In 1945, she became the first Latin American to win the Nobel Prize for Literature. From the 1920s, Mistral lived mostly abroad. Like Neruda, she was named Chilean consul and served as a diplomat in many different consulates, including Naples, Italy; Madrid, Spain; and Lisbon, Portugal. Toward the end of her life she lived in Roslyn, New York.

A greater figure than either Huidobro or Mistral was the Peruvian poet César Vellejo (1892–1938). In 1923, Vellejo left Peru for Europe, where he lived for the remainder of his life. In the 1930s, like Neruda, he became passionately and dogmatically committed to communism, and he supported the Republicans in the Spanish Civil War. However, according to Gallagher, Vellejo did not allow his political views to affect his poetry. Vellejo and Neruda were the two greatest Latin American poets of the twentieth century. Neruda regarded Vellejo as a friend and wrote two poems about him. When the two poets both lived in Paris, they saw each other daily. Vellejo was also a friend of Huidobro.

The Mexican poet Octavio Paz (1914–1998) is another important Latin American poet of the mid-twentieth century. According to Gallagher, Paz's poetry shares with Neruda and Vellejo "the same quest for a better world." Neruda took note of Paz early in the Mexican poet's career, after Paz's first book was published, which Neruda thought very promising. Neruda invited Paz to Madrid in 1937 for an anti-Fascist congress of writers. Paz went on to win the Nobel Prize for Literature in 1990.

In the 1960s, a number of Latin American poets identified themselves with the Third World, especially Africa and Southeast Asia, believing that they had more in common with these colonized people in their struggles for

COMPARE
&
CONTRAST

- **1960s:** Some translations of Neruda's work are published in the United States, but he is still not that well known among the literate public. As a Communist, he is barred from entering the United States, but the ban is relaxed to enable him to attend the thirty-fourth International PEN Congress in New York, in June 1966. Neruda's public reading in New York is filled to capacity. Those who cannot get in watch and listen on closed-circuit television.

  Today: Neruda is an extremely popular poet in the United States. His odes and his love poems are particularly well known. Neruda is depicted in the film *Il postino*, or *The Postman* (1994), about a friendship between Neruda and a postman.

- **1960s:** In the late 1960s, Neruda takes an active role in Chilean politics, campaigning for the left-wing party led by Salvador Allende. After coming to power in 1970, Allende is assassinated in 1973 and a military dictatorship rules Chile until 1990.

  Today: Chile is a stable democracy that is committed to maintaining representative government. It has a market-oriented economy and strong financial institutions.

- **1960s:** Almost all poets in Chile, according to Neruda, are committed to political ideals. They are on the left of the political spectrum, calling for radical reform. Political reform in Chile focuses on land reform. Prior to land reform in the mid-1960s, 4.4 percent of landholders own nearly 81 percent of total farmland. The country is divided into a small number of large farms and a large number of farms whose inhabitants are barely able to eke out a subsistence living. Unproductive large farms contribute to a stagnant economy.

  Today: Chilean poet Carmen Berenguer wins the Ibero-American Pablo Neruda Prize in 2008. Her poetry is considered a voice for the poor people in the southern part of the country. Like much of Neruda's work, her poetry exhibits a concern for Chilean society. She offers a critique of society that questions the process of modernization.

---

freedom than with Europe or the United States. These poets took a revolutionary, socialist stance in their work, supporting guerilla warfare. Writing in 1975, Gordon Brotherston in his book *Latin American Poetry: Origins and Presence*, commented, "Controversial as this emphasis is, not least among the left in Latin America, it has affected recent poetry of the subcontinent deeply and divisively." According to Neruda himself, in an interview with American poet Robert Bly published in 1967, almost all the writers in Chile were on the political left. "We feel supported and understood by our own people. That gives us great security and the numbers of people who support us are very great," Neruda said. He also commented that poets in the 1960s were no longer tied to traditional poetic forms but had the freedom and the confidence to experiment:

> When I was a very young poet I was afraid to break all the laws which were enforced on us by the critics. But now . . . all the young poets come in and say what they like and do what they like.

CRITICAL OVERVIEW

Neruda wrote a total of thirty-five books of poetry, and due to this huge output not every poem he wrote has been discussed directly by critics and reviewers. In the case of "Fully Empowered" most comments refer to the entire book, *Fully*

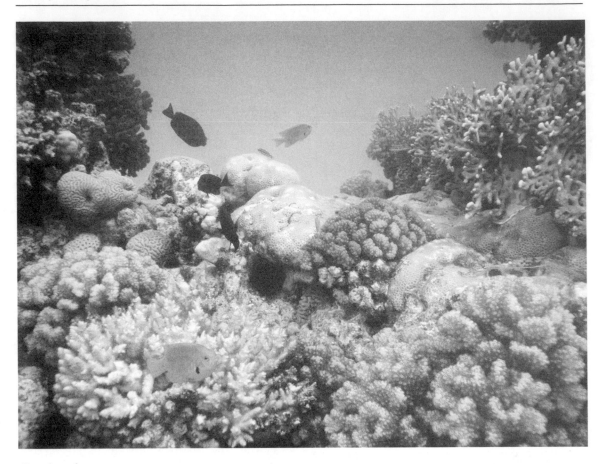

Coral reef (*Image copyright Kochneva Tetyana, 2009. Used under license from Shutterstock.com*)

Empowered, in which the poem appeared. For example, in *Dictionary of Literary Biography*, Eliana Rivero comments, "In this book serenity prevails.... In the thirty-six poems included in the volume, there is a fullness of personal power." Rivero then discusses how Neruda presents the duties and obligations of the poet, and states:

> Ultimately, the poet is the consciousness of mankind, who must try to preserve everything in a meaningful way so it can live eternally. Neruda happily accepts this awesome duty and writes in the ending poem, "Plenos poderes," that "y canto porque canto y porque canto" (I sing because I sing because I sing).

In "Pablo Neruda: A Revaluation," Ben Belitt, who has translated many of Neruda's poems, reaches the same conclusion as Rivero regarding *Fully Empowered*: "This redistillation of serenity clings to the whole of Neruda's *Plenos poderes*, imparting to each of the thirty-six poems that unmistakable 'fullness of power' to which its title bears witness."

In a review of a large collection of Neruda's poems in English, Jay Parini comments in *Nation*, "there are wonders in these pages that will delight readers unfamiliar with the tumultuously varied planet known as Neruda." Parini refers to the "exquisite poems of *Fully Empowered*." In his biography *Pablo Neruda: A Passion for Life*, Adam Feinstein refers to the book as an "eclectic mix," and in a comment that might well apply to "Fully Empowered" states that it is "in some ways, an optimistic book. A theme of rebirth, of daily renewal runs through it."

CRITICISM

Bryan Aubrey

Aubrey holds a Ph.D. in English. In this essay, he discusses "Fully Empowered" as a poem about creativity and the role of the poet.

When Neruda published "Fully Empowered" in 1962 he was no longer a young man.

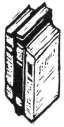

WHAT DO I READ NEXT?

- *Full Woman, Fleshly Apple, Hot Moon: Selected Poems of Pablo Neruda* (1997) translated by Stephen Mitchell, is a collection of nearly fifty poems from Neruda's mature period, including *Canto General, Elemental Odes, Extravagaria, One Hundred Love Sonnets,* and *Full Powers.*

- *The Oxford Book of Latin American Poetry* (2009), edited by Cecilia Vicuna and Ernesto Livon-Grosman, is an anthology that covers five hundred years of Latin American poetry, beginning with the response to the European conquest and continuing through to the experimental poetry being written in the twenty-first century. Over 120 poets are represented, including major figures such as Neruda, César Vallejo, Vicente Huidobro, Octavio Paz, and Gabriela Mistral, as well as many lesser-known poets. Many of the works appear in new translations. The poems are also given in their original languages.

- *Laughing Out Loud, I Fly: Poems in English and Spanish* (1998) by well-known Mexican American poet Juan Felipe Herrera contains poems suitable for younger readers age twelve and older. Each poem is paired with a black and white drawing by Karen Barbour. The collection won the Pura Belpré Award.

- *Neruda and Vallejo: Selected Poems,* (1993) edited with a preface by Robert Bly, is a bilingual edition of selections from Latin America's two greatest poets of the twentieth century. Bly's preface is full of sharp insights into their work.

- Along with Neruda and Vallejo, Paz is one of the major poets writing in Spanish in the twentieth century. His *Selected Poems* (1984) contains sixty-seven poems, rendered into English by a variety of translators, selected from fifty years of the poet's work.

- *How to Read a Poem: And Fall in Love with Poetry* by Edward Hirsch (1999) is an informative and enthusiastic guide to how to read poetry. Hirsch covers a wide range of work, from different periods, nationalities, and styles, ranging from familiar British and American poets such as John Keats, Walt Whitman, and Elizabeth Bishop, to poets from eastern Europe who will likely be new to most readers, and many others. Hirsh's enthusiasm for his subject is infectious and anyone who reads this book will come away with a deeper and richer understanding of the power of poetry.

At the age of fifty-eight, he was entering what has been described as his "autumnal period," often dated from about 1958 to 1970. According to Christopher Perriam, who uses this term in his book *The Late Poetry of Pablo Neruda*, the recurring themes of Neruda's autumnal period are "the land as a source of images and metaphors, the sea as a metaphor for purity, and solitude as a newly sought-after state of mind and being." All of these images and metaphors can indeed be found in "Fully Empowered," and they take some of their force and vitality from the place where Neruda lived for many years, in the house he built at Isla Negra, Chile, which faced the Pacific Ocean. "I live by a very rough sea in Isla Negra—my house is there—and I am never tired of being alone looking at the sea and working there," he told the American poet Robert Bly in an interview published in the collection *Twenty Poems* in 1967.

In "Fully Empowered," Neruda writes of his empowerment as a man and as a poet. By empowerment he means coming into full possession of his knowledge of himself as well as his function and power as a poet. Significantly, this poem is also the title of the collection as a whole;

THE PROCESS BY WHICH THIS POETRY HAPPENS—POETRY THAT IS THE EXPRESSION OF THE FULLNESS OF BEING, EMERGING FROM THAT 'ENCHANTED PLACE' NERUDA REFERRED TO IN HIS NOBEL LECTURE—IS MYSTERIOUS.”

it sums up the message of the whole book. It is also placed last, as if all the poems before it lead up to it in some way and are necessary for that personal empowerment, which arises from the poet's sense that he has fulfilled the role to which he was called. In this collection, Neruda presents a wide range of subjects and themes. Poems such as "Oceans,""Water,""The Sea,"— all favorite images with Neruda that recur in "Fully Empowered"— "Bird," and "Spring" record his exquisite observations of and reflections about nature, as does "Serenade," a poem about the night. There are poems about individuals—an old clock smith the poet knows in Valparaíso, an anonymous poor man who has died and is buried—and about collectives. One of the latter is addressed simply to everyone ("For Everyone"), another, "The People," is a long poem in tribute to all the ordinary working men over the centuries who have built up the American continent. There are some more abstract poems, about sadness, about the power of language ("The Word"), which is especially known to Neruda as a poet, and about his duties as a poet ("The Poet's Obligation")—to cheer those whose hearts are closed up, to bring them a kind of freedom.

All in all, *Fully Empowered* is a varied collection. "I am omnivorous," wrote Neruda in his *Memoirs*. "I would like to swallow the whole earth. I would like to drink the whole sea." It is this fullness of appetite for life, the embrace of all that it offers, that gives to the collection *Fully Empowered* its strength, its wisdom, its understanding, its depth. Much of this wisdom consists of self-knowledge as well as a sense of obligation to humanity as a whole. In the lecture he gave when he accepted the Nobel Prize for Literature in 1971, Neruda spoke about these twin aspects of his poetry: "I believe that poetry is an action . . . in

which there enter as equal partners solitude and solidarity, emotion and action, the nearness to oneself, the nearness to mankind and to the secret manifestations of nature."

He continued:

All paths lead to the same goal: to convey to others what we are. And we must pass through solitude and difficulty, isolation and silence in order to reach forth to the enchanted place where we can dance our clumsy dance and sing our sorrowful song—but in this dance or in this song there are fulfilled the most ancient rites of our conscience in the awareness of being human and of believing in a common destiny.

The element in these descriptions of poetry and the poet that predominates in "Fully Empowered" is self-knowledge, for in order to "convey to others what we are," the poet must first know who he is, and the poem is a highly symbolic presentation of the process by which the poet accesses the "enchanted place" he spoke of in his Nobel lecture. This place is within the psyche of the poet, and it enables him to know all aspects of himself and to sing his own song for the joy of it as well as for the pleasure and enlightenment of others.

"Fully Empowered" is a relaxed, confident, buoyant poem in which the poet is able to access his creativity, the depths of himself, in an easy rhythm that seems to alternate between hard work (he presents himself metaphorically as forging keys and opening doors) and a more passive kind of inward-directed contemplation (described in stanza 6). Many years of writing have shown him the way to navigate the psyche, and he appears to travel it with ease now. He becomes an explorer without ever leaving his own home. Perhaps he resembles the archetype identified by psychologist Carl Jung as the Wise Old Man, a figure who possesses deep insight, who knows the totality of things, and to whom others may turn for knowledge, inspiration, and understanding.

This is a very personal poem. Although the poet does not forget or ignore his connections and obligations to the wider world (expressed in stanza 4 and the first line of stanza 5), he writes primarily about himself. The poem emerges from his solitude—the crowded street of line 1 notwithstanding—and celebrates the inner work that allows him to know himself and to sing his song (i.e., write his poems). The recurring trope (a figure of speech in which a word or expression is used in a way different from the literal meaning) is that of the poet as singer, and this reiterated Orphic "I" puts in mind the American poet Walt Whitman, whose poetry was greatly admired by Neruda. One can almost picture Neruda walking the same metaphorical path Whitman did when Whitman wrote those two celebratory long poems "Song of Myself" and "Song of the Open Road." Whether the bard is Neruda or Whitman, these are the songs (poems) of a man who is self-aware in the deepest sense of the word and is aware also of the invisible threads of life that bind him to the entire universe. This is the connection that Neruda hints at in stanzas 4 and 5 of "Fully Empowered"—the threads that spread out put in mind the activity of Whitman's "A Noise-less Patient Spider," in which the spider, as it puts out its fine silk threads, becomes a symbol for the human soul or spirit in its desire to make connections with its environment. The poet of "Fully Empowered" sings because he can do nothing else, which suggests the indissoluble link between his life and his work. "Poetry is a deep inner calling in man," Neruda wrote in his *Memoirs*. He writes, quite simply, because that is what the being known as Pablo Neruda does; it is as an expression of who he is, and he can no more cease to do it than the sun could decide not to rise or water not to flow. Poetry fulfills his destiny; it is the reason for his being.

The process by which this poetry happens—poetry that is the expression of the fullness of being, emerging from that "enchanted place" Neruda referred to in his Nobel lecture—is mysterious. Even the poet himself cannot explain it, as he clearly states at the beginning of stanza 6. The poem's symbolism suggests that he sinks deeply into his own being, immersing himself in the polarities of life, experiencing the psychic equivalents of land and sea, day and night, light and darkness, in a process that involves both effort and lack of effort and that opens him up to life as well as death, to song and to silence, the silence of what he twice refers to as "non-being." What does he mean by non-being? He is not going to explain it, but it is as if his being unravels and he becomes nothing, or at least nothing that is manifest, and then out of that undifferentiated state he emerges once more, like a song emerging from silence. After all the senses have closed down (note how this process takes place with his eyes closed), they open up again: life emerges from this symbolic death, and does so again and again and again, as

the eternal pulse of life goes on, which is a song, and Neruda the poet catches the rhythms of this song, its melodies and harmonies, as well as its dissonances, and he gives these out for his fellow humans to hear, to know, and to pass on.

Source: Bryan Aubrey, Critical Essay on "Fully Empowered," in *Poetry for Students*, Gale, Cengage Learning, 2010.

Don Bogen

In the following excerpt, Bogen examines the different phases and style changes in Neruda's poetry.

Pity the poets of the New World. If Columbus et al. merely had to subdue the native flora and fauna long enough to set up shop here, the poets had to describe it all. They were stuck with the languages of the Old World—English, Spanish, French, Portuguese—but the literary traditions made about as much sense as a court ball at a trading post. No wonder many of them fell back on the hoariest text of all, the Bible, for a sense of the poet's role. The myth of Adam naming the creatures in the Garden was perfect for a world their languages had not yet touched. Not only did it simplify the task—if you don't know what to call this plant, river or group of people, make it up—it gave the poet a combination of innocence and importance that was hard to resist. In this country that vision ended with the closing of the frontier—Walt Whitman is the last successful exemplar—but it survived longer in Latin America. Describing South America in an interview published in Robert Bly's *Neruda and Vallejo: Selected Poems* (Beacon, 1971), Pablo Neruda noted "rivers which have no names, trees which nobody knows, and birds which nobody has described.... Everything we know is new." The poet's task, as he put is, is "to embrace the world around you, to discover the new world."

> If everything is new and you're the only one who determines what's what, how do you keep your pride at bay, and how do you know when to stop?

The Adamic poet, like his namesake, has a problem: If everything is new and you're the only one who determines what's what, how do you keep your pride at bay, and how do you know when to stop? Both Whitman and Neruda had enormous egos, and neither showed much restraint in output. Because Neruda wrote so much, including weak poems in almost all his more than forty books, it's advisable to start reading him in an edition of selected poems. The best of these, with translations by Anthony

Kerrigan, W.S. Merwin, Alastair Reid and Nathaniel Tarn, has recently been reissued by Houghton Mifflin. The two new translations published by the University of California Press, Jack Schmitt's version of *Canto General* and Margaret Sayers Peden's *Selected Odes of Pablo Neruda*, provide a closer look at the poet's work of the 1940s and 1950s—both its glories and its excesses. This was a pivotal period for Neruda—the culmination of one phase of his career and the beginning of another—and these books are important additions to the body of work available in English translation.

With Neruda it's possible to separate the poetry from the life. Both are huge, protean in their variety and ultimately political Neruda, of course, has a sentimental appeal for anyone on the left. His commitment to the socialist cause and his death in the wake of the U.S.-sponsored Chilean coup can make him seem a literary martyr. But Neruda is more complex than this. While a single presence—expansive, passionate, directly personal—lies behind all his work, his career is marked by distinct changes in style and focus. The Adamic voice and political awareness we associate with him today are not strong elements in his early work. The volume that made him famous at 20, *Twenty Love Poems and a Song of Despair* (1924), is a hybrid of French Symbolist yearning for the ineffable, and earthly Latin American eroticism. In the two major books that followed, *Residence on Earth I* (1933) and *II* (1935), Neruda turned from a young love poet into a surrealist, capturing the alienation he felt as a diplomat in the Far East in bleak monologues with long, fluid lines and torrents of imagery. The end of this period of surreal despair came in the mid-thirties when Neruda was serving in the Chilean Embassy in Madrid. His firsthand encounter with fascism during the Spanish Civil War solidified the basic commitment to the left that infuses all his subsequent work. In 1945 he was elected senator in the Chilean legislature; that same year he joined the Communist Party.

Source: Don Bogen, "Selected Odes of Pablo Neruda," in *Nation*, Vol. 254, No. 3, January 27, 1992, p. 95.

SOURCES

Abrams, M. H., *A Glossary of Literary Terms*, 4th ed., Holt, Rinehart, and Winston, 1981, pp. 127, 195.

Belitt, Ben, "Pablo Neruda: A Revaluation," in *Pablo Neruda*, edited and with an introduction by Harold Bloom, Chelsea House, 1989, p. 155.

Bly, Robert, "Interview with Pablo Neruda," in *Twenty Poems by Pablo Neruda*, translated by James Wright and Robert Bly, Sixties Press, 1967, pp. 102–10.

Brotherston, Gordon, *Latin American Poetry: Origins and Presence*, Cambridge University Press, 1975, p. 169.

"Chile," in *CIA: World Factbook*, https://www.cia.gov/library/publications/the-world-factbook/geos/ci.html (accessed August 5, 2009).

Feinstein, Adam, *Pablo Neruda: A Passion for Life*, Bloomsbury, 2004, pp. 331–32.

Gallagher, D. P., *Modern Latin American Literature*, Oxford University Press, 1973, pp. 10, 67.

Kuhnheim, Jill S., *Textual Disruptions: Spanish American Poetry at the End of the Twentieth Century*, University of Texas Press, 2004.

Loveman, Brian, *Struggle in the Countryside: Politics and Rural Labor in Chile, 1919–1973*, Indiana University Press, 1976.

Neruda, Pablo, *Fully Empowered*, translated by Alastair Reid, Farrar, Straus, and Giroux, 1975, pp. 133–35.

———, *Memoirs*, translated from the Spanish by Hardie St. Martin, Farrar, Straus, and Giroux, 1977, pp. 264, 266, 286–87.

———, "Nobel Lecture," in *Nobelprize.org*, http://nobelprize.org/nobel_prizes/literature/laureates/1971/neruda-lecture-e.html (accessed July 15, 2009).

Parini, Jay, Review of *The Poetry of Pablo Neruda*, in *Nation*, Vol. 277, No. 21, December 22, 2003, p. 44.

Perriam, Christopher, *The Late Poetry of Pablo Neruda*, Dolphin Book, 1989, p. ix.

Rivero, Eliana, "Pablo Neruda," in *Dictionary of Literary Biography*, Vol. 283, *Modern Spanish American Poets*, 1st ser., edited by María A. Salgado, Thomson Gale, 2003, pp. 247–71.

FURTHER READING

Bizzarro, Salvatore, *Pablo Neruda: All Poets the Poet*, Scarecrow Press, 1979.

> Bizzarro analyzes the social and political aspects of Neruda's work from 1936 to 1950, and his later work in the context of his overall development.

de Costa, René, *The Poetry of Pablo Neruda*, Harvard University Press, 1979.

> This is a detailed analysis of Neruda's major works. Costa's aim is to place these works in two contexts, that of Neruda's work as a whole and also that of modern poetry.

Haslam, Jonathan, *The Nixon Administration and the Death of Allende's Chile: A Case of Assisted Suicide*, Verso, 2005.

> This book tells the story of how the Socialist and Communist political parties in Chile gained strength during the 1960s, culminating in the election of the socialist, Salvador Allende, in 1970. The Allende government was overthrown by a military coup in 1973. Haslam describes the numerous ways in which the U.S. government undermined Allende and paved the way for a coup.

Longo, Teresa, *Pablo Neruda and the U.S. Culture Industry*, Routledge, 2002.

> This is a collection of thirteen essays about all aspects of Neruda's work and its reception in the United States. The authors discuss the significance of writing about Neruda and Latin American culture in the United States.

The Hollow Men

T. S. ELIOT

1925

T. S. Eliot and his work were at the forefront of the modernist poetry movement. His lengthy poem "The Hollow Men" was written at both the height of this movement and the height of his career. Indeed, it was published in its entirety only three years after the release of Eliot's most famous epic poem, *The Waste Land* (1922). Parts of "The Hollow Men" were published in the periodicals *Chapbook*, *Commerce*, *Criterion*, and *Dial* from 1924 to 1925. The poem then appeared in its final cohesive form in Eliot's 1925 collection *Poems, 1909–1925*. "The Hollow Men" largely builds on the themes in *The Waste Land*, specifically the need for death to take place as a means to make way for the new. "The Hollow Men" is also written in the same style as its famous predecessor. Both poems additionally share the same source of inspiration: Joseph Conrad's 1902 novella *Heart of Darkness*. "The Hollow Men" also alludes to or is heavily influenced by several works, including Dante Alighieri's fourteenth-century masterpiece *Divine Comedy* and William Shakespeare's 1599 play *Julius Caesar*. A historical allusion to Guy Fawkes Day (a British holiday) also appears in the poem. The density and depth of "The Hollow Men" alone recommend it for further study, as it is not a work that reveals its meaning readily.

The poem remains widely available on the Internet and in collections of the author's works. As of 2009, the 1991 edition of Eliot's *Collected Poems: 1909–1962* remained in print.

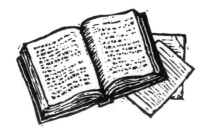

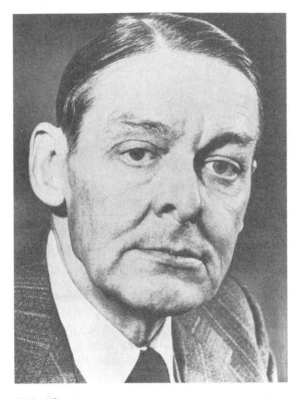

T.S. Eliot

AUTHOR BIOGRAPHY

Born Thomas Stearns Eliot in St. Louis, Missouri, on September 26, 1888, Eliot was the youngest of seven children born to Henry Ware Eliot (president of the Hydraulic-Press Brick Company) and Charlotte Champe Stearns (a schoolteacher and an amateur poet). Eliot's family roots were tied to New England, and he spent his childhood summers there. His interest in literature emerged early, and he was writing short stories by the age of sixteen. In 1906, Eliot attended Harvard University, a family tradition. He graduated with a B.A. in comparative literature in 1909 and an M.A. in English literature in 1910. As a student, Eliot became enamored of the Symbolist movement (a largely French phenomenon), which led him to travel to Paris in 1910. He befriended the artistic and literary luminaries of the day, including Pablo Picasso and Émile Durkheim. The following year, Eliot returned to Harvard to work on his doctorate. Despite completing his dissertation in 1916, he never presented his thesis nor earned the degree.

From 1910 to 1912, Eliot wrote the poems that launched his career, specifically "The Love Song of Alfred J. Prufrock." This poem, however, was not published for several years. After leaving Harvard, Eliot returned to Europe, where he befriended the influential poet Ezra Pound. It was Pound who was instrumental in the 1915 publication of "The Love Song of Alfred J. Prufrock" in *Poetry* magazine. That same year, Eliot met Vivien Haigh-Wood, an English dancer with a history of mental problems. The couple married in June of that year and settled in London. Their marriage was an unhappy one, and they never had children, ultimately divorcing in 1930. In 1917, Eliot began working as an assistant editor for the *Egoist*, an avant-garde magazine based in London. Also that year, Eliot's first collection of poetry, *Prufrock and Other Observations* was published by the *Egoist*. Pound was once again influential in the publication, even financing the endeavor personally.

The following years saw Eliot further ensconcing himself in the society of London's intellectual and literary elite. The release of a second volume of poetry and a volume of criticism further established his literary career. Then, in 1922, Eliot forever secured his reputation with the publication of his iconic epic poem *The Waste Land*. That same year, Eliot also edited James Joyce's novel *Ulysses*. Both works were celebrated as masterpieces and have since been recognized as the iconic works of the modernist movement. Also in 1922, Eliot began working as founding editor of the *Criterion*, a literary magazine that was hailed throughout Europe. Indeed, despite his troubled marriage and his wife's failing health, Eliot's career thrived. Portions of "The Hollow Men" were published in various periodicals from 1924 to 1925; the complete poem appeared in Eliot's 1925 collection *Poems, 1909–1925*. Eliot's tumultuous personal life left him in a spiritual crisis that led him to join the Church of England and become a British subject in 1927.

This period marked a transition in Eliot's life and work, as he published some unpopular conservative criticism and began to move away from the modernist aesthetic for which he had become renowned. His verse also became more explicitly religious, which can be seen in his acclaimed 1930 volume *Ash-Wednesday*. In the latter half of his career, Eliot wrote more plays than poetry, including *The Family Reunion* (1939). His 1949 play *The Cocktail Party* won a Tony Award in 1950. Nevertheless, his poetry was far more acclaimed, especially his 1943 collection *Four Quartets*. In 1948, Eliot was awarded the Nobel Prize for Literature.

Yet, following World War II, none of the poetry Eliot produced was as praised as his earlier successes. In January of 1957, Eliot married Valerie Fletcher (the couple had no children), and finally achieved a measure of personal happiness. He died in London eight years later, on January 4, 1965. His body is buried in Westminster Abbey.

Throughout his career, Eliot supplemented his income by working as a lecturer at universities across the United States, and he also served as literary editor at London's Faber & Faber from 1925 until his death. He has been acknowledged internationally for his work with numerous honorary degrees and commendations, and he remains a pivotal figure in twentieth-century literature.

POEM SUMMARY

I

In a ten-line verse, the speakers claim to be empty yet full, evoking references to the straw men burned in effigy in England on Guy Fawkes Day (a holiday that commemorates the anniversary of the Gunpowder Plot conspiracy to blow up the British Parliament and King James 1st on November 5, 1605). Made of straw, these men are without depth and significance, like the grass in the breeze, or like the movement of rodents over debris in the basement.

The next verse is a couplet in which numerous contradictory terms (such as the idea of being colorless, yet possessing a hue) are introduced. Notably, there is no concrete indication of what these paradoxes are referring to.

In the following six-line stanza, references are made to those who have died and passed on to the afterlife. The speakers declare that the dead may think of them, and if they do, they think of them as empty yet full.

II

This section appears to be narrated by a singular speaker as opposed to the plural speakers in section I. In the first ten-line stanza, the speaker states that in his fantasies of the afterlife, there are eyes he cannot bring himself to look at and that are not present. But in the afterlife, those eyes are like the daylight and there is also a tree that moves. There are words in the breeze that are as somber as a dying star.

In the next eight-line stanza, the speaker says he does not want to get any closer to the afterlife

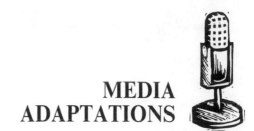

MEDIA ADAPTATIONS

- "The Hollow Men" was set to music and the score was published by Oxford University Press, 1951.
- An audiobook including "The Hollow Men" narrated by Eliot and released by Harper-Collins in 1992 is titled *T. S. Eliot Reads: "Four Quartets," The Waste Land, "The Hollow Men," and Other of His Poems.*

and wants to wear costumes to hide himself from it. He wants to be as elusive as the breeze.

In the section's final couplet, the speaker again notes that he wishes to avoid the ultimate assembly that will occur in the afterlife.

III

In this section, the narrator reverts to the plural voice, but the verses again refer largely to the land of death. In the first six-line stanza of the section, reference is made to that land as a desert. There are also stone statues there, elevated and worshiped by the dead. All of this takes place beneath a dying star. (Here, the reference to the dying star is repeated from the first stanza of section II).

Then, in the second (seven-line) stanza, the speaker indicates that there is another afterlife, and that the previous stanza refers to it. Furthermore, in this second afterlife the dead awake without company, just when they are filled with affection, like mouths meant for kissing. Instead, those mouths beseech the crumbling statues.

IV

The speakers open the section with a five-line stanza that again refers to the eyes that are absent (this image is initially mentioned in the first stanza of section II). In fact the eyes are missing from a vale filled with fading stars. The vale is as empty as the stuffed men (indeed, the same words used to describe them are used to describe the gorge). The vale is also described as the broken jaw of vanished empires.

In the following four-line stanza, this gorge is the final assembly place where the straw men feel their way as one. They do not speak and they come together on the shore of a swollen waterway.

The section's third stanza is comprised of seven lines. In it, the speakers state that without eyes, there is no sight. Should the eyes become present again, they will be an undying star, and a special type of rose representative of the church. This rose is also a reference to Dante Alighieri's *Divine Comedy*. In Dante, the rose symbolizes heaven. For the speakers in Eliot's poem, this rose is the only hope of the hollow men.

V

This section opens with a four-line italicized stanza of a nursery rhyme, an alteration of "Here We Go Round the Mulberry Bush." The mulberry bush, however, is replaced by a cactus plant, again referencing the desert imagery initially introduced in the first stanza of section III.

In the next five-line stanza, the speaker (or speakers, as this is unclear in the poem's final section) says that a shadow lies in the space separating theory and practice, movement and deed.

Between the stanzas an italicized quotation from the Lord's Prayer is set flush with the right margin.

The section's third stanza is made up of five lines. Here the speaker states that the shadow falls in the space separating the idea and the creative act, the feeling and the reaction to it.

An italicized line declaring that life is not short follows, again set flush with the right margin.

In the following seven-line stanza, there are more descriptions of the shadow. It lies amidst the space between yearning and paroxysm, power and being, the core and the fall.

The single line from the Lord's Prayer is repeated.

The section's (and the poem's) penultimate (next to last) stanza is three lines long. Each line is comprised of fragments from the three offset italicized lines that preceded it.

The final stanza is four italicized lines. The first three are identical, and the speaker says that this is how the apocalypse will be. Then, in the final line, the speaker says that the apocalypse will not take place with a great crash but with little more than a quiet moan.

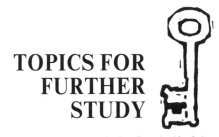

TOPICS FOR FURTHER STUDY

- Use the Internet to research the first half of the twentieth century and the numerous events in the field of poetry that occurred during that period. (Eliot's life and work spanned these years.) Build a timeline or PowerPoint presentation to display the information.

- Much critical discussion of Eliot's "The Hollow Men" centers around his previous epic poem *The Waste Land*. In an essay, compare the two in terms of theme and style.

- "The Hollow Men" is a highly visual poem. It is filled with fantastical and surreal imagery. Make a collage, poster, painting, drawing, sculpture, or other visual representation inspired by the poem. In an accompanying artist's statement, explain how the project changed or enhanced your interpretation of "The Hollow Men."

- Read the 2008 anthology *A Treasury of Poetry for Young People: Emily Dickinson, Robert Frost, Henry Wadsworth Longfellow, Edgar Allan Poe, Carl Sandberg, Walt Whitman,* edited by Frances Schoonmaker, Gary D. Schmidt, Brod Bagert, and Jonathan Levin. With the exception of Carl Sandburg, this collection of classic poetry for young readers includes the work of poets who were essential precursors to the modernist movement. Choose a poem from the anthology and lead a class discussion about the poet's influence on the movement. Be prepared with notes on the poet and the poem, as well as their era.

THEMES

Death

Death pervades "The Hollow Men" from beginning to end. The artificial men are empty yet full. They reference a holiday centered on the tradition of burning an effigy of Guy Fawkes, an act in which death is implicit. A second implication of death is also part of this metaphor. Indeed, the

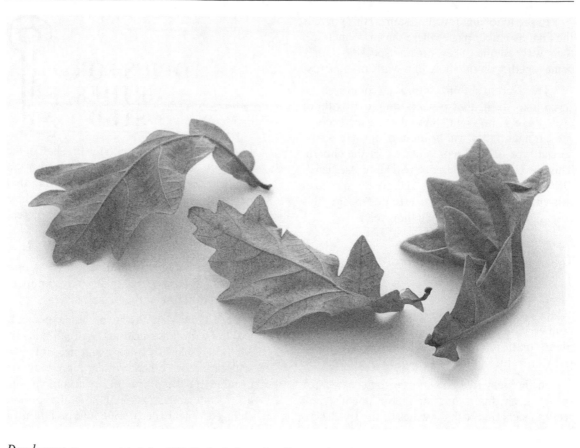

Dry leaves (Image copyright Pefkos, 2009. Used under license from Shutterstock.com)

hollow men of the title call to mind an image of corpses, bodies whose souls have departed. Even the afterlife is a dead place, filled with dying stars and made of a desert landscape. It is also a sightless place, one in which eyes do not exist. In the afterlife, there are crumbling statues and vanished empires. There is a shadow that lies in the space between things. All of these images are of death or are at least deathlike. An extension of this theme is that death is necessary to make way for the new. This death applies to old gods, old religions, and old ideals, all of which will fall by the wayside to make room for new gods, new ideals, new ideas, and the like. This is pointed out by Jewel Spears Brooker in the *Dictionary of Literary Biography*. She says that "Many figures in Eliot's early poems, including all the gods and semigods . . . have to die or be put to death as the condition for the continuation of life. Those who cannot die cannot really live." From there, Brooker goes on to note that "in 'The Hollow Men,' Eliot does not go beyond a presentation of emptiness, but in the act of presenting that, he seems to accept the

death that is the essential step toward his own *vita nuova* 'new life'."

This theme can even be seen in the image of the mouths that beseech crumbling statues. It is further underscored by Eliot's quotations of Joseph Conrad's *Heart of Darkness*, a work that contains a similar, if not identical, theme. Yet, while the old must die to make way for the new, that does not prevent Eliot from using the old as a foundation for the new. This can be seen textually, as the poem (like much of Eliot's work) contains numerous allusions, quotations, and modified quotations from Shakespeare, Conrad, and Dante. Thus, textually, at least, the old does not make way for the new, but is instead used to create it.

Failure of Religion

A secondary theme in Eliot's poem is the failure of religion. Notably, this theme is related to the idea that the old must die to make way for the new. The crumbling statues and the mouths that beseech them specifically seem to reference failed religions, or at least failed prayer. That the mouths were about to kiss and are instead set to a seemingly futile task again seems to speak to the futility of religious ritual. The crumbling statues appear not long before the poem's reference to vanished empires. This latter connection further underscores the idea that the old must disappear to make way for the new. Nowhere in "The Hollow Men" is the failure of religion more clear than in the poem's fifth and final section. The Lord's Prayer is quoted in a chorus-like offset and then rearranged in the main text. The prayer's failure is made clear not only in the way it is rearranged, but also through its pairing with a children's nursery rhyme. It is as if the speaker finds as much solace in doggerel as in prayer. The substitution of one for the other is irrelevant; both are presented in the poem almost as if they are interchangeable. Religion's failure can also be seen in the poem's last line (and perhaps the poem's main theme can be seen in it as well). Indeed, that the world ends in a whimper and not a dramatic or loud display seems to challenge popular religious beliefs regarding the apocalypse. It also once more sets forth that death is itself a failure—the unremarkable denouement at the end of a slow and unremarkable decline.

STYLE

Allusion

An allusion is a reference in a literary or artistic work to another literary or artistic work or to a real-world event or person. In this way, the work grounds itself in the world outside of itself. Instead of becoming a fictional and self-referential construction, an allusive work establishes itself as part of a greater conversation with the events and works it touches upon. For instance, the images of heaven and hell established by Dante are called upon in "The Hollow Men" simply because the poem alludes to Dante's *Divine Comedy*. Thus, Eliot is able to rely on and build upon the reader's previous knowledge of fictional portrayals of heaven and hell without quoting them directly. At the same time, Eliot does directly quote the Lord's Prayer though he does not cite it. This allusion further underscores the religious implications in the poem. The third allusion that can be found in Eliot's poem is to Shakespeare's *Julius Caesar*. In particular, the second, third, and fourth stanzas of the fifth section mention the shadow that lies between theory and practice,

movement and deed, and so forth. This construct is mentioned by Brutus in act 2, scene 1, lines 63–65 of Shakespeare's play. The last notable allusion in "The Hollow Men" is to Guy Fawkes Day. The holiday, on November 5, celebrates the foiling of the Gunpowder Plot of 1605, which was headed by Guy Fawkes. As part of the celebration, stuffed straw effigies of Fawkes are burned on bonfires. This image of straw men and their death is central to Eliot's poem.

Repetition and Chorus

Much of "The Hollow Men" relies on repetition and chorus to underscore its most important images, metaphors, and themes. Descriptions of the straw men as empty yet full are repeated throughout the poem, as are descriptions of the afterlife as a desert. Images of dying stars and lines from the Lord's Prayer also repeat. Notably, the reiterations in the poem often take on a choral or musical aspect, as is the case with the offset italicized lines in the final section. In fact, Eliot's verse was well known for its musical qualities, specifically his later volume *Four Quartets*. The musical aspects in "The Hollow Men" are particularly noticeable in the final two stanzas of the poem. In the penultimate stanza, each line consists of fragments from the three offset italicized lines that preceded it. The final stanza features three identical lines, all repeated in succession. This builds the tension and anticipation relieved by the poem's final line. Ironically, that line states that the end will not deliver a grand finale, only a quiet sigh.

HISTORICAL CONTEXT

Modernism

The modernist style developed in the early twentieth century and was at its most popular when "The Hollow Men" was released. Indeed, no discussion of modernism is complete without acknowledging Eliot's place in it. The movement began in Europe before growing in popularity in the United States, but many of its leading literary figures, such as Eliot, Pound, and Gertrude Stein, were expatriates, Americans living abroad. The movement was not relegated to literature alone, as the visual arts were also an important aspect of the modernist aesthetic.

COMPARE
&
CONTRAST

- **1920s:** Although World War I ended in 1918, Europe is still reeling from the effects, as great social, cultural, and political upheaval follows in its wake. The United States is affected as well, albeit to a lesser extent.

  Today: The Iraq War, spearheaded by the United States, begins in 2003. In 2009, U.S. President Barack Obama declares that all troops will be withdrawn by 2011. Meanwhile, the U.S. military presence in Afghanistan persists.

- **1920s:** The modernist movement is at its peak, led by such poets as Eliot and Pound. Modernist poetry is characterized by a break from traditional poetic language, theme, and form.

  Today: While no one definitive poetic movement exists, new formalism has emerged as one of the more cogent poetic styles of the day. A belated backlash against modernism and the movements that followed it, new formalism is characterized by the reemergence of traditional verse structures.

- **1920s:** Existentialist philosophy is growing in popularity, and its cultural influence can be seen in the art and poetry of the day. Existential ideas regarding the individual as a being apart from society are reflected in the broken traditional art forms that defined modernism.

  Today: As is the case with poetry in the twenty-first century, no definitive philosophical movement exists. The most recent school of thought to emerge is poststructuralism, which was popular during the 1970s.

Several cultural and historical events influenced that aesthetic. At the beginning of the twentieth century, popular belief held that society as a whole was more important than the individual. However, this belief was soon challenged by advances in science and technology. In addition, World War I was the first major conflict in which machinery played a significant role, and the resulting casualties were the largest in recorded history. Thus, the high cost of patriotism and politics came into question, and philosophers and artists alike began to explore the rights of the individual. Rather than being seen as a part of the whole, as was the case previously, individual expression and experience suddenly became worthy of exploration in its own right.

This rather abstract shift in worldview can be seen concretely in the modernist movement, and in the philosophies that preceded it. Existentialist writers such as Jean-Paul Sartre and his predecessor Friedrich Nietzsche questioned the nature of society and man's place in it. Psychologists such as Sigmund Freud and Carl Jung explored the depths of the subconscious, revealing the very foundations of individual identity and its formation. In order to address these new ideas and beliefs, artists broke away from their traditional modes of expression in search of new styles, experimenting with both narrative and visual representations. In prose, straightforward narrative was replaced by stream-of-consciousness, a technique prominent in the works of Stein, James Joyce, and William Faulkner. In art, cubism, imagism, and surrealism evolved, and such styles can be found in Pablo Picasso's work. In poetry, meter and structure were abandoned in favor of free verse. This can be seen in the work of H. D., William Carlos Williams, and W. H. Auden, among others.

Impact of World War I and "The Lost Generation"

Eliot traveled throughout Europe both before and during World War I, which occurred from

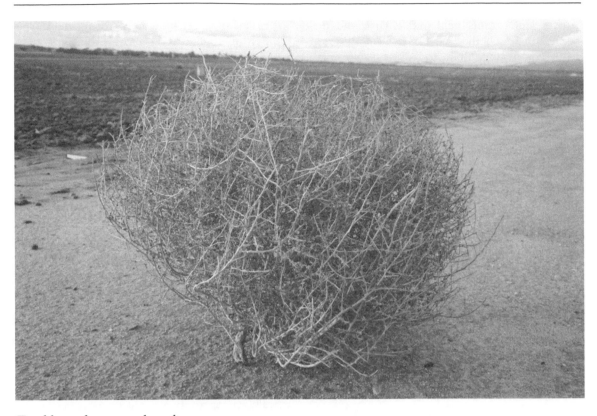

Tumbleweed on a rural road (*Image copyright Michael Ledray, 2009. Used under license from Shutterstock.com*)

1914 to 1918. His decision to settle in England was largely influenced by the war, as his British wife refused to travel overseas to the United States during the conflict. Civilian casualties during the war ultimately were estimated to be around 7 million, while almost 10 million soldiers were killed. The disaffected literature that was produced during and following the war reflects the world's shock at these massive casualties. In fact, many American expatriate writers, like Eliot, felt these atrocities more keenly than their counterparts in the United States. Many of these writers later came to be known as part of "The Lost Generation," a phrase that was coined by Gertrude Stein. Well-known writers typically assigned to this group include Ernest Hemingway, F. Scott Fitzgerald, and John Dos Passos. Notably, although Eliot is not normally considered part of this group, Pound and Stein are. Certainly, the connection between World War I and the dark imagery in "The Hollow Men" is evident, as is Eliot's connection to the literary and intellectual elite who came to be known as "The Lost Generation."

CRITICAL OVERVIEW

"The Hollow Men" was released at the height of Eliot's career, and as such was met with a warm critical reception. Parts of the poem were released in some of Europe's most prominent literary magazines, and thus its final publication was highly anticipated in literary circles. Additionally, the poem was Eliot's first major work after the wild success of *The Waste Land*, and it was read and reviewed in light of that success. Notably, both poems contain similar imagery, language, and themes. In fact, critics have often referred to "The Hollow Men" as something of a sequel to its predecessor. Most contemporary criticism of "The Hollow Men" is devoted to attempts to analyze its many meanings, themes, and allusions. For instance, discussing the conundrum of Eliot's near-constant allusive style in the poem, *Yeats Eliot Review* contributor Joseph Jonghyun Jeon states that "the intelligence of the 'final' section is...not found in profundity of statement; from this standpoint, the poem is not even original. Rather, the tone and affective register of this section are effects of style." Jeon adds that "the strategies of arrangement and collage and the manner in which the poem assembles the borrowed fragments combine to represent a personal struggle. The language here simultaneously reveals and obscures. It cites other contexts by way of allusions, but treats them ambivalently, shedding innocence from the children's song and reverence from the Lord's Prayer fragment."

In a somewhat ambivalent review of the poem, Adam Kirsch writes in *American Scholar* that "The Hollow Men" provides a "vague, portentous thrill ... But the extremity and drama ... do not seem justified if what the poet is talking about is religious doubt." Yet, Kirsch also notes that "Eliot evokes excitement and awe." On the other hand, he also remarks that "the progress of Eliot's poetry from 'Prufrock' to 'The Hollow Men' shows just this process: the sensitive adolescent sheds his humanity and becomes first a cynic, then a fevered nihilist." Jeon, however, is far more forgiving in his assessment, finding that Eliot's poem "offers shadowy expressions of extremely personal emotions" and "reveals the private Eliot through its style." He states that "'The Hollow Men' is a profoundly personal poem without being an autobiographical one." David Spurr, writing in *Conflicts in Consciousness: T. S. Eliot's Poetry and Criticism*, also proffers praise, commenting that "the quality of a poetic style marked by verbal austerity and relentless negation forms a structural counterpart to a thematic strategy that repudiates the validity of human experience at every level."

CRITICISM

Leah Tieger

Tieger is a freelance writer and editor. In the following essay, she discusses interpretations of Eliot's "The Hollow Men" as an autobiographical poem charting the poet's religious struggles.

Eliot was born into a family that was influential in the Unitarian Church. His grandfather was the founder of the Unitarian sect in St. Louis, Missouri, and his uncle founded the Unitarian Church in Portland, Oregon. Yet, as Eliot matured, he rejected his family's beliefs. For much of his early adulthood, Eliot lived without regard to organized religion, a choice that was supported by the modernist milieu in which he lived and worked. Personally, Eliot struggled to reconcile his intellect with his faith and, in 1927,

at the age of thirty-nine, he was baptized in the Church of England. The move took place only two years after the final publication of "The Hollow Men." Eliot's decision to join the Church of England did not endear him to his family, or to his peers. Still, the period in which Eliot struggled with his spirituality also saw the production of three works that are not only religious in content, but also highly prized for their modernist aesthetic, namely, *The Waste Land* (1922), "The Hollow Men" (1925), and *Ash-Wednesday* (1930). In fact, numerous critics have commented on the thematic arc among the three works. According to David Spurr in *Conflicts in Consciousness: T. S. Eliot's Poetry and Criticism*, "'The Hollow Men' replaces the richly chaotic style of *The Waste Land* with an austerity of expression that prepares for the contemplative mode of *Ash-Wednesday*."

Though a great deal of critical attention is paid to the numerous allusions in "The Hollow Men," much attention is also directed toward the poems personal and autobiographical aspects, specifically in regard to its religious content. Even without considering Eliot's personal spiritual journey, the religious tone, content, and imagery in the poem are well worth remaking upon. Quotations from the Lord's Prayer are obviously religious, as are allusions to Dante's *The Divine Comedy*. Yet, the latter does bear some additional exploration. Dante's work is arguably the source of contemporary conceptions of heaven, hell, and purgatory, and Eliot uses these concepts to great effect. The afterlife that Eliot describes is a desert without eyes, watched over by fading stars, replete with crumbling statues and mouths unable to kiss. All of these images take on a quality distinctly reminiscent of Dante's purgatory. Given the belief that souls in purgatory will ultimately be allowed to enter heaven, the idea that Eliot portrays purgatory in the poem is bolstered by the speakers' claim that there is another afterlife, and that there is a final meeting that comes after what would already appear to have been the final meeting.

The absence of eyes in the afterlife, though not an explicitly religious image, is one that many critics have remarked upon in the discussion of "The Hollow Men" as a religious poem. Indeed, according to J. Hillis Miller in *Poets of Reality: Six Twentieth-Century Writers*, "there are no eyes in the hollow valley, and the empty men are bereft of God." In fact, Hillis even goes on to indicate that the absence of eyes in the poem is meant to

WHAT DO I READ NEXT?

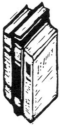

- Modernist poetry paved the way for contemporary poetry; both break traditional forms and topics and tend toward free verse. For an anthology of contemporary poetry specifically geared toward young adults, read *The Invisible Ladder: An Anthology of Contemporary American Poems for Young Readers*, edited by Liz Rosenberg. Published in 1996, the volume includes verse from such notable contemporary poets as Stanley Kunitz, Rita Dove, and Galway Kinnell. The poets also include introductions to their own poems, as well as photographs of themselves as both adults and children.

- The 1999 book *T. S. Eliot: An Imperfect Life*, by Lyndall Gordon, combines two of Gordon's earlier biographies of the poet, *Eliot's Early Years* (1977) and *Eliot's New Life* (1988). In addition to presenting a straightforward account of Eliot's life, Gordon explores Eliot's anti-Semitic beliefs and misogynist tendencies and attempts to reconcile them with the poet's legendary talent.

- Originally published in 1958, Chinua Achebe's *Things Fall Apart* has become a classic young adult novel that also appeals to adults. Just as "The Hollow Men" centers on the death of the old as it makes way for the new, so does Achebe's novel. The plot centers around a Nigerian village and the changes it undergoes in the face of colonialism. Indeed, for both Eliot and Achebe, the death of the old is a necessary mode of progress. Yet, both writers seem to acknowledge that change can be both positive and negative.

- Volume 2 of *The New Anthology Of American Poetry: Modernisms, 1900–1950*, edited by Steven Gould Axelrod, Camille Roman, and Thomas Travisano includes the work of sixty-five American modernist poets, including Eliot, Pound, William Carlos Williams, Wallace Stevens, Gertrude Stein, Hart Crane, Marianne Moore, and Langston Hughes.

- A contemporary and friend of Eliot's, the artist Pablo Picasso was as much a revolutionary in his field as Eliot was in his. For a retrospective of his work, read *Picasso: 200 Masterworks from 1898 to 1972*. The volume was edited by Bernard Ruiz Picasso and Bernice B. Rose and published in 2001.

- Another book that will appeal to both young adult and mature readers is Elie Wiesel's autobiographical novel *Night*. The story follows Eliezer, a teenage Hungarian Jew who survives the Holocaust. Though the book was first published in French in 1958, the horrific events it describes are not dissimilar to the dark imagery in Eliot's poem. Furthermore, Wiesel's protagonist struggles to reconcile his belief in God with the horror he witnesses. This death of God is a common theme in modernist literature, one that is similar to the themes in "The Hollow Men."

signify the absence of the divine gaze. Supporting the idea that the speakers are in purgatory, the critic also finds that "Eliot's hollow men understand dimly that if they endure the death which is prelude to rebirth they have some hope of salvation." *Yeats Eliot Review* contributor Joseph Jonghyun Jeon, however, declares just the opposite: "When the hollow men look to the stars for evidence of divinity and the hope of salvation, they see only more emptiness in places that resemble their own too much to offer any solace. The poem is too committed to demarcating a ground for meaning that the absent divine figure cannot provide." Indeed, Jeon goes on to state that "Eliot makes clear that the hollow men have no agency, and hence are incapable of self-sacrifice. It is central to the poem's project to render such a place as heaven as either inaccessible and inconceivable or proximate, and thus unable to live up to any promise of transcendence." The impossibility of heaven in the poem, to Jeon, is evidenced by sections one through four, which he describes as an "attempt to accord human thought as figured by the hollow men with orthodox belief." Yet, Jeon finds that "the available structures ultimately fold in on themselves. The failure of the many binary differences in these sections also means the impossibility of salvation because an ideal place like heaven and a divine figure become unimaginable."

Certainly, it would seem that religion in Eliot's poem is a dead thing, one that must pass away in order to make room for the new. Yet, Hillis disagrees with this interpretation, observing that "though nature, other people, and God have an almost entirely negative existence in the poem, they do exist as something outside the hollow men." To Hillis, this distinction imbues "nature, other people, and God" with at least one redeeming quality. Regardless, religion's impotence seems to be further indicated in the poem's final section. The juxtaposition (the placing side by side) of the Lord's Prayer with a children's nursery rhyme is a compelling example of this impotence. Another such example can be found in the poem's final line, which asserts that the apocalypse will come quietly, that no grand display heralding the end of the world will be forthcoming. To Jeon, however, this line need not be taken at face value. He states that "the hollow men try unsuccessfully to imagine the existence of a divine and a world that depend on such a figure and, accordingly, their voices fail to register in any effective manner." This failure, then, evokes the whispers referred to in the final lines. Even more remarkably, Jeon declares that Eliot "treats whimpers, not as meaningless utterances that vanish in the abyss between heaven and earth, but as shadowy murmurs that have no meaning until they are considered in relation to one other." He adds: "The key is scale. A whimper among gods is a meaningless sound: a whimper among whimpers is a language."

It is hard to say whether Hillis or Jeon are correct in their varying interpretations; the poem's ambiguous and ambivalent nature implies many possible or plausible meanings. However, Jeon is perhaps most eloquent in his assessment. He finds that "whimpers for Eliot in this poem carry the force of bangs. Whimpers in the end are not retreats." Indeed, if "The Hollow Men" provides any solution to the question of religion,

Jeon asserts: "The answer that this poem provides is that prayer without God is poetry."

Source: Leah Tieger, Critical Essay on "The Hollow Men," in *Poetry for Students*, Gale, Cengage Learning, 2010.

Troy Urquhart

In the following review, Urquhart discusses the interconnection of contrasting ideas in the poem.

In T.S. Eliot's poem "The Hollow Men," the speaker searches for meaning but ultimately fails to strike a balance between the physical world and the abstract. Throughout the poem, the speaker's quest is hindered by his inability to reconcile this existence with "death's other Kingdom," his idea of the afterlife. The poem presents the search for meaning in terms of motion between opposing spheres of existence, yet the speaker's inability to find an acceptable truth creates an image of frustrated inertia. The kinetic images created by Eliot's speaker are immobile, and their tension becomes more pronounced as the poem progresses, emphasizing the speaker's growing dissatisfaction and mental imbalance.

Although images of suppressed motion are present in the first section, the images create a passive, rather than an active, tone. In the first two lines, Eliot's speaker introduces himself by using the first person plural "We" (1,2), which not only indicates the association of other people with the speaker's situation but also suggests a duplicity of character within the mind of the speaker similar to that in Eliot's "The Love Song of J. Alfred Prufrock." The image of "hollow men" (1) who are "Leaning together" (3) is one of immobility. "Leaning" denotes the application of force, but force directed toward a central point and merely providing self-support. The balance of such an arrangement also suggests that it is precarious: should one part change the force with which it leans, the arrangement is likely to collapse. If the speaker's "We" is interpreted as different aspects of one person, the image suggests mental stability that is maintained only through the careful balance of different personas. The "Paralysed force, gesture without motion" (12) confirms this image, for energy is expended without visible result. Further, people who have "crossed / [. . .] to death's other Kingdom" (13–14) do not remember the speaker's "We" "as lost / Violent souls" (15–16), but "As the hollow men / The stuffed men" (17–18). The kinetic energy of this scene is directed inward, and the description of nonviolence suggests that the motion goes unnoticed by those outside the speaker's "We." Throughout the first section of the poem, the speaker's efforts are directed inward and are therefore "meaningless" (7) because they do not influence the outside world.

In the concluding section of the poem, the images of suppressed action reach an almost irrepressible level as the speaker searches for meaning. Through the recitation of rhyme, the speaker returns to his childhood to seek relief from the building tension, but his childhood is a perverted one. In the traditional children's rhyme, the speaker substitutes "the prickly pear" (68) for the mulberry bush, and this substitution connects this section to the "cactus land" (40). Even though the childhood rhyme brings a melodic, chanting rhythm to the poem, the implication that the speaker's childhood resembles the "prickly" cactus rather than the sweet mulberry is unavoidable. The circular motion "round the prickly pear" (68) reiterates the theme of effort without result. It also builds the level of activity: motion has progressed through "leaning" (3), "swinging" (24), "trembling" (49), and "grop[ing]" (58) to the image of a child dancing or running.

The reference to the Lord's Prayer in section 5 ("For Thine is the Kingdom" [77,91]) is in sharp contrast to the motion of the child's rhyme: whereas the rhyme suggests activity, the Lord's Prayer creates an image of kneeling and meditation. Although the contrast of prayer with childhood activity suggests a comparison of contemplation with action, it also implies that the speaker's childhood has become an internal force in his search for meaning. The Lord's Prayer also connects the concluding section to "The supplication of a dead man's hand" in section 3 (43) and therefore suggests that the speaker views himself as dead or dying.

The speaker intertwines pairs of contrasting ideas with these lines, emphasizing the conflict of repressed motion. Through the repetition of "Falls the Shadow" (76,82,90), the "Shadow" becomes the pervading image of the last section, and it suggests something undefined, connecting to "Shape without form, shade without colour" (11). As an indeterminate image, the "Shadow" is neither "the idea" (72) nor "the reality" (73), neither "the potency" (86) nor "the existence" (87), but rather something between the abstract and the physical. It suggests that the speaker vacillates between contrasting interpretations of reality in the search for a balance that exists only outside both the physical and the abstract spheres.

In the final lines of the poem, the energy of the speaker implodes. The thrice repeated line "This is the way the world ends" (95–97), recalls both the chanting of the Lord's Prayer and the children's rhyme and creates an image of stagnation, for although the speaker searches for meaning in the lines, he fails to achieve motion. The inner balance suggested by the "Leaning" figures of the first section is lost in the final line, as the poem ends "Not with a bang but a whimper." The kinetic energy that begins "quiet and meaningless" (7) increases during the poem and peaks in the utterance of the word "bang." The increase in the tension of suppressed motion suggests that the speaker's agitation and mental imbalance increase as the work progresses. However, the speaker remains nonviolent (15–16) even in his state of mental collapse, for he denies the explosion of energy that "a bang" would denote, choosing instead to conclude the world—and the work—with an implosive "whimper."

Source: Troy Urquhart, "Eliot's 'The Hollow Men,'" in *Explicator*, Vol. 59, No. 4, Summer 2001, pp. 199–202.

Michele Valerie Ronnick
In the following essay, the literary allusions in "The Hollow Men" are identified.

Scholars have long endeavored to identify the sources of various images in T. S. Eliot's work, so densely layered with literary allusions. As Eliot himself noted in his essay "Philip Massinger" (1920),

> One of the surest of tests is the way in which a
> poet borrows. Immature poets imitate, mature
> poets steal; bad poets deface what they take,
> and good poets make it into something better,
> or at least something different.

In Eliot's poem "The Hollow Men," several sources have been posited for the "hollow men . . . the stuffed men / leaning together . . . filled with straw" (lines 1–2). B. C. Southam notes three: that the "hollow . . . stuffed men" are reminiscent of the effigies burned in celebration of Guy Fawkes Day; that "according to Valerie Eliot, the poet had in mind the marionette in Stravinsky's *Petrouchka*"; and finally, that the "straw-stuffed effigies are associated with harvest rituals celebrating the death of the fertility god or Fisher King."

In 1963, some years before Southam's summary, John Vickery had proffered an interpretation similar to the third point mentioned. He noted that "the opening lines of 'The Hollow Men' with their image of straw-filled creatures, recalls *The Golden Bough's* account of the straw-man who represents the dead spirit of fertility that revives in the spring when the apple trees begin to blossom." Whereas Eliot may well have had any or all of these ideas in mind, I suggest that there is yet another connection to be made, namely between Eliot's "hollow . . . stuffed men" and the Roman ritual of the Argei.

In 1922, a few years before Eliot wrote "The Hollow Men," W. Warde Fowler described the particulars of this ritual, which was to him a "fascinating puzzle" and "the first curiosity that enticed" him "into the study of Roman religion," in his book *Roman Religious Experience*. The rite according to Fowler occurs

> each year on the ides of May, which is in my view rather magical than religious, though the ancients themselves looked upon it as a kind of purification, [namely] the casting into the Tiber from the Pons Sublicius of twenty-four or twenty-seven straw puppets by the Vestal Virgins in the presence of the magistrates and pontifices. Recently an attempt has been made by Wissowa to prove that this strange ceremony was not primitive, but simply a case of substitution of puppets for real human victims as late as the age of the Punic wars. These puppets were called Argei, which naturally suggests Greeks; and Wissowa has contrived to persuade himself not only that a number of Greeks were actually put to death by drowning in an age when everything Greek was beginning to be reverenced at Rome, but (still more extraordinary to an anthropologist) that the primitive device of substitution was had in requisition at that late date in order to carry on the memory of that ghastly deed. And the world of German learning has silently followed their leader, without taking the trouble to test his conclusions . . . whatever be the history of the accessories of the rite—and they are various and puzzling,—that actual immersion of the puppets is the survival of a primitive piece of sympathetic magic, the object being possibly to procure rain.

Fowler's contemporary Sir James Frazer, whose work *The Golden Bough* greatly influenced Eliot, pointed to aspects of the ritual of purification in river water involved in the rite of the Argei. He observed that

> it is possible that the puppets made of rushes, which in the month of May the pontiffs and Vestal Virgins annually threw into the Tiber from the old Sublician bridge at Rome had originally the same significance [as the Roman festival Compitalia]; that is, they may have been designed to purge the city from demoniac influence by diverting the attention of the demons

> from human beings to the puppets and then toppling the whole uncanny crew, neck and crop, into the river, which would soon sweep them far out to sea. . . This interpretation of the Roman custom is supported to some extent by the evidence of Plutarch, who speaks of the ceremony as "the greatest of purifications."

Frazer also noted that as far as he could "see, there is little or nothing to suggest that the ceremony had anything to do with vegetation," and instead he suggested that the Argei "may have been offerings to the River God, to pacify him."

This motif of sacrificial separation and collective departure at a river's edge then provides a clear thematic link between the "hollow . . . stuffed men," who are "gathered on this beach of the tumid river / sightless" (lines 60–61), and the blind, featureless Argei ready to be tossed away by Roman officials standing on the Tiber's banks. The "tumid river" suggests not only Dante's River Acheron and the souls gathered nearby, as noted by Martin Scofield, but also the waters of Rome's greatest river. For the river into which twenty-four or twenty-seven Argei were hurled on an annual basis was swollen in mid May with spring run-off.

In Rome the ritualized murder of these straw hominids served to absorb evil forces, which rendered them accursed and profane. In Eliot's poem the stuffed men anxiously implore the reader, and "those who have crossed . . . to death's other kingdom" (13–14), to "remember us—if at all—not as lost / violent souls, but only / as the hollow men / the stuffed men" (15–18). Thus the small crowd of rush-stuffed Roman mannikins, who are as clone-like and uniform in their aspect as Scofield once described "the hollow men," find their destiny bound up with a riverside community.

Source: Michele Valerie Ronnick, "Eliot's 'The Hollow Men,'" in *Explicator*, Vol. 56, No. 2, Winter 1998, pp. 91–92.

Charles Sanders

In the following essay, Sanders illustrates the connection between "The Hollow Men" and Heart of Darkness.

T. S. Eliot has openly acknowledged the influence of Joseph Conrad's *Heart of Darkness* on "The Hollow Men" by means of his epigraph, *"Mistah Kurtz—he dead."* The poet has possibly imbibed something more of Conrad in the body of the poem, specifically in the famous conclusion, *"This is the way the world ends/Not with a bang but a whimper"* (*Collected Poems 1901–1962*; New York: Harcourt, Brace & World,

1963). For if we turn to the final scene of Marlow's monologue, in which Marlow lies to Kurtz's Intended, we find him saying, "It seemed to me that the house would collapse before I could escape, that the heavens would fall upon my head. But nothing happened. The heavens do not fall for such a trifle" (New York: New American Library, 1950; p. 157). Of course, we recognize Conrad's meaning immediately: a lie, for Marlow, is tainted with mortality; literally as well as symbolically he carries the sinful burden of Kurtz on his back; in that burden he accedes to his personal mortality. To the wealth of meanings already extracted from Eliot's passage—and without doing violence to any of them—we may now add a further insight: "The Hollow Men," though clearly a contrast to both Marlow and Kurtz (and Guy Fawkes), inherit the double burden. Reduced to childish inarticulation ("For Thine is/Life is/For Thine is the"), they can only sputter their accession in the repetitive rhythm of the nursery or Mother Goose rhyme, "This is the way we wash." They may avert their eyes; they may wear, like the Harlequin, "deliberate disguises"; they may "avoid speech"; but nothing can "wash" away their knowledge, direct or implied, of Kurtz or Marlow. Neither will the house collapse, nor the heavens fall, "with a bang"; the only sound is the "whimper" of a perennially repetitive "papier-mâché Mephistopheles," the all too mortal whimper that the silent wash of the Thames, Congo, or Styx does not obliterate so much as enhance.

Source: Charles Sanders, "Eliot's 'The Hollow Men,'" in *Explicator*, Vol. 38, No. 4, Summer 1980, pp. 8–9.

Everett A. Gillis, Lawrence A. Ryan, and Friedrich W. Strothmann

In the following essay, the authors discuss opposing views of the significance of Eliot's use of the word "empty" in "The Hollow Men."

I

The conventional interpretation of "The Hollow Men" as little more than an extension in mood and imagery of *The Waste Land* has recently been challenged by Frederich W. Strothmann and Lawrence V. Ryan, who contend in "Hope for T. S. Eliot's 'Empty Men'" (*PMLA*, XXXII [September 1958], 426–432) that the poem represents, rather, a transitional stage between Eliot's earlier Waste-Land poems and his later, more affirmative, work: "a long step toward the

> **IN SPITE OF ELIOT'S AVOWED AND DEMONSTRATED INTEREST IN THE RELATIONSHIP BETWEEN POETRY AND MUSIC, IN THE FINAL ANALYSIS THE POEM CAN NOT BE CRITICIZED IN MUSICAL TERMS."**

Four Quartets rather than a very short step out of *The Waste Land*" (p. 227 n).

Their argument rests ultimately on a special interpretation of the word "empty" in the lines "The hope only / Of empty men," which critics heretofore have taken simply as a synonym for "hollow," the epithet applied earlier to the inhabitants of the limbo depicted in the poem. The word "empty" is to be read in the light of the doctrine of the Spanish mystic St. John of the Cross that the soul in its upward journey toward salvation must pass through a spiritual state of absolute quiescence, in which it empties itself—even of hope—as a prelude toward a more active striving. For Professors Strothmann and Ryan, then, the word "empty" signifies a state of grace which though extremely low in the scale, is yet a step forward, and the "empty" men consequently find themselves "journeying through the delectable desert of purgation" (p. 432) that will end at long last in heaven. If one grants their interpretation of "empty," Professors Strothmann and Ryan make an excellent case for their view that the poem ends affirmatively, with a degree of hope for the hollow men. But there are several reasons for disagreeing both with the meaning they assign to "empty" and their conclusion that the poem ends on a "positive note."

The first of these is the basic situation presented in the poem itself, a situation which effectively militates against any possibility of spiritual progress by the hollow men: that of a modern limbo in which exist souls entirely void of spiritual meaning. For the scene and imagery of "The Hollow Men" is based upon the third canto of Dante's *Inferno*, which describes a desolate plain lying between Hell's portal and the river Acheron on which a horde of souls pursue a whirling banner round and round. Because of their miserable condition, says Virgil to Dante—for on earth above they had been neither good nor evil—mercy and justice both scorn them. Thus, totally without spiritual reality, they must remain forever on the plain, barred from crossing over the river (as those "lost / Violent souls" have already done, whose evil has at least a negative spiritual validity) to receive punishment in Hell or reward in Heaven. They are thus, in Eliot's phrase, *hollow* men: in terms of spiritual *value*, "Shape without form, shade without colour, / Paralysed force, gesture without motion," groping together, avoiding speech, on the beach of "the tumid river." In such a state, there is obviously no possibility of spiritual movement or progression such as that vouchsafed Dante, who does cross beyond Acheron, traversing Hell and Purgatory, observing, in the Garden of Eden at the top of the Mount of Purgatory, the triumphal procession of the Church, which causes the Tree of the Knowledge of Good and Evil at its approach to burst into bloom to the accompaniment of hymns. There he likewise sees the eyes of Beatrice reflecting like a mirror the shifting image of a griffin whose alternate forms represent respectively the human and the divine natures of Christ; and he is then carried by Beatrice into Paradise to behold the ranks of the redeemed through which shines God's trinal light—"which in a single star / Givest them all such rapture." These visions, contained in the *Purgatorio,* Cantos XXX–XXXI and the *Paradiso,* Canto XXXI, are obviously the source of the details of Sections II through IV of "The Hollow Men," though perceived by the hollow men only in a feeble and hallucinatory fashion: Beatrice's eyes reflecting the changing image of Christ seeming like "Sunlight on a broken column"; the Tree of the Knowledge of Good and Evil, "a tree swinging," i.e., like a wavering illusion; the hymns sung at the Tree's flowering, as indistinct as the singing of the wind's voice. But even whatever of spiritual validity might possibly exist in such a distorted version of Dante's real and effectual vision is still unavailable to the hollow men, for they lack even a vestige of the necessary spiritual capacity to apprehend it. The question of hope in the poem, then, is purely ironic.

The spiritual situation suggested in the poem is further emphasized by the poem's structure, which is essentially that of a musical composition. Eliot himself in his essay "The Music of Poetry" suggests an analogy between the structure of music and the structure of poetry, and it may easily be demonstrated that *The Waste Land,* which immediately precedes "The Hollow Men," as well as the later *Four Quartets,* follows a sonata-like structure. "*The Hollow Men,*" however, is more of a musical suite, consisting of a series of recitatives and choruses spoken or chanted respectively by the hollow-man leader—the "I" of the poem—and the chorus of hollow men. Controlled specifically by a musical logic, the poem presents its central concept thematically rather than by typical dramatic or narrative methods in which one force tends to triumph over another. The theme of spiritual impotence is initiated in the first movement of the poem by its vivid portrayal of the spiritual emptiness of the hollow men; it is further developed in the three middle movements, which depict the pitiable plight of the prophet or modern Dante in the contemporary world, and the total decadence to which religion has fallen; and is climaxed in the last by a grotesque parody of those formal ritualistic elements associated with the phenomenon of worship. There is thus in the poem, because of the thematic repetition within the different contexts provided by the individual movements, only a deeper concentration on the basic motif of impotence, and hence no form of spiritual progression such as that visualized by Professors Strothmann and Ryan. The presence in the poem of the elements of hope—the "perpetual star / Multifoliate rose"—may seem strange at first sight in a poem so thoroughly devoted to the theme of religious impotency. Yet it has an appropriate role if considered in terms of the musical logic of the poem, namely that of counterpoint. This aspect of musical technique is mentioned by Eliot in his analogy between music and poetry already cited. As counterpoint, the element of hope serves merely by musical contrast to reinforce the basic theme of spiritual inadequacy featured in the poem as a whole.

In addition to the arguments just presented for viewing "empty" as a synonym for "hollow" rather than as a state of grace leading to a positive spiritual condition on the part of the hollow men, we may examine two items of extrinsic evidence supporting the same conclusion. The first of these is Eliot's notable sensitivity with respect to words. His skill in this field is widely recognized by critics; but let us look at a particular example of his selective process at work. In a letter to Ezra Pound in 1922 relative to Pound's excisions of the *Waste Land* manuscript (included in *The Letters of Ezra Pound,* ed. D. D. Paige [New York, 1950], pp. 170–172), Eliot expresses concern regarding a passage which in the final published form of the poem contains the line "And if it rains, a closed car at four" (l. 136). Apparently Pound had made a suggestion regarding the word "taxi," for Eliot replies: "A closed car. I can't use taxi more than once." "A closed car" here is, of course, the inevitable, right word, as "taxi" is in the lines "When the human engine waits / Like a taxi throbbing waiting" (ll. 216–217). It should be admitted here that word repetition does occur in Eliot's verse, but invariably for a special effect. As a matter of fact, "The Hollow Men" itself contains repetition in its opening section, which begins "We are the hollow men / We are the stuffed men" and which closes "As the hollow men / The stuffed men." But as anyone can recognize it is the result of deliberate intention: for the refrain-like quality of the last two lines brings the section to a fitting close.

The other item of evidence is a passage in *The Waste Land* that almost exactly parallels the concluding portion of Section IV of "The Hollow Men" which contains the lines Professors Strothmann and Ryan make so much of. This is a passage in the first section of *The Waste Land* stressing the desolate quality of the waste land landscape: "What are the roots that clutch, what branches grow / Out of this stony rubbish?" After several such lines of descriptive detail, a note of hope is suddenly interjected:

Only
There is shadow under this red rock,
(Come in under the shadow of this red rock);

but one immediately realizes that the comfort promised is not what one has expected—i.e., relief from the heat and glare of the desert—but "fear in a handful of dust." The passage is manifestly ironical, and few critics would suggest that any real benefit has been derived by the waste landers from the promise of shadow under the red rock. Logically, the passage in "The Hollow Men" has the same ironic implications. In much the same manner as the promise of relief in *The Waste Land* is metamorphosized into symbols of desolation and death—"fear in a handful of dust," the "hope only / Of empty men" in "The Hollow Men" is followed by a mordant parody on a service of worship. On the whole, it seems highly probable that Eliot meant the word "empty" to be taken for nothing more than a synonym for hollowness and the degree of grace evident in the limbo of the hollow men as an ironic quality used for rhetorical purposes only.

II

Everett Gillis rests his criticism of our article, "Hope for T. S. Eliot's 'Empty Men'," upon two assumptions that are subject to challenge: he treats the structure of "The Hollow Men" as "essentially that of a musical composition," and he suggests it was simply the author's "notable sensitivity with respect to words" that prevented his repeating the word "hollow" at the end of the fourth section. To support both contentions, he adduces external evidence that appears à propos until one attempts to measure it against the actual text of the poem.

He would regard the work, first of all, as a sonata-like composition, with choral group and leader chanting "a series of recitatives and choruses" in which the theme of religious impotence is presented by musical, "rather than by typical dramatic or narrative methods." In returning to the text, however, one discovers that the so-called "leader," the "I," appears only in Section II. If the poem were a true exercise in thematic variation or musical counterpoint, the "leader" might have been expected to speak at least once more, most appropriately in Section IV. The fact that the "I" occurs only in this one instance and is thereafter dropped suggests, especially if one (rightly) accepts Professor Gillis's contention that Eliot is always meticulous in his use of language, some probable significance in the nonce appearance of an individual speaker. Since we do not find him where he might reasonably be expected to turn up again, it seems quite proper to ask why an apparent "leader" of this supposed chorus of grotesques should appear at all. Without reverting to the discussion of the piecemeal composition of the work, one may note that the "I" occurs only in that section which critics have agreed emphasizes most strongly the unwillingness of the hollow men to confront reality. Professor Gillis himself brings out the "hallucinatory" effect created by Eliot's choice of symbols for the unwanted spiritual fulfillment hinted at in Section II. The "deliberate disguises" and the wish to be "no nearer" may indicate that the "I" serves a peculiar purpose in this passage. For it is within this section that the *hollow* self protests most strongly against making the effort to approach a spiritual reality of which it is dimly aware but which it can not really desire so long as the soul remains in its present distracted state. The self can not actually want spiritual fulfillment so long as it refuses to purge itself of its false desires ("disguises," as they are called in the poem). If Eliot is employing thematic contrast or counterpoint, it would seem to consist rather in a brilliant playing of the egocentric hopelessness of the hollow "I" in the second section against the later hint in Section IV that by overcoming concern for self, the soul can be emptied of its vain longings in preparation for the eventual encounter with spiritual reality. Hence, the contrast between Sections II and IV suggests a development of, rather than a variation upon, the theme with which the poem begins.

The strong emphasis upon the symbolical "eyes," moreover, serves to sharpen this same contrast. Naturally the unprepared, "hollow" speaker of Section II dares not meet the eyes. In his unready state the spiritual realities can not appear except as painful experience or as vague hallucinations. Yet the poem does not say that because they appear fragmentary and unrealized to the unreceptive soul, these spiritual experiences are merely hallucinatory. The complaint of the chorus in the fourth section that "The eyes are not here," that without the eyes "We grope together / And avoid speech," makes it apparent that the "eyes" symbolize a reality positively and truly to be desired. The obvious analogy between the hollow men and Dante's "Trimmers" (*Inferno*, Canto III) need not stand as an obstacle to seeing a glimmer of hope in this climactic section of the poem. A distinction must be made between Dante's and Eliot's "lost" spirits. The Trimmers are dead and without hope in fact; irrevocably they have made "the great refusal" and must remain "sightless" (void of spiritual understanding and fulfillment) forever. The hollow men, though they appear to be destined to a similar end, are nevertheless still alive, are not yet damned. Their present plight is miserable, and if they continue in their despairing state, it promises to be their eternal lot. But in the word "unless" lies their hope; there is a possibility that the "eyes" will reappear provided the necessary condition is met. The necessary condition is that they first take the step, as must all who hope to come to the beatific vision, from hollowness to emptiness.

Eliot's echoes of Dante in this passage require any critic of the poem to ask yet another question. "Why should 'The Hollow Men' apparently embody the same disapproving attitude toward Trimmers as one finds in the *Commedia* unless, as far as the poet is concerned, some positive value inheres in whatever it is that the Trimmers have refused?" If it is bad, or unfortunate, to be a Trimmer or a Trimmer-like hollow man, then must he be fortunate, and certainly not a vain dreamer, who can attain what those undone souls cannot hope to possess. The "perpetual star" and the "Multifoliate rose" must symbolize, for Eliot as for Dante, not a vague, illusory dream of fulfillment, but something truly worth having. It seems unlikely that in this passage Eliot should have accepted the values Dante gives to one set of symbols (the Trimmers) without accepting those he attaches to the other (the eyes, the multifoliate rose).

Nor does Professor Gillis's argument that Eliot is careful not to repeat words except "invariably for a special effect" satisfactorily explain the single appearance in the poem of the word "empty." The statement is, in the first place, highly questionable. One may point, for instance, to Eliot's practice in "Ash Wednesday" of repeating words, phrases, images, often with variations that are slight but full of significance. Granted, these are "special effects"; yet it is difficult to see why "The Hollow Men" should be denied the privilege of embodying similar special effects. The appearance of the word "hollow" at both the beginning and the end (reinforced by the word "stuffed" at the end) of Section I is, moreover, not the only occurrence of functional repetition in the poem. In Section II a similar effect is created by the haunting repetition of the phrase "no nearer." One may raise a more direct objection, however, to the claim that Eliot meticulously avoids repetition wherever he can find an equally suitable synonym. The example of "taxi—car" from *The Waste Land* may not be called in as a proper analogy to "hollow—empty" in the later work. The choice between "car" and "taxi," in the lines cited, while an important esthetic matter, is not crucial within the total context of the poem. Eliot's good taste in substituting "car" in the line in question is evident. Yet *The Waste Land* would have produced much the same effect as a work of art even if the author had followed Ezra Pound's advice on this minor point.

In reading "The Hollow Men," on the other hand, understanding of the relationship between the words "hollow" and "empty" is essential. We agree with Professor Gillis upon Eliot's exquisite sense of words as well as his skill at repetition, often with slight but subtle variation, for special effects. If, then, the repetition of "hollow men... stuffed men" in Section I is effective, why should the author have rejected the word "hollow" at the end of Section IV? It should be noted that the richly suggestive phrase "hollow valley" appears in the same passage. If the author had simply wished to avoid four occurrences of the word "hollow" in the poem, why do we not find here "empty valley" and "hollow men"?

Our discussion earlier in this paper of Eliot's use of Dante's symbolical Trimmers, perpetual star, and multifoliate rose should provide an answer and at the same time free us, we hope, of any charge of begging the question. From the context, the "hollow" speakers associate something positive and greatly to be desired (the "Multifoliate rose") with the condition of "emptiness." Clearly it is something that hollow men are not capable of enjoying. As we insisted in our original article, the thematic development of the poem is made truly effective by the sharp contrast between the despairing repetition of "hollow men . . . stuffed men" in Section I, and the sudden, startling revelation of a possible way out of the dilemma for "empty men" at the critical moment in Section IV.

None of the objections of Professor Gillis adds weight to the conventional interpretation of the poem which our article has called into question. In spite of Eliot's avowed and demonstrated interest in the relationship between poetry and music, in the final analysis the poem can not be criticized in musical terms. No more may the *Four Quartets,* even though the attempt in these later works to draw upon principles of musical composition is evident. The quality and meaning of Eliot's language and imagery, apart from which the rhythmic and harmonic patterns may not be judged without doing violence to his work, are what really matter in his, or in any other writer's poems. In "The Hollow Men," we still contend, the author carefully orders the language, imagery, and harmonies into sharp contrasts so as to make clear that in hollowness lies despair, but that emptiness is a condition of hope.

Source: Everett A. Gillis, Lawrence A. Ryan, and Friedrich W. Strothmann, "Hope for Eliot's 'Hollow Men'?," in *PMLA*, Vol. 75, No. 5, December 1960, pp. 635–38.

Bush, Ronald, "T. S. Eliot's Life and Career," in *Modern American Poetry Review*, http://www.english.illinois.edu/maps/poets/a_f/eliot/life.htm (accessed July 20, 2009), originally published in *American National Biography*, edited by John A. Garraty and Mark C. Carnes, Oxford University Press, 1999.

Eliot, T. S., "The Hollow Men," in *Collected Poems, 1909–1962*, Harcourt, 1991, pp. 77–82.

Flynn, Thomas, *Existentialism: A Very Short Introduction*, Oxford University Press, 2006.

Fraser, Antonia, *Faith and Treason: The Story of the Gunpowder Plot*, Anchor, 1997.

Jeon, Joseph Jonghyun, "Eliot Shadows: Autography and Style in 'The Hollow Men,'" in *Yeats Eliot Review*, Vol. 24, No. 4, Winter 2007, p. 12,

Keegan, John, *The First World War*, Vintage, 2000.

Kirsch, Adam, "Matthew Arnold and T. S. Eliot," in *American Scholar*, Vol. 67, No. 3, Summer 1998, p. 65.

Link, Arthur Stanley, *The Impact of World War I*, HarperCollins, 1969.

Marshall, S. L. A., *World War I*, Mariner Books, 2001.

Marwick, Arthur, *The Impact of World War I: Total War and Social Change; Europe 1914–1945*, Open University Worldwide, 2001.

Miller, J. Hillis, Review of "The Hollow Men," in *Modern American Poetry Review*, http://www.english.illinois.edu/maps/poets/a_f/eliot/hollow.htm (accessed July 20, 2009), originally published in *Poets of Reality: Six Twentieth-Century Writers*, Harvard University Press, 1965.

Monk, Craig, *Writing the Lost Generation: Expatriate Autobiography and American Modernism*, University Of Iowa Press, 2008.

Shakespeare, William, *Julius Caesar*, Barron's Educational Series, 2001.

Spurr, David, Review of "The Hollow Men," in the *Modern American Poetry Review*, http://www.english.illinois.edu/maps/poets/a_f/eliot/hollow.htm (accessed July 20, 2009), originally published in *Conflicts in Consciousness: T. S. Eliot's Poetry and Criticism*, University of Illinois Press, 1984.

Whitworth, Michael H. ed., *Modernism*, Blackwell, 2007.

SOURCES

Armstrong, Tim, *Modernism: A Cultural History*, Polity, 2005.

Bradbury, Malcolm, and James McFarlane, *Modernism: A Guide to European Literature 1890–1930*, Penguin, 1978.

Brooker, Jewel Spears, "T. S. Eliot," in *Dictionary of Literary Biography*, Vol. 329, *Nobel Prize Laureates in Literature, Part 1: Agnon-Eucken*, Thomson Gale, 2007, pp. 402–21.

FURTHER READING

Marino, Gordon, ed., *Basic Writings of Existentialism*, Modern Library Classics, 2004.

> Existentialist philosophy was highly influential to the modernist movement, and this anthology of existentialist writings provides greater insight into that influence. The work of such notable existentialists as Søren Kierkegaard, Friedrich Nietzsche, Martin Heidegger, Jean-Paul Sartre,

and Albert Camus are included in the volume. In addition, introductions to each writer and their life and work are also included.

Miller, Nathan, *New World Coming: The 1920s and the Making of Modern America*, Da Capo Press, 2004.
This book presents a history of the decade in which modernism came of age. It includes discussion of the social, cultural, and political milieu of the day.

Pound, Ezra, *Selected Poems*, New Directions, 1957.
Often credited as the father of the modernist movement, Pound was influential in establishing the literary careers of several important modernist writers. In fact, his work is not hailed nearly as much as his role in the movement. Nevertheless, it is well worth reading, and though this volume was released in 1957, it remained in print as of 2009. This alone is a testament to Pound's lasting contribution to American literature.

Stein, Gertrude, *Selected Writings of Gertrude Stein*, Vintage, 1990.
Another notable modernist writer is Gertrude Stein, one of the few women prominent in the movement. Like Pound and Eliot, Stein was an American expatriate. Her work is best known for its experiments with from and narrative.

I Wandered Lonely as a Cloud

WILLIAM WORDSWORTH

1815

"I Wandered Lonely as a Cloud" is a short lyric poem by the English Romantic poet William Wordsworth. It was written in 1804 and first published in his *Poems, in Two Volumes* in 1807. A revised version, in which the poem was expanded from three stanzas to four, was published in Wordsworth's *Poems* in 1815. The origin of the poem lies in a walk that Wordsworth took with his sister Dorothy in the Lake District in northwest England, where the Wordsworths lived. This was on April 15, 1802, when the Wordsworths were walking near Gowbarrow Park, near Ullswater, and came upon a large number of daffodils near the water. Dorothy described the scene in her *Grasmere Journals*. William did not write the poem until two years later, making much use of Dorothy's account. The poem has always been one of Wordsworth's most popular. Indeed, it is one of the most famous poems in the English language. Quite simple in style, it shows how Wordsworth, like many of the Romantic poets, was inspired by the beauty of nature. It also gives insight into the way Wordsworth composed his poems.

"I Wandered Lonely as a Cloud" is currently available in *"I Wandered Lonely as a Cloud. . ." And Other Poems You Half-Remember from School* edited by Ana Sampson and published Michael O'Mara Books in 2009.

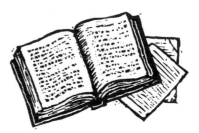

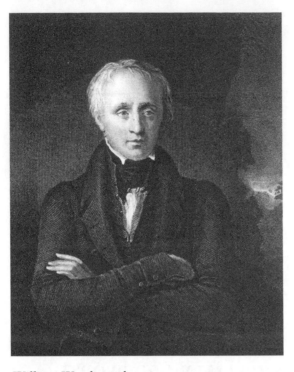

William Wordsworth (The Library of Congress)

AUTHOR BIOGRAPHY

Wordsworth was born in Cockermouth, Cumberland, a small town in the northern part of England's Lake District, on April 7, 1770. His family was quite well off and lived in the best house in town, which was provided for John Wordsworth, Wordsworth's father, by Sir James Lowther, who employed Wordsworth as his legal representative. Wordsworth had three brothers and one sister. His mother died when he was eight, and his father when he was thirteen. Wordsworth spent his first nine years at Cockermouth, and the natural beauty of the region made an impression on him that would inspire his poetry and would endure for his entire life. At the age of nine Wordsworth attended Hawkshead Grammar School and remained there until 1787. Hawkshead was a village near Esthwaite Lake and Lake Windermere. The first books of Wordsworth's long autobiographical poem *The Prelude: The Growth of a Poet's Mind* (1850) describe the blissful days of his childhood and adolescence that he spent exploring nature in and around Hawkshead.

Wordsworth attended St. John's College, Cambridge, in 1787, but had little enthusiasm for his studies. After graduating in 1791, he spent a year in France, during which he became an enthusiastic supporter of the French Revolution, inspired by its ideals of liberty and equality. He published his first poetry, *Descriptive Sketches*, in 1793, about the trip he had made in 1790 to the Swiss Alps. Two years later, when Wordsworth was living in Racedown, Dorset, in southwestern England, he met Samuel Taylor Coleridge, a fellow poet, with whom he was to form a remarkable friendship and creative collaboration. In 1797, Wordsworth and his sister Dorothy moved to Somerset so they could live near Coleridge. Wordsworth began writing *Lyrical Ballads*, with some contributions from Coleridge. The volume was published in 1798 and marks one of the seminal works of the Romantic period, and the beginning of what is sometimes referred to as Wordsworth's great decade, the period during which he wrote most of the poetry for which he is remembered. In 1800, a second edition was published that included Wordsworth's Preface, in which he explained his poetic principles.

Wordsworth, Dorothy, and Coleridge traveled in Germany during 1798 and 1799, and on their return Wordsworth moved back to the Lake District, living in Dove Cottage in Grasmere. In 1802, financially more secure because of a long-delayed inheritance he received from his father, Wordsworth married Mary Hutchinson, whom he had known since he was a child. They were to have five children, two of whom died in infancy. In 1807, Wordsworth published *Poems, in Two Volumes*, which included the first version of "I Wandered Lonely as a Cloud" as well as "Ode: Intimations of Immortality." Wordsworth quarreled with his friend Coleridge in 1810, and nearly two decades passed before they were reconciled.

In 1813, Wordsworth moved to Rydal Mount, Ambleside, a few miles southeast of Grasmere, and was appointed distributor of stamps for Westmoreland (this meant that he collected revenue for the government). Wordsworth was now a famous poet, but the poetry he produced after *The Excursion* (1814) showed a steady decline in quality. He also abandoned the radicalism of his youth and became a political and religious conservative. In 1843 Wordsworth was appointed England's poet laureate.

Wordsworth died at Rydal Mount on April 23, 1850. The final version of *The Prelude*, which he had been revising on and off for years, was published posthumously in 1850.

POEM TEXT

I wandered lonely as a cloud
That floats on high o'er vales and hills,
When all at once I saw a crowd,
A host, of golden daffodils;
Beside the lake, beneath the trees,   5
Fluttering and dancing in the breeze.

Continuous as the stars that shine
And twinkle on the milky way,
They stretched in never-ending line
Along the margin of a bay: 10
Ten thousand saw I at a glance,
Tossing their heads in sprightly dance.

The waves beside them danced; but they
Out-did the sparkling waves in glee:
A poet could not but be gay,   15
In such a jocund company:
I gazed—and gazed—but little thought
What wealth the show to me had brought:

For oft, when on my couch I lie
In vacant or in pensive mood,   20
They flash upon that inward eye
Which is the bliss of solitude;
And then my heart with pleasure fills,
And dances with the daffodils.

POEM SUMMARY

Stanza 1

In "I Wandered Lonely as a Cloud" the speaker describes what he saw one spring day when he was walking in the English countryside. The first two lines state that he was alone as he walked, and he compares himself to a solitary cloud high in the sky. Then suddenly he comes upon a splendid sight: a multitude of daffodils. The daffodils are under the trees and next to the lake. The daffodils sway from side to side, appearing to dance in the breeze.

Stanza 2

In this stanza the poet continues to describe the daffodils. There are so many of them that he compares them to the stars in the Milky Way. The Milky Way galaxy contains billions of stars and forms a band of light when seen at night from Earth. As the poet looks at them, the daffodils continue in an unbroken line at the edge of the bay. He estimates that there must be 10,000 of them, and they are all dancing in the breeze.

Stanza 3

In Stanza 3 the poet continues to describe the daffodils. He notes that the breeze is also making

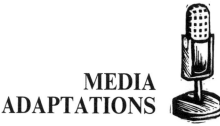

MEDIA ADAPTATIONS

- *Great Poets: Wordsworth*, an audio CD, includes "I Wandered Lonely as a Cloud" in the selection of Wordsworth's poems read by Oliver Ford Davies and Jasper Britton. It was released by Naxos Audiobooks in 2008.

- *William Wordsworth: Poems*, an audiocassette, contains "I Wandered Lonely as a Cloud" in this selection of Wordsworth's poems released by Highbridge Audio in 1998.

the water on the lake move in waves, but the daffodils seem even more joyful than the waves as they dance. In line 3, the poet says that it was impossible for a poet not to be happy when in the presence of such lively and cheerful company as the daffodils. In line 5, he tells how he stood for a long time gazing at the daffodils. But at the time, he adds, he did not fully realize how much the sight had enriched him. That realization would only come later, as the final stanza explains.

Stanza 4

In this stanza the poet reflects on his experience of suddenly coming upon all those daffodils. Some time has passed since he took that walk. Often since then, when he is alone, lying on his couch in a thoughtful mood, or with nothing much going on in his mind, he suddenly sees the daffodils once more in his mind's eye. The memory of the daffodils, and his ability to recreate the vision of them in his mind, brings him great pleasure, and he feels that his own heart is dancing along with the daffodils.

THEMES

Nature

Perhaps the key term in the poem is "lonely," which describes the poet's state of mind as he walks in nature. He does not say merely that he was alone. He refers to a specific lack of a sense of

TOPICS FOR FURTHER STUDY

- Write a short poem that records an experience you had walking in nature. Try to remember a moment when you saw something that surprised or amazed you. In the poem, describe what you saw and how it affected you.

- With another student, research daffodils. How many species are there in North America? Can they be grown throughout the United States? How long is their flowering season? What is the origin of the name? Create a slide show in PowerPoint or similar software program that pictures at least five different types of daffodils, and explain the variations.

- Read the poem "To an Early Daffodil" by the early twentieth-century American poet Amy Lowell, and write an essay in which you com-

pare and contrast it with "I Wandered Lonely as a Cloud." How do the forms of the poems differ? What do the two poems have in common? Which poem do you prefer, and why? You can find Lowell's poem at the Web site Famous Poets and Poems. com, http://famouspoetsandpoems.com/poets/amy_lowell/poems/20005.

- Consult *Poetry for Young People: William Wordsworth*, edited by Alan Liu (Sterling, 2003). Read the biography of Wordsworth and the critical introduction. Referring to this material, write an essay in which you describe how "I Wandered Lonely as a Cloud" embodies the themes that typify Wordsworth's poetry as a whole.

---

community, or connectedness. He is isolated, and in the poem he uses the image of a solitary cloud to convey his mood. He is walking in nature, but he feels a sense of separation from other living things, whether human or natural. But then he suddenly catches sight of the endless line of daffodils, and this changes his mood completely. What meets his eye is not merely a static scene. The wind is blowing, which makes the daffodils seem more than usually alive as they are blown about in the breeze. In this scene of great natural beauty, the poet feels happy and restored to life in a certain way. Before, he was lonely, but now he feels cheerful, moved by the beauty of the scene. It seems to him as if nature, as represented by the daffodils, is alive with joy, and he is able to share that joy. There is therefore a connection between the poet and the daffodils that puts an end to his sense of separation.

It is perhaps significant that the speaker identifies himself (in line 15) as a poet, when he states that such a sight could not fail to make a poet cheerful. He does not say that just anyone would have been affected by the scene, or affected in the

same way. For Wordsworth, a poet was a man of deep sensibilities who was capable of understanding intuitively the connection between man and nature. To be cut off from that feeling could only be experienced by a poet as a painful lack of something vital. The sudden sight of the daffodils in motion, stirred by the wind, jolts the poet into feeling once more the same life that flows through humans and the natural world. It is a moment of true communion with the spirit of nature, and this is why it restores his spirits.

Memory and Imagination

It is important to note that Wordsworth did not write the poem immediately after seeing the daffodils. Two years passed between the time he saw the daffodils and the time he wrote the poem. What prompted the poem, then, was not so much the experience of seeing the daffodils but the memory of it, recreated by the poet's imagination at a later date. What this shows is that for Wordsworth, what he calls in the poem the "inward eye" is in a sense more powerful than the outward eye with which he saw the daffodils.

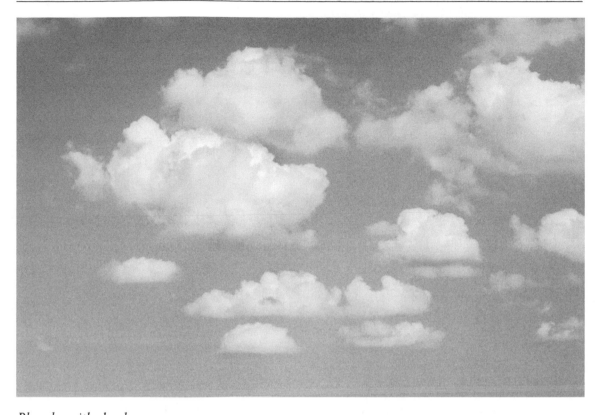

Blue sky with clouds (Image copyright Adisa, 2009. Used under license from Shutterstock.com)

The poet says this quite clearly in the last two lines of stanza 3, which is why the last stanza of the poem focuses not on the daffodils as an immediate sense experience but on the memory of that experience. At the time Wordsworth saw the daffodils, he enjoyed the sight, as anyone would, but he did not realize its true significance until later. In solitude at home, when he is relaxing and in a reflective mood, the sight of the daffodils suddenly comes into his mind again, and once again he experiences a moment of communion with nature; his heart dances with joy just as he remembers the daffodils dancing. The point here is that the really significant moments come not when he is in nature but when he is withdrawn from it. He can recreate the experience for himself without actually going out in nature and seeking a similar sight. The implication is that although nature may, in the poem, be a wonderful sight, the human mind is even more wonderful, since it can summon the experience again when no daffodils are in sight. Indeed, the pleasure afforded by the daffodils, thanks to the power of memory and imagination, has only increased over the intervening two years.

STYLE

Iambic Tetrameter

The poem is written in what is called iambic tetrameter. An iamb is a poetic foot in which an unstressed syllable is followed by a stressed syllable. (A foot, in English poetic meter, consists of two or three syllables, either one strongly stressed syllable and one lightly stressed syllable, or one strong stress and two lighter ones.) The iamb is the most common foot in English poetry. Almost all the lines in this poem are iambic. However, just for variety, the poet does vary the meter in certain places.

At the beginning of stanza 1, line 6, the poet substitutes a dactylic foot for the initial iamb, in the word *Fluttering*. A dactylic foot consists of a strongly stressed syllable followed by two lightly stressed syllables. In stanza 2, at the beginning of line 11, the poet substitutes a spondee (two strong stresses) for the iamb. This has the effect of emphasizing the sheer number of daffodils that he saw, since the stress falling on the first syllable as well as the second makes that foot stand out against the expected iambic meter. This is particularly noticeable when the poem is read aloud, because what we hear (the spondee) is different from what we expect (the iamb). A similar variation occurs in the following line (the last line of stanza 2), in which instead of an iamb the poet uses a trochee, a stressed syllable followed by an unstressed syllable (the opposite of an iamb).

Rhyme

The poet makes use of a regular rhyme scheme throughout the poem. The first line of each stanza rhymes with the third. The second line rhymes with the fourth, and then the last two lines rhyme with each other to form a concluding couplet to each stanza. The words used in the rhymes are mostly simple, consisting of one syllable. The use of rhyme not only supplies an easily identifiable sense of order and structure to the poem but adds pleasure to the reader's experience of it.

Personification

Personification is a poetic technique in which human emotions and feelings are attributed to inanimate objects. For example, the poet states that he is "as lonely as a cloud," which is a form of personification by use of a simile (a comparison of two apparently unlike things in a way that brings out the similarity between them). The poet compares his own loneliness to the loneliness of a single cloud in the sky. A more extended use of personification occurs in the descriptions of the daffodils. The poet describes them as a "crowd," which is a term usually applied to people. Further, the daffodils are described as dancing, moving their heads around almost as if they were human. Dance, however, is a human invention, proceeding according to measured steps. The fact that the daffodils are presented in this light personifies them by attributing to them a human activity. The personification continues when the daffodils are described as gleeful. Glee, which means joy, is a human emotion; presumably, daffodils do not experience joy, and certainly not in the sense that humans do, but the poet is prepared to attribute such joy to them because that is how it seems to him. The personification also has the effect of creating a subtle link, through the spirit of joy, between humans and the natural world.

Alliteration

Alliteration refers to the repetition of initial consonants. Wordsworth does not make much use of alliteration in this poem, but when he does it is with great effect. It occurs in the final line, the repetition of the *d* sound in *dances* and *daffodils*. The word *dance* is a key one in the poem, since it or a variant appears in every stanza. In the first three stanzas, it refers to the daffodils only; in the final line of the last stanza, it refers both to the daffodils and to the heart of the poet. The alliteration gives a pleasing sense of resolution to the poem, suggesting the connection between man and nature that is the theme of the poem.

HISTORICAL CONTEXT

The English Romantic Movement

As a literary movement in England, the Romantic era is often said to have started in 1798, with the publication of Wordsworth and Coleridge's *Lyrical Ballads*, although there were Romantic poems written earlier than that, notably William Blake's *Songs of Innocence and of Experience* (1794). Wordsworth was the leading poet of the first generation of English Romantic poets, which included Coleridge (1772–1834) and Blake (1757–1827). Coleridge is most famous for "The Rime of the Ancient Mariner," which appeared in the 1798 edition of *Lyrical Ballads*, and "Kubla Khan" (written around 1797 but not published until 1816). The leading lights of the second generation of English Romantics were John Keats (1795–1821), Percy Bysshe Shelley (1792–1822), and George Gordon, Lord Byron (1788–1824). There were all born about twenty years after Wordsworth but died young; Wordsworth outlived them all by nearly thirty years. To the second generation also belonged Felicia Hemans (1793–1835) of whom Wordsworth thought very highly, even composing a memorial verse to her following her death.

Wordsworth's Preface to *Lyrical Ballads*, published in 1800, was a seminal document in the theory of Romanticism. Reacting against the formal poetic diction and choice of subject matter in classical eighteenth-century verse, Wordsworth said he wanted to write in a new way, using simple language to reveal the most basic human emotions. He wrote about ordinary country people and everyday incidents in ways that revealed much about their feelings. Unlike the eighteenth-century poets, he thought that social outcasts, such as a retarded boy, a convict, a beggar, and others were suitable subjects for poetry. In placing the emphasis on subjective feeling and emotion, that of the poet and the subject of the poem, Wordsworth marked out a key area of the Romantic spirit.

COMPARE
&
CONTRAST

- **Early 1800s:** Wordsworth spends long hours exploring the Lake District, sometimes walking over thirty miles a day. He advocates for public footpaths in the area and believes that the Lake District is a national treasure that should be preserved. He is therefore one of the first conservationists in England.

  Today: Established as a national park in 1951, the Lake District is England's largest national park, covering 885 square miles. The highest mountain is Scafell Pike at 3,210 feet, and the longest lake is Windermere (10.5 miles). An immensely popular destination for tourists, the Lake District receives 8.3 million day visitors a year.

- **Early 1800s:** From 1803 to 1815, the nations of Europe are engaged in the Napoleonic Wars. These wars pit the French Empire under Napoleon against Great Britain and its allies, which at various times include Prussia, Russia, Austria, and Spain. As the French Revolution is transformed into wars of conquest, the English Romantic poets abandon their earlier support for French revolutionary

ideals. However, poets such as William Blake and Percy Bysshe Shelley remain resolutely opposed to political repression at home.

  Today: There is no political movement in the world that excites idealistic young poets and writers the way the French Revolution excited the Romantics or the Spanish Civil War galvanized many English writers and intellectuals in the 1930s, including George Orwell. In 2003, British writers such as the dramatist Harold Pinter and the poet laureate Andrew Motion publish poems opposing the war in Iraq.

- **Early 1800s:** Wordsworth, a poet of nature, makes the Lake District the setting for much of his work that explores the relationship between nature and the human mind.

  Today: There are many English-language poets and prose writers who take as their subject spirituality explored through nature, including Annie Dillard, Jorie Graham, Wendell Berry, Mary Oliver, Robert Hass, Gary Snyder, and Louise Glück.

The human heart rather than human reason became the touchstone of truth; the authenticity of personal experience was preferred over knowledge passed down by tradition. Because of this emphasis on the subjective rather than objective elements of life, the Romantics excelled at the lyric poem, in which they explored personal thoughts and feelings. This might be considered the major genre of the Romantic period. Along with this emphasis on the subjective came an exalted view of the status of the poet. Shelley famously wrote in his *A Defence of Poetry* that poets were the "unacknowledged legislators of the World." The poet was regarded as a prophet and seer who could discern the truth of things.

The Romantics were explorers in the sense that they wanted to break out of the limitations

imposed by the merely rational elements of life. They explored other realms of the psyche, including dreams and the supernatural (Coleridge's "Christabel" is a good example of the latter) and unusual states of mind (Keats's "Ode to a Nightingale" and Wordsworth's "Ode: Intimations of Immortality from Recollections of Early Childhood"), as well as esoteric systems of thought, which fascinated both Coleridge and Blake. Many of the Romantics were involved in a restless search for the infinite. Their goal was to experience life in a more holistic way, overcoming the separation between subject and object and realizing, at the level of direct experience, the unity of all life. For the Romantics, the agent of this new mode of perception was not reason but the imagination, to which poets such as Wordsworth, Blake, and Coleridge attributed an almost god-like power.

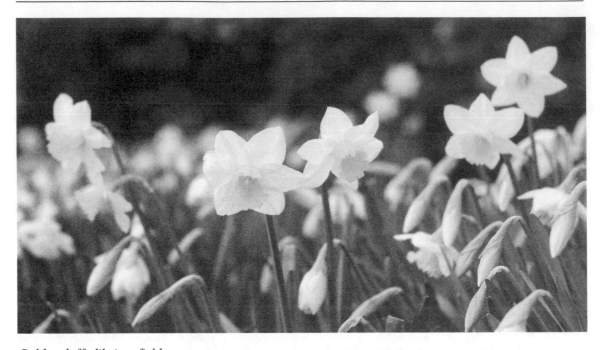

Golden daffodils in a field (*Image copyright Chester Tugwell, 2009. Used under license from Shutterstock.com*)

Many of the Romantics were passionately involved in the social and political issues of their day. The early Romantics were all supporters of the French Revolution, believing that it would usher in a new era of freedom and justice in which man would finally be able to achieve his full potential. Later, the poets would become disillusioned with the course the revolution took, and Wordsworth was subject to conflicted feelings when England declared war on France in 1793. In general, the Romantics supported the ideals of liberty and considered themselves to be radicals, opposed to political repression of all kinds. Byron actively supported the cause of Greek independence from Turkey and died serving it.

The Romantic era is usually regarded as having ended in England in 1832. Although Wordsworth, perhaps the greatest of the English Romantics, would live another eighteen years, his most creative years were long behind him, and he had become a conservative figure. All the other great Romantics were dead. This was also the year that the Great Reform Act was passed, creating fundamental changes in British social and political life.

The Lake District

The Lake District is a rural area in northwest England that is famous for its lakes and fells (mountains), and is forever associated with the name of Wordsworth. Wordsworth lived most of his life in the Lake District, first as a boy in Cockermouth and Hawkshead, then at Dove Cottage, Grasmere, where he wrote many of his most well-known poems, and finally at Rydal Mount, Rydal. His poetry explores the landscape of this region in unique ways, and he knew the Lake District so well that he wrote his own guidebook to it, titled *Guide to the Lakes*, which was published in 1810 and went through five editions by 1835. Even at that time, the Lake District was attracting a burgeoning tourist industry, and in the later years of Wordsworth's life many people came simply to see the places he had written about, and even to visit his home and try to catch a glimpse of the great man himself. Other poets, such as Coleridge and Robert Southey (1774–1843), were also associated with the Lake District. Although not native to the Lakes, Coleridge lived in Keswick, thirteen miles north of Grasmere, for a number of years. Southey was a friend of Wordsworth' and was better known in his own day than in contemporary times. He settled in Keswick in 1803 and remained there until his death in 1843. He was appointed poet laureate in 1813. Contemporary writers coined the term the "Lake School" to describe these three poets, but the term has since been discarded.

CRITICAL OVERVIEW

Although "I Wandered Lonely as a Cloud" has long found favor with critics and readers, it did not meet the approval of Wordsworth's friend Coleridge, who listed in his book *Biographia Literaria* five "defects" in Wordsworth's poetry. The last of these was "thoughts and images too great for the subject," and he chose this poem as one of two examples. Coleridge's point was that the subject of the poem in the last stanza—daffodils remembered—was not weighty enough to supply the kind of bliss Wordsworth described. In Coleridge's view, the "inward eye" is something that occupies itself with more profound thoughts than daffodils waving in the breeze. Later commentators, however, have not endorsed Coleridge's view, preferring to draw out the deeper meanings of the poem. David Ferry, in *The Limits of Mortality: An Essay on Wordsworth's Major Poems*, points out that the loneliness of the speaker at the beginning of the poem "has nothing to do with a separation from the world of men. It is a separation from the harmony of things and the aspect of eternity." This separation is what is addressed in the movement of the poem, which "is a symbol of the poet's relation to eternity (and the difficulty of perfecting that relation)." In *William Wordsworth*, Russell Noyes points out that for Wordsworth the wind metaphorically represents the "creative spirit"; he notes that "the wind's action draws all parts of the composition together and relates them to the whole. It is the breath which, in the climax of recollection, fills his heart with pleasure and sets it to dancing with the daffodils." For Geoffrey Durrant, in *William Wordsworth*, the poem "is only superficially about the daffodils." Instead, it is "an account of the experience of poetic creation." Durrant concludes his analysis by pointing out the following:

> Wordsworth in this poem is describing an experience of which all are capable, but which is increasingly neglected as men become preoccupied with business and professions. It is the imagination that enables man to enter into and give life and significance to the world.

CRITICISM

Bryan Aubrey

Aubrey holds a Ph.D. in English. In this essay he discusses how Wordsworth came to write "I

> **THOSE WHO KNOW WORDSWORTH'S POETRY WILL RECOGNIZE THE DESCRIPTION OF THIS QUIET, TRANQUIL STATE BECAUSE WORDSWORTH MENTIONS IT IN MANY OTHER POEMS, HOLDING IT UP AS AN IDEAL CONDITION OF THE MIND IN WHICH THE TRUTH OF THINGS SPONTANEOUSLY REVEALS ITSELF."**

Wandered Lonely as a Cloud" and what the poem reveals about Wordsworth's theory of poetry.

"I Wandered Lonely as a Cloud" may well be the most anthologized poem in the English language, and generations of school students have been presented with it as an accessible work by one of England's greatest poets. "I Wandered Lonely as a Cloud" may indeed be a simple poem but it is not quite as simple as it might first appear, and it leads the interested reader into a glimpse of the philosophical aspects of Wordsworth's poetry and of his theories about how poetry comes to be written.

The origins of the poem lie in a walk near Ullswater taken by Wordsworth and his sister Dorothy in April 1802. The details of this walk are known because Dorothy kept a journal and recorded the day-to-day activities of herself and her brother. This particular spring day was mild but very windy, so windy in fact that at one point they thought they would have to turn back. But they continued and when they were in the woods they saw a few daffodils close by the lake. Then more and more daffodils appeared, a "long belt" of them stretching along the shore of the lake. Dorothy, whose journals were first published in 1897, long after her death (later published as *The Grasmere Journals* in *The Norton Anthology of English Literature* [1979]), described the sight:

> I never saw daffodils so beautiful they grew among the mossy stones about and about them, some rested their heads upon these stones as on a pillow for weariness and the rest tossed and reeled and danced and seemed as if they verily laughed with the wind that blew upon them over the lake, they looked so gay ever glancing ever changing. This wind blew directly

WHAT DO I READ NEXT?

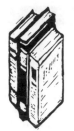

- Wordsworth originally intended his poem "Nutting," to be part of *The Prelude* but decided instead to include it in the second edition of *Lyrical Ballads* in 1800. It is a fairly short poem that gives the flavor of *The Prelude*, telling as it does of one of Wordsworth's quiet adventures as a boy in the Lake District. The poem can be found in *William Wordsworth: The Poems*, volume 1 (1977), edited by John O. Hayden.

- *Black Nature: Four Centuries of African American Nature Poetry* (2009) by Camille T. Dungy contains 180 poems by 93 poets. The poets represented include Phillis Wheatley, Rita Dove, Yusef Komunyakaa, Gwendolyn Brooks, Sterling Brown, Robert Hayden, Wanda Coleman, Natasha Trethewey, Melvin B. Tolson, Douglas Kearney, Major Jackson, and Janice Harrington. The poems are drawn from all significant periods in the history of African Americans, including slavery, Reconstruction, the Harlem Renaissance, the Black Arts Movement, and the contemporary period.

- Samuel Taylor Coleridge's lyric poem "The Eolian Harp" was written in 1795, a few years before Wordsworth began to write his greatest poems. Although it was composed not in the Lake District, but in the southern county of Somerset, it has many of the elements that would later be found in Wordsworth's verse: appreciative description of a quiet scene in nature, followed by some reflections by a tranquil mind about the nature of life and of the interaction between man and nature. Like many of Coleridge's "conversation poems," it has a circular structure, ending where it began but with a deepened understanding of life as a result of the central meditative portion. The poem can be found in Coleridge's *Selected Poetry*, edited by William Empson and David Pirie (2002).

- "To Daffodils," a short and rather mournful poem by the seventeenth-century English poet Robert Herrick, shows that for some, the sight of a daffodil can arouse emotions other than joy. The poem is included in *Selected Poems of Robert Herrick* (2003), edited by David Jesson-Dibley.

- For those who are unable to visit the Lake District in person, the next best thing might be *The English Lakes* (1989) by Robin Whiteman and Rob Talbot, which contains over one hundred photographs of the area, along with an informative introduction and explanatory texts.

- *The Invisible Ladder: An Anthology of Contemporary American Poems for Young Readers* (1996), edited by Liz Rosenberg, contains a selection of poems that were written for adults but are also accessible to young readers. The poets represented include Rita Dove, Galway Kinnell, Maxine Kumin, Nikki Giovanni, and Stanley Kunitz, all of whom write short introductions to their own poems and include black and white photographs of themselves as children and as adults.

- Mary Oliver is one of America's finest contemporary poets; her work is notable for its observation of and reverence for the natural world. Unlike Wordsworth and some other Romantic poets, who often use nature to make grand statements about infinity, eternity, and the human self, Oliver is more content simply to record and enjoy the physicality of nature itself and its recurring cycles. Her *New and Selected Poems: Volume One* (2005) contains a representative selection from her forty-year career as a poet.

over the lake to them. There was here and there a
little knot and a few stragglers a few yards higher
up but they were so few as not to disturb the
simplicity and unity and life of that one busy
highway.

With this description in mind it is easy to see
how the poem came about. Dorothy wrote her
journals not for publication but for the enjoyment
of her brother, and obviously Wordsworth read
this passage and was inspired to write the poem,
perhaps within a few hours of reading it. Two
years had elapsed between the walk and the writing
of the first version of the poem, and the similarity
in choice of words makes Dorothy's influence
clear. She writes that the daffodils "tossed" and
"danced"; it seemed as if they "laughed" and were
"gay," and all these elements make their way into
the poem.

The inspiration for the poem, then, came not
only from nature but also from a literary source.
It is also noticeable that in the interests of his
poetic art, Wordsworth altered some of the
details of the walk. In fact, he was not alone but
with his sister; however, the creation in the poem
of a solitary walker who feels lonely and is then
cheered by the sight of the daffodils creates a
more dramatic contrast than would have been
possible with two walkers. Also, Dorothy reports
a very strong wind, but this becomes a more
gentle breeze in the poem, creating a softer scene
than the one actually witnessed. Wordsworth's
creative reworking of the material, both the original experience and Dorothy's account of it, illustrates the point that poetry is never the mere
recording of facts but the poet's imaginative re-
creation of the scene and its significance.

What is truly fascinating about this poem,
which on the surface appears to be a nature
poem in praise of daffodils, is that Wordsworth's
appreciation of the sight occurs at two removes
from the original experience. First, he is dependent on the literary source in Dorothy's journal.
Second, what most inspires Wordsworth is not
the initial sight of the daffodils. As he states at the
end of the third stanza, he did not realize the full
significance of what he saw at the time. He did not
think much about it. But the experience of seeing
the daffodils worked on him (so to speak) over the
intervening two years, prompted by Dorothy's
description and reaching a new significance not
on Wordsworth's *seeing* the daffodils again but
on *remembering* them, on recreating the sight of
them in the quiet of his own mind when he was
not out in nature at all but comfortable and alone

within the four walls of his home. The poem,
then, is not so much about a sense experience in
nature but rather a mental experience, something
that occurred within the consciousness of the
poet, presumably with his eyes closed or half-
closed to release the "inward eye." This became
a source of pleasure even greater than that provided by the original sense experience. It is the
mental experience that is also the source of poetic
creativity; the writing of the poem came out of
one of these moments, as Wordsworth himself
makes clear in the Preface to *Lyrical Ballads*,
even though that preface was written in 1800,
four years earlier than the poem.

Wordsworth's Preface explains his poetic
practice and gives insight into how he wrote his
poems. He writes that "Poetry is the spontaneous
overflow of powerful feelings." The emphasis here
is on feeling, the subjective realm of the poet's
emotions rather than objects or events in the physical world. Wordsworth continues, "it [poetry]
takes its origin from emotion recollected in tranquility." This is exactly what happened with those
daffodils. In a tranquil state at home, lying on his
couch, relaxed, his mind open, he recalled the
emotions associated with seeing the daffodils,
and this recreates that feeling in his mind, which
is now, as he writes in the Preface, "in a state of
enjoyment." Although the sight of the daffodils
was a pleasurable experience, Wordsworth writes
that even painful experiences, when recalled in a
state of tranquility, can become pleasurable. The
poem that results from this process is intended to
produce in the reader "an overbalance of pleasure."
Wordsworth's poetic technique, then, is intended
to produce pleasure; this is the purpose of poetry
in his view.

Those who know Wordsworth's poetry will
recognize the description of this quiet, tranquil
state because Wordsworth mentions it in many
other poems, holding it up as an ideal condition
of the mind in which the truth of things spontaneously reveals itself. It can be found, for example
in "Lines, Composed a Few Miles above Tintern
Abbey," one of the most celebrated of all Wordsworth's poems, in which he describes in detail a
physiological condition in which the body is
extremely quiet and calm but the mind is highly
alert, able to see into the depth and heart of
things. It is this state of mind that can intuitively
feel the essential unity between man and nature
that was so much a part of Wordsworth's experience, especially in his youth and early manhood,

and on which he based his philosophical beliefs. Many such moments are described in the early books of *The Prelude*, about Wordsworth's boyhood and youth in the Lake District when he felt such deep communion with nature. A description that closely resembles the one found in the last stanza of "I Wandered Lonely as a Cloud" occurs in "Expostulation and Reply" (stanza 6); another example can be found in the final stanza of "The Tables Turned." Both these poems are from *Lyrical Ballads*.

Another key concept in Wordsworth's poetry that is relevant for "I Wandered Lonely as a Cloud" is what he referred to in *The Prelude* as "spots of time." These are particularly vivid moments in the poet's experience, often from early in his life, which he recalls later and which have a power to inspire, to reveal a truth, to restore the mind to a sense of its own vastness and the heart to its deepest feelings. In this sense, Wordsworth is a poet not so much of the present moment but of the past. He is a poet of memory, of the recollected experience rather than the immediate one. It is this sense that those moments during which he gazed at the daffodils became one of the "spots of time," subject to later recall and possessed of a kind of beauty and power that could nourish the poet's inner life long after the daffodils themselves had faded away.

Source: Bryan Aubrey, Critical Essay on "I Wandered Lonely as a Cloud," in *Poetry for Students*, Gale, Cengage Learning, 2010.

Rodney Stenning Edgecombe

In the following review, Edgecombe describes the emotional thought in the lines of "I Wandered Lonely as a Cloud."

Rather as Tchaikovsky incorporated a prelude written by one of his pupils into his opera Opritchnik, so Wordsworth, with due marital pride, implanted the following two lines by his wife in "I wandered lonely as a cloud": "They flash upon that inward eye / Which is the bliss of solitude" (21–22). Either with a mildly malicious purpose, or in ignorance of their source, Coleridge singled them out in *Biographia Literaria* as "mental bombast, as distinguished from verbal" (224). If, he goes on to argue, the memory of daffodils occupies "that inward eye / Which is the bliss of solitude," "in what words shall we describe the joy of retrospection, when the images and virtuous actions of a whole well-spent life, pass before the

conscience which is indeed the inward eye: which is indeed 'the bliss of solitude'" (224)?

This curiously Augustan response inverts and at the same time endorses the belief in decorum that led Johnson to fuss over Lady Macbeth and her knife, and it becomes more than a touch ironical if we set the lines against a passage from *Rasselas* that might well have inspired them:

> I am less unhappy than the rest, because I have a mind replete with images, which I can vary and combine at pleasure. I can amuse my solitude by the renovation of the knowledge which begins to fade from my memory, and by recollection of the accidents of my past life. Yet all this ends in the sorrowful consideration, that my acquirements are now useless, and that none of my pleasures can be again enjoyed. The rest, whose minds have no impression but of the present moment, are either corroded by malignant passions, or sit stupid in the gloom of perpetual vacancy. (534)

Mary Wordsworth seems to have remembered Imlac's juxtaposition of amusement and solitude in formulating the "bliss of solitude." Her husband, in the course of embedding them into a poem about the renovating power of the imagination, seems himself to have recalled the melancholy of Imlac's sic transit reveries ("sorrowful consideration" and "pensive mood" are cognate states) and also supplanted Johnson's "of perpetual vacancy" with Romantic pre-creative indolence ("In vacant or in pensive mood"). Furthermore, in virtual refutation of Lockean images that "fade" from the mental tabula, he deploys the forceful verb "flash," one that combines both motion and intense color. Coming to the poem from the same point of departure (for it seems probable that he too has Imlac's discourse subliminally in mind), Coleridge claims to find these un-Johnsonian adaptations of a Johnsonian sentiment indecorous, for why else would he blame Wordsworth for replacing the conscience—"by recollection of the accidents of my past life"—with a sensuous eidolon?

Source: Rodney Stenning Edgecombe, "Wordsworth's 'I Wandered Lonely as a Cloud,'" in *Explicator*, Vol. 60, No. 3, Spring 2002, pp. 134–36.

Matthew C. Brennan

In the following review, Brennan reviews the explication by some scholars of "I Wandered Lonely as a Cloud."

Shortly after *Poems in Two Volumes* (1807) appeared, Wordsworth worried about readers misinterpreting "I Wandered Lonely as a Cloud" (Letters 174, 194–95). Still concerned in 1815, he attached a note to the poem in his first *Collected Works*. "The subject of these stanzas," he asserted, "is rather an elementary feeling and simple impression [...] upon the imaginative faculty, than an exertion of it" (qtd. in Stillinger 539). Some critics have basically followed Wordsworth's lead: To Jack Stillinger the mental experience embodied by the poem is simple and ordinary (544), and to John Milstead the first three stanzas exemplify merely "a physical stimulus-and-response mechanism" through which the poet remains "passive" (89).

Nevertheless, in the preface to the 1815 collection Wordsworth not only argues that the imagination is ruled by "sublime consciousness" (Stillinger 486), but he also places "I Wandered" among poems categorized by "Imagination." Indeed, many critics ignore Wordsworth's comments on the poem and instead read it as representing a moment in nature of spiritual insight that recurs during a later imaginative re-creation (Joplin 68–69, Stallknecht 81–82, Hartman 5). More precisely, though, "I Wandered Lonely as a Cloud" dramatizes an experience of the sublime in its first three stanzas, which the poet recollects and re-experiences as a "spot of time" in the last stanza.

Like other sublime passages in *The Prelude* and "Tintern Abbey," this one draws on Edmund Burke's as well as Wordsworth's ideas of the sublime. Burke's thoughts in his *Philosophical Enquiry* are especially recalled in the lines that Wordsworth added for the 1815 republication:

> Continuous as the stars that shine
> And twinkle on the milky way,
> They stretch in never-ending line
> Along the margin of a bay:
> Ten thousand saw I at a glance,
> Tossing their heads in a sprightly dance.
>   (7–12)

For one thing, by stretching in a "never-ending line" the daffodils embody the sublime idea of vastness, in particular "vastness of extent" or length. Compared to the sublimity of the "Simplon Pass" or "Mt. Snowdon," these flowers surely seem simple and ordinary, but that is partly because, as Burke explains, vastness of height and depth are more striking and grand than vastness of extent (72).

Another conventional cause of the sublime this stanza exhibits is infinity. The host of flowers appears infinite, hence Wordsworth's impression of their uncountable profusion, "Ten thousand saw I at a glance." As Burke remarks, when "the eye" cannot "perceive the bounds of" things or when they are "continued to any indefinite number"—as with the daffodils—"they seem to be infinite, and they produce the same effects as if they were really so" (73). Moreover, because Wordsworth stresses that the daffodils are "[c]ontinuous" they also constitute what Burke terms "the artificial infinite." This condition applies, Burke explains, through "succession," in which "parts may be continued so long, and in such a direction, as by their frequent impulses on the sense to impress the imagination with an idea of their progress beyond their actual limits" (74). In other words, the flowers are so numerous and extend so far from the poet's vantage that when he suddenly glimpses them, his "sublime consciousness" imagines them as infinite. Significantly, this numerousness of the daffodils leads Wordsworth to compare them to "stars," which because of their profuse number evoke for Burke yet another cause of sublimity: magnificence. Associating the shining profusion of stars with the flowers clearly lends them a similar magnificence and thus evokes a response from the poet akin to his traveler's in "A Night Piece" where "multitudes of stars" and an instantaneous gleam of the moon trigger a sublime vision.

Besides illustrating many of Burke's ideas of the sublime, "I Wandered Lonely as a Cloud" also encompasses Wordsworth's chief elements of the sublime as he defines it in his own unpublished essay "The Sublime and the Beautiful" written in 1811–12. Here Wordsworth divides the sublime into two types: one that is negative and thus similar to Burke's, which hinges on terror; and one that is positive and produces what Wordsworth calls in "Tintern Abbey" "the blessed mood." Both types, Wordsworth emphasizes, create a sense of "intense unity, without a conscious contemplation of parts" ("The Sublime" 354). Clearly, "I Wandered" depicts the positive sublime, which reveals unity by rousing "us to a sympathetic energy" through which the mind participates with the "force which is acting upon it" (354). Through his sublime consciousness the poet perceives the unity of not only the dancing flowers themselves but also the entire scene, which includes both "the waves" dancing "beside them" and himself as he "gazed—and gazed." In this moment of sublime vision, his imagination sympathetically unites him and the scene "in such a jocund company." During the moment itself he does not think; he is "without a conscious contemplation" of the elements unified by his sublime perception. But afterward when he recollects it and re-experiences it as a "flash upon that inward eye"—the agent of sublime consciousness—he recognizes that, like the waves, he too "dances with the daffodils" while part of the interpenetrating "jocund company." This repetition of dance rhetorically enacts the unification of flowers, waves, and poet. The poem opens with the poet lonely, disconnected from his environment, and ends with him connected to it, enjoying "the bliss of solitude" through the unifying flash of sublime consciousness.

Though Milstead interprets the poet's gazing at the daffodils as unimaginatively passive and David Joplin construes it as intensely active because trance-like, the quality of Wordsworth's vision in fact falls somewhere between the purely sensory and the transcendentally spiritual. As we saw, Wordsworth's own note to the poem qualifies the experience as imaginative but one in which he does not exert his imagination. In other words, the poem appears to illustrate what he calls in "Expostulation and Reply ... a wise passiveness." In this passive state he remains receptive to nature's powers, which both "Tintern Abbey" and "The Sublime" testify can produce the sublime; and through "wise passiveness" Wordsworth insists we can feed the mind, even without fully exerting the imagination. Thus, his gazing at the daffodils' dance brings him "wealth" and feeds his "inward eye" despite his unconscious passivity.

Stallknecht's explanation of the various levels of Wordsworth's intuition of "the unity of Being" overlooks the sublime but helps show how the experience of the daffodils evokes sublime consciousness: Although Wordsworth's mystical or intuitive consciousness of "the unity of Being" often followed "robust" imaginative activity, this consciousness "was also sometimes induced by 'wise passiveness'" (9, 12). Because, as Stallknecht writes, this passive state resembles the more active imaginative ones in allowing the "depths of consciousness to manifest themselves" (12), I think we can equate "wise passiveness" with experiences ruled by the sublime consciousness of "intense unity." Wordsworth unfolds just such a sublime experience in the poet's wisely passive vision of the daffodils in "I Wandered Lonely as a Cloud."

Source: Matthew C. Brennan, "Wordsworth's 'I Wandered Lonely as a Cloud,'" in *Explicator*, Vol. 57, No. 3, Spring 1999, pp. 140–44.

David Joplin

In the following essay, Joplin explains the use of "host" in the poem, "I Wandered Lonely as a Cloud."

Although a "nature" writer like Thoreau is widely recognized for his wordplay, his English counterpart Wordsworth is much less so. As often as not, his style tends more toward an Arnoldian "high seriousness" than toward a playful tour de force of language such as Thoreau offers. Nevertheless, Wordsworth is certainly not without his paronomastic moments. One such moment, heretofore unrecognized, may be the pun on "host" in "I Wandered Lonely as a Cloud." Careful attention to host shows how Wordsworth, in a manner anticipating Hopkins, has brought together a number of meanings that help us understand how deeply the daffodils affect the poet's mind.

"Host" appears in the familiar first stanza, which I quote in full:

> I wandered lonely as a cloud
> That floats on high o'er vales and hills,
> When all at once I saw a crowd,
> A host, of golden daffodils;
> Beside the lake, beneath the trees,
> Fluttering and dancing in the breeze.

The comma after "host" serves as emphasis, making us reconsider how Wordsworth intends its meaning. The most apparent needs only brief mention: The "host" is a "crowd" of flowers. The OED (Compact Desk Edition) lists host in this sense as "a great company; a multitude; a large number."

To understand how Wordsworth carries "host" beyond a mere "crowd" through wordplay, one must first note how the crowd affects the poet. In the penultimate stanza Wordsworth describes himself "gaz[ing]" at the daffodils: "I gazed—and gazed—but little thought / What wealth the show to me had brought" (17–18). The repetition of "gazed" indicates an intense activity, almost as if the poet were in a trance. Such an event bespeaks a shift in consciousness, what Owen Barfield would call a "felt change of consciousness" (p. 48). The final stanza emphasizes much the same experience, only this time it occurs through memory—the poet lies on his couch and recalls the "host," which then triggers the mind's reaction. The daffodils, therefore, affect the poet directly and indirectly through his eyes and his mind.

Now to circle back to the wordplay. Because the "host" initiates the effect, it is, as the OED suggests, the agent that "entertains." Or as the American Heritage Dictionary puts it, a "host" is the "one who entertains guests, a master of ceremonies." Wordsworth's reference to his experience as a "show" incorporates this second meaning. The pun, therefore, allows us to see the "host"—the daffodils—as a "master of ceremonies" or guide who treats the guest—Wordsworth—to a "show," which is both the "dancing" flowers and their effect on the poet.

The punning grows more complex as we delve deeper into the nature of the show. On one level, the flowers simply bring psychological ease: The lonely poet sees the "jocund company" and becomes happy. But on another level, the event moves through a transposition into a spiritual experience. For one thing, the intent gazing signals a meditative moment akin to spiritual activity: As he drinks in nature's beauty, the poet attains an elevated state of mind. And the last stanza repeats the experience through memory. But in the latter case, the effect is produced only when the flowers "flash upon that inward eye." Although the "inward eye" is generally taken to be the imagination, it also has a metaphysical application. Ananda K. Coomaraswamy traces the image of the eye to a tradition that links it with the eye of God (50). This line of thought allows the "inward eye" to be seen as the spiritual center of the mind. From such a perspective, as images of the daffodils open his "inward eye," Wordsworth experiences a transcendental moment similar, at least in kind, to the one in "Tintern Abbey," when the temporal gives way to the eternal so that he sees "into the life of things" (48). The initiating "host," therefore, comes through wordplay to occupy the role of initiating priest.

This carries the pun even further into religious contexts. One is the "Biblical and derived" usage that describes a "multitude of angels" (OED). The golden daffodils fit this image insofar as their beauty invokes a correspondent spiritual beauty, as a heavenly host of angels would. Thus, the angelic "host" of flowers enables the poet to participate in a kind of spiritual beauty associated with nature. From here it is not a long step to the narrow liturgical sense of host as the "bread in the Eucharist" (OED). In that connection, the "host" functions as a symbol that transports Wordsworth, so to speak, to a higher level. The pun thus expands to include its full biblical and liturgical connotations.

Yet a final pun occurs through a shift in grammatical function. Host functions first as a noun, but it can also be a verb: "to play the host" (OED). Juxtaposing the nominal and verbal uses, one can see that it is the "host" that "hosts" the event. Thus, the noun host doubles, at least semantically, with the verb's meaning. Such linguistic doubling corresponds to the "layered" effect nature has on the poet.

When Thoreau, the consummate linguist, puns on host, his wordplay seems but yet another instance of his conscious manipulation of language. But I wonder if, in the case of Wordsworth, the pun is more of an unconscious event, one of those in which, as Erich Neumann might suggest, the poet unconsciously engages the archetype. In any event host does carry several semantic possibilities, each of which resonates with and amplifies the others, much as carrion does in Hopkins's wonderfully wrought "Carrion Comfort." These layers of "hosting" help us understand how deeply—and doubly—daffodils affect the poet's mind.

Source: David Joplin, "Wordsworth's 'I Wandered Lonely as a Cloud,'" in *Explicator*, Vol. 56, No. 2, Winter 1998, pp. 67–71.

Bernard Richards

In the following essay, Richards writes about the phonetic significance of the words in the poem.

> The waves beside them danced, but they
> Out-did the sparkling waves in glee:—
> A poet could not but be gay,
> In such a jocund company;
> I gazed—and gazed—but little thought
> What wealth the show to me had brought:

In his essay "A Touching Compulsion, Wordsworth and the Problem of Literary Representation," published in *The Georgia Review* (vol. 31, summer 1977), Geoffrey H. Hartman offers the following interpretation of lines 17–18:

> When Wordsworth writes: "I gazed—and gazed—but little thought / What wealth the show to me had brought," our ear may be justified in adding "I grazed—and grazed." Touch, or materiality, returns to the phantom of sight. The ear develops the image in its own way. (352)

He obviously has not had second thoughts about this reading, inasmuch as the essay has been reprinted in *The Unremarkable Wordsworth* (London: Methuen, 1987).

Consider the following groups of words: pied, pride, plyed; pate, prate, plate; paid, prayed, played; fame, frame, flame; bead, breed, bleed; baize, brase, blaze; pays, praise, plays; fees, freeze, fleas; cock, crock, clock; band, brand, bland; bent, brent, blent; goes, grows, gloze. In each case they would be perfect homophones, were it not for the difference of a letter, the letter being either *r* or *l*. With the difference being so tiny, should one not regard all these words as similar and interchangeable? After all, what's in a letter? The answer is, of course, a colossal amount, and slight as it may seem, there is an enormous difference between goes and grows. The whole evolution of a communal and functional language has depended on precisely these apparently infinitesimal differences, and it is the duty of language users and commentators on language to preserve them if language is to continue to have any kind of utility. To this list one could add gazed, grazed, glazed.

There are considerable differences among gazed, grazed, and glazed. They are separate, and they should be kept separate. "The ear develops the image" says Hartman, but only an ear stuffed with physical and figurative wax could do such a thing. The figurative wax is a cast of mind that approaches a text with a predetermined thesis, insisting on associating the thesis with the text, irrespective of whether or not the text invites or sustains it. Hartman has made a critical move that is completely unwarranted; indeed, to call it "interpretation" is to misuse the term. It is more like creative vandalism. The essay is dominated by some concept of touch in Wordsworth, a sense that is undoubtedly present in many poems, but not in this one at this point, and the ear has no justification in performing the addition. If the ear did in fact confuse the words, then some other mental faculty should come into play to censor it out, and such a discriminatory function should have operated long before the so-called interpretation reached the printed page. Hartman should have had the sense and the humility in 1977 not to offer such an illicit extension of the lines; ten years later he should have had them in extra measure. It is a kindness to call it "criticism" or "explication"; but whatever it is, it should be strenuously resisted.

Source: Bernard Richards, "Wordsworth's 'I Wandered Lonely as a Cloud,'" in *Explicator*, Vol. 48, No. 1, Fall 1989, pp. 14–16.

SOURCES

Coleridge, Samuel Taylor, *Biographia Literaria*, edited by George Watson, Dent, 1984, pp. 258–59.

Durrant, Geoffrey, *William Wordsworth*, Cambridge University Press, 1969, pp. 20, 25.

Ezard, John, "Poet Laureate Joins Doubters Over Iraq," in *Guardian* (London, England), January 9, 2003, http://www.guardian.co.uk/uk/2003/jan/09/iraq.writersoniraq (accessed July 1, 2009).

"Facts and Figures," in *Lake District National Park*, http://www.lake-district.gov.uk/index/learning/facts_and_figures.htm (accessed July 2, 2009).

Ferry, David, *The Limits of Mortality: An Essay on Wordsworth's Major Poems*, Wesleyan University Press, 1959, p. 10.

McCracken, David, *Wordsworth and the Lake District: A Guide to the Poems and Their Places*, Oxford University Press, 1984.

Noyes, Russell, *William Wordsworth*, Twayne's English Author Series, No. 118, Twayne Publishers, 1971, p. 136.

Pinter, Harold, "God Bless America," http://www.haroldpinter.org/politics/god_bless_america.shtml (accessed July 1, 2009).

Shelley, Percy Bysshe, *A Defence of Poetry*, in *Shelley's Poetry and Prose*, selected and edited by Donald H. Reiman and Sharon B. Powers, W. W. Norton, 1977, p. 508.

Wordsworth, Dorothy, *The Grasmere Journals*, in *The Norton Anthology of English Literature*, 4th ed., edited by M. H. Abrams, W. W. Norton, 1979, p. 322.

Wordsworth, William, "I Wandered Lonely as a Cloud," in *William Wordsworth: The Poems*, Vol. 1, edited by John O. Hayden, Penguin, 1977, pp. 619–20.

———, Preface to *Lyrical Ballads*, in *William Wordsworth: The Poems*, Vol. 1, edited by John O. Hayden, Penguin, 1977, pp. 886–87.

FURTHER READING

Abrams, M. H., *Natural Supernaturalism: Tradition and Revolution in Romantic Literature*, W. W. Norton, 1971.
This classic work is one of the best studies of Romanticism ever written. Abrams discusses English and German literature and philosophy, bringing out the parallels between different writers in terms of subject matter, themes, imagery, structure, and other literary elements.

Gill, Stephen Charles, *William Wordsworth: A Life*, Oxford University Press, 1989.
This well-researched biography is particularly strong on connecting Wordsworth's life with his work. Gill also makes use of some Wordsworth family papers that were not discovered until 1977. He argues that there was more continuity in Wordsworth's political and social views than has usually been thought, and that Wordsworth's achievement in his later years, long after his greatest poetry was written, deserves to be respected.

Pottle, Frederick A., "The Eye and the Object in the Poetry of Wordsworth," in *Wordsworth: Centenary Studies Presented at Cornell and Princeton Universities*, edited by Gilbert T. Dunklin, Princeton University Press, 1951.
This is a classic essay and one of the most detailed studies of "I Wandered Lonely as a

Cloud." Pottle examines the poem in the light of Wordsworth's Preface to the *Lyrical Ballads*, concluding that Wordsworth's subject is not so much the physical object but a mental image; he is therefore not a descriptive poet but an imaginative one.

Roe, Nicholas, ed., *Romanticism: An Oxford Guide*, Oxford University Press, 2005.

This collection of forty-six essays is one of the most thorough and up-to-date introductions to all aspects of the literary and historical contexts of Romanticism.

Jazz Fantasia

CARL SANDBURG

1920

"Jazz Fantasia" was written by Carl August Sandburg in 1919 and published in 1920, at a time when jazz, the first truly American form of music, was being born. This was also the dawn of the Roaring Twenties and Prohibition. Jazz and blues were played in honky-tonks and speakeasies (types of legal and illegal nightclubs), where bootlegged alcohol flowed freely. Jazz involves loud, lively musical instruments, rhythm, and fun. "Jazz Fantasia" is about the celebratory sounds of jazz instruments, along with soulful sounds of the blues, embodied in a Mississippi steamboat. A fantasia is a literary or musical work that evokes the imagination through fanciful, supernatural, or unnatural devices.

It is speculated that Sandburg got the idea for this poem while watching a minstrel show. According to Bill Kirchner in *The Oxford Companion to Jazz*, Sandburg said in *All the Young Strangers* that whenever minstrel shows came to town, he always had "two bits for a ticket to the top gallery." Minstrel shows found large audiences and positive reviews. "Most important," Kirchner writes, "they stimulated an attitude indissolubly linked with jazz. They seemed to urge wild, spontaneously, sympathetic movement among singers, players, and audiences alike." It was jazz rising, before it was known as jazz.

The poem first appeared in a collection titled *Smoke and Steel*; the collection is about Chicago, the city where jazz got its name, although this

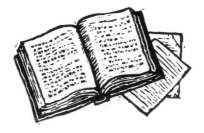

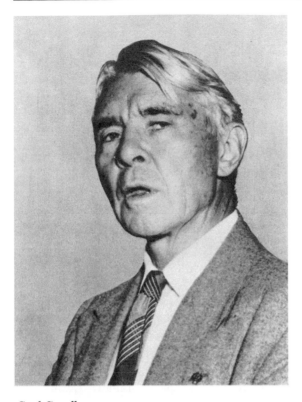

Carl Sandburg (*The Library of Congress*)

form of music actually began in New Orleans. Sandburg traveled around the Midwestern states at the age of eighteen as a hobo, hopping into railroad boxcars, riding the small platforms between cars and stowing away on steamboats. He is known today as the "People's Poet," writing about the daily life and hardships of the poor in their own language. Music plays an integral part in his poetry, and he is remembered as a balladeer who sang his poems and prose, accompanying himself on a banjo.

Though the poem was relatively obscure during Sandburg's lifetime, "Jazz Fantasia" has gained a great deal more attention as the popularity of jazz has grown and flourished. Artists may perform it now as a stand-alone rhythmic poetry reading or with jazz accompaniment. It can be found in the *Complete Poems of Carl Sandburg* (1969), published by Harcourt Brace.

When "Jazz Fantasia" was first published, it was not considered representative of the poetry of the times because of its free verse style, unexalted themes, and the inclusion of coarse slang. These were not valued traits, and this poem was overlooked in favor of other poems, such as "Fog," probably Sandburg's most famous work.

Today, "Jazz Fantasia" is lauded for its genius. It is at once a poem, a musical composition, and an ethereal image of moon, river, and phantom musicians.

AUTHOR BIOGRAPHY

Sandburg was born on January 6, 1878, to Swedish immigrants August and Clara Sandburg in Galesburg, Illinois. His father was a blacksmith's assistant for the Chicago, Burlington, and Quincy Railroad. Times were hard for the family, and as the second of seven children, Sandburg learned the importance of work. One of his first memories was digging in the family garden for vegetables. He went to school through the eighth grade but had to drop out to help support the family. Working dozens of odd jobs (such as bottle-washer, tinsmith's helper, barber shop porter, and painter's apprentice) gave him a lifelong connection to common people and a passion for portraying their plight. Determined to be a poet or a hobo, he left home at age eighteen and experienced the hardscrabble life of a vagrant, working only to pay his passage or for a small portion of food. He learned to love the Midwest and its people, picking up folk stories, jokes, and slang and listening to the music and sound of the cities like Chicago. He made a banjo out of a box and taught himself to play it.

When the Spanish-American war broke out, Sandburg enlisted and was sent to Puerto Rico. After six months, he returned and enrolled in Lombard (now Knox) College in Galesburg, where he first began dabbling in poetry. An admiring professor encouraged him and even published some of Sandburg's poems at his own expense. Sandburg never graduated but spent his next years writing and editing for newspapers and magazines, always composing poetry on the side. He met Lilian Steichan in Milwaukee, Wisconsin, where he was the editor for the *Social-Democratic Herald*. She sympathized with his ideas for social and labor reform, and they were married in 1908. His *Chicago Poems* was published in 1916. In 1917, he began writing for the *Chicago Daily News*. That year, Harcourt, Brace, and Howe published his collection of articles, *The Chicago Race Riots*, which presented a sympathetic viewpoint toward the prejudices endured by blacks in the city.

Meanwhile, his poems were becoming more widely known, as the collections *Cornhuskers* (1918), *Smoke and Steel* (1920, which included "Jazz Fantasia"), and *Slabs of the Sunburnt West* (1922) were published, making him a recognized poet of American western life. His poetry began to take on the mantle of the commonest of people, and not everyone knew how to interpret his slang and his murky images of reality. His *Rootabaga Stories* (1922) showed his love for telling stories to his daughters, and his *American Songbag* (1927) demonstrated his passion for American folk songs and ballads.

Sandburg had a fascination with the life of fellow Illinoisan, Abraham Lincoln. Besides his poetry, he is probably best remembered for his biographies of that president. Sandburg told of Lincoln's disdain for the sale of slave girls in New Orleans; this incident may have informed Sandburg's reports of the prejudices against blacks in Chicago. He received the Pulitzer Prize in History in 1940 for the four-volume *Abraham Lincoln: The War Years*. He also won the Pulitzer Prize for his *Collected Poems* in 1951. He continued to write prolifically; he was named the poet laureate of Illinois in 1962 and received the International Poets Award of Honorary Poet Laureate of the United States in 1963. He died in Flat Rock, North Carolina, on July 22, 1967, at the age of 89.

POEM SUMMARY

Line 1

"Jazz Fantasia" begins with the drums, the instrument most critical to any jazz musical performance. The drums lead the music by their steady rhythmic beat. They set the tone and mood: the cadence of a dance or shuffle. The rhythm of the first part of the fantasia starts out a steady andante (moderate) jazz tempo. Line 1, if spoken in a standard 4/4 time signature (four beats in a row), should have a strict rhythm. In jazz, the first beat is always given more emphasis than the rest; it is stronger than the rest and serves as the downbeat. This convention is helpful in establishing the rhythm of the piece, and it also gives direction as how to dance or march. The repetition of *d's* makes the tongue a percussion instrument on the roof of the mouth, just as the *b's* make a drum of the lips.

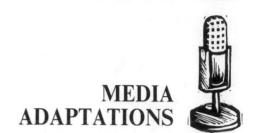

MEDIA ADAPTATIONS

- A free MP3 download of a Librivox recording featuring more than fifteen artists' readings of "Jazz Fantasia" is available online through Internet Archive (http://www.archive.org) as a public domain text (2006).

- Track six on the CD *Back to Japan and China* is titled "Jazz Fantasia" and is performed by the Luther College Concert Band. It is available as an audio CD conducted by Frederick Nyline and produced by Luther College Recordings in 2005.

- *Samba Jazz Fantasia* by Duduka Da Fonseca is an audio CD of a seven-piece jazz/samba ensemble with vocals. It was nominated for the 2003 Grammy Awards for Best Latin Jazz Album. River Sound Studios recorded it in New York in March 2006.

- *Fantasia 2000* is an animated film sequel to the 1940s Walt Disney Pictures *Fantasia*. It was released in December 1999 and features the Chicago Symphony Orchestra and Philharmonic Orchestra. The classical music combined with Disney animation provides a good illustration of the musical form of fantasia.

Lines 2–3

The saxophones now join the ensemble with a wail. Jazz saxophones usually have a sad, beautifully mournful sound. The description of them is like the ripples of high tenor sax notes rushing over, wrapping smoothly over the notes in a gentle massage. However, this passage almost demands the addition of an alto or even lower pitched saxophone, twisting and sustaining. These saxophones are longer and lower to the floor and have a curved shape. Sandburg seems to break up the rhythm with this phrase with a ritardando (slowing) in an improvisational style. He places a bird's eye (musical symbol meaning to hold) at the end of the line, telling the instruments to take a little break. Then, as if he is the master of ceremonies at a jazz concert, Sandburg exhorts his musicians to play. If he were introducing the origins of rock and roll, he would say "Go, Johnny, go!" He introduces this new music genre to the literary world. As the curtain opens, the anticipation rises.

Lines 4–6

The percussion section emerges, and the tempo and mood become lively. A poor street musician would use anything available as an instrument. A tin pan made an excellent tambourine, but without the shakers, it would give more of a light knocking as knuckles rolled and thumped across it. It was an embellishment to the drums, which kept the steady beat, and it gave sixteenth-note jazz rhythms in quick syncopation, emphasizing fast beats not accented in the straight 4/4 time (repetition of four beats in a row). The accent is spoken on the letter *p*, which gives a percussive pop of the lips when read aloud. The trombones come in next and seep their way into the piece. A lower-pitched brass instrument, the trombone has a slide that allows the artist to move directly from note to note or slide smoothly in continuous resonance to the next pitch. The sliding gives the impression of an oozing of sound rather than the strict adherence to intonation that a piano might have. This sliding was very popular when performing while marching. Sandpaper was applied to blocks of wood that were brushed against each other to obtain the repetitive *sh* sound that Sandburg describes. These blocks are also a percussion instrument, and they provide the shuffle sound, like the brushes on a cymbal. When the poem is read aloud, the lungs and throat produce a soft pop of air on the accent beat, and air rushing through the teeth on the *sh* at the end of the word creates a swishing sound. In this case, the first *hu* sound gets an accent, the second one gets a small accent, and the third gets the strongest. The rhythm would span six beats, with *sh* sound getting one beat, *a* getting one beat, the next *sh* one beat, *a* one beat, and the last *sh* being held for two beats. The repetitions of *s* sounds evoke the warning of a spitting snake throughout the phrase. Then, the accent on the *p* produces another percussive pop.

Line 7–11

The mood becomes increasingly more anxious now compared to the simple contentment of line 5, and the whining sound is high like the tender wail of a tenor or soprano saxophone. These

saxophones can have a mournful, aching tone, and they can sound soft but urgent. Unlike the large, curved saxophones mentioned in line 2, these instruments are shorter, and the soprano sax has no curve at all. They are the most expressive of the sax family and can easily replicate the sound of a whine high up in the trees, and at the same time cry out intensely over the absence of a lost loved one. The image rises to a fever pitch as a screaming trumpet play a squeal like that of a fast car fleeing a pursuing motorcycle cop with sirens blasting. With sadness there is now danger: gunfire erupts as the drums fire rapidly, loudly, piercing the ears. The entire ensemble of instruments blasts in unison, and more violence ensues. Two people are clawing at each other, fighting and scratching at each other's eyes, tumbling in a ball to the foot of a staircase. The instruments wail and shriek, smash and crash, pound and batter as the combatants exchange blows.

Line 12–15

Sandburg shouts out to shut up, like an aggravated neighbor in the apartment next door with paper-thin walls and a baby fitfully sleeping. "Shut up in there!" he bangs on the plaster. "That's enough!" It is the sound of fifty thousand blacks from the South crammed into Chicago in the span of just four years, from 1916 to 1920. Chicago is not the utopia they thought it would be: Jobs are scarce and living conditions deplorable. It is a hardscrabble life, and the music portrays the frenzy. A welcome contrast is introduced, and contrast is critical to jazz. It can soothe and calm, like a mother reading bedtime stories. Sandburg pushes on to the night sounds and images with a Mississippi steamboat chugging up the river at night. A bass saxophone bellows out the three low notes of the pervasive fog horn. Its *whoo-whoo-whoo-oo* echoes on the banks. There is a pause, and rich imagery appears again to end the poem: The lights on the boat rise up to the heavens, meeting the sight of the moon, red with sunset, rising to the tops of the hills.

THEMES

The Jazz Age

The 1920s were the beginning of the Jazz Age, when musicians were experimenting with the earliest forms of jazz music. The sound came with the blacks migrating from New Orleans and mixed with the already established ragtime style. In

TOPICS FOR FURTHER STUDY

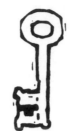

- Select a group of vocalists to perform the poem for the class. Be creative with the arrangement. Assign some voices to mimic instruments or the sounds of the steamboat. Add different pitches to the spoken words (thirds, fifths, or minor sevenths for a jazz sound). Have some voices echo others.

- If you play an instrument, compose and perform a piece that has a jazz feel and represents the different sections of the poem. Pay close attention to the moods of the poem, when the rhythm picks up and the volume changes. Remember that you are trying to replicate the sounds of the city, with wild clamorous music and the night sounds of a slow steamboat chugging down a winding river. Burn a CD of the piece to play for the class.

- Write a poem about jazz. It can be about a concert you attended, a CD you listened to, or something you heard on the radio or performed in band. Pay close attention to rhythm, mood, sound, and imagery. Read it aloud, emphasizing these components.

- Rewrite "Jazz Fantasia" as a rap song. If possible, have other students join you as you perform it, to accompany you with beat box, drum, or dance. If you do not feel comfortable performing live, have someone record it with a video camera.

- Choose a poem from the collection *The Jazz Poetry Anthology* (1991) compiled for a young adult audience by Sascha Feinstein and Yusef Komunyakaa. Compare its themes and style to "Jazz Fantasia" in an essay.

- Read the Coretta Scott King Author Honor winner *Becoming Billie Holiday* by Carole Weatherford and Floyd Cooper. Compare the story of Holiday's rise to jazz fame through pain, poverty, and discrimination to the joy of discovering jazz. Give a PowerPoint presentation about Holiday's life and her importance in jazz history. Add pictures and sound to the slides.

"Jazz Fantasia," Sandburg praises musicians of 1920, who had just begun to play what was recognized as jazz. His recognition of the genius of the movement and the obstacles it had to overcome compels him to press for more, to congratulate the artists, and to exhort them to play on. Of course, Sandburg can take no credit for the jazz movement, but it is notable that a Swedish American poet would grasp the brilliance of the music that would affect nearly every aspect of modern American music from 1920 to present day. As a poet, he loved the way the music could summon images, evoke strong moods, and soothe the soul.

Urban Life

In his poem "Prairie," Sandburg prophesies the coming of bigger cities with skyscrapers and a change from a rural to an urban society. In his *Chicago Poems* and *Smoke and Steel*, in which

"Jazz Fantasia" was included, there are volumes of poems such as "The Harbor," "The Halstead Street Car," "Subway," "Skyscraper," "Work Gangs," and "Broken Face Gargoyles," which depict the sights and sounds of the city life of the new industrial America. His poem "The Windy City" portrays the growing pains of Chicago in 1920.

In "Jazz Fantasia," the sounds are those of the back streets of Chicago. The reader imagines a fight breaking out in a honky-tonk, while all the percussion instruments bang and clamor in a frenzy.

Injustice

In *Sixteen Authors to One*, David Kasner writes that "Sandburg recognizes political material in . . . shovel stiffs, . . . politicians, diplomats, and the honky tonk." Sandburg began his identification with the black man during his years as a

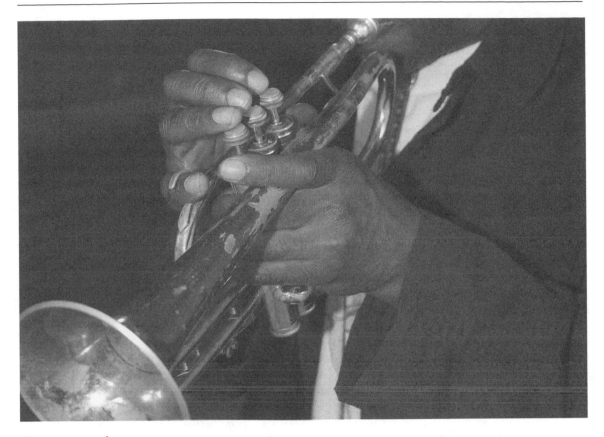

Jazz trumpet player (*Image copyright Karla Caspari, 2009. Used under license from Shutterstock.com*)

hobo, working alongside them as bootblacks (shoe shiners), porters, icehouse workers, and water boys. Harry Hansen, in *Midwest Portraits*, explains that they "seemed most addicted to balladry. Any outstanding catastrophe would lead some improviser to throw together a dozen or more clumsy quatrains telling the story of the event." Sandburg saw the genius in this and adapted it to his folk song telling of stories that he later performed with his banjo. He is faithful to making a social statement with his poetry, and he firmly protests injustice, as he did when he covered the Chicago race riots. He also does this in "Jazz Fantasia." Sandburg tells the jazzmen that because of their music, social equality is waiting for them.

STYLE

Onomatopoeia

Onomatopoeia is the use of a word that imitates the sound it makes. It gives richness and sensory perception to the poem as the word sound is its own meaning. Words such as *clang, crash, bang,* and *boom* demonstrate the sounds they indicate. The clanging of the tympanic percussionists voices the cacophonous sounds associated with a back-street fight that ends crashing down the stairs. The owl sound and the bee sounds are other examples of onomatopoeia. "Jazz Fantasia" makes use of the device in a musical fashion.

The word *drum* sounds like the noise the instrument makes. Banjoes can bang or strum. A tin pan can pound or swish. A bass drum can fire off booms like a bang of bullets from motorcycle or a loud backfire of exhaust.

Free Verse

The poem is written in free verse, which means there is no strict rhyming or meter, a style characteristic of poetry before this time. Other poets who used free verse were Walt Whitman, Ezra Pound, T. S. Eliot, and others who were considered modern poets. North Callahan quotes Sandburg in *Carl Sandburg: His Life and Works* as saying,

Free verse is the oldest way. Go back to the Egyptians, the Chaldeans. The ancient Chinese were writers of free verse.... Read the orations of Moses, the Proverbs and Ecclesiastes for free verse. The Sermon on the Mount is one of the highest examples.

Much of the poetry written today is in free verse style. It allows for more emphasis on mood, imagery, and use of words that can create a tone. However, because "Jazz Fantasia" is about music, and Sandburg was also a musician, there is a rhythm associated with the poem that cannot be analyzed by poetic meter.

Alliteration and Assonance

Alliteration is a poetic device that uses the repetition of consonant sounds that appear close together in the poem. It is similar to rhyming, but the sameness of sound appears at the beginning of the word rather than at the end. This technique gives interest and delight upon reading aloud. Sandburg's writing is designed to be read aloud—he uses alliteration in the consonants of repeated stressed syllables. The letters *b*, *d*, and *s* are prominently used in the alliteration of this poem. Assonance, or the repetition of a vowel sound, is often combined with alliteration. In this case, *u* is used after *d*, *a* is used after *b*, and *i* is often used after *s*. When the poem softens in tone and the sound of the blues sets in, *t* is used after *s*.

Personification

Personification is a figure of speech in which inanimate objects or abstractions are treated as if they have human attributes or feelings. In "Jazz Fantasia," the saxophones are wailing and the trombones are weeping. The treetops are whining, a racing car screams, and the green lanterns on the steamboat appeal to the stars.

Simile

A simile is a device used in literature in which one thing is seen as similar to something else, often by the use of the word "like" or "as." Sandburg tells the jazzmen to groan like the wind in autumn and to scream like a racing car evading a motorcycle cop. He compares the booming of the drums and other loud percussion instruments to two people fighting, tearing at each other and scrambling down stairs.

Sound and Silence

Sandburg uses sound in his poetry, and in "Jazz Fantasia" he wants his reader to hear a jazz song.

Music has to have contrast in intensity, rhythm, and mood to be compelling. The volume of the poem shifts from moderate to loud to soft. Lines 1–6 are moderately loud, lines 7–12 rise from moderately to very loud, and lines 13–16 wind down softly. In a musical piece, the score would be marked *mezzo forte*, *fortissimo*, and *pianissimo*. The saxophones, banjoes, trombones, and sandpaper blocks contrast with the clamor of the percussion instruments, clanging the sounds of the city. The mood and image change quickly with the riverboat's eerie night owl song.

HISTORICAL CONTEXT

Industrialism

The first line of Sandburg's poem "Chicago," published in *Chicago Poems* (1916), depicted the city as the world biggest slaughterhouse. This was a shocking description of the city to people who saw it as a rising industrial urban power in the United States. Sandburg did not intend to besmirch the city's image but rather to describe it in simple terms, in the vernacular of the common people, about whom he was obsessively concerned.

Chicago established itself early as a trade center, processing the products of the prairie, packing meat, milling flour, milling lumber, and transporting the products via its sophisticated rail systems. However, from 1870 to 1930, Chicago became a quintessential industrial center in America. With the rapid growth of the city, construction jobs and industry-creating construction materials began to abound. Artisan workshops were turned into manufactories, where skilled laborers taught apprentices to practice their trades. With the necessity to get work done faster and more cheaply, it was found that keeping the cost of labor down was paramount. The division of labor into small parts in order to reduce costs became the premise of industrialization. If a job once done by a master craftsman could be done in steps by unskilled laborers, the product could be produced much more cheaply. It also gave more power to the employer, who could control wages, labor market supply, advances in technology, and labor uprisings.

Chicago in the 1920s was the model for industrialization, with central access and models for meatpacking, garment-making, and machinery manufacturing. As labor unions and populations grew, the landscape and steel skyscrapers

COMPARE
&
CONTRAST

- **1920s:** Sandburg's free verse style of poetry is not appreciated by most critics, as previous poetry was governed by rhyme and meter. His use of slang language in poetry is considered unfit for poetry, even though it is widely used by common people.

  Today: Sandburg's free-verse, unrhymed, imagery-filled poetry is very much in keeping with today's poetry. As Sandburg did, today's poets make use of the fundamental element that links poetry and culture: music. Today's "People's Poets" are musicians working in rap, rock, hip-hop, country, and other popular styles. No language is off-limits, and rhythm—though not necessarily a regular meter—is imperative.

- **1920s:** Jazz music is considered the music of the black working class, played in honky-tonks or by street musicians. The term *jazz* is not yet universally used, and the sound is still very close to that of ragtime. Wilbur Sweatman and his Jass Band made the first true jazz recording by African American artists in 1916. A notable recording had been made a few years earlier by the all-white Original Dixieland Band, but it is not considered the first jazz recording, only a copy of what was heard in the African American culture.

  Today: Jazz is one of the most widely enjoyed genres of music. It has evolved from its roots in blues and ragtime and spun off dozens of new genres, including swing or big band, cool jazz, bebop, pop, hip-hop, rhythm and blues, smooth jazz, soul, acid jazz, rap, and neo-lounge jazz. Jazz is commonly considered America's classical music.

- **1920s:** The images of the Mississippi steamboat in "Jazz Fantasia" portray the leading means of transporting goods in America. The first steamboat, the *Claremont* (built by Robert Fulton), had been put into use in 1807. The depiction of the steamboat in the poem is somewhat romantic, as more progressive means of transportation are becoming more prevalent.

  Today: Planes, trains, and automobiles have replaced the steamboat as means of transportation. Today, steamboat rides are available as nostalgic excursions, especially on the Mississippi and Colorado Rivers.

---

changed the face of America. Sandburg's images of skyscrapers and the steel structures rising into the sky do not detract from the cityscape, but are inspiring depictions of the changing landscape of America. In "Prairie," from *Smoke and Steel*, he writes that steel is made with a man's blood, and the residual smoke that is released is the spirit leaving his body.

Poverty

Having been born into a poor Swedish immigrant family, working alongside the poor in the most unexalted tasks gave the young Sandburg an immediate camaraderie with the most underprivileged of the working class. As he became educated and respected as a writer, he never forgot that he was one of those people.

Much of the dire poverty in Chicago was found in the slums of the black belt, the segregated area relegated to the black population, which had doubled in size in just four years to 190,000. Ramshackle living conditions, overcrowding, and crime were rampant. Residents of this area desired equal access to jobs and to comfortable housing alongside whites, but deep resentment and prejudice prevented this. They were made to feel unwelcome if they crossed over their boundaries, and they were sometimes attacked and beaten. Most of the houses in the slums of the south side of Chicago had at least six people in a one-bedroom apartment, often with no plumbing. Police felt that controlling crime in this district was a low priority, and they left the area virtually unprotected. Because most of the population of the Great Migration from the South had been sharecroppers who were poorly educated, they found it difficult to compete for jobs. Immigrants from other countries, such as Ireland, were flooding the city as well, and they were given preferential treatment. Blacks were not able to work in civil service jobs, and labor unions did not want to hire them, supposedly because they did not like to pay labor dues. Most blacks had to settle for domestic and personal service jobs, such as elevator operators, doormen, bootblacks, and servants. The most prestigious job was as a rail car porter for the Chicago-based Pullman Company. Union officials who manipulated the animosity between white union labor workers and often brought in blacks as strike-busters. Ultimately, when the strikes were settled, the blacks lost their jobs.

Sandburg chose to work alongside poor black men, doing the same jobs: bootblack, rail yard worker, and gatherer of scrap metal. When he began to write, he became their voice and champion and ultimately was known as the People's Poet. As Hansen notes in *Midwest Portraits*, Sandburg writes about ordinary people. He recalls in listening to Sandburg that he talked of the letters sent to him from quarry workers, men in prison, a black man attending Harvard, sorority girls, the president of an insurance company, and the secretary of a labor union. Hanson recalls how he loved the poor; as Sandburg wrote,

> And then one day I got a look at the poor, millions of the poor, patient and toiling, more patient than crags, tides, stars; innumerable, patient as the darkness of night. And all broken humble ruins of the nations.

Racial Tension

The second assignment that Sandburg received as a reporter for the *Chicago Daily News* was not an easy one. It was to be a series of articles concerning the social significance of the poor black neighborhoods in Chicago, which were bursting at the seams with those who had fled the South. It seemed a logical fit for him because of his concern for the downtrodden and unfortunate. He fairly reported that the situation was of great concern; the overcrowding, high rent for scant accommodations, crime, and poor job opportunities were serious concerns. He tried to appear optimistic as he praised the community for its racial pride, contributions to the war, educated leaders promoting social and economic institutions, cleanliness, and attitude toward progress. He argued that the goals of this community were just: equal access to jobs, education, and fair treatment. Race riots broke out in the city when a young black boy was stoned to death after crossing a segregated line at a city beach. Sandburg's "The Chicago Race Riots" was published in the *Chicago Daily News* in 1919. He described the injustice in the events that had occurred as a multifaceted problem. The police officer who arrived at the scene refused to make any arrests. He said the policeman represented a government blind to Abraham Lincoln and the Emancipation Proclamation, a struggle that had been won "sanctioned and baptized in a storm of red blood." He added that another crucial cause of the incident was the place where it had occurred. Packingtown, where most of the white rioters were from, was an impoverished area of white laborers where crime was rampant. Sandburg divined that what had started as a racial crime had ended in a riot over labor. White union bosses were prejudiced against blacks and said they did not want to pay union dues. This problem intrigued Sandburg so that he spent many years working in and with labor unions to promote equality and solidarity.

CRITICAL OVERVIEW

Sandburg traveled extensively in the United States, reading and singing his poetry. In an anonymous article that appeared in 1921 in the *Lombard Review* titled "Carl Sandburg Reads Poems to a Large Audience," the writer reports, "Probably the most enjoyable was 'Jazz Fantasia'" (quoted in William A. Sutton's *Carl Sandburg Remembered*). The reporter attributes the poem's popularity to the fact that it was not heavy or obscure. The inflections in Sandburg's voice when making the sounds of the instruments were so close to the sound of a jazz orchestra that it made the writer want to dance. Glen Pinkham, a speech professor at Sterling College in Kansas, writes, after watching Sandburg recite "Jazz Fantasia" to the university in 1931, "The hard jazz of

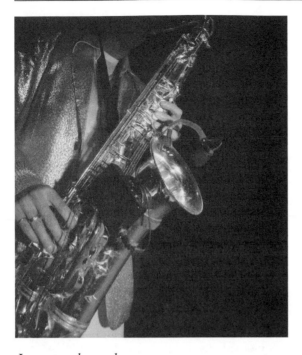

Jazz saxaphone player (*Image copyright Stavchansky Yakov, 2009. Used under license from Shutterstock.com*)

the 1920s from Chicago came alive" (quoted in William A. Sutton's *Carl Sandburg Remembered*). He remembers it as the sounds of a big band orchestra heard through the voice of Sandburg.

According to Sutton, "Jazz Fantasia" has been described as the perfect example of the romantic voice and sense of hearing that Oscar Wilde calls the "lying," the telling of beautiful things with "Vocal Imagination" to convey "Poetic Art."

Harry Hansen reports in *Midwest Portraits* that some people have said they found no beauty or music in the reading of Sandburg's poetry, but when read by Sandburg, with the rich intonation of his deep voice, the beauty was audible, and musical imageries resonated in it. He surprised the audience and carried them with him through his love lyrics, fantasies, grotesques, humoresques, and ballads to the city of smoke and steel.

Sandburg was criticized for his use of free verse by the classicists when *Chicago Poems* was published, but since then he has been cited as the most accomplished poet using free verse. According to Hansen in *Midwest Portraits*, Sandburg was put off by the judgments and set out to defend himself against scholars who said poetry must fit into a traditional mold.

In *Carl Sandburg: His Life and Works* North Callahan recalls that Maxwell Bodenheim, who had previously criticized Sandburg's work wrote to him and said that *Smoke and Steel* was "ten hundred and ninety-three miles above" his other books. He had previously compared Sandburg's poetry to a giant who had ripped apart a sunset and patched the holes in his dirty clothes.

Sandburg had been praised by writers H. L. Mencken, Theodore Dreiser, and Sinclair Lewis; painter Georgia O'Keeffe; and architect Frank Lloyd Wright. However, Sandburg did not always receive the acclaim from critics and poets that he did in popular circles. Joseph Epstein in *Pertinent Players* writes that Ezra Pound, the leader of the modern movement in poetry, reluctantly invited Sandburg to contribute to an anthology. He wrote sarcastically to Sandburg that he was not sure whether *Chicago Poems* would not be better received if it "began six lines later and ended five lines sooner." The New Criticism, a scholarly movement that came into prominence in 1940 and that focused on narrow readings of literary works, could not appreciate Sandburg's rolling rhythms and colloquialisms. His reputation and popularity lagged, and his pocketbook and mental health suffered.

Today, Sandburg has been rediscovered and has regained popularity. Poets and musicians alike now applaud "Jazz Fantasia." It has been recorded, rapped, and danced, and it has been accompanied by jazz musicians. It is read aloud in classrooms, choreographed, and performed in poetry slams. For works such as "Jazz Fantasia," Sandburg holds the title of the People's Poet in perpetuity.

CRITICISM

Cynthia Gower

Gower is a novelist, playwright, and freelance writer. In this essay, she shows that "Jazz Fantasia" by Sandburg was the first poem ever published about the true spirit of jazz.

Langston Hughes has been widely acclaimed as the first true jazz poet, and there is little argument among critics that this is true. Hughes, a black poet of the Harlem Renaissance, wrote poetry unrivaled in its proliferation and depiction of jazz in the early 1900s.

WHAT DO I READ NEXT?

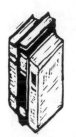

- "Fog" is probably Sandburg's most famous poem. It contains his rich imagery and urban theme but strays from his usual free verse. "Fog" and all of Sandburg's poems can be found in *The Complete Poems of Carl Sandburg* (2003).

- *Hip-Hop Poetry and the Classics* (2004) by Alan Lawrence Sitomer and Michael Cirelli won the Pulitzer Prize in 1974. This one-of-a-kind workbook compares the writing styles of hip-hop artists with classic poets who have been studied for generations. Percy Bysshe Shelley is compared to the Notorious B.I.G. and Shakespeare to Eminem. Motifs, themes, and literary devices are studied with the goal of showing students the significance of classic poets on today's lyricists while giving educators an appreciation for poetry they may have largely ignored.

- *From Totems to Hip-Hop: A Multi-Cultural Anthology of Poetry across the Americas 1900–2002* (2002) presents poetry from many racial and cultural backgrounds. This work, compiled by Ishmael Reed and edited by Francis Murphy, spans from pre-Columbian American works to modern hip-hop lyrics and features authors from Gertrude Stein to Askia Toure and many others.

- *Jazz: An Introduction to the History and Legends behind America's Music* (2007), by Bob Blumenthal, is a concise paperback chronicling the jazz movement. It is a place to start for the unschooled but curious jazz enthusiast. Highly respected by important jazz artists such as Branford Marsalis, Blumenthal is an expert who writes from the perspective of the artists and their musical motivations.

- *Paint Me Like I Am: Teen Poems from WritersCorps*, edited by Bill Aguado and Richard Newirth (2003), is a collection of verse written by at-risk and underprivileged teens. Like those of Sandburg, the poems depict a common-person approach to composition: there are rants (like his against the blights on the poor), raw themes that broach unpopular social problems, and rich metaphors. Titles such as "My Names Is Furious" and "I Am the Broken Pieces on the Floor" reveal the intensity and pathos of the adolescent mind.

Hughes came upon the heels of Sandburg, encouraged by the publication of "Jazz Fantasia" to extend the form of jazz poetry. His first publication appeared in 1926, five years after the publication of "Jazz Fantasia," and he drew inspiration from it as the poem that first celebrated the true spirit of jazz.

Sandburg has been classed with poets such as Vachel Lindsay and Edgar Lee Masters, who were considered the voices of Chicago but not poets of jazz. Neither of these writers, nor any before them, wrote anything that referred to jazz as poetry or music, or the power jazz has to conjure deep emotion and express the soul. "Jazz Fantasia" does exactly that. Jazz was not a standard, recognized term until 1920, the same

year that the poem was published. No one had had the courage to present a work with that word in it to any publisher. It was considered vulgar, base, and inappropriate. In fact, "Jazz Fantasia" might never have been published had it not been hidden away in the collection *Smoke and Steel*. This collection followed Sandburg's *Chicago Poems*, which also dealt with Chicago in the Industrial Age. Becoming a published writer was a privilege afforded Sandburg after he abandoned his days as a hobo and became a newspaper reporter, covering the Chicago race riots and writing essays about Abraham Lincoln. Unfortunately, at that time this opportunity would not have been given to Langston Hughes, as a poor black man.

Percy H. Boynton, in *Some Contemporary Americans*, writes, "I remember vividly the mixture of disgust and contempt with which an official in an old eastern public library handed me a copy of Carl Sandburg's *Chicago Poems* just after the publication in 1916. He resented having to include it in the American poetry section."

This sentiment was shared by many, and Sandburg's insistence on using what was considered crude, "brutal" language that connected him with the poor and common people was not readily embraced. Sandburg was poor, and his boxcar travels as a hobo throughout the Midwest were literally hand-to-mouth, throwing him in the company of the poorest of the poor, including many blacks. He was the friend to the downtrodden, and he keenly felt the injustice toward the poor. In his book *Midwest Portraits*, he tells of working alongside blacks and the friendships he had with them, recalling their names and those in the rail yards that he worked alongside. Here he first heard songs such as "Boll Weevil" and was so enraptured that he tried to imitate the voice of the black man in his poetry. He sat with blacks in the highest segregated balconies and soaked in every word and tune in the minstrel shows. "Jazz Fantasia" is a bold attempt to legitimize this musical genre.

Sandburg defined poetry as being about moods, noises, jumbles, and images of the city. This is the essence of "Jazz Fantasia." Jazz today transcends the descriptions of a music style that swings, improvises, and adheres to a certain rhythm. It is more about mood, imagery, urban life, the rise of a culture, and music that gives wings to the soul.

Today, *jazz* describes a musical genre that is emotional, soulful, and wildly improvisational, one that is intrinsically American, imbued with the passions and agonies of African American history. It is a distinct sound, played by particular instruments, and its roots run deep into the red clay of southern people who went north in hopes of a better life. Jazz was born in New Orleans and migrated north to Chicago at the end of the 1800s, when the red light district around 22nd Street in New Orleans, where many music clubs were located, was closed. Many bands resurfaced in Chicago, such as the Tom Brown Band, but they were not allowed to associate their music with the term jazz. Many sources trace the origin of the word to New Orleans. At the time, it was spelled *jas* or *jass*. The term was slang for *sex* and had inappropriate and seedy connotations with it.

The story goes that in 1915, the Tom Brown Band took a job playing in Lamb's Café. In Chicago, labor unions ruled, and the band had not obtained permission from the local union official to work there. In an attempt to smear the band's reputation, labor representatives spread a rumor around that jazz music was being played at Lamb's Café. The plan backfired when the word got around. People swarmed the club because they were curious about what this music really was. Of course, this was just the beginning of the music that has shaped the United States for over a century without taking a breath. Today, jazz encompasses many subgenres, such as blues, bebop, hip-hop, rap, and even beat box.

"Jazz Fantasia" has gained more popularity today than ever in its history. Jazz clinicians take the poem with them when they travel to teach the essence of jazz. It is a favorite piece in poetry slams. Vocal artists accompanied by jazz musicians have recorded it multiple times. There are audio downloads of "Jazz Fantasia" available as a vocal reading by dozens of artists, all with differing interpretations. Music teachers use it as a vocal class project, assigning the vocal sounding of the jazz instruments to some and echoes of the sound words in dual pitches to others, while one student reads the text. The poem has been incorporated into samba music. "Jazz Fantasia," written in 1919 and published in 1920, was a visionary prophecy of an art form that would be prominent in twentieth- and twenty-first-century American poetry, music, and culture.

Source: Cynthia Gower, Critical Essay on "Jazz Fantasia," in *Poetry for Students*, Gale, Cengage Learning, 2010.

Bernard Duffey

In the following article, Duffey compares the poetry of Carl Sandburg with that of his contemporaries.

No one of the three notable poets spawned by the Chicago literary renaissance of the second decade of this century can be said to have fared very prosperously at the hands of later times. Vachel Lindsay, haunted during his life by a resonantly idealistic vision of possibilities inherent in American life, now seems a proclaimer of apocalypse too unreal for more than rhetoric and gesture. Edgar Lee Masters (the reportorial impulse of *Spoon River Anthology* apart) is surely a failed poet, one lost in a cloud of variously colored romantic posturings, a writer to whom his work was more self-indulgence than either art or expression. Carl Sandburg, in comparison,

"

NATURE IN HIM HAS BECOME SIMPLY
LANDSCAPE, AND, APART FROM THE DISTANCE, THE
REMOTENESS OF ITS BEAUTY, IT IS MADE TO
SUGGEST NO REDEMPTION. EQUALLY IN
SANDBURG TIME IS NO HEALER."

seems more durable. He is in print. His memory has called forth centenary observance. He has had a special stamp struck off in his honor. He is something, at least, of an institution.

But even this degree of survival presents something of a puzzle. He is, in a predominating view, no more than a schoolroom poet, "populistic," "sentimental," and yet one who affords leads to suggest to the children that poetry may be contemporary in interest and personal in form. His work is visibly there, on the map of American literature, yet it is hard to call to mind any criticism of it that has succeeded in giving it major character. Allowing for all this, and conceding that few feel any pressing need for a Sandburg revival, I want nevertheless to take some exception to our willingness to give his poetry a no more than marginal place in our sense of twentieth century writing. Sandburg certainly stands wide of the major thrusts of both the writing and criticism of poetry in our time. . . . He was engaged in the same pursuit of the native which occupied his two Chicago contemporaries, but I want in fact to argue that unlike them he located a poetically constructive imagination of the land in and for which he wrote. His voice gains authenticity when it is considered across its breadth of utterance, and I would find it difficult to make this claim for either Masters or Lindsay. Unlike the latter, his is only occasionally the effort at poetic beatification, and unlike the former he is largely guiltless of ingrown maundering. Instead, I shall argue, though Sandburg shared a certain tentativeness and openness with his contemporaries, he in fact fashioned and for the most part held fast to a close and living sense of the native, one congruent, finally, with his land's own aspect.

What emerges from the whole poetry, in this view, is wholeness of perception, one rooted in a consistent feel for a land conditioned by a problematic history and filling a landscape difficult to redeem by transcendental gesture. His scene is peopled with the kind of minor movers and doers who in fact have so largely occupied it, and who have little choice but to take their character from the land's own spatial and temporal indeterminateness. (pp. 295–96)

In place of the anthology favorites, it is the total fabric of the poems that might now claim attention, beginning with the sense of historical time that prevails in it. Unlike the Whitman he admired, for example, Sandburg's history is one that has no sequential redemptions built into it except, perhaps, for the isolated figures it throws forth from time to time (Lincoln is the great case). Even here, however, history seems to have left him with no more than Eliot's *Quartets* also says it leaves, a symbol only, a remembered reality for our possible use rather than any guarantee of redemption. (p. 296)

The *Complete Poems*, from beginning to end, is studded with observations of place that, across their breadth, can best be characterized negatively, as the absence of any romantic power in nature resembling, say, Emerson's feeling for spirit; and the absence also of the historically bred sense of homeland, of place that has been given its character by deep, repeated actions of will. Landscape for Sandburg is most often simply here, or there, and no more. Instead of the rooted place, there is the open Midwestern landscape known to every eye. It appears most often as prairie. The occasional drama of hill, or forest, or river is seen only seldom. Habitation, rather than dwelling, is the rule. Apart from prairie, and unpredictably, an empty and ever shifting waste of water takes a large place in the poet's work; and he is fascinated over and over again by the palpable impalpable presence of mist. All present themselves as what may be called durations of space, something stretching out in undetermined vectors of distance.

Perhaps the commonest humanizer of landscape in Sandburg is that of response to its beauty, but if we are to understand the sense of beauty that moves him we should beware of easy responses. His is perhaps a little nearer to the negative sense of the sublime than to the beautiful itself, to that which confronts observation almost as an alien realm to be tested in a tremor of mind and feeling rather than received in congenial warmth and pleasure. He seems more often to be haunted by the land than at home in it, and his verse becomes that of a man against the sky to whom connections and relations are inapplicable. . . . The aesthetic in Sandburg is a mode of seeing and feeling that by its nature precludes other participation. It is a mode that asserts itself by negating action or ready involvement, and the poet can be explicit on the point. (p. 298)

But it is a third aspect, the problem of action that must engage us especially, a question that in Sandburg and across the breadth of much of what is called "modernist" poetry raises complicated questions stemming from the fact that the poetry of our time, like so much of its fiction and drama as well, has been a literature of what is felt to have happened to us rather than of what we have done. In this regard, Sandburg seems distinct from his contemporaries most plainly by reason of his own willingness to build whole sections of his poetry upon action in the world. The characteristic of our times, however, has been a contrary one, seeking decision for the poet rather *in* his action as poet. To swing sharply away from the Chicago ambience, we think of Sandburg's contemporaries like Pound, Eliot, Crane Stevens, of Williams as devisers of poetics almost as much as achieved poets. Each of them puts a major effort into the theory of poetry, their deep involvement in what it is to act as a poet.

Sandburg's concerns, to the contrary, flowed almost entirely into practice so that poetry for him became simply expression rather than the act of its definition. It is expression that his own slender essays, "Tentative (First Model) Definitions of Poetry," or the "Notes for a Preface" to the *Complete Poems*, largely insist on. As a result, action in Sandburg has largely to inhere in what he could find to be action outside his poetry, in his own witnessing of action; but such witnessing could only be structured on what were two impediments to active fulfillment and meaning, those of indeterminate time and indeterminate space. (p. 299)

The land of Sandburg's expression is undetermined in time and space alike. It is widely open and calls out for filling. But the actions which the poet seeks in it can only share the fate of the land itself and so share in the indeterminateness of history and landscape. (p. 300)

Rather than action, Sandburg's land is supplied most often with potentialities of action, and often with potentiality that is explicitly arrested. His interior distance, again, is that of standing at some remove, of finding the land which has encompassed him and generated his poems to be itself less than encompassable, a milieu in which he can resume motion only toward his own indeterminate ends. (p. 301)

What emerges from all this I want to suggest is a poetic vision seeking escape from easy idealism, from resolution by willed environment. Such direction sets Sandburg apart not only from his Chicago fellows but, if I may risk such generalization, from any of the prevailing poetic imaginations of America. In our national history there have been three reliances or references poetry has chiefly invoked to resolve the scattered picture the land presents. The first may be called resolution by landscape, or more properly, by a spiritually informing nature. This is the way, most familiarly, of the Emerson of such essays as *Nature* itself or of "Self-Reliance." The second is resolution by time. It is the resolution most fully invoked by Whitman and given its fullest statement in the reliance of "Song of Myself" on the evolution of a self, standing outside of culture in its democratic openness, away from the tentativeness of its beginnings and toward self-reliance and a reliance of selves on each other, but all in turn relied upon through faith in the material thrust of reality, of time's passage toward resolution. The third is that of action, voiced variably across our writing but one presenting great difficulties to the modern. In the poetry of our times, it has most notably found expression in the poet's feeling for his art itself as redemptive act. This, at any rate, would seem to be the resolution sought by Hart Crane in *The Bridge* and alternately sought for and despaired of by William Carlos Williams in *Paterson*.

Sandburg, I suggest is a fourth case, that of recognizing and instituting the undetermined itself. Nature in him has become simply landscape, and, apart from the distance, the remoteness of its beauty, it is made to suggest no redemption. Equally in Sandburg time is no healer. The redemptive hope on which Whitman rested his vision of evolution has become the reiteration of something that now is felt to be no more than process, action subsumed by time and space, which, in themselves, afford no definition. (pp. 301–02)

Perhaps no one could wish really to classify Sandburg as a naturalistic writer, but I may conclude by suggesting that his sense of time, space, and action, all three, forms a sort of protonaturalistic poetic vision, a landscape in which event and endurance provide the basic parameters of his vision as, he suggests, they provide such parameters for existence in his world. He holds back from willed ideality in favor of shaping that world close to the spectacle it most commonly presents. (p. 303)

Source: Bernard Duffey, "Carl Sandburg and the Undetermined Land," in *Centennial Review*, Vol. 23, No. 3, Summer 1979, pp. 295–303.

Gay Wilson Allen

In the following excerpt, Allen examines the literary reputation of Carl Sandburg.

In 1950, at the age of seventy-two, Carl Sandburg published a collected edition of his poetry called *Complete Poems*. It was a heavy volume, running to nearly seven hundred large pages and spanning a generation of poetic output, from "Chicago," first published in Harriet Monroe's *Poetry* in March, 1914, to the great elegy on Franklin Roosevelt, "When Death Came April Twelve 1945." In his "Notes for a Preface" Sandburg wrote, "It could be, in the grace of God, I shall live to be eighty-nine, as did Hokusai, and speaking my farewell to earthly scenes, I might paraphrase: 'If God had let me live five years longer I should have been a writer.'"

Sandburg's most severe critics would probably grant that he is a "writer," even a gifted one, but whether he deserves to be called "poet" is still disputed. (p. 315)

The "puzzlement" experienced by critics thirty years ago becomes even more persistent now after Sandburg has completed his fourscore of years. To some extent this is the natural consequence of the shift in sensibility of both poets and critics during the past three decades, but it is also in part the result of the literary role that Sandburg chose for himself at the beginning of his career, as the reception of his *Complete Poems* demonstrated. It was widely and prominently reviewed, but reviewers betrayed by their words that they had not read the book; indeed, had hardly read Sandburg since the 1920's or 1930's, for the man they wrote about was the theatrical, self-conscious "Chicago poet" and the optimistic affirmer of *The People, Yes*. There was one exception; Louis D. Rubin, Jr., began his perceptive critique in the *Hopkins Review*:

> It seems to me that the critics who most dislike the poetry of Carl Sandburg do so for precisely the wrong reasons, and that those who praise Sandburg's work do so for equally mistaken

reasons. What is bad in Sandburg is not his poetics, but his sentimentality. And when he is good, it is not because he sings of the common people, but because he has an extraordinarily fine gift of language and feeling for lyric imagery.

This is an admirably clear statement of the problem. And readers will either learn to distinguish the poetry from the propaganda and sentimentality or Sandburg's name will fade from the history of twentieth-century poetry. In old age he is still one of the most vivid personalities on the American scene, but his reputation has suffered in almost direct ratio to the rise of Eliot's and Pound's, both members of his own generation; and this is unfortunate, for he has written some poetry that deserves to live.

Sandburg's early role as the poet of Chicago and the sunburnt Midwest helped him gain quick recognition. What might now be called the "Midwest myth" was then in formation, and he found it both convenient and congenial. In part this myth was the final phase of American romantic nationalism. Emerson, in his historymaking "American Scholar" address, called for literary independence from Europe; in the twentieth century a group of Midwestern writers adapted this threadbare doctrine to mean liberation from the cultural dominance of the Eastern United States. There were, of course, new experiences and environments in the region demanding newer literary techniques and a retesting of values and standards, and in the novel especially these needs were met with Realism and Naturalism which yielded stimulating and beneficial results. (pp. 316–17)

Here is the myth: other cities are "soft"; Chicago is brutal, wicked, and ugly, but to be young, strong, and proud is more important. In the first place, Chicago was not unique in its brutality or virility. For social and moral degradation, New York, Boston, or San Francisco could equal it, . . . and for business enterprise and physical expansion, Cleveland, Dallas, Seattle, and a dozen other cities were as dynamic. However, for the first three decades of the twentieth century the Midwest did produce more writers (notably, Anderson, Hart Crane, Dreiser, Fitzgerald, Hemingway, Masters, Lindsay, Frank Norris) than any other region of the United States, thus supporting the notion that the East was effete and that cultural vitality was shifting to midcontinent.

A more unfortunate influence on Sandburg's poetry than his acceptance of the Midwest myth was his own private myth, in which only the poor and oppressed have souls, integrity, the right to happiness, and the capability of enjoying life. There are only two classes in Sandburg's *Chicago Poems*, day laborers and "millionaires." He is contemptuous of the millionaire's "perfumed grief" when his daughter dies, but "I shall cry over the dead child of a stockyards hunky." Certainly a poet has a right to his sympathies, perhaps even a few prejudices—in which no poet could rival Pound. What is objectionable in Sandburg's attitudes and choice of subject in his early poems is his use of stereotypes and clichés. In "The Walking Man of Rodin" he finds "a regular high poem of legs" and praises sculptor for leaving "off the head." This is one of Sandburg's worst stereotypes, leaving off the head, "The skull found always crumbling neighbor of the ankles." Consequently, in the 1930's, when proletarian sympathies were valued more than artistry or universal truth, Sandburg's reputation as a poet reached its highest point.... In the 1950's, when social protest was less popular or even suspect, most serious critics simply ignored Sandburg. Perhaps, however, this is the most propitious time for a re-evaluation, for discovering exactly what as a poet he is or is not.

Sandburg is not, whatever else he may be, a thinker like Robinson or Eliot; not even a cracker-barrel philosopher like Frost. So far as he has a philosophy it is pluralistic, empirical, positivistic. He loves "facts," and has made a career of collecting them to be used in journalism, speeches, biography, a novel, and poetry. Yet he is in no sense a pedant; his facts (when they are facts and not prejudiced supposition) are alive and pertinent, and he is usually willing to let them speak for themselves. "What is instinct?" he asks in "Notes for a Preface" (and the title itself is characteristic). "What is thought? Where is the absolute line between the two. Nobody knows—as yet." He is still, he says, a "seeker." He might be called a pragmatic humanist. Certainly he is not a Naturalist, who believes that human nature is simply animal nature; or a supernaturalist, who has an equally low opinion of mankind. Among his new poems is a satire on a contemporary poet, probably Eliot, who believes that "The human race is its own Enemy Number One." There is no place for "original sin" in Sandburg's theology.

From first to last, Sandburg writes of man in the physical world, and he still regards the enemies of humanity as either social or political. Man's salvation, he thinks, is his instinctive yearning for a better world; in the practical sense: idealism, the "dream."

Source: Gay Wilson Allen, "Carl Sandburg: Fire and Smoke," in *South Atlantic Quarterly*, Vol. 59, 1960, pp. 315–31.

William Loeber

In the following excerpt, Loeber argues against the critics who classify Sandburg's poetry as insensitive.

Snobbishness is so characteristically an imperishable human trait, it is high time it came to be listed among the virtues. Even so universal an appreciation as the appreciation of literature is touched and tainted by this dry-rot of the critical attitude.

Last week I read a paragraph by Dr. Felix E. Schelling, Phi Beta Kappa senator or whatever those elders are called, and luminary of the Department of English, University of Pennsylvania. His statement in substance was a tilt of the academic nose. He declared that Carl Sandburg need trouble no one especially; that Carl Sandburg represented the intellectual Tough, and that we could ignore him as we can ignore the Tough on the streets. "... he is just a man who sets out to find ugly things and to tell about them in an ugly way."

Perhaps, Mr. Sandburg would thank me but little for being irritated by such dusting of sensitive hands; perhaps he would prefer that I forget Dr. Schelling and his dusting; perhaps Mr. Sandburg welcomes the name of Tough. I don't know. Better than that, I don't care. For the moment I am interested in that kind of snobbishness in more or less authoritative pedagogic circles which tilts a nose at any literary expression which does not very obviously carry on the tradition of dead and honored writers.

I suspect that Dr. Schelling spied the word "hog-butcher" and was shocked into a conviction which he could not change though he read every poem Carl Sandburg has ever written. We acquire our attitudes that way. Believing this, I reread Sandburg's three volumes, *Chicago Poems*, *Cornhuskers*, and *Smoke and Steel*. I assumed that Dr. Schelling was willing to dust Sandburg off his hands because of the words Sandburg used and not because of his ideas and imagery. Consequently, if a poem held words or combinations of words like "traffic cops," "soup," "shoe leather," "Philadelphia," "mister," "coffee cups," "summer shirt sale," "scissors," "cheap at the price," words most pertinent to life but, to the professors, quite out of place in an emotional reflection of life, I checked off the poem as a tough-ugly poem.

The result was interesting. Out of the 441 poems in the three books, 199 were tough and 242 could not, I think, even by Dr. Schelling, be considered as tough. I tried to be careful. It frightened me, I was so careful. If a word suggested the least toughness, it threw out the entire poem. In *Chicago Poems*, I learned that only 45 out of 101 were tough; in *Cornhuskers*, 53 out of 103; in *Smoke and Steel*, 104 out of 192. Mr. Sandburg seems to be growing tougher with each book; but my research shows him still on the side of the academic angels.

The point of the matter is, I think, this: it would be absurd for Mr. Sandburg to adopt a set of words foreign to the life he is attempting to express. It is indicative of a rare sincerity that he courageously uses those very words which vitalize his images. And it is ridiculous for his admirers to apologize for him—and some of them do—because it is believed he sometimes writes under the influence of the "he-man" "eater-of-raw-meat" dramatization of his personality. I have the conviction that Mr. Sandburg writes just how it feels for him to be alive. As far as it is humanly possible, he uses those words which are for him the most expressive of his inspiration. And if his choice of words shocks the sensitive, it discloses not so much a lack in his ability to make poems as a limitation in the ability of the academically sensitive to read them.

Whatever the frock-coats think of the clothes Mr. Sandburg's poems wear, there is in the heart of each of them, as Sherwood Anderson has suggested in a recent *Bookman*, the "sensitive, naive, hesitating Carl Sandburg, a Sandburg that hears the voice of the wind over the roofs of houses at night, a Sandburg that wanders often alone through grim city streets on winter nights," a Sandburg that knows and loves his people and their cities. It smacks of an alopogy for what the literary touch-me-nots name the "hairy Sandburg," to mention the "sensitive Sandburg." But I am not apologetic. (Opposing for a moment an attitude, I am forced to divide a poet up.) In all of Mr. Sandburg's poems, those which I like and those which I do not understand, I find the poet Sandburg—essentially the only Sandburg—gripped by indignation, sense of beauty, joy, grief. And that crystal quality of the penetrating poet-eyes, of the warm poet-heart, lifts him quite out of any torpid, heavy-shouldered, thick-necked Tough class,

whether he hog-butchers or waves a lily, whether he jingles "loose change" or whispers....

Unfortunately, you see, for the hand-duster, Carl Sandburg is human, like the rest of us, too human for academic exclusiveness to welcome as poet; especially since, even as poet, he must talk like the particular kind of human being he is—his language so deeply a part of him, he cannot change it to suit the conventions of the classroom, and do it honestly. Best of all, if he can, he defiantly refuses to change it for special occasions, for special ears.

Consequently, it seems to me, he becomes a kind of precious thing to people; because he is able to talk for them and in the words of their mouths. When people go hunting for an expression of those dreams and hopes and beauties they are less articulate over than "home and mother" conventionalities—and it is only a minority who ever do—I have an idea they can come to know Sandburg better than any other of today's poets. If they *try* to meet him. Hand-dusters—and it is painful that so many of them are in a position to present their attitudes to the gullible with as much authority as impunity—insinuate that he is a Tough—a literary Tough, not altogether the proper sort to meet. There is something grossly humorous about it, and something bitter.

Source: William Loeber, Review of *Chicago Poems*, in *Cornhuskers*, Vol. 3, No. 14, February 1922, pp. 105–107.

Paul L. Benjamin

In the following excerpt, Benjamin classifies Sandburg as an everyday poet.

The poetry of Carl Sandburg, the poet who loves the common folk, and who weaves into the meshes of his song the simple, homely things of life—the Kansas farmer with the corn-cob between his teeth, the red drip of the sunset, the cornhuskers with red bandannas knotted at their ruddy chins—cannot be shredded apart from Carl Sandburg, the man. Indeed, as I write I seem to be chatting with him about his work and about the moving things of life, the deep, rich things, of running waters, of companionship with birds and trees, of love and tenderness, of life among those who sweat and toil—those secret, hidden things which only those who are ambassadors to men can truly know and understand.

I see him leaning across the table in the little Italian restaurant, the most human, the most intensely alive man I have ever known. It is his

> **IT IS, HOWEVER, THIS POETRY OF THE COMMON-PLACE, THIS ABHORRENCE OF BOOK-LANGUAGE, THIS RELIANCE ON FOLK IDIOM, THIS PICTURING OF THE SIMPLE, HOMELY THINGS THAT INTERESTS US NOW."**

face that is arresting beautiful as the faces of strong men are beautiful, as Lincoln's is—a brooding face—gnarled and furrowed—cleft chin—a mouth that loops itself into smiles or that booms with deep laughter—"granite" eyes that glow—steel gray hair. Though strong and compelling, and though inevitably the conversation whips about him he has something of the artlessness of the child combined with that uncanny directness and simplicity which children possess.

As he talks you feel the touch of greatness upon this modest, lovable companion; you feel that he is one of those rare spirits who know back alleys, newsboys and farmhands, the crooning of the prairie, and the dust of the long road. You see him leaving school at thirteen to be buffeted by the prairie blizzards as he drives a milk wagon, toiling in brick-yards, swinging a pitch-fork in the husky gang of the threshing crew, shoveling coal, washing dishes, soldiering during the Spanish war, working his way through Knox College. These vignettes of his life quiver in your mind as he talks—and what an infinite range of subjects it is. "Poetry," I hear him say, "is written out of tumults and paradoxes, terrible reckless struggles and glorious lazy loafing; out of blood, work and war and out of base-ball, babies and potato blossoms. For me there is a quality of poetry in: 'Quiet as a wooden-legged man on a tin roof' or 'Busy as a one-armed paper-hanger with the hives.' That glove working woman the *Survey* featured once, talked a speech as vivid as Irish or Chinese poetry at its best. Something like, 'When I look out of the window at night the evergreens look like mittens.' She put a fine, wonderful, vividness of gloves and mittens en masse oppressing her life. One felt humdrum choking a soul of art—and so—tragedy."

There are flashes in his conversation that tell of the painstaking, persistent effort that has given him a mastery of his tools; the growth from the rondeau stage to the perfecting of a gesture of his own, the critical judgment which has led him to discard a mass of his work, publishing only a modicum of what he has composed, the quiet determination to give his own imaginative treatment to the life about him, the compressing of limber words into creative art during the odd snatches of a busy journalistic career.

All this is reflected in his two volumes of poems, *Chicago Poems*, and *Cornhuskers* (Henry Holt and Company), and in his magazine verse, for few persons present their slants at life so fully as does he in his work.

One would hardly suspect this lover of vagabonds and of children, this journalist who writes with a tang and a verve, whose industrial studies and articles on the Chicago race riots have won wide recognition, this delightful companion with his genuine touch of humor, this scoffer at those who strut and preen themselves, of being one of our great American poets. Louis Untermeyer, one of the outstanding critics of contemporary poetry, considers that he ranks with the three greatest poets in these states—the other two being Robert Frost and E. A. Robinson. It is this same Sandburg who in 1914 won the Levinson prize offered through Poetry, and who in 1918 shared with Margaret Widdemer the five-hundred dollar prize of the Poetry Society of America.

To those readers of the *Survey* who in English "Lit" have dissected poems with a forceps or measured them with a calipers, or who have been lulled by the tinkling of certain poets, much of Sandburg's verse may not seem to possess the divine afflatus. Such readers may be bound by the inhibitions of culture. But come with an open mind and a love of freshness and vigor and kindly treatment and you will find that his poems possess a moving rhythm, a rhythm that brawls and roars at times, and then that can be infinitely tender and exquisitely sweet. He does not shrink from using limber words, from using the idiom of the alley, the racy slang of the cornfield, or the argot of the steel-mill. They have the rhythm of life, with deep undertones, with delicate shadings, soft melodies that stir an inner sense of beauty, emotional connotations that express profoundly more than the nice use of words or their masterly groupings, rhythms that suggest intimations of subtle music, melodies that haunt like stirrings among the leaves on autumn nights. . . .

Somewhere Whitman says: "But I am that which unseen comes and sings, sings, sings." So, those who feel melody which "unseen comes, and sings, sings, sings" will turn with recurring frequency to Sandburg. They will discover that there are certain poems; such as "Loam," "Gone," "The Road and the End," "The Answer," "The Prairie," "At a Window," "Joy," "Between Two Hills" and many others which will become part of the dear, remembered things, some of them touched with heartbreak or a mist of tears.

Though written in the so-called "new" forms these are handled with a masterly technique, particularly in the nice use of words, for it is evident that Sandburg loves words; he can caress them, make them rasp and burr, go on velvet feet, cry like the aching call of a bird to its storm-lost mate, or whisper like the flutter of hidden wings. But the words are only a part of the pattern. One might as well brush the dust from a white moth's wing or catch the elusive charm of a young girl's loveliness as separate the words from the poem, no matter if done with consummate skill.

It is, however, this poetry of the common-place, this abhorrence of book-language, this reliance on folk idiom, this picturing of the simple, homely things that interests us now. With it, and this is probably most significant to readers of the *Survey*, is the humanness and simplicity of Sandburg, his use of social material for so many of his themes, his infinite pity and tenderness, his stripping bare of social injustices, and his love of the common folk. Edith Wyatt in a letter expresses much of it in the apt phrase, "Indeed he is a species of nature student of city life." Many of these poems, "Cripple," "Anna Ihmroth," "Population Drifts," "Mill Doors," "They Will Say," although for me not among his most delicate, beautiful pieces, are the ones which most justify an account of him here.

Together with rhythm and a sympathy and understanding of life, is his ability to chisel a picture with a few bold, swift strokes, with a compactness and compression of language, with an intensity and singleness of vision, with an economy of words which gives a peculiar, at times startling effect to his images, an almost biblical brevity. . . .

After all, Sandburg's books are to be lived with, to finger over, to love as one does the faces of children or the caress of chubby fists, to go to when disillusionment threatens, to feel the great, throbbing, singing heart of America through all the inquisitions and repressions, to whiff the pungency of new-mown hay or the fragrance of the furrow turned by the plow, to catch the sweep of the prairie or the tang of the woods, or to see "the grey geese go five hundred miles and back with a wind under their wings." A glimpse of the real Sandburg is a paragraph in his review of Ransome's book on Russia, written for the *Chicago Daily News*: "And then going on as though the human race is essentially decent and sweet and out of the trampling of this vintage of blood and tears, out of a brute earth of cold and hunger, we will yet come through clear-eyed with an understanding of what we want to make of the world we live in."

Source: Paul L. Benjamin, "A Poet of the Common-Place," in *Survey 45*, October 2, 1920, pp. 12–13.

SOURCES

Boynton, Percy H., "The Voice of Chicago," in *Some Contemporary Americans*, University of Chicago Press, 1924, pp. 50–71.

Callahan, North, "The Poetry," in *Carl Sandburg: His Life and Works*, 4th ed., Pennsylvania University Press, 1986, pp.80–103.

Epstein, Joseph, "Carl Sandburg, 'the People's Poet'" in *Pertinent Players*, W. W. Norton, 1937, pp. 332–48.

Hansen, Harry, "Carl Sandburg: Poet of the Streets and of the Prairie," in *Midwest Portraits*, Harcourt, Brace, 1923, pp.15–91.

Karsner, David, "Carl Sandburg," in *Sixteen Authors to One*, Lewis Copeland, 1928, p. 145–55.

Kirchner, Bill ed., *Oxford Companion to Jazz*, Oxford University Press, 2000, pp. 3–5, 7–15, 39–51, 53–61, 148–61, 559–64, 734–43, 766–89.

Lowell, Amy, "Edgar Lee Masters and Carl Sandburg," in *Tendencies in Modern American Poetry*, Houghton Mifflin, 1917, pp. 139 –232.

Sandburg, Carl August, "Man Child" and "The Auditorium," in *Always the Young Strangers*, Harcourt, Brace, 1952, pp. 15–30, pp. 270–79.

———, *The Complete Poems of Carl Sandburg*, rev. and expanded ed., Harcourt, Brace, 1969, pp. 3, 5, 7–8, 16, 33, 79, 175, 179, 271.

Sutton, William A., "A Host of Encounters," in *Carl Sandburg Remembered*, Scarecrow Press, 1979, pp. 75–273.

Untermeyer, Louis, "Carl Sandburg," in *The New Era in American Poetry*, Henry Holt, 1919, pp. 95–109.

Yanella, Phillip R., "Sandburg in 1919," in *The Other Carl Sandburg*, University Press of Mississippi, 1996, pp. 122–50.

FURTHER READING

Bolin, Frances Schoonmaker, and Steven Arcella, *Poetry for Young People: Carl Sandburg*, Sterling, 1995.

This collection of Sandburg's poems is specifically geared to ages nine through twelve. It is illustrated with surreal drawings in ethereal shapes and warm tones that aptly depict the rich imagery of Sandburg's poetry.

D'Alessio, Gregory, *Old Troubadour: Carl Sandburg*, Wallace, 1987.

This is an entertaining recollection of Sandburg's last years. It depicts the aging poet as a member of the New York Classic Guitar Society by his friend of twenty years, syndicated cartoonist and guitarist Gregory D'Alessio. It includes anecdotes of Sandburg's friendships and encounters with the architect Frank Lloyd Wright, guitarist Andres Segovia, and actress Marilyn Monroe.

Golden, Harry, *Carl Sandburg*, University of Chicago Press, 1988.

A memoir and biography of Carl Sandburg, this book heaps lavish praise on him as a poet and biographer. Golden portrays Sandburg as a patriotic, down-to-earth author who has been overlooked by modern critics because of his forthright, direct approach to poetry.

Sandburg, Carl August, *Abraham Lincoln: The Prairie Years and the War Years*, Harcourt, 1939.

This biography won the Pulitzer Prize for History in 1940. Sandburg's research began as a passionate admiration for the sixteenth president after listening to old Illinois prairie men telling stories about Lincoln as a country lawyer. It is considered to be the most comprehensive and authoritative text on the beloved president.

The Lotus Flowers

ELLEN BRYANT VOIGT

1987

Ellen Bryant Voigt's "The Lotus Flowers" is the title poem in her 1987 collection. Both the collection and the poem focus on Voigt's rural upbringing in Virginia. All the included poems are relatively short and filled with imagery related to nature. Most are also narrative poems, seemingly telling a story with a clear beginning, middle, and end. In this manner, "The Lotus Flowers" is a fitting title poem; it represents all of the stylistic and thematic qualities inherent in the collection in which it appears. In fact, "The Lotus Flowers" is also representative of the major themes that appear throughout Voigt's entire body of work. These include the loss of innocence, fate, mortality, and the beauty and threat of nature. Stylistically, "The Lotus Flowers" (and the collection in which it appears) stands apart from Voigt's work. Where "The Lotus Flowers" and its eponymous collection are narrative (containing a story arc), most of Voigt's work is lyric (less structured and more musical). Her narrative poems have been favorably compared to those of Robert Frost.

Appearing in the third of seven poetry collections, "The Lotus Flowers" was written at the height of Voigt's career. Her work was best known during the late 1980s and into the 1990s and is read by students of contemporary poetry. A 2000 edition of *The Lotus Flowers*, released by Carnegie-Mellon University Press, remained in print as of 2009.

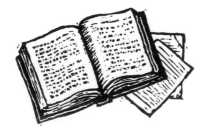

AUTHOR BIOGRAPHY

Voigt was born Ellen Bryant in Danville, Virginia, on May 9, 1943. Her mother, Missouri Zue Yeatts Bryant, was an elementary school teacher, and her father, Lloyd Gilmore Bryant, was a farmer. Voigt was raised on the family farm. From an early age, she exhibited a great deal of musical talent and became an accomplished pianist. Critics would later note the musical quality of her poetry. Voigt attended Converse College in South Carolina as a music major, but soon switched to literature, graduating with a bachelor of arts degree in 1964. The following year, on September 5, 1965, she married Francis George Wilhelm Voigt, a college dean and educator who was also a corporate executive. The marriage produced two children, Julia and William.

Voigt next attended the University of Iowa, earning her master of fine arts degree in both music and literature in 1966. While she was a student there, Voigt worked as a technical writer for the University's College of Pharmacy. She then taught at Iowa Wesleyan College from 1966 to 1969. The following year she went to teach at Goddard College in Plainfield, Vermont, where she created a low-residency M.F.A. in writing program. The pedagogical approach was quite successful, becoming the model for similar programs at Bennington College and Vermont College. Also while at Goddard, Voigt released her first poetry collection, *Claiming Kin*, in 1976. The book immediately secured Voigt's reputation as a talented poet. After leaving Goddard in 1979, Voigt taught creative writing at the Massachusetts Institute of Technology, a post she held until 1982. In 1981, she also served as visiting faculty at Warren Wilson College in Swannanoa, North Carolina, where she taught in an M.F.A. program similar to the one she had designed at Goddard.

In 1983, Voigt released her second poetry collection, *The Forces of Plenty*. She also won a Pushcart Prize that year. In addition to her academic and writing career, Voigt has been a concert pianist and also a guest teacher at writing conferences, including the renowned Bread Loaf Writers' Conference. Her third collection, of which "The Lotus Flowers," is the title poem, was published in 1987, the same year she was honored with the Emily Clark Balch Award from the *Virginia Quarterly Review* in recognition for her work. Five years later, Voigt released her fourth book of poetry, *Two Trees*. It was followed in 1995 by *Kyrie*. The book is arguably

one of Voigt's most successful collections; it was nominated for the National Book Critics Circle poetry award that same year. Her acclaimed essay collection *The Flexible Lyric*, was published in 1999.

Voigt was named Vermont State Poet, a post she held from 1999 to 2003. She was also a Lila Wallace-Reader's Digest Fellow from 1999 to 2001. During this time, Voigt published her sixth collection, *Shadow of Heaven* (2002), which was also nominated for a National Book Critics Circle poetry award. From 2002 to 2005, Voigt was chancellor of the American Academy of Poets. Then, in 2007, Voigt's sixth collection, *Messenger: New and Selected Poems, 1976–2006*, was published. The volume was a National Book Award finalist. As of 2009, Voigt continued to write poetry and resided in Vermont.

POEM TEXT

The surface of the pond was mostly green—
bright green algae reaching out from the banks,
then the mass of water lilies, their broad round
    leaves
rim to rim, each white flower spreading
from the center of a green saucer.   5
We teased and argued, choosing the largest,
the sweetest bloom, but when the rowboat
lumbered through and rearranged them
we found the plants were anchored, the
    separate
muscular stems descending in the dense water— 10
only the most determined put her hand
into that frog-slimed pond
to wrestle with a flower. Back and forth
we pumped across the water, in twos and
    threes,
full of brave adventure. On the marshy shore, 15
the others hollered for their turns,
or at the hem of where we pitched the tents
gathered firewood—
this was wilderness,
although the pond was less than half an acre 20
and we could still see the grand magnolias
in the village cemetery, their waxy,
white conical blossoms gleaming in the foliage.
A dozen girls, the oldest only twelve, two sisters
with their long braids, my shy neighbor, 25
someone squealing without interruption—
all we didn't know about the world buoyed us
as the frightful water sustained and moved the
    flowers
tethered at a depth we couldn't see.

In the late afternoon, before they'd folded 30
into candles on the dark water,

I went to fill the bucket at the spring.
Deep in the pines, exposed tree roots
formed a natural arch, a cave of black loam.
I raked off the skin of leaves and needles,   35
leaving a pool so clear and shallow
I could count the pebbles
on the studded floor. The sudden cold
splashing up from the bucket to my hands
made me want to plunge my hand in—   40
and I held it under, feeling the shock that
    wakes
and deadens, watching first my fingers,
then the ledge beyond me,
the snake submerged and motionless,
the head propped in its coils the way a girl   45
crosses her arms before her on the sill
and rests her chin there.
Lugging the bucket
back to the noisy clearing, I found nothing
    changed,
the boat still rocked across the pond,   50
the fire straggled and cracked as we fed it
branches and debris into the night,
leaning back on our pallets—
spokes in a wheel—learning the names of the
    many
constellations, learning how each fixed   55
cluster took its name;
not from the strongest light, but from the
    pattern
made by stars of lesser magnitude,
so like the smaller stars we rowed among.

POEM SUMMARY

"The Lotus Flowers" consists of two long stanzas and is written in free verse. Each long stanza, however, is divided, roughly in the middle, by an offset or broken line. In fact, in both stanzas, the broken lines occur between the eighteenth and nineteenth lines. The first stanza consists of twenty-nine lines, and the second of thirty. One of the poem's central images, that of the water lilies, refers to the poem's title (lotus flowers are a type of water lily).

Stanza 1

LINES 1–5

The speaker describes a pond's surface as being of a greenish hue. Algae of a vibrant green color stretch away from the shore and the expansive, rounded leaves of the water lilies touch across the pond. The flowers themselves are white and sit atop the leaves like cups on saucers.

LINES 6–10

In line 6, the speaker indicates that she is not alone, that there is a group of people who are bickering and teasing one another. Finally, they decide upon the biggest and most fragrant water lily. A few members of the group go out in a rowboat to retrieve it, rustling their way through the dense pond. However, they find that the lilies are rooted deeply to the bottom of the pond and the stems are incredibly strong.

LINES 11–15

The speaker then says that only the most resolved of the girls (here the gender of the group is revealed for the first time) dare to put their hands in the murky water in an attempt to wrench the flower from its stem. Without mentioning whether or not the girls were successful in their endeavor, the speaker then observes that they all row to and fro across the pond. They do so in small groups of two or three, taking turns. The girls are courageous and adventurous as they stand upon the muddy shore.

LINES 16–20

The other girls call for their turn on the rowboat. Some of the girls are picking up wood for the fire over by the spot where they set up their tents. (It now becomes clear that the girls have gone on more than just an afternoon's outing.) This is also where the line break occurs, between the mention of picking up firewood and the statement that they are in the backwoods. The implication here is that the girls are as wild as the woods that surround them. And yet, the pond is small. Here, the speaker seems to indicate that as wild as things may seem, the pond itself is somewhat tame; it is not as big or impressive as it seems.

LINES 21–25

From their vantage point at the pond, the girls can still see the large magnolia trees that grow in the town cemetery. The large, cone-shaped flowers on the trees are white and easy to spot among the greenery. Thus, the speaker's assertion that they are wild, or in the wild, is immediately contradicted by the mention of visible signs of civilization. The speaker notes that there are twelve girls and that the oldest girl in the group is twelve years old. The speaker's quiet neighbor is also there, as are a pair of sisters who wear their hair in braids.

LINES 26–29

One of the girls keeps shrieking without stopping. The girls are held up and floated by their own innocence, by their ignorance of the world and how it works, just as the frightening water in the pond holds up the lilies. And yet, those lilies are tied to the bottom of the pond; a bottom that the girls cannot catch sight of. Given the half-completed comparison between the girls and the lilies, there is an implicit question: The flowers are held up by the water but deeply rooted in its bottom, and the girls are held up by their innocence, but to what are they rooted?

Stanza 2

LINES 30–34

It is now late in the afternoon, just before the lilies close up for the day. For the first time the speaker refers to herself in the first person. She says that she went to the spring to fill up the bucket. The spring is nestled below the pine trees and bubbles below their exposed roots. The roots form a sort of cave that is filled with black mud.

LINES 35–39

The speaker states that she skimmed the pine needles and leaves from the top of the spring. Once the muck has been removed, she finds a crystal clear, shallow pool. It is so clear that she can see every rock at the bottom, could even count them if she wished. She then describes the shock of the cold water on her hand as it splashes onto her from the bucket.

LINES 40–44

The cold makes her want to stick her hand into the pool, and she does so. She holds her hand there; at first the cold comes as a shock, and then it numbs her. She gazes at her fingers and then at the pool's edge. (Here, the speaker seems to indicate that her numb fingers have become something apart from her, something she looks at with indifference, just as she does the pool's edge.) Yet, there on that ledge lies a snake. It is just beneath the water and is not moving.

LINES 45–49

The speaker says that the snake is coiled up, resting its head on its body just as a girl would rest her head on her arms. Here, the second line break occurs, and the speaker states that she is carrying the bucket back to the raucous campsite. No mention is made of the snake or of whether or not it

attempted to strike. Nevertheless, it is clear that the speaker has returned to her group unharmed. At the campsite, she finds that all is the same. This statement seems to imply, however, that the speaker has experienced an internal change, one she (mistakenly) expects to find reflected in the world around her.

LINES 50–54

When the speaker returns to her group, she finds that the boat is still moving over the pond. When the speaker rejoins the other girls, she no longer refers to herself in the first person, but only as a part of the group. The campfire roars and spits as the girls throw trash and wood into it and into the darkness. They are lying back on their sleeping bags, arranged like so many parts of a wheel.

LINES 55–59

The girls are looking up at the night sky and learning what each constellation is called. They are also learning the myths behind each name. The speaker notes that the constellations are not derived from their brightest star, but from the lesser stars and the form they take as a group. These dimmer stars, the speaker finds, are much like the lilies through which they rowed their boat.

THEMES

Innocence

Innocence and its loss are a major theme in "The Lotus Flowers." This innocence is underscored in numerous ways, particularly in the natural surroundings in which the girls find themselves. The poem could be an idyll, a short verse or painting depicting the virtues of rusticity. The term *idyllic* is derived from this art form, and Voigt's poem is nothing if not idyllic. There is an idealized innocence to the water lilies and to the girls' attempts to pick them. The girls believe themselves to be great adventurers out in the wild. Yet the town cemetery and its magnolia trees are within sight. This contrast between belief and reality also belies the girls' innocence. The girls' hollering for turns on the boat, their gathering of firewood, their campsite, and their discussion of the constellations, are all idyllic and filled with innocence. Furthermore, the girls are no older than twelve, some even with their hair in braids. They are decidedly children,

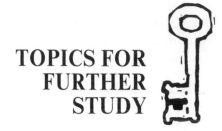

TOPICS FOR FURTHER STUDY

- Use the Internet to research Ellen Bryant Voigt and other contemporary women poets. How does Voigt's life and work compare to that of her peers? What influenced each to write poetry? Do they share themes and styles? What subject matter seems to be common among them? Report your findings to the class in a PowerPoint presentation.

- Read any of the *The Sisterhood of the Traveling Pants* young-adult novel series. Think about how the girls' adventures help them grow as friends and as individuals. Compare and contrast the novel to Voigt's poem in an essay.

- Read the entirety of Voigt's book *The Lotus Flowers*. Prepare an oral report in which you discuss how the title poem plays a part in setting the tone for the entire collection.

- Interview women in your family, school, and neighborhood. Focus your discussion on times these women have spent with other women—how is it different from the time they have spent with their families or with men? Compile your findings in a detailed report written in an interview format.

albeit on the cusp of adolescence. As the speaker points out, their innocence and their ignorance of the way the world works allow them to float like the lilies in the pond.

Nevertheless, there is also a darker undertone to the poem. The pond is murky; it is covered in algae and its water is black. Only the most courageous of the girls dares to stick her hand into it. While the girls are young, the oldest among them is nearly an adolescent, which signifies an impending loss of innocence in the face of aging, maturity, and burgeoning womanhood. The foreboding image of dark or black water is repeated again when the speaker travels alone to gather water. The spring, which is pure and clear, lies beneath black mud, beneath dead leaves and discarded pine needles. Here the contrast between pure and impure (innocent and not) is clear. More important, the snake that the speaker encounters recalls the snake in the biblical story of Adam and Eve. In that story, the snake is the corruptor, the active agent in Adam's and Eve's loss of innocence. Here, the snake lies motionless, a harbinger of that loss. That the speaker is changed by her encounter with the snake is implicit in her observation that nothing at the campsite has changed.

Mortality

Just as the poem is a depiction of innocence about to be lost, so too it is a meditation on mortality. Aging and loss of innocence go hand in hand, and what is aging if not evidence of mortality? Fate is also entwined in this thematic interpretation; loss of innocence, aging, and death are the fate of all of the girls. In fact, the only evidence of civilization in the poem is the cemetery. This is a striking choice, one that certainly underscores the overall sense of decay that permeates the poem. The water imagery in the poem also emphasizes this sense of decay, a decay that certainly signifies, or at least hints at, mortality. The pond is murky and black, even described at one point as frightful. Its depths cannot be seen. The spring, which is pure, a source of life, is nevertheless buried in black scum, a mulch of dead things that must be scraped away before its clarity is revealed. Nevertheless, while the spring is clear, its water is so cold it numbs the speaker's hand, deadening it and draining the life and feeling from it. Even the danger inherent in the snake's presence underscores the speaker's burgeoning sense of her own mortality. The snake is motionless but coiled, and thus could easily strike. In fact, when the snake is compared to the innocent image of a girl resting her head on her arms, the incongruous simile makes the threatening nature of the snake all the more apparent. Even the stars and constellations seem to hint a mortality. Where they are lasting, the girls are not. Even the idyll of girls camping is doomed to pass away. They will age but the stars will not.

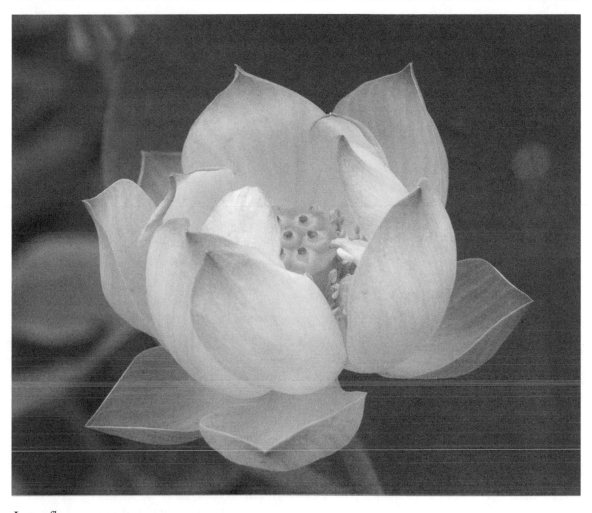

Lotus flower (Image copyright qingqing, 2009. Used under license from Shutterstock.com)

STYLE

Imagery

Because "The Lotus Flowers" is set in nature, it is largely filled with descriptive language and imagery pertaining to those surroundings. It begins with a description of the vibrant green algae in the pond. The reader's eye is led then to the blooms and leaves of the water lilies that float in the pond and to the waxy magnolia blossoms in the nearby cemetery. The description of the speaker's solitary excursion to fetch water from the spring among the towering pines sets a different tone; all of the imagery during this section of the poem is dark and foreboding.

Simile

A simile is a literary device in which one thing is compared to another, usually through the use of such linking words as *like* or *as*. The central simile in the poem occurs when the speaker spies a snake lying motionless with its head resting on its coils. She compares the snake to a young girl crossing her arms on a windowsill and resting her heard on her arms. The speaker also employs a simile when she says that the girls' innocence holds them up just as the water holds up the lilies. Another simile occurs at the end of the poem when the speaker compares the girls laid out on their pallets to spokes in a wheel.

Metaphor

Unlike a simile, a metaphor does not compare two things to one another. Instead, it attempts to make one thing into another. The lilies are described as teacups atop green saucers (their leaves). Later in the afternoon, as the flowers close for the evening, they are turned into candlesticks. In the last line of the poem, the lilies are stars.

Point of View

While the point of view in the poem is entirely in the first person, it is mostly expressed by the plural pronoun "we." The speaker is part of a group of girls and refers to herself almost exclusively as such. She refers to herself as "I" only when she separates herself from the group and goes alone to find water. This interesting stylistic device underscores the tension between the speaker's group mentality and her growing sense of herself as an individual. This assertion is proved by the speaker's observation that nothing has changed upon her return to the camp site. Yet, the implication in this statement is that something has changed—the speaker herself.

Narrative Verse

Put simply, a narrative poem is a poem that has a plot. Or, at the very least, it has a discernible beginning, middle, and end. At its most basic level, "The Lotus Flowers" tells the story of a group of girls who go camping. They arrive during the day, set up camp, gather firewood, row across the pond, and attempt to pick water lilies. In the evening, they gather around the campfire and stare at the constellations. In the midst of this story is another story; that of the speaker, the girl who breaks away from the group in search of water. This is the story of a girl who strips away the flotsam atop a pure spring, who fills her bucket and numbs her hand in the frigid water, a girl who spies a snake and walks away unharmed.

HISTORICAL CONTEXT

Feminism

While Voigt's "The Lotus Flowers" is not a feminist poem per se, it nevertheless portrays a group of girls participating in stereotypical male activities. Voigt was born in 1943, a time when millions of women worked outside the home for the first time in defense related industries. She reached adulthood in the early 1960s as more women began to question their roles and positions in the home, workplace, and society. She held significant positions in the literary and academic world at a time when it was largely dominated by males. The second half of the twentieth century saw the advancement of women's equality in all aspects of society, and Voigt experienced many of these milestones.

Although the first wave of feminism began in the late nineteenth century with the suffrage movement (securing women's right to vote), it was not replaced by the second wave until the 1960s. That second wave lasted until the 1980s, the same period of time during which Voigt established her literary reputation. Second-wave feminism focused on women's equality in society and also on sexual equality. The sexual revolution was in no small part spurred by this; women's desires were examined in light of the fact that they were increasingly seen as equal to men. Women at this time fought for equality and recognition in the workplace and also in the household, where women's roles and contributions had largely been taken for granted. Furthermore, second-wave feminism made great strides in assuring equal access to education for women, as public funding for single-sex schools was abolished.

In the 1990s, third-wave feminism emerged to address the remaining iniquities between men and women. One such persisting issue is wage disparity. However, the movement itself is largely at a crossroads as to its future. Some contemporary feminists believe that the movement has mostly catered to the needs of the middle class, particularly middle-class Caucasians, and that it thus overlooks specific issues relevant to minority groups.

Narrative Poetry

While narrative poetry is a specific style of poetry, it is also a poetic tradition steeped in history. In fact, narrative verse is probably the oldest form of poetry. Before the advent of the written word, stories were committed to memory and transmitted orally. To aid in this endeavor, they were set to verse and even to music. Thus, the earliest known literary works owe their provenance to narrative verse. Take for instance Homer's epics, the *Iliad* and the *Odyssey*, which date from roughly 800 BCE. Other ancient examples of narrative verse include the epic *Gilgamesh*; the earliest written version dates back to around 700 BCE.

Narrative poetry was also prevalent in medieval Europe; one English example of this is Geoffrey Chaucer's *Canterbury Tales*, which was written in the fourteenth century. Other well-known literary figures to employ narrative verse include William Shakespeare, Robert Browning, and Robert Frost. Narrative verse can also be used in plays, as in Shakespeare' works and in ancient Greek drama, and it is employed in such poetic forms as idylls and ballads.

COMPARE
&
CONTRAST

- **1980s:** Although Voigt's work is not explicitly feminist, her poem portrays only girls, and she herself is remarkably successful in a male-dominated field. Supporters of women's rights in the 1980s are known as second-wave feminists. First-wave feminists won suffrage (women's right to vote, established by the Nineteenth Amendment to the U.S. Constitution), and second-wave feminists focus instead on cultural discrimination, including wage disparity.

  Today: Feminism has not taken any cogent form since the establishment of third-wave feminism during the 1990s. If anything, feminism continues to struggle to define itself given the social, cultural, and political strides women made into the twenty-first century.

- **1980s:** Women's Studies becomes an accepted field of study in major universities across the United States and a few begin to establish feminist research institutes. Scholarly journals begin to write about feminist

theory and by the end of the 1980s the U.S. Congress declares March to be National Women's History Month.

  Today: By 2000 more than 700 universities offer Women's Studies programs and the field of study expands to other countries in Latin America, Asia, and Eastern Europe.

- **1980s:** The influence of confessional poetry, which was at its most popular in the 1950s and 1960s, can still be felt. Free verse and first-person speakers remain popular stylistic devices. However, verse in the 1980s stands out in that it features a plethora of female and minority poets.

  Today: Although no definitive poetic movement has emerged in the early twenty-first century, free verse poetry continues to be a popular form of expression. It is rivaled by New Formalism, which heralds the return of more traditional and formal metric verse structures.

CRITICAL OVERVIEW

Although "The Lotus Flowers" has not been widely reviewed, the collection in which it appears has been. For the most part, critics have been laudatory in their assessments, pointing out Voigt's pet themes and the characteristic attention to detail with which she addresses them. In the *Dictionary of Literary Biography*, Laura B. Kennelly concludes that in *The Lotus Flowers*, "Voigt writes with richness and maturity of her familiar concerns: the rural Virginia of her childhood home, the paradox of good and evil, and the relationships between mortal creatures who know they must die." Additionally, Kennelly goes on to state that "stylistically Voigt's poems are traditional in that she describes a scene or an image in musical phrases and lines." Yet more praise is extended by Edward Hirsch in the *New*

York Times Book Review. He calls the collection "a book of fierce regard and passionate attention" and adds that "Voigt's poems increasingly meditate not only on what passes away but also on what survives, how the past determines and informs the present, how it infuses and complicates our adult experience." He applauds "her complex allegiance to the dual countries of childhood and adulthood."

Some critics, such as *Poetry* contributor Peter Campion, have found Voigt's style somewhat stagnant. He writes that "the short-story-like poems in *The Lotus Flowers* (1987), while cunningly constructed, seem to repose beneath a glaze. Voigt's big temptation is to rely on her own mastery, to speak from above, instead of from inside, experience." Thus, he concludes that "despite some enthralling moments...these poems suffer too often from such knowingness."

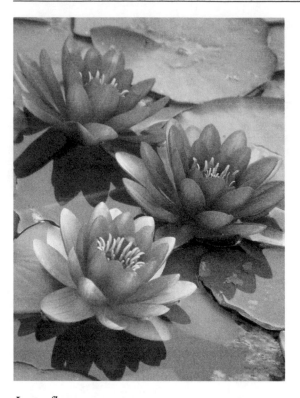

Lotus flower *(Image copyright Tatiana53, 2009. Used under license from Shutterstock.com)*

Even Kennelly notes that Voigt's style is secondary to her themes. She remarks that "fashioning the questions [Voigt] asks in her poetry seems more important to her than achieving new heights of technical virtuosity." Despite this seeming complaint, however, Kennelly declares that "women, in particular, should see themselves as free to write in any tradition, feminist or not.... The positive critical reception of *The Lotus Flowers* suggests that Voigt has taken advantage of such freedom."

CRITICISM

Leah Tieger

Tieger is a freelance writer and editor. In the following essay, she discusses the structure, themes, and symbolism in Ellen Bryant Voigt's "The Lotus Flowers." In particular, she provides a textual explication of the poem.

Textually, Ellen Bryant Voigt's "The Lotus Flowers" is a rich poem. Its diction (use of language) reveals its underlying themes, and its

structure shapes its meaning. Although the poem is written in free verse, it is divided into two long stanzas of almost identical length (the first stanza is twenty-nine lines; the second is thirty). Both stanzas however, feature a broken line just past their first half, between their eighteenth and nineteenth lines. In the first stanza, the break occurs between the statement that the girls are gathering firewood and the statement that they are in the backwoods (a statement that later found to be erroneous). In the second stanza, the line break occurs between the observation that the snake is like a girl resting her head on her arms and the statement indicating that the speaker is carrying the bucket back to the campsite. In each case, the line break is disorienting. Furthermore, the breaks indicate a falsehood or at least an omission. In the case of the first stanza's line break, the statement that the girls are in the wilderness is soon revealed to be untrue. They can see the magnolia trees in the town cemetery from the pond. The latter line break is somewhat more complex in what it attempts to obscure. When the threat of the snake is introduced, it is immediately downplayed by the simile comparing it to a mere girl. Then follows the immediate scene change, brought on by the speaker's statement that she is taking the bucket back to the other girls. This change is made all the more disorienting by the line break. Furthermore, the speaker's ensuing statement that she has found nothing changed indicates that something has changed, just not the other girls or their camp. The sense of disorientation brought on by the line break extends to this seemingly innocent remark—especially because it is not innocent at all.

The structure of the poem is also misleading in that it is fairly regular. The line lengths (barring the aforementioned exceptions) are much the same, as are the enjambments (the line breaks occurring amid the same complete thought/sentence). Indeed, the poem is set at a natural rhythm. When read aloud, the line breaks occur at the end of a phrase or where one would naturally take a breath before continuing. For this reason, the speaker appears trustworthy; the seemingly simple and idyllic tale of girls camping is taken at face value. Where enjambment can often alter the poet's intended meaning, or allow for numerous meanings to coexist, line breaks in "The Lotus Flowers" tend to avoid such confusion. In fact, the enjambment in the poem only alters meaning in the aforementioned line breaks and again when the speaker goes off by herself to get water. Thus, the breaks in the poem's regular and measured

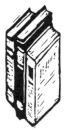

WHAT DO I READ NEXT?

- The 2005 edition of *Read and Understand Poetry, Grades 5–6+* by Linda Armstrong and Jill Norris provides reluctant readers with insight into poetry and how to interpret it. This classroom aid is appropriate for middle grade and young-adult readers, and it provides an easy-to-read refresher for all students of poetry.

- Flora Davis's 1999 book, *Moving the Mountain: The Women's Movement in America since 1960*, presents an in-depth look at the second wave of feminism in the United States. She also explores the rise and fall of first-wave feminism as it pertains to the rise of the second wave. Issues regarding female sexuality and women in politics are also explored. The book features a detailed bibliography as well as interviews with numerous feminist activists.

- Given that Voigt's verse has been compared to Robert Frost, another book appropriate for young-adult or reluctant readers is *Poetry for Young People: Robert Frost*. Edited by Gary D. Schmidt and Henri Sorensen, this 2008 edition of Frost's poetry features twenty-five poems divided into sections inspired by each of the four seasons. Watercolor illustrations of pastoral New England scenes accompany the verses, as do notes on possible meanings and interpretations to be gleaned from each poem. A biographical profile of Frost is also included.

- Homer's *The Iliad* is a classic example of narrative poetry. The 2003 Penguin Classics edition, edited by E. V. Rieu, D. C. H. Rieu, and Peter Jones, is particularly well suited for students. Set during the Trojan War, the story portrays Greek heroes Achilles, Odysseus, and Agamemnon, as they fight the Trojans to reclaim Helen, Agamemmnon's sister-in-law, from the Trojan prince Paris. Themes of mortality and fate akin to those in "The Lotus Flowers" can also be found in this epic poem.

- A multicultural approach to narrative verse can be found in the 2004 edition of the anthology *Get Your Ass in the Water & Swim Like Me: African-American Narrative Poetry from Oral Tradition*. The anthology, edited by Bruce Jackson, was originally published in 1974 and is a collection of African American verse and folk tales. In particular, the collection is hailed for its inclusion of the African American narrative folk verses known as "toasts."

- Perhaps Voigt's most famed collection of poems is her 1995 volume *Kyrie*. The book is possibly one of Voigt's most successful collections, and it was nominated for the National Book Critics Circle poetry award in 1995.

---

structure serve to offset the most important and revealing instances of the poem's meaning.

Certainly, the central event in the poem is the speaker's excursion for water. Again, there are textual clues to alert readers to this fact. For instance, the speaker uses the first-person plural pronoun "we" throughout the poem, signifying that she is a part of the group. Yet, when the speaker leaves to get water, she reverts entirely to the first person singular "I," reasserting her individualism apart from the group. The enjambment

in this section, as previously mentioned, plays the most with meaning. For instance, when the speaker plunges her hand into the cold water, she states that the shock of it is invigorating. Yet, in the following line, the speaker says that the shock that enlivens quickly becomes deadening, as her hand is increasingly numbed by the frigid water. In addition, the line breaks become quick and choppy when the speaker spies the snake, and they remain that way as she attempts to mitigate its threatening power by comparing it to an innocent girl. Also, because the poem's main theme pertains to innocence and its loss, the snake's presence in this blameless camping idyll is all the more fraught with symbolic meaning. The snake in literature can never be fully divorced from the story of Adam and Eve. In that parable the snake is the corruptor, the influential factor in Adam and Eve's loss of innocence and their expulsion from the garden of Eden. It's presence here is full of symbolic meaning.

That the snake's presence has influenced the speaker is undoubtedly hinted at when the speaker asserts that nothing at the camp site has changed, seeming to imply that she herself has changed. A similar instance of indirect statement and understatement occurs at the very end of the first stanza as well. There, the speaker declares that the girls are floating, held up by their innocence and ignorance just as the lilies are held up by the water. Two interesting inferences occur here. The water upon which the lilies float is described as murky and frightening. So too, then, is the girls' ignorance. Everything that they do not understand about the world is equally frightening and murky. However, where the lilies are rooted deeply at the pond's bottom, no mention is made of anything that the girls may be rooted to. The omission is a glaring one in that it presents a deep contrast between the rooted but buoyant lilies and the buoyant but unmoored girls.

At the poem's end, the girls lie arranged in their own constellation (in the spokes of a wheel) as they gaze at the stars and name them. Here too they are unmoored. The stars, floating in the ether, are defined by the patterns they make. The dimmer stars in this scenario are deemed as important as the brighter. From this statement, the speaker returns to the lilies, as she notes that they are grouped in the pond in much the same way as the stars (in fact, she even calls the lilies stars). They are all interconnected by their extensive root system, and they form constellations of their own. The poem is brought full circle here as well, as it opens with the girls' attempts to pluck the biggest and brightest of the lilies. In addition, if the girls float in their innocence as the lilies float in the pond, and if the lilies are (or are like) stars, then it follows that the girls also are (or are like) stars.

Source: Leah Tieger, Critical Essay on "The Lotus Flowers," in *Poetry for Students*, Gale, Cengage Learning, 2010.

Steven Cramer

In the following excerpted interview, Cramer discusses with Voigt the influences on her poetry.

> A LYRIC IS ENTIRELY ABOUT INTENSITY. IT'S ABOUT ALL OF IT SPIRALING IN, AND HOLDING THAT INTENSITY, AND NOT RELENTING. AND I THINK AS THE GENERAL POPULATION READS LESS AND LESS POETRY, THAT KIND OF ATTENTION IS HARDER AND HARDER TO PROVIDE."

"I want to bring outdoors inside," says Ellen Bryant Voigt in "Dooryard Flower," a poem published in *The Atlantic Monthly* last March. That extravagant, paradoxical, *impossible* wish gets at the heart of Voigt's poetic project. From her first book, *Claiming Kin* (1976), through each subsequent volume—*The Forces of Plenty* (1983), *The Lotus Flowers* (1987), *Two Trees* (1992), and *Kyrie* (1995)—Voigt's poetry has reflected her restless search for the means to unite two artistic impulses: to sing and to tell stories. And because she never rests satisfied with a form she's mastered, each time she strives to reconcile song and story, she does so in an unexpected way. Lapidary, emotionally charged lyrics; familial, mythic, and historical narratives; meditative poems linked to epigrammatic "variations"; a sonnet sequence scored for multiple voices—Voigt's work as a whole recites the tale of one artist's "will to change." Her subjects are often local—the woods, the backyard, the family plot, children, seasons—but her overriding concern is universal: choice and fate, and the tension between them that constitutes human life.

This month Voigt publishes *The Flexible Lyric,* a collection of the critical essays she has been writing for the past fifteen years. The book is a passionate defense of the richness, variety, and ambition of the lyric mode, but it's much more than that. *The Flexible Lyric* offers a portrait of a reader's mind—one that can reveal the textures of a poem with microscopic precision and derive aesthetic lessons informed by bracing common sense. And it's a celebration of poetic virtues that are also ethical virtues: clarity, strong feeling honed by intelligence, and what she calls a "relentless striving to be accurate."

Born in Virginia in 1943, Voigt grew up on a farm and, from an early age, was a serious student of the piano—elements of her background that contributed to the vivid imagery and musical patterns in her poetry. She attended Converse College and the University of Iowa. She has received grants from the National Endowment for the Arts, the Guggenheim Foundation, and the Lila Wallace-Reader's Digest Fund. *Kyrie* was a finalist for the National Book Critics Circle award. Voigt has taught at Goddard College and M.I.T., and now teaches for the Warren Wilson College low-residency M.F.A. Program for Writers. She lives in Vermont, where she is currently the state poet. Her reputation as a generous, rigorous mentor is matched by her reputation as one of our most reliably memorable poets.

You were trained as a pianist. You write poetry about music; you write about poems in The Flexible Lyric by paying attention to their musical structures, and you've often used musical analogies in making your own poems. Could you talk about how you became a poet when, for a while, you were quite serious about becoming a musician?

I started playing the piano because my older sister did. For a long time I wanted to be my sister, and the form that took was to want to do whatever she did. She started piano lessons when I was four, so I started piano lessons. She didn't ultimately stick with them, but I did. And I did so because essentially I'm a formalist; that's part of my makeup. I don't have much tolerance for disorder, and of course the world is full of disorder. But the impulse for order can't really take its form in language until you have language. So I was very lucky to have music.

Another thing music provided me was solitude. I grew up on a farm in southern Virginia with lots of relatives around from my father's family and my mother's family. It was exceedingly claustrophobic. Both of my parents loved music and had come from musical families. As long as they could hear the music coming from the piano, I was excused from other things. It was really about the only time I could be alone. Playing piano was an occasion for solitude that was socially sanctioned, which I think is really important in terms of my notion of music, or my relationship to it. Now that I've written poetry for this long, I can look back and see poem after poem that takes up the friction between that solitary individual and whatever that social unit is, be it small or large.

Negotiating the right relationship between self and world?

Exactly. When I decided I needed to escape from this little town, I thought music was going to take me out. My lifetime goal was to be a high school band director; I went to school to become one. Most conservatories trained for performance, and I discovered I didn't like to perform on stage. I loved playing for other people; in college, I played for the chorus and for voice and cello lessons, and I played for the swim team. But I didn't have the technique or the temperament to be a concert pianist.

In the meantime, what I was good at—as often happens—I didn't value to the extent I might have. I could sight-read very well, and play by ear—only after thirty years of making poems do I know that my love of music was love of pattern, of harmony and theory. And those were the courses they kept "placing" me out of. Meanwhile I had various terrible jobs playing the piano, including one at a resort, playing junk all night. And then I saw that I was not suited to be a high school band director, because I didn't have enough patience. In the middle of this, a friend who loved poetry read me some poems, and I was stunned. In my high school, in the fifties, we read "The highwayman came riding, riding, riding, up to the old inn door." That was poetry.

Do you remember the poems your friend read to you?

e. e. cummings and Rilke—"The Panther." Having taken mainly music courses, I had a kind of intellectual hunger by that time. So I signed up for the sophomore survey in English literature where I discovered *Beowulf*; and this was it. I fell in love. I didn't have it in mind to write poems; I just wanted to read them. I took more and more English literature and less and less music. And along the way I started writing poems as an act of homage. They hardly made any sense, I can tell you.

Earlier you called yourself a "formalist." Could you explain what you mean by that term? When you say, "I'm a formalist" you don't mean simply "received" forms.

If you see, out of the corner of your inner eye, this shapely, delicate piece of pottery you want to create, and then you go to the store to get whatever materials you need, and you have an excess of them, but put your first allegiance to that palpable shape you have perceived—even if it means that you will use hardly any of these materials—if that's your first allegiance, then I think you are a formalist. The alternative is to have the materials there, and to see what can be made of them, with first allegiance to those materials: you are willing to compromise on what I think of as the balanced relationship of all the parts. That balance is what "form" means to me.

In The Flexible Lyric you write: "poetry's first allegiance is to music." And "Song and Story," the last poem in Two Trees, suggests a tension that figures persistently in your work: the lyric versus the narrative impulse. Can you talk about those two modes—are they in conflict or do they collaborate?

That's the crucial question I've spent roughly ten years thinking about and trying to figure out. The problem for the poet, I think, is to determine what structure is available to accommodate the materials the poem is going to need. I came to see a huge difference between a narrative structure and a lyric structure. The lyric, of course, has always included various parts of what we think of as story. They're sort of "back story." They lie behind every lyric: that sense of an utterance, a character, a voice in a particular circumstance. But with the lyric structure, the arrangement of the materials is very different.

So how you deploy the elements governs whether it's a narrative or a lyric?

Yes, and the definition I finally came up with—which I use in the essays and have used in teaching—has to do with the order in which the materials are released to the reader.

One thing you can do when you finish a book is to set yourself some new challenge. When I started writing *The Lotus Flowers* I wanted to learn how to write a narrative poem, even if only to understand how a narrative differs from a lyric. I don't know that I succeeded in *The Lotus Flowers*. Narrative isn't the structure I see when I look at the world. What drives me most in the world are those things that join us, things we all have in common, which are not many. But they have to do with the emotional life. That does not fuel a narrative. What fuels a narrative are all the ways in which we are different.

But despite this, narrative could be thought of as the more sociable form. There are ways in which it's more accessible because it varies the intensity for the reader or the listener. "Tell me a story," we say, and then listen to the story because

the storyteller has opportunities to vary again and again the story's rate of intensity. A lyric is entirely about intensity. It's about all of it spiraling in, and holding that intensity, and not relenting. And I think as the general population reads less and less poetry, that kind of attention is harder and harder to provide.

When I finished the poems in *The Lotus Flowers*, I came to suspect the orderly structure of narrative—beginning, middle, and end. For about two years I wrote nothing but fragments. I came to think of them as "middles," as having anti-narrative impulses behind them. I also came to think of them as what a painter might produce, what Monet did when he went out to paint the same haystack every day in different light. For me, that meant allowing myself to take on huge subjects—truth, or beauty, or innocence—and go to that subject every day and have the variant be tone. What would be light for a painter would be tone for a poet.

Source: Steven Cramer, "Song and Story," in *Atlantic*, November 24, 1999.

SOURCES

Campion, Peter, Review of *The Lotus Flowers*, in *Poetry*, Vol. 189, No. 4, January 2007, p. 317.

Cramer, Steven, "Song and Story: An Interview with Ellen Bryant Voigt," in *Atlantic*, November 24, 1999.

Freedman, Estelle, *No Turning Back: The History of Feminism and the Future of Women*, Ballantine, 2002.

Hirsch, Edward, "Heroes and Villanelles," in *New York Times Book Review*, August 23, 1987.

Hoagland, Tony, "About Ellen Bryant Voigt: A Profile," in *Ploughshares*, Winter 1996–1997.

Kennelly, Laura B., "Ellen Bryant Voigt," in *Dictionary of Literary Biography*, Vol. 120, *American Poets Since World War II*, 3rd ser., Gale Research, 1992, pp. 307–11.

Scheub, Harold, *The Poem in the Story: Music, Poetry, and Narrative*, University of Wisconsin Press, 2002.

"Women's Studies Timeline," in *San Diego State University Department of Education*, http://www-rohan.sdsu.edu/dept/wsweb/timeline.htm (accessed August 21, 2009).

Voigt, Ellen Bryant, "The Lotus Flowers," in *The Made Thing: An Anthology of Contemporary Southern Poetry*, 2nd ed., edited by Leon Stokesbury, University of Arkansas Press, 1999, pp. 325–26.

FURTHER READING

Frost, Elisabeth A., and Cynthia Hogue, eds., *Innovative Women Poets: An Anthology of Contemporary Poetry and Interviews*, University of Iowa Press, 2006.

    This anthology presents readers with insight into the poetry of Voigt's peers and also includes fourteen lengthy interviews with contemporary female poets.

Shakespeare, William, *The Narrative Poems*, edited by Jonathan V. Crewe, Penguin Classics, 1999.

    This anthology of Shakespeare's classic narrative poems includes "A Lover's Complaint," "The Passionate Pilgrim," "The Phoenix and the Turtle," and "Venus And Adonis."

Voigt, Ellen Bryant, *The Flexible Lyric*, University of Georgia Press, 1999.

    While Voigt's "The Lotus Flowers" is a narrative poem, most of her poetry is written in the lyric form. These nine essays, written by the poet toward the latter part of her career, all explore the art of lyric poetry. Voigt also includes her impressions of numerous lyric poets and their work.

Yapp, Nick, *1980s: Decades of the 20th Century*, Ullmann, 2008.

    This pictorial history is produced by Getty Images and provides an artistic and insightful exploration into the 1980s.

Mushrooms

SYLVIA PLATH

1960

"Mushrooms" is a poem by American poet Sylvia Plath. The poem was published in England in 1960 in Plath's first collection of verse *The Colossus*. An American edition, *The Colossus and Other Poems* followed in 1962. "Mushrooms" is also available in *The Collected Poems*, edited by Ted Hughes in 1981.

The poem has as its main theme the unexpected power of small and seemingly insignificant things, as symbolized by the growth of mushrooms. While showing an intense sympathy toward nature and its processes, "Mushrooms" can also be interpreted as having a feminist message. This aspect of the poem fits Plath's reputation as an early voice in the emerging feminist movement of the 1960s.

Much of Plath's work has an intensely autobiographical aspect. As her journal writings show, she was preoccupied with the question of how she, as a woman, could forge an identity and define herself in relation to society. This preoccupation became a central theme in her only novel, *The Bell Jar* (1963), and in much of her poetry. "Mushrooms" is a seminal work in Plath's lifelong exploration of an issue that is still much discussed today.

AUTHOR BIOGRAPHY

Plath was born on October 27, 1932, in Boston, Massachusetts, the daughter of German immigrant

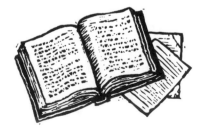

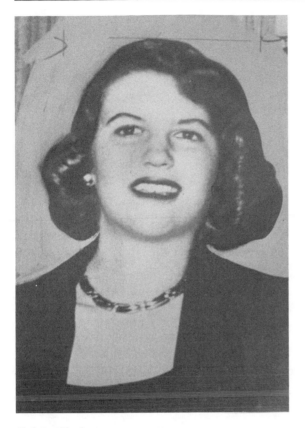

Sylvia Plath (*The Library of Congress*)

Otto Emil Plath, a professor of biology, and Aurelia Schober Plath, a teacher. Plath's father died of diabetes when she was eight years old. Many of her poems focus on her relationship with her father, including "The Colossus," the title poem of the collection in which "Mushrooms" appears.

Plath excelled in her high school studies and published stories and poems in national magazines. She won a scholarship to Smith College and studied there from 1950 to 1955. In 1952 she won a fiction contest run by *Mademoiselle* magazine, and she won a guest editorship to work at the magazine the following year. During this time she began suffering from the depression that would ultimately lead to her death. In a journal entry of June 20, 1958 (quoted by Timothy Materer in *Dictionary of Literary Biography,*), she wrote, "it is as if my life were magically run by two electric currents: joyous positive and despairing negative—which ever is running at the moment dominates my life, floods it." She later based her novel, *The Bell Jar* (1963), on her experiences during this period. On returning home

from New York City, she was given electroshock therapy. On August 24, 1953 she made her first suicide attempt, swallowing sleeping pills. She was hospitalized and physically recovered. After returning to college, she graduated with honors in 1955.

Plath won a Fulbright scholarship to study at Newnham College, Cambridge, England. In February, 1956, she met and fell passionately in love with English poet Ted Hughes. They married on June 16, 1956. Their relationship was tumultuous and Plath often suspected that Hughes was having affairs. After Plath gained her master's degree from Cambridge, the couple went to live in the United States, where Plath taught literature at Smith College. In 1958 they moved to Boston and tried to live off their income from writing. Plath published poems in national magazines but was depressed about a lack of progress in her writing career and publishers' rejections of her first volume of poetry, *The Colossus*.

In 1959 Plath and Hughes moved to England, where Plath had greater success. *The Colossus* was published in 1960 and in the same year, the couple had a daughter, Frieda. Plath later won a Saxton fellowship that enabled her to work on her novel, *The Bell Jar*, and she also wrote large numbers of poems. In February 1962, the couple had a son, Nicholas. That summer, the marriage broke up, and Hughes, who was having an affair, moved to London, leaving Plath to raise their two children. *The Bell Jar*, which tells the story of a young woman's search for identity, her descent into depression, and her subsequent suicide attempt, was published in January 1963 under the pseudonym Victoria Lucas.

Plath struggled with poor health, depression, and the responsibilities of lone parenthood. On February 11, 1963, Plath sealed up the doors of her children's rooms with damp towels, turned the kitchen gas oven on, thrust her head inside, and ended her life. After her death, Plath became an iconic figure for some feminists. They blamed Hughes's treatment of Plath for her suicide. As executor of her estate, Hughes controlled the editing and publication of her work, and he has been criticized for withholding or destroying material that was thought to have reflected badly on him.

Since her death, Plath has become recognized as a major poet of the Confessional School (a school of poetry that deals frankly with the speaker's negative experiences, such as illness, addiction, and relationship problems) and a chronicler of women's search for self-identity and of fascination with death. She was posthumously awarded the Pulitzer Prize in Poetry in 1982 for her volume, *Collected Poems* (Harper, 1981), edited by Hughes, which contains "Mushrooms."

POEM SUMMARY

Stanza 1

On the most literal level, "Mushrooms" is a description of the natural process of the growth of mushrooms. The poem opens with a description of how mushrooms appear seemingly out of nothing, quietly, unexpectedly, and without fuss. They appear overnight. Their white color is noted.

Stanza 2

Using imagery of body parts that normally applies to human beings, the poet describes the mushrooms as pushing through loam, a type of rich, fertile soil considered ideal for growing plants. Having taken possession of one element, the earth, they now emerge into, and take possession of, the air. The stanza makes clear for the first time that the voice of the poem is the first person plural. This means that the poet is speaking as if she is one of the mushrooms.

Stanza 3

The mushrooms grow in secret, with no one noticing their presence. The idea is introduced that some people may want to prevent the mushrooms from growing and treacherously reveal their existence. But this does not happen, and the mushrooms are allowed to progress unimpeded. The grains that make up the soil are portrayed as making space for the mushrooms.

Stanza 4

As in stanza 2, the mushrooms are personified, with the suggestion that they have hands that they use to fight their way out of the earth. There is some effort involved, as the mushrooms have to lift the weight of the soil and other materials that lie on the earth. The soil is described as being covered with pine needles and leaves.

Stanza 5

The mushrooms force their way through or past even the heavy weight of paving stones. They are imagined, metaphorically speaking, as having

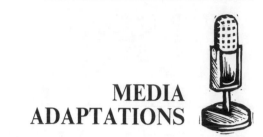

MEDIA ADAPTATIONS

- *Sylvia Plath Reads* (Caedmon, 2000) is an audiocassette of Plath reading her poetry, including "Mushrooms."
- *Voices & Visions: Sylvia Plath* (Winstar, 2000) is a videotape of Plath reading her poetry and speaking in interviews. Commentaries by friends, family, and critics are included.
- *Sylvia* (Universal, 2003) is a biographical film of Plath's tumultuous relationship with Ted Hughes, starring Gwyneth Paltrow as Plath and Daniel Craig as Hughes, and directed by Christine Jeffs.

hammers or rams with which they push their way through obstacles. This image likens them to soldiers laying siege to a fort. The fact that they lack ears and eyes is both a literal and accurate description of mushrooms and (since the personification of the mushrooms has already given them a human aspect) a sinister image, as the idea of a person without ears and eyes would frighten many people. It also, paradoxically, robs the mushrooms of humanity and individuality, as ears and eyes are part of the sensory equipment of human beings.

Stanza 6

The poet returns to the idea introduced in stanza 1 of the quietness of the mushrooms' progress. Not only are the mushrooms, as mentioned in stanza 5, lacking ears and eyes, but they also lack a voice. Again, this is both literally accurate, as mushrooms do not make sounds, and an image that dehumanizes and de-individualizes the mushrooms. It is often said of dispossessed and downtrodden people that they lack a voice, and the poet's portrayal of the mushrooms as voiceless identifies them with these oppressed groups.

In another personifying image using a human body part, the mushrooms are shown pushing their way through holes in an attempt to grow to their full stature. They are successful, as the cracks are forced apart by their efforts.

Stanza 7

In a run-on line (a line that runs from the last line of the previous stanza to the first line of the new stanza), the mushrooms' sparse diet is emphasized. Crumbs and water is the sparsest penitential diet imaginable, but the poet makes it seem even more so by intensifying the idea of crumbs with the insubstantial image of shadows. The blandness of the mushrooms' manner is another factor that emphasizes their ability to fade into the background and not be noticed.

Stanza 8

In another run-on line that crosses stanzas, the poet states that the mushrooms do not ask for much. They are modest and undemanding. Nevertheless, they are successful at multiplying and there are now very many of them. This point is emphasized by the poet's repetition of the second and third lines of the stanza. Repetition used as a literary device is called *anaphora*. The fact that these two lines are also exclamations has the effect of expressing the poet's wonderment at the large number of mushrooms.

Stanza 9

The mushrooms are likened in metaphors to shelves and tables. These are items to which most people give little thought, but people find them useful because they place other items of greater importance on top of them. If the shelves and tables were suddenly removed, the objects they support would crash to the ground. The mushrooms accept this state of things because of their essential humility. The poet is conveying the idea that the mushrooms may be overlooked, but that other things or beings that are given greater status are dependent on them. The final line of this stanza details the way in which other beings depend on mushrooms: the mushrooms are edible and are eaten. This makes the individual mushrooms disappear, as they are consumed.

Stanza 10

The fact mentioned in the previous stanza that the mushrooms are eaten suggests that they disappear, but this stanza makes clear that this is not the end of mushrooms as a collective group. They continue to grow, forcing their way through the earth in their journey of self-realization. They do this in spite of their undoubtedly humble and self-effacing appearance. The final line of the stanza makes clear that the mushrooms have a power that enables them to overcome apparent annihilation: they breed, and rapidly, too.

Stanza 11

The poet ends by invoking the Biblical dictum from Christ's Sermon on the Mount: "Blessed are the meek: for they shall inherit the earth" (Matthew 5:5). While Christian theology often places this event at some point in the distant future, after the Day of Judgment, or in the afterlife, the poet has a shorter timescale in mind: the very next morning. There is a paradox in the fact that something as small and apparently insignificant as the mushrooms can inherit the vast earth. The final line can be taken as a promise or a threat. Like the salesman who sticks his foot in the door to prevent a house-owner shutting him out, so the mushrooms have gained a foothold on world domination.

THEMES

Feminism

The main theme of "Mushrooms" can be seen as the feminist struggle and growth to greater self-awareness. This is treated through the symbolism of the mushrooms, which can be assumed to stand for women.

This interpretation, it might be argued, is the one that is most consistent within the context of the poem. However, symbols frequently have many aspects of meaning and different people interpret the symbol of Plath's mushrooms in different ways. Some essayists have identified the mushrooms with the victims of the Holocaust, jostling for space in cramped conditions; those who suffer mental illness; and even the atomic bomb. The feminist interpretation does not necessarily negate these other interpretations, and the contrary is also true: the other interpretations do not necessarily negate the feminist interpretation.

Life Cycles

"Mushrooms" can be interpreted as a birth myth (a story about the miraculous birth of a hero), or a depiction of death and rebirth. The mushrooms spring into being, apparently out of nothing. This nothingness is the annihilation of being and the death of the spirit, signified externally by their lack of color, voice, eyes, and ears. Inwardly,

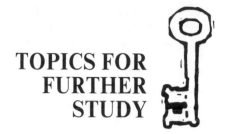

TOPICS FOR FURTHER STUDY

- Research the topic of women's rights before and after World War II in the United States and England. Trace the development and fate of various laws that related to equal rights for women. Make a list of the things that a woman could and could not do in 1930, 1960, 1970, 1980, and 1990, noting if her marital status made any difference. Create a PowerPoint presentation with your findings.

- Write an essay that compares and contrasts Plath's novel, *The Bell Jar*, with her poem "Mushrooms," in terms of themes and authorial voice.

- What relevance, if any, does Plath's "Mushrooms" have to women in today's society? Make a class presentation on your findings in any of the following formats: an oral presentation, a PowerPoint, or a dramatic performance.

- The mushrooms of Plath's poem "Mushrooms" are described as being voiceless. Analyze what it means to lack a voice, either as an individual or a group. Consider such elements as cultural and religious norms; ways of disseminating information, such as the media; poverty; and education. What measures can voiceless people take to acquire a voice in society? What are society's duties and responsibilities in ensuring that people have a voice? Give a class presentation on your findings.

- Read Kashmira Sheth's young-adult novel, *Keeping Corner* (Hyperion, 2007), the story of Leela, a twelve-year-old Indian girl whose husband dies and who encounters Mahatma Gandhi's movement to free India from British rule. Trace Leela's journey of self-discovery and compare and contrast it with the growth process of women as presented in Plath's poem "Mushrooms." Write an essay on your findings.

their blandness, meekness, and discretion contribute to their lack of self-expression and individuality. In terms of the feminist interpretation, these qualities can be seen as having been imposed on women by the expectations of men and society. The poem shows the mushrooms growing and forcing their way into being.

Oppression

The poem's symbolism can also be widened beyond the concept of the feminist uprising to suggest the struggle toward empowerment of all downtrodden and dispossessed people, whatever their gender. There is nothing in the poem that limits its meaning to the female sex. This broader interpretation universalizes the message of the poem and makes a possible thematic link to the civil rights movement, which paralleled the feminist movement after World War II. In this context, the poem is a threat to those in power that the uprising of any previously powerless group of people will come suddenly and without warning.

Self-Examination

"Mushrooms" can be interpreted as detailing women's emergence from invisibility as creatures in their own right. This is not shown as a completed and perfected process but as a work in progress, fraught with challenge and difficulty. Thus the mushrooms are growing but not fully formed. Lacking eyes, ears, and a voice, they resemble embryonic human beings. If it is assumed that the mushrooms represent all dispossessed peoples, then the poem is about the general human struggle for self-identity and self-fulfillment.

Whichever of these interpretations is favored, there is a tension between the desire for growth and individuation and the factors that oppose and oppress these processes. Chief among the opposing factors is the weight of the status quo (a Latin phrase meaning the way things are). The poet makes clear, through references to heaving great weight and vulnerability to discovery and betrayal, that the growth process is onerous and fraught with difficulty. Nevertheless, it ends in triumph, when these small and seemingly insignificant fungi come into possession of the earth.

However, in keeping with Plath's discomfiting voice, this triumph is not expressed in terms of a joyful event. The mushrooms that inherit the earth seem as invasive as salespersons who force a way into someone's home by sticking their foot in the door. The poet does not make clear

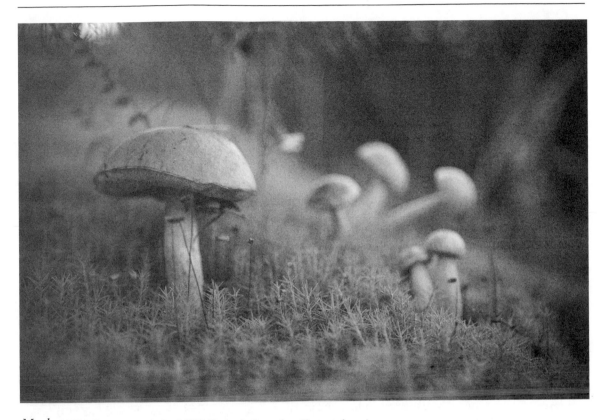

Mushrooms *(Image copyright Barri, 2009. Used under license from Shutterstock.com)*

what happens next, but the symbolism and ominous language suggest that the mushrooms will meet with a hostile confrontation rather than a welcome. The poet suggests that women's self-realization will not be celebrated by all, but instead could be seen as a threat and an alien invasion.

STYLE

Confessional Poetry

In 1958 Plath attended Robert Lowell's poetry seminar in Boston, where she met fellow poet Anne Sexton and became familiar with her work. Plath later identified Lowell and Sexton as poets whose work she admired for what became known as the confessional mode of poetry that they pioneered. The three poets are frequently linked by critics.

Confessional poetry engages in the unabashed exploration of the less salubrious aspects of the poet's life, such as marital difficulties, mental illness, fascination with death, and addiction. It has to do with self-disclosure, without the usual societal filters of discretion or modesty.

While several of Plath's poems fit this mold, the self-disclosure of "Mushrooms" takes a somewhat different form. This is best expressed by Ted Hughes (quoted by Kathleen Margaret Lant in her essay, "The Big Strip Tease: Female Bodies and Male Power in the Poetry of Sylvia Plath"), who noted that Plath shared with Lowell and Sexton not only a similar geographical homeland but also "the central experience of a shattering of the self, and the labour of fitting it together again or finding a new one." "Mushrooms" can be interpreted as detailing the dehumanization and oppression of the female individual and her attempt to build another identity.

Symbolism

A symbol in literature is a thing that stands for or suggests another thing. Often, a visible and concrete thing will be used to suggest something invisible or abstract. Here, Plath uses a visible thing, the growth of mushrooms, to suggest an abstract thing, the feminist uprising and the empowerment of women. (Plath was preoccupied with the journey toward self-identity and self-fulfillment at a time when women did not have rights equal to men. This leads many readers to conclude that the poem is symbolic of the feminist struggle.) More generally, the mushrooms can be said to symbolize any dispossessed group that is growing into its power.

Personification

The symbolism of "Mushrooms" relies upon personification, a literary device in which inanimate or non-human entities (in this case, mushrooms) are given human qualities. The mushrooms are given human-type body parts and behavior, but this stops short of completeness: they are human yet lack ears, eyes, and a voice. This creates a sinister effect and also emphasizes the fact that they are denied full power and complete humanity. This plays into the feminist theme of the poem. While women are portrayed as heavily relied upon for support in the manner of tables or shelves, they are not listened to or credited with full sensory perception. In addition, women who lack eyes and ears might be expected to be blind and deaf to injustices done to them.

There is an implicit question of what would happen to an eyeless, earless, and voiceless woman if she suddenly came into possession of these things. She would be able to see and hear injustice and she would be able to speak about it.

Verse Form

"Mushrooms" is written in a strict and regular verse form which creates an austere impression. There are eleven stanzas of three lines each. Each line has five syllables.

The poet also uses alliteration (repetition of consonants), consonance (repetition of the same consonant two or more times in quick succession), and assonance (repetition of vowel sounds) to enrich the rhythm and meaning. For example, the first line of stanza 2 uses two long *o* sounds (assonance) to reflect the gradual but forceful effort that the mushrooms must expend in their growth.

An example of consonance occurs in the first line of stanza 4, which has four *s*'s. This has the effect of linking the first two words of the line through their *s* sounds with the word *insist*, which has two such sounds. Thus, the entire line adds to the strength of the idea of the insistence of the mushrooms' growth.

The pairing of similar sounds frequently recurs in the poem. In the penultimate (or second to last) stanza the first and third lines use assonance to link words of similar meaning in pairs, reinforcing their significance. The repetition of similar sounds reflects the meaning of the unstoppable multiplication and growth of the mushrooms.

The poem uses eye rhymes, a similarity in spelling between words that are pronounced differently and therefore do not produce an auditory rhyme, to add to the rhythm. The last two lines of the first stanza, for example, each end in a word ending in *-etly*, though the vowel sound of the *e* in each of these words is pronounced differently. The first line, too, ends in the same *-y* sound (assonance). The repetition of these visuals and sounds contributes to the sense of insistent effort and persistence on the part of the indomitable mushrooms.

There are also half rhymes in the poem. A half rhyme is consonance on the final consonants of the words involved. The poet sometimes ties together two stanzas with such half rhymes, as with stanzas 4 and 5. Here, the last line of stanza 4 ends in *-ing*, as does the first line of stanza 5. In this case, the half rhyme, as well as creating auditory rhythm, ties together two words of similar meaning. Both words refer to the material of which the ground is made and through which the mushrooms must push in order to grow.

HISTORICAL CONTEXT

The Women's Rights Movement

Plath wrote "Mushrooms" in post–World War II England. During the war, both in England and the United States, many men of working age went away to fight in the war and women were left to run businesses and work in industry. Furthermore, many men died in combat, so women were needed in greater numbers in the workforce after World War II than they had been before it. These historical events were a major spur for the growth of the feminist movement during the 1960s, 1970s, and 1980s. It was argued that as women were doing the same work as men, they should be paid the same and enjoy equal rights.

During the 1960s in the United States, several federal laws were passed that were designed to improve the economic status of women. The Equal Pay Act of 1963 mandated equal wages for men and women doing equal work. The

COMPARE
&
CONTRAST

- **1960s:** The Equal Rights Amendment to the Constitution, which would have outlawed legal discrimination based on sex, is introduced into every Congressional session, as it has been since 1923. However, state ratification fails and the Amendment is never passed.

  Today: Equality between the sexes is sought in the workplace via the 1964 Civil Rights Amendment, which outlaws discrimination based on race, ethnicity, and gender. While men still earn more than women, this may be due in part to different career choices by women, such as taking time off to have children, or not being willing to travel or relocate.

- **1960s:** In Great Britain, only in 1961 are women teachers granted equal pay with men. The 1960s are marked by a series of strikes by women demanding equal pay with men, ending in the Equal Pay Act of 1970.

  Today: The debate continues over equal pay, with some observers arguing that the real cause of women's lower and unequal pay is job segregation (women tend to favor lower paid careers such as teaching and nursing, and are more likely to work part-time) and the consequent undervaluing of so-called women's skills.

- **1960s:** In the United States, as a result of the activities of the civil rights movement, most of the laws that mandated racial segregation are removed by 1968.

  Today: The remaining barriers to racial integration are mostly social, cultural, and economic. Housing and religion are highly racially segregated.

- **1960s:** Anne Sexton's poetry, published in volumes such as *To Bedlam and Part Way Back* (1960) and *All My Pretty Ones* (1962), helps pioneer the female confessional voice.

  Today: Poets such as Adrienne Rich continue to develop confessional poetry in a way that describes the female experience of life and society.

Civil Rights Act of 1964 outlawed discrimination against women by any company with over twenty-five employees. In 1967 a Presidential Executive Order was issued prohibiting bias against women by federal government employers.

However, discrimination against women in daily life remained. Married women often could not obtain credit cards in their own name. Single or divorced women often could not obtain credit to purchase a house or a car: stories were rife about women having to take along male friends for the purpose of signing the credit agreement, even when they were not the real purchasers.

Even in the area of crime, women were discriminated against. A woman who shot and killed her husband could be accused of homicide, but a man who shot his wife could be accused of a lesser crime of passion. In Pennsylvania, only in 1968 did the courts void a state law that ruled that any woman convicted of a felony should be sentenced to the maximum punishment prescribed by law.

In most states, abortion was only deemed legal if the mother's life was proven to be physically endangered by continuing with the pregnancy. This state of affairs was overturned in 1973 by a landmark case in the Supreme Court, Roe vs. Wade, which ruled that a mother may abort her pregnancy for any reason, up until the point at which the fetus becomes viable.

The Civil Rights Movement

Running parallel with the women's rights movement in the United States was the civil rights movement (approximately 1955–68). The civil rights movement attempted to abolish public and private acts of discrimination on the basis of race, particularly with regard to African Americans.

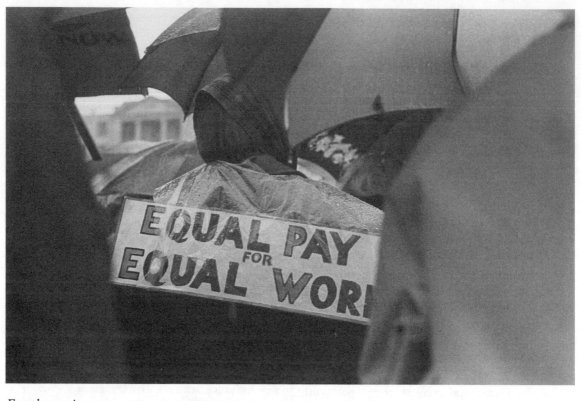

Equal pay sign (Homer Sykes | Getty Images)

The period between 1955 and 1968 was marked by outbreaks of nonviolent protest and civil disobedience aimed at drawing attention to the lack of equity faced by African Americans. One pivotal episode in the civil rights struggle took place on December 1, 1955, when an African American woman and civil rights activist, Rosa Parks, refused to give up her seat on a bus to make room for a white passenger. Her act and the subsequent Montgomery, Alabama bus boycott led to the abolition of segregation on public buses in 1956. In 1960, a student sit-in was held at a Woolworth's store in Greensboro, North Carolina, to protest Woolworth's policy of excluding African Americans. Four African American students from North Carolina Agricultural and Technical College, an all-black college, sat down at the segregated lunch counter at Woolworth's, leaving space for white sympathizers to sit among them. The civil rights movement culminated with the passage of the Civil Rights Act of 1964 and the Voting Rights Act of 1965 which together made discrimination illegal and protected the voting rights of African Americans.

The Treatment of Depression

Electroconvulsive therapy or electroshock treatment was a popular treatment for severe depression in the 1930s, 1940s, and 1950s. Plath was given electroconvulsive therapy for depression, but it only seemed to increase her anxiety. Electroconvulsive therapy is still used today as a treatment for depression, schizophrenia, and bipolar disorder (moods of depression and abnormally elevated mood, or mania). It has gained a controversial reputation due to suggestions that it can cause brain damage. One of its side-effects is memory loss.

The two other main treatments for depression are medication, and psychotherapy, which Plath was treated with. One of the most popular psychotherapies is cognitive behavioral therapy, which aims to change negative thought patterns and behaviors. A commonly prescribed drug treatment for depression is selective serotonin reuptake inhibitors (SSRIs), though controversy has arisen over side-effects said to include suicidal and homicidal ideation (a desire to kill oneself or other people).

CRITICAL OVERVIEW

At the time of her death, Plath was known only to a small circle of other poets. Her fame, and income from her poetry, came later. The collection in which "Mushrooms" was first published, *The Colossus*, was initially rejected by publishers in the United States, but was published in England in 1960.

Because of Plath's relatively modest profile, John Wain was one of the few critics who reviewed the collection. Writing in the *Spectator* in 1961 (quoted in *Modern American Literature*), Wain praises Plath's "care for the springy rhythm, the arresting image and—most of all, perhaps—the unusual word." Wain adds that Plath writes "clever, vivacious poetry, which will be enjoyed most by intelligent people capable of having fun with poetry and not just being holy about it." While Wain notes that Plath had already found "an individual manner," he adds that some of the poems were too derivative of the work of other poets. Roy Fuller, writing in *London* magazine (quoted by Timothy Materer in the *Dictionary of Literary Biography,*), also finds the work "derivative."

Mary Lynn Broe, in her essay, "Protean Poetic: The Poetry of Sylvia Plath," identifies "Mushrooms" as one of several poems of Plath's that "reinforce the ominous power of diminished things ... quiet and discreet, those self-effacing 'Mushrooms' suddenly become threatening despite the cautious syllabics of the poem."

Broe laments the "revisionist" views of the collection that appeared after Plath's suicide, in which critics began to mine *The Colossus* for "the macabre and grisly elements" that might have foreshadowed Plath's suicide: "Now described as a 'breviary of estrangement,' *The Colossus* became a casebook for those seeking evidence of suicidal despair."

Broe writes that after the English poet, writer, and critic A. Alvarez suggested that "the disciplined art of *The Colossus* functioned as a fence to keep psychological disturbance at bay, critics and reviewers jumped on the 'suicide bandwagon' in their eagerness to mythologize Plath." Since these reviewers equated pathology with poetic power, Broe writes, "Any diminished quality of pain or estrangement in the poems hinted that the poet had not yet come to grips with her subject as an artist."

A. Alvarez, in his book, *The Savage God* (quoted in *Modern American Literature*), makes a comment about Plath's work that illuminates the style and subject matter of "Mushrooms." Alvarez believes that Plath thought of herself as a poetic realist, for whom the "extraordinary inner wealth of imagery and associations was almost beside the point." Alvarez explains:

> Because she felt she was simply describing the facts as they had happened, she was able to tap in the coolest possible way all her large reserves of skill: those subtle rhymes and half-rhymes, the flexible, echoing rhythms and offhand colloquialism by which she preserved, even in her most anguishing probing, complete artistic control. Her internal horrors were as factual and precisely sensed as the barely controllable stallion on which she was learning to ride or the car she had tried to smash up.

For Joyce Carol Oates in her 1973 essay, "The Death Throes of Romanticism: The Poetry of Sylvia Plath" (quoted in *Modern American Literature*), Plath's poetry makes personal and accessible the tragedy and spiritual decay of the modern world. In an appraisal of a number of Plath's collections, including *The Colossus*, Oates calls Plath "a tragic figure involved in a tragic action," adding, "her tragedy is offered to us as a near-perfect work of art" in these works.

CRITICISM

Claire Robinson

Robinson has an M.A. in English. She is a former teacher of English literature and creative writing and a freelance writer and editor. In the following essay, she explores how Sylvia Plath's "Mushrooms" functions as a birth myth for the woman of the modern era.

A birth myth or birth tale is a story about the often miraculous birth and infancy of a hero or, in some cases, an entire race of people or a nation. In the case of a hero, the baby is deprived of his true parents and heritage and is cast by fate into a different environment, many times a lowly one, in which he must struggle to survive. The hero is frequently of royal or aristocratic birth but is raised by humble people. This can be seen as giving him a more complete view of the world than he would have had if he had never left his privileged birthright, as well as exposing him to unusual trials that help form his character and prove his worth.

WHAT DO I READ NEXT?

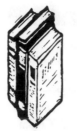

- Plath's *The Bell Jar* (first published in 1963, republished by Harper, 2000), is a heavily autobiographical novel that tells the story of a young woman's mental breakdown and suicide attempt during an internship at a New York-based magazine. It gives an insight into the awareness that gave birth to "Mushrooms."

- Virginia Woolf's nonfiction work *A Room of One's Own* (first published 1929), republished with another of Woolf's works, *Three Guineas*, as *A Room of One's Own and Three Guineas* (Oxford World's Classics, 2008), is closely related thematically to Plath's "Mushrooms." It is a critique of the historical exclusion of women from education and economic independence. In *Three Guineas* (first published 1938), Woolf argues that this historical exclusion could enable women to stand apart from and oppose the drive towards fascism and war.

- *Making Waves: An Anthology of Writings by and about Asian American Women*, edited by Elaine Kim, Lilia V. Villanueva, and Asian Women United of California (Beacon Press, 1989) is a collection of fiction, poetry, and essays by Asian American women. Topics covered include women's search for an identity, feminism, immigration, and prejudice against women and Asians.

- *Pushing the Limits: American Women 1940–1961* by Elaine Tyler May (Oxford University Press, 1998) is Volume 9 of the "Young Oxford History of Women in the United States" series. The book, which is aimed at young adults, considers the stories of prominent women from many different races and cultures in tracing the rise of feminism from the Great Depression to the early 1960s.

- In 1955 the civil rights movement changed forever when an African American woman, Rosa Parks, refused to give up her seat on a bus to a white person. Her autobiography, aimed at older children and young adults and published as *Rosa Parks: My Story*, by Rosa Parks and Jim Haskins (Puffin, 1999), tells the inspiring story of Parks's life and her civil rights activism.

- Betty Friedan's book, *The Feminine Mystique* (first published in 1963, republished by W.W. Norton, 2001), is a seminal work of feminist thinking that depicts femininity as a social and cultural construct. It argues that women, who have no identity except as someone's wife and mother and are denied all creative expression except for giving birth, are manipulated into becoming mere consumers who try to fill the emotional void in their lives by shopping.

- *Silences*, a nonfiction work by the Jewish American author Tillie Olsen (first published in 1978 and available in an edition published by the Feminist Press at CUNY, 2003), analyzes why women are under-represented in literature. Olsen argues that women, especially those of lower socioeconomic classes, are silenced by societal expectations as well as by censorship and self-censorship.

- Plath's poem "Lady Lazarus" (published in *The Collected Poems* by Sylvia Plath, edited by Ted Hughes, Harper, reprint, 1981) is a verse monolog and a life-death-rebirth myth. Voiced by a woman who has survived death multiple times, the poem is inspired by the Biblical figure of Lazarus, a man who was raised from the dead by Jesus Christ. While it is often read as a description of Plath's suicide attempts, it has deeper mythic resonances and deals with themes such as fascination with death, perceptions of the female body, and female power.

> " FOR PLATH, WOMANHOOD ITSELF—NOT SIMPLY THE WAY THAT WOMEN WERE TREATED BY SOCIETY—WAS A BURDEN AND A PRISON: THE DISEASE WAS WITHIN AS WELL AS WITHOUT."

In time, the hero comes of age and reclaims his true heritage and high position in society.

The Biblical stories of Jesus Christ and of Moses are examples of such birth tales, as is the story of the Buddha, the founder of Buddhism, and of Krishna, the god-child of Hinduism. In the case of Jesus Christ, the Bible tells that he was miraculously born of a virgin, though his true father was God. He was born in the humble surroundings of a stable at an inn, which belied his divine origins. Brought up as the ordinary son of a carpenter, he finally became a teacher and leader of men and was acclaimed by his followers as a spiritual savior and the Son of God.

A life-death-rebirth myth or tale is a variation on the birth myth that tells the story of a hero or deity's life, death, and subsequent resurrection. Examples include, once again, Jesus Christ, who, the Bible says, was crucified but rose again from the dead. Another example, from Greek mythology, is Persephone, the daughter of Zeus, king of the gods, and Demeter, goddess of the harvest. Persephone was abducted by Hades, the god of the underworld, who kept her prisoner there. Demeter was so angry that while her daughter was imprisoned in the underworld, the earth ceased to be fertile and winter reigned. Hades was brought to agree to release Persephone back to the earth's surface for a part of the year. When Persephone returned to the earth's surface, fertility returned and plants grew. Thus she was seen as the goddess of fertility and spring.

Sylvia Plath's poem "Mushrooms" is a birth and rebirth myth for the modern age. It is both a personal birth and rebirth myth for the poem's female speaker and, as it taps into widespread female neuroses and concerns, a generic birth and rebirth myth for everywoman.

What is the death that makes rebirth necessary for the modern woman? Joyce Carol Oates writes in her essay, "The Death Throes of Romanticism: The Poetry of Sylvia Plath," that Plath's poetry shows "the pathological aspects of our era that make a death of the spirit inevitable." For Plath, womanhood itself—not simply the way that women were treated by society—was a burden and a prison: the disease was within as well as without. According to Kathleen Margaret Lant, Plath wrote in her journals, "Being born a woman is my awful tragedy. From the moment I was conceived I was doomed ... to have my whole circle of action, thought and feeling rigidly circumscribed by my inescapable femininity." Lant adds that Plath so completely identified power and hope with masculinity that she told a college friend that her ideal family would consist only of herself, her husband, and their magnificently male children. Lant writes that according to Plath's biographer, Nancy Hunter Steiner, "She had decided that her husband would be a very tall man and she spoke, half-jokingly, of producing a race of superchildren, as superlatively large as they were intelligent. The children, she predicted, would all be boys."

"Mushrooms" contains implicitly this death of the female spirit, while describing the rebirth explicitly. The condition of womanhood is portrayed symbolically by the mushrooms. Their birth is shown as sudden and unexpected. Anyone who has observed mushrooms growing knows that they can miraculously appear overnight, seemingly out of nothing. The poet is suggesting in this comparison that women's annihilation has been total and that they have become invisible. Their re-emergence to a position of power will happen without warning, like an ambush. However, even in the rebirth celebrated in the poem, they are still without ears, eyes, and voices, images that connote a being who, like the three wise monkeys of legend, sees no evil, hears no evil, and speaks no evil. These images also bring to mind the clichéd nineteenth-century view of women and children that was preserved, to some extent, until the last decades of the twentieth century: that they should be seen (in a purely decorative role) and not heard. Even the idea that women are visible is qualified, as the mushrooms are white, a non-color that will not, as the old saying has it, frighten the horses.

These ideas are reinforced by the description of the mushrooms' growth as quiet, discreet, and meek. These are all qualities that have been traditionally required of well-brought up women who know and accept an inferior position in society.

The sparse diet of the mushrooms, water and crumbs of shadows, may connote a passage in a seminal work of feminism, Virginia Woolf's nonfiction narrative *A Room of One's Own* (1929). Woolf, in a critique of the denial of a full education to women (most colleges were at that time only open to men), shows her female narrator being denied access to the facilities of a fictional university called Oxbridge, a fusion of the real Oxford and Cambridge Universities. She contrasts this with the freedom of a fictional women's college called Fernham, which, reflecting the real history of women's education, has great difficulties in raising finances to continue operations. Woolf compares the sumptuous dinners served to the male students at the well-financed Oxbridge to the frugal diet of prunes and custard served to the women at Fernham. Both Woolf and Plath are portraying women as second-class citizens who are expected to survive off of substandard fare.

The second stanza of the poem introduces the idea of the mushrooms, and therefore of women, gaining possession of the elements of earth and air. There is a contrast between the smallness and humbleness of the mushroom-women and their grand ambition. This contrast recurs in stanzas 4 and 5, in the opposition of the softness of the mushroom-women's fists and the immense feat of strength that they accomplish in lifting earth and even paving stones. The word fists, used instead of hands, implies a fight.

The idea of combat is carried through the poem in its military metaphors. The second line of the third stanza implies that women's growth to eminence is a secret military siege vulnerable to being betrayed and defeated, presumably by men, the ruling power. The military siege metaphor is taken up again in the fifth stanza, where the mushroom-women are described as having weapons like those wielded by medieval soldiers laying siege to a castle. The implied castle here is male power. Similarly, the mushroom-women's pushing through small holes brings to mind an image of soldiers tunneling into an enemy stronghold, only to pop up unexpectedly within its walls and capture the fort.

In the context of these military metaphors, it is in the mushroom-women's favor to be voiceless, as they are able to accomplish their aims covertly. Thus they are able to turn an apparent weakness into strength. It is perhaps illuminating to bear in mind certain prominent women of history who have carefully constructed a persona of feminine weakness behind which they conceal their formidable strength (Queen Elizabeth I of England, for example). The mushroom-women hide their aspirations to world domination under a bland manner and an avoidance of making demands—again, in line with traditional societal expectations of a decorous woman.

Those readers who like to draw autobiographical parallels with Plath's work may feel that these references are bitter comments on what she saw as an expectation to turn a blind eye to the infidelities of which she accused her husband. But whatever personal relevance these elements of her verse had to Plath, they also have universal application to all women who have felt oppressed by expectations to tolerate behavior that they feel is unacceptable.

The eighth stanza contains an important turning point in the poem marked by the repetition (anaphora) of the exclamations in lines 23 and 24. These lines emphasize the sheer number of the mushroom-women. Suddenly, the mushrooms, which hitherto appear to be determined but vulnerable, appear to possess the strength of numbers. An argument still made today by those seeking equal rights for women is that over fifty percent of the world's population are women, yet in many societies they do not enjoy equity.

The metaphor in stanza 9 that likens the mushroom-women to tables or shelves suggests that women are a vital but overlooked system of support for society. The reference to their being edible has many symbolic resonances. It can suggest that the mushroom-women are consumed by society or by men. Equally, it can suggest that they nourish and sustain society and men, in the same way that tables or shelves support objects that are more valued than they.

The penultimate stanza acknowledges the inherent contradiction at the basis of many women's consciousness: they desire to assert themselves yet feel shame at doing so, leading to the sense that they have to apologize for being as they are and acting as they do. The third line expands on the idea, previously introduced, of strength in numbers. Not only are there many women in the world, but they have a unique power that men lack: the ability to give birth. Thus, by force of sheer numbers and by their ability to multiply, women, like the meek of Christ's Sermon on the Mount, shall inherit the earth.

This grandiloquent prophecy is, however, brought down to earth by Plath's choice of the unheroic image of the humble mushroom to represent women. To portray women as mushrooms shows her ambivalent attitude to her sex and comments wryly on the life-death-rebirth myths of heroes and deities. The mushroom-women, far from appearing as glorious heroes and deities as they reclaim their birthright, remain mere mushrooms, though they are more in number. They are still colorless, earless, eyeless, voiceless, and bland: strange, unformed, and vaguely sinister beings, even to the poem's end. It can be argued that this is how the mushroom-women have been shaped by an oppressive society, so their unprepossessing form and nature is not entirely their fault. But there is to be no final transformation of the mushrooms as they come into their power, no revelation of a beauty that has lain hidden.

The poem also subverts the traditional birth and life-death-rebirth myths in terms of society's response to the reborn hero. The reappearance of the hero is supposed to be greeted by a joyful public. But in the context of Plath's poem, women's reclamation of their birthright will not be welcomed by society. Instead, the last line of the poem likens the victorious mushroom-women to the universally hated figure of the salesman who invades someone's home by planting his foot in the door. Far from being a triumphant resolution, women's victory, it is suggested, is only the start of the real war.

Source: Claire Robinson, Critical Essay on "Mushrooms," in *Poetry for Students*, Gale, Cengage Learning, 2010.

Lisa Narbeshuber

In the following essay, Narbeshuber examines the ways that Plath used public and private connections in her poetry.

Sylvia Plath, in her most ambitious poems, tackles the problem of female selfhood. What is it? Within a world where women are contained by rigid scripts and relegated to silence, how can they revolt? On the one hand, she gives us poems like "The Applicant" and "The Munich Mannequins," where women, reduced to nothing more than commodities, appear robbed of their humanity. On the other hand, in poems such as "Lady

> EACH PIECE OF LADY LAZARUS IS FLAGRANTLY ON SHOW, IN MUCH THE SAME WAY AS THE EARLIEST CONDEMNED CRIMINALS WERE ON DISPLAY DURING PUBLIC TORTURES AND EXECUTIONS."

Lazarus," she presents selves in revolt, resisting assimilation to patriarchal ideals. In both cases, Plath's poetry reacts against the absence, especially for women, of a public space, indeed a language for debate, wherein one might make visible and deconstruct the given order of things. In the following, I argue that Plath deliberately blurs the borders between the public and the private in two of the most celebrated, controversial, and critiqued of her poems: "Daddy" and "Lady Lazarus." Transforming the conventional female body of the 1950s into a kind of transgressive dialect, Plath makes her personae speak in and to a public realm dominated by male desires. Giving the *female construct* voice, so to speak, Plath prefigures recent trends in feminist criticism that read the female body as text. Susan Bordo, for example, sees in the emergence of agoraphobia in the 1950s and anorexia in the 1980s rebellious performances: The public wants to see the woman in the home, so the woman responds by fearing to go out (agoraphobia); the public wants to see the woman thin, so the woman starves herself (anorexia). Bordo summarizes her argument in a language that echoes Plath's poetic desires:

> In hysteria, agoraphobia, and anorexia, then, the woman's body may be viewed as a surface on which conventional constructions of femininity are exposed starkly to view, through their inscription in extreme or hyperliteral form. They are written, of course, in language of horrible suffering. It is as though these bodies are speaking to us of the pathology and violence that lurks just around the corner, waiting at the horizon of "normal" femininity. It is no wonder that a steady motif in the feminist literature on female disorder is that of pathology as embodied *protest—*unconscious, inchoate, and counterproductive protest without an effective language, voice, or politics, but protest nonetheless. (175)

As we will see, in order to bring their private selves into the public realm, the speakers in "Daddy" and "Lady Lazarus" become public performers and rebellious exaggerators, very much like Bordo's agoraphobic and anorexic. They, too, may have trouble communicating (as we will see most obviously in "Daddy"), but this serves to reveal their public voicelessness. Plath's speakers should not be read as pathological case studies; rather it is the culture, written on their bodies, which is exposed as pathological. Likewise, their acts of rebellion almost necessarily contain an unacceptable, self-destructive side. In various ways, Plath brashly pairs the private with the public, to the point where the personal all but dissolves into a ludicrous public performance or event, with the body as displayed object.

This desire in Plath's poetry to trace the connection between the private and the public has not been explored in any depth in Plath criticism. Instead, most criticism reads "Daddy" and "Lady Lazarus" around the psychology of Plath's life, if not exclusively as biography, then as the feminist struggles of a victorious woman over a man or men. For example, critics regard the irrepressible "Lady Lazarus" as "a triumph of vitality" (Broe 175); a journey "from a life of abuse and nightmare to one of liberation" (Markey 122); a wonderful, "searingly self-confident" (Van Dyne 55) exhibition of the speaker's "true identity as a triumphant resurrecting goddess, the fully liberated, fiery true self ... " (Kroll 118–9); an expression of the struggling woman artist's "independent creative powers ... She is neither mad nor 'ugly and hairy,' but a phoenix, a flame of released bodily energy" (Bundtzen 33–4). But such statements are an expression of the commentators' need to find wholeness and steady thought in Plath's poetry, defending her against charges of psychosis, and of a need to identify the emergence of some mighty "Ur-Woman." By focusing on the *conclusion* of such poems as "Lady Lazarus" and limiting their commentary in this way, Plath commentators echo each other's desires to recover some imaginary totality, despite imagery to the contrary. The poems do not bear out the critics' assumptions. When Plath evokes images of wholeness in "Daddy" and "Lady Lazarus," she inevitably undercuts them, emphasizing the systematic play of elements and the constructed ness of meanings. She moves out of the skin of the *individual* and sketches out the social game, the *intersubjective* complexes rather than the *inner strife* that Judith Kroll and other Plath critics focus on. Plath de-

emphasizes identity and emphasizes the roles of various systems. Plath's poetry, then, does not so much demonstrate the crushing of the authentic or "real" self by the patriarchal, as show the role of (social) fantasy in the construction of the subject. More than an attack on the male (or in particular her husband or father), her poetry confronts the mentality of the status quo that accepts the ideology of the individual and notions of the natural, or even the personal, self. She unveils and critiques the private, the hidden, and the normalized by parodying various public discourses of power (gendered male), while portraying her personae as objects of those discourses and, thereby, both the agents and the spectacles of punishment.

Plath creates an arena for public debate in her poetry by relentlessly placing everyday discursive forms (and objects) in quotation marks. She parodies, not just literary form, but everything from machinery to the mythology of the *individual*. But for Plath, ideally, parody does not reform; it destroys. For some critics, Plath's later poetry attempts only an "imitative recasting" (Linda Hutcheon's description of parody). Hutcheon writes how Plath's work "has been seen as a feminist reworking (or parody) of the modes of male modernism which she inherited" (54). But Plath's parodic subversions are not primarily concerned with minor literary debates, such as between the modernist and the romantic. Frederick Buell, for example, writes that, in poems such as "Lady Lazarus," Plath mocks romantic ideas of poetic "incarnation" as "self-destructive unity" (149). Similarly, Toni Saldivar writes how Plath mocks the American literary tradition, perpetuated by Harold Bloom, "of the highly individualistic gnostic imagination that tries to see through the given world in order to see itself in some reassuring self-generated formal identity" (112), while Mary Lynn Broe reads "Daddy" as "pure self-parody," in which "the metaphorical murder of the father dwindles into Hollywood spectacle" (172). These writers are not wrong in their assessments, but, as Hutcheon warns, parody may be limited, in that it often remains conservatively locked within the terms of the discourse it ridicules. Plath sets her sights beyond literary battles or Oedipal struggles.

Not restricting herself to "pure" parody, she attempts to reinvent her world and her place in it. "Daddy," for example, does not so much "dwindle" as explode into Hollywood spectacle, careful to itemize the debris. "Daddy" makes the invisible

visible, the private public, cracking open the interior spaces traditionally designated for women. Plath stages a public trial, turning the commonplace into spectacle, revealing form as deformity, the natural as commodity, domestic life as torture.

It is not surprising, then, that Plath has been lambasted so often for transgressing "good taste." Nevertheless, her "bad form," including her spectacles of abuse, provides a key to understanding her later work. Jacqueline Rose, in her analysis of "Daddy," devotes the entire chapter to the debate over Plath's "inappropriate" use of metaphor. Rose begins, "For a writer who has so consistently produced outrage in her critics, nothing has produced the outrage generated by Sylvia Plath's allusions to the Holocaust in her poetry, and nothing the outrage occasioned by 'Daddy,' which is just one of the poems in which those allusions appear" (205). In defence of Plath's outrageous comparisons, Rose, noting how Plath moves backwards and forwards between the German "Ich" and the English "I," argues that "Daddy" represents, in part, "a crisis of language and identity" (228); after all, Plath was second-generation German: "What the poem presents us with, therefore, is precisely the problem of trying to claim a relationship to an event in which—the poem makes it quite clear—the speaker did not participate" (228). Rose asks in conclusion, "Who can say that these were not difficulties which [Sylvia Plath] experienced in her very person?" (229). In her struggle to show that Plath has "earned" the right to represent the Holocaust ("Whatever her father did to her, it could not have been what the Germans did to the Jews," believes Leon Wieseltier [20]), Rose feels it necessary to turn her into a persecuted German. Her persecution for being a woman (daughter, wife), as the poem would have it, is simply not enough.

James Fenton, although agreeing with Rose, throws out the suggestion that Plath may have believed she actually *was* Jewish:

> Fear of persecution for being a German, whether her own fear or her mother's, would certainly be part of her heritage. And if she thought of her father as a persecuting figure (rightly or wrongly is not an issue), and she knew her father to be Prussian, then it is by no means far-fetched for her to have wondered whether she might not be a Jew (either from her mother's side or through simply not knowing quite what a Jew was, but knowing they were persecuted). (14)

Interestingly, these critics' rationalizations of her Nazi/Jewish imagery return her poems to autobiography, to the private and the individual, even while Plath's metaphors cry out for a broader historical and political context. By radically redefining herself in terms of historically grounded, collective worlds, Plath (whether justified or not) successfully displaces the solitary, private individual. When identifying herself with the concentration camp Jew, she compares herself to a community, just as she identifies her father and husband, who play the tormenting Nazis, as a part of an historical political organization. In all of this, Plath suggests that her own contemporary experience—everyday conceptions of femininity, individualism, and the privacy of the family—conforms to collective patterns. She fights the disappearance of the public, its retreat to the privacy of the home, and "seriality" in general. One cannot see the whole from these little pockets of private perception. Stressing, then, the collective engineering of so-called "private experience," Plath charts a metaphorical map, linking invisible worlds to the cultural processes that inform them.

"Daddy," notoriously, re-stages secret family conflicts between parents and children, husbands and wives. It lifts a veil covering shameful social relations. And just as significantly, Plath "talks back." The opening lines vividly picture a claustrophobic domestic space:

> You do not do, you do not do
> Any more, black shoe
> In which I have lived like a foot
> For thirty years, poor and white,
> Barely daring to breathe or Achoo. (1–5)

This (cultural) space allows for little movement or even speech—she can't "breathe or Achoo." For Plath, the domestic realm stands out in the open, but unnoticed, hidden, or—as the poem suggests—*underfoot*. Plath wants to dismantle the interiority of the "shoe"-house, revealing its contents. As the progression of "Daddy" underscores, her new theatre is external, a decidedly worldly place, full of worldly struggles and a worldly language: "Atlantic" (11), "Polish town[s]" (16), "wars" (13), "Dachau, Auschwitz, Belsen" (33), "[t]he snows of the Tyrol, the clear beer of Vienna" (36), "swastika[s]" (43), "Fascist[s]" (48), and so forth.

In "Daddy," private "family matters" link up with large historical struggles, social organizations, and linguistic systems. Moving from the private, "shoe"-world to the just as stifling political world, consciousness can grasp the machinery that produces and oppresses it. The German language acts like a repressive, mechanical power, bearing down on the collective body:

> And the language obscene
> An engine, an engine
> Chuffing me off like a Jew.
> A Jew to Dachau, Auschwitz, Belsen.
> I began to talk like a Jew.
> I think I may well be a Jew. (30–5)

In general, Plath suggests the power of language ("an engine") to subject the self. But more specifically, she implies that certain styles of discourse violate body and soul more than others. She emphasizes the word "obscene" by placing it at the end of the stanza. To her, German is "the language obscene," but the word "obscene," falling where it does, also introduces her own words: as if to suggest her situation *and* her metaphors are indecent. Through such audacious, dramatic comparisons, Plath pictures human relationships as violent and grotesque *spectacles*, giving individual, private relationships public currency. At the same time, by having to *force* the domestic into the public arena, she highlights how these relationships normally remain serialized and closed off from social life.

Within this world of conflict, Plath, as I suggested earlier, "talks back," fantasizing possible alternatives to the pact of silence common among families. She occupies the position of speechlessness, but she struggles to respond:

> I never could talk to you.
> The tongue stuck in my jaw.
> It stuck in a barb wire snare.
> Ich, ich, ich, ich,
> I could hardly speak. (24–8)

Even though she may stutter—a shameful defect?—the persona does not hide her deficiency but gives voice to her fear and anger. Her fixed "ich" may also be seen to mirror the stuttering repetition of the oppressor's language ("An engine, an engine"), which "chuffs" out the same sound over and over again, revealing itself as a homogenizing, mechanical force. She responds in kind, with her similarly aggressive "obscene" language: She speaks crudely, and in a most unladylike way, of her "Polack friend" (20) and says to her father, "Daddy, daddy, you bastard" (80). By speaking not only "the language obscene" but also the actual German language ("Ich, ich, ich, ich"), the persona demonstrates that, even as she attempts to escape her oppressor's (male) language, it makes heavy

claims on her. It may even suggest her complicity. Her underlying desire to be desired by her father ("[e]very woman adores a fascist" [48]) has caused her, at times, to play along with the terms of his game, living within the rigid configurations of his language. "Daddy" embodies tremendous sociopsychological tension: for Plath utilizes a language of mastery (clarity, directness, multiple worldly allusions) that she simultaneously subverts with her startling array of marginal voices (with nursery rhymes, baby talk, speech defects, "hysteria"). But Plath's parody, while revealing submission to cultural paradigms, transcends ridicule. Plath dramatizes both her imprisonment in the oppressor's script—doing the important work of laying out dominant discursive codes—*and* the important points of resistance, on the margins.

Within these boundaries, her persona fantasizes herself as powerful, overpowering her tormentors, as when she imagines killing them ("If I've killed one man, I've killed two—" [71]), even driving a stake into her father's heart. Significantly, in the final act, she desires a collective judgement of this drama:

> And the villagers never liked you.
> They are dancing and stamping on you.
> They always *knew* it was you. (77–9).

She does not want to be alone in her condemnation of the Other. For Plath, this collective problem deserves a collective response, and she aims to give it one.

It should be noted, especially in the case of Plath, whose biography attracts so much attention, how she moves from the literary universe to the "real world." Jacqueline Rose tells how an "old friend wrote Plath's mother on publication of the poem in the review of *Ariel* in *Time* in 1966 to insist that Plath's father had been nothing like the image in the poem" (229). As this quotation demonstrates, Plath's poems, intentionally or not, perform a sort of "talk back" or "back talk," a rudely public, counter-discourse that rejects the family code of silence. By making feelings and ideas public, Plath risks a great deal. She risks banishment by her family and by a public anxious to preserve the status quo of middle-class family life.

In "Daddy," Plath reframes the private in terms of a public discourse, framing personal, family conflicts within larger cultural processes (language, homogenization, technology, politics). Making abstract processes concrete, she gives human faces to collective activities, forcing them into a dramatic, conflictual dialogue. In much of her late poetry, Plath repeatedly imagines a fragile self (very often *feminized*), subject to inhuman, and specifically modern, processes of rationalization (i.e., where the self is "paved over" by logic, statistics, uniformity, etc., processes that are most often viewed, by her, as patriarchal). For example, in "Face Lift" and "In Plaster," the uniqueness of the old self is literally erased or transformed, while in "Tulips," "The Surgeon at 2 a.m.," and "Three Women: A Poem for Three Voices," the female patient blends into the sterilized, white, homogenous, flat (and patriarchal) surroundings of the hospital, effectively losing her identity or uniqueness. As Renée Curry writes with respect to "In Plaster": "The wintry whiteness of the white walls presses in on the speaker … The pressure results in eradication of herself and obliteration of the volatility of life" (156). Some critics, including Linda Wagner-Martin (64–5), read the white room in "In Plaster" as representing a place of peace, a haven from social obligations, which is disturbed by the emergence of the blood-red tulips. For me, the persona's desire to melt into the white surroundings suggests the seductive nature of the institution, encouraging her to abandon her difference and become "uniform," like the passing nurses. I argue that, for Plath, rationalized worlds eliminate any form of public stage. In "Three Women," conversation retreats underground in the face of the hospital's overarching discourse. The three never speak to each other or, for that matter, anyone else. The poem's sharp stanzaic divisions structurally divide one voice from the next. Against this absence of public forum, Plath, in some of her late poems, exposes and challenges the deep rift between non-public and public types of discourse, between individual and collective experiences and responses.

In "Lady Lazarus," Plath puts her persona on display, in theatrical and carnivalesque fashion, before the "peanut-crunching crowd" (26). The elements of a reified social matrix come alive, transformed into visible actors capable of disrupting the commodified world through dialogue, gesture, and sheer physical presence: through a "theatrical / Comeback in broad day" (51–2). As in "Daddy," the death she transcends is the commodification of her body. First, she again identifies with persecuted Jews, the marginalized and hidden. Secondly, her body has been stolen from her and divided into diverse, saleable objects. These body parts/objects belong to the Nazis, who do with them as they like. Her skin, like an electric light source, shines "[b]right as a Nazi lampshade" (5). The "masters" convert her foot into a lifeless "paperweight" (7) and her face into "a featureless, fine / Jew linen" (8–9). The poem's frequently enjambed lines, which appear to sharply break, and yet link, each stanza of three, reflect these images of broken body parts.

Although Lady Lazarus bears witness to her own perverse commodification (is there any other kind?), her theatrics somehow resurrect a powerful self-possession. She raises the commodity to a sort of blinding "nakedness," so that herstory no longer belongs to the master. The word "nakedness," here, reflects John Berger's use of it; he writes, "To be naked is to be oneself" (54). Lady Lazarus tries to assume herself. She wants to subvert a metaphorical "nudity" that Plath describes in poems like "The Applicant" and "The Munich Mannequins." Berger opposes the terms "nudity" and "nakedness": "To be nude is to be seen naked by others and yet not recognized for oneself. A naked body has to be seen as an object in order to become a nude. (The site of it as an object stimulates the use of it as an object.)" (54). Both "The Applicant" and "The Munich Mannequins" powerfully dramatize their female figures' obscene "nudity." They become pure, voiceless surfaces. In "The Applicant," the wife, literally a piece of property (a "living doll" [33], "*that*" [29], or "it" [34–40]), a "guaranteed" (15), completely obedient slave, awaits purchase by the male customer:

It works, there is nothing wrong with it.
You have a hole, it's a poultice.
You have an eye, it's an image. (36–8)

The parallelism of these lines sets up the male as consumer to her object. The potential wife does not control her own body or actions. In "The Munich Mannequins," Plath takes the image of socially "tailored" woman to its extreme conclusion. The metaphorical mannequins experience no pleasure; they appear only for the pleasure of others—for the tailor who takes apart, dresses, and assembles "her," and for the consumer who watches "her." Not even *living* doll[s]" (emphasis added) that "can sew" (34) or "cook" (34) or "talk" (35) as they do in "The Applicant," these manufactured women appear only for show.

These poems practically explode from the stress imposed on the female selves. Their strangling objectification makes their silence that much more painful: Plath says the mannequins are "[i]ntolerable, without mind" (15). The wife-product and the mannequins are, in a way, invisible spectacles. "To be on display," writes Berger, "is to have the surface of one's own skin, the hairs of one's own body, turned into a disguise which, in that situation, can never be discarded" (54). By removing mind so absolutely, though, Plath puts on display the women's "naked" and twisted corpses,

> So, in their sulfur loveliness, in their smiles
> These mannequins lean tonight
> In Munich, morgue between Paris and Rome, (10–2)

which have been hidden, in part, by the fantasy that she wants it, that she desires the consuming male gaze. Plath leaves the women only "their" bodies, without the pretence of voice or free will, and, by doing so, makes them speak their grotesqueness. The mannequins are "[o]range lollies" (14) (Lolita-like, innocently sexually seductive) on "silver sticks" (14) for men to consume. For Plath, the lack of mind ("Voicelessness" 27, the wifely script) is obscene. How can this object recover itself? Or, as Luce Irigaray puts it, "How can such objects of use and transaction claim the right to speak and to participate in exchange in general?" (84). Plath answers with "Lady Lazarus."

As Susan Van Dyne observes with respect to "Lady Lazarus," "Lazarus is simultaneously the performer who suffers and the director who calculates suffering's effect" (57). Unlike the wife-product or the Munich mannequins, Lady Lazarus plays both subject and object of her own torture, a frighteningly animated (humanized) lampshade, *material witness* of its own production. In *Gender Trouble*, Judith Butler posits that the social construction of gender can be subverted through theatrical or parodic acts. Certainly, in "Lady Lazarus," the emergence of the human face, to face the inhuman, creates an air of instability and scandal. Consistent with Susan Bordo's understanding of the woman who becomes anorexic, a dramatic conflict emerges when the desires of the (female) object arise and revolt against what she is, a sort of envelope of death. Lady Lazarus demands her own exposure, to have the skin-like napkin covering her peeled off:

> Peel off the napkin
> O my enemy.
> Do I terrify?— (10–2)

This public torture both titillates and threatens. Lady Lazarus seductively conflates the prison camp with a pornographic world of male desire:

> The peanut-crunching crowd
> Shoves in to see
> Them unwrap me hand and foot—
> The big strip tease. (26–9)

The crowd has come to witness the effects of her suicide/attempted suicide, "an art, like everything else" (44) that she does "exceptionally well" (45). But far from just watching, they also act upon her, complicit in dissecting her body. Perhaps her sacrifice entails conveying to the disenfranchised crowd (the lower classes in the proverbial peanut gallery) her body as a body of knowledge, their history held up to them.

Plath's drama superimposes a public world over a world that keeps pain and death silent and secret. In this respect, "Lady Lazarus" echoes Foucault's strategic idealization, in *Discipline and Punish*, of pre-modern communal discourse. In light of Foucault's work, one can see "Lady Lazarus" as an attempt to recover the ritual (found in pre-modern models of punishment) displaced by what Foucault describes as the contemporary, "coercive, corporal, solitary, secret model of the power to punish" (131). Plath's poetic arena echoes a return to the earlier, "representative, scenic, signifying, public, collective model" (131). Foucault's extended description and documentation of Damiens, the condemned, details the intense symbolism invested in the prisoner's body. In effect, the condemned man acted out a theatrical battle between the king he had offended and himself. Power displayed itself before the community. According to Foucault, this life-and-death struggle was highly unstable, so that the condemned man, by addressing the crowd, might even persuade them into taking his side and attacking the judges. Similarly, Plath introduces a symbolic ritual wherein she can present the body as evidence, and wherein she can directly address the crowd. Each piece of Lady Lazarus is flagrantly on show, in much the same way as the earliest condemned criminals were on display during public tortures and executions. Rather than being kept quietly contained and hidden, as in modern methods of imprisonment, her torture plays in full view of the public:

> Gentleman, ladies
> These are my hands
> My knees.
> I may be skin and bones,
> Nevertheless, I am the same, identical woman. (30–4)

Executions traditionally allow for the convict's "last words"; and the idea of "last words" has a unique potency here. Like a convict before his execution, Lady Lazarus, under the protection of her own death, can say anything. She has nothing left to lose, since nothing remains of her to punish or prohibit. In this respect, she occupies a position of strength, power, and privilege, which makes her all the more fascinating and attractive to her witnesses. Hence, as Foucault argues, the public execution condemns, while it glorifies, the criminal. The person we watch facing his or her death fascinates on the face of it, while the crime that got him or her there, especially if considered monstrous, suggests the work of an exceptional nature. Foucault clearly prefers the dramatic public nature of the event, the visibility of the players (crowd, judges, criminal, king), and the revolutionary potential of the ritualistic dialogue to the removed, rational procedures of modernity. The witnesses are participants in the execution. They are even "the possible and indirect victim[s] of this execution" (68), as they may admire or identify with the criminal. So just as a whole aspect of the carnival played within the public execution, "which ought to show only the terrorizing power of the prince" (61), the status quo here is put at risk: Authority may be mocked and the criminal transformed into a hero. In the case of Lady Lazarus, she actually orchestrates the public performance of her own death.

Plath's position also bears striking resemblance to the situations of self-flagellating female mystics in the late middle ages. According to Laurie Finke in *Feminist Theory, Women's Writing*, female orthodox mystics would ritualistically inflict excessive pain on themselves, and, in doing so, appropriate cultural representations of their bodies: "She assumes for herself the power to define the authority that represses her sexuality: not man, but God" (96). Just as these mystics claimed divine authority ("'My me is God,' wrote Catherine of Genoa; Hadewijch of Brabant wished 'to be God with God'; Angela of Foligno wrote that 'the Word was made flesh to make me God'" [Finke 94]), so Plath wrote in her diary on 13 November 1949: "I want, I think, to be omniscient … I think I would like to call myself 'The girl who wanted to be God'" (qtd. in Introduction, *Letters Home* 40). This position also resembles Sartre's view that, above all, *man* desires to be God (69–73). Sartre argues that man's impulse to possess a particular woman is a transference of

his desire to lay hold of a world in its entirety. Could Plath's desire, then, to possess herself as "woman" reflect her desire to be God? Like the self-flagellating mystic, she becomes in her poetry both object and subject, both the one scarred and the one who scars. As we saw in "Daddy," for example, she both stutters or speaks the language of the oppressed ("talks like a Jew") and speaks masterfully. Ultimately, like the female mystic, she achieves representational power at the point that she seems ready (at least metaphorically) to annihilate herself. Just as the mystic poached upon the authority of church and state in her self-inflicted torture, so Plath usurps the technologies that control, construct, and harm her represented bodies. Within the context of the poem, it is she who inflicts pain and mythologizes her self, not the larger institutions of, say, marriage or the church. A bit pathologically (and understandably), she resembles the neurotic who identifies with death—either as abject victim or as sadistic destroyer—in order to understand and master it.

Lady Lazarus's potency comes, in part, from her having risked death and, therefore, becoming impervious to the threats of male power; ironically, death is one of her theatrical tricks. It shocks and encourages an audience to read the writing on her body (which one assumes will later be the writing of her poetry). Death is for her "an art" (44), a "call[ing]" (48), which she does "exceptionally well" (45). It brings her body into the "broad day" (52) as spectacle, "the theatrical" (51). In part, Plath achieves this poetically by delivering parallel constructions that encourage each short, quick, condensed line to stumble into the next, mimicking both the hectic intensity of this spectacular event and the power of the persona's thoughts:

> "A miracle!"
> That knocks me out.
> There is a charge
> For the eyeing of my scars, there is a charge
> For the hearing of my heart—
> It really goes.
> And there is a charge, a very large charge
> For a word or a touch
> Or a bit of blood
> Or a piece of my hair or my clothes. (55–64)

This "miracle" of death and rebirth obviously echoes the story of Christ's crucifixion and resurrection. The persona's assertion that

> These are my hands
> My knees.

I may be skin and bones,
Nevertheless, I am the same, identical
    woman (31–4)

echoes Christ's words in the *New Testament*: "Behold my hands and my feet, that it is I myself: handle me, and see; for a spirit hath not flesh and bones, as ye see me have" (*AV*, Luke 24.39). Drawing such parallels, Plath transforms this already spectacular event into the most dramatic, communal, and historical of all public executions. Comparing herself to Christ at the Cross (just as she identified herself with the Jews), she loudly and irreverently forces her personal, private self into the public realm. She is not one person being executed, but a collective, in much the same way that Christ was crucified for the sins of all. Not just one person, but everyone, must take responsibility, especially in this case. Moreover, the story she echoes, like the story of Lazarus, belongs to a patriarchal text, which again emphasizes a certain entrapment (and complicity) in the language and thoughts of her oppressor.

At the same time, Plath gathers power by inverting the Cartesian "I" of traditional poetics. Just as she parodies the Christ story, so she parodies the fully, self-conscious, "male" poet. Instead of thinking in terms of internalized reflections or meditations, Plath begins with the production of her body, its textualization. She first appears as a collection of body parts: "The nose, the eye pits, the full set of teeth" (13). Thereafter, she explores what that body means to her as a thinking person; or more accurately, she lets the body parts speak their meanings ("I have a body, therefore I am"). She plays the actress, the freak, the criminal, the rebel ("Out of the ash / I rise with my red hair / And I eat men like air" [81–3]), and the saint (with her sought-after bodily artefacts). But she also represents the body reduced to statistic, quantity, or elements, as in the following, chilling lines:

Ash, ash—
You poke and stir.
Flesh, bone, there is nothing there—
A cake of soap,
A wedding ring,
A gold filling. (73–8)

Plath's death-camp metaphor (the cake of soap made from the body; the gold taken from the teeth) shows the persona's body as violently disembodied, lacking self-possession or unity. Her body, here, belongs to an exterior power that values it best when dead, whether as fragmented and refashioned into useful commodities (soap, a lampshade, . . .), or as, according to another script, resurrected into martyrdom for the salvation of others. And yet, behind the violent commodification, Plath hints at postmodern, non-serialized social relations: the self-possessed body (behind the "cake of soap"), displays of wealth and status ("[a] gold filling"), and a symbol of community and ceremony ("[a] wedding ring"). She puts on display both commodification and the traces of human community that commodification still allows—that which resists complete assimilation, a counter-memory. Lady Lazarus plays a double role. As a victim, she dramatizes the torture of a woman who has lost her body to an anti-communal, serialized society. But at the same time, she dramatizes the repossession of her body, which partly represents a body of knowledge. This sacrificial body of knowledge offers itself as a gift, a form of recovered memory for the crowds of disenfranchised.

The discourses of both "Daddy" and "Lady Lazarus" attempt to give shape to and make *present* the order of controls, constructed scripts, and stereotypes. The personae expose both the contemporary social organization and themselves as constructed, rather than simply given or natural. Their identities, therefore, have the potential to be countered and reconfigured. The shape and meaning of *human being* is open for debate and change. Like Susan Bordo's agoraphobics and anorexics, "Lady Lazarus" puts a human face on collective and dehumanizing processes, as well as aggressively addressing them. This is not just subject and object coming together, but the silent objectified-oppressed becoming subject and addressing the centres of power. Her body is a collection of social artefacts; her body contains history and addresses history, but not piecemeal. Plath shows that the evidence is there to be dredged up and condensed into a sensible shape. In "Lady Lazarus" that means a human form. Both "Lady Lazarus" and "Daddy" work out where power can be located, as well as pointing out how this society has become a "serial" one, within which the self cannot gain a view of the whole. Plath stands outside, views, and addresses the very community she silently, passively inhabited. The poems confront the community by staging dramas of punishment. These spectacles of torture, although educational, are simultaneously self-destructive, as the speakers in both poems desire their own deaths. And yet, through these self-flagellating, suicidal personae, we may see diverse aspects of constructed female identity.

Source: Lisa Narbeshuber, "The Poetics of Torture: The Spectacle of Sylvia Plath's Poetry," in *Canadian Review of American Studies*, Vol. 34, No. 2, 2004, pp. 185–203.

SOURCES

Alvarez, A., *The Savage God: A Study of Suicide*, Random, 1972, p. 20, reprinted in "Sylvia Plath (1932–1963)," in *Modern American Literature*, edited by Joann Cerrito and Laurie DiMauro, Vol. 3, 5th ed., St. James Press, 1995, pp. 19–26.

Broe, Mary Lynn, "*The Colossus*: 'In Sign Language of a Lost Other World,'" in *Protean Poetic: The Poetry of Sylvia Plath*, University of Missouri Press, 1980, pp. 43–79.

Hoyle, Ben, "Nicholas Hughes, Sylvia Plath's Son Commits Suicide," in *Times* (London, England), March 23, 2009, http://www.timesonline.co.uk/tol/news/uk/article5956380.ece (accessed July 25, 2009).

King James Bible, Matthew 5:5, http://kingjbible.com/matthew/5.htm (accessed July 26, 2009).

Lant, Kathleen Margaret, "The Big Strip Tease: Female Bodies and Male Power in the Poetry of Sylvia Plath," in *Contemporary Literature*, Vol. 34, No. 4, Winter 1993, pp. 620–69.

Materer, Timothy, "Sylvia Plath," in *Dictionary of Literary Biography*, Vol. 152: *American Novelists Since World War II*, 4th ser., edited by James Giles and Wanda Giles, Gale Research, 1995, pp. 194–201.

Oates, Joyce Carol, "The Death Throes of Romanticism: The Poetry of Sylvia Plath," in *Southern Review*, Summer 1973, pp. 501–502, reprinted in "Sylvia Plath (1932–1963)," in *Modern American Literature*, edited by Joann Cerrito and Laurie DiMauro, Vol. 3, 5th ed., St. James Press, 1995, pp. 19–26.

Plath, Sylvia, "Mushrooms," in *The Colossus*, Faber & Faber, 1967, pp. 34–35.

Wain, John, Review of *The Colossus*, in the *Spectator*, January 13, 1961, p. 50, reprinted in "Sylvia Plath (1932–1963)," *Modern American Literature*, edited by Joann Cerrito and Laurie DiMauro, Vol. 3, 5th ed., St. James Press, 1995, pp. 19–26.

Woolf, Virginia, *A Room of One's Own*, edited by Mark Hussey, Houghton Mifflin Harcourt, 2005.

FURTHER READING

Middlebrook, Diane, *Her Husband: Ted Hughes and Sylvia Plath—A Marriage*, Penguin, 2004.
This book is a critically acclaimed account of the relationship between Plath and her poet husband, Ted Hughes. Middlebrook analyzes how each saw the other as a means to becoming the writers they wanted to be.

Plath, Sylvia, *The Unabridged Journals of Sylvia Plath*, edited by Karen V. Kukil, Knopf, 2000.
Though Plath's diaries were originally published in 1982, they were heavily abridged by Hughes. This volume is a full transcription of the diaries that Plath kept during the last twelve years of her life.

Rupp, Leila J., and Verta A. Taylor, *Survival in the Doldrums: The American Women's Rights Movement, 1945 to the 1960s*, Ohio State University Press, 1990.
This accessible overview of the history of the modern feminist movement is designed for use in schools and colleges. It includes an examination of the roles of the Equal Rights Amendment and the 1964 Civil Rights Act.

Wagner-Martin, Linda, ed., *Sylvia Plath: The Critical Heritage*, Routledge, 1989.
This is a collection of contemporary reviews and essays on the work of Sylvia Plath written from 1960 to 1985. It is a useful introduction to Plath's work.

The Old Stoic

EMILY BRONTË

1846

The Brontë family was a remarkable literary phenomenon in the first half of the nineteenth century. The father of the family, Patrick Brontë, was an Irish farm boy who lifted himself up by his own literary and scholarly efforts to become a country parson of the Church of England. The four children who survived to adulthood became important authors. Two of them, Charlotte and Emily, wrote novels considered among the most important in English literary history: Charlotte's *Jane Eyre* and Emily's *Wuthering Heights.* The other two siblings, Branwell and Anne, also made outstanding literary achievements, but all four died young, probably of tuberculosis.

Emily Brontë's "The Old Stoic" is part of the body of poetry produced by the Brontë siblings that has been generally neglected in favor of their famous novels. The poem first appeared in 1846 in the volume *Poems by Currer, Ellis and Acton Bell,* a collection of verse that included poems by all three sisters. "The Old Stoic" is one of the few pieces of poetry by any of the Brontës to go into wide circulation, appearing, for instance, in every edition of the *Oxford Book of English Verse.* The poem is an idealized description of a Stoic philosopher. It expresses his innermost thoughts and ideals as disdain for the common desires of humanity and then as a prayer to the gods.

The literary work of Charlotte, Emily, and Anne Brontë, as well as that of their brother Branwell, grew out of their collaborative childhood writing projects, or juvenilia, in which they built

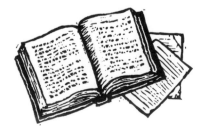

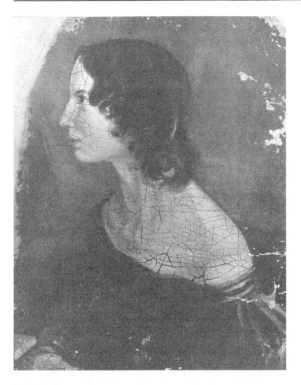

Emily Bronte

up a consistent picture of fantasy worlds of their own creation. Although specific references to the fantasy realms of Angria and Gondal were carefully edited out of the publications, "The Old Stoic" and even *Wuthering Heights* were originally part of, or at least intimately connected to, this fantasy literature produced by the Brontës.

AUTHOR BIOGRAPHY

Emily Jane Brontë was born on July 30, 1818, in Thornton, England. Two years later, her family moved to Haworth in Yorkshire, where she would spend almost her entire life. She had two sisters, Charlotte and Anne, and a brother Branwell. Quite unusually for a middle-class family, the sisters all determined to support themselves through their own labor, never seriously seeking proposals of marriage. Given the limitations placed on English women at that time, they had to work as teachers. Emily served as an ordinary classroom teacher at Miss Pratchett's school in Halifax for almost a year, and later spent a year in Brussels with Charlotte and Branwell, where she both studied and taught piano. At the end of the year,

an inheritance from an aunt made all three sisters self-sufficient without having to teach further. Emily herself continued her studies much further than her sisters, learning Latin from her father and pursuing study as a sort of monomania to the exclusion of other activities and social connections.

As was not unusual in middle-class families of their era, the Brontë children entertained themselves with ambitious literary projects. They wrote copiously, including handwritten and illustrated versions of magazines, and produced plays to be enacted by their toy soldiers and dolls. More exceptionally, their literary productions all had a unified theme, namely the epic saga of the Empire of Angria, a fictitious country they created in central Africa. What was unique was that the Brontës continued to pursue these kinds of projects as adults. They frequently spent evenings reading to each other stories and vignettes set in their fantasy worlds. Emily and Anne later branched off, creating their own Gondal Saga, about a fictitious island in the North Pacific. All of Emily's poetry, including "The Old Stoic," was written as part of this saga. "The Old Stoic" itself was probably meant as a character sketch for use in the fictional world.

In 1845, Charlotte found a notebook with some of Emily's verse in it and conceived of the idea of publishing a volume of poetry by all three sisters. Emily was mortified to have her privacy invaded in this way, but she eventually agreed. Charlotte edited the poems, removing all references to Angria and Gondal, and gave them titles (for this reason, Emily's poem is sometimes referred to by its first line, "Riches I hold in light esteem"). On May 22, 1846, the volume was published, under the pseudonyms Currer, Ellis, and Acton Bell. The volume was in general favorably reviewed but sold only two copies. Nevertheless, the three sisters rushed to publish novels. Still working under their pseudonyms, in 1847 Emily and Anne published *Wuthering Heights* and *Agnes Grey* as a set, while Charlotte published *Jane Eyre* separately. These works met with more success. Branwell was desperately trying to start a literary career of his own, but with little success. In September 1848, he died (possibly of tuberculosis, but he had become an alcoholic and opium addict), and the three sisters attended his funeral. All three caught colds. Emily's case most likely reactivated a latent infection of tuberculosis and she died at home in Haworth, England on December 19, 1848.

POEM TEXT

Riches I hold in light esteem,
And Love I laugh to scorn;
And lust of Fame was but a dream
That vanished with the morn—

And if I pray, the only prayer   5
That moves my lips for me
Is—'Leave the heart that now I bear,
And give me liberty.'

Yes, as my swift days near their goal,
'Tis all that I implore—   10
Through life and death, a chainless soul,
With courage to endure!

POEM SUMMARY

In three stanzas, Brontë's "The Old Stoic," also known by its first line, "Riches I hold in light esteem," briefly invokes several commonplaces about Stoicism (a form of Greek philosophy popular in the Hellenistic and Roman eras), appeals for the grace of Stoic liberty, and seeks to find a type of salvation within Stoicism. The entire text is a quotation from an unnamed speaker, whom Emily's sister Charlotte, when she edited the poem for publication, chose to call an old Stoic, from his central philosophical ideas and his evident nearness to death. However, it is worth noting that there are no clues in the poem as to the gender of the narrative voice.

Stanza 1

Stanza 1 lists a number of ordinary human desires that Stoicism considers to be worthless. The first line addresses the love of wealth. The narrative voice of the poem expresses a complete lack of interest in wealth. The moral perfection and happiness of the Stoic sage (as the ideal archetype of a Stoic philosopher is often called) comes entirely from his own interior psychological condition, so the status of his material possessions and wealth is irrelevant. The Greek Stoic philosopher Epictetus (c. 55–c. 135), whom the Brontës most likely read as the source of their knowledge of Stoicism, advises his students in his *Handbook* to give up all concern for external matters like wealth and property in order to cultivate the tranquility of mind that makes the sage independent of the external world: "If you want to make progress, give up all considerations like these: 'If I neglect my property, I will have nothing to live on....' It is better to die of hunger with distress and fear gone than to live upset in the midst of plenty." He urges his students to tell themselves that poverty (or any other adverse condition they experience) must be ignored since worry about what they cannot control will only cause unhappiness; to tell themselves about not desiring what they cannot control: "'This is the price of tranquility; this is the price of not being upset.' Nothing comes for free." Epictetus does not think much even of the disinterested use of wealth in philanthropy to help one's friends. The difficulty is that pursing money, even for a worthy goal, is viewed as an inherently degrading process. So the person who wants charity is asking the person who gives it to injure his own spiritual condition in order to help the recipient. Such a person must ask himself: "Which do you want more, money or a self-respecting and trustworthy friend? Then help me toward this, and do not expect me to do things that will make me lose these qualities." Wealth, which most people consider to be a great source of happiness, does not concern the Stoic sage because the possession of it is not something that is within his control. Rather, one must usually submit oneself to the control of external forces in order to acquire wealth, and this will inevitably lead to unhappiness.

In line 2, the narrative voice of the poem dismisses love as a matter of serious concern, finding it laughable instead. The meaning of the line is not clear. Brontë may mean love in some general sense, or she may be using the word as a euphemism for sexual desire. In the former case, Brontë is alluding to one of the elements of Stoic ethics strangest to modern feeling. The Stoic feels able to love himself to the degree that he had perfected the Stoic ethical teaching within himself and freed himself from the perturbations of the world, attaining the perfection that naturally belongs to the world itself as a whole. He values other human beings, that is, loves them, not according to any conventional criteria such as blood relation or marriage, but according to the degree they have attained stoic virtue for themselves, that is, to the degree they are like the sage himself. This leads to a somewhat surprising consequence: the sage's concern for even his own children extends only to the degree to which they are able to be taught and are able to put into practice Stoic ethics so that they themselves may become sages. The sage is only able to love others to the degree they resemble himself, or to put it another way, to the degree they both resemble god.

While the sage does not disdain love in this specific sense—indeed, it is among his dearest virtues—he does disdain the conventional signs of love as expressed by most people. This conventional love is what the Brontë character mocks. It is within this context that Epictetus is able to say with almost brutal honesty:

> You are foolish if you want your children and your wife and your friends to live forever, since you are wanting things to be up to you that are not up to you, and things to be yours that are not yours.

And again, "If you kiss your child or wife, say that what you are kissing is a human being; for when it dies you will not be upset." The sage is no more disturbed by the death of his own wife or child than he would be at the death of a stranger's wife or child. All such a death amounts to is that something that was given to him for a brief time by powers beyond his control was taken away again in the same way. Like so much else, the ties of family and friendship are revealed, upon Stoic examination, to be external goods that are beyond our control, and so the sage cannot allow his happiness to depend on them or to become sad when they are lost. If, on the other hand, Brontë is talking about sex, then the matter is even more clear cut. The satisfaction of desire with another person is clearly something that is not within the power of an individual to control, so the sage will find neither happiness nor disappointment in it or its lack. Epictetus teaches:

> At each thing that happens to you, remember to turn to yourself and ask what capacity you have for dealing with it. If you see a beautiful boy or woman, you will find the capacity of self-control for that.

In lines 3 and 4 of stanza 1 of Brontë's poem, the narrative voice says that fame is an illusion no more lasting than a dream. Fame, in a Victorian context, as well as in an ancient one, is more likely to mean a political career and the power and influence that come with it, rather than celebrity from working in the entertainment industry as the word might connote in twenty-first century society. Brontë, throughout the poem, refers to core Stoic ideas. While Stoicism offered what it claimed to be infallible advice for any sage in a position of power, it disdained seeking fame and power as it did anything that entailed a desire for things beyond human control. While many people might consider that fame or power are goods in themselves that would bring happiness, in the Stoic conception, they are external conditions that one cannot be sure of obtaining, so their desire will inevitably lead to unhappiness. Even if one obtains fame, it will only lead to a greater desire for fame. So the only answer is to recognize that fame is something

outside of human control and not desirable. While Epictetus tells his students, "You can be invincible if you do not enter any contest in which victory is not up to you," he also cautions them that the happiness of the philosopher is of a very different and higher order than the happiness that seems to come from those who gain fame and honor from holding high public office:

> For if the really good things are up to us, neither envy nor jealousy has a place, and you yourself will want neither to be a general or a magistrate or a consul, but to be free. And there is one road to this: despising what is not up to us.

This thought leads naturally into the next stanza, concerning Stoic ideas of liberty.

Stanza 2

Stanza 2 of the poem is a prayer directed toward the gods, asking only that they not interfere with the narrator's interior psychological condition but grant him freedom. Despite its mechanistic worldview, prayer is by no means foreign to the Stoics who considered piety to be a natural virtue. In fact, one of the greatest masterpieces of Stoic literature is a hymn to Zeus composed by the second head of the school, the Greek philosopher Cleanthes (c. 330–c. 232 BCE. The fact that the freedom the Stoic asks for is contrasted with the gods possibly intervening in the innermost process of his being suggests what freedom is for a Stoic. It is not license to pursue selfish pleasure. It is not even freedom to speak and act as one wishes, since the Stoic realizes that it is in the nature of things that these will be constrained by forces outside of his control. It is instead the freedom to think in accord with nature and discover by his own experiences and reflection how he can attain happiness and how he can make the right decisions about what is within his control and what is not within his control. He cannot ask the gods to supply this knowledge to him, since it is the ruling principle within himself that makes these decisions and that is, for the Stoic, the irreducible core of human identity. If the gods intervened there, there would be nothing left that was genuinely human. For the Stoic, Epictetus makes clear, the gods have no need to intervene in the interior condition of a human being but only in the affairs of the exterior world.

Stoic piety demands belief that the gods arrange the affairs of the universe justly. Therefore, the Stoic need only live in accord with this divine arrangement of the world. He does not require any help through a special revelation or intervention. While the Stoics certainly believed that the gods communicated with humankind through omens and prophecy, the motions of the stars, and the behavior of birds, these communications concerned only the outside world. If a Stoic receives an unfavorable sign, according to Epictetus, he should tell himself: "None of these signs is for me, but only for my petty body or my petty property or my petty [legal affairs] or children or wife." Since the gods have arranged the world perfectly, it is up to the Stoic to see how any omen, and any outcome of an omen, is actually for the best: "For all signs are favorable if I wish, since it is up to me to be benefited by whichever of them turns out correct." For the Stoic sage, such as the narrator of the poem, who internalized the divine principles within himself and makes the same judgments as the gods, even divine signs are merely another object on which to exercise his judgment. While to truly live in freedom is to be no different than a god, freedom must come from within the individual and cannot be given by any outside condition, even the gods.

Stanza 3

Stanza 3 recapitulates in summary the ideas of the other two stanzas. The narrative voice, even as it sees death approaching, does not wish for a prolongation of life, or for any other apparent good that might not be forthcoming. The narrative voice appears only to live through its innermost self in freedom from desires for the things that are not within its control and the hardihood to endure with indifference circumstances that the world calls misfortunes. The speaker invokes the very factors that elevate the Stoic sage above the world in the only kind of salvation available to the Stoic.

THEMES

Salvation

As positively as Stoicism was viewed by the educated middle class of nineteenth century Britain, that culture was nevertheless a deeply Christian one, and it was quite usual for Christian ideas to insinuate themselves into Victorian endorsements of the ancient philosophy. Brontë does an excellent job of avoiding this temptation, but she moves in that direction in her apparent conception of Stoic salvation when she speaks about death. Her narrator prays for the same indifference to circumstance he knew in life to persist in death. If

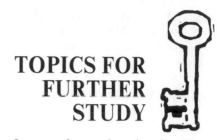

TOPICS FOR FURTHER STUDY

- Think of some of your favorite characters from novels you have read. Write a character sketch of them in the form of poetry. Use descriptive language and a poetic rhyme scheme like the one used in "The Old Stoic."

- The fantasy material the young Brontës circulated among themselves about the worlds of Glass Town, Angria, and Gondal imitated the then newly popular publishing form—the magazine. Read some of young Charlotte and Branwell's Angria articles from *An Edition of the Early Writings of Charlotte Brontë*, edited by Christine Alexander, and *The Works of Patrick Branwell Brontë*, edited by Victor Neufeldt, and republish them in your own words as a blog or Web site.

- Read Epictetus's *Handbook*. Compare its precepts to your own moral beliefs and ideas that guide your behavior. Report to your class on the differences and similarities using a Venn diagram.

- Many Web sites exist to assist authors in creating their own fantasy world-building exercises. Visit some of them and start to build your own world and share the results with your class. Good places to start include The Language Creation Society (http://conlang.org) and the world-building page at the Eclectic Company, which is a well-maintained page of links to further sites at http://www.bmarch.atfreeweb.com/Worldbuilding.htm.

the moment of death is meant, so that the end of life can be met fearlessly, that is not incompatible with Stoicism. But some contemporary readers may not resist the temptation to read the contrast drawn between life and death as being between life and death as the afterlife (which is not a factor in Stoicism). The passionless existence of the Stoic sage was often taken as the model of the existence of the saved Christian in the world to come, as though salvation consists of becoming like a Stoic sage. But the degree to which Brontë herself intended this is debatable.

Stoicism

Brontë's "The Old Stoic" gives a series of private thoughts and mental prayers in the voice of a character devoted to Stoicism and meant to be typical of that philosophy. Stoicism is a system of philosophy devised in the years after 300 BCE by the Greek philosopher Zeno. He was certainly Greek by culture but he came from Citium on Cyprus where much of the population was Phoenician, and sources, which are about 500 years later than his period, suggest he may have been of Phoenician descent. Zeno came to Athens to study philosophy, desiring to live according to the same manner of life as the great Greek philosopher Socrates. Zeno did not study at the Platonic Academy, however, or with the students of Aristotle at the Lyceum, either of which might have been viewed as successors to Socrates, but with the Cynic philosopher Crates of Thebes. The Cynics were concerned exclusively with human behavior and felt that men ought to live in accord with their essentially animal character, hence the name Cynic, which means canine. After a decade of study, Zeno began to teach his own new philosophy at the Stoa Poikile (the porch of the paintings), an Athenian public art gallery from which his school took its name. Zeno's students and immediate successors were Cleanthes and Chrysippus. Stoicism eventually became the dominant form of philosophy in the early Roman Empire. The first-century Greek Stoic teacher Epictetus and the Roman emperor Marcus Aurelius in the following generation are responsible for the only surviving extended treatises of the school, but the thought of the original Stoics are preserved in numerous quotations by later authors such as the Roman orator Cicero.

Stoic philosophy differed from Platonism and Aristotelianism in being entirely materialistic, believing that nothing existed apart from physical matter. The Stoics rejected the idea that whatever faculty of a human being is responsible for thoughts and feelings was some type of nonmaterial entity of a different character than the rest of the world, such as a soul, spirit, or divine spark, but rather were the results of a material process just like anything else that can be observed. Stoics by no means rejected the idea of god, but they held that god was simply the totality of the universe and, in particular, the cause of the universe existing in the best possible way. Just as human beings have reason, god is the reasoning power (*logos*) that arises from the body of the universe. Cleanthes praised this being in his poetic *Hymn to Zeus*, though he insisted that all divine names, not just Zeus, rightly apply to this god.

The Stoics insisted that the universe as a whole was perfect, and that if some condition or event, such as a storm that destroyed farmers' crops or the death of a child, seemed imperfect to the human beings it affected, that was because their limited perspective was incapable of seeing the whole. Cleanthes expressed the idea in his hymn by saying that even what is hated by human beings is lovely in the eyes of god. Accepting the traditional Greek view that matter is composed of the four elements—fire, air, water, and earth—the Stoics held that the universe must exist as part of a greater cosmic cycle. Since fire is the most perfect element, the universe must originally have been all fire. The other elements are produced by the life process of fire, and their creation and recombination brought into being the universe as we experience it. But, since it is necessary for the universe to be as perfect as possible, it will strive to return to the condition of being all fire after many long ages. Then the process will repeat infinitely. Since, according to the Stoics, the universe is perfect, any deviation would be less than perfect, so each universe created between the periods of fire (*ekpyrosis*) will be identical, down to every individual person such as Socrates or Thomas Jefferson living again in exactly the same way they were known to have lived their lives. Thus, everything that happens is preordained and outside of human control. While Stoics did not conceive of any form of human survival after the dissolution of the physical body (since they believed nothing existed that was not material), every human being, would, nevertheless, live again, as it were, in each successive age

Since according to the Stoic view it is impossible to change the state of the natural world, it follows that the best way to live is in accord with nature as it actually exists. A human being must

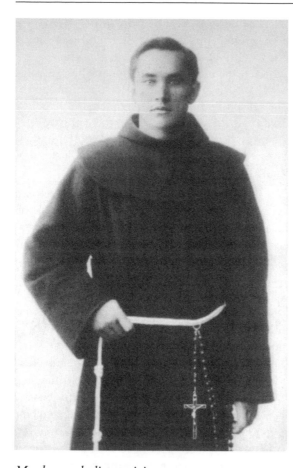

Monks symbolize stoicism (© 2009 / Jupiter Images)

learn to distinguish what he cannot control (external circumstances) from what he can control (his reactions and feelings about external circumstances). Suffering is caused by wishing things to be different than they are and wishing to change what one is powerless to change. The Stoic sage, who has perfected his ethical training, wishes things to be just as they are and completely frees himself from suffering by perfecting his interior psychological composition. He is not emotionless, as is popularly conceived, but rejects those emotions (strong passions) that are not subordinate to reason as though they were a sort of mental illness. In this way, he becomes a god since his reason becomes identical to the right reason that regulates the universe in the best possible way. The sage does not feel any desire to obtain fame, wealth, power, or any of the other things that ordinary human beings are constantly making themselves miserable over.

STYLE

Lyric Verse

"The Old Stoic" is written in traditional poetic form as lyric verse. The poem consists of twelve lines organized into three four-line stanzas. Each line has a specific number of metrical feet, either four (tetrameter) or three (trimeter). A foot is a group of syllables; in this poem, the meter is iambic, which is to say most of the feet are iambs, an unstressed syllable followed by a stressed syllable. The iamb is the most common foot in English poetry. Each stanza has two couplets. The first line of each couplet is a tetrameter, the second a trimeter. The lines rhyme, that is, have the same vowel and final consonant sounds in the last stressed syllable, in the pattern *ABAB* within each stanza. The poem is relatively free of alliteration (repetition of the same sounds), personification (the attribution of human qualities to animals and inanimate objects), and other meaningful poetic devices.

Fantasy World-Building

All four of the Brontë siblings spent their youths and much of their adult lives engaged in writing what is usually called their juvenilia, the creation of complex fantasy worlds documented in various literary forms. Indeed, since even her novel *Wuthering Heights* grew out of this context, it can be said that Emily always remained enmeshed in these fantasy worlds. In June 1826, the four Brontë children (Emily was eight years old) began to collaborate to produce plays in which the leading actors were a set of toy soldiers and various dolls that their father had given them. These soon grew into the Glass Town Saga about an imperialist kingdom carved out of central Africa. The children did not make a single story on this premise, but rather documented the history and culture of Glass Town (later Verdoplis), which was the capital of the Empire of Angria. Glass Town was populated by characters molded after the politicians and authors who filled the pages of *Blackwood's* and *Town and Country* magazines. Indeed, the principle form of documentation for the saga was hand drawn and written versions of these magazines that the children drew and wrote themselves, filling them with illustrations, poems, literary reviews and notes, political news, and every kind of material found in the actual publications, but about events in Glass Town rather than London. As they grew older, the children split: Charlotte and Branwell continued the original fantasy in works generally called the Angria Saga, while

Anne and Emily started over, creating their own world of Gondal, set on a mythical island in the North Pacific Ocean.

This kind of detailed building of a fantasy world, in which there was no coherent story but rather a variety of documents in which stories could be traced from piece to piece with the overall goal to provide a general framework for narrative, was exceptional in the nineteenth century. When the Brontës began to publish, they suppressed the world-building elements of their literature. World building of this kind is now commonplace in the burgeoning publishing market for fantasy literature. During World War I, English writer J. R. R. Tolkien set out to create his own fantasy world, based on his scholarly studies of philology (historical or comparative linguistics), rather than the perusal of magazines devoted to popular middle-class culture. Tolkien proceeded in more or less the same way as the Brontës, building up a world out of a variety of documents that looked more like a complete history of a civilization than a novel. (Branwell had also created an artificial language for Angria, though he never went as far in that direction as Tolkien.) Tolkien tried and failed to publish some of this material, but he eventually brought out a selection of narratives from his world of Middle Earth, beginning with *The Hobbit* in 1937 and followed in 1954 with *The Lord of the Rings*. After the phenomenal success of those works, Tolkien's son Christopher began to publish the original background material and has brought out more than a dozen volumes of his father's notes. In contemporary literature, the writing of narratives set in completely created fantasy worlds is a well-published genre. More remarkably, numerous Web sites exist specifically to facilitate world building whose users are not necessarily aiming at a formal publication but are interested in pursuing the enterprise for its own sake.

HISTORICAL CONTEXT

Pseudonymity

When the Brontës undertook to publish their poetry in 1846, they did so under the pseudonyms Currer, Ellis (Emily's pseudonym), and Acton Bell. Over the next two years, when they brought out their novels, they used the same pseudonyms. The practice of publishing under assumed names was more common in the nineteen century than in modern literature. Certainly it was not a secret to contemporary reviewers

that the given authors were pseudonyms, though none suspected the poets to be women. One reason the Brontës used this screen was because, according to Charlotte (in her introduction to the no longer anonymous second 1850 edition of *Wuthering Heights*), they were "averse to personal publicity." There was a more fundamental reason, however, because they "had a vague impression that authoresses are liable to be looked on with prejudice." This was certainly true, despite the fact that the most eminent novelist of the previous generation was undoubtedly Jane Austen. Women novelists had been a clichéd term for some time, associated especially with Gothic literature and with excessive emotionalism, poor style, and little literary merit.

The Brontës' poems, as well as their initial novels, were all published at their own expense. This was a common practice in the nineteenth century, when Jane Austen, John Keats, and many other leading authors had to pay to publish their own works. Circumstances changed in the twentieth century, however, and today only vanity presses take money from their authors. Given the changes in the publishing industry brought about by the Internet, self-publication may again become a possible outlet for serious literary work.

Epictetus

Epictetus was a Stoic philosopher who lived in the late first century CE. He is almost certainly the source of Brontë's knowledge of Stoicism, through the 1758 English translation of his works by Elizabeth Carter. Epictetus has sometimes been thought to be the old Stoic of Brontë's poem, but her work contains no information that relates to the known facts of Epictetus's life. Epictetus was more concerned with giving advice for practical living, especially for living in a compromised world, than in presenting the kind of systematic philosophy aimed at by the early Stoics.

Epictetus was born as a slave in Hierapolis in Asia Minor (modern Turkey) in the mid-first century CE. Epictetus is not a real Greek name but rather is the word that means "bought." He came to Rome as a slave of Epaphroditus, himself a freed slave of the emperor who worked in the government bureaucracy in the capital. How or when Epictetus learned Stoicism is unknown. But after being freed, he worked as a teacher of the philosophy, first in Rome and then in Nicopolis (modern Bulgaria). Epictetus wrote nothing

COMPARE
&
CONTRAST

- **1840s:** Women writers are dismissed as incapable of producing serious literature because of their gender. The commercial success of women novelists in particular is taken as evidence of artistic inferiority.

  Today: Gender is not a criteria in establishing literary merit. Women writers are judged among the greatest living authors and women frequently win the most prestigious literary awards such as the Nobel Prize.

- **1840s:** The genre of the fantasy novel, in which an entirely fictional reality is created in the most minute detail, does not exist.

  Today: Thanks largely to the work of J. R. R. Tolkien, the fantasy novel is one of the most successful genres, though many literary critics still dismiss it.

- **1840s:** Authors, not only women, frequently publish their work anonymously (or pseudonymously) for various reasons.

  Today: Anonymous publication is rare since authors strive to create name recognition to increase book sales. Pseudonyms may be used by writers wishing to establish separate brands: Nora Roberts writes romances under her own name, but pens mysteries as J. D. Robb.

- **1840s:** Poetry is generally considered more important than prose from an artistic viewpoint, and it has a wide reading public.

  Today: Poetry, though still given critical prestige, hardly overshadows prose, especially fiction, and new poetry is generally read by only a small literary elite.

himself, but attracted many aristocratic students, including Arrian, who eventually became a provincial governor and also wrote an important surviving history of Alexander the Great. Arrian wrote up and published his notes of Epictetus's lectures that filled several books under the title *Discourses*, of which the first four survive. Arrian also excerpted this work into a brief manual known simply as the *Encheiridion* ("handbook"). These publications are the source for knowledge of Epcitetus's thought and are generally published under Epictetus's name. A commentary on Epictetus's lectures by the fifth-century Greek Neoplatonic philosopher Simplicius also survives. The details of Epictetus's life come from this work. The most famous episode of his life is probably fictitious. Supposedly, while he was still a slave, Epaphroditus wished to test how far his Stoic indifference to suffering went and had Epictetus bound and tortured until his leg was broken, but he elicited no greater response than calmly telling Epaphroditus that his leg bone had snapped.

CRITICAL OVERVIEW

The first person to read "The Old Stoic" was Brontë's sister Charlotte when she read the private notebook of poems in 1845. She was impressed enough to reveal her invasion of her sister's privacy, which had a high cost in awkwardness within the family, and to be able to persuade her sister to publish the work. The initial reviews of the poetry volume of all three sisters were generally favorable. The four contemporary reviews are often reprinted, for example, in *The Scribner Companion to the Brontës* by Barbara and Gareth Lloyd Evans. A reviewer in the *Critic* (July 4, 1846) was the most enthusiastic, saying of the collection, "Here we have good, wholesome, refreshing, vigorous poetry—no sickly affectations, no namby-pamby, no tedious imitations of familiar strains, but original thoughts, expressed in the true language of poetry." A reviewer of the same date in the *Athenaeum* singled out Emily's poems (published under the pseudonym Ellis Bell) as superior to her sisters': "[The] instinct of song...[rises] in...Ellis, into an inspiration, which may yet

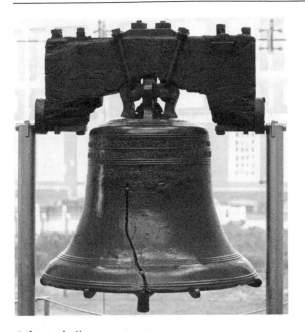

Liberty bell (Image copyright Racheal Grazias, 2009. Used under license from Shutterstock.com)

find an audience in the outer world." A review in the October issue of *Dublin University Magazine* was also favorable, while a reviewer in the *Spectator* (November 11, 1848) found the poems mannered and commonplace in their subject matter, but thought the poets might be capable of improvement to an acceptable standard of writing if their work became more disciplined.

Just as the original reviewers did not single out "The Old Stoic" for special comment, it has received very little attention from modern critics, even among the neglected Brontë poems. However, Margaret Maison, in her 1978 article in *Notes and Queries* pointed out that Brontë's poetry as a whole, not merely "The Old Stoic," shows a knowledge of Stoicism. It is probable that she had read the first-century Stoic Epictetus who was a very popular author in England during the eighteenth and nineteenth centuries. In particular, Maison points out that Elizabeth Carter's 1758 translation of Epictetus was intended for the education of girls and Brontë would almost certainly have used it, both as a student and as a teacher. Barring any additional information being discovered, this translation is the most likely source for Brontë's knowledge of Stoicism.

Patricia Ingham in *The Brontës* treats the appellation "The Old Stoic" given the poem by Charlotte as reflecting Emily's intentions and goes further, adding that it refers to Epictetus as the character described in the poem, thus reading it as unrelated to Gondal. Yet, she also takes the liberty desired by the narrative voice of the poem as expressing Emily's own desire, not for freedom in the Stoic sense, but in the more modern sense of freedom from responsibility. Ingham generally reads the poem as expressive of an illness Emily suffered in 1838, although the poem was most likely composed three years later.

CRITICISM

Bradley A. Skeen

Skeen is a classics professor. In this essay, he explores the context of "The Old Stoic" in the Gondal Saga in relation to the development of the modern genre of fantasy.

The main unanswered question about Brontë's "The Old Stoic" is how it is to be understood in relationship to Gondal, the fantasy realm created by Emily and her sister Anne. The problem concerns all of her poetry, the bulk of which comes from two manuscript notebooks in which she made fair copies in 1844 of older poems that she wished to preserve. One she headed "Gondal Poems" and the other simply with her initials, E. J. B. "The Old Stoic," however, comes from neither source, but from a single sheet dated March 1, 1841, now in the Honresfeld collection kept in private hands by the Law family.

The first critic to seriously consider the Gondal background of Emily's writing was Fannie Ratchford in two studies published in the 1940s and 1950s, especially in *Gondal's Queen*. Since it was acknowledged that even *Wuthering Heights* grew out of Gondal material, she naturally took all of Emily's poetry as related to the cycle of material about the mythical realm. The fact that Emily did not write the name Gondal in the E. J. B. Notebook or on other manuscripts is not a serious objection since it is not known what their original organization might have been, except that Emily's surviving sister Charlotte later destroyed most of the Gondal material, and that many of the surviving scraps of poetry were torn out of larger notebooks at some point in the past, most likely by collectors. Ratchford found that Emily's poetry as a whole could be fit together like broken pieces of a statue, to suggest the original outline of the Gondal Saga without

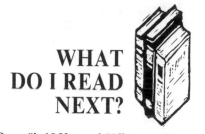

WHAT DO I READ NEXT?

- Charlotte Brontë's 1853 novel *Villette* explores many of the same Stoic philosophical ideas that Emily touched upon in "The Old Stoic."

- The 2003 encyclopedia by Lisa Paddock and Carl Rollyson, *The Brontës A to Z*, gives an introductory treatment of the Brontës' lives and works.

- *Emily Brontë: A Critical Anthology* (1973) by Jean Pierre Petit presents a collection of critical essays on Brontë's work, beginning some of the first reviews of the Bell poetry volume and continuing through modern studies by figures like Virginia Woolf and Sylvia Plath.

- Steve Vine's *Emily Brontë* (1998) in Twayne Publisher's "English Author" series gives a balanced overview of her life and work.

- Lawrence C. Becker's *A New Stoicism* (1998) reinterprets Stoicism as a moral philosophy for use in the modern world.

- Christine Alexander has published two volumes of material relevant to Charlotte's writing about Angria as a young adult in *An Edition of the Early Writings of Charlotte Brontë* (1987, 1991).

- Xavier S. Thani Nayagam compares Indian and Stoic philosophy in his 1962 lecture *Indian Thought and Roman Stoicism*.

- Brontë's *Wuthering Heights* (first published in 1848 and widely available today) is her only novel and is a great story of love and heartbreak that had endured through the years.

---

leaving any part of it unaccounted for. The fact that Emily continued to write new Gondal poetry, even after *Wuthering Heights* was published in 1847, would seem to argue strongly for Ratchford's interpretation. Yet, this view has not found favor with many later critics.

The more recent trend in relating Emily's verse to Gondal, as presented in the article on her poetry

> EMILY AND HER SIBLINGS CAN BE SEEN AS THE FIRST GREAT WORLD BUILDERS, ANTICIPATING THE MODERN EXPLOSION OF THE EXPLORATION OF FANTASY WORLDS AS A NEW POPULAR GENRE."

in *The Oxford Companion to the Brontës*, for instance, has been to separate her verse from Gondal as far as possible. The "purely Gondal reading of Emily Brontë's poems appeared to reduce their significance for many readers, confining them within a self-indulgent childhood fantasy world." Poetry that cannot be detached from Gondal is routinely dismissed as rubbish and melodrama. So critics have "felt the need to clearly divide Emily's poetry into Gondal and non-Gondal categories, and so rescue some of the poems as personal romantic statements." The criteria for division would seem to be between good and meaningful poetry, and poetry that is related to the juvenile (in the more pejorative sense) world of Gondal. The problem with this division is that many of Emily's poems acknowledged as her best work are clearly set in Gondal. For instance, Emily's published poem "The Prisoner" is a fragment from the long poem "Julian M. and A. G. Rochelle" in the Gondal notebook. Critics who try to downplay the importance of Gondal explain this phenomenon with the claim that removing lyric poetry from its specific context in Gondal to an unbounded universal context magically transforms the same lines into more deeply meaningful poetry. It must be noted that the one responsible for this transformation was not Emily herself, but Charlotte, who acted as her editor.

At least part of what explains such seemingly paradoxical criticism is a long-standing academic prejudice against fantasy as a literary theme. This is the same prejudice that prevented the Brontës from ever considering publication of Angria or Gondal material. The same consideration hampered J. R. R. Tolkien in his initial attempts to publish works set in his fantasy realm of Middle Earth. Most critics still wish to dismiss Tolkien, just as they dismiss Gondal, despite the overwhelming popularity of fantasy literature once it became available in commercially published literature. Tom Shippey, in his *J.R.R. Tolkien: Author of the Century*, has made the case that fantasy has become the dominant genre of English literature over the course of the twentieth century, with academic critics fighting against it vigorously. Fantasy suffers from the prejudice that it is unreal and devoted to infantile wish fulfillment, despite the evident fact that even the most realistic novels of Marcel Proust or Ernest Hemingway are set in a carefully constructed artificial world just as much as Middle Earth or Gondal.

A more persuasive solution to the problem of Gondal is to see Brontë as a forward-looking author whose instinct was to anticipate the rise of fantasy. Emily and her siblings can be seen as the first great world builders, anticipating the modern explosion of the exploration of fantasy worlds as a new popular genre. The exploration of the human condition through such a manipulation of authorial reality hardly reduces the meaning of the Brontës' poetry, since its meaning remains the same whatever its context. The creation of a fantastic world as the setting of a work of literature is hardly new with the Brontës. Rather, they found inspiration in the ancient epic poets Homer and Virgil, and in English epics such as John Milton's *Paradise Lost*. What they added to tradition, through their imitation of contemporary popular magazines that gave form to their efforts, was the modern and even postmodern characteristics of play with genre and ironic distancing of the author and reader from the text. Their awareness of the interplay between artistic creation and commercial publication marks their fantasy world as a place of sophisticated literature, possessed of all the serious literary characteristics critics declare lacking in fantasy.

To turn more directly to "The Old Stoic," it is not hard to see how it must have functioned within the Gondal Saga in general, and to make some educated guesses about the specifics. There seems to be little doubt that Emily was acquainted with the writings of the first-century Stoic philosopher Epictetus and that her presentation of Stoicism within the poem is closely based on his works. Epictetus is by far the most accessible surviving source for Stoic philosophy, and all the more so in the nineteenth century for a reader unacquainted with the ancient Greek original since his works were widely translated. In particular, the translation by Elizabeth Carter in *All the Works of Epictetus, which are now Extant; Consisting of His Discourses, Preserved by Arrian, in Four Books, the Enchiridion, and Fragments* was most likely well known to Emily since she was unusually highly educated for a woman of her time, and she also trained and worked as a professional teacher, however briefly. The closest that one can come to confirmation of this is a saying from the *Handbook of Epictetus* that deals in a unified way with precisely the same subject matter as Brontë's poem: the rejection of wealth, love, and fame in a context of Stoic conceptions about salvation. Epictetus imagines a banquet in which all the apparently goods things of life are offered. The proper way to act, he says, is to take each plate as it is passed to you, and not to reach out for it before it comes to you, and not to keep it when it is to be passed on to someone else:

> In the same way toward your children, in the same way toward your wife, in the same way toward public office, in the same way toward wealth, and you will be fit to share a banquet with the gods.

But if you can reject even what is offered to you and partake of nothing, then you will have passed from the companionship of the banquet to join the company of the gods, acting as they themselves do and surpassing the merely human. This is the ultimate goal of Stoic philosophy. In both Brontë and Epictetus, by not only not desiring but by actively rejecting the value of worldly goods, the Stoic proves himself worthy of divine status, though Brontë seems to push this off to an afterlife in the conflation of Stoic and Christian ideas fashionable in the nineteenth century.

Many modern readers take the old Stoic of the title to be Epictetus, as though the ancient philosopher were the speaker of the poem. This is a universalist reading of the poem, meant to make it accessible to readers with no special knowledge of the Brontës' created world, that moves it away from Gondal where Epictetus would not be a possible character. However, the title "The Old Stoic" was given to the poem by Charlotte, not Emily, and can, therefore, hardly be used as evidence for a reading of Emily's intended meaning. The poem is more likely meant to be a sketch of an unidentified character within the Gondal Saga. There is ample precedent for the development of such a character. For instance in William Shakespeare's *Julius Caesar* the character of Brutus has little relation to Caesar's historical friend and assassin Brutus, but rather is a fictionalized character who consistently acts and speaks as a Stoic philosopher would in the situations presented by the plot of the play. Brontë very likely intended something of the same kind.

Thinking along these lines, there is no warrant to accept Charlotte's characterization of the Stoic as old. It is true he speaks of death as swiftly approaching, but this is not most naturally taken as a reference to old age but as a Stoic commonplace. The Stoic viewed death as the only certainty in life and lived ever mindful of it. Even if Emily's Stoic has some definite reason to think he might die soon, there is no reason to think this death would come from old age. Ancient Stoic philosophers were famous for speaking out against political tyranny and oppression, even at the cost of their own lives when the tyrant silenced them through execution. A scene along those lines would offer far more dramatic potential within the Gondal Saga than a mere death from old age. Here is an instance when the original context of Gondal, even if it must be recreated, gives more depth of meaning to the poem, in contrast to the shallowness implicit in the Universalist reading, which would make the poem merely a restatement of Epictetus's own philosophy in old age.

Source: Bradley A. Skeen, Critical Essay on "The Old Stoic," in *Poetry for Students*, Gale, Cengage Learning, 2010.

Maggie Allen

In the following essay, Allen shows the influence of German romantic poets in Brontë's poetry.

The comment by Mrs Gaskell that 'anyone passing by the kitchen door might have seen [Emily] studying German out of an open book', suggests an influence on Emily Brontë by the German Romantic poets.

The great influx of German literature coming into England in the early decades of the nineteenth century brought with it the work of Goethe, Schiller, Tieck, and Novalis, followed later by Eichendorff and Brentano, among others. Their work was frequently published in *Blackwood's* and *Fraser's* literary magazines, and they found support from Thomas Carlyle, Madame de Staël, Sir Walter Scott, and the poets Shelley and Byron.

One factor often mentioned in the popular rise of German literature in England is Madame de Staël's book, *De L'Allemagne*, published in London in 1813. This was '[. . .] a great success and sold out completely in three days'. The book revealed the Germans to be 'civilised by Christianity and their

> THE POEMS OF EMILY ARE PASSIONATE AND SINCERE. HER SOLITARY WALKS ON THE MOORS ALLOWED HER TO BE A ROMANTIC WANDERER, TO BE AT ONE WITH NATURE AND SHARE ITS SECRETS. HER POEMS REPRESENT THE CHANGING FACES OF NATURE, ITS EXTREMES AND COMPLEXITIES."

history is that of the middle-ages, Gothic rather than classical'. The Gothic ingredient found its way into art, architecture, and many facets of English life, but was prominent in literature.

'Gothic' displayed a darker side of Romanticism, whereby writers and poets explored death, often in a nightmare setting. The desolate landscape and atmosphere were all encapsulated into a world of shadows. Even the Gondal poems do not escape the European Romantic and German Gothic influences:

> Emily's powerful women offer female versions of the Romantic exile, that outcast, outlawed, or otherwise isolated figure, the lonely bearer of the truth who rejects or rebels against the society from which she has been exiled.

A good example of 'Gothic' is Emily's poem, "The Prisoner" (1845), where the only escape is death, with its 'dungeon crypts [. . .] year after year in gloom and desolate despair [. . .] the vision is divine'. The poem contains the mystical experience with its loss of consciousness and the descent of peace bringing with it the divine vision, 'then dawns the invisible, the Unseen its truth reveals'.

The influence of Novalis (1772–1801) and his mystical vision can be seen in the poetry of Emily Brontë where consciousness attempts to transcend reality through nature, aiming for that close union with God, freedom, and immortality. The night and yearning for death are familiar themes running through the poetry of both Novalis and Emily Brontë, along with that curious 'visionary' aspect that both poets adopt, which is uncanny; revelations, and visions accompanied by feelings of ecstasy and joy, in an individual and personal response for their own particular need.

"The Visionary" poem by Emily Brontë has its analogue with Novalis's *Hymns to the Night* with its silence and isolation of the poet who awaits the divine vision, accepting that her transcendental powers are 'its guiding star'. Both poets use the silence of the night in which to perceive the spirit world. For both Novalis and Emily Brontë the night brings peace and happiness, as they gaze into the immortal realm.

Hymns to the Night could be described as poems of meditation or reflection on death. They use images of the night to seek the spiritual world, and, like Emily Brontë, the quest for eternity is a powerful force. Novalis states that the night makes us aware of ourselves and nature as one, 'More heavenly than those glittering stars we hold eternal eyes which the Night hath opened within us', compared with Emily Brontë's "Stars", 'And hide me from the hostile light (daylight) / That does not warm but burn'. The poems of Novalis and Emily Brontë are unique for their visionary qualities, but also because they were written at a time when Romanticism gave them the opportunity to develop their innate powers.

Johann Wolfgang von Goethe (1749–1832) captured the essence of man's role in nature when he declared, 'If I work on unceasingly till my death, nature is bound to give me another form of being when the present one can no longer sustain my spirit', which echoes the beliefs of Novalis.

Goethe captured the essence of man's role in nature in his musical poetry, with its addition of Gothic machinery in such poems as "King of the Elves" (Erlkönig), and "Welcome and Farewell" ("Willkommen und Abschied") which has formative links with Emily Brontë's Gondal poems, and their high emotional and musical rhythms.

Goethe's poem "Night Thoughts" has its affinity also with Novalis and Emily Brontë. The poet speaks to the stars as they 'shone in splendour', and the 'sojournless eternal hours [that] lead you', which can be compared with Emily Brontë's "Stars" which have 'glorious eyes' and provide a divine vision, 'I saw him blazing still', while for Novalis the stars were 'making | Signal with voices sweet'.

Friedrich von Schiller, the German Romantic poet and writer, a volume of whose collected works was to be found on the Brontë bookshelves alongside *Deutsches Lesebuch* or *Lessons in German Literature* (London: Duval & Co., 1837) and *Rabenhorst's Pocket Dictionary of the German and English Language* (London: Longman, Brown & Co., 1843), was frequently to be featured in *Blackwood's Edinburgh Magazine*, and was a close friend of Goethe. Together they were the recognized leaders of the German Romantic movement. Schiller produced many ballad-style poems, as well as experimenting with 'fragment' poetry, a feature of the Romantic movement. Similar fragments can be seen in the poetry of Emily Brontë, which have been thought to be a part of other poems, or, merely drafts, but arguably the German Romantic influence can be seen at work, 'What is that smoke that ever still | Comes rolling down that dark brown hill', capturing the mist descending on the moors.

But it was Brussels that was to change the isolated life of Emily Brontë. It was a period of her life that 'had been overlooked by too many students', according to Robert K. Wallace. Emily discovered 'a world of cathedrals and pictures [and] learned to read the masters of French and German literature, all of which led her to producing some of the best work of her life', indicating that her foreign experience was to provide a turning point in her life. Wallace concludes that,

> [. . .] to Beethoven himself it was obvious that music and literature could inhabit the same emotional, spiritual and stylistic realms. In 1823 he declared that his musical ideas are roused by moods which in the poet's case are transmuted into words, and mine into tones, that sound, roar and storm until at last they take shape for me as notes.

Wallace finds many similarities between Beethoven and Emily Brontë as nature provided the inspiration for both in their expression of the Romantic style. Beethoven would have strengthened Emily's links with European culture, and served as a role model on which to base her writing, with music providing a very powerful and emotional language indeed.

Philip Barford, in his study of Beethoven's late piano sonatas, turned to Emily Brontë's poem, "The Prisoner," for a parallel to the spiritual vision expressed by the sublime variations movement that concludes Beethoven's *Opus 109*. The poem is suggestive of the mystical experience, since it is dramatic in its quest for ecstasy and emotional response.

Wallace states that it is no surprise that Beethoven's music was especially taken up by Emily as, 'her assimilation of his music and his legend in the 1840s sets in a new light the time lag between the Romantic equilibrium he achieved at the beginning of the Romantic age in music and she achieved near the end of the Romantic age in literature'.

The German Romantic writers relied upon music as a necessary ingredient of their poetry, and even Goethe has a love—hate relationship with Beethoven, although each admired the talent of the other. Beethoven composed several pieces of music based on Goethe's texts. The poetry of Tieck is also full of musical effects, combining assonance, rhyme and rhythm to evoke the sounds and moods of music. According to James Hardin, 'who else could have conversed with Mozart, Beethoven, Wagner [. . .]'. The poetry of Tieck, with its verbal music was later to influence the German poets Heine and Eichendorff.

The poems of Emily are passionate and sincere. Her solitary walks on the moors allowed her to be a Romantic wanderer, to be at one with nature and share its secrets. Her poems represent the changing faces of nature, its extremes and complexities. Here she could meditate on her own emotional instincts. She shares this with the German Romantic poets, particularly Eichendorff, whose portrayal of the natural world is reminiscent of Emily Brontë's with its aesthetic landscapes, colourful images, and the wandering poet—that ever-Romantic figure who appears in her poems.

The poem "Moonlit Night" by Eichendorff, with its nocturnal, symbolic landscape, 'so starry-clear was the night', has a religious significance; nature is of divine origin which echoes nearness to, and distance from, God, as 'my soul spread/Its wings out wide', and 'flew through the silent regions'. The 'silent regions' suggest a past the poet wishes to leave behind—the flawed world of mankind—in order to reach eternity, the fulfilment of Romanticism.

Poetry shows the relationship between the poets and the discourse of the age. The German Romantic movement was firmly established in Britain at the time Emily Brontë was writing and, despite the differences in country and culture, the poetry of the German Romantics does have an affinity with that of Emily Brontë. There are strong similarities of interest between Emily and poets such as Goethe and Novalis, nature and Gothic, for example, and their imaginative and spiritual vision. The influence of Beethoven on the German Romantic poets and Emily is also strong. In conclusion, while no single definitive factor links Emily Brontë directly to the German poets, the German influence was clearly present.

Source: Maggie Allen, "Emily Brontë and the Influence of the German Romantic Poets," in *Brontë Studies: The Journal of the Brontë Society*, Vol. 30, No. 1, February 2005, pp. 7–10.

Edward Wagenknecht

In the following excerpt, Wagenknecht examines the Gondalan theme used by Brontë in a biography and book of poetry.

Angria was an African kingdom; in the early days all the Brontë children lived there. But when Charlotte went to Roe Head, Emily found it impossible to work comfortably with Branwell; she and Anne therefore withdrew from Angria and betook themselves to Gondal, a large island in the North Pacific. The prose histories of Gondal have not survived, though Miss Ratchford has been able to recover broad outlines by reference to Emily's poems, most, if not all, of which used the same materials. This is the psychological moment, then, for the new and definitive edition of Emily's poems which Mr. Hatfield has just given us, the first that has ever been prepared from Emily's own manuscripts, and which thus definitely supersedes all the earlier texts with their many inaccuracies. Variant readings have been indicated with scrupulous care, the history of the manuscripts is given, the poems themselves are arranged in the order in which they fall in the history of Gondal, and an elaborate series of keys makes it possible for the careful reader to think Mr. Hatfield's thoughts after him. There are still many lacunae in our knowledge of Gondal, however, and neither Mr. Hatfield nor Miss Ratchford has feared to indicate these frankly.

Taken together, these two new volumes of Brontëana deal the popular view that literature is necessarily autobiography the heaviest blow it has sustained in many a year. If ever any writers were noted for their subjectivity, the Brontës have been so noted. And if ever any writers have provided a favorite hunting-ground for Freudian quackery, it has been they. Yet now it is absolutely proved that all the principal matters they are supposed to have derived from personal experience had actually been described by them in another form before the experiences in question took place! This is not a matter of conjecture; we have documentary evidence on the table. Unless we are now willing to admit that imagination is a part of experience—"An imaginative experience," says Walter de la Mare, "is not only as real but far realer than an unimaginative one"—it is going to be pretty difficult to digest the new data.

Of course this does not mean that it is necessary to go to fantastic extremes in the other direction and to deny the connection of literature and life altogether. And of course we must grant that it is possible for a writer to use an imaginatively conceived experience and to color it with what has happened personally to her. But none of this will help the Freudians very much.

Source: Edward Wagenknecht, Review of *The Brontës' Web of Childhood/The Complete Poems of Emily Jane Brontë*, in *Modern Language Quarterly*, Vol. 3, No. 1, March 1942, pp. 139–42.

Augustus Ralli

In the following essay, Ralli discusses how Emily Brontë's personality is incongruous with the work she created.

Emily Brontë is among the great ones whom it is said that we do not know, and the curiosity that seeks to know more of a writer than his works reveal has been condemned as unworthy. We are told that since he has expressed his mind, and so given his best to the world, we should not hunt after mere personal details. That this objection sounds more plausible than it is, and the modern instinct to make biography intimate is not a mistaken one, is the task here set before us to prove.

Let us realize in the beginning that art is a social virtue, that the ultimate reward of all success is social success, and that man is incomplete till he has expressed not only his mind but his personality. The supreme fact of life is personality, and its expression can be attained only by contact with men and women. To win battles, sway senates, discover new lands, write immortal verse: beyond all these, beyond even the mind's satisfaction in exercising its powers, is the approval of such as have done like things, is admission sought and won into the Paradise of this world— the kind glances of fair women and brave men. Disraeli's social success pleased him as much as his political, and there have been great men without personal magnetism, such as the American General Grant, or Jenner of vaccination fame. An aristocracy of pure intellect will never possess the earth, and the unkempt man of genius no longer excites admiring wonder. While man inhabits the earth he consists of body as well as

> THE TRAGEDY OF CHARLOTTE'S LIFE WAS ENFORCED SOLITUDE; WHEREAS EMILY, IF SHE EVER HAD WORLDLY DESIRES—AND WE GATHER FROM HER POEMS THAT SHE HAD—CONQUERED THEM ONCE AND FOR ALL."

mind; the ascetic ideal that despises the body as a clog to the spirit is rejected; and the modern culture of the body implies that it is a means of expressing the soul. Did not Leonardo da Vinci say that one of the two most wonderful sights in the world was the smiling of women?

Plato commended the spoken above the written word, because its meaning is strengthened by change of voice, glance of eye, movement of hand; and we need only revolve in our thoughts a few homely instances to be assured how vain it is to dispart mind and body. A letter cannot compensate for an absent friend, and a bore is a person whose utterances may be foretold. A twice-told tale will weary, and words that passed almost unnoticed may return and rankle in solitude, and again dissolve like a dream when the speaker is beheld once more in the flesh. A child prefers a story told rather than read from a book, and the very word "lecture" is evilly associated. Gloom envelops a company when a person adopts the lecturer's tone, speaking in a manner once removed from the personalities of his hearers, solving the problem by the help of ready made wisdom instead of that generated by the immediate contact of minds. A great orator creates the illusion in each member of his audience that he is spoken to directly; and a letter writer of genius never loses contact with his correspondent, whether his theme be objective or subjective; whether it be Cowper analyzing his religious melancholy, or Horace Walpole describing the Gordon riots.

The conclusion is that mind and body express each other, and we do not know our fellow creatures by one alone. Because of the few surviving details of his life we do not know Shakespeare, though through the mouths of his characters we have his thoughts on every subject in the world and beyond. Much of the cloud of darkness surrounding Chatham has been dispelled by the discovery of his latest biographer, Mr. Basil Williams, that he was exceptionally grateful for acts of personal kindness. Modern critics like Mr. T. S. Eliot and Mr. J. Middleton Murry affirm that every mental process has its equivalent in the world of sense; indeed Mr. Eliot says that *Hamlet* remains obscure because Shakespeare failed to find something in the outer world corresponding to the hero's disgust at his mother's conduct. It pleases us to think that the essence of the immortal biography is contained in Dr. Johnson's stentorian call to his servant Frank for a clean shirt, when Boswell had pleaded successfully with Mrs. Williams and the road to the Wilkes dinner party lay open.

The lack of objective correlatives places Emily Brontë among the unknown. Yet the task must not be abandoned, even if we make only the slight advance of realizing more fully the difficulties that beset us. If personality is the force proceeding from united soul and body made objective by the difficulties which stay it or which it overcomes, we can learn something by inquiring into the nature of the difficulties. We think of Cowper succumbing in his struggle with the wish to believe; FitzGerald self-banished from a world he found too hard; Swift finally baffled in his desire for power and place and retiring to die like a poisoned rat in a hole—to use his own phrase; Charlotte Brontë vainly seeking love as a refuge from hypochondria: and in consequence we know much of all these. Then we turn to Gibbon or Wordsworth, both of whom realized their personalities objectively—the one in his history, the other in contemplating nature and giving to his thoughts enduring form. Again, we have a middle class such as Byron and Carlyle, who achieved great fame but remained miserable— the one because of his lost social reputation, the other through imperfect faith and despair at the condition of the world.

With Emily Brontë there is a break between the operations of her mind as her books reveal it and the few biographical facts that have come down to us. We know that she was the least accessible of the three sisters of genius in the remote Haworth parsonage. She refused all acquaintance beyond her family, and yet was passionately interested in the fortunes of the people about her. As Charlotte says: "She knew their ways, their language, their family histories; she could hear of them with interest, and talk of them with detail, minute, graphic, and accurate; but *with* them she rarely exchanged a word." At school in Brussels she spoke to no one, and although, with Charlotte, she spent her weekly holiday at the house of an English family, she remained throughout impenetrable to friendly advances. Heger remarked upon her capacity for argument, unusual in a man and rare indeed in a woman; adding that hers was a stubborn tenacity of will which rendered her obtuse to all reasoning where her own wishes or her own sense of right were concerned. Mrs. Gaskell described her as reserved in the least favorable sense of the word; that is, indifferent if she pleased or not. When she went as pupil to Roe Head and teacher to a school near Halifax, she succumbed to homesickness, and her year's absence in Brussels was nearly cut short for the same reason. She loved liberty, she enjoyed passionately the lonely moors, and she loved wild animals because they were wild. Even in the small home circle she had a preference, and we doubt if she responded fully to the affection Charlotte lavished upon her. Charlotte described her as intractable, and observed that to advocate one side of a cause would ensure her adoption of the opposite. She began to write poetry without confiding in Charlotte, and was not pleased by Charlotte's chance discovery of her manuscripts. Perhaps her sister Anne, with a lesser mind, had a more receptive nature, and made a better companion to a woman of genius. To the end of Emily's short life the two played the game of make-believe which they called the *Gondal Chronicles*. No summary of facts should omit such harrowing details of her death scene as the silence she opposed to questions as to her state, and her refusal until too late to allow a "poisoning doctor" to come near her.

With every wish to estimate Emily favorably, it is hard to do so with the foregoing facts in mind. Exclusive family affection is not a commending trait, and one who persistently declines friendly advances is apt to forfeit human sympathy. In her last illness, had she no thought for the moral sufferings of her sisters when she refused to answer questions or see a doctor? And yet it is only fair to recall Charlotte's saying that she was full of ruth for others though without pity on herself. If we turn from Charlotte's direct sayings to her fictitious and therefore suggestive ones, we are equally baffled. Shirley Keeldar was supposed to represent Emily in happier circumstances, and yet, while external things such as the rich dresses she wore are much dwelt upon, we are not helped in the ultimate object of our search—a human soul made more beautiful on earth by the body.

There is enough to stimulate but not satisfy the imagination. We can picture the pleased expression on her face in solitude when anticipating her sisters' home-coming, the smile with which she greeted them, the especial look she reserved for Anne when they found themselves alone. On the reverse side we can picture the despair in her eyes when one after another came the harsh reviews of *Wuthering Heights*. But still we lack the actual collision of soul and sense with the outer world to make the vision real.

Life is greater than art, the artist's mind surpasses his work, and the crowd of men, indifferent to art, never desist to seek God in their fellow creatures, though they may know it not. The example of Emily Brontë suggests two problems especially prominent at the present day: personality and hero-worship. Carlyle taught us that hero-worship is the adamant below which unbelief cannot fall; and that if you convince a man he is in the presence of a higher soul his knees are automatically loosened in reverence. Lately Marcel Proust remarked that some people think of society as an Indian caste in which you take your place as you are born, but in reality all is due to personality: the humblest can become the friend of princes, and there are many princes whose acquaintance no one desires.

Carlyle preached the doctrine of work; he predicted a commonwealth of workers, and advised the man who had no work to hide himself; yet he privately admitted true good breeding to be one of the finest things in the world, and remarked the care of well-bred persons to avoid all unpleasant topics in conversation. The two are contradictory, for the effect of strenuous work—other than artistic—is to materialize, and good breeding can only thrive in the soil of leisure. The kind of character developed by the Victorian professional and business man is an answer to those who plead the dignity of work; and the modern desire for education in late life is an attempt to restore the balance of the mind which every profession inevitably disturbs. The duty of work is to overcome difficulties; the powers which it develops are the combative or competitive; whereas the right use of leisure is to promote the growth of the soul—and the greatest soul is that which has the greatest power to love. Good breeding implies that the material struggle has been concluded

generations back, that there is no need to compete with others for means of living and so acquire the habit of preferring things to persons. That a leisured class by attaining a certain mental outlook becomes the symbol of a more perfect life, alone justifies its existence in our distracted modern world, and makes the sight of luxury side by side with poverty at all bearable; and the toiling millions still feel an instinctive respect for those who dress finely and bear themselves graciously and do no work, despite the Communist orator.

That leisure and accumulated wealth are daily put to the worst uses is a truth we will not stay to consider in our search for the conditions in which personality may develop. Something has been said of good breeding, but as the highest beauty lies in expression, and the world soon tires of perfect features that lack it, so the long-solved material struggle does but prepare the ground by eliminating gross desires. We return to Proust's saying, and also remember that Becky Sharp climbed the social ladder to be ultimately bored. The soul uses the refined body to suggest a higher beauty; for man seeks God in his fellow creatures, and it was a doctrine of the neo-Platonists that a beautiful person could not be wicked. Hence are those stories eternally fascinating which tell how gods or angels have come down to live with men.

Thus the world labors to produce a race intermediate between God and man: the body on which generations of leisure have worked as with a chisel, the feelings—when not blasted by pride—responding to the sorrows of the lowest, the mind touched by those arts and philosophies which add thought to beauty. And to become a member of this race is the crown of all earthly effort, including art. Keats and Shelley were two of the most intense lyricists of all time, yet each laid aside his art before the close of his troubled life because the world would not listen. Surely this tribute of art to life proves that man's deepest desire is to be approved by man. And what exists scattered in the mass of men is brought to a focus in this selected intermediary race. Each carries with him the memory of a human friend transfigured, and all moral codes and material considerations shrink to nothing by contrast with the immediate presence of man. He may be thought insincere, for he neither argues nor contradicts, never speaks a distasteful truth, promises what he cannot perform, and will discard a friend for an unlucky word. Yet through this over-value of mankind we see dimly on the outer edge of society something of heaven on earth, of the reign of love. But always the law holds good that heaven reveals itself through the earthly beauty of line and color: and so we end where we began with Leonardo's saying of the smiling of women.

To the opinions of Carlyle and Proust which have been the props of this argument we now add a third. Professor Bradley described the tragic hero as intense rather than extraordinary—as one who thought and acted in a manner little removed from the average person but more energetically. We admire Antony and Cleopatra, for instance, and contemn the politic Octavius and his impeccable sister. The modern craving for personality has displaced the balance too far from mere good breeding to the region of despotic will and tempestuous passion. Never has the lot of undistinguished people been harder, nor the bore more severely let alone. In old days the human race was united by the subconscious thought of the brotherhood of man; but now, in our eagerness to see the vision before the coming of night, we apply widely the mordant remark of Charles Maurras against literary egoists, that not everybody has a soul.

Having rejected the theory that an author's work is his best biography, but convinced that the writer of a great book has a great soul, and that to learn how this soul moved among us in its earthly vestments is to learn something of heaven, we pass on to glean what we can from Emily's books. And they also strike us, as did her life, by other-worldliness, by excess of soul over body. She has been called primitive, a descendent of giants and Titans, and so on, but this is not the emotion that *Wuthering Heights* conveys; she is on the hither side of civilization, not before it begins but where it ends, and what Carlyle called the dim waste that lies beyond creation appears. The wild scenery of Wuthering Heights, the lonely moors impassable in winter, the stony track that leads off the main road to the deserted farm, where the slant of the stunted firs and thorns shows the force of the north wind, the rude furniture of the dwelling, the hard manners of its inmates—all point to something far withdrawn from the world we know. We are on the pinnacles of the moral world, with its restraints and conventions out of sight; the scene is laid in a spot that has not changed since creation, and that symbolizes the end of civilization; and there is

nothing primitive in the souls of those who act out their destinies in these abandoned tracts.

As we approach the stern tale, something of at least the outlying parts of Emily's mind will be revealed. As common traits of the characters we may cite intellectual vigor and sarcastic speech, such as we might expect to find in the Yorkshire farmer or land-worker, out of whom Heathcliff was idealized: the effect of a keen brain and little education, solitude, hard weather, rough work. When old Mr. Earnshaw dies late at night, the messenger dispatched for the doctor and parson returns with the doctor and says the parson will come in the morning. Heathcliff says sneeringly that Isabella Linton married him thinking he was a hero of romance, and at first none of his brutalities disgusted her. "I suppose we shall have plenty of lamentations now!" exclaims Catherine when Edgar at last realizes the mortal nature of her illness. Catherine again is under no illusions as regards her lover; she warns the infatuated Isabella that Heathcliff is a pitiless, wolfish man, not the kind who conceals depths of benevolence beneath a stern exterior. The above saying of Heathcliff leads to a further common trait of Emily's characters: their self-consciousness. Catherine speaks of turning her fits of frenzy to account; Linton Heathcliff admits he has a bad nature and cannot be scorned enough, and is too mean for the younger Catherine's anger; and many other instances spring to the mind. It is the trait which makes Shakespeare's characters psychologically real and individual: from *Richard III*, where it shows rather crudely, to the most consummate examples of his genius: Hamlet, Iago, Falstaff.

Like Shakespeare, Scott, Jane Austen, like all the most creative artists, Emily's characters become objective and self-moved; the one point of contact with her personal nature is sarcasm. But it is a sarcasm bound up with intellectual vigor: the power to foresee clearly, while others, blinded by mere wishes, are dimly groping after truth. Keen untutored brains struggling with hard conditions might foster its growth in her models, but with Emily the cause was excess of spirit reacting on her own powerful mind, making this earth too small a point to see realized the thoughts she drew from the infinite. The note of Charlotte's writings is regret; Charlotte would have been happy in a full family life, in society, in contact with any persons who treated her kindly. The tragedy of Charlotte's life was enforced solitude; whereas Emily, if she ever had worldly desires—and we gather from her poems that she had—conquered them once and for all. No doubt she grieved deeply at the immediate failure of *Wuthering Heights*, and she resigned further literary work, yet the fact remains that the balance is shifted too heavily on the side of soul for us to see her as a glorious earthly figure.

Charlotte describes nature as one who loves the joys of this world; the beauty of her landscapes in dawn or sunset is heightened by the suggestion from her own mind that another day has passed, and her hopes are unrealized, and death will come. Also, the love that she describes, though transcending time and space, is not entirely strange to earth. Most of us when first reading *Jane Eyre* in childhood knew that we were falsely told in the concluding chapter that Jane married Rochester; we felt instinctively that the inner truth of the story was thereby violated, that the poor human institution of marriage was a small thing to two such souls wandering in eternity. And yet for a short spell they might have been happy on earth: Jane Eyre and Rochester at Thornhill, Lucy Snowe and Paul Emanuel in the schoolrooms of Villette. It is otherwise with Catherine and Heathcliff who, as children on the moors, had just a foothold in time, but cannot be imagined living together as man and wife even in the extra-conventional world of the story. But if their love is not of earth still less is it of heaven, and we must search for the true region where their souls have scope.

Many writers have attempted to depict a world beyond this, and none have succeeded like Emily. Haeckel, in the midst of foolish generalizations, did arrest our thought when he asked if we realized what we meant by eternity, and pointed to the profound legend of the Wandering Jew. Yet the desire to persist at least beyond this world is ineradicable, and Emily speaks in accents that convince us a further sphere exists. It comes to us in Mr. Lockwood's dream, and not Clarence's dream in *Richard III*, not the witches in *Macbeth*, not the raising of Samuel by the Witch of Endor, have so true a ring of an actual experience of the soul. The keynote of the dream is subtly struck when sour old Joseph tells the younger Catherine that she will never mend her ways but go right to the devil like her mother before her. It is followed by the discovery of the writing in the old book which affects us strangely because we know that the writer has passed behind the veil. Then comes the dream: the tapping of the branch on the lattice;

the ice-cold hand which seizes the dreamer's; the sobbing voice, "Let me in . . . I'm come home. I'd lost my way on the moor;" the child's face looking through the window; the reiterated cry, "It is twenty years . . . I've been a wait for twenty years;" the effect on Heathcliff of sliding back the panels. . . .

What are the symbols that Emily uses so skilfully as to make us believe that this once-removed world exists? In the first place we have the rude setting of the story, the point in life where all joyful social intercourse has ceased, and human relations are just preserved. It is neither primitive nor return to barbarism, but the end of a world, the dropping one by one of the refinements of life till the soul is naked. The austere moors, the bare dwellings typify it; the coming of a stranger brings it home to us, like one of Shakespeare's underplots which reflect the main action and add a meaning. Such was Hindley Earnshaw's wife who came from no one knew where, without name or fortune, the "rush of a lass" far advanced in consumption, but who was so delighted with the old farm house that she would have nothing changed for her comfort, whose gay heart never failed her till within a week of her death. Catherine said well that she had no more right to marry Edgar Linton than to go to heaven, and her dream taught her how miserable she would have been in heaven. The Linton family does seem an alien presence on the moors, and the interior of Thrushcross Grange, into which Catherine and Heathcliff gaze spell-bound, with its crimson carpet and crimson-covered chairs and white and gold ceiling, so remote as almost to be unreal. Here again we see Emily's soul stronger than that of Charlotte, who described such things with a tinge of regret that she too did not live in splendid places and wear rich fabrics. Heathcliff's brutality is neither that of the savage, the boor, nor the over-civilized man driven mad. When he strikes the younger Catherine he does the easiest thing to gain his object, because nothing else is worthwhile in a perishing world. The manner of his death typifies this world from which life is visibly receding.

But if the soul is thus stripped naked, all the more urgent is its craving for love. It has attained the extreme point of earth, it reaches forward into the abyss beyond, it even exchanges messages with those whom the abyss has swallowed, and always it cries for love. Because of this we feel that the new world, a corner of which is mysteriously revealed, is more good than evil. That much evil remains—above all the sense of sin for earthly deeds—we do not dispute, but that love continues and will eventually triumph over sin, is the last conviction. Catherine's unrestrained childhood, the passionate dispositions of the Earnshaw family, Heathcliff's rough caresses which bruise the arm of his dying love—all these are symbols of the ultimate recovery of the spirit. Edgar Linton finds comfort in books after his wife's death, Hindley Earnshaw, in the same condition, becomes a gambler and raving drunkard. Because the soul is a real thing its conflict with gross matter is terrible: such was Hindley's unreasoning persecution of Heathcliff as a boy. While on earth it may appear worsted in its conflict with evil, but Emily has power to convince that the decision is elsewhere. The device of the Greek chorus has been a favorite one with playwright or novelist; it here finds an unparalleled exponent in the character of Nelly Dean. Catherine confides her spiritual affinity with Heathcliff to be met with the retort: "If I can make any sense of your nonsense, Miss—." As with Thersites in *Troilus and Cressida*, or Apemantus in *Timon*, her very blindness to the wonderland of Catherine's soul must flash something of its glory upon the dullest reader.

Turning from her novel to ask whether her poems will supply the image of an earthly-heavenly creature, again the answer is negative. The balance may be shifted a stage back towards earth, but is still not equal. One cannot but hear the cry of the heart in "*Remembrance*," but there is no means of knowing the proportion of real and ideal. Let us however recall a few of her best pieces and brood over their distinctive charm. Such are "*The Linnet*," "*The Prisoner*," "*The Lady to Her Guitar*," "*How Clear She Shines*," "*Often Rebuked*," "*The Outcast Mother*," "*The Old Stoic*," and the poem already mentioned. Take the last stanza of "The Linnet":

> Blow, west wind, by the lonely mound,
> And murmur, summer streams—
> There is no need of other sound
> To soothe my lady's dreams.

And this from "The Lady to Her Guitar":

> It is as if the glassy brook
> Should image still its willows fair,
> Though years ago the woodman's stroke
> Laid low in dust their Dryad-hair.

And place beside them these lines from Wordsworth's "Highland Reaper:"

> A voice more thrilling ne'er was heard
> In springtime from the cuckoo bird,
> Breaking the silence of the seas
> Among the furthest Hebrides.

And this stanza of Mr. De La Mare's, the effect of snow on fields at break of day:

> It hangs the frozen bough
> With flowers on which the night
> Wheeling her darkness through
> Scatters a starry light.

Differ as may the poet of fairy-land from the poet who, beginning with the beauty of nature, thereafter includes man, and so rises to believe in a divinely ordered universe, they are one in this: their vision of beauty has brought them peace on earth. It is not so with Emily who, though rivalling them in beauty, is at peace only with nature and not with man. The greatest poets carry with them an ideal world which is proof against intruders: thus William Blake, greater of course as mystic than poet, met and saluted the Apostle Paul in the Strand. Emily falls short of supreme greatness in that she is muted by a trespasser in her imaginative Eden. The earth must be delivered from man's presence before she can recognize it as Godlike; she is inspired by night,— especially winter nights, when human activity is suspended for many long hours, or starry nights which suggest remote worlds where perhaps sin is not,—by the barest tracts of the moors where no house can resist the wind, by snow which muffles human footsteps and masks human traces, by time and death which defeat man, and make his mightiest happenings—his battles and empires, his material progress, the voices of orators, even the cry of sufferers—a momentary break in the eternal silence.

In this shrinking from her fellow creatures, in their power to shatter her bright world by their mere presence, lay Emily's weakness. Yet she is stronger than Charlotte, who depended utterly on others, and whose consistent regret for lost happiness sounds in her every page. Had we biographical means to know whether this trait was inborn or developed by circumstances, much of the mystery of her personality would be solved. She confesses in her poems to a fleeting desire for fame, and such a stanza as this from "Remembrance" has an authentic ring:

> But when the days of golden dreams had
>   perished,

And even despair was powerless to destroy,
Then did I learn how existence could be
    cherished,
Strengthened and fed without the aid of joy.

But so have many of Shakespeare's sonnets, over which the battle between evenly-matched commentators has swayed backward and forward for generations. Suffice it that if from the internal evidence of her novel and poems we have realized more clearly what she was not, some slight advance has been made toward conceiving an image of her personality despite a forcedly agnostic conclusion.

Source: Augustus Ralli, "Emily Brontë. The Problem of Personality," in *North American Review*, Vol. 221, No. 826, March 1925, pp. 495–507.

SOURCES

Alexander, Christine, and Margaret Smith, eds., *The Oxford Companion to the Brontës*, Oxford University Press, 2003.

Bock, Carol, "'Our Plays': The Brontë Juvenilia," in *The Cambridge Companion to the Brontës*, edited by Heather Glen, Cambridge University Press, 2002, pp. 34–52.

Brontë, Emily, "The Old Stoic," in *The New Oxford Book of English Verse 1250–1950*, edited by Helen Gardner, Oxford University Press, 1972, p. 677.

———, *Wuthering Heights*, edited by Beth Newman, Broadview Press, 2007.

Carter, Elizabeth, trans., *All the Works of Epictetus, Which Are Now Extant; Consisting of His Discourses, Preserved by Arrian, in Four Books, the Enchiridion, and Fragments*, 3rd ed., J. and F. Rivington, 1758.

Dodds, Madeleine Hope, "Gondaliand," in *Modern Language Review*, Vol. 18, 1923, pp. 9–21.

Epictetus, *Handbook of Epictetus*, translated by Nicholas P. White, Hackett, 1983.

Evans, Barbara, and Gareth Lloyd Evans, eds., *The Scribner Companion to the Brontës*, Charles Scribner's Sons, 1982.

Ingham, Patricia, *The Brontës*, Oxford University Press, 2008, pp. 13–14.

Leighton, Angela, "The Poetry," in *The Cambridge Companion to the Brontës*, edited by Heather Glen, Cambridge University Press, 2002, pp. 53–71.

Maison, Margaret, "Emily Brontë and Epictetus," in *Notes and Queries*, vol. 223, June 1978, pp. 230–31.

Ratchford, Fannie Elizabeth, *The Brontës' Web of Childhood*, Columbia University Press, 1941.

———, *Gondal's Queen*, University of Texas Press, 1955.

Saunders, Jason L., ed., *Greek and Roman Philosophy after Aristotle*, Free Press, 1966, pp. 59–150.

Shippey, Tom, *J. R. R. Tolkien: Author of the Century*, HarperCollins, 2000.

FURTHER READING

Gérin, Winifred, *Emily Brontë*, Oxford University Press, 1971.
    This is the standard biography of Brontë and the usual initial guide to the study of her life and writings.

Gezari, Janet, *Last Things: Emily Brontë's Poems*, Oxford University Press, 2007.
    Although Gezari does not deal directly with "The Old Stoic," she gives a critical treatment to Brontë's badly neglected poetry.

Turner, Frank M., *The Greek Heritage in Victorian Britain*, Yale University Press, 1981.
    Turner discusses the role of Greek philosophy in nineteenth-century British culture.

Winnifrith, Tom, and Edward Chitham, *Charlotte and Emily Brontë*, Macmillan, 1989.
    This book gives a brief overview of the entwined literary lives of the two sisters, and to a lesser degree the other two Brontë siblings.

On My First Son

BEN JONSON

1616

The English author Ben Jonson was one of the most well-respected and popular writers of his day. Best known for dramas such as *Every Man in His Humour* and *Volpone; or The Fox*, Jonson also wrote a significant body of sophisticated and intelligent poetry, including his 1616 folio *Epigrams*. Included in this volume are two of Jonson's most well-known poems, "On My First Daughter" and "On My First Son," epitaphs for two of Jonson's children who died in childhood. Jonson wrote "On My First Son" in 1603, the year King James VI of Scotland ascended to the English throne as James I, and the year that the plague made a return visit to England, killing thousands of Londoners, including Jonson's first son, Benjamin. The short poem is poignant in the grief and sense of loss Jonson expresses. At the same time, however, it is also a statement of Christian consolation; Jonson has faith that his son is in a better place than in the earthly realm. Although first published over 400 years ago, Jonson's poem is still widely available in many anthologies such as *English Renaissance Poetry* (1990), edited by John Williams and published by the University of Arkansas Press. Moreover, although Jonson wrote the poem in a very different time and place, the sentiment expressed in "On My First Son" remains just as compelling in the twenty-first century as it did in England in the seventeenth century.

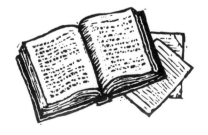

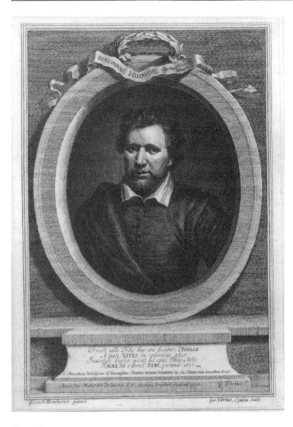

Ben Jonson (*The Library of Congress*)

AUTHOR BIOGRAPHY

Jonson was born around June 11, 1572, near London, England, a month after his father's death. Jonson's father had lost his property under the reign of Queen Mary, and was imprisoned. Jonson's mother later married a bricklayer.

Although poor, Jonson attended St. Martin's Parish School, and subsequently was a student at Westminster School, studying under William Camden, well-known in his time as an antiquarian. This relationship proved to be an influential one for Jonson, who later commented in one of his poems that everything he knew in the arts could be attributed to Camden.

In 1589, Jonson left school to follow his stepfather's trade. It is likely that although most of the students at Westminster would have continued their education at university, Jonson was unable to do so because of poverty. He apparently did not flourish as a bricklayer, because in the early 1590s, he served in the military in Flanders. In 1594, he married Anne Lewis; authorities disagree about

the number of children born to the couple with some claiming at least two and others claiming at least four. He began his career in the theater about the same time, working as an actor and a playwright, although little is known about his life during this period except that he was associated with Philip Henslow's theater company.

In 1598, Jonson's first well-known play, *Every Man in His Humour*, was performed. Also in the same year, Jonson killed the actor Gabriel Spencer in a duel and was charged with murder. He narrowly escaped execution by claiming he was a member of the clergy, proving this by reading scripture in Latin. Jonson also began writing and publishing poems about 1598.

By 1603, Jonson was becoming well-known and enjoying royal patronage from the court of King James I of England. However, in the same year, the plague returned to London, leaving over 30,000 people dead in its wake. Among them was Jonson's son, Benjamin. In response to this tragedy Jonson wrote the poem "On My First Son" in 1603, a poem that later appeared as Epigram 45 in his 1616 collection *Epigrams*.

Jonson presented his first royal masque, *The Masque of Blackness*, for the queen in 1605. The new dramatic genre included singing and dancing with elaborate costumes and set design, and achieved great popularity among the royal court. Jonson collaborated with the designer and architect Inigo Jones to produce some of the best known and most characteristic of the Jacobean masques. At the same time, Jonson reached the peak of his dramatic achievements, producing *Volpone; or The Fox* in 1606 and *The Alchemist* in 1610.

Jonson received several honors during his lifetime. In 1616, King James I appointed Jonson the first poet laureate of England, awarding him an annual pension in return. While on a walking tour of Scotland, the city of Edinburgh made him an honorary burgess. Later, Oxford University presented him with an honorary Master of Arts degree.

Jonson's library was destroyed by fire in 1623, and his dramatic and literary career waned, although a large group of younger poets and writers registered their admiration of Jonson by styling themselves as "The Sons of Ben." In 1628, Jonson fell ill and never recovered, dying on August 6, 1637. He is buried in Westminster Abbey, where the epitaph on his grave reads "O rare Ben Jonson."

POEM TEXT

Farewell, thou child of my right hand, and joy;
My sin was too much hope of thee, loved boy.
Seven years thou wert lent to me, and I thee
    pay,
Exacted by thy fate, on the just day.
O, could I lose all father, now! For why   5
Will man lament the state he should envý?
To have so soon 'scaped world's and flesh's
    rage,
And, if no other misery, yet age!
Rest in soft peace; and, asked, say: Here doth
    lie
Ben Jonson his best piece of poetry—   10
For whose sake, henceforth, all his vows be
    such,
As what he loves may never like too much.

POEM SUMMARY

"On My First Son" is a poem of twelve lines, written in response to the death of Jonson's first son, Benjamin, a victim of plague. The poem is written in couplets, with the following rhyme scheme: *aabbccddeeff*. The poem is also written in regular iambic pentameter. Iambic simply means that an unaccented syllable is followed by an accented one, and pentameter means that there are five such pairs (called feet) of one unaccented syllable followed by an accented syllable in each line of the poem. Iambic pentameter can be represented as follows: da DUH da DUH da DUH da DUH da DUH. This is a fairly natural rhythm in English, often used in oratory.

Lines 1–4

In the first two lines of the poem, Jonson addresses his dead son and says goodbye to him. He affirms that this son had great value for him and gave him happiness. Moreover, the name Benjamin, both the name of the writer and the dead child, means "right hand." Thus, in line one, Jonson is referring to the child's name indirectly by creating this pun. At the same time, the reference to the right hand also reminds readers that as a writer, Jonson's right hand would be very important to him.

In line 2, Jonson chastises himself for having too many ambitions and wishes for the boy. Jonson has invested himself in his son's future to the extent that he now believes he was sinful in doing so. While it is admirable to want good things for one's child, Jonson seems to be saying that he was overly involved in thoughts of his son's future. While modern audiences might not find this sinful, in Jonson's time, putting the love of any human, even a first son, before the love of God would be considered sinful. In addition, the line adds significant poignancy to the poem. Jonson seems to be saying that his grief is all the greater because he loved his son so much.

In line 3, the reader discovers that Jonson's son was only seven years old at the time of his death. In this line, Jonson introduces a financial motif into the poem. He tells his son that the boy was only on loan to his father. That is, although the boy was the father's son, he did not belong to him. And, as with any loan, Jonson must pay back the principle, in this case, the son's life. The last three words of line 3 might seem confusing, as it sounds as if Jonson is saying to his son that he (Jonson) will be repaying the loan to his son. This is not the case. Word order and meaning in early modern English is more flexible than in the English of the twenty-first century; thus, the line actually means "You were loaned to me for seven years, and now I must pay back the loan with your life."

Line 4 continues the sentence begun in line 3. Jonson states that it is providence, or destiny, that requires payment of the loan. Furthermore, Jonson also lets readers know that the day of his son's death was also his son's birthday. The word "just" in this line has multiple meanings. In the first place, it means "exact," as in the expression "just so." So the repayment comes on the exact day of the son's birth. In addition, "just" also carries with it the connotation of justice, as in a just law. Thus, Jonson sees in the coincidence of the child's death on his birthday a kind of divine justice in action.

Lines 5–8

Line 5 begins with a outcry from Jonson, as if he is overcome with grief. He wishes that he could somehow not be the child's parent at this moment. But this is an expression of grief, not of reality. The point here is that if he could somehow not be the child's father, he would not feel so much pain. The interjection of the heartfelt exclamation juxtaposed with the previous line's financial motif makes the outpouring of grief all the more painful. Immediately after the exclamation point, however, Jonson rounds out the line with two words that begin a new sentence completed in line 6. In this sentence, Jonson asks why it is that people feel grief when they know that the loved one will be in a better place.

He continues this thought in lines 7 and 8. Not only will his son be in a better place, he will also escape the pains and sorrow visited upon the body in life. Jonson further asserts in line 8 that even if someone is fortunate enough to escape most of the illnesses and misfortune life offers, there is still the misery of old age. A child who dies young does not have to experience the loss of physical or mental function due to aging.

Lines 9–12

Line 9 contains two phrases often found in epitaphs. Indeed, lines 9 and 10 read as if they could be carved onto the boy's tombstone. In these lines, Jonson wishes for his son peaceful rest. In addition, he asserts that his child is the best of all of his creative works. Line 10 also presents an interesting detail of early modern English. In present-day English, possession is marked by an apostrophe followed by the letter "s." For example, in present-day English, the phrase "the book of Ben Jonson" could also be written "Ben Jonson's book." In early modern English, the same phrase could be correctly written "Ben Jonson his book." (The apostrophe in present-day English stands in for the missing part of the word "his.") Poets in Jonson's time had a choice between using "his" or the apostrophe, depending on what they needed in order to maintain their meter.

Jonson concludes the poem with a promise that he will never indulge himself by caring for another human being as much as he has his son. The lines suggest that Jonson wants to protect himself against future pain, although it is also possible that he is attempting to correct the sin noted in line 2, of having too much hope for his son. In either case, as a reader, it is difficult to imagine Jonson being successful in keeping this vow. The rest of the poem points to a person who experiences grief and life deeply.

THEMES

Grief

In "On My First Son," Jonson provides a glimpse into deep, fatherly grief over the loss of his first child, Benjamin, who died from the plague on his seventh birthday. Through simple, straightforward language, Jonson expresses this grief while, at the same time, attempting to assuage it. In the

first two lines of the poem, Jonson addresses the boy as if he is present, and says goodbye to him, telling him that he was his pride and joy. Indeed, it is as if Jonson blames himself in line 2, saying that it was sinful of him to have so much pride and hope in the boy.

In lines 3 and 4, Jonson turns away from the outright expression of grief in an attempt to explain why the boy has been taken. He uses a financial metaphor, referring to the boy's life as a loan. Thus, Jonson attempts to comfort himself with the knowledge that God had only temporarily loaned the boy to his father, and that now, because it is the boy's time to return to God, the father must repay the debt.

However, no sooner does Jonson make this assertion than the full force of his grief emerges. In line 5, he exclaims that if he could, he would not be the boy's father. He does not mean in this line that he truly would not want to be Benjamin's father, but rather, he does not want to feel the pain a father necessarily feels upon the death of his child. Again, after this outburst, Jonson tries to assuage his own grief by wondering why a person should be so grief stricken when he knows, as a Christian, that his son will be in heaven. He further attempts to comfort himself by saying that his son will not be subject to all the pain and misery the world heaps upon a person, including that of growing old. In other words, his son, having died young, will never know how difficult life can be. He will have gone directly from a young and joyful life to heaven, a place where he will be happy for all eternity.

Jonson seems to come to terms with his grief through the writing of the poem. Yet the very last line suggests perhaps otherwise, depending on the reading. In this line, Jonson says that he is promising on the life of his son that in the future; he will not be overly attached to that which he loves. While this is the apparent meaning of the poem, that one should never love another person more than one loves God, there is also the sense that Jonson intends to use the memory of his grief for his son to harden himself against future losses. By refusing to "like" what he loves, he can perhaps save himself the pain of future grief.

Death

Death is one of the great mysteries of humankind. It can come slowly, or suddenly, but come it will, to every living creature. In act 3, scene 1 of *Hamlet*, written by Jonson's great contemporary

TOPICS FOR FURTHER STUDY

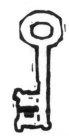

- Read several accounts of the lives of Ben Jonson and William Shakespeare. Prepare an essay in which you compare and contrast the two men, using such criteria as their biographies, their work, and their influence on those who came after. Why do you think that Jonson was considered the finest writer of his age but has not achieved the same level of popularity Shakespeare still has even in the twenty-first century?

- Read the young-adult novel *At the Sign of the Sugared Plum* (2003) by Mary Hooper, a fictional account of two young women's experiences in plague-stricken London during the seventeenth century. With a group of your peers, write a scene from the novel as a play and present your scene to your classmates.

- With a small group of students, research the Black Death by reading articles in books and online. Working as a team, prepare a video or multimedia presentation for your class about what you have learned about the plague. Be prepared to answer questions from your classmates after showing them the presentation.

- An epitaph is a short verse or pithy sentiment that is inscribed on a gravestone. Collect as many epitaphs as you can find online, or by visiting cemeteries. Create a collage of epitaphs to share with your classmates, and write a epitaph for yourself. How would you like to be remembered?

- Ben Jonson often used the epigram as a poetic form for invitations, letters, compliments, elegies, and reflection. Read Jonson's epigram "Inviting a Friend to Supper" several times. Look up any references or words you do not recognize to help you understand the poem. Then write a poetic invitation to a friend to come to your house to supper, modeling your poem after Jonson's.

- Read Jonson's poem "On My First Daughter." What were the circumstances surrounding the death of Jonson's daughter? Write an essay in which you compare and contrast this poem with "On My First Son."

William Shakespeare, Hamlet calls death "the undiscover'd country from whose bourn / No traveler returns." This, of course, is the issue: since no one survives death, there is no one to return to tell people what to expect.

This gap in human knowledge is one that people have tried to fill for millennia, through religion, art, and literature. Jonson, in "On My First Son," does his best to come to terms with the death of his seven-year-old son by relying on standard Christian consolation. In lines 3 and 4, he reports that his child's death has been required by fate, another way saying that the child's death is a part of God's divine providence. Jonson must try to console himself by admitting that his child's life was really only on loan to him, from God, and that it is God's prerogative to call the loan in. These lines, then, suggest that Jonson sees death as not only inevitable, but that each death comes at its own time, no matter how painful it is for those who are left.

The second feature of standard Christian consolation can be found in lines 6 through 8. In these lines, Jonson questions why someone should be unhappy over the death of a child, when through that death, the child not only achieves heaven, he or she also escapes all of the trials and tribulations of living. Such thoughts were common in Jonson's time; Shakespeare gives voice to something similar in Hamlet's act 3, scene 1 soliloquy: "To die, to sleep— / No more, and by a sleep to say we end / The heartache and the thousand natural shocks / That flesh is heir to; 'tis a consummation / Devoutly to be wish'd." Death, then, becomes the passage out of a painful life and into eternal bliss. And yet, for

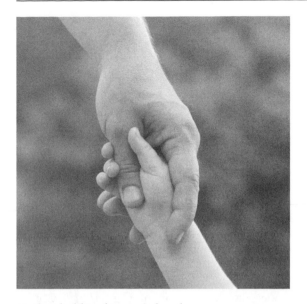

Father holding his son's hand (Image copyright Vita Khorzhevska, 2009. Used under license from Shutterstock.com)

Jonson, this explanation does not seem to sit comfortably. In the last line of the poem, he suggests that he will have to guard his feelings so that he does not have to suffer so much pain in the future at the death of a loved one. While he pays lip service to Christian consolation, it appears that he remains unconsoled.

STYLE

Epigram

"On My First Son" is included in Jonson's 1616 collection *Epigrams*, and is a good example of the genre of epigrams. The word "epigram" comes from two Greek words that mean "to write on" or "to inscribe." In the Classical world of Greece and Rome, an epigram was literally an inscription, often serving as an epitaph for the dead. The greatest writer of epigrams in the Classical world was Martial, a Roman writer who lived during the first century CE. His work in Latin was well-known among English writers of the Renaissance.

By Jonson's time, an epigram meant a pithy saying, characterized by precision, economy of language, balance, wit, and polish. It could also be a short poem with the same characteristics. Jonson used Martial's work as a model, and most scholars cite Jonson as the greatest writer of epigrams in English.

Epigrams are often satiric or humorous, and Jonson wrote many such epigrams. However, Jonson also expanded the genre, and used the epigram to write invitations, epistles, reflective poems, compliments, and eulogies. He also used the epigram in its original sense, that of the epitaph.

While not humorous, "On My First Son" meets the requirements of the genre: it is short, highly polished, and tightly constructed. In addition, it is witty without being funny. Jonson uses puns throughout the poem, including the allusion to his son as his right hand—Benjamin means "right hand" in Hebrew. In addition, when he calls his son a piece of poetry, he is punning on the Greek word for poetry, *poesis*, a word that originally meant "making." A poet, then, is a maker, and his poem is something he made, just as a father makes a son.

Another characteristic of Jonson's epigrams and of later epigrams in English is the use of closed, rhyming couplets. Couplets are simply two contiguous lines of poetry that rhyme at the end. This, and the regular use of iambic pentameter in "On My First Son" provides a tightly controlled structure through which Jonson can express his grief.

Elegy and Epitaph

The word "elegy" comes from the Greek *elegos* meaning "lament." Usually, an elegy is a reflective meditation on a particular death, although in English, elegies can also be meditations on death in general, or on war or love. Indeed, the Elizabethans frequently called their love poems elegies. Later, however, elegy came to be strongly identified with mourning.

A second word associated with writing that concerns death is "epitaph." An epitaph is generally an inscription on a burial marker, and often begins with the words "here lies." The purpose of an epitaph is to name the person who is buried, and provide some pithy information about the person. Jonson's epitaph on his tomb in Westminster Abbey reads simply, "O Rare Ben Jonson." (Visitors to Westminster will note that Jonson's name is spelled incorrectly on his grave as "Johnson.") Jonson's epitaph illustrates particular economy and wit. Many scholars assert that it is a pun; *orare* in Latin means "pray for."

"On My First Son" demonstrates the characteristics of the elegy in that it is a reflective poem about a death that meditates on the nature of death itself. At the same time, it closes with what is clearly an epitaph, in that it uses the words "here lies," referring to the burial of Jonson's son. In addition, the epitaphic ending provides closure to the earlier meditation on the nature of death.

Thus, Jonson's poem "On My First Son" qualifies as an epigram, an elegy, and an epitaph. Jonson's skillful use of these literary forms demonstrates keen wit, careful use of language, and the balanced phrases he pioneered in the early seventeenth century.

HISTORICAL CONTEXT

Plague in England, 1600–1604

Bubonic plague is a bacterial disease present in rodents that is spread by fleas that bite an infected rodent, and then bite a human or other susceptible animal. Once infected, humans and other animals can spread the disease through exposure to bodily fluids. The lymph glands swell dramatically, forming "buboes." In the modern world, bubonic plague can be treated with antibiotics; left untreated, it is very often fatal.

In 1348 and 1349, bubonic plague swept all over Europe in an epidemic known as the Black Death. It is difficult to even imagine the devastation that this disease caused. By 1350, as much as half of the human population of Europe had died; in some areas, the death toll was as high as 70 percent. And then the deaths slowed, and stopped. It appeared that the plague was over.

Such was not the case, however. According to John Kelly in his book *The Great Mortality*, a "new epidemic, which began in 1361, marked the beginning of a long wave of plague death that would roll on through more than three centuries."

Jonson's son Ben died in one such wave of plague that spread through England between 1600 and 1604. While not as widespread or as devastating as the earlier epidemics, the mortality rate was still high. Moreover, the continuing incidences of epidemic plague reminded the population that life was fraught with uncertainty, and death could call at any moment. In 1665 alone, the Great Plague of London, chronicled by the writer Daniel Defoe, killed some 100,000 people in London and the surrounding area, according to A. Lloyd Moote and Dorothy C. Moote in their 2004 book, *The Great Plague: The Story of London's Most Deadly Year*. It is little wonder that thoughts of death were never far from people's minds.

England in 1603

1603, the year of Jonson's composition of "On My First Son" was a year of great transitions. Most importantly, the long reign of Queen Elizabeth I came to an end.

Elizabeth, born in 1533, was the daughter of King Henry VIII and his second wife, the commoner Anne Boleyn. Catholics in England and throughout the world did not believe that the union between the king and Boleyn was legitimate: it was only made possible by Henry's ultimate break with the Catholic Church in Rome and his formation of the Church of England under the Archbishop of Canterbury. Consequently, Elizabeth herself was regarded was an illegitimate child by many people. When the king had Boleyn executed in 1536, Elizabeth was no longer regarded as a princess and was removed from the line of succession.

When Henry died in 1547, he was succeeded by his young son, Edward VI. A sickly boy, Edward died at fifteen, in 1553. Edward, a Protestant, and his advisors did not want the throne to go to Henry's other remaining child, the Catholic Mary, daughter of Henry's first wife, Catherine. After Edward's death, his advisors plotted to put Lady Jane Grey on the throne, a position she held for just nine days before Mary took her rightful and legal place as the Queen of England. Queen Mary, known among some as "Bloody Mary" for her persecution of Protestants, ruled England until 1558. During part of this time, Elizabeth was under house arrest.

Upon Mary's death, Queen Elizabeth I ascended to the throne. She was a Protestant, but worked toward a middle way, neither welcoming nor persecuting (for the most part) Catholics. Under Elizabeth, English culture flourished. In addition, with the defeat of the Spanish Armada, a naval fleet sent by King Philip of Spain to invade England, England quickly established itself as a world power under Elizabeth's rule.

Elizabeth did not marry, however, in spite of many political maneuvers and intrigues. As she grew older, this became increasingly worrisome for the English. They feared social upheaval and political instability as the long-reigning queen neared the end of her life. Ultimately, it was decided by Elizabeth and her ministers that

COMPARE
&
CONTRAST

- **1600s:** Plague continues to resurface in Europe throughout the seventeenth century. In 1665 alone, 68,596 Londoners die of the disease.

  Today: According to the Centers for Disease Control, human cases of bubonic plague in the United States in the twenty-first century average between 10 and 15 cases per year, and there are virtually no recorded cases anywhere in England in this century.

- **1600s:** One in five children die before they reach the age of ten in seventeenth-century England, according to Patricia M. Crawford

and Laura Gowing in *Women's Worlds in Seventeenth-Century England* (2000).

  Today: About 6 children in 1,000 die before the age of five in England.

- **1600s:** By the time of his death, Ben Jonson is, according to his biographer David Riggs in his 1989 book *Ben Jonson: A Life*, the most famous poet of his age, and is viewed by his contemporaries as the finest writer of the time.

  Today: William Shakespeare, Ben Jonson's contemporary, is far more popular than Jonson, and most scholars consider him the greatest writer in the English language.

King James VI of Scotland had the best claim to the throne.

Elizabeth's death in 1603 came after a rule of 45 years. During her reign, men from humble beginnings such as Jonson were able to achieve great fame and notoriety for their artistic efforts. For those long accustomed to Elizabeth's rule, the accession of James the VI of Scotland as James I of England must have seemed strange indeed.

What Jonson could not have known in 1603, however, was that King James I would be even more amenable to the theater and to his plays and poetry than Elizabeth had been. If the English language flourished under Elizabeth, Jonson's fortunes flourished under James. Despite the terrible outbreak of plague in 1603, the year marked an upward movement in the arc of Jonson's career.

CRITICAL OVERVIEW

Jonson enjoyed a great deal of popularity in his own day, primarily for his plays such as *Every Man in His Humour* and *Volpone; or The Fox*. In addition, his poetry was so well thought of in his

own day that the next generation of poets styled themselves as "Sons of Ben."

Jonson's 1616 collection *Epigrams*, the collection that includes his 1603 poem "On My First Son," contains some of Jonson's very best work. This collection, and particularly "On My First Son," continue to attract significant critical attention.

Wesley Trimpi, for example, in his classic book *Ben Jonson's Poems: A Study of the Plain Style* (1962), argues that the relationship between the father and son is the most important thematic concern of the poem. He writes, "The theme is rather the relation between father and son than the death of a child." Likewise, Claude J. Summers and Ted-Larry Pebworth in their 1979 book *Ben Jonson* also focus on the relationship between father and son as well as noting that the poem is specifically about "the reconciliation of a father to the loss of a son. This relationship is strikingly underlined by allusions, witty in their subtlety, but never indecorous."

In a 1972 study appearing in the journal *ELH*, Arthur F. Marotti comments on Jonson's economy of words in "On My First Son." Marotti writes, "When we read the epitaph [Jonson] composed for the boy, we are struck as much by

---

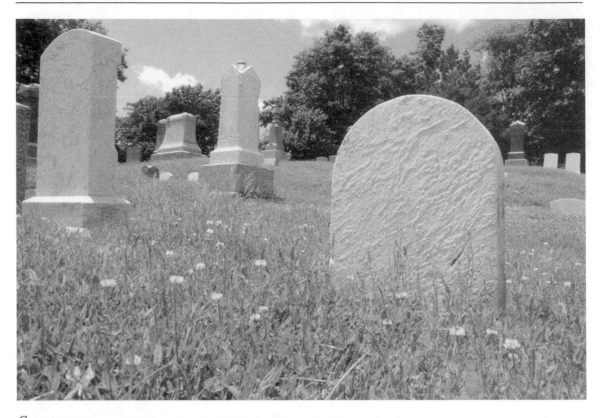

Cemetery *(Image copyright Brittany Courville, 2009. Used under license from Shutterstock.com)*

what he does not say as by what he does. . . . The epigraph's miniature form (small in comparison to the formal elegy) interacts with the large emotion it adumbrates." Marotti argues that Jonson emphasizes the emotional content of his grief by condensing the poem to its most potent parts, leaving out nearly all imagery and emotion.

Several scholars relate the story of Jonson's dream while he is away from London avoiding the plague. In the dream, Jonson sees his son's death. When he awakens, he is relieved to know that it was only a dream. However, just a little later, he receives a letter from his wife relating the death of their son in precisely the same manner he has foreseen. David Lee Miller, in particular, writing in a 1994 essay appearing in *Desire in the Renaissance: Psychoanalysis and Literature*, finds significance in the dream. He argues that such dreams (and by extension, such poems) are "the essential dream[s] of a culture founded by Abraham and refounded by Jesus on the sacrifice of the son's body to the Father's word."

Scott Newstok takes a different approach in his analysis of "On My First Son." Newstok, in

his article "Elegies Ending 'Here': The Poetics of Epitaphic Closure" (2006), makes a distinction between the elegy and the epitaph, noting that an epitaph refers directly to the tombstone. He also notes that epitaphs can occur within an elegy, and provide closure for the poem, and for the life it commemorates. He cites Jonson's "On My First Son" as a "paradigmatic instance" of this maneuver; according to Newstok, "The early, mournful address to the deceased child eventually shifts to a terminal epitaph."

Finally, Eric Haralson, in his chapter "Manly Tears: Men's Elegies for Children in Nineteenth-Century American Culture" in *Boys Don't Cry? Rethinking Narratives of Masculinity and Emotion in the U.S.* (2002), discusses the "gender divide" between elegies written for girls and those written for boys. He argues that "in the Anglo American tradition, the gender divide in child elegies might conveniently be traced back to the pairing 'On My First Daughter' and 'On My First Son.'" Haralson further argues that Jonson misses his son more than he does his daughter, and that his son is "instrumental to the poet's very identity as a maker."

CRITICISM

Diane Andrews Henningfeld

Henningfeld is a professor emerita at Adrian College where she taught literature and writing for many years. She continues to write widely about literature for a variety of educational publishers. In the following essay, she examines Jonson's transformation of two distinct traditions in English poetry, as represented by "On My First Son."

David Riggs, in his fine biography of the playwright and poet Ben Jonson, *Ben Jonson: A Life* (1989) writes, "By the time of [Jonson's] death . . . he had become the most celebrated poet of his age, a man who outshone even Shakespeare and Donne in the eyes of his contemporaries." Jonson's popularity in his own time was such that King James I made him the first poet laureate of England, providing him with a pension for his work as court poet.

While Jonson's reputation has faded in subsequent centuries, any examination of the history of English poetry will reveal his considerable importance to the development of the short lyric. His influence was felt during his own lifetime; as Gamini Salgado, writing in the 1991 *Reference Guide to English Literature*, argues, "Contemporary practitioners of verse esteemed him so highly that a group of them, which included Herrick, Suckling, and Carew, styled themselves the Sons of Ben and produced a commemorative volume *Jonsonius Virbius* after his death in 1637."

His contemporaries and modern scholars hold something in common: the recognition that Jonson's epigrams, in particular, demonstrate a shift in the style and structure of the short poem. Jonson inherited two very different traditions of poetry in English, and through his impressive learning, clear language, and deep understanding of the human condition, he was able to transform both traditions, melding them together into a style and vocabulary still recognizable today.

The first tradition that Jonson inherited is what the scholar Wesley Trimpi, in his seminal *Ben Jonson's Poems: A Study of the Plain Style* (1962), and John Williams, in his introduction to the second edition of *English Renaissance Poetry: A Collection of Shorter Poems from Skelton to Jonson* (1990), identify as the native tradition. Williams argues that the native tradition in Elizabethan poetry is a direct descendent of medieval poetry. Further, he identifies several important

> IN THE END, THE TOOLS JONSON USED WERE THOSE HE INHERITED FROM BOTH THE NATIVE AND PETRARCHAN TRADITIONS; THE ARTISTRY OF USING THOSE TOOLS, HOWEVER, WAS UNIQUELY HIS OWN."

characteristics of poetry written in this tradition: "The subject of the Native poem is usually broad and generic and of . . . persistent human significance; the purpose to which the subject is put is instructive or informative or judicial . . . the Native poet speaks from his own intelligence."

Thus, a poem such as John Skelton's "Upon a Dead Man's Head" offers a good example of this style. Written in the late fifteenth century, this poem addresses the most significant of all human concerns, the awareness of the inevitability of death. The situation of this poem is that of the poet contemplating a skull. Skelton describes in simple but graphic and dreadful terms the way the body disintegrates upon death. He informs his readers that death is universal, and will come to every human being; no one can escape the fate of bodily corruption. Finally, he instructs readers to set their thoughts on Jesus and the Virgin Mary, rather than on the things of the world. Only through steadfast belief in Jesus will the reader's eternal soul be rescued from the horrors of bodily death. The style of the poem is straightforward, and not in the least sophisticated. Its content takes precedence over its style, and the very short lines bump along to the inevitable end rhyme.

Williams also notes that while the native tradition matures and finds fine voice in later poets such as Walter Raleigh, it retains some essential characteristics. According to Williams, "the diction is deliberately plain, almost bare, and subservient to the substance or argument of the poem. The syntax moves toward simplicity, most units being straightforward and declarative." In other words, poetry written in the native tradition tends to use a plain, not embellished, vocabulary; the words used in the poem are less important than the message of the poem; and the syntax, or word order, of the

WHAT DO I READ NEXT?

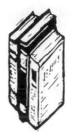

- Debra Johanyak's 2004 *Shakespeare's World* provides a great deal of information about the social and cultural milieu of Jonson's time. In addition, the book offers a closer look at William Shakespeare, Jonson's friend and contemporary, providing a contrast between the two writers.

- Gary Soto's 2003 young-adult novel *The Afterlife* tells the story of a seventeen-year-old Latino boy named Chuy who is killed in a men's room at a dance hall as the book opens. The story is told from Chuy's point of view, and reveals how much his family loves him and grieves for him, among other thematic concerns.

- The Northern Irish poet Seamus Heaney's collection *Death of a Naturalist*, first published in 1966, and available in a 1999 paperback edition from Faber, includes two poems thematically connected to "On My First Son." "Digging" is about writing and the relationship between father and son, while "Mid-term Break" is a poem about a young boy's death, and the grief his father and sibling feel.

- A. E. Houseman's poem "To An Athlete Dying Young," published in *A Shropshire Lad* (1896), tells the story of a young man who dies at the peak of his prowess, before he must witness his records being broken and experience his body aging.

- *The Lovely Bones* (2002) by Alice Seabold tells the story of a young girl who is murdered and her family's grief over her death.

- Like Ben Jonson, his contemporary William Shakespeare also lost a son, Hamnet. Bill Bryson's 2007 biography of Shakespeare, *Shakespeare: The World as Stage*, is an accounting of Shakespeare's life, including a discussion of the death of his son.

---

poem is straightforward and simple, written as declarative sentences, without embellishment.

The second tradition that Jonson inherits goes by several names. Some scholars call it the Petrarchan style, others the courtly style, and still others, the gilded style. Petrarch was a fourteenth-century Italian poet who wrote, among other things, a series of beautiful sonnets about love. In the 1530s, the English courtier and poet Thomas Wyatt visited Italy, and brought Petrarch's sonnets back with him to England, where he began translating them. The poems became very popular in England among the courtly class, and soon young poets were all emulating the style.

Unlike the native tradition, Petrarchan poetry is, according to Williams, "suggestive and indirect." Further, in this style, it is the vocabulary and use of language that is paramount, rather than the message. They are filled with references to beautiful, idealized women, and elegant appeals to the Muses, Greek goddesses of the arts who were often invoked by artists, musicians, and writers. In addition, as Williams notes further, "The relationship between the syntactical unit and the poetic line is a great deal more flexible and varied, with syntactical units frequently running abruptly over the line and completing themselves at odd and unexpected positions." What Williams notes here is that in the Petrarchan style, sentences and phrases are not necessarily attached to a particular line. Rather, a sentence can stop abruptly midline, or spill over into the next.

By the end of the sixteenth century, the conventions of Petrarchan poetry are so well-known, and so often badly executed, that poets such as Jonson's contemporary William Shakespeare can parody the work in their own sonnets. For example, in Shakespeare's Sonnet 130, "My Mistress' Eyes Are Nothing Like the Sun," Shakespeare juxtaposes the description of a real-life woman with the silly, idealized, and, by now, clichéd descriptions of Petrarchan poetry.

Thus, by the very early years of the seventeenth century, Jonson has before him both the direct language of the native style and the flexibility and beauty of the Petrarchan style at his disposal. No other poet before him was able to meld so well the two traditions. Trimpi's term for Jonson's style is the classic plain style, referencing Jonson's close familiarity with classical writers such as Seneca and Martial, while Williams calls it simply plain style. In either case, as Williams argues, Jonson's poetry "is the first in English . . . that is really capable of comprehending the extreme range and diversity of human experience, without falsifying that experience or doing violence to it."

"On My First Son" supports Williams's arguments. Jonson's vocabulary in this poem is largely based on Anglo-Saxon words, as opposed to Latinate forms. In addition, his diction, or word choice, is plain and simple, devoid of the artificiality that marks so much of the Petrarchan poetry. Like the best native poetry, "On My First Son" is instructive as well as informative. Jonson tells his reader that his son has died, that he is grieving, but that he can be consoled by knowing his son is in a better place and that he has been spared the ravages of age. By placing his own experience as a model, others might learn how to cope with extraordinary grief.

The flexibility introduced into English poetry by the incursion of the Petrarchan model is also evident in this poem. Although the poem is regularly metered, it does not have the heavy stresses of the native style. In addition, lines 5 and 6 illustrate both caesura (a break that occurs midline) as well as enjambment (the carrying over of a thought from one line to the next without a pause at the end of the line). Neither of these stylistic devices was available to a writer in the strictly native tradition.

Thus, while Jonson is also clearly referencing his training in the classical writings of the ancient Greeks and Romans in this poem, he is filtering it through the native sensibility as well as the stylistic devices of Petrarchan poetry. His subject and his style are in perfect balance, neither taking precedence over the other. Such a melding of styles allows for greater subtlety and sophistication than either tradition was able to accomplish on its own.

In addition, Jonson's transformation of the traditions he inherited allow him to speak directly to the reader about his own personal experience in clear, economical, and moving phrases. As James Loxley writes in *The Complete Critical Guide to Ben Jonson* (2001), the poem is "a mapping of grief which traces the complexities of a psychological state claimed, unequivocally, for the poet himself. Guilt and shame mingle with the attempts at self-consolation."

Finally, in poems such as "On My First Son," Jonson demonstrates his supreme balancing of not only subject and expression, but also of emotion and intellect. As Claude J. Summers and Ted-Larry Pebworth note in their book *Ben Jonson* (1979), "On My First Son" "recognizes conflicting impulses in the response to loss. Again, there is tension between intellectual and emotional reactions."

It is a testament to Jonson's great skill as a writer that he is able, in the twelve short lines of "On My First Son," to express deeply felt grief directly to the reader, offer a form of consolation and instruction, and produce a beautifully worded poem. In the end, the tools Jonson used were those he inherited from both the native and Petrarchan traditions; the artistry of using those tools, however, was uniquely his own.

Source: Diane Andrews Henningfeld, Critical Essay on "On My First Son," in *Poetry for Students*, Gale, Cengage Learning, 2010.

Joshua Scodel

In the following excerpt, Scodel explains the literary and historical context of "On My First Son."

"On My First Sonne," Ben Jonson's most compelling short poem, has received much excellent commentary, yet critics have not thoroughly explored the most relevant literary and historical contexts for understanding the poem. Jonson does not simply attempt to confront and conquer his grief over the loss of a son. He transforms a traditional generic combination, the elegy with a final epitaph, in order to bury and commemorate his son properly. Residing in Huntingdonshire during the 1603 London plague with his mentor William Camden and Sir Robert Cotton, Jonson, after premonitions of his son's death, learned in a letter from his wife that his son had died. Jonson had probably been estranged from his wife and therefore away from his children since 1602. By contemporary standards, Jonson had certainly neglected his patriarchal obligations in the summer of 1603: it was considered the particular responsibility of the male head of a household to look after his family in time of plague. Jonson could not have attended the burial of his son, which would have taken place quickly after death. He thus failed to pay his final debt to his son. He could not have been satisfied with the burial his son received: during plague, funeral ceremonies were sharply curtailed, and most of the dead, instead of being buried in the consecrated ground of churches or churchyards with burial services, were quickly "covered simply with a winding-sheet, and flung without burial rites into pest-pits." Jonson's son, as a Catholic child, would have had even less chance of being properly buried. In "On My First Sonne" Jonson provides a compensatory burial ritual and an individualizing, immortalizing gravestone inscription for the boy who was in all likelihood unceremoniously buried in an unmarked grave. The poem thus implicitly asserts the power of poetry's verbal rituals and constructs: poetry can provide a proper burial for the dead without a body or a priest and a worthy monument to the dead without a material tomb.

Source: Joshua Scodel, "Genre and Occasion in Jonson's 'On My First Sonne,'" in *Studies in Philology*, Vol. 86, No. 2, Spring 1989, pp. 235–59.

J. Z. Kronenfeld

In the following article, Kronenfeld argues that "On My First Son" can be viewed as more than a theological work.

> Farewell, thou child of my right hand, and
> ioy;
> My sinne was too much hope of thee, lou'd
> boy,
> Seuen yeeres tho'wert lent to me, and I thee
> pay,
> Exacted by thy fate, on the iust day.
> O, could I loose all father, now. For why
> Will man lament the state he should enuie?
> To haue so soone scap'd worlds, and fleshes
> rage,
> And, if no other miserie, yet age?
> Rest in soft peace, and, ask'd, say here doth
> lye
> BEN.IONSON his best piece of *poetrie*.
> For whose sake, hence-forth, all his vowes
> be such,
> As what he loues may neuer like too much.

Critical understanding of poetry normally involves an attempt to see it in relation to culturally available beliefs and attitudes. However, the

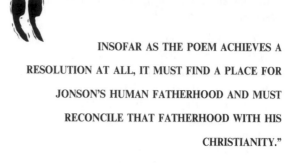

INSOFAR AS THE POEM ACHIEVES A RESOLUTION AT ALL, IT MUST FIND A PLACE FOR JONSON'S HUMAN FATHERHOOD AND MUST RECONCILE THAT FATHERHOOD WITH HIS CHRISTIANITY."

decision that a particular framework is relevant must be based on the fullest possible understanding of the text and of the range of available beliefs—explicit or implicit; frameworks used in too doctrinaire a manner may mislead rather than illuminate.

The only two detailed critical treatments of Ben Jonson's extremely moving Epigram XLV consider the poem in terms of a particular theological framework—one that firmly distinguishes love of the human or temporal from love of the divine and eternal. This perspective, which at first appears to illuminate the problem of the poem's speaker and to point to its solution, is, in fact, misleading. Both critics too readily turn to a particular doctrine to define the concerns of the poem. They do not look closely enough at the statements the poem itself makes for indications of its specific use of available beliefs and attitudes, and for indications of the kind of theological solution it ultimately reaches—which is actually much less dogmatic than they would have it. My reading, therefore, must begin with an explanation of why these readings, and the theological distinction on which they are based, subtly but significantly misconstrue the subject and resolution of the poem, failing to account precisely for its language and tone, and failing to account for its total effect.

Francis Fike and W. David Kay agree that the crux of the poem is Jonson's "confession" (l. 2) that he has misplaced metaphysical hopes for his own immortality or blessedness on a transitory human object—his child. For Fike, Jonson had "placed hope in his son . . . to the point of sinful idolatry—to the point, perhaps, that the child Benjamin and not God had become the ground of his hope for deliverance from death" (208–9). His idolatry took the form of "inordinate affection" (210). Similarly, for Kay, Jonson has failed to observe a traditional distinction such as Augustine's: we should "use" (or "enjoy *in God*") the temporal, but only "enjoy" the eternal for its own sake. According to Kay, Jonson confesses that he had not "enjoyed his son 'in God,' but had 'placed his hope of blessedness' in the child alone" (134). These readings make the subject of the poem the Christian's relationship to his God—a relationship that has been endangered by a willful confusion of the love appropriate for the temporal with the love appropriate for the eternal—rather than the father's relationship to his son.

While showing that there exists an ample tradition of solutions to the problem of the misapplication of metaphysical expectations, Kay and Fike do not convincingly establish that the poem actually concerns such expectations. Because they interpret line 2 as a confession of the sin of idolatry, they cannot satisfactorily avoid the implication that Jonson almost immediately confesses that he has in some sense loved his son too much. Consequently, these critics too quickly resolve, and, in part, misconstrue, the persistent conflict between the loving father and the Christian. These readings fail to explain why a frank and unmitigated expression of love, and even of parental pride, co-exists with the recognition of a "sinne" of "too much hope." They are forced to regard the final vow (ll. 11–12) as a redressing of the presumed sin of idolatry and thus to misinterpret it. Finally, they preclude the recognition that the poem actually achieves a genuine emotional reconciliation of its conflicting claims, rather than a victory of the Christian over the father.

The theological framework that underlies such readings insists on a firm subordination of love of the temporal to love of the eternal; in fact, within this framework, ordinary human affection is not considered a form of Christian love at all. For Augustine, God alone may be "enjoyed"— since He is perfect Being and the end of all desires; men may only be enjoyed "in God," or, more properly, "used." Thus, man is not to be loved "for his own sake" but because we love God and would enjoy Him. Although Kay's argument depends on such an equation, Augustine's appropriate love or "use" of humans is not really equivalent to ordinary human affection; it is Christian love of neighbor—"either because [he is] righteous or in order that [he] may be righteous"— which is in itself subordinate to love of God, but is in no sense "an extension of family affection." For Augustine, the private, natural human affections "based on natural relationships, whether of family or friendship or of a common humanity" are forms of "carnal" or worldly love.

According to Kay, then, Jonson confesses that he has "enjoyed" man, or placed "too much hope" in him; we must note that this interpretation has the specific theological sense of expecting man to fulfill metaphysical hopes for a final good. But even if the Augustinian distinction is not literally applicable—since appropriate love or "use" of humans is not concerned with ordinary familial affection—it strongly suggests that ordinary human affection may be over-extended, that one may love one's friends or children in the wrong way, or too much, with an "inordinate affection" (Fike, 210; Kay, 134, n. 20). Indeed, in the sixteenth-century literature of consolation "too much hope" seems very much like "too much love." As Miles Coverdale says in his *Treatise on Death* (c. 1550), when warning us to avoid making man an "idol," "God himself will be he, of whom all good things undoubtedly must be hoped and looked for; and unto his dishonour it serveth, if the heart cleave not only unto him. . . . [B]lessed is the man that setteth his love, comfort and hope upon the Lord." Another passage implies that ordinary human affection is not under consideration, as in Augustine: we are enjoined to love our friends "not for affection to them" but because "God hath commanded [us] to love them." But even here a marginal note warns us not to lay out hearts, "love and affection *too much*" on the transitory humans we love (III.ix.127, my italics).

Thus the critics are assuming the relevance of a framework which is either literally irrelevant to ordinary human affection, or which defines it as a false or inferior form of love that must be contrasted to true love, love of the divine. Unless love of the human shows the marks of containment or control, it must be idolatry. And they further assume that Jonson himself explicitly shares this framework and interpretation, that the excessive hope in l. 2 can only refer to such a sin.

However, the central question that the poem poses is not "what is the true relationship of man to God?" but "what is the relationship of father to son?" Jonson knows intellectually that the rational or Christian solution to the problem of his grief is that the father must be subordinated to the Christian or, more than subordinated, lost, or loosed, as in "O, could I loose all father, now." As St. Jerome said to Paula in his consolation on the loss of her daughter, "I pardon you the tears of a mother, but I ask you to restrain your grief. When I think of the parent, I cannot blame you for weeping; but when I think of the Christian . . . the mother disappears from my view." But Jonson cannot draw the line between temporal fatherhood and the proper attitude of the Christian. To paraphrase lines 6–7 loosely and in their context as illustration: "O, could I only discard the feelings of a father, now that I have returned what I fully understand was only lent to me, now that the temporal object of those feelings is gone. After all, for what reason (for what purpose, to what end?) will man lament the state he should envy?" Although the form of the latter question suggests that it is not rational to do so, it honestly recognizes that man indeed *will* lament the state he should envy. He cannot "loose all father." Jonson cannot stop feeling like a parent, as Jerome urges Paula to do, even though his son is dead. As temporal father, he feels that he has lost his child. He still feels humanly related to something now missed, although there is nothing to relate to—he is not really "related" to a child returned to God, and there is no point in thinking in terms of such a relationship. Thus a theological framework requiring that the father be lost or completely shed is just what Jonson's analysis reveals he cannot accept; it is hardly a solution to the problem of grief, but a source of grief in itself. Consolation in accordance with such a framework essentially denies the persistence and legitimacy of Jonson's feelings as father and the father's extremely high valuation of his earthly creation—"his best piece of poetrie"; it gives no place to them. In a genuine emotional consolation, these feelings that persist *after* the loss of their object would be given a rationale, rather than merely suppressed.

On the other hand, within the theological framework, resolution of the poem requires a pulling back from a "sinne" of "too much love" and consequently "a protective avoidance of grief" (Kay, 134, n. 20). As Coverdale in fact says, "If we fasten our hearts . . . upon our children and friends, that is, *if we love them too much*, and not God above all things; then hath our sorrow no measure as ought, as they are altered or taken away" (III.ix.127–8, my italics). But even if these emotional attitudes may be found in the consolation literature, they cannot be found in the poem. The concluding vow—"As what he loues may neuer like too much"—does not in the least suggest any plans for the mitigation of love in the future.

Let us see what happens when we try to read the final vow in terms of the distinctions made in Augustine, the consolation literature, and the critics' arguments. Let us suppose that the crucial distinction is here made in terms of two attitudes toward the same temporal object; we shall assume, for the moment, that the poet is concerned with the difference between "using" someone for the sake of God, and "enjoying" someone for his own sake, or, to speak in the terms of the consolation literature, that he is concerned with the difference between "appropriate love" and "too much love." We immediately confront the significant problem of seeing "love" in Jonson's line as parallel to "using" or "enjoying *in God*," that is, to "appropriate love" or "not too much love." The line does not qualify "love" or refer it to a context, or indeed state anything about it except its existence, while the theological arguments, which are concerned with marking the distinction between the divine and the human, are totally concerned with qualification. The "love" Jonson talks about here implies the very opposite of mitigation, reserve, or control; it is inevitable, unquestioned. The syntactic shape of the line takes its existence for granted, allowing for no qualifiers: "As what he loues, may neuer like too much." If the theological distinction is at all relevant to Jonson's words, it is closer to his implicit distinction between "liking" (possibly a form of appropriate love) and "liking too much" (an inappropriate love). It is liking that Jonson promises to control; he vows not to allow himself to become too pleased with what he loves. But to construe Jonson's "love" as equivalent to "appropriate love" is to misrepresent the line. A distinction between the right amount of love and too much love, or between "using" something and "enjoying" it for its own sake, is neither equivalent to, nor has the same effect as, the statement Jonson makes; he says that one may be pleased by something or be pleased by it too much, but will inevitably love it.

The theological framework posited by the critics, then, seems to lead the reader away from the precise language and the tone of the poem. Another context can be provided, however, which eliminates the misleading equation of "too much hope" with "too much love" and which permits an emotional reconciliation of the conflicting claims of the loving father and the Christian. We shall move, as the poem does, from Jonson's positive love of his human child, which is not qualified in the way the critics suggest, to his love of the child as God's gift (that is, in his true place in the scheme of things), and finally, and only implicitly, to his love of God.

Jonson certainly begins his attempt at self-consolation in accordance with the purpose of Stoic consolation: the curing of grief, a disorder of the soul. "[T]he passions of man [must be] brought vnder the obedience of reason." In addition, he seems to have conceived his poem in accordance with the manner of comforting in Wilson's *Art of Rhetorique* that applies to those cases where we show "either they should not lament at al, or els be sorie very little . . ." (p. 65). The first four lines attest to the determination of the father to return without grudging what he knows was only a temporary loan and to draw the appropriate lessons from his loss. Nevertheless, these lines do not subordinate or reject his human love of the child, but maintain it, alongside a recognition of the fallibility of his human hopes.

When Jonson names Benjamin and directs attention to the positive connotations of his name by calling him "thou child of my right hand," he is saying something more than what he would have said by using the phrase "child of the right hand" or "son of the right hand" (the literal meaning of *Benjamin*). The difference between the two expressions lies in the emphasis on the father as the transmitter of the fortunate or auspicious qualities (masculine strength, goodness, etc.) almost universally associated with the right hand as opposed to the left. Seen in this light, the phrase does emphasize the relationship of father to son, and does suggest the role of the father as giver or creator, in a purely biological or temporal line of transmission, a suggestion reinforced by the allusion to the son as something he made in line 10. Thus, readers who have detected a note of parental pride in the phrase are not without justification. The first line of the poem does suggest Jonson's earthly delight in his son, and that delight is at least in part grounded in the son as an extension of the father.

It is not at all necessary to assume that the poem makes a judgment against this kind of feeling. "My sinne was too much hope of thee" obviously co-exists with the re-assertion of the poet's love in the immediately following "lou'd boy," which phrase does not necessarily mean "boy who was loved," but "beloved boy," boy who is still loved. Similarly, this admission of guilt or fault need not undermine or even seriously

qualify the first line of the poem with which it co-exists, but may describe a sense not pertaining to feelings of love, joy, and reasonable parental pride in which Jonson was at fault. Jonson has not come close to wrecking his life on the illusion that the mortal may be equated with the eternal, as Fike suggests (219); he has not expected that his son was immortal—even in an emotional sense—or that he might achieve immortality through his son, but has rather erred in his expectations of what was his *earthly* due.

An understanding of this crucial distinction must begin with the recognition that Jonson's poem concerns "unseasonable death," the death of a young boy. As Plutarch says in his "Consolation to Appollonius," "we meet with some persons who affirm that the death of everyone is not to be lamented, but only of those who die untimely; for they have not tasted of those things which we call enjoyments in the world. . . . It is for the sake of these things that we condole with those who lose friends by untimely death, *because they were frustrated of their hopes* . . ." (my italics). Or, as Jeremy Taylor, the Anglican divine, says, "[some] can well bear the death of infants [having understood little, they lost little], but when they have spent some years of childhood or youth, . . . when the parents are to reap the comfort of all their fears and cares, then it breaks the spirit to lose them." Now timely and untimely death may both teach the vanity of placing "too much hope" on the earthly. To live either as if one's children were immortal or as if they were given to us for an assured, though finite, period is to be confused about the nature of the temporal. But one can see the crucial importance of the distinction. It is one thing to expect to satisfy *immortal* goals with mortal things—this alone is Augustine's false "enjoyment"—and another to expect, however improperly, one's full or due mortal share of mortal things, that is, that one's children will attain maturity.

One may indeed accept mortality and yet not accept "unseasonable death." The consolation literature reminds the bereaved that there "really" is no difference—while making clear that the general human perception of difference is well recognized. As Miles Coverdale says, "we think the death of children to be unnatural, even as when the flame of fire through water is violently quenched. The death of the aged we think to be natural, as when the fire quencheth itself . . ." (III.x.128, "Of the Death of Young Persons in

Especiall"). In all cases, then, the advice is similar. "[T]his shortening of their days is an evil wholly depending upon opinion: for if men did naturally live but twenty years, then we should be satisfied if they died about . . . eighteen; and yet eighteen years now are as long as eighteen years would be then" (Taylor, 109). "We must remember that God knoweth much better than thou and we all, when it is best for every one to die" (Coverdale, III.x.129).

Thus, the implicit question answered by "My sinne was too much hope of thee, lou'd boy" is not really "why did he die?," even though there are contexts available in the consolation literature that interpret death of the loved object as a punishment for sin, or as a warning against excessive attachment to creatures. The question is "why am I grieving so much?" in the sense of "why am I surprised by death?" And the answer is: my sin was a false expectation of my earthly due, literally "too much hope," in this sense. Jonson's lines point to a sin in not having allowed for God's ultimate control over human events, to his having had a false expectation of the "natural" life of children, rather than to an idolatrous confusion of the heavenly and the earthly, or an "inordinate affection." Thus, they carry no implication that he has loved the child whom he unabashedly and un-self-condemningly prizes in the wrong way, or too much.

Lines 3 and 4 express the father's knowledge of and determination to accept the consolatory commonplace concerning human life as a loan, given for no assured time: "Seuen yeeres tho' wert lent to me, and I thee pay / Exacted by thy fate, on the iust day." These lines follow logically, and indeed seem to be more fully integrated into the poem, when we read the "sinne" of "too much hope" as a sin of false expectations concerning the "natural" life of children. Kay is certainly right in pointing to the additional stresses in the lines, as well as to the role of a victim hinted at in the harshness of "*exacted* by thy fate," as indicators of the emotional cost of the attitude the father knows he must take and determines to take: "and I thee pay." "Exacted" does suggest a *forced* payment, and as such further strengthens the argument for the relevance of the topic of unseasonable death. As Coverdale says, the death of young persons is comparable to "unripe apples, that with violence are plucked off the tree" (III.ix.128). Even if these lines do not convey a complete emotional acceptance, however, Jonson's use of the word "just" does imply that he

has renewed his understanding of the terms on which heaven's gifts are given, and it does imply his belief in Providence: "God knoweth . . . when it is best for every one to die" (Coverdale, III.ix.129). The classical consolations similarly stress that fortune has made no promises, but their overall implication is that it is unreasonable to expect reason from an irrational force. "Fortuitous things," including children, "depend[ ] upon uncertain and fickle chance" (Seneca, *De Consolatione ad Marciam*, X.i). "[T]hings deserved and undeserved must we suffer just as [Fortune] wills" (*ibid.*, X.6).

In these lines, then, Jonson's human fatherhood and his Christianity tensely co-exist. The full emotional recognition of the conflict, indeed, of the apparent inefficacy of reasonable or Christian consolation, bursts forth with "O, could I loose all father, now." While the classical prose consolations, particularly as practiced by Seneca and Cicero, begin with sympathy for the loss (if any sympathy is expressed at all) and work up to precepts on the proper attitude to take, Jonson begins with as much Christian resolve as he can summon, but admits, almost despairingly, that his Christian understanding still leaves his emotions as temporal father of a dead son without a rationale or resting place. Lines 7 and 8 also admit doubts about the Christian perspective, while still trying to attain it. They do further define the falseness of hopes concerning a "natural" length of life. Had his son lived, what would he have gained? Sin, the world's buffeting, and the miseries of age. Yet, these lines also convey a note of purely human, personal feeling which qualifies Jonson's Christian understanding that his son has, as the commonplace puts it, escaped unscathed the tarnishing he would receive in the world. The phrase, "And, *if no other miserie*, yet age," does hint at the difficulty Jonson has in conceiving of even the hypothetical sinfulness of his child.

Insofar as the poem achieves a resolution at all, it must find a place for Jonson's human fatherhood and must reconcile that fatherhood with his Christianity. Such a reconciliation cannot be achieved in Jerome's manner, reminiscent of Augustine: "Too great affection towards one's children is disaffection towards God" (*St. Jerome: Letters*, 53). But Jonson's "sinne" has been shown not to be the extreme one—idolatry; the poem need not speak from the Augustinian position that all love is rightly God's, that any love not initially referred to God is false. Jonson's clearly maintained love of his child and high estimation of his worth need not stand in the way of resolution. In fact, while in some passages the Christian consolation literature is Augustinian, in others it explicates the idea of the gifts of God in terms strongly suggesting the *connections* between natural love of the human, love of God, and God's love of man. "For as for father and mother, brother and sister, wife and child, friend and lover, yea, and all other things that we have, what are they else but lent goods and *free gifts* of God...." (Coverdale, III.i.113, my italics). The implications of "free gifts" are clearer in the following passage in which Coverdale uses the metaphor of a man's refusing to return a costly table which has been lent by a great lord: "Is that now my reward for lending you so costly a table, *which I did of love, undeserved on your part*, that ye might have commodity and pleasure thereof for a while? Yea, the more worthy the gift was that I lent you to use, the more thankful you should be unto me" (*ibid.*, my italics). The very worth of the thing lent, then, is a measure of the magnitude of God's unconstrained love for unworthy mankind. To grudge the return is a failure to understand the true nature and value of the gift, amazing even as a loan, as well as the nature of mankind, intrinsically undeserving, even of such loans. "[B]lessing[s] . . . but lent" ("Elegie on the Lady Jane Pawlet") inspire not simply a just or fair attitude on the part of the receiver, as should the gifts of Fortune (cf. Seneca, *De Consolatione ad Polybiam*, X.2); they inspire gratitude and love of God. This Christian context of the idea of the gift, then, makes it possible to connect the worthiness of the thing received and the human love it *appropriately* inspires with the love of God for man and, implicitly, with the love of man for God. It is in terms of these connections between love of the human and love of the divine, rather than in terms of the attempt to mark the distinction between them, that the poem and its resolution are best explained. And it is the epitaph in lines 9–10, when considered for its implications, that addresses itself to the questions raised by the poem, and indeed answers them in human terms, which are also divine.

These lines work in two ways which are intrinsically related to each other. On the one hand, Jonson humbles his estimation of his poetic creation in favor of his human creation; "his best piece of poetrie" gives enormous value to the

temporal reality of his son. The very great emotional intensity of this line, the conviction it gives of Jonson's great love of his *earthly* son, surely stems from his evaluation of a perishable, transitory human reality, that has in fact departed (the lines refer to the human reality), as a creation clearly surpassing "immortal verse," the Renaissance assurance against oblivion and the ravages of time. Some of the classical consolations at times show a tendency to console by stressing values other than the unique value of the thing lost; they urge that the mourner turn to the writing of immortal literature, to other friends or children. There is even a certain tendency to discount the value of the thing lost, to belittle it. Children, along with wealth, honors, and so forth, are externals, "borrowed trappings" (Seneca, *Ad Marciam*, X.2); extended grief for externals is ignoble, especially to the Stoic. Even the Christians move in this direction: the death of a child brings release from a burden as well as freedom from the temptations to sin in order to provide for it (Coverdale, III.iii.118). It is with such tendencies to console by distracting the mourner from the missed object or by diminishing its value that Jonson's consolation contrasts.

But this very elevation of transitory human flesh—of nature—over potentially immortal art necessarily implies that a simultaneous step be taken; the nature of this best achievement, Jonson claims, requires that he deny all title to it. To call his son the best thing he ever made (literally, via the pun on the etymology of "poetrie") is to call attention to the difference between his making of children and his making of poems (even if both are not ultimately his doing alone). Insofar as he did make his son, he is the best thing he ever made. But in what sense can he have, literally, created him? What is it, as the poem has asked all along, to be biologically related, to be a "father"? "We do not call parents the creators of men; nor farmers the creators of corn—although it is by the outward application of their actions that the goodness of God operates within for the creating these things...." If his son is much more valuable and perfect than any creation of his own art, finally that can only be because what he is comparing to man's art is God's. God writes in things, not words. The epitaph communicates Jonson's intense earthly love of his child, his great sense of its worth, and at the very same time allows for only one source of that worth, which merits so great a human love, for only one source of all "free gifts" given out of "undeserved" and immeasurable love.

The parent's sense of the unsurpassable value of a human creation is necessarily a sense of powers beyond his control. The two-line epitaph embodies the emotional realization of the attitude Jonson willed to take in lines 3 and 4 when he spoke of his son as something lent to him, not his to claim. It is here that the resolution of the dilemma of the father and Christian begins. It is human love for the human child that leads to an acceptance of the will of the God who alone can create so valuable a gift.

When we look at the concluding lines of the poem, we face a genuine ambiguity concerning the referent of "for whose sake" in line 11. If the antecedent of "whose" is Ben Jonson (as only Fike suggests), we do have the advantage of no change in referent from "whose" to the following "his" and "he," as well as the advantage of the apparent plausibility of vows taken for the sake of Ben Jonson rather than for the sake of his son. We may then understand that Jonson now vows to amend his own life by vowing to make parental love rest on an understanding of the nature of God's gifts. His understanding and acceptance, achieved through love, may allow him to live in accordance with God's will in the future, that is, more readily to accept and prepare for God's ultimate control of human events.

However, the ambiguity is indeed genuine. It is also plausible that the referent of "whose" is the entire phrase "BEN. IONSON his best piece of *poetrie*," that is, his son. Just as the epitaph pays tribute to "his best piece of poetrie," even though that human creation no longer exists, so the vows may be understood as a tribute to the departed, as vows taken "for his son" in the sense of "for the memory of his son." Although his vows seem to apply to the future ("henceforth," "may never") and to other experiences with loved things, they may still be understood to resolve the problem of the place of his fatherly affections in relation to his religious beliefs. They make possible the appropriate attitude towards his son's memory. He has already emotionally realized the sense in which his son is not his achievement, not something he owns which may please him as something he has made might please him, but a loving gift of God which inspires love both for the child and for God; now he must love the child accordingly.

However we understand the grammar, the nature of the vow itself actually makes it serve both Jonson and the memory of his son. The difference between "love" and "liking too much" in the last line is not the difference between an appropriate affection stopping short of idolatry that is *less* than one's love for God, and an inappropriate affection that results from loving humans as one should love only God. The emphasis falls on love; no reservations are expressed about it; it is inevitable. Rather, what "love" means is human love, the love of parents for children, which is inevitable, but can be extended and continues to exist, even for a dead child (the father is not "lost" or "loosed"), because the love of that child is recognized as an appropriate response to a worthy gift of God. This is a love which can transcend the child's death, because it is, at its best, unselfish, concerned with the child's ultimate welfare. It is not the concern of the poem to distinguish such love from "true love" or love "in God." The experience of human love, the tremendous valuation of the human child as best earthly creation, and even the sense of loss that re-confirms value, need not be suppressed. They themselves lead to an understanding of transcendent love, that is, the Creator's love for unworthy mankind, expressed in the form of such valuable gifts. That understanding makes possible human transcendent love: love of God, and love of the child *as soul*, not earthly creation. In contrast with this, "liking too much" simply represents an attitude more earth-centered and selfish, an attitude associated with the thought of the child as a human creation that merely pleases its earthly maker, an attitude incapable of accepting loss. The poem concerns the difference between an expanded human love that avoids "liking too much" and a limited human love that does not; it does not concern the difference between love of children and love of God.

We may now more fully understand the sense in which Jonson's vows are made for the sake of his son. The classical consolations stress that memory allows things once possessed to remain with one indefinitely, that love continues to exist in spite of the loss of the loved one when that love takes into account the departed's true value and welfare and the fact that he would not want one to grieve. The state of mind permitting peaceful and pleasant contemplation is completely antithetical to the urge to excessive grief. The resolve embodied in Jonson's vows will make it possible for the father to exist in a new form, to be able to contemplate and cherish the memory of his son because it is not painful to him. And the memory will not be painful because the understanding and acceptance of his son's true welfare are achieved through his love and high valuation of his son—understood in their proper context—not *in spite of* his love for his son. True parental love continues to exist, but is transformed; it may overcome the broken spirit which is the first reaction to the loss of its temporal object. Jeremy Taylor comments on those whose spirits are broken: "This is true in many, but this is not love to the dead, but to themselves; for they miss what they had flattered themselves into by hope and opinion; and if it were kindness to the dead, they may consider that, since we hope he is gone to God and to rest, it is an ill expression of our love to them that we weep for their good fortune" (108). There may seem to be a resemblance, even in this passage, to that reading which stresses false hopes, in the sense of idolatry. But recall that Taylor goes on to categorize the idea that unseasonable death is an "evil" as "wholly depending upon opinion," that is, a false expectation of the "natural" life of children; he makes no mention of anything that can be construed as idolatry. The point is that this passage, like Jonson's poem, concerns the continuation and extension of human love in a divine framework, not the sharp distinction of love of the human and love of the divine. It is a matter of loving the human in accordance with its ultimately divine source, not of avoiding love for the human because it is not divine. Insofar as a calming of emotion is achieved in Jonson's poem, it is not arrived at through the mere intellectual acceptance of the supremacy of transcendent or non-earthly values, as the detailed critical treatments suggest; the conflict between the speaker's emotions as a father and his desire for the appropriate Christian resolve is the subject or problem of the poem. Rather, the consolation is achieved through love, of his temporal son, of his son as God's gift, of his son returned to his Creator, and implicitly of the Creator. This reading has the advantage of providing a bridge between the temporal and the transcendent, rather than demanding the rejection of one for the other. Thus, it fully takes into account the father's intense love of his human child, about which the poem makes no apologies, as an integral part of its total meaning.

Source: J Z. Kronenfeld, "The Father Found: Consolation Achieved Through Love in Ben Jonson's 'On My First Sonne,'" in *Studies in Philology*, Vol. 75, No. 1, Winter 1978, pp. 64–84.

SOURCES

Crawford, Patricia M., and Laura Gowing, eds., *Women's Worlds in Seventeenth-Century England*, Routledge, 2000.

Evans, Robert C., "Ben Jonson," in *Dictionary of Literary Biography*, Vol. 121, *Seventeenth-Century British Nondramatic Poets*, 1st ser., edited by M. Thomas Hester, Gale Research, 1992, pp. 182–212.

"Great Plague of London," in *Encyclopedia Britannica Online*, 2009, http://www.britannica.com/EBchecked/topic/243560/Great-Plague-of-London (accessed July 25, 2009).

Haralson, Eric, "Manly Tears: Men's Elegies for Children in Nineteenth-Century American Culture," in *Boys Don't Cry? Rethinking Narratives of Masculinity and Emotion in the U.S.*, edited by Milette Shamir and Jennifer Travis, Columbia University Press, 2002, pp. 88–123.

Jonson, Ben, "On My First Son," in *English Renaissance Poetry: A Collection of Shorter Poems from Skelton to Jonson*, 2nd ed., edited by John Williams, The University of Arkansas Press, 1990

Kelly, John, *The Great Mortality: An Intimate History of the Black Death, the Most Devastating Plague of All Time*, HarperCollins, 2005.

Loxley, James, *The Complete Critical Guide to Ben Jonson*, Routledge, 2001.

Marotti, Arthur F., "All About Jonson's Poetry," in *ELH*, Vol. 39, No. 2, June 1972, pp. 208–37.

Miller, David Lee, "Writing the Specular Son: Jonson, Freud, Lacan, and the (K)not of Masculinity," in *Desire in the Renaissance: Psychoanalysis and Literature*, edited by Valeria Finucci and Regina Schwartz, Princeton University Press, 1994, pp. 233–61.

Moote, A. Lloyd, and Dorothy C. Moote, *The Great Plague: The Story of London's Most Deadly Year*, The Johns Hopkins University Press, 2004, pp. 1-50.

Newstok, Scott L., "Elegies Ending 'Here': The Poetics of Epitaphic Closure," in *Studies in the Literary Imagination*, Vol. 39, No. 1, 2006, pp. 75–100.

Riggs, David, *Ben Jonson: A Life*, Harvard University Press, 1989.

Salgado, Gamini, "Ben Jonson: Overview," in *Reference Guide to English Literature*, 2nd ed., edited by D. L. Kirkpatrick, St. James Press, 1991.

Shakespeare, William, *Hamlet*, edited by Susanne L. Wofford, Bedford Books of St. Martin's Press, 1994.

———, "My Mistress' Eyes Are Nothing Like the Sun: Sonnet 130," http://www.poets.org/viewmedia.php/prmMID/15557 (accessed August 17, 2009).

Skelton, John, "Upon a Dead Man's Head," in *English Renaissance Poetry: A Collection of Shorter Poems from Skelton to Jonson*, edited by John Williams, 2nd ed., University of Arkansas Press, 1990, pp. xi–xxxv.

Summers, Claude J., and Ted-Larry Pebworth, "Chapter Five: The Poetry," in *Ben Jonson*, Twayne Publishers, 1979, pp. 138–57.

Trimpi, Wesley, *Ben Jonson's Poems: A Study of the Plain Style*, Stanford University Press, 1962, pp. 180–85.

Williams, John, ed., Preface to *English Renaissance Poetry: A Collection of Shorter Poems from Skelton to Jonson*, 2nd ed., University of Arkansas Press, 1990, pp. xi–xxxv.

FURTHER READING

Harp, Richard, and Stanley Stewart, eds., *The Cambridge Companion to Ben Jonson*, Cambridge University Press, 2001.
> This is a useful collection of articles ranging from the historical background of Jonson' work to insightful critical analyses.

Houlbrooke, Ralph A., *Death, Religion, and the Family in England, 1480–1750*, Clarendon Press, 1998.
> Houlbrooke provides a clear and interesting historical context for the thematic concerns of Jonson's "On My First Son."

Jonson, Ben, *Volpone and Other Plays*, edited by Michael Jamieson, Penguin, 2004.
> Jonson's satiric plays offer a vivid contrast to poems such as "On My First Son" and allow the student to appreciate the full range of the writer's talent.

Maclean, Hugh, *Ben Jonson and the Cavalier Poets*, W. W. Norton, 1975.
> Maclean offers a collection of Johnson's work along with that of poets who came to be known as the "Sons of Ben" and provides a useful historical introduction.

Martin, Randall, ed., *Women Writers in Renaissance England*, Longman, 1997.
> This book is an anthology of writings by female contemporaries of Jonson. Their works includes elegies, epistles, poems, and prose, providing an interesting contrast with Jonson's work.

Shoulders

NAOMI SHIHAB NYE

1994

Naomi Shihab Nye had been publishing poetry for fourteen years before "Shoulders" appeared in the 1994 collection *Red Suitcase*. Like most of her poetry, "Shoulders" presents a slice of life in which an everyday, simple act—in this case, a man carrying his son on his shoulders across a street—becomes a metaphor for something much larger than itself.

Unlike some poets, Nye seeks to say exactly what she means so that the reader understands her message precisely. Her themes of love and people caring for each other are understood in virtually any culture, a fact that pleases Nye since she is herself a product of two cultures, Palestinian and American.

"Shoulders" is immediately accessible and can be understood on a first reading, but closer examination is also rewarding. A second reading reveals carefully chosen words that paint for the mind's eye a picture rich in color, sound, and texture. The simplicity of the poem's form and meaning are a result of the care with which Nye constructed this work.

Because of its message of human kindness and caring, "Shoulders" has appeared in the anthology *In the Arms of Words: Poetry for Disaster Relief* (2005/2006), the proceeds of which are donated to an international relief fund.

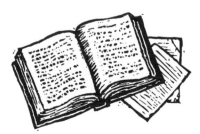

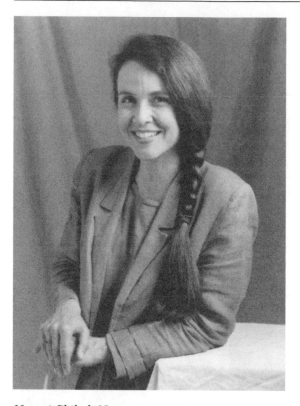

Naomi Shihab Nye (*Reproduced by permission*)

AUTHOR BIOGRAPHY

Nye was born in St. Louis, Missouri, on March 12, 1952. Her journalist father was Palestinian, and her mother was a Swiss-German American teacher. With them and her brother, she spent her high school years in Jerusalem and in San Antonio, Texas. A self-proclaimed poet since the age of six, Nye eventually earned her bachelor of arts degree in English and world religions from Trinity University in San Antonio, the city she calls home. She used her degree to land several teaching jobs over the years. Nye has taught at the University of California, Berkeley, the University of Texas at San Antonio, and Our Lady of the Lake in San Antonio.

Nye's first collection of poems, *Different Ways to Pray*, was published in 1980. Her interest in exploring the differences and similarities between various cultures was evident in this first collection, and themes of multiculturalism have continued to flow through her work. Nye won the Voertman Poetry Prize for this collection, and she won it again for her third poetry collection, *Hugging the Jukebox*, two years later.

Nye has continued to publish collections of poetry for adults and children, as well as picture books, throughout the 1990s and into the twenty-first century. *Red Suitcase*, which contains the poem "Shoulders," was published in 1994. Her work has earned numerous awards, including four prestigious Pushcart Prizes. The Pushcart Prize is the most honored literary project in America, and many famous authors were first recognized by it: John Irving, Raymond Carver, and Tim O'Brien, among others. Nye was awarded a Guggenheim Fellowship in 1998. The money from this award allowed her to teach less and write more.

In addition to writing poetry and children's picture books, Nye has published essays in a variety of periodicals, including *Atlantic*, *Atlanta Review*, and *Ploughshares*. She has edited several poetry anthologies, including the award-winning *This Same Sky*. Her 2002 poetry collection, *19 Varieties of Gazelle: Poems of the Middle East*, was a finalist for the National Book Award for poetry.

Nye's work has been featured on National Public Radio, and she has been included on two Public Broadcasting System (PBS) poetry specials, *The Language of Life with Bill Moyers* and *The United States of Poetry*. She has also appeared on the PBS show *NOW with Bill Moyers*.

Nye's love of language translates into song as well. She is a songwriter and folk singer who considers poetry and songs to be cousins.

In addition to writing, Nye is active in promoting international goodwill through the arts. In that capacity, she has traveled to the Middle East and Asia as a representative of the United States Information Agency (USIA) three times. The function of the USIA was, in part, to advocate America's official policies overseas, in language and terms that were meaningful to those specific cultures. The USIA was abolished in 1999, when most of its functions were transferred to the Under Secretary of State for Public Affairs and Public Diplomacy.

Nye has written and edited more than twenty volumes of poetry and fiction. For more than thirty years, she has conducted writing workshops in schools, an activity she considers food for writing. In an interview with Rachel Barenblat at *Pif* magazine, Nye explains, "Writing travels the road inward, teaching, the road out—helping others move inward—it is an honor to be with others in the spirit of writing and encouragement."

POEM SUMMARY

Lines 1–5

In the first lines of "Shoulders," Nye gives the reader a focal point: a father carrying his sleeping son on his shoulder in the rain. He looks both ways and carefully crosses the street. The reader immediately knows he is a gentle and careful father, protective of his son. He is aware of both what he can and cannot see, and he will let no harm come to his boy. Readers are focused on the father.

Lines 6–9

The reader's attention shifts to the child. The boy is the most precious cargo in the world, yet nowhere is he obviously marked as such. This section of the poem reflects Nye's belief in the value of children, as well as the father's feeling. The reader is again told beyond doubt that the child is both precious and fragile.

Lines 10–12

In writing about Nye for *The Progressive*, journalist Robert Hirschfield says her poetry is characterized by a "deep listening quality." The center section of "Shoulders" is an illustration of this quality. In lines 10–12, Nye brings the man and boy together in the reader's eye as she blends senses: The father hears his son's breathing. The boy hums as he dreams. The reader can almost hear as well as see these three lines because Nye has infused them with a sensual quality.

Lines 13–18

A major shift occurs in these final lines as Nye writes in first person and thereby draws the reader into the scene she has created. The man is no longer just one man, nor is his son just one son. They represent every individual in the world. Nye's core message appears in this section: People must be willing to go out of their way to help one another or they cannot survive. Without human kindness, life's journey will be long and fraught with one obstacle after another.

Reaching out to help and love each other is, in "Shoulders," what makes life worth living. More than that, it makes life possible.

Nye relies on literary technique to convey this message. The tone of the poem changes at line 13, making the reader aware that this is new

territory; the real message of the poem lies ahead. Whereas lines 1–12 make careful use of imagery and sound so that the tone is almost a whisper, lines 13–18 do not use either. Nye uses abrupt words and hard consonant sounds such as *t* and *d*. In doing so, she startles the reader out of the lull that she creates in the previous twelve lines, as if to say "Wake up!"

THEMES

Universal Love

Much of Nye's poetry is about humanitarianism and people caring for one another. "Shoulders" is no exception. A father carries his son across the street. He looks both ways, twice. He is very careful to get his boy safely to the other side. In lines 13–16, Nye says that people must be willing to care for and protect one another when such benevolence is required because there will always be hardship, and life's journey is long.

The poem is only eighteen lines long, yet within that framework Nye has made her point clear: Life is not just about the individual's needs and desires. It is about caring for others, going out of one's way to see that they are protected and their needs are met.

Trust

The father in the poem has been entrusted with his son's care. The small boy knows he is in good hands. He is comfortable enough to fall asleep, even as rain falls upon him. Nye indicates the boy's breathing is regular, a hum. It is an easy sleep, deep enough that he dreams. His father, knowing he is responsible for caring for his son, protects him from splashes, from traffic, and from danger. Knowing his son is fragile and needs the father in order to grow up, the father faces the rain, ignoring his own comfort, and focuses on getting his son to safety and warmth. He will do this thousands of times throughout the boy's life, if not literally, then figuratively.

Nye underscores this theme of trust in her word choice. She emphasizes the fragility and vulnerability of the child, using words that would apply to something of value that is being sent out into the world. That value is ascribed to the child in the poem, and lines 4 and 5 suggest the father's awareness of the value as well as his son's trust in him.

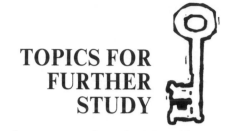

TOPICS FOR FURTHER STUDY

- Find other poems written by Nye. Choose one that addresses the same themes as "Shoulders," but in a different way. In an essay, compare and contrast the two poems, describing their similarities and differences.

- Draw or paint a picture of what you see when you read "Shoulders." Choose colors that reflect or represent the feelings you get from the poem. Explain your selections in a short essay on the back of the picture.

- Poetry is just one form of art; music is another. If you play a musical instrument, write a tune to accompany this poem. What is the tone of the music? Is it fast paced or slow paced? Do you hear it being played solo, or by a larger musical group? Play the song for the class.

- Read the Robert Frost poem "The Road Not Taken." Compare his road to the one Nye describes in "Shoulders." How do they differ? How are they similar? Write your own poem using the road as a symbol for your life.

- Using the Internet, research a culture other than your own. Familiarize yourself with elements of its language, customs, social norms, and values. Then write a poem about your own life using techniques that would allow a person from that culture to identify with your poem's theme(s). For example, you could use dialect or slang from that culture in your poem to help the reader understand your message.

- Read Nye's young-adult novel *Habibi*. Pay special attention to the imagery used in descriptions of Jerusalem. Following Nye's lead, choose a place you have been to and describe it in an essay using vivid imagery.

Individual Responsibility

A single person not only can but *must* make a difference. This is a strong message in Nye's poem. It is up to each person to take responsibility for the well-being of others. The boy is tired; he is fragile, and so the father helps him and protects him. Nye says if people are not willing to reach out and give of themselves, no one will survive.

Throughout her career, Nye has attempted to use poetry as a means of cross-cultural communication. While recognizing the needs and rights of individuals in society, her poetry—"Shoulders" included—stresses the idea that all concerns are universal. In this instance, *all* children are important and fragile. They must be handled with care on an individual basis, as well as at a societal level. In lines 13–16, Nye switches from singular pronouns to plural, applying the individual example to all of us.

STYLE

Symbolism

Nye's poem is a word picture of one very brief moment in time: A father carries his son across a street to safety. But everything in that slice of life is representative or symbolic of something bigger. The father is Everyman (the representative of humankind in medieval morality plays). He is every person in the world, just as his son is every child or weaker person in need of human kindness.

The act of carrying the boy across the street is symbolic of any act of kindness, be it carrying someone, caring for someone in time of sickness, teaching a child a new skill, or anything else. The road in this poem is life's journey, which Nye is saying will always be wide, never easy, and not something one can travel alone. The rain symbolizes the hardship and obstacles every person faces in life. There will always be rain; there will always be hardship.

Free Verse

"Shoulders" is written as free verse: It does not rhyme, and there is no consistent meter or rhythmic pattern. By choosing to write the poem in this style, Nye allows herself and the reader to focus on language rather than form as a way to understand the poem's meaning without being preoccupied with rhythm or line length. Instead, she uses specific words to make the reader feel the scene she is portraying.

Varied Points of View

"Shoulders" begins with the third-person point of view. Nye tells the reader what is happening. In line 13, she switches to first person plural,

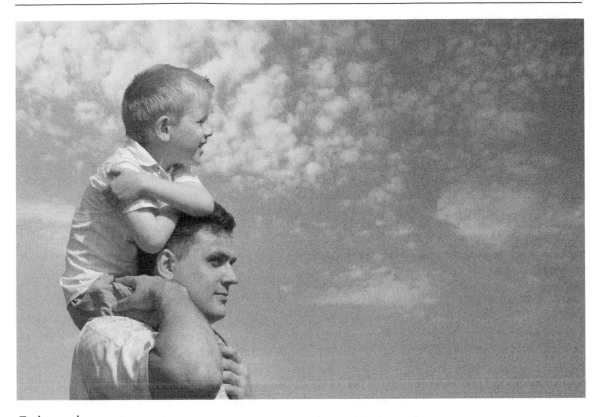

Father and son (*Image copyright Vadim Ponomarenko, 2009. Used under license from Shutterstock.com*)

thereby involving the reader and herself in the scene. By implementing two points of view, she is forcing the reader not only to accept what she is saying but to claim ownership, in a way. She is saying, in effect, "Here's how it is. If you aren't part of the solution, you're part of the problem." The reader is no longer watching the scene unfold, but is actually participating in it.

Synesthesia

Synesthesia is a condition in which one's senses are blended. For example, music has both a sound and a color associated with it. Food has a taste and a color. For some synesthetes, every letter of the alphabet appears in a particular color. Nye blends the senses in her poem. The man uses sight to look up and down the street. He hears his son's breathing and feels the rain falling. By incorporating several of the senses, the reader has a vivid image of the father carrying the son across the road.

Poetry as Conversation

In an interview with Teri Lesesne for *Teacher Librarian*, Nye explains that "poetry is the closest genre to the way we think, in images with leaping connections, metaphorically, sometimes in fragments. We should feel very at home with it." Her understanding of poetry as a way of seeing and saying something is what makes her poems accessible. "Shoulders" uses no difficult words that must be looked up in a dictionary to understand. There is no rhyme or technical format. Nothing about the poem is forced. Each line just is what it is, in tone and in length. It is a perfect reflection of what Nye means when she describes poetry as the closest genre to the way people think.

HISTORICAL CONTEXT

Multiculturalism

"Shoulders" was written in 1994, when multiculturalism (the idea that different cultures can peacefully coexist) was at the forefront of social and academic thought. One of the poem's themes, universal love, hinges on the idea that humans must be willing to help anyone, anywhere in the world, if they are to survive together as a species. Unsaid but implied is the idea that differences of any kind do not matter.

The poem, however, is timeless. The scene Nye depicts could take place anywhere in the world, at any given time. This ambiguity is another facet of multicultural thought.

International Discord

Because Nye is both Palestinian and American, she grew up with an acute sense of the differences between the two cultures. Her poetry became a way to bridge the gaps between cultures, generations, and races.

In 1991, during the Persian Gulf War, she was the visiting poet at a school in Dallas, Texas. She brought to class some poems written by Iraqi poets. In a 2005 interview with Bryan Woolley of the *Dallas Morning News*, Nye described the experience. The poems were not about war but about fathers and children, mothers and their daughters. "And kids were saying things like, 'Gee, I never thought about there being children in Iraq.'" Hearing that response, Nye feels those poems made a difference.

In large part because of the Gulf War and the ongoing violent struggles against apartheid (social policy of legal, economic, and political discrimination against non-whites) in South Africa until 1994, cultural and ethnic conflict were uppermost in people's minds in the early 1990s despite the fact that America was experiencing its own serious economic recession. Nye's 1994 poetry collection, *Red Suitcase*, included poems depicting life in all its glory and ugliness.

The poems in *Red Suitcase* include "How Palestinians Keep Warm," "Someone Is Standing on the Roof of the World," and "Holy Land." The poem "For the 500th Dead Palestinian, Ibtisam Bozieh," is about a thirteen-year-old girl who was murdered at gunpoint simply because she was Palestinian. In the poem "Jerusalem," Nye writes about a place in her brain where hate is not allowed to grow.

"Shoulders" that was chosen to end the book. Without depicting a specific place or time, it is a perfect poem to wrap up a collection that has focused a tender eye on the uselessness of discord and disruption, death and hate, war and exile. It is a poem of hope, one that beseeches the reader not only to care, but to act on that feeling. Written in a time of international upheaval and local uncertainty, "Shoulders" carries the rest of the book on its back.

CRITICAL OVERVIEW

Nye is regarded as one of the leading female poets of her generation in the American Southwest. So highly respected is her work that she was invited to read at the Library of Congress and the White House during Bill Clinton's presidency.

In 1995, veteran journalist Bill Moyers shone a spotlight on Nye when he made her the first featured poet of his new PBS poetry series *The Language of Life*. A hectic schedule of speaking engagements and book tours followed for the Texas-based poet.

Her poem "Shoulders" was included in an anthology of poetry titled *In the Arms of Words: Poetry for Disaster Relief* (2005/2006). All of the proceeds from the sales of the book went directly to AmeriCares, an international relief organization.

Because of Nye's multicultural heritage, much of her work (poetry, prose, and lyrics) explores race relations in terms of finding peace and making room for differences. "Shoulders" is one of her rare pieces that does not concern itself with a multicultural theme. The man and child featured in the poem could be of any race; it simply does not matter. By not specifying ethnicity or race, Nye has made a pointed choice to portray the father and son as anyone and everyone.

The bulk of Nye's poetry brings an energy to local life and daily events, small moments that, when strung together, make up a life. "Shoulders" does just that as it focuses on a father and son crossing the street. In her essay for *The Women's Review of Books*, journalist Alison Townsend judges the collection of poetry in *Red Suitcase* to be an "intersection of private and public history." She interprets Nye's focus to be on "the contribution individual histories make to world history" and points to "Shoulders" as the poem that makes that point best.

Although Nye's poetry appeals to people because of its accessibility and simplicity and its refusal to be esoteric or too intellectual, a review in *Publishers Weekly* found the book—and "Shoulders" in particular—lacking. "The final poem strains to carry both a child and the book on its back.... Nye's strength is her ability to express subtle emotions; weightier issues overwhelm her small, clear voice."

COMPARE
&
CONTRAST

- **1990s:** This decade sees the rise of the Spoken Word movement. Although poetry has always been an oral art form, the invention of the printing press made publishing poetry more immediately important than reciting it. There was a renewed interest in oral poetry in the 1960s, as there is again in the 1990s. Concurrent with this most recent interest in oral poetry is the explosion of the rap music scene. Technically speaking, rap is considered a form of spoken word. In an interview with Sharif S. Elmusa of *Alif: Journal of Comparative Poets*, Nye expresses an appreciation for the way rap music plays with words. Elmusa agrees and explains the role of rap in trying to make poetry vital for his son: "I encouraged him to listen because I liked the way rappers played with words. Rap seemed like the next-best thing to poetry."

  Today: At the turn of the twenty-first century, poetry as it is generally written and read is ready for something new. John Barr, president of the Poetry Foundation, explains in an article for *Poetry Magazine* that a new kind of poetry is necessary "because the way poets have learned to write no longer captures the way things are. . . . The art form is no longer equal to the reality around it." Poetry is, generally speaking, losing its audience as other art forms come to the forefront. Poets strive to bring their art to a younger audience.

- **1990s:** Multiculturalism—the idea that varied cultures can coexist peacefully and in equality—reaches its zenith in the 1990s. Everything from literature to curriculum to politics includes a multicultural aspect. For Nye, who is both Palestinian and American, multiculturalism is at the heart of her poetry. She uses that poetry to try to bridge cultural gaps and bring together people from all walks of life.

  Today: The terrorist attacks on New York's World Trade Center and Washington, D.C.'s Pentagon building in 2001 deal a serious blow to the idea of multiculturalism in America. At the end of the first decade of the twenty-first century, society struggles to maintain respect for the individual in society while finding acceptance and tolerance for social groups organized around culture, gender, nationality, race, and other factors.

- **1990s:** The early years of the decade are ones of economic strain in America as the Persian Gulf War is fought, oil prices and the federal budget deficit increase, and America's gross national product falls. Unemployment is high, and many families struggle just to keep from losing their homes. Experts cite the resulting increase in adult stress levels as a primary influence on the increase in child abuse and substance use. Nye's poem is a reminder that children are precious and need to be nurtured.

  Today: America's economy is once again turbulent. The federal government has intervened in business by financially helping major companies, such as banks and automobile manufacturers, to keep them from going bankrupt. Unemployment is high, and homes across the country are going into foreclosure, leaving millions homeless and jobless. As adults frantically worry how to live from one paycheck to the next, the needs of children are easily overlooked. Nye's poem, with its message of responsibility, perhaps rings even more true today than it did when it was written.

Booklist reviewer Donna Seaman praises Nye's poetry in general. In 2005, she likened Nye's poetic collections to water "because her poems are clear, flowing, essential, and capable of not only keeping one afloat but also slipping into even the most tightly closed corner of her mind."

Nye expresses the philosophy that poetry can bridge cultural gaps by providing details because people are people, regardless of background. "My poems simply try to remember that," she explains in an interview for *Writing!* magazine. "Poems respect details. Hopefully, those details can help us enter one another's worlds and imagine them."

CRITICISM

Rebecca Valentine

Valentine is a freelance writer and editor who holds a bachelor's degree in English with an emphasis on literary analysis. In this essay, she considers Nye's poem "Shoulders" in terms of its musical devices.

In addition to being a poet, Nye is a song-writer and singer. In her poem "Shoulders," Nye employs several musical devices to develop the tone and message of her words.

Upon a first read, Nye's poem seems to be very simple—little more than a thought jotted down on paper. But even the simplest poems are created with purpose. In "Shoulders," Nye uses her songwriting techniques and knowledge to paint a word picture whose meaning relies as much on hearing as it does on understanding the words.

Throughout the first twelve lines, Nye uses soft consonants and blends. The words are quiet, and their sounds are soothing. Especially if read aloud, these lines of poetry give the reader a sense of tranquility.

That peaceful feeling is abruptly and starkly broken beginning with line 13. From that point on, Nye uses words with hard consonant sounds such as *t*, *g*, and *r*. These sounds are more gutteral; they do not flow softly off the tongue. Considered in contrast to the preceding twelve lines, the harsh sounds of lines 13–18 are startling.

Along with the shift to hard consonants comes a change to short words. Throughout the first twelve lines, Nye uses multisyllabic words more often. Lines 13–18 rely primarily on monosyllabic words to reinforce their message. Of a total of thirty-five words in those lines, twenty-seven have just one syllable. The sound of these words being read can be called staccato. Their sound is rapid and hard, much like the sound of an automatic weapon being fired.

This staccato sound is unpleasant, especially after the lull of the longer, softer words in the first twelve lines. Nye's message—we will perish if we cannot help one another—is underscored by her word choice. It is an urgent message, one not to be ignored. The reader has no choice but to notice it because Nye has made it blare out, like a car horn in the solitude of night.

Consonance is another musical device used in the construction of "Shoulders." Consonance is the repetition of the same sound in short succession. Within the first five lines, Nye uses the soft blend *sh* three times. In a similar vein, she uses *th* twice in a three-word span. In lines 10–12, the reader hears the sound *h* five times. The soft sound of that consonant is almost like a lullaby, and readers let down their guard down just as Nye is about to assault them with the core message of her poem.

Nye foregoes the use of rhyme in her poem. Rhyming tends to give a poem a more lighthearted and frivolous quality. Nye's tone in "Shoulders" is serious, almost reverent. She indicates her attitude toward the subject—father and son—with words denoting vulnerability and fragility. Rhyming has no place in this particular poem.

An alternative to rhyme is assonance, a technique in which vowel sounds are repeated in neighboring words. This stylistic choice adds to the flow of a poem or song. Lines 10 and 11 of "Shoulders" use the long *ea* sound four times in the scope of fourteen words. As she does with consonance, Nye uses assonance in this passage directly preceding her message, highlighting that message and making it all the more agitating.

Nye's poetry, including "Shoulders," is not difficult to understand. But the reason for this is not because it is basic or simplified. Nye has managed to fuse her musical sensibility into her poetry. Good music and good poetry share a dynamic that makes them intriguing and meaningful to both read and hear. Nye's poetry shines because it can be felt—by the brain, the heart, and the ear. It is a sensual experience built by an artist who appreciates her craft as much as her end product. *Booklist* contributor Pat Monaghan said it well in a review of *Red Suitcase*: "Nye is a fluid poet, and her poems are also full

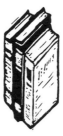

WHAT DO I READ NEXT?

- Nye's *A Maze Me: Poems for Girls* (2005) is a collection of poetry geared toward teenage girls. The poems touch on everyday experiences of girls from all cultures.

- The 2001 young-adult novel *A Step From Heaven* is author An Na's story of a Korean girl who emigrates to California when she is just four years old. The cultural differences set Young Ju's family on a path of disintegration and force the family to find a way to blend the old with the new.

- Alan Sitomer and Michael Cirelli's 2004 interactive workbook titled *Hip-Hop Poetry and the Classics* compares contemporary hip-hop with more traditional poetry and shows students the two are not so different after all. The authors provide in-depth analysis of poetic literary devices, writing activities, and more.

- Written for grades seven and up, *You Hear Me?: Poems and Writing by Teenage Boys* is a collection of poetry edited by Betsy Franco and published in 2001. Some explicit themes, such as drugs, AIDS, and sex, give this book a more raw urgency than found in the average young-adult work, as its poems give voice to the hopes and fears of young men from a variety of cultures.

- *Paint Me As I Am: Teen Poems from WritersCorps* (2003) is a collection of poems written by disadvantaged youth. WritersCorps is a program that allows established poets to share their skills and motivation techniques with at-risk youth. Poet Nikki Giovanni provides the foreword to this collection edited by Bill Aguado and Richard Newirth.

- Jaime R. Wood's *Living Voices: Multicultural Poetry in the Middle School Classroom* (2006) introduces students to a form of literature that often causes anxiety in young readers. The book contains step-by-step lesson plans and provides examples of student writing. A chapter of accessible resources is included at the end.

---

of the urgency of spoken language. Her direct, unadorned vocabulary serves her well."

Source: Rebecca Valentine, Critical Essay on "Shoulders," in *Poetry for Students*, Gale, Cengage Learning, 2010.

Robert Hirschfield

In the following article, Hirschfield examines how Nye's Palestinian background has influenced her life and poetry.

> Why are we so monumentally slow?
> Soldiers stalk a pharmacy:
> big guns, little pills.
> If you tilt your head just slightly
> It's ridiculous.

The words are those of Naomi Shihab Nye, from her poem "Jerusalem."

Her father, a middle-class Palestinian from Jerusalem, lost his home and everything he owned in 1948. He put down roots in St. Louis, Missouri, where, in 1952, Naomi Shihab was born.

"My first images of Palestine were the thin blue air-letter sheets that he would mail to Palestine, then receive in the mail," his daughter recently recalled. "How the light would come through those translucent pages! There was something magical about words that had travelled so far."

The author of many books of poetry and young adult fiction, Nye was a National Book Award finalist for *19 Varieties of Gazelle: Poems of The Middle East*, and twice has won the Jane Adams Children's Book Award.

One of her young-adult novels, *Habibi* (available through the AET book club as is her *Space Between Our Footsteps*), is based on her experiences as a teenager in the West Bank in the mid-1960s, when her father decided to return to live in his native land. (The outbreak of the Six-Day War in 1967 sent him back to America to stay.)

"I had a rebellious streak, as teenagers have," Nye explained. "I had no patience at all with the conservative Old World culture, yet I loved how tuned-in my grandmother and cousins were to every little detail of daily life. So very much like poetry."

Nye has been back many times since then. Like any ordinary Palestinian—even one from San Antonio, Texas, where she now lives with her family the poet is in possession of a hidden cargo of occupation horror stories.

"I was sitting once with my grandmother, when she was about 103, and my child was with me," she told the *Washington Report*. "Suddenly, bursting into the house, was the son of my cousin. The Israelis broke into his house while he was in the shower and brutally beat the boy. Both his eyes were blackening. He said, 'They think I know a boy who threw some stones last week, but I don't know him.'

"I sat there thinking, If someone beat up my son, what would I be inclined to do?"

Other times, while walking in her grand-mother's village with old Palestinian men, she would find Israeli guns pointed at them.

"I would say in English to the soldiers, 'We are not fighting you. We are just out for an evening walk. Why are you doing this?'" Nye said. "They would be furious, and ask to see my passport."

Her contact with Jews, since her teens, has mainly been as friends. There was their shared Semitic background, their shared conflict— bloodlines and bloodshed.

"There is a scene in *Habibi*, at the dinner table," Nye said, "where the girl asks her father, 'Is this irrevocable? Do we all have to fight forever? Or is it just that we fight the way families fight?'"

The poet writes about the Southwest, a lost parrot, an old love, Mother Teresa and other subjects, as well as about Palestine and the Palestinians. She sees her words as her contribution to Palestinian resistance.

"Many people would say that words do nothing," she noted. "Others, like myself, believe that language, whether it be poetry, like [Mahmoud] Darwish's poetry, or song, can fortify and rejuvenate the spirit."

What poetry can do, Nye believes, is to transport people "across the gap," beyond tribal borders. Israeli poets Yehuda Amichai and Dahlia Ravikovitch are long-time residents in her pantheon of poets who matter. "Presence and truth" were the checkpoints they had to pass through to get there.

Nye closely monitors the pollution of political language in America. "George Bush said, when Hamas won the election: 'You cannot be a partner in peace if you've got an armed wing.' He should talk!" his fellow Texan said. "He has an armed wing, an armed tail feather, and another armed wing. He has every armed wing there is."

As an Arab-American, Sept. 11—and the reaction to Sept. 11—wounded her two hearts (three, if you count Darwish's "land of words" as a third body).

"9/11 was horrific," Nye stated. "I think all the civilian deaths in Iraq are equally horrific. I think the unspoken, undescribed oppression of Palestinians for 58 years is horrific. I think the suicide bombings of Israel are horrific."

In her open letter "To Any Would-Be Terrorists," written after 9/11, Nye begins by saying how very much she hates using the word "terrorists."

"Do you know how hard some of us have worked to get rid of that word, to deny its instant connection to the Middle East?" she writes. "And now look. Look what extra work we have. Not only did your colleagues kill thousands of innocent, international people in those buildings and scar their families forever, they wounded a huge community of people in the Middle East, in the United States and all over the world. If that's what they wanted to do, please know their mission was a terrible success, and you can stop now."

A scolding mother, she mentions her own American mother, who has worked so hard in her life to undo people's poisonous stereotypes about Arabs.

In tones of an exhausted friend, Nye ends her letter by saying, "We will all die soon enough. Why not take the short time we have on this delicate planet and figure out some really interesting things we might do together? I promise you, God would be happier."

She suggests they read Rumi, even American poetry, and quotes the Arab-American writer Dr. Salma Jayyusi: "If we read one another, we won't kill one another."

Nye detects an edge of rage in some of her own post-9/11 poetry. It doesn't please her. She likens poetry to a lever that keeps trying to flip up a lid so one may discover what lies beneath it. Rage, she knows, kills wonder.

Source: Robert Hirschfield, "Naomi Shihab Nye: Portrait of a Palestinian-American Poet," in *Washington Report on Middle Eastern Affairs*, Vol. 25, No. 6, August 2006, pp. 73–74.

Joy Castro

In the following interview with Castro, Nye discusses her writing background, politics in poetry, and multicultural literature.

Naomi Shihab Nye is best known for her six volumes of what William Stafford has called "a poetry of encouragement and heart." These, together with her widely anthologized short stories and luminous nonfiction, have earned her four Pushcart Prizes, the I.B. Lavan Award from the Academy of American Poets, two Voertman Awards from the Texas Institute of Letters, a Guggenheim Fellowship, and a Witter Bynner Fellowship from the Library of Congress.

For the past decade, she has also been winning recognition for a sizable oeuvre of multicultural literature for young readers, all of which is infused with a direct, determined commitment to peace and cross-cultural understanding. As a Palestinian American who spent part of her childhood in Jerusalem and as a long-time resident of San Antonio, Nye focuses on both Arab American and Latino issues in her books for young readers. Her edited collections, which emphasize visual as well as literary art, include This Same Sky: A Collection of Poems from Around the World(1992), which the American Library Association named a Notable Book,The Tree Is Older Than You Are: A Bilingual Gathering of Poems & Stories from Mexico with Paintings by Mexican Artists(1995), andThe Space Between Our Footsteps: Poems and Paintings from the Middle East(1998). Her original works for children include two picture books for young readers:Sitti's Secrets(1994), which won the Jane Addams Children's Book Award from the Women's International League for Peace and Freedom, and the lyricalBenito's Dream Bottle(1995). Her 1997 novel for young adults,Habibi, was named an ALA Best Book for Young Adults, an ALA Notable Book, a New York Public Library Book for the Teen Age, and a Texas Institute of Letters Best Book for Young Readers. Called by one critic "the work of a poet, not a polemicist," it received

> MY GOALS HAVE ALWAYS BEEN TO MAKE WONDERFUL VOICES AVAILABLE TO MORE READERS, TO PROMOTE POEMS OF HUMANITY AND INTELLIGENCE THAT EXTEND AND CONNECT US ALL AS HUMAN BEINGS, TO ENLARGE READERS' HORIZONS—INCLUDING MY OWN, AS I WORK ON THE BOOKS—AND TO HELP CONNECT PEOPLE."

both the Judy Lopez Memorial Award for Children's Literature and the Jane Addams Book Award.

Joy Castro: The direct, courageous expression of simple truths about family, friendship, and compassion seems to work well for your characters. In Habibi, for example, Liyana yells down the Israeli guards in order to visit her imprisoned father, a Palestinian American doctor: "Her throat felt shaky. But she didn't turn. . . . "Of course it's possible!" she said loudly. "He is my father! I need to see him! NOW! PLEASE! It's necessary! I must go in this minute!" (228). Liyana succeeds; the guards let her in. In your bio note at the end of the paperback edition of Sitti's Secrets, which is about young Mona's visit to her Sitti, her grandmother, in a Palestinian village, you write, "If grandmas ran the world, I don't think we'd have any wars." Can you talk further about your vision of the way in which personal connections function in the struggle for political peace?

Naomi Shihab Nye: Well, most of us aren't politicians, so personal connections are all we have. I guess I've always wished that people could speak up with their honest, true, insightful feelings and needs when they have them—but of course, it's not always so easy in real life: inhibitions confound us, expectations hinder us. We have all lost many opportunities to speak out about crucial issues we believe in. I have probably been guiltier than most since I have so many generous occasions on which I am invited to express my opinions. This is a luxury writers can never take for granted.

In books, I hope that my characters are brave and strong. I want them to use their voices. I want young people to be reminded, always, that voices are the best tools we have. In whatever seemingly personal venues we may find ourselves, voices matter. A voice may stir up little waves that reverberate out and out much farther than we could ever imagine. I hope this is true. It has seemed to be so in my experience.

Castro: I remember during your rending here at Wabash last fall, you described your "Nye dinner," in which you invited all the Nyes in the San Antonio phonebook, sight unseen, to your house for a meal. For days after you left, people from the audience were buzzing about the risky generosity of that action: welcoming complete strangers into your home. It's the kind of action that occurs at the end of Habibi, when Liyana's Palestinian family hosts Omer, her Jewish friend, in their home—not without some accompanying tensions. What kinds of risks are involved in cross-cultural understanding, and how, in your fiction for children and young adults, do you encourage readers to prepare for and face those risks?

Nye: Thanks for remembering that offbeat Nye-family story of ours! Well, people who consider the world an interesting place filled with delicious variations always hope to get to know many other people who are unlike themselves in certain ways: different colors or cultures or food-preferences or song-styles or religions. You know, I've never understood the impulse to be with people only like ourselves. How dull that would be.

Sometimes it's comforting to be with one's own crowd for a *little* while, sure. Next weekend, for example, I'll be attending the largest annual gathering of Arab Americans in the United States in Washington, DC and it's always fun, like finding out you have this enormous family. But then you go back to your own neighborhood filled with so many different backgrounds and feel even *more* interested in all the possibilities and styles.

Sometimes appetites need to be whetted. I would hope that writing for young people might serve as an invitation to *get to know* some of those other slightly different folks out there in the world—without fear, without ever thinking of "otherness" as a threat. It's a glory, not a threat. We'd have fewer school shootings if kids could remember this. Those people unlike us: how to have empathy with them, for them? Those lives seemingly unlike our own: how are we connected, ultimately? We all sleep, eat, have dreams and loves and hopes and sorrows. I want writing to be connected to all of this.

Castro: Habibi and Sitti's Secrets seem like two different versions of a similar story: one for older, one for younger children. Can you talk about the autobiographical elements of that story, and how you decided to move aspects of your own childhood experience into the realm of fiction? What were some of the challenges of doing so? I noticed that the chronology, for example, was updated.

Nye: Well, we're stuck with ourselves, aren't we? You're right, of course, in noting this. Someone I don't know sent me an e-mail from California: "Do you realize you have recycled some of the same material in various books of yours?" She had a rather snippy, academic tone. I wrote her back, "Yes, indeed, I am filled with shame," and never heard from her again. The truth is, we should not be filled with shame! We're like our own old grandpas telling the same stories. But I wasn't through with this material, I guess.

I updated it because I wanted to write it as closely-to-the-minute as I could—never an easy thing when dealing with the Middle East and its fluctuations. One must hope to find some deeper, timeless place when one writes, even though our stories are *set* in time. We all write out of what we know toward what we want to find out.

Anyway, I never met Omer, in *Habibi.* He's a totally made-up guy. My next book, I'm happy to report, contains many characters and events I have never met in my life. I wish they'd show up, though.

Castro: In writing about the Palestinian American experience, do you feel you were charting territory that really hadn't been explored in US publishing for children and young adults?

Nye: I would not be so brazen as to say "charting new territory," but I think there is much room for more Arab American perspectives in work for young people. Librarians have told me that, for one. And I am very happy each time I see a new book appear that conveys this perspective. For people interested in finding more books with a Middle Eastern connection, write an organization called AWAIR (awair@igc.org) and ask them to send their fine catalogue of listings.

Castro: Did you have the conscious sense while you were working on Habibi that you were writing against American stereotypes about Arabs and Arab Americans?

Nye: I would say it was both conscious and unconscious. When one lives in the United States, one cannot help but be aware of the general media stereotyping against Arabs that goes on—things have gotten much better in this regard in recent years, surely, more balanced—but it is certainly still a live wire in many places. Here on the very table next to me I have Professor Jack Shaheen's book called *Arab and Muslim Stereotyping in American Popular Culture*—he has helped document patterns of recent ugly images in TV and film, as well as in political reporting and op-ed pieces, as has my friend Ali Abunimah of Chicago, who has taken on NPR and other media entities in full force in recent years.

When, for example, do Americans hear the word "terrorist" applied to others as often as it's applied to Arabs? I remember when that crazed Zionist gunned down the men and boys in the Hebron mosque as they were praying—our newspaper here in San Antonio never once referred to him as a terrorist; they actually called him a "good doctor." Sheesh! I have been writing letters to the editor about this stuff all my life. So have all the other Arab Americans I know.

So I would have to say that the sense of wanting a positive image of Palestinians or Palestinian Americans to come forth through the simple story and appealing characters in *Habibi* was definitely part of my writing consciousness—but I didn't want it to be rhetorical, or a soapbox, or a didactic position, simply an intrinsic one. There's a great quote from Marcel Khalife, the beloved Lebanese singer, about Israeli occupation of his own country: "We fought an occupier that stole the details of our lives. We were forced to protect our sleep, our air, and the pound of flour with blood and steel."

I salute the work of the Seeds of Peace camp in Maine—there's also a branch in Jerusalem now—which brings together Arab and Israeli young people every summer, hoping to build a sense of enlarged humanity in the region's future. I think we'll have to count on young people. The older ones haven't done so well. That's another notion that wove through *Habibi* for me.

Castro: Many writers who explore ethnicity in their work—I'm thinking here of Bharati Mukherjee and Lan Samantha Chang, for example—have been pressured to commodify their ethnicity for publication (exoticized jacket photos, explicitly "ethnic" cover images, etc.). Have you experienced such pressure? Is there a difference between children's publishing and publishing for adults in that regard?

Nye: No such pressures have ever been exerted on me. You're right, this may be a difference between books for young people and books for adults—thank goodness. Writers for young people may enjoy more freedom from marketing niches, etc. I must always thank my terrific editor Virginia Duncan, who used to work at Simon & Schuster and is now at Greenwillow, Harper/Collins, for her guidance in all matters—she is the best editor there could ever be. Her instincts are a keen compass on a true, true road. She is not swayed by hype, jive, or anybody else's pressures.

Castro: Most of your multicultural books for younger readers, both the edited collections and the original works, are very visual in their appeal—Habibi, I think, is the only exception. Was that a deliberate choice on your part from the inceptions of the projects, or did the focus on art evolve gradually?

Nye: Well, we all love art and we always wanted the books to look appealing. I live with a terrific visual artist, photographer Michael Nye, whose portraits appear in *What Have you Lost?* [a 1999 poetry anthology Nye edited]. Virginia cares a great deal about matching the visual and textual elements—she has let me have a say-so in the selection of all artists and art for our books. I can't imagine working with an editor who operates otherwise, though apparently many writers do. This is far more important to me than royalties because it creates the whole ambiance and personality of a book. I couldn't live with a book that had art I didn't care for.

Castro: Nancy Carpenter did a beautiful job with the illustrations in Sitti's Secrets. Several incorporate surreal imagery—deserts superimposed onto hanging bedsheets, an ocean in the sky above the young protagonist—while others do not. Readers have to search carefully, look for unexpected magic. Can you talk about the way in which that process relates to the story you're telling in Sitti's Secrets, and to the larger story about intercultural relations that all your books for young readers seem to offer?

Nye: Yes, I love Nancy's work! She experimented with her paintings for *Sitti's Secrets*, painting directly onto maps, using collage-effects in those desert scenes. We are doing another book together, called *Baby Radar*, and I'm thrilled she said yes to it.

And yes, I think readers (and human beings, in all the moments of their daily days) should always be on the lookout for layerings, tucked-away bits of magic, that help our scenes to glisten—they're there, it's just that sometimes we don't see them. This is what poetry urges us to do: pay that kind of attention. Unfortunately, international relations often hinge on Bigger Talk,

Political Language, Generic Public-Speak, that is less intimate or endearing than a bucket, a swing, a jug of water, a sprig of mint. We have to reclaim those things ourselves, for sustenance. Kids are closer to this than adults. That's one reason I like to write for them.

Castro: Do you have in mind a particular child—or a type of child—as an ideal reader when you write for children?

Nye: Hmmmm. An open-minded one? I like to think most kids are open-minded.

Castro: Benito's Dream Bottle, a picture book, is dedicated to your son Madison. Children have such fresh and startlingly profound ways of looking at things, as you recorded in the poem from Fuel (1998), "One Boy Told Me," which is made up entirely of quotations from Madison and which got such a warm reception when you read it here last fall. The whole concept of a dream bottle that young Benito comes up with—"It's inside every body, between the stomach and the chest. At night, when we lie down, it pours the dreams into our heads" (10)—reminded me of my own son's patiently repeated explanation of his many-chambered stomach (we'd been reading about cows) that, oddly enough, allowed him to be full of his dinner after only half a plate while still leaving plenty of room for dessert. His "dessert chamber" became a much-used expression among our extended family. Do any of the images in Dream Bottle come directly from Madison?

Nye: The image of the swivel cap that opened and closed by itself, and the way the dreams would pour out when a person lies down and go back in when the person stood up: all that came from him.

Castro: Were there any challenges in transposing elements of the story onto a Latino family's experience? Did you have any concerns about effecting that cultural translation successfully?

Nye: Truth is, I never thought of it as a Latino family—just a Latino neighborhood. I realize "Benito" is a Latino name, but here in San Antonio, I know more than one Anglo Juan, for example. Name cross-overs, experience cross-overs: you show me one culture that doesn't dream and then I'll start worrying. A few critics of that book said, "These characters look like Asian-Latinos!" which made me laugh since Yu Cha Pak, the artist, is a Korean now living in Houston. I did not have a specific cultural intent with that book. It was *very* important for me to use the name Mr. Laguna, because he was our beloved ninety-five-year-old neighbor and he really wanted to see his name in a book before he died.

Castro: The central idea of Benito's Dream Bottle—the restoration of imaginative freedom, spontaneity, creativity to an older person by the care and concern of an innocent child reminded me very much of narratives by Frances Hodgson Burnett, as does the spunk of characters in other books, like Liyana in Habibi. I remember that Mary in The Secret Garden and Sara in A Little Princess both negotiate the move from colonized India back to an England that is supposed to be home but is actually strange to them. Was Hodgson Burnett a writer you read when you were growing up?

Nye: I do not recall reading Hodgson Burnett when I was growing up, though I certainly liked *The Secret Garden* as an adult. I appreciate your mentioning the spunk factor very much. Nothing matters more. Spunk is number one.

Some of my favorite authors as a kid were Margaret Wise Brown, E.B. White, Carl Sandburg. Louisa May Alcott, Langston Hughes, and the list continues evolving through reading to this day! Some of my favorite current authors include Karen Brennan, Mary Ann Taylor-Hall, W.S. Merwin, Larry Brown, Reginald Gibbons, Edward Hirsch, Lucille Clifton, Jane Hirshfield—well, I have many, many, and I read widely in the Books for Young People field, too. I just loved Louis Sachar's *Holes*, as did millions of other people in the U.S.

Castro: You've edited three wonderful collections of multicultural literature for young adult readers. Can you explain your goals for those projects?

Nye: My goals have always been to make wonderful voices available to more readers, to promote poems of humanity and intelligence that extend and connect us all as human beings, to enlarge readers' horizons—including my own, as I work on the books—and to help connect people. My friend Wendy Barker, a fine poet, once called me a human switchboard. I think that was the greatest compliment I ever received.

Castro: In the introduction to The Tree Is Older Than You Are, you respond to anticipated criticism of your role as a non-Mexican editor of Mexican text. The passage reads:

> Now I live in one of the most Mexican of U.S. cities, in an inner-city neighborhood where no dinner table feels complete without a dish of salsa for gravity, and the soft air hums its double tongue. For some, this may not qualify me to

gather writings of a culture not in my blood. I suggest that blood be bigger than what we're born with, that blood keep growing and growing as we live; otherwise how will we become true citizens of the world? For twenty years, working as a visiting writer in dozens of schools in my city and elsewhere, I have carried poems by writers of many cultures into classrooms, feeling the large family of voices linking human experience. We have no borders when we read. (7)

Can you talk further about the politics of ethnic difference—territoriality, the commodification of ethnicity, cultural appropriation?

Nye: All I can really say about this is I think we all need to be both bigger and smaller than we are. We are uplifted by one another's cultures, infused, enlarged. Cultures by necessity blend and commingle and enrich and flavor one another.

If I were to present myself as an expert insider in the Mexican American community, people might take issue with that, but as an anthologist and lifetime reader and traveler in the region who simply appreciates Mexican poetry and visual art, I feel equipped to choreograph a book of the same. We may all appreciate one another's cultural traditions and help to be vehicles of traditions not originally our own by blood without having to feel guilty for it. But I guessed some people might ask, "Hey, who's she to talk about this?"—you know, can't there be Anglo experts on the blues? Sure, why not? Some of the best talks I've ever heard about Japanese poetry were by Anglo-Americans.

We are who we are, but we're not stuck there. I *love* it when a non-Arab serves me hummus, believe me!

Castro: Has being a Poet in the Schools affected your writing and editing for younger readers?

Nye: Being a Poet in the Schools is a fabulous pleasure, responsibility, blessing, experiment, and ongoing discovery for everyone who ever participates in such a program. It takes enormous energy reserves and flexibility. Being a nomad-by-nature helps too! It has inspired, uplifted, and challenged all of us who do it. And I keep running into kids, ex-students, who say how much it mattered to them too. My most recent anthology, *Salting the Ocean: 100 Poems by Young Poets* [2000], is a collection of some favorite student writings from over the years. I planned to work as a visiting classroom poet for two years when I started and have now been visiting schools for twenty-five years. I don't do many long-term

ongoing workshops the way I used to do, however. Usually my visits now are one or two days long. Sometimes I miss the longer stints. There are lots of good people doing that work.

Writing projects for teachers in various states—the New Jersey Writing Project, for example, and many others—have encouraged teachers to make creative writing an essential part of the curriculum. They've done so much good. I'm always shocked, however, at how many classrooms in the United States this wisdom hasn't reached yet. Bravo to Teachers & Writers Collaborative and the Writing Project at Columbia University for all the work they've done in this field, too—bravo to everybody. But no bravo to teachers who still imagine that occasional writing—for tests and official "assignments"—will ever be enough.

Castro: What has the reaction to the edited collections been from bookstores and educators? Do you know if the books are being used in schools, or if most of their readers just discover them privately on bookstore shelves?

Nye: People have been very kind and welcoming to these books. I'm happy to report that the books *are* being used in many schools and *The Tree Is Older Than You Are* has been warmly received by ESL teachers as well as Spanish teachers. Also, it ended up being distributed in Mexico by the Sanborn Company, which made me glad.

Castro: Do you have any other multicultural editing projects in mind for the future?

Nye: Yes I do, but first I have to finish this endless second novelito I'm working on! It is set in San Antonio, titled *Florrie Will Do It.* Also I am working on new poems, new essays, new picture books, and trying to improve upon my garden. After twenty-one years in the same house, wouldn't you think I'd have a beautiful yard by now? But I'm still working on it. Like writing does if we do it often enough, my yard seems to have taken on a life and directions of its own—I walked outside one day and there was this *enormous* bed of blossoming yellow and orange nasturtiums all around the mailbox. I have no memory of ever planting them.

Source: Joy Castro, "Nomad, Switchboard, Poet: Naomi Shihab Nye's Multicultural Literature for Young Readers: An Interview," in *MELUS*, Vol. 27, No. 2, Summer 2002, pp. 225–37.

SOURCES

Barenblat, Rachel, "Interview with Naomi Shihab Nye," in *Pif*, http://www.pifmagazine.com/SID/240/?page = 1& (accessed July 16, 2009).

Barr, John, "American Poetry in the New Century," in *Poetry Magazine*, September 2006, http://www.poetryfoundation.org/journal/article.html?id = 178560 (accessed July 17, 2009).

Colloff, Pamela, "Naomi Shihab Nye: Her Poetry Finds Meaning in the 'Gleam of Particulars,'" in *Texas Monthly*, September 1, 1998.

Elmusa, Sharif S., "Vital Attitude of the Poet: Interview with Naomi Shihab Nye," in *Alif: Journal of Comparative Poetics*, 2007, pp. 107–108.

Hirschfield, Robert, "A Poet Walks the Line (Naomi Shihab Nye)," in *Progressive*, November 1, 2006.

Kavanagh, Meg, "Everywhere Impulse, Devotion, Everywhere: A Conversation with Naomi Shihab Nye," in *Cooperative Children's Book Center, School of Education, University of Wisconsin-Madison*, 2003, http://www.education.wisc.edu/ccbc/authors/experts/nye.asp (accessed July 16, 2009).

Lesesne, Teri, "Honoring the Mystery of Experience," in *Teacher Librarian*, Vol. 26, No. 2, November 1998, p. 59.

Matthews, Tracey, ed., "Nye, Naomi Shihab," in *Concise Major 21st-Century Writers: A Selection of Sketches from Contemporary Authors*, 3rd ed., Thomson Gale, 2006.

Miazga, Mark, "The Spoken Word Movement of the 1990s," in *Michigan State University*, https://www.msu.edu/~miazgama/spokenword.htm (accessed July 17, 2009).

Monaghan, Pat, Review of "Red Suitcase," in *Booklist*, Vol. 91, No. 4, October 15, 1994, p. 395.

"Naomi Shihab Nye," in *Poets.org*, http://www.poets.org/poet.php/prmPID/174 (accessed July 16, 2009).

"Naomi Shihab Nye," in *Steven Barclay Agency*, http://www.barclayagency.com/nye.html (accessed July 20, 2009).

Nye, Naomi Shihab, "Shoulders," in *Red Suitcase*, BOA Editions, 1994, p. 103.

———, "'We Need Poetry Ever' More Than: Talking with Poet Naomi Shihab Nye about Writing, Identity . . . and Cars," in *Writing!*, October 1, 2007.

Review of "Red Suitcase," in *Publishers Weekly*, Vol. 241, No. 39, September 26, 1994, p. 59.

Seaman, Donna, Review of *You and Yours*, in *Booklist*, August 1, 2005.

Townsend, Alison, Review of *Red Suitcase*, in *Women's Review of Books*, Vol. 13, No. 3, December 1995, pp. 26–28.

Woolley, Bryan, "Poet Builds Bridges, Line by Line," in *Dallas Morning News*, September 24, 2005, http://www.dallasnews.com/sharedcontent/dws/fea/life/stories/DN-NSL_nye_0925liv.ART.State.Edition1.20612533.html (accessed July 20, 2009).

FURTHER READING

Barry, Lynda, *What It Is*, Drawn and Quarterly, 2008.
School Library Journal gave this book a starred review. Barry has filled each page with drawings, photographs, and paintings to accompany this collection of philosophical questions for teens to ponder. She encourages readers to explore their own creativity through writing in a way that appeals to students who prefer art to writing or who do not believe they have what it takes to write.

Digh, Patti, *Life is a Verb: 37 Days to Wake Up, Be Mindful, and Live Intentionally*, skirt!, 2008.
Digh's stepfather was diagnosed with lung cancer and died thirty-seven days later. She continually asked herself what she would do with her life on any given day if she knew she had but thirty-seven more left to live. The resulting humorous book is part meditation, part memoir, and part workbook to help interested readers find more meaning in their daily existence.

Hamby, Zachary, *Mythology for Teens*, Prufrock Press, 2009.
Written by a high school communications arts teacher, this book relates ancient stories to modern culture for teens. Readers are encouraged to question and deconstruct issues such as revenge and forgiveness, the meaning of life, and the role of women in society.

Nye, Naomi Shihab, *Habibi*, Simon Pulse, 1999.
This young-adult novel tells the story of a fourteen-year-old in an Arab American family that moves from St. Louis, Missouri, back to Jerusalem, Israel. When Liyana falls in love with a Jewish boy, she challenges cultural and traditional norms. The background is one of violent conflict between Palestinians and Jews.

The Poetry Center and John Timpane, *Poetry for Dummies*, For Dummies, 2001.
This guide explores five thousand years of verse and seeks to demystify poetry for those who fear it most. The text provides a variety of definitions of poetry according to some of the most celebrated poets of their time. Readers will have the opportunity to master three steps of interpretation and participate in individual writing exercises.

Wooldridge, Susan G., *Poemcrazy: Freeing Your Life with Words*, Three Rivers Press, 1997.
This is a "how to" book for people who do not yet know they are poets. Wooldridge helps readers learn to create images, use metaphor, and find poetry in everyday life.

Sympathy

PAUL LAURENCE DUNBAR
1899

"Sympathy" was published in *Lyrics of the Hearthside* (1899), Paul Laurence Dunbar's fourth book of poems, one of the six major volumes he would complete in his brief thirty-three years of life. Though he also wrote novels, short stories, songs, and plays, he is remembered chiefly as a poet. Before writing "Sympathy," he was already famous and known as the Negro Poet Laureate, having toured the country performing his dialect poems about the plantation days. By 1899, the year "Sympathy" was published, he was discouraged that the public did not seem interested in his other works written in standard English. He wrote his serious poetry, like "Sympathy," in literary English, on a variety of subjects in addition to black themes. He had a lyric gift, but critics said his standard English poems were imitative and praised only the poems in dialect, which they believed to be more genuinely expressive of the Negro. The poem "Sympathy" is one of his most famous statements about racism. He did not feel free to write as he wanted and compared the feeling to being a bird in a cage.

The son of slaves, Dunbar felt the continuing legacy of slavery in a time of rampant racism in the United States. Dunbar's struggle to become the first recognized African American author continued even after his death in 1906. Later readers accused him of catering to whites with his poems depicting slaves on the plantation. In the modern age, he has taken his place as one of the founders of African American literature, and his poems

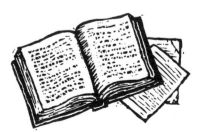

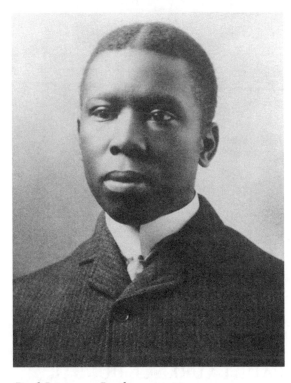

Paul Laurence Dunbar (The Library of Congress)

have been memorized by generations of African Americans and other Americans alike. Though he felt like a failure, he inspired the writers of the Harlem Renaissance in the 1920s to use their vernacular speech as literary expression. "Sympathy" can be found in the *Collected Poetry of Paul Laurence Dunbar* (1993), published by the University Press of Virginia.

AUTHOR BIOGRAPHY

Dunbar was born June 27, 1872, in Dayton, Ohio, to Joshua Dunbar and Matilda Burton Murphy Dunbar, a widow with two sons by her previous slave marriage. Dunbar's parents had both been slaves in Kentucky. After the emancipation, thousands of freed slaves moved north, and Matilda took her young sons to Dayton and became a laundry woman, until she met and married Joshua. Joshua was an alcoholic, and Matilda obtained a divorce and custody of Dunbar, her sickly son, of whom she was protective. Dunbar was the only black student at Dayton Central High School, but he was accepted and excelled.

Dunbar began to write seriously at the age of sixteen and published some of his poems locally. His first real encounter with racial discrimination came after high school in 1891. He could only find menial work as an elevator boy. However, when the Western Association of Writers met in Dayton in 1892, Dunbar was invited to give the welcome, which he composed and recited in verse. He made such a positive impression on the group that he found supporters to help him publish his first collection of poetry, *Oak and Ivy*, in 1892. The volume contains black dialect poems inspired by the dialect work of James Whitcomb Riley. In 1893, Dunbar went to Chicago, Illinois, to work at the Haitian Pavilion at the Columbian Exposition. There he met abolitionist and author Frederick Douglass who recognized his talent and employed him.

With the help of patrons, Dunbar published his second volume, *Majors and Minors*, in 1896. It was favorably reviewed in *Harper's Weekly* by William Dean Howells, a leading American writer and critic at the time. Dunbar became an overnight celebrity as the first nationally known black writer in American society. With his charm, manners, talent, and musical voice, his readings electrified audiences. In 1896, *Lyrics of a Lowly Life* was published by Dodd, Mead in New York.

In 1897 Dunbar worked as a clerk in the Library of Congress. He married another black author, Alice Ruth Moore in 1898 at the height of his fame and productivity. He published his first novel, *The Uncalled*, and first collection of short stories, *Folks from Dixie*, in that same year. *Lyrics of the Hearthside*, containing "Sympathy," was published in 1899.

Dunbar became gravely ill in 1899 with tuberculosis. The Dunbars moved to Denver, Colorado for his health, where he published his second novel, *The Love of Landry*, and a collection of short stories titled *The Strength of Gideon* in 1900. His third novel, *The Fanatics*, was published in 1901, and his last novel, *The Sport of the Gods*, was released in 1902.

Also in 1902, Dunbar and Moore separated because of his alcoholism. He spent his last days in Dayton with his mother, still producing until the end: *Lyrics of Love and Laughter* and *In Old Plantation Days* (both 1903); *The Heart of Happy Hollow* (1904); and *Lyrics of Sunshine and Shadow* (1905). He died of tuberculosis on February 9, 1906, at the age of thirty-three. Many of his poems, essays, and plays were collected and published posthumously.

POEM TEXT

I know what the caged bird feels, alas!
When the sun is bright on the upland slopes;
When the wind stirs soft through the springing
   grass,
And the river flows like a stream of glass;
When the first bird sings and the first bud opes,   5
And the faint perfume from its chalice steals—
I know what the caged bird feels!

I know why the caged bird beats his wing
Till its blood is red on the cruel bars;
For he must fly back to his perch and cling   10
When he fain would be on the bough a-swing;
And a pain still throbs in the old, old scars
And they pulse again with a keener sting—
I know why he beats his wing!

I know why the caged bird sings, ah me,   15
When his wing is bruised and his bosom sore,—
When he beats his bars and he would be free;
It is not a carol of joy or glee,
But a prayer that he sends from his heart's deep
   core,
But a plea, that upward to Heaven he flings—   20
I know why the caged bird sings!

POEM SUMMARY

Stanza 1

LINES 1–3

"Sympathy" is a lyric in iambic tetrameter, seven line stanzas of four metric feet per line. The last line of each stanza is shorter, with three feet. The first line establishes the poem's controlling metaphor of the caged bird looking at a spring day, which mirrors the speaker's situation. The speaker ends the line with an exclamation that suggests a sigh of regret. Although the main rhythm of the poem is iambic (alternating unstressed and stressed beats), many spondees (two strong beats together) are used for emphasis.

The next few lines create a contrast between the cage and a beautiful spring day. The bird would especially feel restrained on a day when the sun is shining outside on the meadows and hills. In line 3, the image of wind blowing through fresh grass creates a feeling of refreshment and freedom, denied to the caged bird. The rhyme scheme of this stanza is *ABAABCC*. Lines 1, 3, and 4 are connected through end rhyme, which helps create the melodious singing sound of wind and the river in the next line. The alliteration (repetition of initial consonants) in lines 2, 3, 4,

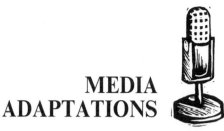

MEDIA ADAPTATIONS

- *The Paul Laurence Dunbar Collection* is a package of three DVDs and three audiotapes with top African American storytellers reading stories and poems by the poet. It was produced by Cerebellum Corporation in 2008.
- *The Poetry of Paul Laurence Dunbar*, narrated by Bobby Norfolk, produced in 2004 by August House, is available as an audio download or audio CD from LearnOutLoud.com.

and 5, reinforces the flowing sounds of wind and water.

LINES 4–7

In line 4, the river, like the wind, is another image of movement. This dynamic quality of the landscape would make anyone inside a small space feel restless. The first bird singing in spring, depicted in line 5, and the first flower opening express hope ordinarily, but to one shut up, it would be torture not to share the joy of expansion, to be a mere onlooker.

The perfume from the flower is delicate and subtle, like a bird's song. The suggestion in line 6 that the perfume actually sneaks out of the flower cup when no one is looking (through alliteration) is another image of the natural expression of living things that cannot be denied or shut off. The thought breaks off with a dash creating suspense before the last line of the stanza. The expansion of the previous line is brought to a sudden halt in line 7 with the return to the image of the caged bird. The rhythm and rhyme of the poem establish the nature of life to sing out.

Stanza 2

LINES 8–10

In line 8, the speaker says he understands why the bird beats its wing inside the cage. The spondees emphasize the useless flapping of the bird's wings. In the next line, the bird continues hopelessly to beat its wings on the cage bars until it bleeds. The repeated alliteration in lines 8 and 9 create a feeling of restraint. The cage metaphor suggests the former slave status of black people, but it also signifies a current restraint. The poet's wife, Alice Dunbar, says he wrote the poem when he was working all day in the Library of Congress in Washington, D.C., looking out the barred windows to the green grass and trees. He felt imprisoned, doing menial work, when he wanted to be writing. In line 10, the bird flaps his wings but instead of getting anywhere, it must return to its perch. The spondee in the middle of the line recreates this image of the flapping wings pushing the bird back to its perch.

LINES 11–14

In line 11, the speaker expresses what the bird wants to do. Instead of clinging to a perch, it wants to be on the swinging branch of a tree. Both a perch and a bough are made of wood, but one is alive with movement, and one is dead and artificial as part of a man-made birdcage. It is apparent in line 12 that the bird has obviously repeated this action many times because it has scars from previous attempts to free itself from its cage. The fact that the scars are very old, however, could also suggest the legacy of slavery. The current pain of facing racism and restriction evokes the old historical wound that is still bleeding.

Each time the bird tries to get free and is thwarted, the pain in its wings hurts more. Line 13 ends with a dash, like hitting a brick wall. The pressure of the emotion has built up in this stanza without any resolution. To underscore this lack of movement forward, the concluding couplet is not CC but again, *AA* (the stanza's rhyme scheme is *ABAABAA*). Lines 8, 10, 11, 13, and 14 all rhyme. There are only two rhymes in this stanza, *A* and *B*, as though the bird is only allowed to sing one or two notes. Line 14 is a concluding shorter line and echoes line 8, which is a variation of the refrain of the poem.

Stanza 3
LINES 15–17

In line 15, the speaker says he understands why the bird in the cage sings, and again utters a sigh of sadness. The bird's wing is injured and its heart is sore, in line 16, and yet the bird sings. Its heart is not in the song, and yet it still sings. This is what people want from a caged bird: a song.

There is "B" alliteration in lines 16 and 17 as the speaker describes the bird once again beating his wings to get free. The "B" is a sound that stops as it is articulated. It suggests that the power of the bird's song is stifled. This line could also paradoxically explain the fact that the only freedom the bird or speaker feels is in singing, even if constrained.

LINES 18–21

Lines 15, 17, and 18 rhyme, but the lyrical effect is muted in this stanza, with darker images and harsher sounds. In line 18, the speaker says that the song the bird sings is not joyful. The song the bird sings is a spontaneous prayer from its heart. The feeling that the bird has reached its limit is recreated in the three strong beats together at the end of line 19.

In line 20, the bird's song is also described as a plea, a begging to a higher power for relief. This tentative prayer ends with a dash at the end of the line, showing that it is inconclusive. The rhyme scheme of this stanza is the same as the first stanza (*ABAABCC*). It explains that the speaker understands why the bird is singing despite its imprisonment.

THEMES

Racism

The central metaphor of the caged bird in "Sympathy," with the bird forced to perform within confinement, could be taken as suggesting the slavery African Americans endured in the United States for two and a half centuries. Though Dunbar lived after the emancipation, the legacy of slavery continued through various social, legal, and psychological constraints. He was refused white collar or journalistic work because of his race, forced to work in the confinement of an elevator and the barred library stacks that were the inspiration for the poem. Dunbar was a brilliant and creative man, but he struggled to overcome the racial stereotype of blacks as slow, lazy, and child-like. The blacks he portrayed in his dialect poems, singing and dancing on the plantation, were part of the folklore of the past to him, like the Midwestern folklore used in James Whitcomb Riley's poems. He heard stories of the Old

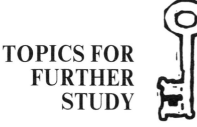

TOPICS FOR FURTHER STUDY

- James Whitcomb Riley (1853–1916) was an influence on Dunbar's decision to write local color poems using dialect. Choose one student in class to recite Dunbar's dialect poem, "When De Co'n Pone's Hot," celebrating a Southern black meal. Another student can perform James Whitcomb Riley's Hoosier dialect poem, "When the Frost Is on the Punkin." Discuss the scenes and characterization of each poem in class. How do the poets preserve regional folk life in their poems?

- Alice Dunbar (later known as Dunbar-Nelson), the poet's wife, was also a well-known black author. Read Alice Dunbar's poems "Rainy Day" and "Cano—I Sing" and contrast the messages of those poems to Dunbar's "Sympathy." Write a paper comparing and contrasting their poems in content and style.

- Research the influence of Dunbar on poets of the Harlem Renaissance, such as Langston Hughes, and report to the class in a PowerPoint audio and visual presentation, using poem selections of both authors to illustrate your points.

- Dunbar's poems "Sympathy" and "We Wear the Mask" are often taken as statements of the difficulties African Americans have faced. Use these poems as points of departure to critique the statement of another work of African American poetry or fiction of your choice in an essay.

- African American poetry is influenced by such oral forms as spirituals, sermons, jazz, work songs, gospel, and blues. Apply this idea to the dialect poems of Dunbar. First have the class read one of Dunbar's poems such as "An Ante-bellum Sermon" or "A Negro Love Song" on paper and then have it performed aloud by a practiced reader. In an in-class essay explain what you heard from the music and rhythm of the poems that you did not see while reading it on paper.

- Compare and contrast the theme of freedom in "Sympathy" with the freedom represented in the Pearl Buck novel *The Good Earth*, (1931) suitable for younger readers. Present your conclusions in an essay.

South from his mother and had a talent for reproducing accent, phrasing, and characterization. Dunbar was also highly educated. He saw himself as middle class, urbane, worldly, and able to meet other artists from around the world.

Though Dunbar never denied his race, and in fact, made many statements on racial injustice, he did not feel he should be tied down to black dialect poems. He was interested in art and experimented with many genres and ethnic voices. He used both white and black characters in his fiction. Dunbar wrote serious literary pieces in the tradition of Lord Alfred Tennyson, Henry Wadsworth Longfellow, John Keats, and Percy Bysshe Shelley. Dunbar became famous as an African American poet but few understood the range of his accomplishments or regarded his many talents as important. His dialect poems imitating the speech of southern plantation blacks were what made him popular, and people wanted to see him perform what they thought was authentic black speech. Like a bird in a cage, he felt he had to produce what audiences expected of a black man.

Dunbar never felt he had accomplished what he wanted. Critics have since interpreted his frustration in many ways; for instance, that he was unable to find an authentic black voice within white culture. The poem "Sympathy" is often taken as a statement of this dilemma, where the poet feels hemmed in and unable to be himself. The old scars that the bird carries from beating his wings on the bars could symbolize the scars of the black race that Dunbar also must carry, for though Dunbar lived a comparatively privileged life, moving freely in both black and white society, he was not free of being typecast. Similarly, much was expected of him as a symbol of his race. He was rarely allowed to be an individual publically. Other Dunbar poems that comment on racism include "The Haunted Oak,""We Wear the Mask,""The Poet,""Right's Security,""The Warrior's Prayer,""To the South on Its New Slavery,""Frederick Douglass," and "Ode to Ethiopia."

Freedom

A bird is a frequent poetic symbol for freedom since it can fly. It is also a common symbol in poetry for the poet. The yearning of the bird for its freedom in "Sympathy" is graphically portrayed when the bird sees the landscape outside. It hears other birds sing and the wind and river rushing and responds by beating its wings against the cage, trying to get out. The urge for freedom is so compelling that the bird endures pain again and again trying to fly, only to be beaten back. By presenting the contrast between the cage and the spring day, it is obvious that a cage is a cruel perversion of life. Whether meaning a literal cage, as slavery, or a psychological one, as Dunbar and many black artists have felt, Dunbar protests that it is wrong to thwart the potential of any living being. It is natural for every creature to express its life and want its freedom. In this poem, the bird, and by implication the speaker, is denied what is natural. The speaker has sympathy for the bird, so the poem is from the point of view of the one without freedom. An onlooker might think that the bird should be quiet, or that the speaker should be content. From the interior point of view, racial prejudice causes extreme suffering and damage. The poet emphasizes a sense of sympathy for the prisoner. Other Dunbar poems on the theme of freedom include "Emancipation,""Ode to Ethiopia,""Justice,""Differences," and "Lincoln."

The Nature of Poetry

Bird song is a metaphor for poetry. There are several implications about poetry in the poem. First, a poet is a person with sympathy. Sympathy means to feel with another being, to put oneself in the place of others. Dunbar's writings, both poetry and prose, do exhibit such sympathy with a variety of characters from all cultures. For instance, his short story "The Lynching of Jube Benson" shows insight into both black and white psychology. He depicts African Americans in his dialect poems with humor and insight ("The Party" and "When Malindy Sings").

Dunbar was influenced by Romantic literature for his serious poems and by regional local color writing for his dialect poems. His underlying aesthetic in the standard English verse is romantic in his choice of subject matter (love, great lives, art, freedom, injustice) and form (odes, ballads, sonnets, and lyrics). Romantic poets celebrated nature as Dunbar does in the first stanza of "Sympathy." The poet, being sensitive, feels with all creatures, and sees and records beauty as well as injustice. While in his fiction Dunbar experimented with realism, for instance in his novel *Sport of the Gods*; in his poetry he holds romantic tenets, showing his talent as a great lyricist.

Freedom is essential for creativity to flow. A bird may sing in a cage, but it is not the same as the bird singing unfettered in nature. In fact, one cannot put restraint on song, for it is a spontaneous welling up of the impulse of life. This is brought out in the first stanza with the image of the perfume sneaking out of the flower cup. It is so delicate an expression that one might hardly notice how the perfume is emitted, but certainly, one could not stop a flower from putting forth its scent. It is part of the identity of the flower. Similarly, it is in the nature of a bird to sing or a poet to write. One does not tell the river how to flow or the bird how to sing. When society shuts down creativity or the voice of anyone trying to speak his or her truth, it is against nature, the nature of the individual, and of nature in general.

The song of a bird or poet comes from a deep place. Whether in joy or pain, the poet/bird sings from the heart about the origin of its song. If restrained, the singer will not produce a happy song, but it is important to note that the desire to sing is so strong that even pain will not stop the singer from singing. In fact, it can make the song more poignant. This idea of the sorrow of African American song is inherent in the blues, and Dunbar believed that rich lyric sorrow was the essence of African music.

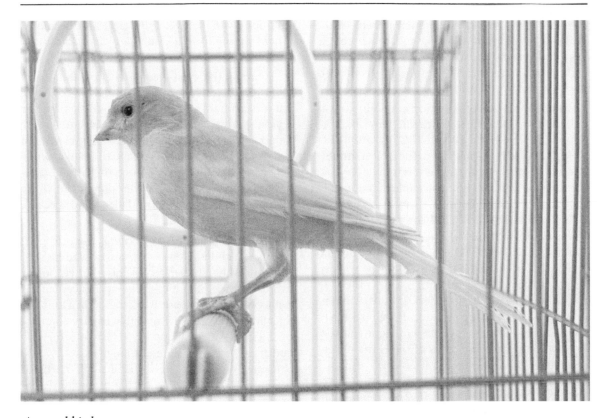

A caged bird (Image copyright Vinicius Tupinamba, 2009. Used under license from Shutterstock.com)

STYLE

Personal Lyric

Lyric poetry is an ancient genre, popular from classical times through the present, in almost every culture. Lyric means song and was originally a song sung to an accompanying lyre or stringed instrument. A lyric poem is short and musical rather than narrative or dramatic, expressing emotions or thoughts. A personal lyric represents the subjective experience of one speaker. The speaker may or may not have the same feelings as the poet, but it is the representation of a speaking person's thoughts on a particular subject, for instance, love. Dunbar was influenced by the lyric poetry of Tennyson, Keats, Shelley, Longfellow, and Edgar Allan Poe. Famous lyric poems include Tennyson's "Now the Crimson Petal Sleeps" and Poe's "To Helen."

The fact that lyrics predominate in Dunbar's poetry is illustrated by the fact that several of his volumes have the term lyric in the title: *Lyrics of Lowly Life*, *Lyrics of the Hearthside*, *Lyrics of Love and Laughter*, and *Lyrics of Sunshine and Shadow*. The lyric or song was flexible enough to accommodate both Dunbar's poems in literary English and his dialect poems. He put the two types side by side in the later volumes, so that one might see "In the Morning," written in humorous dialect, alongside the serious "The Poet," expressing in standard English his concern that he had failed as a writer.

Protest Poem

Dunbar was no doubt inspired by two of his favorite American poets, John Greenleaf Whittier and Longfellow, who wrote protest poems against slavery before the Civil War as part of the abolitionist movement. It was not necessary for Dunbar to depend on white models, however, for the history of African American oral traditions shows an emphasis on protest. The enslaved Africans kept up their spirits with encoded messages in their songs and spirituals. Such familiar religious spirituals as "Get on Board, Little Children" and "Go Down, Moses," were a way to talk about freedom and slavery in Biblical terms or to warn about an impending escape attempt. The song "Oh, Freedom" is another that was sung at secret meetings on the plantations. It became an anthem of the civil rights movement. The fact that these protests were coded indicates something important about early African American literature. It was dangerous to express protest too openly.

In the post-Reconstruction era, Dunbar was still writing in a time of racial tension. Like fiction writer Charles Waddell Chesnutt (1858–1932), Dunbar learned to write for a double audience, with protest generally muted or told through indirection. Some notable exceptions to this are Dunbar's famous racial assertions in "The Haunted Oak," "We Wear the Mask," and "Sympathy." "Sympathy" protests the racist conditions under which Dunbar had to write and live, though his argument is cleverly worded through metaphor. He symbolically refers to the pain of slavery that generations of Africans must still carry as the scars on the caged bird's wings. Those scars would be enumerated more bluntly in the protest poems of the Harlem Renaissance in the 1920s and 1930s in such examples as "Incident" and "Saturday's Child" by Countee Cullen. Langston Hughes's "I, Too, Sing America" asserts more boldly than Dunbar dared, that the black voice is part of the American voice.

The protest poems of the 1960s centered around the civil rights movement; for instance, "The Ballad of Birmingham" by Dudley Randall recounted the bombing of children in a church. Compared to the later more aggressive protest poems written by black poets, Dunbar has been accused by modern critics of being an Uncle Tom, accommodating white tastes with black stereotypes in his dialect poems. This is an incorrect assumption, for Dunbar did protest injustice in both his poetry and prose.

African American Poetry

Slave poets Lucy Terry, Jupiter Hammon, and Phillis Wheatley published works even before the American Revolution. Phillis Wheatley (1754–1784), the child prodigy slave of the Wheatley family who produced polished eighteenth-century verses, was the first well-known African American author, traveling abroad to promote her work and the work of abolitionists.

African American poetry refers to the writings of those people who were brought forcibly to the United States from Africa and kept in bondage for two and a half centuries. It was forbidden for slaves to learn to read or write, and yet they did both. At first they continued their native oral tradition with songs, spirituals, and sermons. After learning to write, many ex-slaves like Frederick Douglass wrote slave narratives.

During the post-Reconstruction era, from about 1870 to World War I, published black authors primarily produced journalistic prose or fiction, or single poems. Dunbar's ambition to be an accepted mainstream poet led him to write in standard European and American poetic forms. When inspired by James Whitcomb Riley's example to write poetry in regional dialect, he wrote poems in black southern dialect and became famous for it.

Dunbar preferred to write literary English poems, which he felt most expressed who he was. Yet his white audience felt his dialect poems expressed the authentic black experience and his publisher favored these works as well. Dunbar's dilemma was a crucial moment in the development of African American poetry. He wrote for two audiences with two different languages. "Sympathy" partly describes this dilemma of the black writer who writes against such a heavy burden of expectations.

Dunbar's experiments inspired later poets such as Hughes, James Weldon Johnson, Cullen, Claude McKay, and Jean Toomer during the Harlem Renaissance to integrate these separate modes of expression into an English language that could distinctively express the African American voice. It was the revolution of the 1960s that garnered African American literature, like other minority literatures, praise and respect. With black writers being taken seriously and winning Pulitzer and Nobel prizes, their work could no longer be denied its place as part of mainstream American literature, and black authors felt free to use whatever language their imaginations could invent.

HISTORICAL CONTEXT

Failure of Reconstruction

Reconstruction is the period after the Civil War (1865–1877) in which the United States tried to restructure American society by abolishing slavery and amending the Constitution (precisely the 13th, 14th, and 15th amendments) to give civil rights to four million former slaves. While federal troops were stationed in the South, state governments were organized to give blacks the right to vote and schools and positions in government. By

COMPARE
&
CONTRAST

- **1900:** Only a handful of African Americans, such as Alice Moore Dunbar, go to college.

  Today: Although underrepresented in terms of total college population, millions of African Americans enroll in higher education and earn college degrees.

- **1900:** There are few published African American writers, especially outside of black journals and magazines.

  Today: African American writers win the highest literary prizes (Pulitzer, Nobel), write best-selling novels that are made into films, and are studied as part of the American literary canon.

- **1900:** Jim Crow laws, which legally separate the races in public settings in southern

states, regulate the lives of African Americans. These laws disenfranchise African Americans, who are not considered part of the democratic process.

  Today: African Americans have full political rights, and the first African American U.S. President, Barack Obama, is inaugurated in 2009.

- **1900:** Tuberculosis (TB), the cause of Dunbar's death, is almost always fatal, with no treatment available except bed rest in a mild climate.

  Today: TB can be cured with anti-TB drugs, although it has made a comeback recently, because it has become resistant to some traditional medications.

1877, however, white supremacists in the South had reasserted their power and states' rights to enact Jim Crow laws that led to segregation of the races and deprived blacks of their civil liberties. Peonage, the practice of creditors forcing debtors to work for them, was common in the South and was criticized in Dunbar's poem "To the South on Its New Slavery." Full citizenship for African Americans did not come about until almost a century later during the civil rights movement in the 1960s. Black historians have called the period from 1877 to the end of World War I the "nadir" of race relations in America.

Black Migration to Northern Cities

After the Civil War, the United States changed rapidly from an agrarian economy to industrial capitalism. With the emancipation, blacks began migrating from the South to escape poverty and racial violence to the North where there were jobs and more opportunities. The largest migrations happened after Dunbar's death, but even during his life he witnessed and even worried about African Americans moving from a country life in the South to ghettos in the northern

cities. In *The Sport of the Gods*, he pictures a black family ruined by moving to New York. Dunbar was one of the first to see that racism could be as virulent in the North as in the South.

Racial Discrimination and Racial Violence

The terrorism the Ku Klux Klan and other hate groups inflicted on blacks in the late nineteenth and early twentieth century was largely countenanced by both southern and northern whites. D. W. Griffith's film *The Birth of a Nation*, released in 1915, clearly casts the Ku Klux Klan as heroes restoring order to the South and shows blacks as evil. W. E. B. Du Bois, the black activist whom Dunbar admired, objected to this piece of hate propaganda accepted as mainstream. In the 1890s, when Dunbar was beginning his career, there were hundreds of lynchings in the country. Dunbar was so appalled by this unpunished practice of mob violence that he wrote a poem, "The Haunted Oak," and the short story, "The Lynching of Jube Benson," in protest. Although Dunbar was luckier than many of his race, Dunbar did deal with racial discrimination, even in Ohio. He was unable to realize his dream of going to Harvard Law School and had to be satisfied with a high school education. He was forced into taking menial jobs and told flatly that newspapers and other businesses did not hire minorities.

Racial Stereotypes: Minstrelsy and Uncle Remus

Minstrel shows were a form of popular musical and comedy entertainment after the Civil War, lampooning blacks as stupid and superstitious. At first the parts were played by whites in black-face, but later, by blacks themselves in "Amos and Andy" routines, with stock characters like Jim Crow, Jim Dandy, and Mr. Bones. They sang and danced and spoke in southern black dialect. Even the most liberal newspapers and magazines of the day spread racist caricatures of African Americans in articles and cartoons. Popular myths about the "good old South" were spread in the Uncle Remus stories (1881) by a white journalist, Joel Chandler Harris, who used black folklore and dialect. As Dunbar also used life on the plantation and black dialect for his dialect poems, he was later criticized for portraying slavery in a comic and acceptable light. That this was not his intent or the result of his works has successfully been argued by many recent critics. The Uncle Remus stories were stereotypes; Dunbar's folk poems transcend such images.

Rise of the Black Middle Class

In spite of tremendous opposition, African Americans found ways to become educated and succeed, becoming lawyers, doctors, business entrepreneurs, actors, and artists. Dunbar is praised as the first black professional author in America, able to earn a living by writing and speaking. The strategy for raising blacks to the middle class was hotly debated among black activists. Booker T. Washington (1856–1915) was a slave, but he became an educator and leader of the African American community after the Civil War. He pleaded with middle-class whites to let the black race develop along separate lines to develop the industrial skills they needed to support themselves economically. He was accused later by W. E. B. Du Bois (1868–1963), a black scholar and political advocate, as an accommodationist (compromiser). Though Washington won white support for blacks, he did not push for black college education and equal rights as Du Bois did.

Du Bois's famous statement that a black man lives in double consciousness, having to switch between white and black expectations, is often applied to Dunbar's situation of trying to please both white and black audiences. Du Bois was a founder of the National Association for the Advancement of Colored People (NAACP) and was the first African American to earn a Ph.D. from Harvard University. He began the push for civil rights which was later taken up by Dr. Martin Luther King, Jr.

In spite of Dunbar's early poverty, he grew up in a town that was more integrated than most. Dayton, Ohio, was an end point of the Underground Railroad and in Dunbar's youth, ten percent of the population was black. Dunbar graduated from a white high school, and he was even the editor of the school newspaper. He was proud to live a middle class life with his wife, Alice, in Washington, D.C., with other black professionals, a life he describes in his essay, "Negro Society in Washington" in the *Saturday Evening Post* (December 14, 1901). The black middle class at this point was still segregated, however.

CRITICAL OVERVIEW

When Dunbar published his second collection of poems, *Majors and Minors* (1896), a famous actor, James Herne, sent his copy to novelist and critic William Dean Howells, who reviewed it in *Harper's Weekly* on June 27, 1896, reprinted in Peter Revell's *Paul Laurence Dunbar*. It was Dunbar's twenty-fourth birthday, and overnight he found himself famous as the first genuine Negro poet of America. Howells compares him to Robert Burns in his use of dialect, saying that Dunbar "has been able to bring us nearer to the heart of primitive human nature in his race than anyone else has yet done." Though Howells made Dunbar famous, the praise did a certain amount of damage, for Howells pronounces Dunbar's standard English poems to be inferior to his dialect pieces. Dunbar was never able to influence the public to take his standard English poems (such as "Sympathy"), or his prose, seriously. He established his fame as a performer of his dialect pieces.

When "Sympathy" was published in *Lyrics of the Hearthside* in 1899, critics echoed Howells's earlier statements. In a review for the *Baltimore Herald* (March, 1899) reprinted in E. W. Metcalf,

Jr.'s *Paul Laurence Dunbar: A Bibliography*, a contributor comments: "Mr. Dunbar's choice of words is happier when he is writing in the musical speech of the Negro." Also reprinted in Metcalf's work, a contributor to the *New York Mail and Express* (April 8, 1899) praises the standard English poems as "amateur excellence," but the dialect poems as proving "his eminence among the dialect writers of America." Many critics of the time saw his standard English poems as imitative.

After Dunbar's death, his widow, Alice Dunbar, also an author and critic, attempted to correct the idea that the dialect poems express the poet. Quoted by Revell in Twayne's "United States Author" series, Alice states: "it was in the pure English poems that the poet expressed *himself*. He may have expressed his race in the dialect poems; they were to him the side issues of his work." The controversy picked up in the 1920s with the new emphasis on black pride in the Harlem Renaissance making it appear that Dunbar catered to whites. According to Revell, Dunbar's friend and fellow writer James Weldon Johnson, in his anthology, *The Book of American Negro Poetry*, defends Dunbar as the first to use dialect "as a medium for the true interpretation of Negro character and psychology." In the first known balanced and serious criticism of Dunbar, *Paul Laurence Dunbar: Poet of His People* (1936), Benjamin Brawley claims that Dunbar was a genius who was constrained by the racism of his time from speaking as he wanted to, but also that he created a landmark for other black authors with his work.

Nevertheless, the 1940s and 1950s were low points in the appreciation of Dunbar. In *Dunbar Critically Examined* (1941), Victor Lawson declares: "In his poems in dialect Dunbar stood as the conscious or unconscious apologist of the plantation." This image of Dunbar was gradually erased with the revival of interest at the Centenary Conference on Dunbar in Dayton in 1972. In a contribution to *A Singer in the Dawn: Reinterpretations of Paul Laurence Dunbar* (1975), Darwin Turner provides an opinion similar to Howells's original evaluation: "[Dunbar's] unique contribution to American literature is his dialect poetry."

In hindsight, the criticism comes full circle, but with the addition of understanding both the racism Dunbar fought and his contribution of the black vernacular as legitimate poetic speech. In addition, new previously unpublished Dunbar manuscripts reveal his breadth and experimentation in various genres. Despite critical debates, Dunbar's poems entered the oral traditions of African Americans from the beginning, and they are often memorized by school children. In the 1980s, black poet Herbert Woodward Martin traveled with a one-man show, reciting Dunbar's dialect and standard poems to receptive audiences, illustrating their power when performed. Dunbar is now considered a mainstream American poet who was black, instead of a segregated Negro poet. This is what he had hoped for, but it took him a century to achieve this goal.

CRITICISM

Susan Andersen

Andersen is a writer and college English teacher. In this essay, she considers Dunbar's poem "Sympathy" as a symbol of the African American poetic tradition.

Dunbar was often called the Negro Poet Laureate at the beginning of the twentieth century, but by the 1950s he was seen as an embarrassment to many readers because his dialect poems called up plantation stereotypes of African Americans. In his day, white readers embraced his dialect poems ("The Party," "When Malindy Sings") as the authentic voice of a Negro poet, while his standard English poems, such as "Sympathy," were seen as imitative. Forced to continue writing and performing the dialect pieces due to public opinion, he feared that he had failed as a writer, as is evident in his poem, "The Poet." Beginning in the 1970s, there has been an ongoing reassessment of his contribution to the American literary canon. Critics have pointed out his difficult but crucial position between black and white cultures. How could he speak in a true voice using either standard English or a black dialect? Dunbar had to forge a tradition of African American poetry that did not exist; the caged bird metaphor in "Sympathy" can be seen as a symbol for that tradition, and it yields both positive and negative implications.

Dunbar had dual aspirations from his youth to be a voice for his people and to be accepted as an American author without racial consideration. He thought of being a journalist at first. He had been the editor of his high school newspaper, thoroughly accepted for his literary talents in an all-white high school in Dayton, Ohio. Perhaps Dunbar thought of that experience as

> DUNBAR HAD TO FORGE A TRADITION OF AFRICAN AMERICAN POETRY THAT DID NOT EXIST; THE CAGED BIRD METAPHOR IN "SYMPATHY" CAN BE SEEN AS A SYMBOL FOR THAT TRADITION, AND IT YIELDS BOTH POSITIVE AND NEGATIVE IMPLICATIONS."

proving that his integration into the mainstream of American literary life was possible. He continued writing journal articles throughout his life, and many of his strong opinions against racism were printed in leading newspapers and magazines. His interest in writing poetry and literature, however, prevailed as his choice of career. As is quoted in Benjamin Brawley's *Paul Laurence Dunbar: Poet of His People* (1936), Dunbar told a white sponsor, Dr. H. A. Tobey, that his life ambition was "To be able to interpret my own people through song and story, and to prove to the many that after all we are more human than African."

In *Figures in Black: Words, Signs, and the "Racial" Self* (1987), Henry Louis Gates, Jr., points out that literacy was a matter of life and death for blacks in this country, the only way they could prove they were human and not primitive animals: "each piece of creative writing became a political statement." Dunbar's statement of purpose is thus necessarily both ambitious and defensive, for he has something "to prove to the many." In the same work, Gates describes "the subtext of the history of black letters as this urge to refute the claim that because blacks had no written traditions they were bearers of an inferior culture." Dunbar began his career then with a huge burden to carry, like the bird with scarred wings. He had to express his racial self and his literary self, but in a manner that would pave the way for other African Americans without offending the dominant culture. His sponsors and audiences were mostly white in an era of high racial tension. He wanted to justify and interpret his people but also to be respected as an artist above all. By being accepted in the same spirit of the great poets he loved (John Keats, Percy Bysshe Shelley, Lord Alfred

Tennyson, Edgar Allan Poe, and Henry Wadsworth Longfellow), he would in one stroke accomplish something for his race and himself: "I consider that a colored poet of sufficient ability to make a name for himself would do more to enlighten and encourage the ambition of the multitude of colored people in America than almost anything else," quotes Felton O. Best in *Crossing the Color Line: A Biography of Paul Laurence Dunbar 1872–1906* (1996). Dunbar made it clear, however, that he did not want to be just a curiosity—a Negro poet—he wanted equal respect: "He felt that he was first of all a man, then an American, and incidentally a Negro," Brawley states.

By being stereotyped early on as that great anomaly, a black poet, who could only properly interpret his race through dialect, Dunbar felt like an animal in a zoo. He was a prolific author in his brief thirty-three years. He was a journalist. He experimented with lyrics in standard English, southern black dialect, and white dialects, such as Irish American and German American. He was a librettist for an operetta and composed lyrics to popular songs in both dialect and standard speech; he was the author of four novels, some with white characters. He wrote short stories and plays, including one play in the form of an eighteenth-century English comedy of manners ("Herrick"). Many of his manuscripts were unpublished in his lifetime because the publishers only wanted the black dialect poems that sold well, about life on the old plantation. As these poems were often humorous, they reminded white audiences of the minstrel shows with blackface comedians making fun of the black race. Myron Simon, in a contribution to *A Singer in the Dawn: Reinterpretations of Paul Laurence Dunbar* (1975), quotes Dunbar's response to this confusion: "I am sorry to find among intelligent people those who are unable to differentiate dialect as a philological branch from Negro minstrelsy."

Yet if he composed in standard English, Dunbar was accused of imitation. William Dean Howells had set the tone from the beginning in his 1896 review by saying that only Dunbar's dialect poems were original. The cry was picked up by every reviewer after that; the standard English poems were considered weak. After his death, the poet's wife, Alice, defended the standard English poems, saying that they were the poems that contained his own voice. By 1899, when he published "Sympathy," Dunbar felt

WHAT DO I READ NEXT?

- *A Hope in the Unseen: An American Odyssey From the Inner City to the Ivy League* by Ron Suskind (Broadway Books, 1998) is a nonfiction book for young adults widely read in modern-day schools. Journalist Ron Suskind tracked the progress of Cedric Jennings out of an inner city high school in Washington, D.C., to Brown University. The work is the true story of how one courageous teenager fought his way out of poverty and violence to realize a dream that Dunbar was denied.

- The longest short story Dunbar ever wrote was originally published in *The Strength of Gideon* (1900). "One Man's Fortune," reprinted in *The Paul Laurence Dunbar Reader* edited by Jay Martin and Gossie H. Hudson (Dodd, Mead, 1975) details the racist treatment of Bertram Halliday, a young black college graduate. In the story Dunbar demands equal treatment of blacks.

- *The Betrayal of the Negro: From Rutherford B. Hayes to Woodrow Wilson, Vol. 1* by Rayford Whittingham Logan, (Perseus, 1997) was first issued in 1954 and is a classic historical study of the racism of the post-Reconstruction era. A scholar at Howard University, Logan was in President Franklin D. Roosevelt's Black Cabinet.

- Young-adult novel *Mexican WhiteBoy* by Matt de la Peña (Delacorte, 2008) depicts biracial Danny Lopez's dilemma of not belonging to either the white American or Mexican culture. Dialogue includes street vernacular and Spanish words.

- *Give Us Each Day: The Diary of Alice Dunbar-Nelson*, edited by Gloria T. Hull (W. W. Norton, 1984), is the journal of Dunbar's widow for 1921 and 1926–1931. It gives a glimpse of the life of an intellectual black woman, writer, and political activist during the Harlem Renaissance.

- Jean Wagner and Kenneth Douglas's 1973 work *Black Poets of the United States: From Paul Laurence Dunbar to Langston Hughes* provides both a historical and biographical review of black poetry and major African American poets from early slavery to the Harlem Renaissance. Originally published in France in 1963, it provides a broad perspective.

---

imprisoned in many ways. He was making little progress in his career because of prejudice about the type of poetry he should produce. He was also working a menial job as a clerk in the Library of Congress. The inspiration for the caged bird in "Sympathy" came from looking out the barred windows of the library to the trees outside. In a 2006 contribution to *Pacific Coast Philology*, Camille Roman remarks on the symbolic irony of Dunbar trying to write African American poetry while imprisoned in the Library of Congress with the white man's books that were the legacy of his oppressor.

However, in *The Signifying Monkey: A Theory of Afro-American Literary Criticism* (1988), an important work on African American literary theory, Gates describes a practice of the African oral tradition called "Signifyin(g)" that illuminates Dunbar's poetry. Signifyin(g) is defined as wordplay using "repetition and reversal." Even slave songs "signified" on the oppressor by taking phrases and reversing the meaning. Gates finds this principle of irony to be one of intertextuality, where one text comments on a previous text by playing upon a given phrase or idea. This oral tradition from Africa is at work in American jazz, the blues, spirituals, ragtime, hip-hop, and rap, and it occurs as well in written African American texts.

Using this information, a reader can see new meaning in "Sympathy," which could at first glance seem imitative. For instance, in the first stanza, Dunbar introduces the bird in spring-time, a standard image from Romantic poetry to suggest the poet. Both Keats and Shelley used bird song as a metaphor for the spontaneity of the creative act. Shelley's ode "To a Sky-Lark" and Keats's "Ode to a Nightingale" are major statements of their poetic philosophies. Shelley compares the song of the skylark/poet to natural processes such as the wind spreading around the perfume of a flower. This image of scent coming out of a flower is also apparent in the first stanza of "Sympathy," making it seem like a repeat of Shelley's idea. In Dunbar's version, however, the image is ironic with the perfume stealing out of the flower. This stealthy poetic act "signifies" on Shelley's and Keats's ecstatic and unfettered birds. Dunbar's bird is crippled in a cage of racism and sings in spite of pain. That the caged bird symbol seemed right for African American literature is affirmed by poet Maya Angelou, who used Dunbar's line for the title of her autobiography, *I Know Why the Caged Bird Sings* (1970).

Dunbar's essay "Negro Music," written the same year as "Sympathy," could serve as a commentary on his poem. In the essay, reprinted in *In His Own Voice: The Dramatic and Other Uncollected Works of Paul Laurence Dunbar* (2002), Dunbar describes an insight he had when he heard some Africans singing at the Columbian Exposition in Chicago, Illinois, in 1893. He thought to himself: "It is that heritage." Immediately, he connected to something in the African song and saw how it had become the heritage for African American artists. African music had "rich melody" and "mournful minor cadences" that touch the heart. The African "startles us," but because the tradition had taken on a new depth in America, the "negro American thrills us." Though white critics had accused him of being an imitator, he turns the tables by asserting the originality of African song: "With the black man's heritage of song has come the heritage of sorrow, giving to his song the expression of a sorrowful sweetness which the mere imitator can never attain." One thinks of spirituals and the blues, of all the great singers—Bessie Smith, Billie Holiday, Ray Charles, and James Brown. Dunbar calls the strain in all black music "running like the theme of a symphony—the strain a supplication to God for deliverance." This statement describes the last stanza of the poem accurately, when the bird's song is described as a prayer.

The caged bird as a symbol for African American artists thus is positive and negative. Though enslaved, African Americans did not stop singing or creating beauty out of their pain. Dunbar is able to feel a positive continuity with ancestral song for the African American writer. This legacy he passed on to others to work out more fully. In a contribution to *Post-Bellum, Pre-Harlem: African American Literature and Culture 1877–1919* (2006), Caroline Gebhard points out that black literature is not the creation of one artist alone, and that Dunbar was only the first to tackle the problem of dialect versus standard English. Later writers in the Harlem Renaissance learned to blend vernacular speech and standard English seamlessly together to carry on Dunbar's experiment with voice. In an interview reprinted in *In His Own Voice*, Dunbar insists he has the right to move between languages as a poet: "I hope you are not one of those who would hold the negro down to a certain kind of poetry." He further explains in the same interview, "The races have acted and reacted on each other." Far from seeing literature as a segregated affair, he insists on the healthiness of intertextuality.

Dunbar is one of the first African American artists to create a double voice in his poetry, to appeal to two audiences at once. Blacks understood the irony of "When Malindy Sings" in its praising blacks as better singers than whites; whites understood the music of the dialect, which Dunbar reclaimed as legitimate poetic speech. In the introduction to *The Complete Poetry of Paul Laurence Dunbar* (1992), Joanne M. Braxton observes Dunbar's growth as a poet by comparing the two poems he called "Sympathy." The first by that title appeared in *Oak and Ivy* (1892), his first collection. It is stilted and was not reprinted in later editions. The "Sympathy" written in 1899, Braxton states, "moves away from the imitation of European models and toward a strong poetic voice of his own." In *Crossing the Color Line*, Best points out that no matter what critics have said, other black writers have consistently seen Dunbar as "the pioneer who paved the way for black writers to enter the literary profession."

Source: Susan Andersen, Critical essay on "Sympathy," in *Poetry for Students*, Gale, Cengage Learning, 2010.

Charles Eaton Burch

In the following critique, Burch maintains that Dunbar's poetic forte is humorous dialect poetry, with a few standard English standouts.

If Paul Laurence Dunbar is to continue to have a place in American literature, it seems to be fairly well agreed that it is to be accorded to him largely because of his poetry written in the Negro dialect. While such a statement is true in the main, it does not define the range of his work. His poetry in literary English has sufficient merit to warrant attention and study; and no survey of his poetry can be considered complete which totally ignores his English verse....

A few admirers of the poet's work have endeavored to establish the fact that his English verse is "pregnant with a depth of thought." To many, however, the application of this view, to the greater portion of his poetry is too sweeping. It is only for a very small part of his verse in literary English that such a claim can be made. For Dunbar's lack of broad literary training prevented him from accomplishing any sustained flights in the established media of the language. (p. 469)

"The Mystery" and "The Dirge" may ... be included in this small group of selections....

Paul Dunbar was at home in dealing with rollicking humor. His dialect poems show him at his best in this field. However, his English humorous verse is interesting. One might with some justice claim that in dealing with Negro plantation life he was furnished with a wealth of humorous material. But since he had no such help in his English humorous verse, we are forced to conclude that he was of an essentially humorous nature. "At Cheshire Cheese" is indicative of what he was capable of doing at times. (p. 470)

Our author was on his own ground when he turned to genuine pathos. His way was not strewn with roses. The few years of domestic happiness were soon overshadowed by the loss of companionship of the one who had exerted a real influence on his life and work. And when we add to this misfortune an enfeebled body it is not difficult to account for a portion of this poetry of pathos. However, there is a danger of overstressing the influence of these circumstances on his poetry. For many poems of this character were written before these forces began to operate in his life. Among the many poems of this character his "Ships That Pass in the Night" is perhaps his best effort. It is truly a modest contribution to the world's literature of pathos. (pp. 470–71)

Dunbar had a true appreciation for the beauty of external nature. In our day when the poetry of nature has come into its own and can claim some of the world's greatest poets, there is a tendency to overlook the nature poetry of some of the lesser lights.... Dunbar, in his English verse, seldom sounded any new notes; his nature poetry generally follows the paths so well begun in the latter half of the eighteenth century. That he was capable of writing the poetry of the commonplace in nature may be determined from his treatment of Southern plantation life in his dialect poetry. Yet a few nature poems in literary English are worth mentioning. There is a touch of nature in "The Poet and the Song." (p. 471)

"The Drowsy Day" is full of suggestions of the gloomy mood of nature....

"The Sailor's Song" breathes something of the rugged yet fascinating life of the ocean.... (p. 472)

Dunbar was not only the first American Negro to gain a fairly large degree of recognition for his work in creative literature, he was also the first to give a true lyrical expression of the life of the Negro of the plantation. In examining his verse in literary English, one discovers the Dunbar who is proud of the struggles and aspirations of the "New Negro," just as truly as his dialect poetry reveals his sympathy with the lowly life of his people. He never allows any of the larger happenings of his people to pass unnoticed. Often he is found paying a tribute to the departed Negro who has labored in behalf of his people; at times he exults in the victories of the colored soldiers of America, or proudly raises a song in honor of his race. "The Ode to Ethiopia" is perhaps better known among the masses of the colored people of America than any other one of his English poems. (pp. 472–73)

Dunbar did not produce any great poems in literary English; however, he did add a few charming poems to the native literature. His was not the role of the great master with the mighty line. But his simple lay is so full of melody, so full of heart, that the lover of literature often leaves the major poet to spend many pleasant moments with him. (p. 473)

Source: Charles Eaton Burch, "Dunbar's Poetry in Literary English," in *Southern Workman*, Vol. 50, No. 10, October 1921, pp. 469–73.

Joseph G. Bryant

In the following critique, Bryant compares Dunbar's poetry to the poetry of Robert Burns, based on their similarities regarding dialect poetry.

[The] sparkling wit, the quaint and delightful humor, the individuality and charm of Dunbar's poetry are not excelled by any lines from the pen of a Negro. No person can read his verse without being forcibly impressed that he is a remarkable man, a genius demanding attention. The New World has not produced a bard like him. Although distinctively American by birth and education, as well as a Negro, yet his prototype is on the other side of the Atlantic. Robert Burns and Dunbar, in many important particulars, are parallel poets. They seem to have been cast in the same mould; with limited educational advantages, both struggled up through poverty, and each wrote largely in the dialect of his clan. He is strong and original, and like Burns, lyrical in inspiration. Probably there never were two men of opposite races, so widely separated by time and distance, and yet so much alike in soul-qualities. With no desire and no doubt unconsciously, he has walked complete in the footprints of the eminent Scottish bard; has the same infirmity, animated by the same hope, and blessed with the same success. (p. 256)

In Dunbar there is no threnody, not even distant clouds arch the sky. Hope and joy are the dominant notes of his song. No poet more effectively warms the cold side of our life and sends sunshine into grief-stricken souls than he. He laughs sorrow away; he takes us into the huts of the lowly and oppressed. There we find, amidst poverty and illiteracy, unfeigned contentment and true happiness; a smile is on every face, and hope displays her brightest gifts. No matter how sorrowful, who can read without considerable emotion "When de Co'n Pone's Hot," "The Colored Band," "The Visitor," "The Old Front Gate," "De Way Tings Come," and "Philosophy." But not all his poetry bubbles with fun, at times he is a serious poet, and appeals strongly to the serious side of life, as does his "Weltschmertz." It is full of tender sympathy; it touches chords which vibrate throughout the poles of our nature; he makes us feel that he takes our sorrows and makes them his own, and helps us to bear up when burdened with woe. "The Fount of Tears," "Life's Tragedy," "The Haunted Oak," and the fifth lyric of "Love and Sorrow" reveal a high order of poetical genius; he reaches the deepest spiritual recesses of our being. (pp. 256–57)

I prefer "The Rugged Way" to Lowell's "After the Burial." "The Unsung Heroes" has all the imagination and pathos of Bryant's "Marion's Men;" "The Black Sampson of Brandywine" will live as long as his "African Chief." Read Bryant's and Dunbar's "Lincoln"—the black poet does not

suffer by comparison. I do not in the least wish to convey the impression that Dunbar is a greater poet than Bryant; they move in different parts of the poetical firmament. Each is a master in his respective sphere. As a writer of blank verse Bryant has no equal in America; and as a lyrical poet with a large vein of rich humor Dunbar is without a peer in the Western Continent. (p. 257)

Source: Joseph G. Bryant, "Negro Poetry," in *Colored American Magazine*, Vol. 8, No. 5, May 1905, pp. 254–57.

W. D. Howells

In the following review, Howell's critique of the dialect Dunbar uses in his poetry explains how dialect became a milestone for the poet.

[Howells was the chief progenitor of American Realism and one of the most influential American literary critics of the late nineteenth century. He wrote nearly three dozen novels, few of which are read today. Despite his eclipse, he stands as one of the major literary figures of the nineteenth century: he successfully weaned American literature away from the sentimental romanticism of its infancy, earning the popular sobriquet "the Dean of American Letters." Through Realism, a theory central to his fiction and criticism, Howells sought to disperse "the conventional acceptations by which men live on easy terms with themselves" that they might "examine the grounds of their social and moral opinions." To accomplish this, according to Howells, the writer must strive to record impressions of everyday life in detail, endowing characters with true-to-life motives and avoiding authorial comment in the narrative. In addition to many notable studies of the works of his friends Mark Twain and Henry James, Howells reviewed three generations of international literature, urging Americans to read the works of Émile Zola, Bernard Shaw, Henrik Ibsen, Emily Dickinson, and other important authors. Dunbar was another writer that Howells introduced to the reading public. In the following excerpt from *Harper's Weekly*, he reviews *Majors and Minors*, praising Dunbar's dialect verse. This review proved to be a milestone in the poet's career. A year later, however, Dunbar sadly remarked: "I see now very clearly that Mr. Howells has done me irrevocable harm in the dictum he laid down regarding my dialect verse."]

[Mr. Dunbar] is a real poet whether he speaks a dialect or whether he writes a language. He calls his little book *Majors and Minors*, the

Majors being in our American English, and the Minors being in dialect, the dialect of the middle-south negroes and the middle-south whites; for the poet's ear has been quick for the accent of his neighbors as well as for that of his kindred. I have no means of knowing whether he values his Majors more than his Minors; but I should not suppose it at all unlikely, and I am bound to say none of them are despicable. In very many I find the proofs of honest thinking and true feeling, and in some the record of experience, whose genuineness the reader can test by his own....

Most of these pieces, however, are like most of the pieces of most young poets, cries of passionate aspiration and disappointment, more or less personal or universal, which except for the negro face of the author one could not find specially notable. It is when we come to Mr. Dunbar's Minors that we feel ourselves in the presence of a man with a direct and a fresh authority to do the kind of thing he is doing....

One sees how the poet exults in his material, as the artist always does; it is not for him to blink its commonness, or to be ashamed of its rudeness; and in his treatment of it he has been able to bring us nearer to the heart of primitive human nature in his race than anyone else has yet done. The range between appetite and emotion is not great, but it is here that his race has hitherto had its being, with a lift now and then far above and beyond it. A rich, humorous sense pervades his recognition of this fact, without excluding a fond sympathy, and it is the blending of these which delights me in all his dialect verse....

Several of the pieces are pure sentiment, like "The Deserted Plantation"; but these without lapsing into sentimentality recall the too easy pathos of the pseudonegro poetry of the minstrel show....

Mr. Dunbar's race is nothing if not lyrical, and he comes by his rhythm honestly. But what is better, what is finer, what is of larger import, in his work is what is conscious and individual in it. He is, so far as I know, the first man of his color to study his race objectively, to analyze it to himself, and then to represent it in art as he felt it and found it to be; to represent it humorously, yet tenderly, and above all so faithfully that we know the portrait to be undeniably like. A race which has reached this effect in any of its members can no longer be held wholly uncivilized; and intellectually Mr. Dunbar makes a stronger claim for the negro than the negro yet has done....

I am speaking of him as a black poet, when I should be speaking of him as a poet; but the notion of what he is insists too strongly for present impartiality. I hope I have not praised him too much, because he has surprised me so very much; for his excellences are positive and not comparative. If his Minors had been written by a white man, I should have been struck by their very uncommon quality; I should have said that they were wonderful divinations. But since they are expressions of a race-life from within the race, they seem to me indefinitely more valuable and significant. I have sometimes fancied that perhaps the negroes *thought* black, and *felt* black; that they were racially so utterly alien and distinct from ourselves that there never could be common intellectual and emotional ground between us, and that whatever eternity might do to reconcile us, the end of time would find us as far asunder as ever. But this little book has given me pause in my speculation. Here, in the artistic effect at least, is white thinking and white feeling in a black man, and perhaps the human unity, and not the race unity, is the precious thing, the divine thing, after all. God hath made of one blood all nations of men; perhaps the proof of this saying is to appear in the arts, and our hostilities and prejudices are to vanish in them.

Mr. Dunbar, at any rate, seems to have fathomed the souls of his simple white neighbors, as well as those of his own kindred; and certainly he has reported as faithfully what passes in them as any man of our race has yet done with respect to the souls of his. It would be very incomplete recognition of his work not to speak particularly of the non-negro dialect pieces, and it is to the lover of homely and tender poetry, as well as the student of tendencies, that I commend such charming sketches as "Speakin o' Christmas," "After a Visit," "Lonesome," and "The Spellin' Bee." They are good, very good....

Source: W. D. Howells, "A Review of *Majors and Minors*," in *Harper's Weekly*, June 26, 1896, p. 630.

SOURCES

Best, Felton O., *Crossing the Color Line: A Biography of Paul Laurence Dunbar 1872–1906*, Kendall/Hunt Publishers, 1996, pp. 44, 110.

Brawley, Benjamin, *Paul Lawrence Dunbar: Poet of His People*, University of North Carolina Press, 1936, reprint ed., Kennikat Press, 1967, pp. 4, 37, 76.

Braxton, Joanne M., Introduction to *The Collected Poetry of Paul Laurence Dunbar*, University Press of Virginia, 1993, p. xxi.

Dunbar, Paul Lawrence, "Negro in Literature," in *In His Own Voice: The Dramatic and Other Uncollected Works of Paul Laurence Dunbar*, edited by Herbert Woodward Martin and Ronald Primeau, Ohio University Press, 2002, pp. 206–207; originally published in *New York Commercial* 1898, Paul Laurence Dunbar Collection, reel IV, box 16, Ohio Historical Society.

———, "Negro Music," in *In His Own Voice: The Dramatic and Other Uncollected Works of Paul Laurence Dunbar*, edited by Herbert Woodward Martin and Ronald Primeau, Ohio University Press, 2002, pp. 184–85; originally published in *Chicago Record*, 1899, Paul Laurence Dunbar Collection, reel IV, box 18, Ohio Historical Society.

———, *The Collected Poetry of Paul Laurence Dunbar*, edited by Joanne M. Braxton, University Press of Virginia, 1993.

———, *The Paul Laurence Dunbar Reader: A Selection of the Best of Paul Laurence Dunbar's Poetry and Prose, Including Writings Never Before Available in Book Form*, edited by Jay Martin and Gossie H. Hudson, Dodd, Mead, 1975.

Gates, Henry Louis, Jr., *Figures in Black: Words, Signs, and the "Racial" Self*, Oxford University Press, 1987, pp. 25–26, 29.

———, *The Signifying Monkey: A Theory of Afro-American Literary Criticism*, Oxford University Press, 1988, p. 66.

Gebhard, Caroline, "Inventing a 'Negro Literature': Race, Dialect, and Gender in the Early Work of Paul Laurence Dunbar, James Weldon Johnson, and Alice Dunbar-Nelson," in *Post-Bellum, Pre-Harlem: African American Literature and Culture 1877–1919*, edited by Barbara McCaskill and Caroline Gebhard, New York University Press, 2006, pp. 162–78.

Hudson, Gossie H., "The Crowded Years: Paul Laurence Dunbar in History," in *A Singer in the Dawn: Reinterpretations of Paul Laurence Dunbar*, edited by Jay Martin, Dodd, Mead, 1975, pp. 227–42.

Lawson, Victor, *Dunbar Critically Examined*, Associated Publishers, 1941, p. 78.

Metcalf, E. W., Jr., *Paul Laurence Dunbar: A Bibliography*, Scarecrow Press, 1975, pp. 131–33.

Revell, Peter, *Paul Laurence Dunbar*, Twayne's "United States Author" series, No. 298, Twayne Publishers, 1979, pp. 90–91, 93, 190.

Roman, Camille, "The Caged Bird's Song and Its (Dis)Contents," in *Pacific Coast Philology*, Vol. 41, 2006, pp. 32–38.

Simon, Myron, "Dunbar and Dialect Poetry," in *A Singer in the Dawn: Reinterpretations of Paul Laurence Dunbar*, edited by Jay Martin, Dodd, Mead, 1975, p. 121.

Turner, Darwin T., "The Poet and the Myths," in *A Singer in the Dawn: Reinterpretations of Paul Laurence Dunbar*, edited by Jay Martin, Dodd, Mead, 1975, pp. 59–74.

FURTHER READING

Alexander, Eleanor, *Lyrics of Sunshine and Shadow: The Tragic Courtship and Marriage of Paul Laurence Dunbar and Alice Ruth Moore: A History of Love and Violence among the African American Elite*, New York University Press, 2001.

> Alexander chronicles the difficult marriage of the Dunbars and why they separated due to drinking and domestic violence. She also discusses other middle class African American marriages showing sociologically how the pressures of race and gender at the turn of the century eroded relationships.

Brown, Fahamisha Patricia, *Performing the Word: African American Poetry as Vernacular Culture*, Rutgers University Press, 1999.

> Brown focuses on the features of African American oral traditions that appear in vernacular speech and modern poetry. For instance, the call-and-response repetition, preaching, and the boast are highlighted in the works of various black poets.

Du Bois, W. E. B., *The Gift of Black Folk: The Negro in the Making of America*, 1924, Square One Publishers, 2009.

> Sociologist, scholar, and civil rights activist Du Bois documents the contributions of African Americans in an attempt to counter negative stereotypes. He shows black Americans as explorers, inventors, artists, soldiers, and farmers. The book was reissued to mark the centennial of the National Association for the Advancement of Colored People, which Du Bois helped to found.

Dunbar, Paul Laurence, *The Sport of the Gods*, Dodd, Mead, 1902, Signet Classic, 1999.

> This realistic novel was ahead of its time in describing a southern black family moving to New York City and facing the same forces of racism as in the South because blacks had no legal protection.

Two Eclipses

SHMUEL HANAGID

C. 1044

"Two Eclipses," is the English translation of the title of a poem written in Hebrew in 1044 by the Spanish poet Shmuel HaNagid. The poem documents two eclipses, one lunar and one solar, that occurred in the month of Kislev that year. In the Hebrew calendar, Kislev is the third month of the civil year and the ninth month of the religious year; it usually corresponds to a thirty-day month that falls in November December. The lunar eclipse occurred on November 8, 1044, between 11:00 in the evening and 2:00 in the morning; the solar eclipse took place on November 22 from 8:00 to 11:00 in the morning.

"Two Eclipses" was included in *Ben Kohelet,* one of HaNagid's three collections of poetry. This title means "After Ecclesiastes" referring to the twenty-first book of the Old Testament, or the Hebrew Bible, though sometimes HaNagid's collection is referred to as "The Little Book of Ecclesiastes," reflecting the title HaNagid's son gave to it after his father's death. The poems in this collection, including "Two Eclipses," are regarded as HaNagid's most mature poems; they consist of epigrammatic verses that describe natural phenomena ("Gazing through the Night,""The Earthquake") or offer meditations on death ("You Felt the Fear of Death,""Ask the Dead and They'll Tell You"). By titling the collection "After Ecclesiastes," one of the more philosophical books of the Old Testament, HaNagid announced that the poems would be meditative reflections from a philosopher rather than a statement of religious

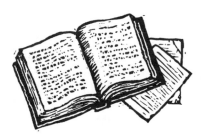

doctrine from a rabbi or theologian. Perhaps, taken together, they would reflect Ecclesiastes 1:4: "A generation goes, and a generation comes, but the earth remains forever."

AUTHOR BIOGRAPHY

HaNagid was a poet, statesman, merchant, and military leader. Western writers often alter the Hebrew "Shmuel" to "Samuel," sometimes Ishmael, and his last name is variously written as HaNagid, ha-Nagid, Hannagid, and ha'Nagid. He was born in 993 as Shmuel ben Yosef ha-Levi to a prominent Jewish family in Cordoba, Spain, and received a classical education, studying Hebrew, Greek, and Arabic, including the Quran, the sacred scripture of Islam. Not a great deal is known about his early life. As a young man he probably earned his living in the spice business and in international trade.

When the Berbers, an invading tribe from North Africa that had recently converted to Islam, overthrew the Islamic caliphate of Cordoba in 1013 after a three-year civil war, HaNagid, along with many others, fled. (A caliphate is a unified Muslim territory, similar to a nation or empire). He settled in the port city of Malaga, Spain, where he again engaged in trade. According to tradition, he was approached by a maidservant at the court of Habbus, the Muslim king of Grenada, who asked him to write letters for her to her master, the king's vizier. (*Vizier* is an Anglicized form of the Arabic word *wazir* and simply means "high official.") Habbus eventually saw the letters and was impressed by HaNagid's wisdom and his skill with Arabic calligraphy. Accordingly, he gave HaNagid a position first as a tax collector (based probably on the belief that a Jew would find it easier to collect taxes from other Jews than would a non-Jew), then as secretary, then as assistant vizier, and finally as vizier. He became embroiled in a dispute that led to his dismissal, but he later returned to court as the assistant to the king's vizier.

Spanish Jews were proud of HaNagid's success, so they elected him "Nagid," or governor of Spain's Jewish community, in 1027; in this way Shmuel ha-Levi became Shmuel HaNagid, or Samuel the Governor (or Samuel the Prince). He continued to play a prominent role at court, and when King Habbus died in 1037, his son and successor, King Badis, promoted HaNagid to the position of chief vizier of Granada. The king also put HaNagid in charge of the Muslim army. In the years that followed, he served as a military leader in battle and in a role analogous to today's minister or secretary of defense. As part of King Badis's administration, he played a key role in turning Andalusia, the southernmost region of Spain, into one of the wealthiest and most powerful regions. (Andalusia is a large region consisting of several provinces, including Cordoba and Grenada; complicating matters is that Cordoba and Grenada are also the names of the capital cities of the provinces by the same names.)

HaNagid also wrote a Hebrew grammar, commentaries on the Old Testament and Jewish law, and poetry, though the dates when he completed his three collections of poems are not known. He was widely known throughout the Jewish community for his generosity and his willingness to provide support, both moral and material, for students and scholars. Through his many accomplishments, he came to be regarded as one of the most powerful and influential Jews in medieval Spain. He died in 1056, probably from the effects of exhaustion after leading yet another military campaign.

POEM TEXT

My friend, are you sleeping?
Rise and wake the dawn,
look up at the sky
like a leopard skin strippled above us,
and see the moon where it should be full,   5
go dark like a kettle, or kiln,
like the face of a girl—
half of it flushed,
the other darkened in shadow.
Return and glance at the sun,   10
brought to the end of the month in dimness,
its halo of light on the darkness,
like a crown on the head of a Libyan princess,
and the earth whose sun has set,
reddened—as though with tears.   15

Both of the beacons were stricken
in the space of a single month
by Him whose dominion is splendor and
    strength;
He covered the moon with His circle of earth,
and the sun with His moon: 20
this is the work of the Lord who toys with
    creation.

He fashioned patches of dark in the moon,
and the sun He created clear,
therefore I liken them now

in their dimness against the dark,   25
to women bereaved:
the face of the one is bruised,
the other both bruised and wounded—
the light of day on a day gone dim,
and the light of night darkened at evening   30
during the watch.
Like an angry king who brings trouble
on his lords in their own domains,
first He struck the brightness of night,
and afterwards blotted the daylight,   35
like a king who prepared a poisonous cup
for his mistress, and then for his queen.
Behold what happened—look closely in
     wonder,
study it well, and read:

Yours is the greatness,   40
who brought the light in its weight and
     measures,
and darkened the moon at its cycle's center,
like a bird caught in a snare.
You'll do it again in five months more;
looking onto the earth,   45
you'll make it reel like a drunkard.
You've ordered the moth and it eats
the Bear and Orion in great constellation;
you fixed for the living among them
a place like a shield;   50
and all when you rule will be trodden as one,
though not with a shout in a winepress.

Yours is the glory, yours entire,
every horse and chariot houghed.
It's you who brings on heat in winter,   55
and winter, at summer's height;
you who upends the abyss,
who brings affliction into the sea
like a woman in labor;
you who'll cast toward all the living—death,   60
as the arrow flies to its target;
you on the bitter and great
and terrible day of judgment
who will wake me and judge
all who've forsaken the statues,   65
commandments, and Law.

When you place my deeds in judgment's scale,
may the side of evil, lighter, rise.
On the day you lift me up from my dust
I'll turn and my spirit in fear of your wrath   70
will flee, and you'll say:
"Peace be upon you; be still, and do not fear."

If there remains not a trace of my righteousness,
may your mercy be near.

POEM SUMMARY

Lines 1–15

The speaker in "Two Eclipses" begins by addressing an unseen friend who appears to still be
sleeping in the morning. He urges the friend to
wake up, to wake up the dawn, and to look at the
sky, which has the mottled appearance of the skin
of a leopard. He notes that the moon is supposed
to be full but that it is going dark, and he compares it to a kiln, a kettle, and a girl's face, part of
which is blushing. He notes that half of the moon
is darkened, as if in shadow. The speaker then
draws the friend's attention to the sun, which later
in the month became dim. He describes a full
solar eclipse, where the sun is darkened but a
rim of light filters out around the edges. He compares the sight of the sun in eclipse to a crown on
the head of a princess from Libya (a nation in
North Africa). The result is that the sun has set,
casting a reddish glow. He compares the effect to
the earth being in tears.

Lines 16–21

In stanza 2, the speaker notes that both of these
sources of light, which he compares to beacons,
were darkened in the same month. He does not
use the word "God," but he makes it clear that
God, a source of power, majesty, and brilliance,
was the source of the two eclipses. In one case
God used the earth to cover the moon; in the
other he used the moon to cover the sun. The
speaker concludes the stanza by noting that the
two eclipses were the work of God and that God
plays with the worlds he created.

Lines 22–39

The speaker begins stanza 3 by noting that the
moon was made with darker portions but that
the sun was made entirely clear and uniform.
This prompts the speaker to draw a comparison
between the dimmed sun and moon on the one
hand and grieving women on the other. One of the
women has a face that appears to be bruised,
presumably like the sun; the other woman's face
is both bruised and injured, presumably like the
moon. The speaker then notes that the sun provides daytime light but that the day has gone dim.
Similarly, the moon is a source of light at night, but
it too has been darkened in the evening, just at the
time that guards begin to watch over the city. In a
new sentence, the speaker compares God to a king.
Just as an earthly king might become angered and
direct his wrath against lords who rule territories
within the kingdom, so God, the heavenly king,
turns his anger against day and night. With a lunar
eclipse, he strikes a blow against the night's source
of light, then with a solar eclipse he blots out the
daylight. The speaker then compares God's ctions

to those of a king who gives poison first to his mistress, then to his wife, the queen. The speaker then urges the listener to see what happened, to examine the phenomena closely, and to read the lines that follow. The stanza ends with a colon rather than a period, suggesting a change in the poem.

Lines 40–52

With stanza 4, the speaker is no longer addressing the friend. He is now addressing God, and it is these lines that the speaker urges his friend to read at the end of the preceding stanza. Accordingly, the stanzas that follow are written in the second person, with "you" and "your" referring to God. He begins by noting that God's greatness enabled him to create light, but it is that same greatness that enables him to darken the moon at the middle of its cycle. He then compares the darkened moon to a trapped rabbit. The speaker then notes that five months later there will be another lunar eclipse—which in fact turned out to be true; on May 3, 1045, a lunar eclipse occurred from 7:00 to 10:00 in the morning. God then will look at the world he created and cause it to become dizzy as though drunk. At this point, the speaker becomes slightly obscure. He makes reference to a moth, but this is an alternative meaning for the word *Ash*, which is the name of a star mentioned in the biblical book of Job. The star/moth is then said to consume star constellations called the Bear (Ursa Major, the constellation that includes the Big Dipper) and Orion (a prominent constellation named for the hunter by the same name in Greek mythology). Within the star constellations God created the earth, where living things could exist. The speaker concludes the stanza by acknowledging the power of God, who can tread upon all of his creation. In the same way, people tread upon grapes in a winepress in the process of making wine. When they do so, they shout, perhaps in triumph and joy. When God treads on his creation, there will be no shouting.

Lines 53–66

In stanza 5 the speaker continues to pay tribute to the glory of God. He says that this glory belongs entirely to God and that it is recognized by every horse and chariot that has been houghed. This word refers to the severing of tendons on the back legs of captured horses in ancient times. It is possible that the speaker's references to horses and chariots are references to constellations of

stars. "Horse" would possibly refer to Pegasus, named after a winged horse in Greek mythology, while "chariot" would possibly refer to Auriga, the Horse Driver, a constellation named after the mythological figure who invented the chariot because his feet were deformed and he was lame. The speaker goes on to note that God can turn the weather hot in winter and cold in summer. God can also turn the oceans upside down and bring turmoil to the seas, which he compares to a woman in the pains of giving birth. Ultimately, God can cause all living things to die, throwing death at them in the same way that an arrow finds its target. The speaker says that on Judgment Day God will awaken him—just as the speaker awakened his friend at the beginning of the poem—and will pass judgment on everyone who has broken God's commandments and Jewish law. The repetition of awakening suggests that the eclipses are a form of God's judgment, prefiguring the greater judgment that will take place when a person dies.

Lines 67–72

The penultimate stanza continues with the theme of judgment. The speaker says that God will weigh his actions, and he expresses hope that the evil side of the scale will be lighter and will therefore rise under the heavier weight of the side of the scale filled with good; the scale the poet envisions is a beam scale with pans hanging on each side. The speaker goes on to say that on that day God will raise his soul from the dust of his body but that the speaker will attempt to flee because he fears God's anger. He expresses hope, though, that God will offer him peace and comfort and will urge him not to feel fear.

Lines 73–74

The final stanza of the poem consists of just two lines. The speaker acknowledges the possibility that on the Day of Judgment, God will find no righteousness in his soul. He hopes, then, that God will show mercy toward him; God's mercy at the end of the poem is thus a counterpoint to his anger.

THEMES

God

The central theme of "Two Eclipses" is the power and majesty of God. The poem begins as the speaker sees a lunar eclipse, then describes a

TOPICS FOR FURTHER STUDY

- Write a poem based on your observations of an astronomical event: an eclipse, a meteor shower, a phase of the moon, a rainbow, or the conjunction of planets in the sky. Pictures and illustrations of astronomical events are available on many Web sites or in books about astronomy. In your poem, include not just observations but your sense of the meaning or significance of the event.

- A great many astronomical observations were made in the medieval Arabic world, particularly during the Golden Age when HaNagid lived. Conduct research into the history of medieval astronomy. Who were some major astronomers? What discoveries did they make? What words derived from Arabic are still used in the field of astronomy? Present your findings in an oral report, using as many visual aids as possible.

- In the biblical Old Testament—the scripture that HaNagid would have studied and learned—eclipses were often seen as tokens of God's anger. Using the Internet, conduct a search for references to eclipses in the Old Testament. Prepare a list of the eclipses (and perhaps other astronomical events as well) and the reactions of people to them. What significance did the writer of the biblical book attach to the eclipse or other heavenly event? Present your findings in an essay.

- Using the Internet, conduct research into Cordoba, Spain, where HaNagid was born and spent his early years. Many of the buildings and monuments from that time survive. Imagine that you are a tour guide. Download pictures of medieval Cordoba and, using PowerPoint, take your classmates on a virtual "walking tour" of the city that HaNagid would have known. Be sure to explain to your classmates what you are showing them and why it is significant for an understanding of medieval life at that time and in that place.

- In contemporary life, hostility between Muslims and Jews often erupts into violence. In medieval Spain, though, Muslims and Jews lived side by side, and although HaNagid was a Jew, he served in the court of a Muslim king. Conduct research into the history of Jewish-Muslim relations during the medieval period. To what extent did the two communities cooperate? To what extent did they compete? What impact did Christians living in Muslim-Jewish lands have, if any? Present your findings in a written report.

- Imagine that you are a translator, trying to translate a poem such as "Two Eclipses" from medieval Hebrew into modern English. With every word and phrase, you would have choices to make. Thus, for example, the opening lines of HaNagid's poem might have been translated as: "My friend, as you still asleep? / Get up and awaken the morning, / look up to the heavens / like the mottled skin of a leopard over our heads." Use synonyms to write an alternative translation of the poem and be prepared to explain how your "translation" creates a different effect on the reader.

- Denise Levertov was a modern American poet who wrote both for adults and young adults. Locate her poem "Flickering Mind," found in her 1959 collection *A Door in the Hive*, and compare the nature of her religious experience with HaNagid's in an essay.

---

solar eclipse during the same month. In biblical tradition, eclipses were seen as a sign of God's wrath. God was presumed to be angry at humans for transgressing his laws, so he in a sense inverted the natural order by blotting out the sun or the moon, striking fear into the hearts of people who witnessed these unusual events. That both of these events would occur in the same month would at any time be highly unusual, and during the medieval period it would have been a sure sign of God's displeasure. The speaker of the poem goes on to call the reader's attention to the greatness of God, his strength and brilliance. God is so powerful that he can move planets and thus play with his creation. Clearly God is like an angry king when he toys with his planets and stars.

The second part of the poem, beginning with the fourth stanza, is then addressed directly to God, who holds power over light and dark, over the planets and all the constellations of stars. He created the earth as a place that would shield living things, but he is so powerful that he can tread on all of his creation whenever he wishes. The speaker goes on to note further instances of the majesty and power of God, which every captive horse and chariot (perhaps a symbolic allusion to other constellations of stars in the heavens) recognizes. God has power over heat and cold and can invert them, just as he can toy with the arrangement of planets and stars. He can cause turmoil in the oceans. Ultimately, he has the ability to impose death on every living creature. Death, then, at least for humans, entails judgment, and the speaker fears that day because he, along with other humans, has not always followed God's law. God has the ability to raise the speaker's soul from the dust he leaves behind—his body—and when the speaker stands before God, he will tremble with fear. The poem, though, ends on an optimistic note, for the speaker says that God *will* soothe him and allay his fears. God can be an angry God, but he can also be merciful, and that mercy is just as much part of God's majesty as is his wrath.

Sin

A theme closely related to the power of God is that of the sinfulness and failures of humans. In the Jewish biblical tradition, the Jews and God enjoy a special relationship with each other. The covenant God's chosen people have with God imposes responsibilities on each. Humans, though, because of their sinfulness and imperfections, often break the covenant. They fail to follow God's laws, such as the Ten Commandments. The poet also makes reference to Law, which likely means Jewish law. This law, called the Halakha in Hebrew, consists of the total body of Jewish law contained in the Old Testament, particularly the first five books, which Jews refer to as the Torah. In these books are 613 *mitzvot*, or laws and principles of ethics every Jew is to follow. Added to the *mitzvot* is the Talmud, or Talmudic law, which is a record of discussions by Jewish rabbis that expand on and interpret Jewish law. This body of law applies not only to a Jew's religious life but to his everyday life as well.

Following biblical tradition, the poet in "Two Eclipses" regards eclipses as a sign of God's anger. The eclipses represent God's judgment on his people, causing fear and consternation. The darkness caused by the eclipses prefigures the darkness of death, when God will awaken the poet—just as the poet awakens his friend to the lunar eclipse at the beginning of the poem—and judge him. The poet recognizes his own human sinfulness but expresses hope that on the Day of Judgment, the scales in which his deeds are weighed will show that good has outweighed evil. Nevertheless, the poet expresses fear of facing God on the Day of Judgment, though he also describes his confidence that God will calm his fears and, perhaps, show mercy for the poet's lack of righteousness.

Nature

In the modern scientific era, the tendency is to think of humans as somehow separate from the natural order. The natural order is something that humans aspire to control in order to conquer hunger, cold and heat, disease, and ultimately death itself. The modern scientific method turns nature into something "other," something outside of humanity to be studied and understood. The medieval religious outlook, however, saw nature in a very different light. Medieval philosophers tended to accept the Hellenistic (ancient Greek) concept that the natural order was governed by immutable laws; one of these laws was that the natural order consisted of four elements: earth, air, fire, and water. This point of view is hinted at in "Two Eclipses" with its reference to the dust of the earth, the heat and cold of the air, the fire of the sun that reddens the earth, and the waters of the ocean.

Jewish thinkers, though, were steeped in the traditions of the Old Testament and of rabbinical literature, which placed less emphasis on immutable laws and more on the concept of a divine creator who directly regulates events for a divine purpose. Astronomy was a particularly fertile field

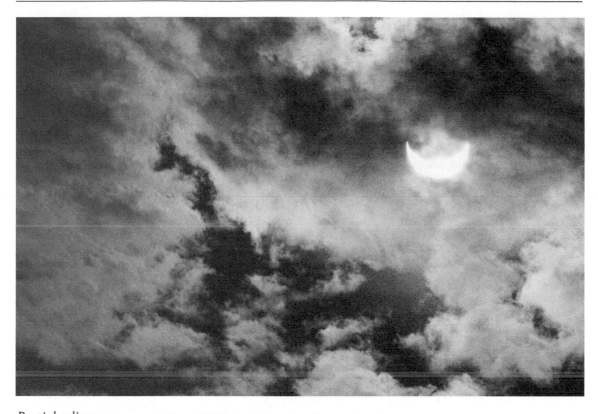

Partial eclipse (Image copyright Vasca. 2009. Used under license from Shutterstock.com)

for this line of thought, for through astronomical observation the medieval philosopher—someone like HaNagid—was able to reconcile the two views of nature. On the one hand, the regular, predictable movements of the planets and stars—a regularity that enabled HaNagid to predict the eclipse that would occur five months hence—suggested that the universe operated according to immutable laws, much as the Greeks had thought. On the other hand, following Jewish tradition, these regularities were a certain sign of a creator whose creation was a physical expression of his power and greatness. Thus, the eclipses that form the center of HaNagid's poem are not simply natural phenomena to be studied and understood. Rather, they are manifestations of a divine will to which humans have to submit.

STYLE

Simile and Metaphor

A primary poetic device HaNagid uses in "Two Eclipses" is simile, the comparison of otherwise unlike objects using words such as "like" and "as." Early in the poem, for example, the sky is said to have the appearance of a stippled leopard skin. Because of the eclipse, the sky goes dark and is explicitly compared to a kettle, a kiln, and a girl's face. The solar eclipse created a ring of light that is compared to a crown of light on a dark-skinned Libyan princess's head. The eclipse is said to redden the earth, and a comparison is drawn with a face reddened by tears. Because of the eclipses, the sun and the moon are compared to women who are mourning. God is likened to an angry king who sows trouble among his lords and who offers a poisoned cup to his mistress and to his queen. The eclipsed moon is compared to a rabbit caught in a trap, and when the poet predicts the future eclipse, he says that God will make the earth dizzy, like someone who has had too much to drink. When God brings turmoil to the sea, the sea is like a woman in pain from giving birth. When God brings death to people, it is likened to an arrow finding its target.

In addition to simile, HaNagid also uses metaphor, the comparison of otherwise unlike things by seeing them as equivalent. Thus, at the start of the poem, the dawning day is said to be awakening. The sun and moon, and sources of light, are equated with beacon lights. The dark patches of the moon are bruises. Metaphors of weighing and scales are also used. God created the light and weighed and measured it, and later, on the Day of Judgment, God will weigh the poet's deeds on a scale; the poet expresses hope that the side of the scale containing good is heavy enough to outweigh the side containing evil, which will rise, just as the poet's soul will rise out of the dust of his body.

Meter

One of the chief difficulties of translating poetry is retaining some sense of the prosody of the original—that is, the original's regular metrical (rhythmic) patterns. These patterns are particularly important for medieval Hebrew poetry, for it was commonplace for poets such as HaNagid to adhere to the metrical forms used throughout much of the Old Testament. The chief characteristic of these forms is that they were based on a hierarchy of elements. The most elemental was the verset, consisting of two or three stress units. Two or three versets made up a poetic line, two or three lines made up a strophe, and two or three strophes made up a stanza. Stanzas would be combined into sections, and the poem as a whole would comprise sections. In "Two Eclipses," HaNagid generally follows this tradition. Thus, for example, the first line of the poem consists of two stress units, the second of three, the third line two, and the fourth line three. Lines within each stanza form natural groupings. Thus, in the first stanza, lines 1–9 form a strophe, as do lines 10–15. Overall, the poem consists of seven stanzas. The first three form one section of the poem, and the next three form a second section. The final stanza, consisting of just two lines, forms a kind of coda that balances God's mercy with his anger. It should be noted that HaNagid does not adhere to this metrical form in a rigid manner. The translation has more of a free verse quality, with lines of alternate lengths, stanzas of alternate lengths, and so on. Nevertheless, the poem's metrics retain the metrical feel of the Old Testament poetry that HaNagid would have known intimately.

Imagery

The author ties "Two Eclipses" together with patterns of imagery. These patterns impose unity on the poem, linking one part in parallel fashion with other parts. Chief among these patterns of imagery is that of light and dark, as would be expected in a poem about the sun and the moon. At the beginning of the poem, the moon goes dark, and the speaker says that it is darkened like the face of a girl who is blushing. The ring of light that escapes around the edges of a solar eclipse contrasts with the darkness of the head of a princess from Libya. The sun and the moon are compared to beacons, which shed light. The moon is said to have been created with dark patches, as opposed to the clearness of the sun, and during the eclipses, the sun and the moon are dim, surrounded by darkness. Lines 29 and 30 explicitly refer to the light of daytime and light shed by the moon at night, but both became darkened. God created the light and dark, so God has dominion over them; he created the light of the moon by striking it, as a metalworker would strike an object in a forge.

Similar patterns of imagery unite the poem, although HaNagid does not use these patterns as extensively. The imagery of faces is used twice, once in suggesting that the darkening moon resembles the face of a blushing girl, once when he compares both eclipses to the face of bereaved women. Imagery associated with royalty is also used. During the solar eclipse, the ring of light that surrounds the moon is seen as a crown on the head of a princess, and God is repeatedly described in terms that suggest royalty, particularly in being an angry king who is the cause of trouble among the lords that rule God's domains.

HISTORICAL CONTEXT

Muslim Spain

The early medieval period was a tumultuous one in Spain. Muslim Arab forces crossed the Mediterranean Sea in 711, landed on the southern tip of the Iberian Peninsula (Spain and Portugal), and conquered the peninsula within a period of just a few years. This conquest expanded the scope of the growing Muslim empire. In 750, civil war resulted in the end of the Umayyad Caliphate in Damascus, Syria, which had ruled

COMPARE
&
CONTRAST

- **1040s:** Hebrew poetry tends to be biblical poetry, drawing on themes, styles, and particularly the language and vocabulary of the Old Testament.

  Today: Modern poets writing in Hebrew continue to link their verse to biblical traditions but draw on a wider, more contemporary vocabulary and style that reflect the concerns of modern life.

- **1040s:** The kingdoms of Spain are under the control of a Muslim dynasty, though the region has large Jewish and Christian populations.

  Today: Spain is largely a Catholic country, though many of the monuments that Muslims built in the Middle Ages still exist and

are regarded as important parts of the nation's heritage. Muslims make up just over 2 percent of the population are are a growing population in Spain.

- **1040s:** Religious writers regard natural phenomena such as eclipses as the work of God and manifestations of God's power and greatness; natural disasters or unusual occurrences are often regarded as a sign of God's anger.

  Today: While many people still see the hand of God in the natural order, most regard eclipses, along with natural disasters and other natural phenomena, in a scientific rather than a religious light.

---

the Islamic empire. ("Umayyad" is the family name of the ruling dynasty at the time.) It was replaced by the Abbasid Caliphate, which ruled from Baghdad (now the capital of Iraq), launching what came to be called the Golden Age of Arabic culture—a time when the arts and sciences flourished. One survivor of the Umayyads, though, fled to Cordoba, Spain, where he established a caliphate that in time rivaled that of the Abbasids. A major project he undertook was the construction of the Great Mosque of Cordoba. In particular, he established a court where scientists and men of letters gathered, resulting in the emergence of secular poetry written both in Arabic and in Hebrew. Cordoba grew in power and became renowned for its art, letters, textiles, architecture, libraries, and sophistication. This was the environment in which HaNagid lived and wrote.

Biblical Poetry

A medieval Jew writing in Hebrew, including such figures as HaNagid, wrote poetry that had

firm links with the Old Testament, particularly the Torah, the first five books of the Old Testament (Genesis, Exodus, Leviticus, Numbers, and Deuteronomy). Hebrew poetry during this time period drew heavily on the themes, style, metrics, and language of the Old Testament, much of which was written in verse form. The purpose of poetry was not to explore the state of mind of the individual but to see creation as a manifestation of the greatness and power of God. Accordingly, medieval biblical poetry dealt with such topics as creation, the patriarchs, the history of the Jewish people, prophecies, and the like. When such a poet examined a natural phenomenon such as an eclipse, the purpose of the poem was not to make minute observations, nor was it to explore the psychological state of mind of the poet in response to the event. Rather, it was to see the event in the context of man's relationship with God. In this sense, medieval biblical poetry is very different from modern confessional poetry, which is far more introspective and far more focused on the psychology of the poet.

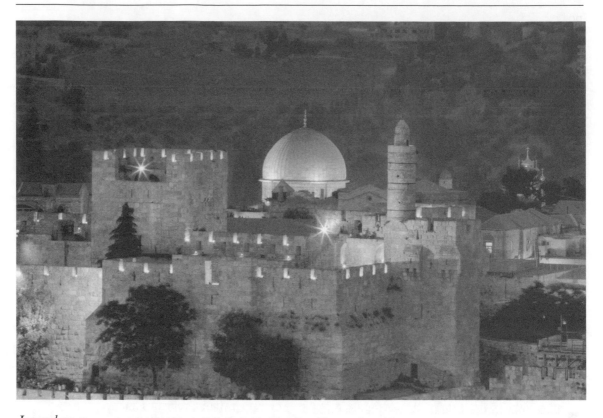

Jerusalem *(Image copyright Mikhail Levit, 2009. Used under license from Shutterstock.com)*

CRITICAL OVERVIEW

Little direct commentary on "Two Eclipses" exists, but there is more on HaNagid's corpus of poetry. One of the earliest comments is from Moshe Ibn Ezra, a poet who lived in Grenada, Spain, and was one year old when HaNagid died. About HaNagid, he writes: "His poems . . . are various and full of color, powerful in their contents, fine in their form, original in their ideas, and clear in their rhetoric. All that pertains to his compositions and works and letters is known to the uttermost edges of east and west and across the land and sea" (quoted by Peter Cole in *Selected Poems of Shmuel HaNagid*). Early in the twentieth century, *The Jewish Encyclopedia* is less kind: "Samuel's poetic compositions are distinguished for their elevation of thought; but they are devoid of elegance of form. It became proverbial to say: 'Cold as the snow of Hermon, or as the songs of the Levite Samuel'." (Levite refers to one of the biblical tribes of Israel; the Levites were regarded as teachers and rabbis.)

Modern critics have in a sense rediscovered HaNagid. Two lines of thought about the poet and his work can be found. One focuses on the aesthetics of his poetry. Cole, the leading translator of his poems, says approvingly in *Selected Poems of Shmuel HaNagid*: "HaNagid was able to fuse Hebrew and Arabic, given and personal, lyric and epic dimensions in what we now think of as his signature manner. Throughout the three books his poetry presents a compelling forward thrust and relative simplicity of diction, yoked by artifice to complexity of texture and thought." Similarly, Raymond P. Scheindlin, in *Wine, Women, and Death: Medieval Hebrew Poems on the Good Life*, sorts HaNagid's poems (and the poems of other medieval writers in Hebrew) according to their thematic content and concludes that HaNagid "set the standard" in incorporating elements of Islamic art in their poetry. He notes that HaNagid wrote "gnomic" poetry, meaning poetry that has the characteristics of maxims or aphorisms, and he refers to HaNagid as a "great" poet of the Golden Age of medieval Spain.

The other strain of modern criticism focuses more on the interconnectedness of HaNagid's poetry with his life. A good example of this type of biographical criticism can be found in Ross Brann's *The Compunctious Poet: Cultural Ambiguity and Hebrew Poetry in Muslim Spain*. Brann notes that "upon a first reading, the Nagid's verse sparkles with all the audacity and temerity we might expect of a Dionysian, no trivial accomplishment for a rabbi of the eleventh century!" ("Dionysian" refers to the ancient Greek god Dionysius and is used to suggest a frenzied or abandoned quality, as opposed to calmness.) He goes on to note, though, that "the Nagid was a man possessed of inflated designs and driven by a grand vision of himself. At times, he seems obsessed by his own unique career as a man of letters, politician, and Jewish communal leader." In praising the poems, Brann says: "The Nagid's Arabic-style Hebrew verse, despite its diction, allusions,... and the names of its collections is not a revivified corpus of Temple hymns, but an innovation, both in form and in content, of a new school of Hebrew poets."

CRITICISM

Michael J. O'Neal

O'Neal holds a Ph.D. in English literature. In the following essay, he examines Shmuel HaNagid's "Two Eclipses" as part of a tradition of Hebrew biblical poetry.

The version of "Two Eclipses" reproduced here is a modern English translation of a poem written by a Spaniard in Hebrew a millennium ago. Any translator of such a poem has to make a number of decisions and compromises in making it accessible to a modern reader while retaining essential qualities of the original. One alternative is to attempt a literal, phrase-by-phrase, line-by-line translation. This alternative rarely works, for the English version is likely to sound awkward and forced. Further, the grammars and sound systems of English and Hebrew are different, making a unit of language that sounds perfectly normal in one sound awkward in the other. In translating poetry, the translator can try to maintain the rhythm of the original, but doing so requires taking considerable liberties with the original language. Or the translator can try to maintain the tone of the original, which again requires compromises with language and meter along the way. Or the translator can focus on the imagery of the original, but doing so might entail

ignoring rhythm. Any translation, then, is a series of compromises, but the translation of poetry is far more problematic than that of prose because of the more rigorously formal nature of poetry.

A translator of HaNagid's poems—as well as the translator of those of most of his contemporaries—can rely on one element of the poems to serve as a kind of glue, or as a set of girders that support the poems. Any reader of HaNagid's "Two Eclipses" who is versed in the Old Testament would readily recognize the links between the poem and the poetry of various biblical books. Some two thirds of the Old Testament is written in verse rather than prose. Some of these books, such as Psalms and Proverbs, are recognizably in verse and are studied today as examples of biblical literature; in this regard, the most recognizably literary book of the Old Testament is the Song of Solomon, which consists entirely of lyric poetry. Other books, though, that are not thought of as "poetry" were in fact written in a poetic style. Genesis is usually translated and printed as prose, but in fact in its original form, it is far more poetic than is usually thought. It was customary—indeed, almost obligatory—for a medieval poet writing in Hebrew to draw on the language and style of the Old Testament. A Jewish philosopher, poet, and scholar like HaNagid saw his life and circumstances as part of an unbroken chain of events in Jewish history, a chain that reached back to the historical events recorded in Genesis and Exodus and that extended through the present on into a future. This chain of events represented the working out of the Jewish nation's covenant with God as God's chosen people. Accordingly, a poem such as "Two Eclipses" would in effect be regarded as an extension of and gloss on the truths of the Old Testament, made manifest in HaNagid's life in medieval Spain.

So far, the emphasis has been on the Hebrew Bible. HaNagid, though, lived in a Muslim community and was fluent in Arabic. He studied the Quran, the scripture of Islam, and he was surrounded by a "Golden Age" of Arabic and Islamic art, including not only architecture and ornamentation but poetry as well. Like the Hebrew poets, Arabic poets linked their poetry to the Quran, using its metrics and vocabulary as the raw materials out of which they shaped their poetry. (It should be noted, however, that Islam is divided on the question of whether the Prophet Muhammad allowed poetry; some passages of

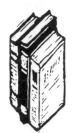

WHAT DO I READ NEXT?

- Another medieval Jewish poet was Abraham Ibn Ezra (1092–1167). His poems "I Have a Garment" and "My Stars" both deal with observations of the heavenly bodies. These and other poems can be found in *Twilight of a Golden Age: Selected Poems of Abraham Ibn Ezra* (1997), translated by Leon J. Weinberger.

- Readers interested in Hebrew poetry from a range of authors in medieval Spain can find a collection in *The Dream of the Poem: Hebrew Poetry from Muslim and Christian Spain, 950–1492* (2007), translated by Peter Cole.

- Readers interested in more modern Hebrew poetry might turn to the nineteenth-century work of Hayim (often spelled Chaim) Nahman Bialik in *Songs from Bialik: Selected Poems of Hayim Nahman Bialik* (2000), translated by Atar Hadari. Bialik is regarded by many as one of the most important Hebrew poets and one of a handful of late nineteenth- and early twentieth-century Jews who resurrected the Hebrew language.

- For information about the Umayyad and Abbasid Dynasties of medieval Islam, a good starting point is chapter 5 in Michael J. O'Neal's *The Crusades: Almanac* (2005).

- Readers interested in the state of astronomical knowledge in medieval Spain can consult Julio Samsó's *Islamic Astronomy and Medieval Spain* (1994).

- "On an Eclipse of the Moon" (1846), a brief lyric poem by British writer Walter Savage Landor takes a very different view of the phenomenon of a lunar eclipse.

- "Peace on Earth" (1913) by American poet William Carlos Williams is a brief lyric poem that references Orion, the Bear, and other constellations of stars.

- Readers interested in poetry about astronomical phenomena can find a wide-ranging collection of such poems by writers from all eras and cultures at "Nox Oculis: Astronomical Poetry," at http://pages.infinit.net/noxoculi/poetry.html.

- Marge Piercy is a Jewish poet who writes poetry suitable for young adults, including *The Art of Blessing the Day: Poems with a Jewish Theme* (1999).

- To read other examples of HaNagid's poetry relating to God and nature, try "The Earthquake" and "The Miracle at Sea," both in *Selected Poems of Shmuel HaNagid,* translated by Peter Cole (1996).

---

the Quran are critical of poets, others seem to admire poets and poetry. Many Muslims reject categorically any notion that the Quran is poetic, but it does not follow that others do not find poetic elements in the Quran.) One of the techniques of Islamic poetry is the use of Quranic language as a kind of inlay, similar to mosaics. Islamic architecture and ornamentation did not allow for the representation of living things, especially humans, so it focused instead on color and bravura geometrical effects. This aesthetic was transferred to poetry by the use of language from the Quran that was "inlaid" into Arabic

poetry. HaNagid would have been familiar with much of this poetry, which reinforced a similar aesthetic in Hebrew poetry. Hebrew authors used the word *shibbuts* to refer to this technique, in which biblical language is "inlaid" into poems.

This connection with the Old Testament can be found at nearly every turn. In line 2, for example, the speaker urges his friend to awaken from sleep and to awaken the dawn. The line virtually quotes Psalm 57:8, "I will awake the dawn!" The poet's comparison of the sky to a leopard skin echoes Jeremiah 13:23, where the writer asks whether a leopard can change his spots. The suggestion in the poem that the earth is reddened as though tears are flowing echoes Job 16:16: "My face is red with weeping." When the poet says that God has covered the moon with a circle of earth, he echoes Isaiah 40:22: "It is he who sits above the circle of the earth." When the poet compares the face of the moon to a face that is wounded and bruised, the line is inspired by Isaiah 1:6: "From the sole of the foot even to the head, there is no soundness in it, but bruises and sores and bleeding wounds." The poet's odd image of the moth eating the Bear and Orion was likely inspired by Isaiah 50:9: "Behold, all of them will wear out like a garment; the moth will eat them up." This image is continued in Isaiah 51:8: "For the moth will eat them up like a garment." Numerous other instances of these kinds of biblical echoes can be found from other Old Testament books: the Song of Solomon, Jeremiah, Chronicles, Samuel, Zechariah, Daniel, Joel, Malachi, Deuteronomy, Nehemiah, Joshua, Samuel, and Judges. These echoes continue to the end of the poem, when the poet envisions that God will allay his fear on Judgment Day, reflecting Isaiah 7:3–4: "And the Lord said to Isaiah, 'Go forth to meet Ahaz . . . and say to him, 'Take heed, be quiet, do not fear, and do not let your heart be faint.''"

At issue is not whether the poet quotes the Bible. Sometimes he did, lifting verses or phrases from the Old Testament and using them almost word for word. Usually, though, the poet who wrote in the biblical tradition used the vocabulary and imagery of the Bible. The Bible became in effect the poet's lexicon, his dictionary and phrase book. His readers, who likely read and studied the Old Testament and had likely committed large portions of it to memory, would have immediately recognized the biblical language. This language was the structuring principle of HaNagid's poems, including "Two Eclipses," and any translator of his poetry would likely work to preserve that biblical language in bringing HaNagid's work to new generations of readers.

Source: Michael O'Neal, Critical Essay on "Two Eclipses," in *Poetry for Students*, Gale, Cengage Learning, 2010.

Jay Ladin

In the following review, Ladin discusses Selected Poems of Shmuel HaNagid *and the challenges of translation.*

> THE STRUGGLE TO RECONCILE SENSE WITH SENSIBILITY HAS NO DOUBT CHECKED THE SLEEP OF EVERY TRANSLATOR OF POETRY. BUT MEDIEVAL HEBREW POEMS PRESENT A UNIQUE AND PROBABLY INSURMOUNTABLE OBSTACLE. AS SCHEINDLIN'S LUCID, INSIGHTFUL COMMENTARY MAKES CLEAR, THE COURTIER-RABBIS LIVED PROFOUNDLY HYPHENATED LIVES."

News flash: The Vatican has announced that the Pope and other ranking church clergy have begun writing secular poetry in Latin, warping the ancient phrases of Vulgate and Mass into stylish, sophisticated odes to wine, women, and song. . . .

Impossible, surely. But at the onset of the last millennium, this is what happened, albeit among rabbis rather than cardinals, in Hebrew rather than Latin, and in Muslim-controlled Andalusia—then the cultural and religious center of the Jewish world—rather than the Holy See. In the mid-tenth century, one Dunash ben Labrat brashly set the Hebrew tongue, for centuries reserved for prayer and sacred study, to the quantitative meters and distinctly secular themes of classical Arabic verse, then the sine qua non of literature. Dunash touched off a literary wildfire that blazed several hundred years and became known, in retrospect, as the Golden Age of Hebrew poetry. The cream of the Jewish community—courtier-rabbis who shuttled between Muslim palaces and Jewish yeshivas—started writing poems about brimming crystal goblets, the luscious girls and boys who filled them, and a host of other distinctly non-spiritual subjects that hadn't been hymned in Hebrew since before the fall of Rome:

> . . . Bring me wine from a cup
> held by a girl,
> who excels on the lute;
> a mature vintage, made by Adam,
> or new, from Noah's fields.
> Its hue like living coral
> and gold, its bouquet
> like calamus and myrrh—

like David's wine that queens prepared,
impeccably, or graceful harems . . .

(from "Your Years are Sleep")

These lines by Shmuel HaNagid, considered the first great Golden Age poet and one of the greatest Hebrew poets of any era, echo the Biblical books of Genesis, Samuel, Ezekiel, Psalms, and, faintly, Job, all in the course of rifting on one of the wine-song themes of Arabic meistersinger Abu Nuwas. The tongue is the tongue of the Torah, but the images are pure pleasure-palace.

Medieval Hebrew poetry steered a course between piety and blasphemy that probably cannot be mapped on modern charts—imagine, if you can, a Papal sonnet starting "Hail Marian full of grapes," and the Catholic world treating it not as a case of demonic possession, but as a glorification of their holy tongue. The Arabic poets whom the Golden Agers adopted as models made a great point of demonstrating, through virtuosic versifying, the purity and potency of the language of the Koran. The courtier-rabbis, with the over-achieving minority's chauvinistic pride, were determined to trump their Muslim counterparts and prove the Torah's Hebrew a poetic medium as fit or fitter than scriptural Arabic. If only contemporary Arab-Jewish conflicts could be so bloodlessly and ravishingly resolved.

As we dip our toes into our own new millennium, it is fitting that interest among English-speaking readers in this poetic treasure-trove from the last seems to be growing, to judge by the recent publication of Peter Cole's *Selected Poems of Samuel HaNagid*, and the upcoming appearance of a new translation of HaNagid's sometime protege and fellow Golden Age luminary, Solomon Ibn Gabirol. Medieval Hebrew poetry is what we would now call a triumph of multiculturalism. Admitted to and tolerated (if not welcomed) in the upper echelons of Muslim society, ambitious Andalusian Jews steeped themselves in Arabic language, literature, philosophy, and science. But rather than assimilating, the Jews of the Golden Age—and this is what made it a Golden Age—took the siren song of non-Jewish culture as a wake-up call. The result was a renaissance that included unparalleled achievements in philosophy, philology, and, of course, literature, as Hebrew leapt the margins of prayerbooks and scrolls and reentered the alleys, palaces, and boudoirs beyond them.

The variety and vividness of this verse may startle those who think of learned, devout Jews as pallid, angst-ridden yeshiva bochers bowed, like the soul of Cynthia Ozick's hapless "Pagan Rabbi," beneath towers of musty tomes. Shmuel HaNagid, for example, chronicles earthquakes, conjures up scent-soaked gardens, gloats over fallen rivals, seduces coquettish serving boys and girls, cossets and lectures his son Yehosef, and strolls among slaughtered livestock:

> I crossed through a souk where the butchers
> hung oxen and sheep at their sides,
> there were birds and herds of fatlings like squid,
> their terror loud
> as blood congealed over blood
> and slaughterers' knives opened veins.
>
> In booths alongside them the fishmongers,
> and fish in heaps, and tackle like sand . . .

(from "The Market")

HaNagid's poems have an earthiness without equivalent in the liturgical Hebrew verse that flourished before, during, and after the secular Golden Age. But despite the strikingly observed images, medieval Hebrew verse was courtiers' poetry, bred (and inbred) in the hothouses of luxury, sophistication, and intrigue that were the Andalusian Muslim courts. Written by and for a small elite of men who had received identical educations, attended the same parties, read the same books, were subject to the same social pressures, and subscribed to the same values, this poetry, like that of the Elizabethan courtiers, is largely a matter of convention and wit, brimming with highly wrought phrases, ingeniously deployed cliches, oblique allusions, and formal tours de force. Even the brutal realism of HaNagid's market scene is a play on Ecclesiastes, and its grim meditation on death ("And my heart . . . asked: / Who are you to survive? What separates you from these beasts?") an occasion for spectacular artifice. As in many medieval Hebrew and Arabic poems, each line shares the same rhyme-syllable, in this case "dam," Hebrew for "blood"; mortality, as represented by its most vivid metonym, tolls at the terminus of every line.

Medieval Hebrew poetry was a performance art, and showmanship was as important to Golden Age poets as it is to contemporary slam competitors. In the Andalusian Muslim courts, poetry was simultaneously a revered art form, a popular pastime, and a means of climbing the social ladder. Bravura displays of poetizing had the same effect on reputation as sharpshooting feats in Hollywood Westerns. Improvisational contests were common, and, if the stories are true, men could rise from obscurity to power by spontaneously composing poems that met seemingly insuperable thematic and formal challenges.

The poetry that flourished under these conditions looks rather repetitive when judged by contemporary standards. Golden Age poems are composed largely of stock phrases, stock sentiments, stock characters, and stock images. Much of their brilliance, originality, and resonance are lost on those unversed in the arcana of classical Arabic poetics and sacred Hebrew texts.

Hebrew readers can, at least, appreciate the word-play of these poems without being medievalists. English versions cannot even hint at the sonic and semantic splendor of the originals. Imagine a prose crib of Gerard Manley Hopkins, or a Shakespeare sonnet stripped of puns, rhymes, and iambs, and you get the idea. And yet, translators cannot afford simply to throw in the musical towel, as Leon J. Weinberger's Jewish Prince in Moslem Spain, an early 1970s attempt to make Shmuel HaNagid's verse accessible to English readers, demonstrates in page after wooden page:

> My God, pray change the heart of the young
> dove who stole
> My sleep that he may give back but a little of
> it to my
> eyelids.
> My beloved, who came with solemn oath
> and gave to me
> His heart's love as a gift, without compulsion,
> Has betrayed me. But then all young lovers
> are unfaithful.
> And so do forgive him his sins, or failing
> that, punish me
> instead.

("All Young Lovers")

Like the other ninety-four in the collection, this translation is lexically faithful yet poetically DOA. Golden Age poems, like jazz, the twentieth century's most spectacular example of highly conventionalized improvisational art, don't mean a thing if they ain't got at least a bit of that swing. Raymond Scheindlin's rendering in *Wine, Women and Death*, his introduction to what he calls *Medieval Hebrew Poems on the Good Life* sacrifices accuracy in a bid to suggest the scintillating word-play of the original:

> Change, my God, the heart of that chick that checked
> My sleep, and make him give it back to me;

> A fawn who swore by Your name to give
> His love to me, a gift of his own free will,
> And then betrayed me; lovers all betray.
> Forgive his sin—or wipe me out, I pray.

Both the virtues and drawbacks of Scheindlin's approach to translation are apparent in the first two lines. Far livelier than Weinberger's "the young dove who stole," the phrase "that chick that checked" aptly renders the rhythmic bounce and vocalic play of HaNagid's punning phrase, "gozal asher gazal."

But Scheindlin pays a poetic price for substituting "chick" for "dove." Chicks rank distinctly lower than doves in the pecking order of ornithological imagery, and "chick," thanks to its previous career as Sixties slang, comes perilously close to making the poem sound like the prayer of an aging, insomniac hippie. Worse problems arise from the jazzy but inaccurate switch from "stole" to "checked." "Stolen" sleep can presumably be "returned," as the speaker demands in the original; since "checked" sleep, whatever that is, cannot, the word blurs the poems sophisticated play on the notion of romantic give-and-take.

The struggle to reconcile sense with sensibility has no doubt checked the sleep of every translator of poetry. But medieval Hebrew poems present a unique and probably insurmountable obstacle. As Scheindlin's lucid, insightful commentary makes clear, the courtier-rabbis lived profoundly hyphenated lives. For these poets and their contemporary readers, Hebrew was the language through which they praised, petitioned, and strove to penetrate the will of God—and it was emphatically not the language in which they transacted business, flattered their Muslim rulers, argued with their wives, or muttered to themselves when they woke in the middle of the night.

No English can convey what the secular use of Hebrew meant to Golden Age poets. The ironies inherent in yoking together Jewish and Muslim worlds are implicit in every Hebrew syllable they fitted, with courtiers' self-conscious flourishes, to Arabic literary conventions—and they become startlingly explicit, when sacred phrases are transposed into profane songs.

Of course, when your lexicon is the Bible, every word is a reference and a quotation; the most straightforward request for illumination can easily come out as "Let there be light." But in many poems, these secular shocks are as crucial as plays on the language of love are to

Shakespeare's sonnets. In the poem quoted above, for example, HaNagid turns direct address to God—the rhetorical mode is that of the most intimate prayer—into the vehicle for a witty, homoerotic complaint. In English, the poem hovers uneasily between blasphemy and bathos. In Hebrew, the word-play fuses the two into a self-lacerating critique of the courtier-rabbi's love affair with secular Muslim culture.

The hinge is the line Scheindlin renders as "lovers all betray." "Lovers" in the Hebrew is tzvi, which literally means "gazelle," but which, in medieval Hebrew poetry, is the stock phrase used for the comely young boys hired to serve and flirt at the wine parties that Golden Age poets, Muslim and Jewish, frequented and frequently wrote about. HaNagid draws attention to this word by making a point of avoiding it in the first line, substituting and playing on the idiosyncratic "ghozal" instead. "Tzvi" also means "ornament," "beauty," or "glory," a multiple entendre which unites the poet and his love-object as betrayers—the poet betrayed by the tzvi (young lover) is himself a betrayer, in using the sacred tongue for the sake of tzvi (poetic ornament, secular beauty, personal glory).

The last line, which mimics Moses' plea to God to forgive the Israelites for making the Golden Calf ("Now, if You will, forgive their sin—if not, erase me from the Book you have written!"), trumpets the identification between poet and tzvi—in both senses of the word. The Israelites' sin was fashioning and worshipping a figure that conformed to forbidden, non-Jewish conventions; part of their penance was "stripping themselves of their finery." Read with this resonance in the ear—and it cannot be, in English, for annotation of a reference does not produce the same frisson as does instantaneously recognized quotation—the poem is at least as much about the moral and spiritual complexities of writing secular Hebrew poetry as about love. The final outburst—"Forgive his sin—or wipe me out, I pray"—is simultaneously guilt-ridden and sardonic, self-humbling and unmitigatedly chutzapadik. Whether or not the sin of tzvi was forgiven, HaNagid and his fellow secular Hebrew poets clearly chose to risk being blotted out of God's Book rather than renounce their own.

Shmuel HaNagid's poems account for an extraordinary amount of the gilt of the Golden Age. Generally acclaimed as one of medieval Hebrew poetry's four greatest poets—the others are Solomon Ibn Gabirol, Judah HaLevi, and Moses Ibn Ezra—HaNagid pioneered many of what became its standard practices, and audaciously experimented with unusual meters and modes. A poet with the technical command and influence of Auden at the height of his powers, he was also a field general roughly as renowned as Patton, the local Muslim ruler's chief of staff and confidant, a famous Talmudic authority, and undisputed head of the Andalusian Jewish community. In his own eyes, and in the cultural pantheon of the Golden Age, HaNagid—a title that means "leader"—was a latter-day King David, a warrior-poet-priest-prince who personified the glory of the Jewish people.

Before the publication of Peter Cole's translations, HaNagid was hard to find in English. Weinberger's 1973 translation is a good sampling of HaNagid's oeuvre, and, with its facing Hebrew texts, is invaluable for the English-speaking reader who has enough Hebrew to get by with help from a literal trot. And Scheindlin's mid-Eighties bilingual anthology includes a number of HaNagid's poems. But Scheindlin's stated goal is to introduce readers to the typical features of medieval Hebrew poetry, not to spotlight its most distinctive achievements; his translations are instructive exempla, not poems in their own right.

Cole's collection is the first to translate a broad swath of HaNagid's work into a modern poetic idiom. Cole has attempted, as he puts it, to "conduct the poet's quality of emotion and movement of mind. When the voice in the Hebrew is ambitious or subtle or aggrieved, or where the verse is particularly musical, inventive, or sublime, I try for a similar sense of the English...." Cole's attentiveness to HaNagid's voice shows. One of the strengths of his anthology is the abundance of passages in which HaNagid's varied tones snap and swagger across the centuries. We hear his tough-minded realism ("They bake, they eat, they lead their prey; / they split what's left to bring home" ["The Market"]), intellectually nuanced faith ("God restores what He levels / though He keeps His secrets and erases His ways" ["The Miracle at Sea"]), snide superiority ("One needs, it seems, only fringes, a turban, and beard / to head the Academy now" ["House of Prayer"]), rabbinic wisdom ("It's heart that discerns / between evil and good, / so work to develop your heart" ["It's Heart That Discerns"]), courtier's cynicism ("The king's fickleness /

resembles the drunk's" ["The King"]), unblinking contemplation of his own mortality ("Heart says: you'll live forever— / and death as it speaks / grasps you with claws" ["Soul Opens Inside You"]), chest-thumping pride ("No good could come of one / who exalts himself over my family, / no peace to him who threatens my city" ["The War with Yadir"]), and unassuagable grief ("By the life of the Living / God, for the world / he'll be in my blood / like fire, / until I'm dust / in the dust at his side" ["On the Death of His Brother Isaac"]).

Cole makes a point of arranging his selection along the lines of HaNagid's original collections. He even includes the peculiar prefaces written by HaNagid's chief scribe, his son Yehosef, who notes for posterity that "I wrote these out in my own hand when I was eight and a half years old, it being that my birth, according to my father's precise records, may God sustain him for me, took place at three hours and four fifths of an hour exactly, on the night of the third day of the week...."

Such astrological particulars don't tell us much about HaNagid, but the structure of the diwan (as Golden Age oeuvres are known) does. The titles of HaNagid's three collections—*Ben Tehillim* ("After [literally, "Son of"] Psalms"), *Ben Mishle* ("After Proverbs"), and *Ben Kohelet* ("After Ecclesiastes")—frame his distinctly worldly poems as offspring of the Biblical Hebrew canon. This seemingly defensive maneuver audaciously transforms holy writ into literary precedent. The title *Ben Tehillim*, for example, points up the fact that, like HaNagid's collection, the Book of Psalms is an eclectic anthology which ranges from the intimately personal to the die-stamped formulaic, from vivid narratives to brief lyrics, from ecstatic boasts to heartbroken confessions. It also underlines the parallel between HaNagid and David, the poet whose personality and lyric prowess dominate the Book of Psalms, and whose trademark poetic move is to present his secular endeavors as sacred dramas—a canny, tacit justification for HaNagid's own poetic undertaking.

Ben Tehillim was a groundbreaking book: HaNagid's drinking poems, love poems, boasts, friendship poems, and so on consolidated many of medieval Hebrew poetry's basic genres. It also contains some of the Golden Age's most unique works. HaNagid experimented with epic storytelling, represented in Cole's selection by "The

Miracle at Sea," a yarn (though some scholars think it is intended as a factual account) of HaNagid's deliverance from a sea-monster, "its head huge as a galley with oars, / its face haughty, like a hill, / its eyes like pools...." He tracked what we would now call the stages of grief in an intimate, "In Memoriam"-like sequence of elegies (excerpted and rearranged by Cole), charting his responses to the illness and death of his brother Isaac. And he resurrected Hebrew war poetry in pieces like "The War with Yadir," a pugnacious, consciously Davidic melange of religious self-justification ("I trust in the Lord who humbled my foes"), strategic play-by-play ("Two of the Spanish princes were there, / and the Zemarite troops, and they seized the city"), editorial ("He was a foe in the line of my king— / and the evil of strangers pales / beside the evil of kin"), and metaphoric filigree ("We slew them two against three, / like long vowels against short in a word").

Ben Mishle is, as the title suggests, a collection of proverbs, many of them rephrasings of chestnuts from Arabic and Hebrew wisdom literature. Where the Biblical Book of Proverbs is presented as paternal advice, HaNagid's is what we would now call mentoring. As befits the most successful Jewish courtier since Joseph, he sardonically spotlights for his junior colleagues the discrepancies between public and private, deed and thought, appearance and reality, which no ambitious Golden Age Jew could afford to ignore:

The rich are small in number,
and the brilliant likewise are few;
and the number of each is further reduced
when they step side by side into view.

HaNagid's last, and possibly posthumous, collection, *Ben Kohelet*, though not as dazzlingly variegated as *Ben Tehillim*, is much more diverse than *Ben Mishle*. In addition to proverbs, it includes narratives, descriptions of eclipses and earthquakes, and, as one would expect from the title, down-in-the-mouth meditations on death. Ecclesiastes was an ideal model for the aging HaNagid: The Biblical Kohelet rambles between proverb, rant, carpe diem-style injunctions, and bitter boasts of evanescent triumphs. HaNagid, too, had seen the glorious come and go:

You whose souls on earth were exalted,
will soon rise over all—
and be remembered in the world ever after
as a dream when it fades is recalled.

(from "Know of the Limbs")

Cole writes that he "tried to account for my understanding of the poet's distinctive combination of pathos and wit, his integration of artifice and the steady pressure of the personal in his lines." Not surprisingly, Cole is more successful at translating HaNagid's "pathos" than his "wit." Existential despair travels remarkably well across languages and centuries:

> Earth to man
> is a prison forever.
> These tidbits, then,
> for fools:
> Run where you will.
> Heaven surrounds you
> Get out if you can.

HaNagid's "wit" and "artifice," however, are much more culture-bound, a matter of conventions nearly a millennium out of date. Cole comes closest to "accounting" for both in HaNagid's most personal epigrams, like those above, whose wit is built into their concision, and whose artifice is readily denoted by a hint of meter and a bit of rhyme. Second-best are those that yoke proverbial injunction to chiseled images, and that attest to the ironic, unblinking intelligence behind the generalities:

> Delay your speech
> if you want your words
> to be straight and free of deceit—
> as a master archer
> is slow to take aim
> while splitting a grain of wheat.

But there was no Golden Age Ezra Pound to instill fear of generalities into medieval Hebrew poets. Many of HaNagid's bons mots sound, to contemporary ears, too much like Polonius and too little like Hamlet. It is hardly Cole's fault that he cannot breathe poetic life into such homilies as "If you're finding the good at fault, / you're in the dark all alone; / if you can't see the kindness of others, / there isn't much hope for your own."

The biggest problem with Cole's translation, however, is that in poems more than a few lines long—that is, in much of this book—he has not found ways to bridge medieval Hebrew and contemporary English poetics. Cole nods toward HaNagid's formal intricacies with sound- and word-play when he can, but his primary means of effecting what he calls "sustaining poetic reality" is enjambment:

> Your years are sleep,
> their fortune's wheel a dream;

> best, my friend, to shut your
> eyes and ears—God
> grant you strength—
> and leave the hidden things
> around youto one
> who's good with clues.
> Bring me wine from a cup
> held by a girl,
> who excels on the lute . . .

(from "Your Years are Sleep")

Here and throughout this book, Cole relentlessly breaks, indents, and otherwise chops up HaNagid's lines in ways which are alarmingly at odds with the flow of the original poems, gambling that abrupt linebreaks can transform leaden medievalisms into edgy, personal-sounding utterances with the feel of living poetry. The gamble only occasionally pays off. Here, for example, the first line's accusatory tone grabs the reader by the collar. By the second line, though, this grip is already slackening: "their fortune's wheel a dream" is too abstract to sustain the first line's urgency. "Best, my friend," makes another stab at directness, but Cole blunts the effect by breaking the line after "your," a disorienting, Williamsesque move that he repeats in the next line, presumably to defamiliarize the pious interjection "God grant you strength." The constant enjambments shatter the sentence into brief, intrinsically meaningless phrases whose syntactical and logical ligaments can barely be discerned. The return to clear, direct address in the second stanza (Cole's innovation— the original is not thus divided) is refreshing but inexplicable, a momentarily welcome but ultimately confusing shift that adds to the sense that the poem is a string of gnomic non sequiturs.

It is easier to appreciate what Cole is doing—and failing to do—by comparing his rendition to Weinberger's literal version:

> My friend, all your years are sleep
> Both good and bad are dreams.
> Therefore shut your eyes and ears
> (May the Lord give you strength!)
> And leave the hidden things
> In your world to those who understand
>   them.
> Rather, give me a cup of old wine to drink
> From the hand of a young maid skilled on
>   the 'alamot.

Cole knows what Williams knew: that syntax-defying line-breaks can turn the simplest statements into series of enigmatic fragments. But the complexities that Cole's layout introduce have nothing to do with HaNagid's gorgeous weave of sound and sense, and completely eclipse the already obscure conventions with which HaNagid is playing. As Scheindlin notes in his commentary, "The opening sententious reflection ... [is] a parody of pietistic verse ... [that] is really advising the listener to censor bothersome reflections ... If life is nothing but sleep, then sleep! Leave the thinking to God, and drink up." What was, to HaNagid, a mock-sermon admonishing drinkers to drink more seriously becomes, in Cole's enjambing hands, a mordant cryptogram.

Such long-dead conventions as the wine-party poem certainly require some sort of poetic resuscitation for contemporary readers, but Cole's enjambment strategy is self-defeating: It renders individual lines intriguingly obscure, but prevents them from coalescing into structure, sense and, since HaNagid was not writing postmodernist pastiche, poetry....

In some poems, Cole's search for le mot juste leads him to lexical choices which, while not exactly wrong, draw too much attention to themselves for the good of the poem. The word "contortions," for example, seems a bit extravagant in the midst of a conventional rhetorical question like "How could a person sin when he sees / the contortions of each man's journey?" ("The Earthquake"). And what epigram could survive the wedging of the word "vitae" into this crucial slot: "Ask the dead and they'll tell you: Come / look at your vitae's secret and sins" ("Ask the Dead and They'll Tell You")?

The Talmud quotes a certain Rabbi Tarfon as saying, "Do not shy from the unattainable." Cole certainly has not. His versions of HaNagid may well be definitive in the sense of proving that, pending some improbable change in the way we read and write poetry, you can't get here from there. But we are indebted to Cole for reminding us of the days when poems were the very coin of social capital, when poets were princes, warriors, and sages who knew all there was to know about living and dying, and weren't afraid to proclaim it:

> And they said: Who are you ...
> And I answered ...
> my songs surpass even those of the Levites,
> even those of the close-cropped priests.
> Coffers of gold are within my dominion,
> and chests of the finest clothes.
> In my presence the experts go dumb,

and scholars as though they were guilty ...
They stand there in silence before me—
even the movers and shakers;
I reveal to them marvelous things, of hidden interests,
"obscure"—and fashion my difficult rhymes,
which know no peer in creation.

(from "How I Helped the Wise")

Source: Jay Ladin, "The Prince and the Paupered: Medieval Hebrew Poetry Meets the Twenty-First Century," in *Parnassus: Poetry in Review*, Vol. 25, Nos. 1–2, 2001, pp. 109–24.

Robert Alter

In the following review, Alter examines the translation problems associated with Selected Poems of Shmuel HaNagid, *in which "Two Eclipses" appears.*

The life of Shmuel HaNagid, a figure scarcely known outside Hebraist circles, would make an extraordinary story even if he were not one of the great European poets of the medieval period. Born in Cordoba in 993, he fled to Malaga at the age of 20, when his native city fell to the Berbers. Like many economically privileged Jewish males in Andalusia in this era, he had been given a double education: in Bible and Talmud (among many other projects, he would publish a work of authoritative erudition on talmudic law), and in philosophy, the natural sciences and Arabic literature. He appears to have been successfully involved in commerce early on; and within a few years the kingdom of Granada, which controlled Malaga, appointed him tax-collector and then governor or regent (the meaning of the Hebrew term nagid) of the Jewish community of Granada.

In 1037, apparently because he had the wit to back the right claimant to the throne in a succession struggle, he was elevated to vizier of Granada and commander-in-chief of its army. The majority of the Granadan population, it should be said, was probably Jewish, and the ruling elite, which was Berber, may well have felt it could trust a Jew in this high office more than an indigenous Arab. Beginning in 1038, HaNagid went out on military campaigns at the head of the Granadan army and recorded his experience in the first battle poems written in Hebrew since biblical times. He continued these expeditions, together with all his other political

" FOR ALL THE FLAWS OF HIS RENDERINGS, HOWEVER, PETER COLE HAS PERFORMED A REAL SERVICE TO ENGLISH READERS IN MAKING THIS GENEROUS SELECTION OF HANAGID'S POEMS AVAILABLE, AND AT LEAST SOME OF THE TIME PRODUCING ENGLISH VERSIONS THAT SUGGEST THE BEAUTY, THE WIT AND THE VITALITY OF THE HEBREW."

and cultural activities, until shortly before his death in 1056.

HaNagid came of age just a few decades after a momentous innovation in the cultural life of Andalusian Jewry: the adaptation to Hebrew of the norms and the conventions of Arabic poetry. Formally, this meant composing verse in Hebrew in an intricate system of strict quantitative meters with an elaborate deployment of often hyperbolic imagery (in many ways analogous to the "conceited style" of Renaissance English sonnets). Substantively, since the new Hebrew poets embraced virtually all the Arabic genres, this meant that secular poetry was being written in Hebrew for the first time in well over 1,000 years—erotic verse, drinking poems, philosophical reflections, intimate epistolary verse, poetic riddles, satires, panegyrics, nature poetry and confessional or autobiographical poems.

When Shmuel HaNagid began to write poetry, probably around 1013 or somewhat before that pivotal date in his life, the new literary movement had developed a good deal of momentum in the Andalusian Jewish social elite. In an odd coincidence of destiny and talent, however, this man who would achieve such a remarkable political career also turned out to be the first true master of medieval Hebrew poetry. He would be followed by three others whose greatness is undisputed: his younger contemporary Shlomo ibn Gabirol and, two generations later, Moshe ibn Ezra and Yehuda HaLevi. The poetic movement he helped to shape would continue to flourish for another

seven centuries, spreading to a number of Mediterranean countries, reaching as far as Yemen and showing the greatest vigor in Italy, where it was introduced by the itinerant Avraham ibn Ezra (Browning's Rabbi Ben Ezra) in the twelfth century.

Although readers of Hebrew never entirely forgot the great Spanish-Hebrew poets, this large body of vibrant, sensuously rich verse has really been rediscovered in our century. Treasure-troves of manuscripts have been unearthed (we now possess eight times the number of authentic poems by HaNagid than were known before 1934); scholarly editions of the major poets have been established; scrupulous historical and philological investigations have been undertaken. Especially worthy of mention is the illuminating work of the late Dan Pagis (himself a fine Hebrew poet), which did much to clarify the formal conventions and the distinctive aesthetics of the medieval tradition. Hebrew readers now have the poems available in a new abundance, with greatly enhanced textual reliability, and they also have the critical tools to read the poems in clear focus, with heightened appreciation.

Conveying this poetry in any language but Hebrew is quite another matter. There are four significant aspects of the medieval poems that create nearly insuperable difficulties for the English translator: the elegance of the complex quantitative meters, for which there is scarcely any English equivalent; the concomitant concision of idiomatic usage and the compression of syntax the poets adopted to suit the meters; the predominant use of monorhymes, to which Hebrew and Arabic lend themselves, but which are unfeasible in an English poem that is much longer than a couplet; and the pervasive deployment of biblical locutions, sometimes with the most complex evocation of the original biblical contexts for a readership that would have been familiar with the entire Hebrew Bible almost verbatim. Rendering in English a poem by HaNagid or ibn Gabirol is a little like trying to translate Pope's heroic couplets into a language that has no notion of rhyme or accentual-syllabic meter for an audience totally ignorant of the Greek and Latin poets that Pope invokes or parodies.

This stubborn resistance to translation, in the language and the formal structures of the medieval poems, should be kept in mind in assessing Peter Cole's efforts in this interesting new book. His performance as a translator seems to me extremely uneven, though there are moments of real felicity. It would require astounding virtuosity, which he does not possess, to produce truly satisfying English approximations of these wonderfully poised and eloquent Hebrew poems.

Cole has done his homework on the subject with admirable care. His introduction on medieval Hebrew poetry and HaNagid is intelligent, helpful to the general reader and aptly informed by the best modern scholarship. At the back of the book, he provides nearly eighty closely printed pages of notes on the poems to instruct the English reader about their intricate line-by-line deployment of biblical—and rabbinic—allusions. His selection of poems is judicious and should give English readers a representative sense of HaNagid's handling of all the principal poetic genres of the period. Cole's book also enables one to see how certain personal preoccupations of the poet run across the boundaries of genre and even sometimes reshape genre.

Let me give a central instance. HaNagid is a poet who, in the full tide of a spectacularly active life, is spooked by mortality, haunted by visions of the body mouldering in the grave: "and my tongue which has told of my life / will be in its box / like a stone in the heart of the sea". These broodings on death appear in the sort of poems where you would expect them, such as his aphoristic wisdom poems that he called "After Ecclesiastes," or his stunning cycle on the death of his brother Isaac, or the memorable ubi sunt poem grounded in his military experience, which begins with the following lines:

I quartered the troops for the night
in a fortress
which soldiers destroyed long ago,
and they fell asleep at its walls and
foundations
while beneath us its masters slept on.
And I wondered: what had become
of the people who dwelled here
before us?
Where were the builders and soldiers,
the wealthy
and poor, the slaves and their lords?

But mortality also proves to be a kind of counterpoint to the generically dictated exuberance in many of HaNagid's drinking poems. Thus, one of them begins with the somber

words, "Your years are sleep, / their fortune's wheel a dream" and then boisterously invokes the immemorial practice of wine-drinking— "Bring me wine from a cup / held by a girl, / who excels on the lute; / a mature vintage, made by Adam, / or new, from Noah's fields."—and then concludes with an injunction for all good drinkers to "keep the laws of Kohelet, / fearing death, / and the fury to come." ("Kohelet" is the Hebrew name for "Ecclesiastes.") These words are virtually a HaNagid signature: no other poet of the period superimposed tombstone on wine-cask in this fashion, and in a genre meant to be playful and celebratory.

The lines I have quoted from "I quartered the troops" and "Your years are sleep" are representative instances of Cole's competence as a translator. Their rhythmic integrity and their expressive directness give you some sense of what is going on in the original, even if they lack the virtuosic sound-play and word-play repeatedly manifested in HaNagid's Hebrew. At times Cole shows real flair, as in these lines, enlivened by alliteration and vivid diction, from the feistily self-assertive poem HaNagid wrote when he left Cordoba:

And the friends who fray me,
their fine physiques and
slender thinking,
thinking it's ease or gain
that drives me,
pitching from place to place,
my hair wild, my eyes
charcoaled with night—
and not a one speaks wisely,
their souls blunted, or blurred,
goat-footed thinkers.

Cole's versions can also be quite effective in capturing HaNagid's descriptive vigor, as in these lines from a poem on an earthquake that shook Granada in 1047:

He when He pleases who brings out
the sun
and lights the hills with fire,
ripples the mountains like wind
rippling spikes of wheat in a field.

Finally, Cole is often surprisingly good in rendering the sharp bite of HaNagid's brief aphoristic poems (in the Hebrew, many are mere couplets), sometimes using rhyme, as does the original, to snap shut the structure of emphatic utterance:

Delay your speech
if you want your words
to be straight and free of deceit —
as a master archer
is slow to take aim
while splitting a grain of wheat.

Unfortunately, Cole's translations are not consistently this effective. He tends to wobble between taking liberties—usually understandable liberties—with the original and an excessive literalism. The result is an abundance of lines and locutions that don't quite sound like English, such as this brief sequence from the cycle on the death of the poet's brother: "who'd herd as one the heifer and bear, and none devour, / and none make prey," or this reference to the obedience of his troops, "they're willingly drawn in my cord," or this praise of God, "justice shapes your mouth and heart." Cole's sense of appropriate diction sometimes slips, as when, in an exquisite nature poem, he renders remes (the biblical "creeping things") as "bugs," or when he translates a reference to the lovely light of the moon as "glare," and some of the poems are marred by anachronistic terms that would have never occurred to an eleventh-century person: "You flaunt your phallic soul," "briefings," "movers and shakers," "debunks."

The most regrettable lapses in these English versions are when Cole, apparently reaching for a fancy poetic effect, becomes simply unintelligible. In some of these instances, even a look at the Hebrew did not help me see what he was trying to say: "and the God of sentence / send aegis," "I act the horizon," "you'll move toward peace through my promise," "smothered their hearts with lids," "a stone to start trouble." A few of these puzzlers reflect misconstruals of the Hebrew. In a battle poem, HaNagid is made to say of the fearsome enemy, "In their might . . . the parable makers were richly endowed." This obscures the plain sense of the Hebrew, which is that the makers of parables or bywords of valor would coin their parables in the image of these fierce warriors. Among the other lines just quoted, the enigmatic phrase "move toward peace through my promise" derives from a misreading of the last word of the poem, mavtihi, which has nothing to do with "promise" (as in modern Hebrew) but means instead "he who makes me safe," that is, God; so the actual sense of the line is "I trust you will go in peace to my God."

For all the flaws of his renderings, however, Peter Cole has performed a real service to English readers in making this generous selection of HaNagid's poems available, and at least some of the time producing English versions that suggest the beauty, the wit and the vitality of the Hebrew. I must confess, however, that a sampling of translations by Hillel Halkin in an essay on HaNagid ("The First Post-Ancient Jew," Commentary, September 1993) seems to me consistently superior to Cole's versions in their control of poetic diction and in a general sense of refined expression.

Compare these two treatments of a brief poem that is an elegant variation on the convention which combines the pleasures of drinking with the pleasures of sexual desire. First Cole:

I'd give everything I own for that gazelle
who, rising at night to his
harp and flute,
saw a cup in my hand
and said:
"Drink your grape blood against my lips!"
And the moon was cut like a D,
on a dark robe, written in gold.

This works well enough, and is another illustration of Cole's clear competence, though the idiomatic usage is a shade off in the line about drinking the blood of the grape, and the "D" sticking out at the end of the line seems too obtrusively English an equivalent for the little curved Hebrew letter yod. (Cole's line-breaks, moreover, are quite eccentric, and reflect nothing in the Hebrew.) Here is Halkin:

What would I not do for the youth
Who awoke in the night to the sound
of the skilled flutes and lutes,
And seeing me there, said to me,
"Here drink the grape's blood from
my lips."
Oh, the moon was a comma writ small
On the cloak of the dawn in watery gold.

There is a nice stylistic fluency in that version (compare Halkin's opening line with Cole's) and a sense of finely elevated poetic utterance ("the moon was a comma writ small") that bring us closer to the perfect pitch of HaNagid's exquisite Hebrew. Halkin's last line, moreover, manages to include "dawn" and "watery," both present in the Hebrew and essential to the delicate pictorial effect, both unaccountably omitted in Cole's version.

But translating these poems steeped in the aesthetic of a distant age and marked with such a dazzling otherness of linguistic texture is an endless task, for which there is no perfect solution. Even in English approximation, however, one can sense an extraordinary poetic vitality that flows from the shifting interplay between the polished artifice of convention and the resonance of individual experience. Dan Pagis, the leading critic of this whole body of poetry, offered an account of it that moved from one side of the dialectic to the other: in his weighty Hebrew studies, he stressed the intricacies of convention and in a slim English volume, published posthumously, he reconsidered the same poets and detected the affecting lineaments of individual experience.

Here is a haunting case in point. Poems about the fleeting span of human life and the inexorability of aging reflect a set convention of wisdom poetry in the Spanish medieval period. A more technical convention is a recurrent structure of challenge and response: a poem begins with the words, "he said," followed by a challenge to the poet's views or actions, and the poet in turn offers a vigorous rejoinder. But consider the following poem, which I quote in my own inadequate English version. It is not just a gesture of convention, since it marks a real date—1043—in the life of Shmuel HaNagid and expresses a very personal, and characteristic, brooding over life's ephemerality and the nature of time. In this instance, moreover, the challenge is delivered, exceptionally, by a woman—a young woman, one suspects—and, as one critic has noted, HaNagid swerves from the convention of response, slipping instead into an interior monologue, as though the speaker felt there was no point trying to explain to her what fifty years could mean to him. Across the gap of centuries, the poem still poignantly speaks to anyone who has reflected on the ambiguities of life in time.

> She said, "Be glad that through God
> you have reached
> full fifty years in your world." And
> how could she know
> There's no difference for me between
> my days now passed
> and Noah's days of which I've heard
> told?
> I have nothing in the world but the hour
> in which I am—
> it pauses a moment, and then like a
> cloud moves on.

Source: Robert Alter, "The Jew's Last Sigh," in *New Republic*, Vol. 214, No. 19, May 6, 1996, pp. 30–34.

SOURCES

Brann, Ross, *The Compunctious Poet: Cultural Ambiguity and Hebrew Poetry in Muslim Spain*, Johns Hopkins University Press, 1991, pp. 48, 53.

HaNagid, Shmuel, *Selected Poems of Shmuel HaNagid*, translated by Peter Cole, Princeton University Press, 1996, pp. xvii, xix, 145–47.

May, Herbert G., and Bruce M. Metzger, eds., *The Oxford Annotated Bible*, New York: Oxford University Press, 1962, pp. 628, 698, 823, 831, 870, 886–87.

"Samuel Ha-Nagid," in *Jewish Encyclopedia.com*, http://www.jewishencyclopedia.com/view_page.jsp?artid = 183& letter = S&pid = 0 (accessed September 2, 2009).

Scheindlin, Raymond P., *Wine, Women, and Death: Medieval Hebrew Poems on the Good Life*, Oxford University Press, 1999, p. 137.

FURTHER READING

Frank, Daniel H., ed., *The Cambridge Companion to Medieval Jewish Philosophy*, Cambridge University Press, 2003.
> This volume examines Jewish thinkers who lived in Islamic and Christian lands during the Middle Ages (ninth through the fifteenth centuries) and wrote philosophy about God, creation, and similar theological matters—the type of matters that HaNagid incorporated into his poetry.

Gerber, Jane S., *Jews of Spain: A History of the Sephardic Experience*, Free Press, 1992.
> Gerber's volume traces the history of Judaism in Spain, with emphasis on the Golden Age and its accomplishments in literature, philosophy, science, and other disciplines. This volume introduces readers interested in the poetry of HaNagid and his contemporaries to the cultural milieu in which they wrote.

Nirenberg, David, "What Can Medieval Spain Teach Us About Muslim-Jewish Relation," in *CCAR Journal: A Reform Jewish Quarterly*, Spring–Summer 2002, pp. 17–36.
> This article looks at contemporary problems between Muslims and Jews through the lens of Muslim-Jewish relations in medieval Spain. It raises for consideration the nature of the historical relationship between these two groups, with implicit suggestions for lessening modern tensions between them.

O'Callaghan, Joseph F., *A History of Medieval Spain*, Cornell University Press, 1975.

This volume is a good starting point for readers interested in the social, political, and cultural milieu in which HaNagid lived.

Septimus, Bernard, "Hispano-Jewish Views of Christendom and Islam," in *In Iberia and Beyond: Hispanic Jews between Cultures*, edited by Bernard Dov Cooperman, University of Delaware Press, 1998, pp. 43–65.

This article provides insights into the position of Jews in medieval Spain and how Judaism interacted with Islam and Christianity during the era in which HaNagid lived.

Upon the Burning of Our House, July 10th, 1666

ANNE BRADSTREET

1678

Anne Bradstreet, a seventeenth-century New England colonial woman, achieved fame when a family member had her privately circulated poems published in England. The collection, *The Tenth Muse Lately Sprung Up in America*, was published in 1650 and won Bradstreet so much critical and popular acclaim that her *Several Poems Compiled with Great Variety of Wit and Learning, Full of Delight*, published in 1678, was warmly received as well. This later collection, which was published after the poet's death, includes poems that are more personal in nature than those that appeared in the 1650 volume. "Upon the Burning of Our House, July 10th, 1666" is a poem in this later, more personal style. It is elegiac in tone (an elegy is a poem of mourning), in that its focus is on the sense of loss the poet experiences following the destruction of her home. In the poem, Bradstreet strives to uphold a Puritan response to the tragedy, to view it as God's will, and as a moral lesson. This Puritan element is a major theme of the poem. At the same time, Bradstreet struggles with powerful emotions, including deep sorrow and intense feelings of loss. The conflict between Bradstreet's instinctive emotions and her intellectual, religious response creates a palpable tension in the poem.

Bradstreet's "Upon the Burning of Our House, July 10th, 1666" was originally published in *Several Poems Compiled with Great Variety of Wit and Learning, Full of Delight* in 1678. It is

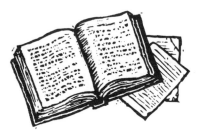

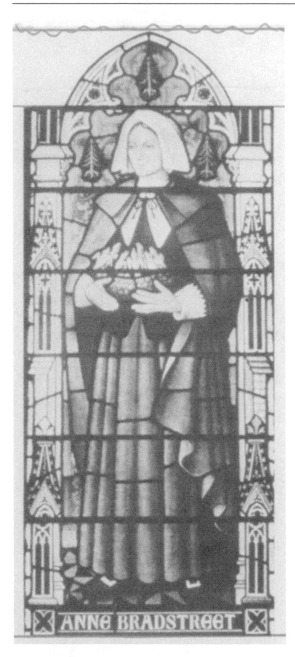

Anne Bradstreet

available in *The Works of Anne Bradstreet*, edited by Jeannine Hensley, and published in 1967 by the Belknap Press of Harvard University Press.

attend school but was privately instructed by her father, who worked as a steward for the Earl of Lincoln from 1619 to 1630. At the age of sixteen, she was stricken with smallpox, but survived. Shortly afterward, she married Simon Bradstreet, whom the family had known since Anne was a young child. In 1630, when she was eighteen years old, she and her husband and parents traveled with a group of Puritans to Massachusetts to begin a new life in the American colonies. Arriving in Salem, they moved throughout the colony, to Charleston, to Newton (which later became Cambridge), and to Ipswich. In 1645, the Bradstreets eventually settled in Andover, where they raised a family of eight children. Their first was born in 1633, the last in 1652.

Bradstreet wrote poems prolifically during this time period and copied her verses for circulation among family members. In 1650, Bradstreet's brother-in-law returned to England with a copy of the poems in hand, and, without Bradstreet's knowledge, had them published as *The Tenth Muse, Lately Sprung up in America*. Bradstreet later revised this collection. The revised works from *The Tenth Muse*, combined with new poems, including "Upon the Burning of Our House, July 10th, 1666," resulted in the volume *Several Poems Compiled with Great Variety of Wit and Learning, Full of Delight*. Bradstreet, however, would never see this book in print. The poet died of tuberculosis in Andover, Massachusetts, on September 16, 1672, and the volume of poetry was published in 1678.

The poems in the new volume were more personal in nature than the works on more academic topics that appeared in *The Tenth Muse*. In poems such as "Upon the Burning of Our House, July 10th, 1666" Bradstreet recorded events in her life, and her emotional responses to them. Her poetry is extensively influenced by her Puritan faith, and spiritual themes, such as salvation and the nature of God's will, are incorporated into simple domestic verses as well as into poems more overtly spiritual. What little information is possessed about Bradstreet's life has, to a large degree, been gleaned from her poetry.

AUTHOR BIOGRAPHY

Bradstreet was born Anne Dudley to Thomas Dudley and Dorothy Yorke Dudley in 1612 in Northampton, England. Bradstreet did not

POEM SUMMARY

Lines 1–6

Bradstreet's "Upon the Burning of Our House, July 10th, 1666" is not formally broken into stanzas. (A stanza is a unit of poetry, or a grouping of lines that divides the poem in the same way that a paragraph divides prose. Bradstreet's poem appears on the page as a fifty-four-line poem without any stanzas.) However, each six-line subset of the poem roughly functions as a stanza in that it typically focuses on one idea. In the first six lines, Bradstreet opens the poem by setting the stage for the events of the night of July 10, 1666, observing that when she went to bed that night, she could not expect the sorrow she was soon to experience. She describes waking to loud noises and voices shouting. The sixth line of the poem in particular is open to dual meanings. In this line, Bradstreet speaks of her desire to keep her fear of the fire hidden, implying that if her faith were stronger she would not have been so afraid. Alternately, the line may be interpreted as suggesting that Bradstreet's desire is to experience this trial, that she welcomes the impending tragedy as an opportunity to strengthen her faith.

Lines 7–12
In the next six lines, Bradstreet describes seeing the light of the fire for herself and praying to God to strengthen her, to help her during this time of need. Exiting her home, she begins to see the full view of what is happening and describes the flames consuming her home.

Lines 13–18
Bradstreet relates watching the house burning, how she stared until she could look no longer. At that moment, when she looked away, she praises God as one who both gives and takes, as the one responsible for leaving all of her possessions in the dust. She claims that God's actions are just, that it is his will that must be done and not her own. With the superiority of God's will asserted, Bradstreet tells herself that she must not worry or be discontented in the aftermath of the fire.

Lines 19–24
While God may have left her family bereft of its possessions, his actions, Bradstreet repeats, are just. Bradstreet further insists that God provides what is sufficient and necessary. She speaks of how later, after the fire, she passed the ruins of her home and was overwhelmed with sorrow at seeing what little remains of the places where her days were spent, where she used to sit and sleep.

Lines 25–30
The lamentation for what is lost continues, as Bradstreet recollects the treasured pieces of furniture that have been destroyed, a favorite trunk, a chest. All her cherished possessions, she observes, are now ashes, and she can no longer look upon or touch them. No longer will guests visit her in that house, or sit and dine there.

Lines 31–36
The cataloging of loss continues in these lines, as Bradstreet notes that no visitors will gather and tell stories. No longer will candles warmly light her home. Bradstreet recalls treasured events that took place in her home. The mention in this section of the voice of a bridegroom in the house is a reference to her son on his wedding day, according to the critic Josephine K. Piercy in her 1965 study of Bradstreet's poetry, titled *Anne Bradstreet*. Her home, she reveals in lines 21 through 36, was more than just a container for her property. The structure housed experiences, celebrations, conversations. In line 36, Bradstreet says farewell to all these things and attempts to brush off her attachment to the home and its contents as mere vanity.

Lines 37–42
Next, Bradstreet begins to scold herself, questioning where true wealth really resides. She asks herself whether or not she should have placed all of her hopes and dreams in the mortal world, in physical items, which have now succumbed to ruin. She admonishes herself to look heavenward, above the blowing dust and ashes that were once her home, and consider the house that God has built for her in heaven.

Lines 43–48
Reminding herself of how glorious heaven will be, Bradstreet also notes that her home in heaven will be permanent and will not be able to be destroyed like her home on earth. Alluding to the Christian notion that Jesus died for the sins of the faithful, Bradstreet describes her home in heaven as being paid for already by God.

Lines 49–54
In the final lines of the poem, Bradstreet continues to speak of the high price of her heavenly home, that price being the death of God's son. But God's gift to his people, the sacrifice of his son Jesus, provides her with enough wealth that she needs nothing more. Once again, she bids

farewell to her home and her possessions. In the final two lines of the poem, Bradstreet prays to be released from her love of this world. She reassures herself that all her hopes and wealth are to be found in heaven.

THEMES

Loss

Bradstreet's "Upon the Burning of Our House" is concerned primarily with the poet's great sense of loss, along with her attempt to mediate this pain through her faith in God. Throughout the middle third of the poem, Bradstreet offers an emotional itemization of her material losses and suggests the psychological toll such losses have taken. The physical items that have been destroyed by the fire are described as her goods, her wealth, her treasures, and she draws specific attention to favorite items, including a trunk and a chest. She speaks often of such pieces being left in ashes, in ruins, as dust. In addition to listing to the objects she cherished, Bradstreet catalogues the memories her home enshrined. Recounting guests at her table, candles shining throughout the home, stories being told, Bradstreet emphasizes that the loss she is experiencing is significant. She has not merely been left without a few of her favorite things, objects that could probably be replaced. As a seventeenth-century mother and wife, she has lost her home, her sphere of influence. Her life and work—not just domestic chores, but the work of raising a family, running a household, entertaining guests, educating and nurturing her children—all occurred within the home that is now in ashes. In the fire she lost a part of her self. She attempts to minimize her sense of loss by viewing the objects that have burned as things to which she was vainly attached.

Faith

Bradstreet's Puritan faith is an integral part of her poetry, and "Upon the Burning of Our House" is no exception. She uses her faith as a means of coping with her fear during the fire and with her intense feelings of loss in the aftermath of the fire. In the first third of the poem, Bradstreet reveals her terror and describes the way she turns to God for aid; she cries out for help, for the strength to see her safely through the immediate danger. Once she has left the house, Bradstreet is able to fully assess the scope of the tragedy. At once, she reminds herself that God

takes as easily as he gives, and she blesses his name for doing so. At times, she finds comfort in reminding herself that God's will takes precedence over her own. At other times, she scolds herself for her the pleasure she has taken in material things. She believes she has been vain to cling so much to worldly possessions. Bradstreet uses approximately the last third of the poem both to chide herself for mourning and to discuss the salvation that God has provided through the sacrifice of his son. She reflects on the heaven that awaits her, and in contemplating her permanent home with God in heaven, refers to the ashes of her own burned home as the dust from a heap of dung. Whether or not Bradstreet is successful in consoling herself through her faith is unclear. It is certain that she attempts to do so, for her poetry in general, while at times revealing her struggle with Puritanism, is not thought to be overtly ironic. Her effort at assuaging her pain through her faith must be viewed as an earnest one, but in the closing lines of the poem she asks for assistance in her efforts when she prays to be released from her love of the world and its attractions.

Throughout the poem, one has the sense that Bradstreet pits her sorrow and mourning against her Puritan faith. She allows herself to feel grief only briefly before chastising herself. Her mourning, after she has lovingly and sorrowfully begun to consider what she has lost, is attacked in the final third of the poem as human weakness, something to be despised, a reminder of unworthiness. After itemizing her losses, she similarly recounts to herself the reasons she should learn from grief: God has sacrificed his son for her sins, and a home awaits her in heaven.

STYLE

Lyric Poetry

"Upon the Burning of Our House" is considered a lyric poem. A lyric poem is one in which the poet explores personal feelings and thoughts rather than telling a story. Typically short in length, lyric poems do not necessarily adhere to any formal structure. Modern lyric poems may be written in unmetered, unrhymed verse, or free verse, whereas earlier poems, such as Bradstreet's "Upon the Burning of Our House" are often more structured. Bradstreet's lyric does not contain stanzas. A stanza, or a grouping of lines in a poem, divides the poem into sections

TOPICS FOR FURTHER STUDY

- Bradstreet's Puritan faith plays a prominent role in much of her poetry and is at the heart of the conflict in "Upon the Burning of Our House." Using online and print resources, research seventeenth-century New England Puritanism. What role did women play in the church? Who were prominent leaders in the church during Bradstreet's lifetime? What did the Puritans believe about heaven, and who was considered saved (that is, eligible for heaven, rather than condemned to hell)? Create either a written report or a PowerPoint presentation compiling your findings. Be sure to cite all sources used in writing your paper or presentation.

- In 1658 Bradstreet wrote a lyric poem about the family she reared in the home that burned in 1666. Titled "I Had Eight Birds Hatcht in One Nest," the poem explores the joys and pains of family life. Compare this poem with Bradstreet's "Upon the Burning of Our House." Are the structures similar? What rhyme scheme and meter does Bradstreet employ? To what extent does Bradstreet's Puritanism come into play in the earlier poem compared to the later one? How do the respective tones of the poems differ? Write a comparative essay in which you share your interpretations and your conclusions.

- Bradstreet was the first American female poet, and she wrote at a time when women were not typically encouraged to express themselves. Using resources such as Laurel Thatcher Ulrich's *Goodwives: Image and Reality in the Lives of Women in Northern New England, 1650–1750* (published by Vintage in 1991), research the roles and daily lives of women during this time period in American history. What were society's expectations of women? How did the domestic and social roles of men and women differ? What were society's views on the education of women? Incorporate your findings into a written report or a PowerPoint presentation, or write and recite a poem about what your life might have been like if you had been a woman in the New England colonies in the seventeenth century.

- The ruined physical structure of Bradstreet's home is, in effect, the setting of her poem "Upon the Burning of Our House." The poem identifies some of the contents of the home but provides little information on the structure itself. Research the architecture of seventeenth-century New England, using as resources such books as *American Home: From Colonial Simplicity to the Modern Adventure* (by Wendell D. Garrett, David Larkin, Michael Webb, et al., and published by Universe in 2005). The first several chapters of this book discuss the architecture of early American homes and include images of period buildings. How rustic were the homes of Bradstreet's day? How much variation in style was there in the architecture of this time? Incorporating images you find in print and online sources (images that you properly cite), create a presentation in which you discuss your findings. As an alternative assignment build a diorama of the house and the surrounding grounds.

- Read Chapter 3 of *The Colonial Mosaic: American Women 1600–1760* (1995) written by Jane Kamensky for young-adult readers. Compare what you have learned about Anne Bradstreet's family life with the description of family life in this chapter. Construct an essay that compares and contrasts the lives of Bradstreet and other colonial women.

---

the way paragraphs divide prose. The groupings typically display a repeated pattern in terms of number of lines and rhyme scheme. Bradstreet's

"Upon the Burning of Our House" does not contain a stanzaic structure, but rather consists of 54 lines of rhymed verse. While not divided

---

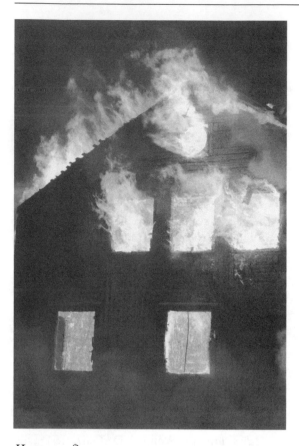

House on fire *(Image copyright stocksnapp, 2009. Used under license from Shutterstock.com)*

into stanzas, the poem contains 27 couplets, or pairs of rhymed lines. Each couplet features the same metrical pattern. Meter is the pattern of unaccented and accented syllables in a line of poetry. A metrical unit consists of at least one unaccented syllable along with at least one accented syllable and is called a foot. The type of meter is described in terms of the number of feet per line of poetry. The pattern of accented and unaccented syllables in Bradstreet's poem is iambic, a pattern consisting of an unaccented syllable followed by an accented syllable. There are four such units in each line. Therefore, the poem is said to be written in iambic tetrameter. Within the confines of the formal structure of the poem, a structure consistent with the conventions of the time period, Bradstreet explores her emotional responses to the tragedy of losing her home and possessions.

Elegiac Poetry

An elegy is a poem of mourning. Most often, elegies depict grief related to the loss of a loved one, but the designation of elegy is also applied to poems such as Bradstreet's "Upon the Burning of Our House" that focus in a meditative fashion on other types of losses, or are used as expressions of solemnity or somberness. In Bradstreet's elegy, the poet mourns the loss of her home, her favorite possessions, the place where happy memories have been created. In the elegy, Bradstreet plumbs the depths of her grief, exploring the particulars of the general loss of her house. For example, it is not just the loss of the physical structure, the shelter provided by her house, that is mourned. Rather, Bradstreet mourns the loss of individual objects and specific activities, such as dinner with guests, storytelling, the sound of voices in the home. The poet furthermore examines her response to her own grief, chastising herself for experiencing feelings of loss and attempting instead to feel comforted by her faith.

HISTORICAL CONTEXT

Seventeenth-Century Colonial Puritanism

Seventeenth-century Puritans were a sect of English Protestants who believed that the Church of England, although it had split from the Roman Catholic Church in the sixteenth century, still needed to be "purified" from practices associated with the Church of Rome. Wishing to preserve an English Protestant faith untainted by Catholicism, some fought for change in England and were subsequently persecuted for their efforts. In 1630 and in the following years, many Puritans fled to the English colonies in America in order to escape violent punishments and death. Once in the colonies, Puritans embarked on a life lacking in many of the comforts enjoyed in England. As Rosamond R. Rosenmeier explains in an essay in *Puritan Poets and Poetics: Seventeenth-Century American Poetry in Theory and Practice*, edited by Peter White and Harrison T. Meserole, and published in 1985, the Massachusetts Bay Colony Puritans were settling a land still considered a wilderness. They also believed themselves to be living in the last days on earth before God's final judgment on mankind and the return of Jesus to the world. Given the gravity of their situation as they understood it, the community felt it crucial that believers properly prepare themselves for Judgment Day. But as Rosenmeier further points out, an examination of Bradstreet's writing reveals evidence of the conflict within the Puritan

COMPARE
&
CONTRAST

- **1660s:** Seventeenth-century American colonists, as subjects of the English Crown, do not have a central governing body that presides over the colonies as a whole. Rather, individual colonies are ruled by governors. Bradstreet's father, Thomas Dudley, serves as a governor of the Massachusetts Bay Colony for a time, as does her husband, Simon Bradstreet.

  Today: Today the United States government is organized around three individual branches, designed to balance the power held by any one person or group. The three branches are the legislative (which includes Congress and the House of Representatives), the judiciary (the federal courts), and the executive (the offices of the president, vice president, and cabinet members). Each state is governed by its own legislative, judiciary, and executive branches.

- **1660s:** Religious groups in the American colonies include the Protestant sect known as the Puritans, as well as Quakers and Baptists. Many practitioners of these faiths fled England, where punishments for nonconformity to the Church of England included violent beatings, maiming, and death.

  Today: The most prominent religion in the United States, according to a 2007 study by the Pew Forum on Religion and Public Life, is Protestantism, a designation that, in the Pew survey, includes, among many, Baptists, Lutherans, Methodists, and modern evangelical Protestants. The next most prominent religion in the United States is Catholicism.

- **1660s:** American poetry is formal in structure, containing regular rhyme patterns and metrical structure. The works of such early American poets as Anne Bradstreet and Edward Taylor are largely religious in nature and are often viewed as devotional pieces to God.

  Today: Much of modern American poetry is free verse poetry, poetry without set metrical structure or rhyme patterns. No subject is off limits to modern American poets, who write freely about religion, sexuality, war, and everyday life, among other topics. Other poets devote themselves to the more formal poetic structures of the past. This movement, known as New Formalism, began in the 1970s and remains popular today. Twenty-first century New Formalist poets include such writers as Dana Michael Gioia and Rachel Hadas.

community regarding the best way to approach their faith in the new land. Conflict within the community stemmed from disagreements about biblical interpretation, the nature and proof of salvation in church members, as well as church organization and the relationship of the church to the larger secular community. In general, Puritans focused on a strict moderation and regulation of their earthly desires, and their relationship with God was the supreme guiding force in their lives. Nothing in one's personal life—not relationships, possessions, or vocation—was supposed to interfere with one's devotion to God. Suffering and hardships were paths toward God, lessons in personal humility, and faith in God's justice.

Seventeenth-Century Colonial Women

Women in colonial New England helped to settle a land that bore little resemblance to the established communities in the England they had left. Elaine Showalter, in her 2009 examination of the American women writers, *A Jury of Her Peers: American Women Writers from Anne Bradstreet to Annie Proulx*, describes Bradstreet's life as one of "extraordinary danger and deprivation." In discussing the physical tasks required of the women of the Massachusetts Bay Colony, Showalter itemizes the household duties that were required of women, tasks that included all of the cooking, cleaning, sewing, and laundering. Showalter also observes that women faced the challenges of giving birth and nurturing infants and children "in the wilderness." Similarly, Adrienne Rich, in her foreword to *The Works of Anne Bradstreet*, edited by Jeannine Hensley and published in 1967, describes the New England colonies in the early 1600s as "a time and place in which heroism was a necessity of life." Rich further delineates Bradstreet's challenges as a female author living in colonial America when she praises Bradstreet's exceptional poetry, which was written, she states, while Bradstreet was "rearing eight children, lying frequently sick, keeping house at the edge of wilderness." Compounding the normal daily struggles faced by a mother of eight in frontier Massachusetts were the additional spiritual challenges faced by Puritan women. According to Susan Pérez Castillo's 1990 essay on gender roles and conflict within the colonial Puritan community, (an essay published in the Portuguese journal *Revista da Faculdade de Letras Do Porto: Linguas e Literaturas*), Puritan women were viewed as "irresponsible minors" and subject to punishment by their husbands for violating both civil and religious law. Castillo goes on to identify other oppressive regulations of female behavior, noting that women were not allowed to vote or to ask questions during church gatherings and were viewed as individuals likely to tempt men into illicit actions. Colonial New England Puritans, according to Showalter, clung to the notion of male intellectual superiority, yet women such as Bradstreet were nevertheless encouraged in their writing rather than punished.

CRITICAL OVERVIEW

The known early criticism of Anne Bradstreet's poetry centers largely on the 1650 edition of *The Tenth Muse Lately Sprung Up in America*. The contemporary opinions regarding her work appear to have been largely favorable. For example, Jeannine Hensley, in her introduction to the 1967 *The Works of Anne Bradstreet* speaks of the "general approval" Bradstreet's first volume of poetry received. In Rosamond Rosenmeier's introduction to *Anne Bradstreet Revisited*,

her 1991 study of Bradstreet and her work, the critic observes that Bathsua Mankin (a female English writer and critic who lived during the same time period as Bradstreet) ranked Bradstreet as an "excellent Poet." Rosenmeier also finds that, Bradstreet's work seems to have been highly regarded during the next century as well; she cites the praise lavished on Bradstreet by the New England Puritan minister and writer Cotton Mather (1663–1728) as evidence of Bradstreet's reputation as an admired poet.

More recent criticism explores individual poems in depth. Criticism of Bradstreet's "Upon the Burning of Our House" focuses heavily on the tension between the poet's response to her tragedy and her Puritanism. Jim Egan, in his 1999 *Authorizing Experience: Refigurations of the Body Politic in Seventeenth-Century New England Writing*, explores the way the conflict between the experience of grief and the reassurances offered by the Puritan faith are mitigated in Bradstreet's "Upon the Burning of Our House." In examining the poem, Egan finds that Bradstreet strives "to redirect longing away from family and toward God," but that despite her efforts, "Bradstreet persists in distrusting experience" as a means of preparation for "spiritual existence." Mitchell Breitwieser, in his 2007 *National Melancholy: Mourning and Opportunity in Classic American Literature*, examines Bradstreet's elegies as explorations of loss and as challenges to Puritanism. Breitwieser describes "Upon the Burning of Our House" as "Bradstreet's boldest defense of mourning," in that the poem features not a person, but a material object—Bradstreet's home—as "the lost object of love." Similarly, Elaine Showalter, in her 2009 study of American female authors *A Jury of Her Peers: American Women Writers from Anne Bradstreet to Annie Proulx*, emphasizes that Bradstreet's "Upon the Burning of Our House" reflects the emotional distress the poet felt in spite of her attempts "to interpret the catastrophe as a divine warning against vanity and materialism."

CRITICISM

Catherine Dominic

Dominic is a novelist and a freelance writer and editor. In the following essay, she studies the transitions in Bradstreet's "Upon the Burning of Our

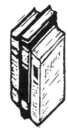

WHAT DO I READ NEXT?

- *To My Husband and Other Poems*, published in 2000 by Dover Publications, is a collection featuring Bradstreet's best-known and highly regarded poems, including romantic verses to her husband. The collection also includes a selection of poems on motherhood and domestic life, and on the deaths of her parents and grandchildren.

- *Mistress Bradstreet: The Untold Life of America's First Poet*, published in 2005 by Little, Brown, is a biography of Anne Bradstreet by Charlotte Gordon. Gordon explores Bradstreet's life and work within the context of the hardships endured by the settlers of the Massachusetts Bay Colony.

- *An American Triptych: Anne Bradstreet, Emily Dickinson, and Adrienne Rich*, written by Wendy Martin and published in 1984 by the University of North Carolina Press, studies Bradstreet, Dickinson, and Rich as examples of feminist poets from three different time periods. Martin explores the way each woman's society and culture shaped her views and her poetry.

- *The Account of Mary Rowlandson and Other Captivity Narratives*, edited by Horace Kephart and published by Dover Publications in 2005, is a collection of captivity narratives (accounts, sometimes fictionalized, of early colonists being captured by Native Americans), including Rowlandson's, which is among the best known of such narratives. Rowlandson, a contemporary of Bradstreet, was held captive by the Narragansett Indians in 1676, and her account of the experience (*A True History of the Captivity and Restoration of Mrs. Mary Rowlandson*) was published in 1682. The work describes the hardships she endured and also contains her observations on daily life in a Native American community.

- *The Puritan Dilemma: The Story of John Winthrop*, written by Edmund S. Morgan, was originally published in 1958; a third edition was published by Longman in 2005. The work describes the experiences of Winthrop, who led English Puritans to New England in 1630; the Bradstreets sailed with him on the journey. Morgan's work provides a young adult audience with the historical and religious background of the time period.

- *The Witch of Blackbird Pond*, written by Elizabeth George Speare, was originally published in 1958 and was reissued through Laurel Leaf in 1978. The book, which takes place in the Colony of Connecticut in 1687, is considered a classic young adult novel of historical fiction. The Newbery Award–winning novel explores, through the character of a young girl and the Quaker widow she befriends, the religious and political conflicts in New England Puritan communities. For the student of Bradstreet's work, the novel provides a glimpse of the changes and developments in Puritan society.

- *I, Too, Sing America: Three Centuries of African American Poetry*, edited by Catherine Clinton and illustrated by Stephen Alcorn, is a collection of poems by African Americans. Some of the poems were written as early as the 1700s, offering students of Bradstreet's poetry a look at the way poetry developed in colonial America (and beyond) among individuals with a different perspective. Targeted at young adult readers, the book was published by Houghton Mifflin Books for Children in 1998.

House, July 10th, 1666" that reveal the tension between the dictates of the poet's Puritan faith and her natural need to grieve in the aftermath of the tragedy. She argues that the persistent shifts in focus, from faith, to grief, and back again, reveal the highly personal nature of the poem as well as *demonstrating the emotional effects of the unresolved internal battle Bradstreet endures.*

Bradstreet's "Upon the Burning of Our House, July 10th, 1666" swings like a pendulum between Bradstreet's Puritan beliefs and her deep emotional turmoil regarding the loss of her home. While it is tempting to try to assess whether or not Bradstreet's sorrow is successfully mitigated or addressed by her faith, such an exercise would not only be highly subjective, but would also be misguided. It will always be debatable whether or not there is a clear winner in the conflict between grief and faith in the poem; rather, what is most significant is the nature of this battle. The poem's final lines emphasize the futility of attempting to draw definitive conclusions about any resolution Bradstreet may have been conveying. In these last two lines, Bradstreet divulges her desire for her spiritual beliefs to be sufficient to see her through her life so that she may one day reside in heaven. Of crucial importance here is that Bradstreet ends the poem with a prayer for assistance; she asks to be relieved of her love for her life on earth. The only certainty "Upon the Burning of Our House" offers is that Bradstreet longs for her faith to satisfy her emotional and spiritual needs. Whether or not it possesses that ability or even that potential is not conveyed; there is no resolution for Bradstreet. However, an examination of the poem's twists and turns, of the way the battle between grief and faith is waged, illuminates the poet's sense of longing, mourning, and conflict and aids in the reader's understanding of the poem's resultant tension.

"Upon the Burning of Our House" shifts repeatedly from the poet's extreme emotional distress to her grasping at the structures of her Puritan faith for support. In the poem's first seven lines, Bradstreet describes the scene of waking from sleep during the night to the terrifying noises and sights of the house fire within which she finds herself. In these moments of horror, she turns to God, making the first of many transitions in the poem from her emotional suffering to her seeking of strength in her faith. Lines 8 through 10 mark her first appeal to God; they are a simple request for emotional and spiritual support. Bradstreet turns quickly back to the trial at hand in lines 11 through 13, where she watches the flames devastate her home. Her phrasing in these lines suggests she is almost unable to look away from this horrifying scene,

> THE ONLY CERTAINTY 'UPON THE BURNING OF OUR HOUSE' OFFERS IS THAT BRADSTREET LONGS FOR HER FAITH TO SATISFY HER EMOTIONAL AND SPIRITUAL NEEDS. WHETHER OR NOT IT POSSESSES THAT ABILITY OR EVEN THAT POTENTIAL IS NOT CONVEYED; THERE IS NO RESOLUTION FOR BRADSTREET."

but when she does, in line 14, it is to praise God, and to remind herself that God both gives and takes. Bradstreet spends less time than before in the spiritual world of her faith, unable in the immediacy of the tragedy to take any comfort in God. Although she has sought God's aid, the most solace she can glean from her faith at the moment is the acknowledgement of God's ability to take away some of the gifts he has blessed her with—her home and her possessions. In line 15, Bradstreet focuses on what God has done, stating that it was God who rendered all her personal belongs into dust.

Just as instinctively as Bradstreet turns to God for comfort, she also posits blame for the tragedy with him. Yet her shame in doing so springs up just as quickly, in lines 16 through 18, revealing a new dimension to her faith. In these lines, Bradstreet insists it is God's will, not her own, that is just. Deferring to God's judgment, Bradstreet chastises herself for having felt wronged by God's actions. She reminds herself that she should not complain. Lines 19 and 20 indicate the poet's insistence that God is just, and that he has left her family with what they need in life, nothing more. In her emphasis on being provided with what God has determined to be sufficient, Bradstreet suggests her own guilt in having wanted more than what God has determined she needs.

Despite the poet's guilt in having wanted more than God deemed necessary, in having desired more than God thought she deserved, Bradstreet nevertheless returns to the subject of what she has possessed, belongings she has cherished, items she no longer has. Lines 21 through 35 represent Bradstreet's extended exploration of her loss and grief. She allows herself for the first time a space of uninterrupted mourning. For fifteen lines, Bradstreet does not interrupt her grief with her self-admonishment regarding her need for greater faithfulness. She ceases blaming herself for wanting material possessions, and she relinquishes, for a short while, the scolding and shaming. Bradstreet tenderly lays to rest a past lived in what appears to have been a pleasant and joyful home. One can intuit from these lines that to this point Bradstreet's life, whatever its tragedies, was also filled with joy and love. The depth of her sorrow at her loss suggests how truly she must have enjoyed a happy and loving home before the fire. Bradstreet offers equal tribute to the home's contents, its former guests, the stories told, and the memories her family created there. She speaks of favorite things and pleasantries, dinners shared and stories swapped. Her images capture not just objects, but the subtleties of what constitutes a home. Bradstreet grieves, observing that all such memories have been silenced.

The next line of the "Upon the Burning of Our House," line 36, marks the poem's the next transition, and is jarring in its abruptness. Bradstreet first bids farewell, in French, to the remains of her beloved home, and in the next breath disregards the entire construct of home—her memories, her belongings—as a representation of her vanity. In characterizing so much as so little, Bradstreet shows the extent of her guilt regarding her attachment to her material possessions. From lines 36 through 52 she continues this process of devaluing the objects and concepts that she has just mourned. She chides and scolds herself for not trusting God and derides her belongings as meaningless. Perhaps the most visually startling example of the poet's expressed contempt for her material wealth is her comparison of the ash from her burned home with the dust rising from a heap of dung. This characterization is so drastically different from what she has conveyed in the previous lines that one can either begin to doubt the poet's sincerity or pity her for her faith-inspired need to deny her genuine feelings of loss and grief. The extreme way in which Bradstreet attempts to renounce her attachment to her home and her treasures is a clear demonstration of the conflict her faith has generated within her. While Puritanism has taught her that nothing should be an obstacle in her devotion to God, her life experiences, as this poem suggests, have been so overwhelmingly positive that her

duty to her faith was extremely difficult to fulfill. In the poem, Bradstreet characterizes trials and suffering as instructive. Loss of personal items, as her lines indicate, should be viewed as a punishment for vain attachments to earthly possessions, and as a lesson that greater and permanent spiritual wealth awaits the faithful. To this point, Bradstreet has not only expressed heartfelt sorrow regarding her loss, she has conveyed extreme frustration with her own emotional reaction. She has loved deeply and, consequently, she mourns deeply. Compelled then to deny her bereavement, Bradstreet reveals the turmoil wrought by the Puritan notion that grieving for one's loss suggests that one bears too strong an attachment to material possessions and that such intense feelings regarding worldly objects and relationships impede the journey toward God.

The last two lines of the poem reveal much about the poet's attempts to place the fullness and richness of her life within the proper spiritual context. They are lines pregnant with doubt, confusion, and longing. After bidding farewell again to her possessions in line 52, lines 53 and 54 suggest her yearning for release from her worldly desires. Bradstreet seeks in these lines the ability to value her impending heavenly rewards more highly than her life in this world; she pleads to be allowed to possess this attitude. In making this request, it seems apparent that while she longs for the ability to see her life in this faithful way, she does not yet possess the proper Puritan attitude. At the heart of this poem is the turmoil in Bradstreet between what she should feel and what she does feel. The poet seeks an attitude, a Puritan mindset, in which the world is renounced in favor of God. At the same time she mourns for what she has lost, she grieves for her things, her memories, her past, her home. At the end of the poem, Bradstreet seems to be grieving precisely because she grieves at all for her loss.

Source: Catherine Dominic, Critical Essay on "Upon the Burning of Our House, July 10th, 1666," in *Poetry for Students*, Gale, Cengage Learning, 2010.

Tom Sleigh

In the following excerpt, Sleigh explains Bradstreet's view of "American" in American poetry.

As a boy, I remember one of the few Sundays that our family went to church. Our regular attendance was partly hampered by the fact that one Easter Sunday my older brother, on a dare from Weegee Hansen, hit Reverend Fox in the back of the head with a water balloon: you can imagine the withering effect this might have on tender religious feelings, especially when Reverend Fox turned up at our house later that afternoon, seeking, as he put it, "to wring that little sinner's neck." But on the particular Sunday I have in mind, Reverend Fox recounted the story of Saul on the way to Damascus, in which God knocks Saul, the Christian persecutor, off his horse and he rises up from the dust as the apostle Paul. The miracle of the conversion went right by me. All that I could think about was the fate of the horse: Was Paul a better master than Saul? When God knocked Saul into the dust, did the horse also feel the blow? What kind of fodder did the horse get that evening in Damascus? The fact that my mind focused on the horse first, and Saul second, indicates how far I am from comprehending the mind of a truly religious sensibility, for whom Paul's conversion would have been a template: the fallen consciousness is brought to God's light by the fire of faith, and the self that suffers the flames is all the better for the scorching.

Although my sympathies may lie with the horse and not with God's implacable heat, implicit in this conversion story are questions about identity, how it gets established, and what forces are sufficient to sponsor it. In the realm of poetry cocktail parties, you get to hear your share of conversion stories: cocktail parties being what they are, no one is under oath. And so I once witnessed a poet undergo multiple conversions in a single evening: depending on the confessor's faith, this Paul/Saul claimed to be an autobiographical poet one moment, a L=A=N=G=U=A=G=E poet the next, a narrative poet after that. Totally apart from whether or not these professions were sincere, is the question as to why a poet shouldn't be able to inhabit all these positions at the same time. And it's an interesting question as to why this kind of fluidity causes such unease in the poetry world, as well as in the realm of cultural debate. If you claim to be in league with the aesthetics of poet X, then you can't possibly like the work of poet Y.

One aspect of this unease is the ongoing and inevitable debate about the place of subjectivity in art. What are its limits and possibilities, its responsibilities and risks? The varying camps of cultural and critical theory in which "I" is both a grammatical project and projection of systems of power, and the almost pre-literate hostility that some poetic scribblers feel toward any attempt

> **ABSTRACTED FURTHER AND FURTHER FROM ITS DIVINE SOURCE, BRADSTREET'S VERSION OF A RELIGIOUS SELF GIVES WAY TO THE EMERSONIAN SELF, THE WHITMANIAN SELF."**

to call the authority of "I" into question, makes for a lot of noise—some of this noise is what a friend calls "a tempestio in a teapotio," the usual jockeying for audience that every generation is heir to, while some of it harks back to a reigning and basic question that underlies American imaginative writing from its beginning in Anne Bradstreet and Edward Taylor. Emerson formulated it when he asked what was "American" about American poetry, and what and whom should American poetry serve. But it exists in embryo in Bradstreet, when she declares that she wants no "Bayes" of laurel as handed down by tradition, but is content with a home-grown "wholsome Parsley wreath. . . ."

While the poem seems like a form of obeisance to God's inscrutable will, the poem seems to hint that all is not right in the New World's dunghill mists. Bradstreet's admission that the voices calling out "Fire" dovetail with a secret desire of her own makes one wonder about Bradstreet's hidden tendencies toward the community: is she a kind of spiritual pyromaniac wrestling with her more saintly self over how best to burn down God's house? Of course I realize that one of Bradstreet's aims is to use her own persona as a vehicle to proselytize. And from that point of view, her self-admonishments are both exemplary to others as well as sincerely felt. I suppose what I'm talking about is a kind of historical sixth sense that the poem exudes to a secular reader like myself. In Bradstreet's New World, the tenor of religious feeling is undergoing a subtle shift: because there are no rose windows and high-flying spires to buttress your belief, to a sincere Puritan like Bradstreet, God's personal presence begins to imbue everything, from a chest or a trunk to a burning house. And as God's personal involvement in your life increases, so too does His responsibility for your fortunes. And that level of personal intimacy is bound to have serious psychological consequences.

As I said before, I realize that my horsy loyalties may reflect my own secular shortcomings in understanding an intelligence like Bradstreet's. Nonetheless, when Bradstreet shifts from "I" to "thine" toward the end of the poem, I sense the ground of being shifting as the pronouns shift: this division of soul is finding expression on the level of grammar. Bradstreet's ambivalence about losing "that store I counted best" is subtly signaled by her use of the second and third person pronouns to address the "mighty Architect" and keep him at a slight grammatical remove. In contrast, she lavishes affection and regret on her burned out house by addressing it as "thee." And in the final couplet, Bradstreet's teethgritting resignation is likewise undercut by a subtle shift in pronouns in the last third of the poem. Once she learns that her house is on fire, she goes from addressing the Lord as "my God" in the eighth line, to calling on God in the third person, even while she tries to bless "His name that gave and took." Of course, one wonders why she should need to bless His name at all. Shouldn't she be the one asking for His blessing?

Further evidence of this psychic strain is the way she addresses herself in a strangely disassociated second person, which at first seems like a form of self-address, but in fact is an address to her house. When she says, "Under thy roof no guest shall sit," the psychic blurring between herself and her "pleasant things" that "in ashes lie" signals the spiritual depths in which she now burns. It's as if the shift in pronouns signals a clandestine desire to cut loose from the Puritan God and explore her own peculiar psychological mechanisms. She splits off from the sorrowing self in order to admonish that self, and in the process the "I" sanctioned by the divine principle has begun to split along the grain. The more Bradstreet exhorts herself to see in her personal tragedy a divine lesson, the further she ventures into her own subjective wilderness. Apparently obedient, her mind may be the horse ridden by God, but it harbors animal tendencies to rear up and throw Him.

Abstracted further and further from its divine source, Bradstreet's version of a religious self gives way to the Emersonian self, the Whitmanian self. For the self in American poetry has usually been dependent on some sponsoring transcendental source, even in a poem like "The Waste Land" with its reflexive inclusion of personified spiritual qualities of Datta (give), Dayadhvam (sympathize), and Damyatam (control) from the Upanishads, not to mention the weird, oneiric Christ-like figure wandering in the desert who sinisterly invites the reader to "Come in under the shadow of this red rock." Since its inception in Bradstreet, American poetry has never been content to let the self hang in the wind, subject to the uncertainty of its own status, but able to experience that uncertainty in its own independent way. And this seems as true to me now as it was to those in the seventeenth century.

When I mentioned this view to a friend of mine, he thought it was a pretty strange claim, since in his mind any poetry that wasn't overtly devotional more or less had to be based on epistemological uncertainty. And I don't disagree. Maybe what I'm talking about is more an attitude of inquiry, a special attentiveness to this metaphysically weightless condition. The image I have in mind is of a poet in a spacesuit, crossing the void with a little jet pack, and when that fails, behaving like Milton's Satan as he fights his way through chaos, who "With head, hands, wings, or feet pursues his way." In other words, to make that uncertainty a place to explore so that the poet doesn't try to vanquish it by falling back on universalizing abstractions—which are, as always, in abundant supply. In our age, God the supreme authority has been displaced by secular abstractions like "hegemonic discourse"; or if you are a semiologist, the "transcendental signifier." And the poetic doctrine of "deep image," which saw consciousness as a set of images pre-existent to tainted history, looks to Jung's notion of the collective unconscious as its sponsoring, transcendental authority. Even theories of poetry that stress language's primacy seem based on a displaced passion for the assertion in John: "In the beginning was the Word." And aesthetic stances like objectivism, imagism, and followers of projective verse tend to treat the world's surface as a kind of phenomenological absolute. We may give lip service to human subjectivity as its own self-sufficient cause for being, but even the scientific assumptions surrounding neurological research, such as the right-brain/left-brain structures of consciousness, have been enlisted as a way to root the self in something outside its own waveringly subjective force field and experiential flow. This scientific way of explaining consciousness as brain function resembles a kind of Cartesian variant: "If my mind is structured like this and perforce must think like that, therefore I am the projection of that structure that I think of as if it were my self."

Shifting from an epistemological to an historical perspective about the place of the self in American poetry, we return to the questions Emerson asked: what makes American poetry "American" and not European; and whom or what should American poetry serve. Frost's half-joking line, "The land was ours before we were the land's" points to not only the irony of a colonial situation in which the colonists, fleeing the oppression of their mother country, feel alienated in the promised land, but their unconscious arrogance in assuming that the land is theirs while being blind to their own murderous intention to take the land by force from its Indian inhabitants. Of course the ironies I'm deploying here are more mine than Frost's, since he did read the poem at John F. Kennedy's inauguration, hardly the venue for revisionist thoughts about the United States' westward expansion.

But if you squint at those lines from a certain historical perspective, Frost's repetition of "we" implies a queasiness about who this "we" really is, in which ethnic and class divisions are elided so that "we" may possess, and become possessed by, the land whose price "was many deeds of war." The answers to these questions about American poetry's status as American—which seem narrowly chauvinistic at worst, and at best a goad to make a "nation language" that isn't cowed by what Seamus Heaney once called "the Absolute Speaker" of bureaucratic and technocratic officialdom—don't seem to have entertained the notion that American poetry could be a force in its own right, a self-sufficient category of human consciousness. Either its purpose was to serve God in the New World theocracy; or, as democracy replaced theocracy, it must serve, according to Whitman, as a prophetic source for the ever renewing energies of democratic experiment.

But to return to Bradstreet: as Puritanism became less and less the attempt to fathom the mystery of God's grace in the New World wilderness, and more and more focused on individual salvation and self-scrutiny for the purpose of exposing sin, the native skepticism of such scrutiny inevitably turned against its transcendental author, the hitherto unimpeachable "I am that I am." Belief becomes non-belief through Puritanism's own genius for self-scrutiny and self-doubt,

and so the grounding authority of the self is forced to find new ground: Emerson floats the concept of the Over Soul, a version of God as human and human as God, but all so undifferentiated that the self begins to blur into universal consciousness: it becomes wispy, thin, fog that mists a mirror. And then Whitman attempts to clean the mirror by focusing on the body: this seems like a promising direction, to ground the self in the universality of sexual feeling; he calls this "adhesiveness," but his missionary zeal about eros as a democratic force doesn't take into account how oblique sex is, how opaque, how irremediable to generalization—people actually having sex in Whitman is too often a question of hygiene, physical and mental, and too seldom a matter of "sharp-toothed touch." Whitman's intuition of the self grounded in sexual pleasure smudges out into his proselytizing zeal to make us all into mothers and fathers of clean-limbed sons and daughters of the Republic.

After Whitman's vision of democracy based on the body gets trampled under by the Civil War and the national psyche splits into North and South; after the Robber Barons who endow our major museums cement the divisions between the classes; after advertising seduces the language of private desire into the language of consumerism; after Eliot and Pound explode the remnants of the self into the many voices of "The Waste Land," and the historical perspectives and personae of the *Cantos*; after New Criticism puts pressure on the work and begins to displace the author as the subject of literary study; after autobiography becomes just another form of psychological and historical projection; after "confessional poetry" becomes simply a blanket term of disapproval of certain kinds of done-to-death subject matter; after the death of the author, both as a joke and as a serious challenge to the myth of authorial mastery over language; after re-readings of cultural icons like Shakespeare, such that Shakespeare's heroes are removed from the realm of action in the world, and made into specular instances of various schools of psychoanalytic and cultural critique; after media conglomeration and the proliferation of "real time," "real life" news coverage and television shows, such that the self observing the self impersonating the self becomes the most current form of naturalism; after a sense of time as serial begins to fragment into a sense of time as discrete, so that the actual moment of writing becomes part of the drama of writing, as in Beckett's speakers who make the phenomenon of their own vocalizing the focus of the story; after all this, who would dare claim that the "I" isn't a phantom and a projection of language, a mere grammatical convenience? Add to all this the lingering prestige of the Tel Quel group declaring that writing (as Italo Calvino informs us in his essay, "Cybernetics and Ghosts") no longer consists in "narrating but in saying that one is narrating." According to this idea, the immediate claim of sympathy on the reader by an "I" confident of its status as not only a linguistic entity, but as a flesh and blood speaker whose fate is of intrinsic interest, has come to an end. What one says becomes identified with the act of saying. The psychological person is really a grammatical person, defined by its place in the discourse.

But I balk at this—there is something a little canned about all of it, a little too symptomatic of a kind of expected, "with it" theorizing that ignores what I feel when I write. And so I don't quite know how to take my own list...is it merely poetry gloom, culture gloom, spleen? Or in a more serious vein, could the list be symptomatic of a desire to make up stories that would join in the weave of stories that blanket all earth's creatures in an atmosphere of compassion and intelligent concern—what Teilhard de Chardin called the noosphere? If this notion seems a little too idealized, its hard-headed corollary would be a pluralist, quasi-anthropological way of understanding the world, in which there are many different cosmologies and cultures all functioning with equal authority, if not equal in their political and economic status.

Both of these models pose a quiet challenge to what vestiges of the Whitmanian self remain. After all, when Whitman says, "I do not ask the wounded person how he feels, I myself become the wounded person," underneath the well-meant identification, a certain violence is being done in that omission to ask. Yes, the poet is identifying with the wounded, but the identification is also a kind of erasure of that person's local cultural and historical circumstances. So is there a way of allowing the voice of the wounded to speak through the poem, while preserving the right of the poet to make the kind of confident self-assertions that Whitman makes? In other words, how can the poet make the partiality of "I" into an interesting formal feature among many, as opposed to the be-all end-all of

lyric utterance? More importantly, how can the solitary singer's story participate in the larger story, as Wallace Stevens puts it, "of the planet of which it was part. . ."?

My notion of the "I"'s partiality depends to a certain extent on understanding the range of solutions to the problem of solitary singing and its potential participation in the larger story of the planet. One of the most prevalent solutions has been to favor dissolution of the teller of tales into a tale telling itself, language out on its own space walk, floating through referentiality, as opposed to being anchored in it. You might call this a constructivist perspective, in which words have their own autonomy and plasticity, and meaning doesn't depend upon a solitary singer, but is the result of the poet's exploratory relationship to many different lexicons, ranging from the slogans of advertising to political rhetoric to the whisperings of private feeling. Of course the danger here is relegating the singer to a language prop, or what one critic dubbed the "subjectivity effect."

And then there's Allen Ginsberg's notion of poetry as "first thought, best thought." This approach makes the solitary singer's song the by-product of a meditative practice of mindfulness that would release us from the world of illusion to the eternal truths behind the veil of Maya. To further that recognition, Ginsberg was willing to sacrifice what he called "the whole boatload of sensitive bullshit" that undergirded the myth of poetic mastery. A poem's *raison d'être* is to serve as a prayer wheel whose mind-expanding spin helps us contemplate the inexhaustible forms of reality, and of the unity behind those forms. His poetry of swift notation proposes that the self is nothing more—or less—than the ebb and flow of perception, in which perception is a springboard to comprehending the Oneness of the universe.

Another tack is Robert Duncan's practice of poetry as composition by field: the page is a field of possibility and the words are actions on that field. That the actions are of consequence becomes a matter of knowing when the self is at the right spiritual pitch to plot a significant course in words, the words open to the accident of inspiration at every moment of composition. There is no perfected "form" for the poem to take on, no conventional adherence to beginnings, middles, or ends. Every poem the poet writes is really the sign of a continually unfolding revelation that only comes to an end at the poet's death—and not even then, because the story is taken up by other poets, and in Auden's phrase, "modified in the guts of the living."

And now I hesitate. My sense of the dilemma that faces contemporary poets and how they represent "I" might simply boil down to this: no matter how fragmented words appear on a page, they will tell a certain story, if only as the trace of the mind that willed them onto the paper. And so the "I" is still intact, if not as a personality in words, then as words diffusing the traces of a personality, a doppelgänger projected outward from the page. And so the mere presence of a poem suggests that the poet is also a subjective presence, if only as a projection of the operations of language. Well, and so what? Who didn't know that if you saw marks on a page that someone put them there? But is that really as obvious as it sounds? Well, yes—provided that you're willing to grant those marks the provisional status of "author"—but if you aren't, or if your initial reaction is to think this is writing, *l'écriture*, an inheritance of the tribe's codes and customs, as opposed to thinking this is the texture of an individual mind, then the question of the authority of who is speaking becomes important in our experience of these marks.

Most serious readers float somewhere halfway between these two shores and reserve judgment about the issue of authority until they are well into the experience of reading. But this very reservation of judgment is also a hesitation that affects writers: I can identify at least three tendencies in American poetry that this self-consciousness has engendered: the fact that "I" has been impeached as too confident in its pronouncements has forced some poets to adopt the tone of self-reflexive irony and jokiness that undercuts the commitment of the voice to any particular tone, stance, or provisional stab at truth. This is an extremely popular stance, and amounts to a widespread period style. Another strategy is to adopt the tone of phenomenological inquiry, but to do it in such a way that suggests an obsessive temperament relentlessly interrogating perception: the stance here is that the obsession flows from an obsession with "truth"—a truth that may already be discredited as merely a projection of human desires, but is better than nothing. When this stance amounts to more than a surface manner, it can produce poems of great power and integrity, as in the

work of Frank Bidart, or in the best poems of John Ashbery. But all too often, it degenerates into the third tendency: an armored, "smart" sounding vocabulary that steers back and forth between the referential and the hiply non-referential, a kind of brainy, process-is-all surrealism that at its best promises verbal innovation, and at its worst feels utterly formulaic in its disjunct leaps of association—a more complex variant of the above mentioned joky ironist, but who as an undergraduate read a smattering of Lyotard and Baudrillard and picked up their tone of philosophical inquiry.

But let me put my cards on the table and suggest another way of thinking about the impeached "I." What I'm proposing is not to be taken as a manifesto, but a speculation on how the self in poetry is a kind of self-impersonation, the subject of a voice, or voices, that are always aware of their own provisional status. As I mentioned earlier, I want to incorporate that provisionality into the poem's formal structure. The shortcoming in Whitman's stance toward the wounded, in which Whitman desires to be the wounded person, is that he seems unconscious of his own limited subjectivity. The verbal formulas Whitman resorts to, the catalog, the relentless parallelisms, speak to the automatic nature of Whitman's response. And the difference between a poem like "The Waste Land" in its multiple voicings and many-eyed perspectives, and my speculation, has to do with Eliot's manipulation of the voices in the poem. Great a poem as it is, there is something faintly imperious about Eliot's virtuosity, the sense of a puppet master deploying the materials of his poem with just a touch too much certainty. The material, for all its portents of chaos, never really seems on the verge of spinning out of control. And it's precisely this sense of the material beginning to get away from the poet, the sense that the voices in the poem have an autonomy beyond the authorial presence, that interests me. And from a reader's viewpoint, I mean more than the fact that poems often bear contrary meanings to their authors' overt intentions, as in the case of Blake reading Milton and saying that Milton was of the Devil's party, but without knowing it. In my scenario, the poet is deeply attuned to the paradoxes and contradictions inherent in having both devils and angels whispering in his ear: the poet must express, simultaneously, the many ways that such opposing and unruly recognitions might function in a poem.

Many contemporary writers have responded to this question of self as self-impersonation, but what do I mean by that phrase? Of course, it's a truism that the first thing any writer does is impersonate whoever the "I" is that does the writing. Italo Calvino, in an essay on the levels of reality in literature, creates a flow chart that starts with Gustave Flaubert, the author of various books who then impersonates the author of the book he is currently working on, in this case, *Madame Bovary,* who then projects himself into Emma Bovary who then projects herself into the Emma Bovary she would like to be. The salient thing about this flow chart is that it works in reverse as well, with each link in the chain reaction transforming, both forwards and back, all the other links. So when Flaubert says, "Madame Bovary, c'est moi," the question arises as to how much of the "I" who shapes the characters is, in fact, an "I" who has been shaped by the characters. In American literature, this way of thinking has been taken to an extreme point by a poet like James Merrill in "*The Changing Light at Sandover,*" in which the poem's author, James Merrill, is also the speaker of the poem who also becomes a character denominated in his speeches by the initials, JM, even as the entire poem's cosmological machinery is made present to the author/character through the oracular voicings of a Ouija board. This is obviously a radically different and mischievous way of thinking about writing than the myth of the writer as a little god or as a master of language who "treats" his material by giving it style. But you don't have to go as far as Merrill does in order to see that this flow chart notion of intersubjectivity upends the traditional hierarchy of author set above his so-called "characters."

How seriously do I mean all this? I don't for a moment imagine that anyone will sit down with this model in their head and apply it systematically. But what I'm interested in is finding a way of talking about the slippery transactions that go on between whoever "I" is and the words that "I" is putting on the page: the old model of revision as the writer working toward a formal unity seems to me far too limiting a description of the possible ways of writing poems. And since one of the crucial determinants in how you think about the art is the way you envision embodying the self in language, I'm interested in putting forth a new description that opens up the old model, if not exactly exploding it. The various levels of reality that interact in the creation of art, the empirical, psychological, supernatural, aesthetic, mythic, all of which sort together in a play like *Hamlet* (*e.g.*, the political rottenness of

Denmark; Hamlet's state of mind; Hamlet's father's ghost; the play within the play; and the actors killed off as characters and resurrected as themselves at the curtain call), suggest just how insufficient and blinkered this all too settled notion of "I" is.

But how would a poet actually write the kind of poem I envision? Let's imagine P walking down the street to do some shopping, his own internal monologue fissioning off in various directions: PTA, long-ago memories of late-night heroin parties, a fantasy about the Medal of Honor being given to John Waters, a plan to set aside certain hours in the afternoon to re-read Paul Valery's musings on the character of Monsieur Teste, that monster of abstraction who knows the plasticity of thought because everything Monsieur Teste thinks his mind obligingly performs. P has a little notebook in his pocket, and suddenly these random thoughts begin to suggest words: the words keep getting distracted by a not-too-original erotic fantasy, a sort of bookmark that marks off the page of desire that P is currently perusing. But brushing away the thought, P sits on a bench, takes out the notebook, all the while feeling a little foolish to be doing this outdoors at a bus stop rather than at home at his desk: but the words are beginning to announce themselves: "The window is stuck. First tragedy of the day." And suddenly P is no longer P, he is stretched between his various thoughts and roles, he is stepping out of his skin and plunging into the currents of language. As P scribbles though, he begins to be aware of other P's that want to say things: the P that doubts that windows are tragedies, the P that wants to salvage that sense of tragedy by turning it into a joke, the P that begins to feel despair that any of these words will ever make it into a finished poem, let alone get published in a book of poems. And then P has a savage turn against the "I" that is writing the poem and puts down the notebook in disgust, suddenly torn between his sense of real tragedies, what he knows is the political awareness of the poem, and his desire to insist on the window's stuckness as indeed feeling like a tragedy, a metaphysical condition he can't escape from. And so the poet is stretched between politics and transcendence, and feels a growing hostility toward any settled position, and more and more desperate to be affected by, and responsive to, all positions at once. In Seamus Heaney's words, the poet is disposed to be "negatively rather than positively capable."

And then he begins to pull away from the window and to try to view it from the farthest reaches of space, or to view it from as great a temporal distance as possible, in order to give that negative capability free play. Now he is channeling the spirit of George Herbert in which a human being "is a brittle crazie glass"; and as he peers through that glass he's also looking through Larkin's high windows, meditating on the "sun-comprehending glass, / And beyond it, the deep blue air, that shows / Nothing, and is nowhere, and is endless," and suddenly he is taking out his pencil again and writing a very different kind of poem: a poem that might say "I," but in which a "self-forgetful, perfectly useless concentration," in Elizabeth Bishop's phrase, has taken over all the anxieties, the hesitations and squirmings. And what to say about his concentration except that it seems neither an act of the self or the product of the many different voices that consciousness is woven from. It speaks, as Kafka says, with the voice of an alien stranger, but a stranger whose voice seems to resonate inside P, if not exactly belonging to P. And of course that voice keeps diffusing into voices: the voice of tradition that Herbert and Larkin represent, the voice of the social world that P inhabits, the voice of English itself in the way it inflects, reflects, and projects outward the words flowing from that "self-forgetful, perfectly useless concentration," in which will and imagination are involved in a call and response of completely mutual entailment.

I realize that this description can be dismissed as mere soft-focus blur—but that blur seems more true to the actual process of writing a poem than a more coherent laying out of terms and principles based on a myth of mastery of language. Of course, allowing yourself such permeability is its own talent. I see in that talent a kind of transcendent achievement that nevertheless has nothing to say definitively about the transcendence of the self. Of course, much contemporary academic criticism has focused on calling into question the notion of a transcendental self, and in the process tries to eliminate the concept of individual authorial genius as a necessary criterion of literary and cultural value. These attitudes are expressed in the various HOW TO READ theories, in which an interpretive grid is laid on top of a poem so that it produces certain kinds of meanings in relation to that grid. My focal point is somewhat different, in that I am not so much interested in how

we read, as in the experience of understanding what happens to us as we read. And since I'm a writer, I take the further step of trying to account for what happens to us as we write. If that's your point of entry, then what you are doing is trawling through your own unconscious processes for some glints and gleams that might prove useful to others when hauled up into the light. So when I say that the myth of mastery over language is insufficient and blinkered, I'm not doing so to undermine the difficulty of the art of poetry, and how the genius of individual poets negotiates that difficulty. What I am doing is hoping to find some inklings and intuitions that will suggest a more comprehensive model of subjectivity for the working artist.

I want poetry to be as complex, as resistant to easy generalization, and as humanly capacious as Proust's *Remembrance of Things Past* (one of the obvious models for Merrill's "The Changing Light at Sandover"). The many levels of reality the novel occurs on are paralleled by how the "I" can be split into a number of voices, all working under the aegis of the Argus-eyed Marcel: the narrator who writes the work (or rather complains about not writing the work), the sufferer of the narrator's tale who lives out what the narrator is nerving himself up to write, the social commentator of drawing rooms and bedrooms, the cultural historian of a bygone era. This many-eyed way of seeing many-leveled reality suggests, for poetry, the obvious analog of many different kinds of speech sorting together, with no self-consciousness about juxtaposing wildly differing lexicons and forms of diction. And this is precisely the procedure of John Ashbery. But Ashbery's is not the name that seems to exemplify in the fullest way possible the potentialities of a multiply overlapping "I." In fact, Ashbery's multi-vocal, multi-perspectived way of writing a poem isn't so much a form of provisionality as a settled stance. In other words, the formal inventiveness in Ashbery has crystallized beyond the point where the formal structure of the poem is being called into question. Despite the associative movement that Ashbery has perfected, his poems as formal structures are fairly static. A reader knows more or less the linguistic territory Ashbery will inhabit, and from that settled perspective there is capacious, often brilliant insight into the "solving emptiness" that underlies daily life. But despite the standard critical line that Ashbery is a poet of ceaseless transformations, what I feel in his poems is a fatalist at work. Ashbery's ingenuity as a rhetorician doesn't extend to wanting to ground the "I" in a unitary identity, so as to call that identity into question, to explode it, to deny its existence, to diffuse it into the quietly rebellious pronouns at work in Anne Bradstreet's poem, or the myriad other operations you can perform. In other words, Ashbery assumes the multiplicity of "I," but never does that enter into his poems as a process of ongoing revelation. Consequently, Ashbery represents what Elizabeth Bishop once called "the mind at rest," as opposed to "the mind in motion."

Source: Tom Sleigh, "Self as Self-Impersonation in American Poetry," in *Virginia Quarterly Review*, Vol. 82, No. 1, Winter 2006, pp. 174–89.

William J. Scheick

In the following excerpt, Scheick examines the aesthetic dislocations in Bradstreet's verse.

. . . Arguments particularly fail to account for the aesthetic dislocations in Bradstreet's verse. These moments are too peculiar to be designated as the result of convention or tradition. Consider, for instance, the private and posthumously published poem "Upon the Burning of Our House, July 10th, 1666," in which a number of critics (e.g., Stanford, "Dogmatist"; Wess; Martin) have detected a tension between emotion and belief. This verse commences by recalling in detail many of the poet's prized material possessions lost in the fire. During most of the poem Bradstreet intently revisualizes these lost objects, only to stop the enumeration abruptly, *as if* some part of her mind had suddenly realized the impropriety of such a recollection. Indeed, before this brusque halt, the implicit direction of her poem threatens to unleash her anger at the deity, who ultimately is responsible for her loss. She halts this dangerous veering of her verse by interjecting, "Adeiu, Adeiu, All's Vanity" (237).

The explicit sentiment of this line, safely ventriloquized in the language of Ecclesiastes 1:14, can readily be explained by arguments for the poet's application of literary and heuristic conventions. Turning to scripture, as if to prayer, to thwart insurgent sentiment is culturally prescribed for a Puritan. What cannot be explained by these arguments is the aesthetic effect of this maneuver. To put the matter simply, something aesthetically disjunctive occurs in this short, stifled line when compared to what has preceded it in the poem. There is no "poetry"

in this formulaic line, no detail, which is another way of saying that its alleged instruction does not inhabit the emotion-laden, well-furnished house of the poem as the poem has been constructed up to this point. The line is devoid of the harmony of aesthetics and emotion that has been evident until this line appears.

Instead of reflecting the poetic embodiment of literary and rhetorical conventions—say, the decorum of imperfection (Mignon) or the logogic site (Scheick, *Design 2*)—this particular line of verse records the sudden intrusion of an ideological convention from *outside* the aesthetic/domestic feelings, from *outside* the authorial presence, previously evident in the poem. As a site of logonomic conflict, the disruptive nature of this line may represent some theocratic ideal, but it also signals the flight of the poet from her potentially rebellious sentiment, as if the house of her emotion-full verse were also dangerously on fire.

The poem, in fact, now disintegrates into a "heap" of routine religious questions. These questions are "narratively" designed, with or without the poet's conscious consent, to suspend and contain the feelings featured in the first part of her poem. These concluding questions reveal a bifurcating tension in the poet and her verse, whether or not she is aware of it. They indicate, finally, just how difficult it is for Bradstreet, at an unconscious level at least, to renounce her secularly valued material possessions and her secularly defined identity expressed in a smoldering anger over temporal losses.

"Upon My Son Samuel His Going to England, Novem. 6, 1657," another private and posthumously published verse, likewise conveys "a hint of the struggle" between emotion and belief (White 309). It does so, narratively at least, by fissuring in a manner similar to "Upon the Burning of Our House." This later poem opens with Bradstreet's indication of the ways she will praise God if her son safely returns to her after his perilous transatlantic voyage. After sixteen well-managed lines of this sentiment, the poet abruptly interjects an extremely terse introduction of the other possibility: "If otherwise I goe to Rest, / Thy Will bee done, for that is best." Again the poet follows the cultural prescription to turn to scripture, this time the Lord's Prayer (Luke 11:2), to counter unsanctioned sentiment. And again there is an aesthetic price. The abbreviated and formulaic manner of these lines, akin to the sudden line of emotionally-vacant formula in "Upon the Burning of House," intimate the flight of the poet from her poem, no longer a safe vessel of her emotion.

Cast adrift, the poet's abandoned feelings need mooring, and so in the next two concluding lines of her poem she asks the deity to "Perswade [her] heart" to accept divine will should this terrible event occur. The request for persuasion is also clearly an indication of her need to be persuaded. If the possible loss of her son is a thought Bradstreet must entertain, it is not a possibility that she can naturally accept, whatever the authority behind it. Foundering on this discord, the poem (over-freighted with both disclosed and undisclosed feelings) can find no satisfying theocratic port. The poem is, accordingly, abandoned as the poet withdraws her emotional and aesthetic presence from the compromised vessel of her verse.

Such a performance in this poem and in "Upon the Burning of Our House," among many others, does not successfully conform to, or revise, or ironically engage any Renaissance literary tradition. If intended as hagiography in conformity with Reformed tradition, such a performance is likewise badly flawed because the idealized example of the second part is so pale, so flat, and so impoverished in aesthetic and emotional register when compared to the individualized fervid example of the first part. One readily wonders what normal reader would prefer this second voice to the first. Is it not altogether likely that the more human voice would continue to linger, like an elegiac ghost, in the memory of the reader even after this voice had been hagiographically banished at the end of these two severely bifurcated poems?

The disruptive lines in "Upon the Burning of Our House" and "Upon My Son Samuel" indicate some deep conflict that cannot be perfectly negotiated by the application, revision, or ironic articulation of any literary convention or tradition available to the poet. The displacement of sincerity, sentiment, and aesthetics by arid formula results in the fracturing of both poems into two disjunctive pieces that the poet, much less the reader, cannot satisfactorily associate. Disclosure of feeling becomes non-disclosure, and this development signals a progressive atrophy of sincerity, sentiment, and artistry.

How much of this disjunction was perceived by the poet remains uncertain. Although both poems exist in manuscript only in her son Simon's hand, it is probably safe to assume that Bradstreet left them substantially as they are and so possibly did not quite see the effects of this conflict on her art. Today, for that matter, the fissures that result from the seismic activity of constrained resistance and declared conformity beneath the surface of Bradstreet's art are visible to many readers. For our purposes, finally, two observations are important: not everything in Bradstreet's verse can be identified as authorially deliberate, especially apropos tradition or convention; and occasionally her poems reveal unwittingly expressed instances of logonomic conflict.

Source: William J. Scheick, "Logonomic Conflict in Anne Bradstreet's 'A Letter to Her Husband,'" in *Essays in Literature*, Vol. 21, No. 2, Fall 1994, pp. 166–84.

Montgomery P. Sellers
In the following excerpt, Sellers discusses the historical significance of Bradstreet in American literature.

[Though Anne Bradstreet] wrote some prose, it is as a poet only that she is known, and while she was not a great poet in any high sense of the word, in some of her work there is the true poetic spirit. The lack of surrounding literary conditions, and the strictness of her religion, as well as her remoteness from a great center of culture, shut her out from the inspiring influences of the great Elizabethan literature. Yet we find that in her verse which places her above the other versifiers of colonial times.

The plan of the greater part of her writings is very simple, without any stress being laid upon the poetical quality of the verse. In the "Four Monarchies," "Four Elements." and the "Four Seasons," each monarchy, element and season, as the case may be, comes up and says what it can for itself. There is a great deal in the way of natural history, the history of nations, and of medical and scientific knowledge, all in the style of the verse of the time, which was not very elevated, and had Anne Bradstreet written these only, her name would not now be held in so much honor. She has lines to match even the very worst of the other versifiers of her day. But when we strike such a passage as this:

> Sometime now past in the autumnal tide
> When Phobus wanted but one hour to bed,
> The trees all richly clad, yet void of pride,
> Were gilded o'er by his rich golden head—

we come into the very atmosphere of the poetic spirit. We have heard nothing like it earlier in the history of American literature. What a contrast to the rude hymns of the "Bay Psalm Book," Michael Wigglesworth's "Day of Doom," and all the memorial verses of that time! Written in the later years of Anne Bradstreet's life, at her home near Andover, we see in them an expression of the true poetic feeling in the presence of nature. "Contemplations," for it is the first four lines of that we have just quoted, is not only the very best of Anne Bradstreet's poems, but is the true beginning of poetry in America....

"Contemplations" is the first true American poem. It is to Anne Bradstreet's honor that amid all the rubbish of colonial verse she has given us a breath of the spirit of true poetry. And we should honor her, too, for her place in our history of literary culture, as the pioneer of American poets.

Source: Montgomery P. Sellers, "New England in Colonial American Literature," in *New England Magazine*, Vol. 28, No. 1, March 1903, pp. 100–107.

SOURCES

Baer, William, "Appendix IV: The Formalist Revival," in *Writing Metrical Poetry: Contemporary Lessons for Mastering Traditional Forms*, Writer's Digest Books, 2006, pp. 236–40.

"Biography," in *AnneBradsteet.com*, http://www.annebradstreet.com/Default.htm, (accessed on July 9, 2009).

Bradstreet, Anne, "Here Follows Some Verses Upon the Burning of Our House, July 10th, 1666," in *The Works of Anne Bradstreet*, edited by Jeannine Hensley, Belknap Press of Harvard University Press, 1967, pp. 292–93.

Breitweiser, Mitchell, "Early American Antigone: Anne Bradstreet," in *National Melancholy: Mourning and Opportunity in Classic American Literature*, Stanford University Press, 2007, pp. 57–83.

Castillo, Susan Pérez, "Gender and Dissent in Colonial New England: Anne Hutchinson and the Antinomian Controversy," in *Revista da Faculdade de Letras Do Porto: Linguas e Literaturas*, 2nd ser., Vol. 7, 1990, pp. 225–36.

Egan, Jim, "The Insignificance of Experience," in *Authorizing Experience: Refigurations of the Body Politic in Seventeenth-Century New England Writing*, Princeton University Press, 1999, pp. 82–94.

Hensley, Jeannine, ed., "Introduction: Anne Bradstreet's Wreath of Thyme," in *The Works of Anne Bradstreet*, Belknap Press of Harvard University Press, 1967, pp. xxi–xxxv.

Heyrman, Christine Leigh, "Religion, Women, and the Family in Early America," in *Divining America: Religion in American History*, National Humanities Center, http://nationalhumanitiescenter.org/tserve/eighteen/ekeyinfo/erelwom.htm (accessed July 15, 2009).

"Key Findings and Statistics on Religion in America," and "Appendix 2: Classification of Protestant Denominations," in *The Pew Forum on Religion and Public Life: U.S. Religious Landscape Survey*, http://religions.pewforum.org/reports, (accessed July 15, 2009).

Martin, Wendy, "Anne Bradstreet," in *Dictionary of Literary Biography*, Vol. 24, *American Colonial Writers, 1606–1734*, edited by Emory Elliot, Gale Research, 1984, pp. 29–36.

Piercy, Josephine K., "The Craftsman," in *Anne Bradstreet*, Twayne Publishers, 1965, pp. 74–101.

"Religion and the Founding of the American Republic: Crossing the Ocean to Keep the Faith," in *Library of Congress*, http://www.loc.gov/exhibits/religion/rel01.html, (accessed July 13, 2009).

Rich, Adrienne, "Foreword: Anne Bradstreet and Her Poetry," in *The Works of Anne Bradstreet*, edited by Jeannine Hensley, Belknap Press of Harvard University Press, 1967, pp. ix–xx.

Rosenmeier, Rosamond, "The Wounds Upon Bathsheba: Anne Bradstreet's Prophetic Art," in *Puritan Poets and Poetics: Seventeenth-Century American Poetry in Theory and Practice*, edited by Peter White, Pennsylvania State University Press, 1985, pp. 129–46.

———, "Introduction: The Critical Sources," in *Anne Bradstreet Revisited*, Twayne Publishers, 1991, pp. 1–13.

Showalter, Elaine, "A New Literature Springs Up in the New World," in *A Jury of Her Peers: American Women Writers from Anne Bradstreet to Annie Proulx*, Alfred A. Knopf, 2009, pp. 1–14.

"U.S. Federal Government," in *USA.gov*, http://www.usa.gov/Agencies/federal.shtml, (accessed July 15, 2009).

FURTHER READING

Archer, Richard, *Fissures in the Rock*, University Press of New England, 2001.

Archer explores the social life and structures of New Englanders in the seventeenth century and includes discussions of family life, the economy and politics of New England communities, and religion.

Fitzmaurice, James, Carol Barash, Eugene R. Cunnar, and Nancy A. Gutierrez, eds., *Major Women Writers of Seventeenth-Century England*, University of Michigan Press, 1997.

The editors of this collection provide an introduction to each of the female authors whose work is represented in the volume and also provide a general critical overview to women's writing in England during the seventeenth century. The collection offers the student of Bradstreet's works the opportunity to assess the writings of the poet's English contemporaries, including the playwright Aphra Behn, the poet and essayist Margaret Cavendish, and the poets Anne Finch and Mary Wroth.

Miller, Perry, ed., *The American Puritans: Their Prose and Poetry*, Columbia University Press, 1982.

Miller's collection features journal entries, essays on history, religion, and philosophy, and on the poetry of American Puritans, providing a broad sampling of the thought and intellectual Puritan culture of the seventeenth century.

Vaughn, Alden T., *New England Frontier: Puritans and Indians, 1620–1675*, 3rd ed., University of Oklahoma Press, 1995.

Vaughn provides a detailed historical examination of the interactions between Puritan settlers and Native Americans during the seventeenth century and maintains that the early relations between these two groups were largely peaceful.

What For

GARRETT KAORU HONGO
1982

Garrett Kaoru Hongo's "What For" appeared in the 1982 collection *Yellow Light*. This poetry collection was Hongo's first volume of poetry that was all his own. It reveals much about who Hongo is as a poet and what his unique perspective is. The book explores Hongo's family and his past. It is a sort of collage of places he has lived, people he has known, stories he has heard, and who he understands himself to be. "What For" is one of the family poems in the collection. The speaker recalls his childhood self and the things he loved most. He mentions magic, religion, his grandparents, and his physical surroundings.

But "What For" is primarily about the speaker's father. The child anticipates his father's return from a hard day of physical labor and enjoys the little time they spend together. As a child, the speaker wanted to heal his father and make him feel better physically. He imagines what it would be like to play catch among the papaya trees together, but he settles for the dream of bringing magic and healing to his father. The title points the reader to the speaker's multiple statements about what he "lived for" when he was six years old. These were the things that were most important and exhilarating to him. "What For" is a poem of innocence and childhood longing. It also touches on some of the themes that run through Hongo's work, such as family, generational ties, love of homeland, and joy in the everyday.

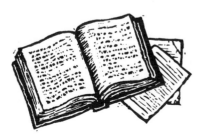

AUTHOR BIOGRAPHY

Hongo was born in Volcano, Hawaii, on May 30, 1951. While Hongo is considered an important voice among post-World War II Japanese Americans, he is more than just a niche poet. His work resonates with a wide and diverse audience of readers. Hongo's style is considered postmodern, as it utilizes a variety of techniques and sources. Hongo draws from his personal experience, his studies of Japanese literature, the music he loves, and his family's own history. He has been awarded fellowships by the Guggenheim Foundation, the National Endowment for the Arts, and the Rockefeller Foundation; his 1988 book *The River of Heaven* was a finalist for the Pulitzer Prize.

When Hongo was eight months old, his family moved to Oahu, and when he was six, they went to California. His high school had one-third Caucasian and Chicano students, one-third Japanese American students, and one-third African American students. This experience gave him a unique view of the challenges and opportunities involved in bringing different cultural backgrounds together. After graduating with honors from Pomona College in 1973, he spent a year in Japan on a Thomas J. Watson fellowship. He began graduate study in Japanese language and literature at the University of Michigan, but then, wanting to get back to the West Coast, he moved to Seattle, where there was a community of Asian American writers.

While in Seattle, he held the position of poet-in-residence for the Seattle Arts Commission and founded a theater group called The Asian Exclusion Act. In 1978, he brought his affinity for community to the collaborative poetry anthology *Buddha Bandits Down Highway 99*. Hongo completed an M.F.A. in Creative Writing at the University of California, Irvine, in 1980.

In 1982, two significant events took place—*Yellow Light* (the collection that includes "What For") was published, and Hongo married Cynthia Anne Thiessen, a violinist. The couple has two sons, Alexander (1984) and Hudson (1987). During the 1980s and early 1990s, Hongo taught at the University of Washington, the University of California, Irvine, and the University of Missouri; he also served as the poetry editor for the *Missouri Review*. In 1988, his second collection of poetry, *The River of Heaven* was published. Critics note that this volume reflects Hongo's desire to tap into ancestral wisdom and inspiration. In the second part of the volume, he writes about Los Angeles in a way that focuses the reader's attention on the humanity of the people who live there. In 1995, Hongo and his wife separated; they divorced in 2000. As of 2009, he is a professor of creative writing at the University of Oregon.

Hongo's third book, *Volcano*, was published in 1995. Here, the poet turns his attention to his connection to his father, his community, and the land. The motif running through the book is that of a journey, both literal and figurative.

As a poet, Hongo has created a body of work that brings ethnic issues to light without being combative. He is largely optimistic, and his depiction of family, community, and culture are affectionate. In addition to developing his own writing, Hongo works to encourage other Asian American writers in their work, and in helping them get published. The sense of community and brotherhood that is evident in his poetry is also evident in his actions.

POEM TEXT

At six I lived for spells:
how a few Hawaiian words could call
up the rain, could hymn like the sea
in the long swirl of chambers
curling in the nautilus of a shell,   5
how Amida's ballads of the Buddhaland
in the drone of the priest's liturgy
could conjure money from the poor
and give them nothing but mantras,
the strange syllables that healed desire.   10

I lived for stories about the war
my grandfather told over *hana* cards,
slapping them down on the mats
with a sharp Japanese *kiai.*

I lived for songs my grandmother sang   15
stirring curry into a thick stew,
weaving a calligraphy of Kannon's love
into grass mats and straw sandals.

I lived for the red volcano dirt
staining my toes, the salt residue   20
of surf and sea wind in my hair,
the arc of a flat stone skipping
in the hollow trough of a wave.

I lived a child's world, waited
for my father to drag himself home,   25
dusted with blasts of sand, powdered rock,
and the strange ash of raw cement,
his deafness made worse by the clang

of pneumatic drills, sore in his bones
from the buckings of a jackhammer.   30

He'd hand me a scarred lunchpail,
let me unlace the hightop G.I. boots,
call him the new name I'd invented
that day in school, write it for him
on his newspaper. He'd rub my face   35
with hands that felt like gravel roads,
tell me to move, go play, and then he'd
walk to the laundry sink to scrub,
rinse the dirt of his long day
from a face brown and grained as koa wood.   40

I wanted to take away the pain
in his legs, the swelling in his joints,
give him back his hearing,
clear and rare as crystal chimes,
the fins of glass that wrinkled   45
and sparked the air with their sound.

I wanted to heal the sores that work
and war had sent to him,
let him play catch in the backyard
with me, tossing a tennis ball   50
past papaya trees without the shoulders
of pain shrugging back his arms.

I wanted to become a doctor of pure magic,
to string a necklace of sweet words
fragrant as pine needles and plumeria,   55
fragrant as the bread my mother baked,
place it like a lei of cowrie shells
and *pikake* flowers around my father's neck,
and chant him a blessing, a sutra.

POEM SUMMARY

Stanza 1

The speaker of "What For" recalls the things he loved and looked forward to when he was six years old. In the first stanza, he describes his childhood sense of magic: a few Hawaiian words had the power to make it rain and sang through the nautilus like the sound of the sea. The Amida Buddha (the main Buddha in the Pure Land sect of Buddhism) had the power—through the liturgy of a priest—to satisfy the poor with words (mantras) while they offered what little money they had.

Stanzas 2 and 3

In the next two stanzas, the speaker talks about his grandparents. First, he remembers how he looked forward to the war stories his grandfather told while playing *hana* cards (Japanese cards). He remembers his grandfather playing cards and slapping his cards down with a short martial arts-type yell. Readers may notice that

the speaker says he looked forward to his grandfather's stories, but the description makes it evident that he looked forward at least as much just to being with his grandfather.

In the next stanza, the speaker's attention turns to his grandmother. He remembers her in the kitchen, cooking a curried stew. As he lived for his grandfather's stories (surely filled with excitement and intrigue), he also lived for his grandmother's songs, which were likely soothing and carefree. The grandmother's domestic life is underscored by the fact that while she cooks, she also weaves mats and sandals. The religious motif appears again here, as the design she is weaving is Japanese calligraphy of Kannon's love. Kannon is a bodhisattva, a being whose compassion leads him or her to desire the state of spiritual enlightenment known as Buddha-hood for all living beings.

Stanza 4

The speaker says he lived for the red dirt that stained his feet, and also for the salt from the sea and the wind that got in his hair. He recalls how he loved finding a smooth, flat stone he could skip in the trough of a wave. All of these things demonstrate the speaker's deep love for the setting and place of his childhood, for the specific natural features that he loved and that became part of him.

Stanzas 5 and 6

In the next two stanzas, the speaker takes the reader into part of his daily routine as a child. He tells how he anticipated his father's return from work, exhausted and dusty. The description of the father's physical appearance and fatigue imply that the father works at a construction site or in a mine. It is hard work that is physically demanding. In fact, the father is already at least partially deaf, and the drills and jackhammers worsen the condition.

The speaker continues his memories of his father at the end of a hard day of work into stanza 6. He handed his dented lunch box to the speaker, and then the boy unlaced the military boots his father had been working in all day. This interaction conveys how completely exhausted the father was; he sat down without even taking his lunch box to the kitchen, and his young son worked at the laces to remove his boots. Then the father heard the new name the boy had made up at school that day and allowed him to write the name on the newspaper. As tired as the father was, he had patience for his young son. When the father touched the child's face, his hands felt like a gravel road. They were rough and calloused. Only then did the father tell the speaker to run along and play, so he could get up and set about scrubbing all the dirt from his face. The speaker describes his father's face as resembling koa wood, a Hawaiian wood with a rippling grain.

Stanza 7 and 8

The speaker takes the reader into his emotional life as a child in the next two stanzas. He saw his father's pain and fatigue at working so hard, and he wanted to make the pain go away. Specifically, he wanted to make his legs and joints feel good again, and he wanted to be able to give his father back his hearing. He even describes what it might be like if his father could hear by referring to the delicate sound of crystal wind chimes.

The eighth stanza continues describing how the child wanted to heal his father. He was aware that his father had wounds from his past and present—from the war and from work. The speaker imagines that if he could heal him, his father's shoulders would not ache, and the two of them could play catch together with a tennis ball. Regardless of whether the scene is a memory or a fantasy, the son longs to play with his father the way other boys do. By referring to the papaya trees, Hongo brings in the tropical setting he loves. In both of these stanzas, the speaker wants to be the one to heal and provide relief for his father. His desire is not just for his father to be healthier—he himself wants to be the agent of that relief. It is an active rather than a passive desire.

Stanza 9

In the last stanza, the speaker connects his train of thought from the previous two stanzas back to the first stanza. In the first stanza, he spoke of magic and religion. Here, he applies those beliefs to the desire to heal his father. He says at the beginning that he wanted to be a doctor (a healer) of pure magic (effortless, innocent power). He reiterates the language motif of the first stanza by explaining that he wanted to make his father a necklace of words that smelled of trees, flowers, and freshly baked bread. Hongo uses synesthesia (mixing the senses so that one object is described with the sensory information of another; here the words have scent). This

creates an interesting dynamic that supports the innocence of the child's perspective. In the last image, the speaker imagined himself putting a shell and flower lei on his father and speaking a blessing over him. The speaker refers to a sutra, which is a Buddhist scriptural saying.

THEMES

Innocence

"What For" portrays the heart of a child. The speaker recalls the things he lived for as a child, and the things he wished desperately he could make happen. They are all innocent things, and Hongo makes it easy for the reader to connect with the innocence in the way he captures details. The poem opens with comments about magic and Hawaiian incantations against a background of Buddhism. The child believed that uttering the right words could make magic happen. There is nothing dark about this magic at all; it is the innocent fantasy of having the power to control one's world. The example the child considers is making rain.

Even when the child discusses religion, there is nothing jaded or zealous in it. In the first stanza, when he mentions the priests getting money from the poor and offering little in return, it does not come across as critical. In the final stanza, the child's innocent grasp of religion becomes part of his love for his father. He wants to chant a blessing for his father as an act of love.

The other things the child lives for evoke childhood innocence, too. He describes his grandparents, busy doing things that grandparents do. The grandfather tells war stories and plays cards, and the grandmother sings while she cooks and weaves. Hongo captures a sense of nostalgia in these images, as if to take the reader back to a simpler time in everyone's life. The speaker lived for these simple interactions with his grandparents.

The fifth stanza begins with the statement that he lived in a child's world, waiting for his father to come home from work. The thing the speaker was most concerned with as a child (according to the poem) was his father's sore, wounded body. His concern came from compassion and love for his father, and his wish that things were different. He enjoyed simply unlacing his father's boots, but he secretly wished that his father was strong enough to play catch in the

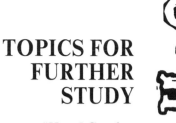

TOPICS FOR FURTHER STUDY

- Read Marilyn Chin's poem "How I Got that Name." With respect to family, Chin has a very different point of view in this poem than Hongo's speaker has in "What For." How do you account for the differences? Consider ethnicity, gender, geography, and other elements that make writers unique. Create a chart to help you identify the similarities and differences.

- Mitali Perkins' novel *Monsoon Summer* follows fifteen-year-old Jasmine as she explores her dual heritage by accompanying her mixed-race parents to her mother's homeland of India. Jasmine grapples with finding her own identity, as all teens do, but the process if both complicated and deepened by two cultures that define her. Write a poem in the style of "What For" that reveals something about Jasmine's relationship with her parents.

- Go back and read "What For" again, marking all descriptions of the physical setting and landscape. How clear a picture does Hongo create for the reader? Why do you think he chose these particular features for the poem? Look for three or four paintings or photographs that depict this setting, and create a PowerPoint presentation using the images and lines from the poem. You may choose a video-editing program, a photo-editing program, or anything else that suits your vision for the project.

- How well do you know your grandparents? Using the basic structure of the second and third stanzas of the poem, write about your own grandparents in a way that reflects your own perspective and experiences.

- The speaker recalls wishing he had the power to heal his father's injured body. When you were a child, what was something you wished you could transform in some way? Write a diary entry from your perspective as a child, describing your desire to change something. Take your time so you can get back in touch with the thoughts and feelings of your childhood.

- The poem has a number of Buddhist references. Read about Buddhism with special attention to the references in the poem. How does this enhance your understanding of the speaker and his family? Share what you learned by writing footnotes for the poem to illustrate the Buddhist references.

---

backyard without pain. This is a telling desire of a child's heart; he wants more from his relationship with his father. When he was a child, this desire manifested itself in a dream of playing catch. Since the speaker is writing in the past tense, the reader can assume that the speaker's desires have gotten more complicated and heavy over the years, but he still remembers vividly the innocent desires of his heart as a child.

Father-Child Relationships

Although the speaker writes about his grandparents and the natural setting of his childhood, the poem is really about the little boy and his father. The first four stanzas begin with simple statements about what he lived for—spells, war stories, his grandmother's songs, and the red dirt in his community. But in the fifth stanza, he makes a broader statement that he lived in a child's world, and then he tells the reader that he waited every day for his father to drag himself home from work. This is the thing the little boy looked forward to most, and it did not matter that his father was tired and dirty. It was not that he wanted his father to do much of anything; he just wanted to see him and be around him. The little boy is glad to take the lunch box and put it away, and then to unlace the military boots his father wore to work. This is not exciting stuff, but it was what the speaker most looked forward to every day.

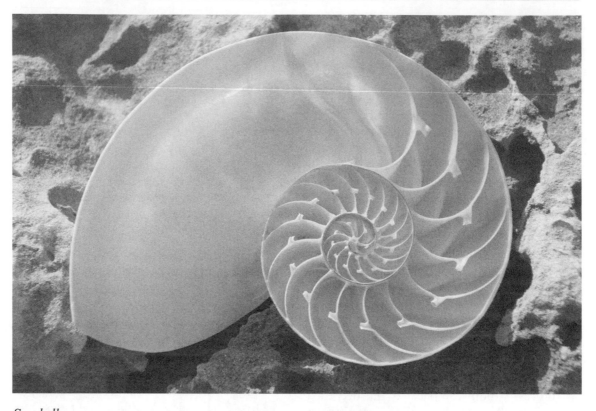

Seashell (*Image copyright Geanina Bechea, 2009. Used under license from Shutterstock.com*)

The speaker reveals that his deepest desire as a child was to be able to take all the pain, soreness, and deafness away from his father. He wanted to see his father at his strongest and healthiest for two reasons. First, he did not like seeing his dad suffer. Even though he was just a child, he could see that his father dragged himself home and was dirty and sore from the heavy work he did all day. Second, he wanted to be able to play with his father. He imagines what it would be like to play catch carefree among the papaya trees, without his father hurting. Because of the son's compassion for his father, the pain he knows his father suffers interferes with the son's pleasure in the time they are spending together. Still, he feels no disappointment or resentment toward his father. Rather, he is unhappy with the situation. His love for his father gives him pity beyond his years.

Because Hongo does not give the father's side of the story, there is less to go on with regard to the father-son relationship. Hongo gives enough, however, to demonstrate clearly that the father deeply loves his family and has a special relationship with his young son. The father

works a grueling job to take care of his family. He is wounded, scarred, sore, and deaf, but he gets up every morning and works a long, hard day so his family's needs will be met. When he comes home from that job, he does not demand to be left alone. He humbly sits down and hands his son his beat-up lunch box and lets his son take off his boots. Then he indulges the little boy as he tells his dad made-up names, and he even allows the child to write on his newspaper. Before sending the little boy on his way, he rubs his little face. This is a tender moment, and one that reveals the heart of the father toward the son.

Family History

By including the grandparents and the religious references, Hongo gives the poem an added generational dimension. As a child, the speaker loved his grandfather's war stories, and he loved watching him play cards with such fervor. He also loved hearing his grandmother sing as she made stew and wove mats and sandals. These are very ordinary, routine things the speaker describes, which indicate that the little boy saw his grandparents regularly. They probably lived nearby, and the child saw his grandparents in their everyday lives. He loved them, and he loved the things they did. Three generations are portrayed in this poem, and Hongo is clear that there is a great deal of love across all three.

The fact that the grandmother is weaving a Buddhist image into her work suggests that religious devotion is important to her. That the child mentioned Buddhist elements in other stanzas, apart from the third stanza (the one about the grandmother), lets the reader know that religion has been passed from one generation to the next. It is something significant that the generations share, and an important area of teaching in this family.

STYLE

Parallelism

Hongo uses parallelism in several ways in "What For." In the first stanza, the speaker says that when he was six, he lived for magic. He gives a few examples such as how saying certain Hawaiian words would bring rain or how a priest's words would heal the desires of the poor. In the last stanza, Hongo returns to the idea of magic, but he personalizes it. At the end of the poem, the little boy no longer worries about the rain or the poor; he is only worried about his father. He is still the same child who lives for magic, but Hongo revisits the topic in a new way. This ties the poem together and also shows progress as the child has taken the idea of magic and folded it into his fantasy of healing his father.

The other way Hongo utilizes repetition is by using anaphora (the repetition of the same word or phrase at the beginning of two or more lines) to give the poem cohesion and structure. The first five stanzas begin with "I lived," and they all form a unified section of the poem describing the various things this six-year-old lived for in his daily life. This consistency is a useful guide for the reader through the speaker's recollections. These particular repeated words ensure that the reader understands the significance of the five things the speaker has chosen to share.

The last three stanzas all begin with "I wanted to," and these stanzas describe what the speaker wished he could change. The first part of the poem is about what he thought was ideal when he was a child, and these last stanzas are about what was not ideal at all. Again, Hongo uses anaphora to give these three stanzas presence and relationship to one another.

Imagery

Perhaps because setting and personal experience are so important to Hongo, this poem includes imagery throughout to bring the memory pictures to life. Hongo calls on all the senses in his imagery, which signifies that the speaker' memories of his life when he was six are vivid. In the first stanza, we hear a hymn from a nautilus, ballads of a Buddha, the drone of a priest, and strange Hawaiian syllables. In the second stanza, the sounds of the grandfather playing cards include the slap of the cards and the martial arts yell he delivers as he plays. The third stanza brings the scent of curry stew simmering and the song the grandmother sings. In the fourth stanza, the surroundings are described in the red of the volcanic dirt, the salt and wind in the air, and the sight of a stone skipping through a wave. In the fifth stanza, the father is described in terms of his physical appearance after working on a construction site all day. The sound of the drills is expressed in the onomatopoetic clang, which is juxtaposed with the deafness of the speaker's father.

In the next stanza, the father's hands are likened to gravel, a very descriptive portrayal of the touch. The father's face is likened to koa wood, a Hawaiian wood with wavy grain. The use of simile to describe the father's physical appearance is very effective. Onomatopoeia is used again in the seventh stanza, where the speaker remembers wishing he could heal his father's deafness. The speaker considers crystal chimes, and the words Hongo chooses sound like a breeze going through them. He describes the "fins of glass that wrinkled and sparked the air," creating the tinkling sound of the wind passing through crystal chimes.

The last two stanzas explore the child's wish to heal his father. A carefree image of playing catch in the backyard reveals the heart of the child, and the imagined necklace for the father is full of sensory images (words, shells, flowers, and scents).

HISTORICAL CONTEXT

Yonsei

Hongo is *Yonsei*, meaning he is fourth-generation Japanese American. Like other ethnic groups, Japanese Americans have made a place in American culture and society. The first-generation Japanese Americans held more closely to the traditions of Japan than have successive generations. For many *Yonsei*, identity is a difficult issue because they want to honor and identify with their Japanese roots but, like Hongo, they know that they are profoundly influenced by American life. In fact, since the 1960s, the percentage of marriages between Japanese and non-Japanese spouses has risen consistently. In many *Yonsei* households, being Japanese is only expressed in celebrating certain festivals, eating Japanese food, and perhaps giving children Japanese first names or middle names.

While earlier generations spoke Japanese as a first language and English as a second, most *Yonsei* speak English as their first language. Some do not even learn Japanese. In Hawaii, where there is a larger Japanese population, more current-generation Japanese Americans learn Japanese. As is the case with most Asian cultures, Japanese Americans tend to prioritize education and emphasize it in their homes. The most common religions practiced in Japanese American homes are Buddhism, Shinto, and Christianity. In areas with a large Japanese American population, it is not uncommon for the major Buddhist festivals to become community events.

For Japanese Americans who were in America during World War II, the subject of internment is still painful. Because America was at war with Japan, many Japanese Americans were forcibly relocated to internment centers until the alleged danger was deemed neutralized. Entire families were forced into internment camps, and it is a chapter in American history that is difficult to face, especially for those who were impacted. Of course, *Yonsei* like Hongo were not affected by this event, as it took place in the time of their parents or other relatives. The degree to which the internment is part of their identity is very individual because the degree of discrimination felt by prior generations is less of an issue.

Buddhism

Buddhism is practiced in many Japanese homes, and there are multiple references to it in Hongo's "What For." Buddhism is based on the teachings and sayings of Buddha (Siddhartha Gautama). Buddha was born in what is now known as Nepal, and is considered a teacher who possessed divine knowledge and insight to share with the rest of the world so that others could understand the cycles of rebirth and escape from suffering. Buddha taught on the Indian subcontinent until his death in approximately 483 BCE.

Although there are differences among types of Buddhism, the basic beliefs remain consistent. Buddha teaches the concepts of rebirth and reincarnation. The concept is not about an individual eternal soul, but rather about the process of rebirth itself moving toward perfection. Once a being achieves a high level of maturity and self-lessness, he or she attains nirvana, a state of perfect peace and freedom from suffering. This is the salvation taught by Buddhism, and many of the practices of devotees are designed to support the individual on his or her path to nirvana. Among these are meditation, moral living, exercise for the mind and body, participating in ceremonies, and invoking bodhisattvas (such as Kannon in Hongo's poem). Bodhisattvas are beings that are wise, enlightened, and so compassionate for mankind that they wish for all to attain Buddhahood. While not exactly parallel, they are similar to the saints to whom Catholics pray. The cycle of rebirth and suffering is moved by the energy of karma, which refers to the actions a person takes and his intentions behind them. A person's actions produce positive or negative consequences that appear in the current or a future life.

The Four Noble Truths of Buddhism address the subject of earthly suffering. The Truths teach that life leads to suffering; there is a cause of suffering, and it is rooted in self-centeredness; there is an end to suffering in letting go of desire and replacing it with enlightenment; and to attain enlightenment, one must follow the Eightfold Path set forth by Buddha. The components of the Eightfold Path fall into three categories: prajna, which is for enlightenment (proper understanding of the Four Noble Truths and seeing life as it really is, wise thinking, and renunciation of earthly things); sila, which is for morality (proper use of one's speech, proper use of one's actions through adherence to the Five Precepts, taking care of one's own livelihood without harming anyone else); and samadhi, which is for meditation (good thoughts and intentions, self-awareness, practicing meditation to arrive at higher states of consciousness).

Similar to the Judeo-Christian Ten Commandments, Buddhism has the Five Precepts, which require people to abstain from killing, stealing, lying, misusing sexual activity, or partaking of alcohol. There are additional precepts for Buddhist monks.

COMPARE
&
CONTRAST

- **1980s:** In 1982, more than 533,000 people obtain legal permanent resident status. Immigration rates during the 1980s come close to those of the turn of the twentieth century. All told, more than six million people immigrate to the United States during the 1980s, most of them young and pursuing the American dream.

  Today: In 2008, more than 1.1 million people are granted legal permanent resident status. The topic of immigration is hotly debated as a recession strains the economy and the issue of illegal immigration has no clear solution.

- **1980s:** In 1980, Congress establishes the Commission on Wartime Relocation and Internment of Civilians. The purpose is to determine the impact on those interned during World War II (who were primarily Japanese Americans), and also to reexamine the relocation of Alaskan Aleuts. The commission works on this project for three years.

  Today: The commission found that there was no justification for interning Japanese Americans during the war, and a formal apology has been issued, along with reparations. In the twenty-first century, sentiment is largely on the side of the Japanese Americans, and people criticize the dishonorable treatment they endured.

- **1980s:** As of 1982, only one winner of the Nobel Prize in Literature is Japanese, Yasunari Kawabata, in 1968.

  Today: As of 2008, two winners of the Nobel Prize in Literature are Japanese, Yasunari Kawabata in 1968 and Kenzaburo Oe in 1994.

CRITICAL OVERVIEW

Hongo's first volume of poetry, *Yellow Light*, was published to critical acclaim, marking the author almost instantly as an important contributor to Asian American literature. In *MELUS*, Mary Slowik discusses the work of Hongo and three other poets at length. Of Hongo, she notes that he strives to connect with his heritage, but in America "the heritage is fragmented, broken, silenced." She adds,

> If Hongo wants to reroot Asian culture in America, he first must discover the missing American story. His growing awareness of the suppressed American history leads him to angry outburst against both his Japanese family and the Anglo culture that has so injured them.

Slowik sees an agenda for his people in Hongo's work as a poet. She writes, "Hongo also aspires to be a priest for his generation and those before him, a task which complicates and historicizes the voice in his poems." Similarly, George Uba in the *Journal of Ethnic Studies* notes that *Yellow Light* "grapples with...the problem of an ethnic group whose own identity remains ill-defined." He sees Hongo striking a balance between individual experience and cultural identity, summed up as "the quest for a personal identity and the desire to build and retrieve a collective identity by sifting through the past." According to Uba, Hongo is interested in neither the Japanese experience nor the American experience, but the unique experience of Japanese people in America. He concludes,

> Hongo applies wit, intelligence, and craftsmanship to his serious theme as few others have been able to do. His book is certain to gain a privileged station in Asian American literature courses, as well as to fuel the continuing controversy over enlarging the American literary canon.

Diane Wakoski gives an enthusiastic review of *Yellow Light* for the *American Book Review*. She deems the volume "one of the most exciting

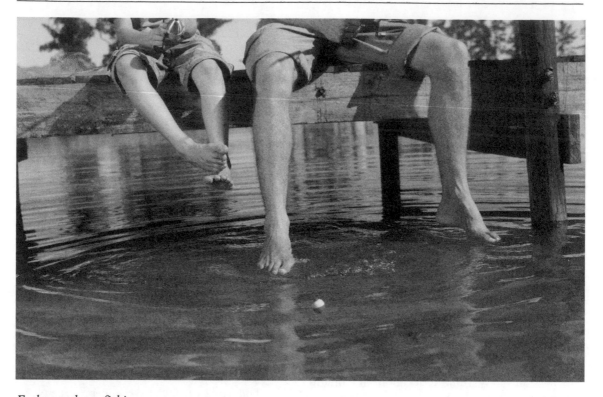

Father and son fishing (© 2009 | Jupiter Images)

books of poems I have read in recent years," describing Hongo's language as "sensuous" and his accomplishment as "astonishing."

CRITICISM

Jennifer Bussey

Bussey is an independent writer specializing in literature. In the following essay, she comments on how Garrett Hongo's "What For" gives insight into what matters most to the Hawaiian-born Japanese American poet.

After one collaboration, two volumes of poetry, and a memoir, Garrett Hongo is an established voice in Asian American literature. His postmodern style variously utilizes different techniques, voices, sources, and forms. Hongo is more concerned with exploring and voicing his personal experience and the collective experience of Japanese Americans than he is with adhering closely to a regimented style of writing. He is especially concerned with the experience of non-first-generation Japanese Americans, like himself. He is *Yonsei*, which is fourth generation,

and thus his identity is different from that of his grandparents. To Hongo and others in his situation, the issue of identity is not simple. Through Hongo's poetry, he works through the nuances of this—and many other—aspects of his experience. In "What For," a poem that appeared in his first volume of poetry, the 1982 *Yellow Light*, the speaker goes back into his childhood memories to recall what was most important and exciting to him when he was six years old. It is a moving and sensitive piece that goes much deeper than nostalgia. Based on the rest of Hongo's canon of work and his vision as a poet, it is likely that this poem reveals what is really important to Hongo himself in terms of his Japanese and Hawaiian roots.

Over the course of the poem's nine stanzas, the speaker brings up magic, religion, language, nature, grandparents, and his father. In the first and last stanzas, he tells that he lived for magic. He says that a few Hawaiian words could bring rain or make music in a nautilus. He says that a priest's Buddhist liturgy has the power to "conjure" money from the poor but still leave them satisfied by his words. In the last stanza, the speaker returns to this idea of magic, which he

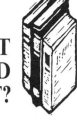

WHAT DO I READ NEXT?

- *Culture Shock and Japanese-American Relations: Historical Essays* (2007), by Sadao Asada, takes a look at the history of relations between Japan and the United States, including such hot topics as the bombing of Pearl Harbor and the atomic bomb. Asada examines what relations are like today, and how each culture views the other.

- Marilyn Chin's 2002 poetry collection *Rhapsody in Plain Yellow* expresses the poet's concerns about identity and heritage with her modern sensibility. Her poems touch on traditional themes but discuss them in modern contexts and with modern subjects with which readers can more readily identify.

- Edited by Sari Grossman and Joan Brodsky Schur, *In a New Land: An Anthology of Immigrant Literature* (2007) compiles various genres of literature from writers of divergent ethnic backgrounds. Their works reflect the difficulties of being part of two or more cultures, and the promise of a new beginning.

- Hongo's *The River of Heaven* (1988) was a Pulitzer Prize finalist. Scholars and admirers of Hongo's poetry find it a fascinating work in which the poet deepens his vision of the places he has been, the people he has known, and stories he has heard.

- Graham Salisbury's novel *Under the Blood-Red Sun* (2005) tells the story of a hard-working Japanese family living in Hawaii at the time of the bombing of Pearl Harbor. Thirteen-year-old Tomi faces the traumas of war, racism, family struggle, and self-reflection in this historical novel.

- Dale Ann Sato's *Japanese Americans of the South Bay* (2009) relates the history of Japanese Americans in Los Angeles County. Sato explains why they settled in this area, how they established their own communities, and the struggles of the generations that came after them as they set about preserving Japanese traditions while embracing American culture.

> 'WHAT FOR' IS A POEM WITH EMOTION, LONGING, AND REMEMBRANCE, BUT LIKE MOST OF HONGO'S POETRY, IT WORKS TOWARD FOCUSING THE POET'S IDENTITY. HE VISITS HAWAIIAN AND JAPANESE CULTURES IN THIS POEM, PICKING UP CERTAIN ELEMENTS AS IMPORTANT AND SETTING OTHERS ASIDE."

interweaves with religious elements. He wants to use pure magic to heal his father and then chant a sutra to bless him. A sutra is a saying or discourse attributed to Buddha. Hongo chooses to begin and end the poem with the idea of magic and religion, and it is clear that what this represents to the child is simply power. Being a child can be a powerless feeling, so the child in the poem wants to draw some power and a sense of control (over the rain, or over his father's health) by mastering magic. That he includes Buddhism in this demonstrates that the child has not internalized his faith, but regards it as an external thing. His grandmother weaves calligraphy about Kannon, a bodhisattva, into her work. A bodhisattva is a being who has so much love and compassion that he or she strives for enlightenment that will benefit others. This tells the reader that Buddhism is part of this family's identity, and the child is probably being educated in it. Perhaps because of the child's young age, however, he has categorized it in a different way.

It is important to remember that this poem is the recollection of a grown man. He necessarily sees things through the lenses of his memory and his experiences since the time of that memory. There is nothing in his words or tone that suggest he still believes in magic, and the tenderness he brings to other parts of the poem are absent in his passing references to religion. He understands that to others, faith is important and comforting. The desires of the poor he mentions in the first stanza are healed, and his grandmother clearly has a personal connection to her beliefs. But the speaker does not reveal any similar feelings. This suggests that, of all the things about his Japanese heritage that are meaningful to him, Buddhist devotion is not one of them.

In the fourth stanza, the speaker recalls how he lived for the unique elements of his natural surroundings. He loved the red volcanic dirt that stained his skin, and he loved the salt from the sea that stuck to his hair. From the way he describes these things, it is clear that he loved having the place physically become part of him. They were not annoyances in the least. He loved being physically changed by being out in nature. This indicates the importance of place and homeland to Hongo, and the ways he interacts with it. The boy in the poem literally wants his homeland all over him.

The speaker remembers fondly what he loved about his grandparents. The details demonstrate that he watched them closely and appreciated their quirks. He remembers how he lived for the war stories his grandfather told them while playing Japanese cards. He remembers that his grandfather played with gusto, slapping the cards down with a martial arts-style yell. His grandmother sang, and he lived for her songs. He remembers her cooking curried stew and weaving grass into mats and sandals. These details enable the reader to connect with the speaker's love for his family. In the descriptions of his grandparents, he includes a Japanese card game and ethnic food, but these elements are only meant to give depth to the portrayals of his grandparents. Like the religious references, these are not things that seem particularly close to his own heart, even though they are aspects of his heritage.

The real thrust of this poem is the young son's love for his father. He lives for his father coming home, dirty and tired from a long, hard day of work. The son loves the brief time he spends with his father, and he wishes he could heal the aches and the pain that are the result of the harshness of his life. These are not passing wishes, but a dream with a lot of emotion and detail. They are the heart of the poem and reveal much about the son's character at such a young age. The detail with which he describes the pain can only be coming from the adult speaker, remembering anew his father's aches and pains. A child would not possess that level of sensitivity and insight, although the child knew enough to know he wanted to make it better. And the son knew enough to know he really wanted his father to be able to play catch with him like any typical

father and son. But the son—as a six-year-old or as an adult—is not resentful toward his father or the hard life that made him the way he was. The same love seems to have been consistent throughout the speaker's life.

In the discussion of the grandparents and of the father, the speaker makes it very clear that family is the single most important thing to him. Given the scope of Hongo's work beyond this poem, it is fair to extrapolate that Hongo felt the same way about his family. His interest in his family encompasses the generations before him, his own identity as a Japanese American born in Hawaii, and the generation after him that includes his two sons. This is an important element in Japanese culture, and that sense of family loyalty seems to be embraced by Hongo, even if it is Westernized by the addition of deep, heartfelt emotion.

One other aspect of the poem speaks very loudly as being important to the speaker and certainly to Hongo, and that is the presence and power of language. In his comments about magic and religion, the speaker locates the power in the words. A few Hawaiian words (not dances or music or ceremonies) create rain, and a Buddhist ballad spoken to the poor heals the desires of their hearts. The speaker loves his grandfather' stories, and his grandmother's songs—all words. The interaction with the father is almost silent, save for the son's sharing a made-up name from school, and the silence is a haunting reminder that the father's deafness is a cruel irony to a son who places so much importance on words. But as the poem gains momentum toward its close, the speaker describes wanting to make the father a necklace of what? Of "sweet words." And the words capture the other senses because they have scent, which the father can experience. In the final line of the poem, the son remembers wanting to speak a blessing to his father. No longer wanting to invoke magic to make something exciting happen, he merely wants to express love to his father in a spoken blessing.

"What For" is a poem with emotion, longing, and remembrance, but like most of Hongo's poetry, it works toward focusing the poet's identity. He visits Hawaiian and Japanese cultures in this poem, picking up certain elements as important and setting others aside. Although the speaker refers to Buddhism, Japanese games, and ethnic food, these are background to what

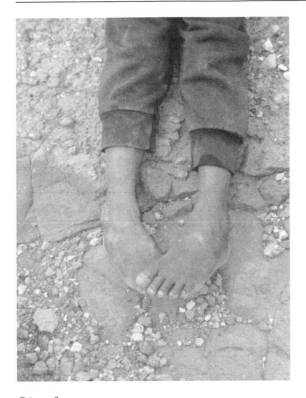

Dirty feet (Image copyright Humberto Ortega, 2009. Used under license from Shutterstock.com)

really matters to Hongo's speaker. And what really matters is generational ties, immediate family, and words.

Source: Jennifer A. Bussey, Critical Essay on "What For," in *Poetry for Students*, Gale, Cengage Learning, 2010.

Alice Evans

In the following interview with Evans, Hongo discusses the craft of writing and the role of his family history in his poetry.

[Alice Evans]: At a craft workshop recently, you talked about how important it is for the individual to act as a witness to history. Witnessing appears to be a primary directive in your work. How would you describe the poet's role as historian, from both a broad view and a personal one?

[*Garrett Hongo*]: As poets we need to portray the events of the world from our own point of view. We need to be attached to the events of the world in our own lives. Sometimes history passes us by and we don't know it. I believe that poets must speak as witnesses to historical events. I don't believe in [the official version of]

American history; I believe in what we've witnessed as the travesties in American history.

I try to be faithful to the history of Japanese in America and write from it, and I've made it my responsibility to know everything that I can about it. It's like Czeslaw Milosz says about Lithuania: "If there is no singer there is no history." That's how I go into the world: if I don't write it, it's not going to get written, and I don't want people to stop that. I see that the person in my way who is causing me difficulty is also repressing the expression of the history of my people.

I have a lot of pride. It comes from my people, my whole family. I had a very proud grandfather and grandmother whose pride was taken away because of World War II. You don't forget it.

Tell me about your own history. What were the forces that produced an acclaimed poet? How did the doors open for you?

The reason I'm doing anything at all is because I'm an individual who is part of a corrective process in American history. I got educated because Governor Pat Brown funded a program for poor kids to study at the best universities in California. So I was given an academic scholarship to go to a very elite school, Pomona College. Because this education came from a political circumstance of opportunity and empowerment, it's not hard for me to believe the thing that I believe. And I never give a damn about making it.

You say you don't give a . . . about making it, but you have made it. You've been very honored as a poet. What has that meant for you?

It's not a question of making it. It's a question of standing up and honoring a past which I feel was dishonored. It's on those principles that I carry myself forward.

Yes, I've been honored, and I'm happy for that, for complicated reasons, I suppose. One of the nice things about that is it gives me more opportunity to address my subjects. Honors, insofar as that's concerned, are very good. They endorse my projects and they give me the opportunity to address my subjects. They also are great medallions and great weapons in the fight to get that story told.

I wish my grandfather had been honored, but this country did not do that to him, so I do it.

Your poetry shows great depth of feeling, a characteristic I find unusual for a man.

Maybe it's a human characteristic. Most males are not human any more. I like that joke in the book *Little Big Man,* where the Cheyenne call themselves human beings and they call the other people ghosts—or the "white man." Maybe male culture—I don't want to offend anybody—but maybe people have forgotten how to be human beings.

My grandfather was not this way, my father was not this way, Hawaiians are not this way. We have a lot of *aloha*—spirit, love, trust. When I moved from Hawaii to Los Angeles there was no *aloha* in Los Angeles. Man, there was a lot of brutality. But it's good that I learned about that too, because you have to ward things off. Tenderness is a very underrated emotion. It's also much attacked and maligned. So I've made it my job to learn a vicious kind of tenderness.

Could you elaborate?

James Wright's tenderness I believe in. You know the poem, "To a Blossoming Pear Tree"— "the dark blood in my flesh drags me down with my brother"—that's the kind of tenderness I believe in. I love you because I know we're both going to die. I love you because everyone else is trying to beat us up. "Flayed without hope, I held the man for nothing in my arms."

A lot of people were excited about having you come to teach at the University of Oregon. What kind of teacher are you? What do you emphasize and what ticks you off?

The kinds of things I might criticize a student for are a lack of commitment, a lack of concern for the reader, obscurity. I like things to be reasonably clear. I don't go in for a lot of verbal pyrotechnics, but there's always a Gerard Manley Hopkins out there, or a Hart Crane, or a Charles Wright. You've got to worship them.

I care a lot about self-knowledge, knowing what you're going to write about, knowing what you sing, knowing what you like to sing about, and helping the students connect with that.

I guess I'm still a Confucian. I believe that people are basically good, not basically bad. So I believe that if they learn to trust their nature, something good will emerge out of it, even if it's an angry nature. You know, people aren't angry for no reason, they're angry for a reason usually. And poetry is a loving craft, so even angry poems are in the service of some love.

You talked at the craft workshop about poetry being treated as an elite practice. You mentioned being turned off by literary aloofness, obscurity, a system of privileged meaning accessible only to those initiated into that system. What kind of emphasis do you put on technique?

Technique can show a commitment, technique can show energy. Technique shows you've invested. Also candor shows you've invested, you've invested in trust.

The thing I work to build first in the workshop is trust. Not only that the students trust me, but that they trust each other, because the thing that kills expression and creativity is a lack of trust, an environment of hostility. And the workshop's primary function to me is to give people a sense of a sympathetic yet creatively critical audience. That's the main job.

I've been in some very destructive workshop situations.

Well, it's easy to be destructive—to be critical and careless. It's harder to be critical and supportive. There are not too many people who have shown the ability to do that in our history. Some of my heroes are people who have been great teachers—Bruce Lee, Theodore Roethke, Philip Levine. When I interviewed for this job, and people asked me why I wanted to do this, I said: because this is a self-assignment for me. I believe in the craft, I believe in the profession, I believe in the cause, and in my own mind I'm not going to be significant in terms of my people unless my work is shown to be valuable, in that it helps better the world. In the martial arts, as in anything, the final requirement of someone in the profession—in the art—is that they start a school that lives beyond their own life, that they help people find what is valuable in the art, that they inspire people not only to do well but to try to do well for others. And that's what's left for me to do yet. That's the reason I came here. It was an opportunity for me to test and extend myself, but also to contribute.

We have to increase the opportunity for people to have free voice, free expression, and that's what I hope for here.

Poetry—creative writing—is free speech. That's why Jesse Helms wants to shut us down. There are very strong forces in play right now that want to shut down the National Endowment for the Arts, because the understanding is that it is a forum for free speech in America. It really is

I have a friend who's a legal scholar, in what they call critical legal studies. She did an article on poetry—particularly women's poetry—as an alternate system of jurisprudence to the law, and I think that's the reason why people are so upset by it. That's why poetry is so threatening and why it's practiced by so many people who are outside of economic and political power. Because it's our system of jurisprudence. Poetry is another judgment.

And speech with devotion to private moments of emotion also has a place in poetry as well as speech about unauthorized history. After all, that's what the Old Testament was about. And the New Testament. They're unauthorized histories.

Donald Barthelme said, "Do you think the Bible would have been written if people thought they were writing the Bible?" That's pretty good, I've got to say. Barthelme inspired me a lot, and his confidence that this could be done helped me. . . .

Let's talk a little about your writing habits now. Are you a disciplined writer, do you write every day?

I'm an actor as a writer. I prepare the character, you know, like Stanislavsky.

So the idea of the character dictates the poem?

Not really, no. The gut, the feeling, the emotional and narrative core of the book does.

I was talking to Barry Lopez and asked him how it was to work with a certain editor. He said "I don't know yet, I haven't shown her anything." He's been working on this book for two and a half years—three years almost—and said, "I don't know, I don't know this book very well yet." I said "huh?" and he kept talking: "the way

I do things, I never show an editor anything until I get at least a complete draft done, and then I'll go over it line by line." He's still kind of putting the book together and doesn't know what kind of a book it is, what the personality of it is, what's going to go in it. He *lives* the book; he's preparing it.

That's the way I do it too, but I don't know what I'm doing. He knows what he's doing, For him it's a method. For me it's floundering.

It was great to hear him tell me that because when I write my book of poems I kind of run into the poetry, I run into the book. Like, I was writing and it didn't really come together, but I just kept living with this feeling of trying to capture the love, the *aloha* [a word of welcome], the commitment to democracy my father had, because I knew I didn't have what he had. So that was my *koan* [a prayer of meditation], that was my problem with *The River of Heaven*. And once I got it, once I felt "in the feeling," then the poems started to come, one by one, then more, then more and more and more and more.

Every time I extended myself I realized something new, and I pushed myself to the next level; the last poem I wrote for the book was "The Pier," a long poem at the end of *The River of Heaven*. It's a democratic statement. My father had those beliefs. He's a Hawaiian Democrat.

He was active politically?

Every Hawaiian is active politically. You know, equal rights, enfranchisement for all peoples, and Go For Broke. And that's kind of, like, you talk that way, you think that way on the mainland—especially in Orange County at the "University of Apartheid"—you're ostracized, you're looked upon as some kind of dirty, rotten ethnic. So I wanted to do something that might blossom, because they're trying to take that belief away from me. It's like a religion. You kill the religion first and it's easy to have the people die.

I wanted to bring the religion back in me and there were certain fathers behind it also, not just my own flesh fathers, but William Butler Yeats and his great poem, "Among Schoolchildren," and William Wordsworth, in "The Immortality Ode." "Among Schoolchildren" is a model behind "The Pier." Instead of schoolchildren it's Cambodians and Vietnamese that I see. Those two poems are ghost poems behind "The Pier."

So I took on as much as I could, I took on my father's life and his democratic principles, and I wished to critique the oppressive ideology of white racism and to invoke the great fathers of mystic revelation and poetic power, William Butler Yeats and William Wordsworth—and I tried to put it together in "The Pier."

My working method is to let the meditation grow. I guess it's kind of Eastern, but it's also like Wordsworth. He walked all over the Wye Valley, meditating, ruminating, and he'd come back and then write the poem about it after his long walks. I don't have a craftsman-like, disciplined daily writing method.

The River of Heaven came together at the MacDowell Colony in six weeks, I read somewhere.

It wasn't only those six weeks, though they were crucial. MacDowell helped a lot and going to Hawaii helped a lot. Just before I was at MacDowell I was in Hawaii with my friend Edward Hirsch. I was running around, I was showing Hawaii to this person, who wanted to know me and my history and he appreciated it so much. It inspired me, his love for my people's way, it inspired me to share more of my heart through poetry with the rest of the world.

Tell me about the book you're working on now, Volcano Journal.

It's a book of retreat and return, meditation on going home to a home I never knew, which is this volcano. And coming back to it, to the history of my family, coming back to that culture, the biology, the *biota* [the animal and plant life of a particular region considered as a total ecological entity], the rainforest, the volcano itself. It's nonfiction, not like John McPhee, more like Thoreau.

When you read from that book the other night, you mentioned that you needed to experiment with form. Could you talk about that?

In writing this book, the poetic form needed to expand for me. What I found to be the form was the Japanese *nikki*. It's a travel diary, poetic prose. We have examples in American literature in *Moby Dick* and *Walden*. In that vein I write this book.

You were eight months old when your family left Volcano. What took you back there?

I was invited, when I was about 31, to give a couple of readings in the islands and was invited to give a reading in Volcano, where they have an art center.

What happened for you there?

I knew that that was it. I knew I had to go back. I knew I wasn't finished with it. I knew there was something. And I was true to it. I was true to that little insinuation, and it's made all the difference in my heart. It's made all the difference in the soul of my family. My boys love it, my wife, everything. So I didn't ignore my calling.

It seems that in Volcano you found yourself as a writer.

That's right. In geography and geology, you know, when lava comes out of the earth it's not magnetized, and the way they can map continental drift is by tracing the magnetic fields, because after the lava is emitted and solidifies, then it's magnetized, and it's magnetized according to our orientation to magnetic north. So there's something to that, the first time you come into the world. Many people are magnetized. You get your little stratigraphy, that kind of thing. I feel perfect there, I can't tell you. It's always a good day in Volcano.

I have a friend, Native American poet Ray Young Bear. When I met him I was nothing, I was completely shiftless. He had a feeling for his ancestors, he had a feeling for his tribe and his people, he knew where he stood, he walked with the grandfathers. I took that as a criticism of my own psyche and soul. When we were eighteen, I didn't have that. When I was eighteen, I was like the "stolen child." But I have that now. I walk with my grandfathers and have absolutely complete confidence. I'm their grandson. It took me a lot longer than Ray, but I got there.

In Yellow Light, you write about returning to Japan to find your family's name. Are you talking about your natal family?

Everybody. I'm talking about those that the literature has forgotten, those that the culture has forgotten. It's important to me that we be remembered, that there be a literature for us, that we be sung about, that there be songs for the lives that my people have lived. That's why the poetry of Philip Levine inspired me so early—"Vivas for those who have failed," the names of the lost.

I said in an interview somewhere, sometime, part of the motivation behind my first book was to recuperate or reinscribe our name in the registry, the list of names in Japan, the list of names in Hawaii.

So not literally Hongo, but the lost names of all your people.

There's a serious pun in that, because my name means homeland. Hongo means homeland.

I was a little confused because there was some mention of changing names, or taking on a new name.

A lot of Japanese did that. Like people coming through Ellis Island, they just changed their names.

Tell me about the use of oral history in your poetry. You write very eloquently about people not directly connected to you.

You write the history of the tribe and you sing from sources. I used the Oral History Project of the Ethnic Studies Department at the University of Hawaii, God bless them. We need to be liberated, the love of oral history needs to be liberated, the love of our people needs to be liberated. We're a colonized place, culturally colonized.

This is our pride, this is our history, this is our identity. We're a colonial people. We're like the blacks in southern culture. I mean, politically we're a canceled culture. We're like the copper miners in Chile—there's no difference. We're like the students in Tiananmen.

So you're trying to reawaken. . . .

I'm not trying, I have to. It's a compulsion with me. I don't have a choice. If I'm going to be what my grandfather was, I have to do it this way. For me to be a person in my eyes, this is what I have to be.

Your mother's father is the one who was taken away?

That's right. It's like Indians say: you have ghosts, you have your *aumakua*. I have my *aumakua*, I have my guardian spirits.

Tell me more about your work habits. When you're in Eugene, are you able to write?

No—impossible.

That's what I thought. You need the open time that a Guggenheim provides; you need NEA [fellowships]. If you wanted to now, could you earn your living solely as a writer?

I could probably get an advance, but I don't know if I could live on it. I'm still learning to be a prose writer and still learning what kind of a prose writer I am. I'm enjoying the experience, finally.

I'd like to get back to your writing question. I like to write seven pages every day except weekends, which I like to spend with my family.

Sometimes I just get a page. I just get a bad page. I get a lot of pages that are real lousy but I've started working on a problem, or a theme, a beat, narrative or emotional, and the next pages are really . . . I just trash it and I find my way into the subject. I'm enjoying myself, so I write between a page and seven pages a day, single-spaced.

You work first thing in the morning?

Pretty much.

Your poetry is very songlike at times, it's very lush. You've described your style as narrative, Whitmanesque. You relate oral history, you talk about your roots, both family personal and family historical, and it seems to me you go all the way back to the universe itself. Your work has lots of references to the universe.

Thank you. I've looked down into the middle. You stand over a pond of lava boiling up, or you stand on the top of Mauna Kea and you look up at a star, it's impossible to think anything else.

Well, it's a very expansive view. A lot of poetry is focused only on the personal these days, only on the wounds the person has suffered. Yours branches out into the universe.

There are so many things to wither the soul, and poetry does the opposite. I won't let my poetry wither my soul, poetry has to enhance it. I don't believe in poetry as a discipline, or a narrow field, or an elite practice. I believe in poetry as empowerment. *Singing for Power*, you know, that great book by Ruth Underhill about the Papago Indian ceremonies. I mean, I like those ideas that poetry is like singing for power, trying to find, crying for your own vision. Every one of us finds it in our own way, if we're worth anything. But one of the things I like about being a poet, is that I get to do that. I don't always have it, but I get to do it every now and then. I like it.

I feel privileged to be able to do this. I feel very grateful to be able to do it. At the same time I feel proud. I've sacrificed. I haven't cared about cars, or career, or those kinds of things. I've been caring for the singing. I mean, I've had great teachers—like Bert Meyers, like Charles Wright—great, scrupulous, ethical, dedicated artists who have helped me feel the right way, who have confirmed my intuition and instincts and who fostered my loyalties. I needed those teachers to help me along, I did, I did.

To help you find your song?

Yeah, particularly my man, Charles Wright.

What did he teach you?

To believe in my poetry, to let my poetry lead me into my life, not the other way around.

Who's helped you the most with craft?

Well, with the technique, I can help my own self. What I needed help with was to believe in my spirits and to confirm my impulses and to deepen them, and also to challenge me to be loyal to them. C. K. Williams was the most instrumental. I brought a poem into class, the one about the woman on the bus, "Stay With Me." C. K. looked at me like this, he drilled me with his eyes. "This is the real thing," he said. "If you can write like this, I don't understand why you write all that other stuff." He was working on "Tar," a breakthrough poem for American literature. It's no wonder how passionate he was. He said, "I don't see why you waste your time, and what's more, I don't see why you're wasting *mine*." The next week I wrote "Yellow Light," then "Off from Swing Shift." All the poems in *Yellow Light* were written under C. K. Williams and Charles Wright.

C. K. taught me to write from a grander state than the mundane, to take the big thing and put all of it in the poem, not to divide it off into short story or essay. He confirmed me in my devotion to writing my own thing. He pounded me on top of my head until I got mad and charged. He motivated me. If it weren't for him I don't know if I would have had the guts. I can't slack off from that level of vision.

Source: Alice Evans, "A Vicious Kind of Tenderness: An Interview with Garrett Hongo," in *Poet & Writers Magazine*, Vol. 20, No. 5, September-October 1992, pp. 37–46.

George Uba

In the following review, Uba asserts that the main concerns of Yellow Light *are personal identity and use of the past to build a collective identity.*

A few years back a popular weekly newsmagazine ran an article on Japanese Americans, treating them as an American success story. The article was headlined—"Outwhiting the Whites." Garrett Kaoru Hongo's book of poetry, *Yellow Light*, demolishes the onesidedness of such headlines and grapples with the underlying problem toward which they unintentionally point: the problem of an ethnic group whose own identity remains ill-defined.

Not that Hongo merely trumpets the familiar tune of ethnic pride. Rather, he excels at balancing a passionate interest in ordinary working-class people performing ordinary activities, with a deep-felt concern over what they are often the unknowing victims of. In the title poem, "Yellow Light," for instance, an unidentified Los Angeles woman returns with a load of groceries to her "neighborhood of Hawaiian apartments, / just starting to steam with cooking" but fails to observe the "war" being waged between the "dim squares" of kitchen light in the barrio and the "brilliant fluorescence" emanating from the wealthy Miracle Mile district. Neatly skirting both the sentimentality and the obvious partisanship that this scenario invites, Hongo concludes the poem without even a glimmer of awareness on the woman's part of the class conflict to which she seems heir, but instead with a riveting, ambiguous image of the yellow moon, at once minatory and transfiguring, that devours "everything in sight." In "Off from Swing Shift," one of several fine poems written about his father, Hongo combines an incisive portrayal of a factory worker who, only within the safe confines of home, dares remove "the easy grin / saying he's lucky as they come," with a genuinely moving depiction of hope seasoned with despair, as the man, a Japanese American war veteran gradually growing deaf "from a shell / at Anzio," listens for the late race results on the radio.

The balance Hongo strikes between the individual's private experience and the larger cultural matrix of which the individual constitutes a part refers the reader to the principal concerns of the book as a whole: the quest for a personal identity and the desire to build and retrieve a collective identity by sifting through the past. In his search for personal identity, Hongo not only jockeys back and forth through time but also through space, traveling from California to Japan and back again. In Japan he finds himself inescapably the outsider, reduced, at least at first, to writing "postcards" back home. But these "Postcards for Bert Meyers" are not filled with the banalities of the ordinary tourist; instead, they define both what has been lost and what has been retained in modern Japan's headlong rush for technological advance. At one point the poet is the bemused foreigner caught in the literal crush of rush hour commuters, able to recover his equilibrium only at the moment when the train stops "And lets out a small puff / Full of tiny Japanese people" ("Yamanote Sen"). At another point he is a lone human figure magically transformed in an urban landscape itself transformed by a sudden rain: "All around me / the ten thousand things / of the universe go slack / in the day's new lagoon / and I seep out of myself like / water from the soaked earth..." ("Alone in a Shower"). Gradually, the poet achieves a harmony with that part of the Japanese past that remains alive to the mutual imagination of its descendants on both sides of the Pacific.

Throughout the book, Hongo's wit and humor leaven the more programmatic elements of his quest. In "Crusing 99," even as he journeys toward the California town called Paradise, he playfully admits that he is inclined to allow his "mind to wander" and at one point even grumbles that the "Dodgers / haven't made it to Vero Beach." And in the marvelous, whacky tour de force, "Who Among You Knows the Essence of Garlic," he savages the pretensions of foreigners by converting their interest in exotic foods into a weapon turned back upon them.

While Hongo's personal quest carries him afar, his attempt to build a collective identity leads him to concentrate wholly upon the Japanese experience in America. Except for the long, hortatory poem "Stepchild," Hongo resists the twin temptations to script an Asian American history at a single stroke and to lash out at those elements of American culture that have worked to deprive Japanese Americans not only of their identity but, more insidiously, of their awareness of their need for one. Instead, he concentrates on individuals and on fragments of lives, and allows their interconnections steadily and silently to accumulate. Within this compass, Hongo ranges widely, from a memorable portrait of a hard-drinking plantation laborer in Hawaii named Kubota who "laughs and lights a cigarette, / breathes out a wreath of smoke / for his funeral, fifty years away" ("Kubota") to an evocative description of a visit to the Nippon Kan in Seattle's Astor Hotel, where yellowing programs and an "open tray of greasepaint," lonely artifacts from a final stage performance in the fall of 1941, help lead to a surrealistic epiphany, a moment of total engagement within the past ("On the Last Performance of *Musumé Dojoji*..."). "And Your Soul Shall Dance" is a hymn to the artist and writer Wakako Yamauchi, who, as a child, yearns so intensely to escape the unpoetic confines of her environment, a "flat valley grooved with irrigation ditches," that when she enters the schoolyard her "classmates scatter like chickens, / shooed by the storm brooding" on her horizon.

Occasionally, Hongo slips. The poem "Roots," which celebrates the links the poet has forged with his Japanese past and the self which has come into his possession, is overburdened finally by the weight of its message. Simply to affirm that there is "a signature to all things / the same as my own" is not enough when the reader expects to be shown that this is so. The long "Crusing 99" suffers from the opposite problem: despite its boisterous humor, it is never completely clear of purpose and ultimately grinds to a halt before a mystifying "scarecrow / made of tumbleweeds" and its own disconcerting mixture of poetic styles. And perhaps more poems on the war-time internment of the Japanese on the West Coast are in order too, given Hongo's avowed concern with curing the condition of "amnesia" within Japanese American culture. Nevertheless, this is an excellent volume of poetry, make no mistake. Hongo applies wit, intelligence, and craftsmanship to his serious theme as few others have been able to do. His book is certain to gain a privileged station in Asian American literature courses, as well as to fuel the continuing controversy over enlarging the American literary canon.

Source: George Uba, "A Review of *Yellow Light*," in *Journal of Ethnic Studies*, Vol. 12, No. 4, Winter 1985, pp. 123–25.

Diane Wakoski

In the following review, Wakoski lauds Yellow Light *as an exciting book of poetry.*

In the spring of 1963, Gilberto Sorrentino, primary book reviewer for *Kulchur* magazine, reviewed my second appearance in print, a book called, as a joke by its editor LeRoi Jones, *Four Young Lady Poets.* In his review, Sorrentino said,

> Diane Wakoski is the least interesting of the four poets presented.... Essentially, this is middle-class poetry.... Miss Wakoski's poems

are disguised in the "modern" trappings but she is as superficial as Edward Albee, another middle-class product.

Of the three other poets, Carol Berge has gone on to become an interesting avant garde fiction writer; Rochelle Owens, an impressive avant garde playwright; and, until recently, Barbara Moraff had more or less disappeared from the literary world, to my knowledge not having published any books for the past 10 years. For better or worse, I have published 13 collections of poems, numerous small press "slim volumes," and a bit of writing on contemporary American poetry.

I have begun my review with this painful memory, never quite healed, to say that I vowed when reading that unthinking and condescending view of my work (though, I must say, I am a deep admirer of Albee's plays, but I am afraid that our work has little in common, not even middle-classness, for when Sorrentino was writing those lines he had obviously not investigated my life. I come from the lower classes, with virtually uneducated poverty-line parents) that I would never so thoughtlessly review young writers, first books, new work. The three books of poems I want to talk about here are very fine examples of poetry and authors whose work I am thankful to talk about. I would like to say things about Hongo, Luhrmann, and Williamson that I wish had been said about my early work, for I feel great affinities with all these poets, each so different but each working in the strength of "American grain."

It was not entirely gratuitous of me to quote Sorrentino's words about my early poems. For something he said as condemnation—"Middleclass"—is now, 20 years later, something we must reckon with as mainstream reality. And for better or worse, we have made a middleclass art in America, to serve I suppose, the first genuine middle-class country where, according to the authors of *Megatrends*, there are now more white collar workers than blue, and information is our new industry.

When we use words like "academic," "middleclass," and "bourgeois," as pejorative now, I think we all sound a little dated and out of touch. There *is* a new American poetry which comes out of comfortable orderly lives. It is written by the Kinnells, Staffords, Levertovs, Creeleys, Kumins, Rothenbergs, and even Ginsbergs. The "men in Brooks Brothers suits" are no longer the enemies. In fact, we live in a decade where it is hard to identify the enemy, though many of the predictions of Orwell's *1984* have come true. Self-destruction seems far more a hazard of our society than either a Big Brother or a Gestapo-style police.

It is to these problems that Tom Luhrmann addresses himself in *The Objects in the Garden*. Like most of us, Luhrmann is a member of the American middle-class who perceives inherent difficulty and pain in the comfortable, even beautiful way of life we have achieved....

In contrast to *The Objects in the Garden*, Garrett Hongo's *Yellow Light* could originate in another world. And perhaps it does. Hongo is first generation American, with Japanese parents. Some part of his childhood was lived in Hawaii, and most of his poems are located in Southern California. This is a dull way to introduce what I think is one of the most exciting books of poems I have read in recent years. It was love at first reading, that had me walking through the midwestern streets of East Lansing, Michigan, dreaming of Southern California, thinking of Rexroth's poems, feeling the spice of crossing two cultures and having the riches of both. Hongo's language is more sensuous than Kinnell's or Levertov's or Lorca's, at his best. Not to slight those poets, all favorites of mine, but Hongo is astonishing. After reading "Who Among You Knows The Essence of Garlic?" I may give up writing food poems, for this one tops everything I have seen in my *Feastletters* search.

> Flukes of giant black mushrooms
> leap from their murky tubs
> and strangle the toes of young carrots.
>
> Broiling chickens ooze grease,
> yellow tears of fat collect
> and spatter in the smoking pot.
>
> Soft ripe pears, blushing
> on the kitchen window sill,
> kneel like plump women
> taking a long, luxurious shampoo,
> and invite you to bite their lips.
>
> Why not grab basketfuls of steaming noodles
> lush and slick as the hair of a fine lady,
> and squeeze?
>
> Two shrimps, big as Portuguese thumbs
> stew among cut guavas, red onions....

It is an amazing piece of descriptive writing. But that is the least of Hongo's skills. He has written the best poem I have ever seen on the American treatment of native Japanese during the Second World War, because it is not really written about that subject, nor does it preach or editorialize in any way. It is a poem called "Off from swing shift," which is about his father coming home from work and getting involved with his passion of gambling, in this case, the home races. He ends the poem,

> There are whole cosmologies
> in a single handicap,
> a lifetime of two-dollar losing
> in one pick of the Daily Double.
>
> Maybe tonight is his night
> for winning, his night
> for beating the odds
> of going deaf from a shell
> at Anzio still echoing
> in the cave of his inner ear,
> his night for cashing in
> the blue chips of shrapnel still grinding
> at the thickening joints of his legs.
>
> But no one calls
> the horse's name, no one
> says Shackles, Rebate, or Pouring Rain.
> No one speaks a word.

It is true, when one has a rich ethnic background, full of unusual customs, interesting foods, a different language or perhaps even religion that there might be something richer in a person's life to write about. Perhaps Sorrentino's dismissal of the middle-class was a feeling that there could be nothing to write about in the uniform lives of the suburbs compared to the slums of big cities. Yet, John Updike has magnificently disproved that in his Rabbit series. The one difference I see between Hongo and Luhrmann's middle-classness, has nothing to do with richness of materials, for both have immense imagination and sensuous powers of description. No, the difference is that Luhrmann's poems are shadowed with a sense of impending crisis, both social and personal (because the social will affect us all), and Hongo's poetry simply is filled with a—what shall I call it—*joie de vivre? Elan?* Somehow there is no contemporary word, but there is an enthusiasm which simply cannot be suppressed. In a long poem, "Cruising 99" the reader can feel the spirit of life itself moving from rhythmic incantation to prophecy. But unlike Luhrmann's prophecy, Hongo's comes from the persona of a wayside palmist who tells him,

> Look at your hand now.
> You can see yourself dancing
> on the hell just above the wrist.
> You must be a happy man.

> You'll be born again and again,
> get to the threshold of Heaven,
> never enter but keep coming back,
> here, for fun, for friends,
> until this will be Paradise,
> and Paradise just an old resort
> the highway's passed by.
> Well have a nice trip.
> You'll make it yet.
> Says so right in that curvy line
> around the Mount of Venus,
> that thumbstump there,
> right where the long straight line
> cuts across like an interstate.

Contrast this with Lurhmann's lines in "Hurricane Weather,"

> The hurricane has come
> and overturned the Ferris wheel.
> It has covered the bugle with dust
> and set the rocking horse on fire.
> It has mated the ostrich and the rhino
> and made one of us think he's in Heaven.
> And no wonder words don't work.

Perhaps I love Luhrmann's poems for their sense of doom, just as I love Hongo's for their insouciance. What the truth of American poetry today is, is that both Hongo and Luhrmann came through middle-class college educations, Luhrmann at Sarah Lawrence and New College, Hongo at Pomona College; and both have MFA degrees in writing, from Columbia and UC, Irvine, respectively. And they have personal individual visions, not some stereotype we must label and reject as "middle-class."

Source: Diane Wakoski, "A Review of *Yellow Light*," in *American Book Review*, Vol. 6, No. 2, January-February 1984, pp. 4–5.

SOURCES

Drake, Barbara, "Garrett Hongo," in *Dictionary of Literary Biography*, Vol. 120, *American Poets since World War II*, 3rd ser., edited by R. S. Gwynn, Gale Research, 1992, pp. 133–36.

Fonseca, Anthony J., "Garrett Hongo," in *Dictionary of Literary Biography*, Vol. 312, *Asian American Writers*, edited by Deborah L. Madsen, Thomson Gale, 2005, pp. 117–22.

Slowik, Mary, "Beyond Lot's Wife: The Immigration Poems of Marilyn Chin, Garrett Hongo, Li-Young Lee, and David Mura," in *MELUS*, Vol. 25, nos. 3-4, Fall-Winter 2000, p. 221.

Uba, George, "A Review of *Yellow Light*," in *Journal of Ethnic Studies*, Vol. 12, No. 4, Winter 1985, pp. 123–25.

Wakoski, Diane, "A Review of *Yellow Light*," in *American Book Review*, Vol. 6, No. 2, January-February 1984, pp. 4–5.

FURTHER READING

Cheung, King-Kok, ed., *An Interethnic Companion to Asian American Literature*, Cambridge University Press, 1997.
Frequently referenced by scholars of Asian American literature, this volume contains essays on topics pertinent to studying literature in this area. In addition to considering literature by ethnicity, the editor includes essays that compare works across ethnicity to uncover similarities in theme and style.

Filipelli, Laurie, *Garrett Hongo*, Boise State University, 1997.
Filipelli's book is the only book-length biography to date for Hongo. It is part of the Western Writers series, and is referenced often in studies on the poet.

Hongo, Garrett, *Volcano: A Memoir of Hawaii*, Vintage, 1996.
Using a strong journey motif, Hongo explores the people and places of his childhood, seeking his roots both figuratively and literally. Critics find this book interesting on its own, but particularly interesting for readers of Hongo's poetry.

Houston, Jeanne Wakatsuki, and James A. Houston, *Farewell to Manzanar*, Houghton Mifflin, 1973, reprint, 2002.
Japanese American writer Jeanne Wakatsuki Houston and her husband describe her experiences at the Manzanar, California internment camp during World War II. Rather than giving an overview, they offer a personal account that makes the dishonor of internment accessible to a young-adult audience.

Woman Work

MAYA ANGELOU

1978

By the time Maya Angelou wrote "Woman Work" in 1978, she had already published three volumes of prose in addition to two previous collections of poetry. It is for her prose that she is most highly praised but her poetry—and "Woman Work" in particular—explores themes such as exploitation and self-identity in an intimate and immediate way that cannot be achieved in prose. Poetry is by its nature more personal and in most cases, relies heavily upon the meaning and value of every single word. Feelings, nuances, and emotions must be inferred or explained in a more economical format, making every word matter.

Angelou's identity as an African American, a woman, and an African American woman influences much of her poetry. This is true of all the poems included in the collection *And Still I Rise* (republished in 2001 as *Still I Rise*). The theme of self-identity in "Woman Work," is especially interesting because the poem allows for two related but differing interpretations. Using imagery and rhythm, Angelou provides the reader with details of her speaker's workaday world, a world in which every day is like the last, and relief is found only in communing with nature. Angelou's masterful manipulation of words presents two possible scenarios: the narrator is a slave or she is representative of any woman whose daily life is dedicated to caring for others.

"Woman Work" was published in a decade when poetry was more mainstream than

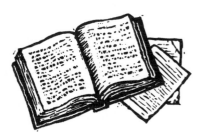

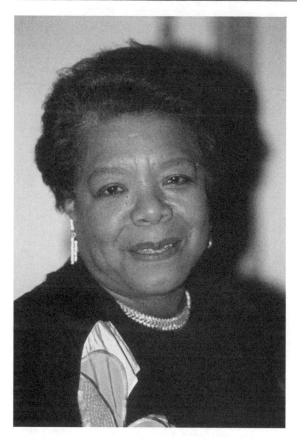

Maya Angelou *(Getty Images)*

it is in the twenty-first century. The 1970s were years of self-exploration for women but also for young people in general. This was a transitional decade marked by the end of the controversial Vietnam War, the increasing momentum of the Feminist Movement, and a shift in how Americans considered themselves and their place in society as social norms and values changed. The cultural focus became one of individualism, and the increased interest in self-analysis and understanding manifested in an surge of self-help books and self-awareness discussion groups.

Poetry was the ideal literary form for the decade because it could have structure or not; it could rhyme or not; it could be specific or general. In other words, poetry was a personal expression that could take virtually any shape and still be a legitimate literary form. People who might not write an essay or an article could express themselves in poetry. And so, poetry in the 1970s was used as a vehicle to explore one's self in relation to the world. "Woman Work" does that.

AUTHOR BIOGRAPHY

Maya Angelou was born Marguerite Ann (or Annie) Johnson on April 4, 1928, in St. Louis, Missouri. Her parents divorced when she was just three years old, and she and her brother (who nicknamed her Maya) were sent to live with her paternal grandmother in the poverty-stricken rural town of Stamps, Arkansas. The children called their strict but loving grand-mother Momma and spent those Arkansas years in relative calm.

At age seven or eight, while visiting her mother in St. Louis, Angelou was raped by her mother's boyfriend. When she told her uncles what had happened, they murdered him. Ange-lou felt responsible and suffered extreme feelings of guilt. She ceased talking and was returned to Momma in Arkansas.

Angelou was mute for five years, during which time she developed a love of language and, ironically, the spoken word. She memorized poetry and secretly—for white authors were forbidden by Momma—read William Shakespeare, Charles Dickens, and Edgar Allen Poe. At twelve, Angelou began to speak again.

Momma and the children moved to San Francisco, where Angelou's mother was living, in the 1940s when the presence of the Ku Klux Klan made Stamps a dangerous place to live. Angelou graduated from high school at seven-teen and soon gave birth to a son she named Guy. She held various jobs in those early years, including dinner cook and night club dancer. In the early 1950s, Angelou married a white man named Tosh Angelos. The marriage did not last, and after the divorce she studied dance and joined the cast of a touring production of *Porgy and Bess.* Angelou continued to dance professionally throughout the decade.

After another brief marriage that took her and Guy to Egypt, Angelou moved to Ghana, West Africa, in 1962. She earned a living as a freelance writer and feature editor. Returning to the United States in the mid-1960s, Angelou took a position as a lecturer at the University of California in Los Angeles and continued act-ing. She began writing her first autobiographical volume, which was published in 1968. Nomi-nated for a National Book Award, *I Know Why the Caged Bird Sings* remains Angelou's most famous and beloved work. She eventually pub-lished five more volumes of her autobiography.

Angelou turned her sights to poetry and published her first collection in 1971. *Just Give Me a Cool Drink of Water 'fore I Diiie* earned its author a Pulitzer Prize nomination and was followed by two more volumes that decade, the second of which was *And Still I Rise* (1978), in which "Woman Work" appears. Angelou married once more, in 1973; the union ended in 1980. By 2009, Angelou had published more than thirty best-selling volumes of poetry, fiction, and nonfiction. In addition, she has written plays, children's books, essays, film and television scripts, and dozens of articles for various journals and periodicals.

In addition to writing, dancing, acting, and teaching/lecturing, Angelou's career includes civil rights activism (with Malcolm X and Martin Luther King, Jr.), singing, and film directing. Highlights include an invitation to compose and read a poem at President Bill Clinton's inauguration in 1993 and a seat on two presidential committees.

Angelou's work and efforts have been honored with countless awards, including three Grammy Awards, the National Medal of Arts (2000), the Lincoln Medal (2008), and more than thirty honorary degrees from universities across the country. In 2009, Angelou was featured as one of *Success Magazine*'s top five women who wield extraordinary influence through their work. Cited especially for her efforts to combat racism and injustice, Angelou credits her self-directed education for empowering her to incite change. In the interview with Erin Casey, Angelou explains how education "liberated me from some of the ignorance that can make a person mean and cruel and prejudiced and stupid. Education has helped me understand that this is my world, but no more mine than yours."

POEM TEXT

I've got the children to tend
The clothes to mend
The floor to mop
The food to shop
Then the chicken to fry   5
Then baby to dry
I got company to feed
The garden to weed
I've got the shirts to press
The tots to dress   10
The cane to be cut
I gotta clean up this hut
Then see about the sick
And the cotton to pick.

Shine on me, sunshine   15
Rain on me, rain
Fall softly, dewdrops
And cool my brow again.

Storm, blow me from here
With your fiercest wind   20
Let me float across the sky
'Til I can rest again.

Fall gently, snowflakes
Cover me with white
Cold icy kisses and   25
Let me rest tonight.

Sun, rain, curving sky
Mountain, oceans, leaf and stone
Star shine, moon glow
You're all that I can call my own.   30

POEM SUMMARY

Lines 1–14

This first stanza of "Woman Work" is the most important in the poem because it is here the reader could infer that the woman speaking is a slave.

Lines 11 and 14 talk about crops that need tending. These are not just any crops, but those grown in the Deep South and traditionally harvested by African American slaves. Cane and cotton were two of the most profitable crops in the Antebellum (pre–Civil War) South, and plantations relied on them for profit. The most economical means of harvesting them was through free—slave—labor.

Once that fact is established, the first stanza takes on new meaning. The chores listed are not necessarily—or even probably—the woman's own. Whose children is she tending, whose clothes need mending? Is the floor that needs mopping her own? Surely not, since line 12 tells the reader she lives in a hut. Would she be having company? Probably not, but wealthy plantation owners often entertained guests. Most, if not all, of the first stanza refers to activity that is imposed upon the woman for the benefit of others. Nowhere does she talk about herself except in relation to the responsibilities she is expected to fulfill.

Conversely, some readers might interpret this first stanza to be a description in the life of any hardworking woman in a domestic situation. Until the late 1940s and early 1950s, African

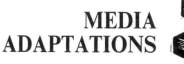

MEDIA ADAPTATIONS

- Maya Angelou reads an abridged version of *And Still I Rise* on audiocassette, produced by Random House Audio in 1996.
- Random House Audio Voices released an unabridged version of *And Still I Rise* on CD in 2001. The author reads her own work.
- An audio download of 13 selections from *And Still I Rise* is available at http://www.audible.com. The poem "Woman Work" is included.

Americans often found work as sharecroppers in the south; they worked and lived on the land as tenants. In return, a certain percentage of the harvest was given to the landowner. Cane and cotton were prominent crops in the American South and needed someone to tend to them.

Read from this perspective, the woman's life would be very similar to that of a slave because much of her daily work is done for the benefit of someone else, though to a lesser extent. Her housing would still be shabby, accurately described as a "hut," perhaps with wooden floors that required mopping.

Lines 15–30

The remaining four stanzas can be analyzed together because they work as one unit. Whereas the first stanza, which is nearly four times longer than each of the remaining four, concerns itself with what the woman must do on a daily basis for someone else, the remaining sixteen lines are all about what nature can do for her.

Lines 15–18 invoke the sun's warmth and the rain's dewy moisture to cool her brow.

Lines 19–22 beseech the storm and its wind to blow her across the sky, far from where she is, so that she might find rest.

Lines 23–26 rely on gentle snow to cover and comfort her so that she can rest her weary body and mind.

The final stanza, lines 27–30, acknowledges that the woman owns nothing but nature's elements, and even that ownership is figurative rather than literal. Every moment of the woman's life is spent in service to others, and when at last she is done at the end of a long and tiring day, all she has left is the natural world surrounding her: sun, sky, mountain and stone, stars, and moonlight.

These last four stanzas are all about finding comfort and release, stolen moments of peace from the monotonous and never-ending routine of her daily life. Nature is the source of this woman's strength. The idea that the woman speaking is a slave is reinforced in the final line of the poem.

While lines 11, 14, and 30, support the idea that the speaker is a slave, so does the placement of the poem in the collection *And Still I Rise*. "Woman Work" is situated between "To Beat the Child was Bad Enough" and "One More Round." The former is about child abuse; the latter about slavery. Both surrounding poems explore themes of bondage and abuse, and "One More Round" discusses the "daily grind" of slavery, suggesting a routine of toil and exploitation. It would make sense that "Woman Work" examine a similar topic.

THEMES

Slavery

Upon first read, "Woman Work" may seem like a poem written about any woman with a family to care for. Lines 11 and 14 clearly change that impression because most women in modern America do not cut (sugar) cane or pick cotton. These two chores indicate that the woman is a slave.

Considered in this light, the reader understands that the bulk of the chores that make up the woman's day are not self-serving; they are chores she must perform for her master. The children belong to him. The floor that needs mopping in line 3 is probably not hers, since she lives in a hut. The company she must feed? It is probably not hers. Although some of what she must accomplish may be for herself, most of it is not.

Line 12 suggests the woman is a slave. Most people, even those living in abject poverty, would not refer to their homes as huts. The

TOPICS FOR FURTHER STUDY

- Choose a poem from the "Thorns" section of Pat Mora's collection titled *My Own True Name: New and Selected Poems for Young Adults*. Compare the imagery in one of these Latina poems with that used in Angelou's "Woman Work." Make a Venn diagram to illustrate how the imagery is similar and how it is different. How does the imagery used help the reader "see" Mora's poem?

- Using marker, paint, or colored pencils, draw a picture to represent each of the five stanzas in "Woman Work." Be sure the colors you choose reflect the feeling each stanza inspires in you. As an alternative, find images and create a PowerPoint slide presentation to present the feelings each stanza inspires.

- Read Angelou's poem, "Phenomenal Woman." How does it compare to "Woman Work"? Write a brief report on how the poems are alike and how they differ. Include in your report mention of themes and literary style.

- Read the poem once with the idea that the woman is a slave. Read it again with the idea that she is just an ordinary woman. How does the meaning of the poem change upon these two readings? Write an essay using specific lines from the poem to support your ideas.

- Consider an aspect of your own life and write a poem about it. Try to use sound, imagery, and other style techniques to make your poem come to life. Read the poem aloud to the class.

- Using your own words, rewrite "Woman Work" as an English sonnet. The English sonnet is a 14-line poem that uses an *abab cdcd efef gg* rhyme scheme. How does changing the structure of a poem change its meaning and how it affects the reader?

woman in the poem lives in a hut—a small, crude shelter. Most slaves lived in shacks and huts while their masters lived in great, sprawling mansions. It is possible that the woman is simply poor, but this line, taken along with the others, strongly suggests she is a slave.

The final line of the poem also makes clear that the woman is a slave. By claiming only nature as her own, she acknowledges her lack of control or ownership over the rest of her life. At the end of a long, back-breaking day, this (slave) woman takes comfort in the sun and the rain, the stars and the moon. They assuage her sadness and soothe her spiritual emptiness. They are all she owns in the world.

Those readers who interpret the poem to be about women in general rather than those within the confines of slavery might substitute the slavery theme with one of work. Lines 1 through 14—nearly half the poem—examine this theme by listing chore after chore after chore. The reader quickly understands that the woman's life revolves around the duties she must perform.

Self-Identity

The poem is an exploration of self-identity. This particular woman identifies who she is by what she does: She works for—is owned by—someone else. She is a slave. She is a tired woman who wants nothing more than to rest. Lines 22 and 26 support the idea that her world is a weary one.

There is no evidence throughout the poem that the woman identifies herself using any other means of measurement. She makes it clear in line 30 that she owns nothing more than her natural surroundings. She lives without. She is nothing more than her role allows her to be.

Self-identity is a theme of the poem regardless of reader interpretation. Even if the speaker is not a slave, she clearly considers her life in terms of its drudgery and daily routine. Enjoyment is found only when the work is done and she can rest.

African American Culture

The institution of slavery is a major, if not the primary, factor in understanding the African American culture and experience in America. Because "Woman Work" explores the theme of slavery, by extension it explores the theme of African American culture.

Gender Roles

"Woman Work" examines what it meant to be an African American woman in a slave culture. If this poem were about a man, the first 14 lines would read quite differently, with the exception of lines 11 and 14. Although male slaves cut cane and picked cotton alongside the women, the bulk of their chores were different, perhaps not so mundane.

In that same vein, there is no way to know if line 15 through 30 would have been written as they are if the person speaking was male. Historically, women have been more connected to nature (Mother Earth) and its physical aspects; their work has centered around natural functions: caring for children and the sick, preparing food and cleaning up afterward, even the act of sex has been, historically, an obligation for women. Men interact with nature in a more exploitive way, generally speaking. Their interaction with the physical aspects of the earth has historically been to take what they need or want by hunting, mining, drilling, logging, and so on.

That the woman in the poem finds comfort in nature is a natural extension of her traditional gender role. Were the speaker a man, those four stanzas would create a completely different message because of their traditional gender role and relationship to nature.

Exploitation

To be exploited is to work excessively hard for someone else's benefit. The first stanza of this poem explores the theme of exploitation whether the woman is understood to be a slave or simply representative of most women. The list of chores never ends; as soon as she completes the last one, the cycle begins again. She is overworked, exhausted, and weary, but all the effort expended is for someone else's benefit.

Nature

The four shorter stanzas consisting of lines 15–30 concern themselves with nature as a source of comfort and rejuvenation. For the woman whose life is defined by what she must do, the peaceful qualities found in nature—gentle snowflakes, curving sky, cooling dewdrops—are gifts she relies upon to provide respite from her activity-filled days.

Transcendence

Despite the obvious repetition of the chores described in lines 1–14, "Woman Work" is about transcendence, or rising above and beyond the limitations imposed upon the speaker. Lines 15–30 find her engaged in a sensual (meaning of the physical senses), almost spiritual experience as

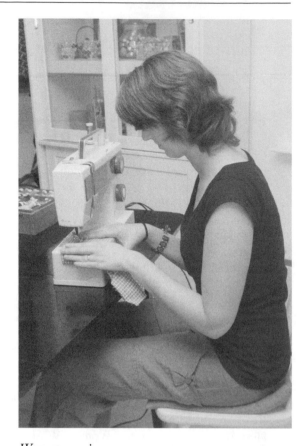

Woman sewing (Image copyright Gertjan Hooijer, 2009. Used under license from Shutterstock.com)

the dew cools her brow and the winds carry her across the sky. She is communing with nature and finding peace and even a kind of balance in her dreary life.

STYLE

Rhyme

Rhyme is a technique that often lends a singsong quality to a poem. Angelou's use of rhyme in much of her poetry is one aspect critics tend to criticize because they believe it makes her poetry sound juvenile.

Angelou's use of rhyme in the first 14 lines of "Woman Work," however, is appropriate and underscores the meaning behind the stanza. By developing the stanza using rhyming couplets (every pair of lines rhymes), the poem shows that the work is mundane. That rhyming quality makes the stanza seem more like a list whose items must be checked off every day. The woman's frustration can be felt as she reels off the list of activities she must complete.

Rhyme is used but more loosely in the four shorter stanzas and not to the same effect. Instead, the end rhyme is a means of pulling together each stanza to present a complete image in the reader's mind.

Imagery

Imagery is descriptive language that evokes a sensory (sight, smell, taste, sight, and sound) experience. The poem's four shorter stanzas, in which the speaker refers to nature and its elements, uses imagery to convey meaning. For example, in the third stanza, lines 19–22, she uses words and phrases that force the reader to envision what is happening: storm, blow, fiercest wind, float.

Likewise, lines 23–26 rely on imagery: Snowflakes fall gently, giving cold, icy kisses. The reader can actually *see* these images as the speaker describes them.

Rhythm

Angelou does not use a consistent rhythm throughout the poem or even throughout each stanza, but she uses it in much the same way she does rhyme: to underscore the meaning of her message.

In lines 1–14, the lines are relatively short—4 to 7 syllables. Nearly every word in those lines is one syllable. These two features considered together give the stanza a choppy feel, even as the aforementioned rhyme lends a singsong quality. The brevity of both words and line length add to that feeling of the speaker checking off each activity as its listed or reeling off the (seemingly) endless list quickly before she forgets something.

Repetition

Repetition is used only in the first 14 lines. Like the rhyme and rhythm techniques, this repetition lends itself well to the point of the stanza. Lines 1, 7, 9, and 12 begin with some form of the word "I," a reminder that the speaker is burdened with this laundry list of chores. Lines 2, 3, 4, 8, 10, and 11 begin with "the." Again, this repetition adds to the singsong rhythm that serves this stanza so well. Lines 5, 6, and 13 begin with "then." First the speaker must do this, this, and this, and then she must do that, that, and that. Repetition

emphasizes the endlessness of the responsibilities shouldered by the woman.

Alliteration

Alliteration is the repetition of consonants, and Angelou employs alliteration all the way through the first stanza, or 14 lines. She uses hard consonant sounds, primarily "c" and "t." These give a harsh, angry tone to the words of the stanza. This harshness is emphasized by the short length of the words: tots, cane, cut, hut, sick, pick, mop, shop.

Personification

Objects are personified when they are given human characteristics. Although Angelou does not use personification very much, she does use it when talking about the woman's interactions with nature.

In lines 17 and 18, the dewdrops cool her brow. Usually, the idea of cooling one's brow involves one person comforting another. In lines 23–25, the snowflakes cover the woman with kisses. Again, this is an act of comfort, one usually involving humans.

This use of personification emphasizes the important role nature plays in the speaker's life. Nature relieves and comforts, restores and provides. It acts as a sort of soul mate in the life of a woman who has spoken not one word of having a partner or husband or even friend.

Spoken Word

All of the style techniques mentioned previously are more obvious if the reader reads this poem aloud. Angelou writes in the oral tradition, meaning she intends for her work to be spoken aloud. By speaking the lines, the reader more clearly hears the rhythm, the rhyme, the repetition, and alliteration. Sounds of letters and words support the imagery. The combination of sound and voice intonation brings this particular poem to life.

HISTORICAL CONTEXT

The 1970s were a decade of social and cultural transition in the United States. America was well into the Vietnam War, and the country found itself divided according to political ideology. The 1960s, known as a period of great social activism owing in part to the war, faded as the 1970s

COMPARE & CONTRAST

- **1970s:** The social and cultural focus is on women's rights as women seek equality in the workplace and beyond.

  Today: Women have made great progress since the 1970s, but they still make only seventy-eight cents for every dollar earned by men. Although more men stay home and take care of household chores than ever before, cooking, cleaning, and tending to children is still largely considered women's work.

- **1970s:** There is an outpouring of new work regarding the history of slavery in the American South. Landmark studies and research lead historians to reassess and reinterpret that era in American history.

  Today: Slave narratives are accepted as legitimate texts in the American literary canon.

American culture recognizes the injustices of the institution of slavery, and the federal government makes a formal apology but does not pay slavery reparations.

- **1970s:** The trend in poetry leans toward confessional (the sharing of intimate details of one's life), surrealistic (dream-like imagery to represent the subconscious), and multicultural (voices from a variety of cultures). There is a strong interest in the voices of African American women.

  Today: Poetry is in a transitional state. As an art form, it is embraced more academically than it was in previous decades. And yet, the existence of blogs, social networking sites, and zines makes poetry more accessible to the masses than ever before.

---

morphed into a culture of self-absorption. As the war came to an end, the Feminist Movement came to fruition and gained momentum. As women challenged traditional societal expectations and gender roles, the emphasis shifted from what America was as a society to who Americans were as individuals and what they needed and wanted. It became a decade of psychological analysis and self-awareness.

Social Movements

Three social movements defined the 1970s: Environmentalism, Feminism, Gay Rights. Major environmental legislation was passed, most notably the establishment of the Environmental Protection Agency in 1970, followed by the Clean Water Act of 1972 and the Endangered Species Act of 1973. As concern for the environment and its resources increased, so did the interest in nuclear power. When the Three Mile Island nuclear plant meltdown in 1979 made headlines across the country, opposition to nuclear power intensified.

The women's rights movement known as the second wave of feminism gained momentum throughout the 1970s. Women demanded equal consideration and treatment and joined the workforce in numbers never before seen in America. Women's groups—such as the National Organization for Women—that were formed in the 1960s increased their memberships as women sought both social and political balance in their lives. By the mid-1970s, many federal laws had been passed promoting equality for women. Title IX of the Education Amendments of 1972 made discrimination on the basis sex illegal in any educational institution that received federal funds and opened the way for greater opportunities for women. Military academies began accepting female students. The most controversial case ever to appear before the Supreme Court made legal a woman's right to have an abortion. *Roe v. Wade* was decided in 1973 and remains at the forefront of political and social issues even in the twenty-first century.

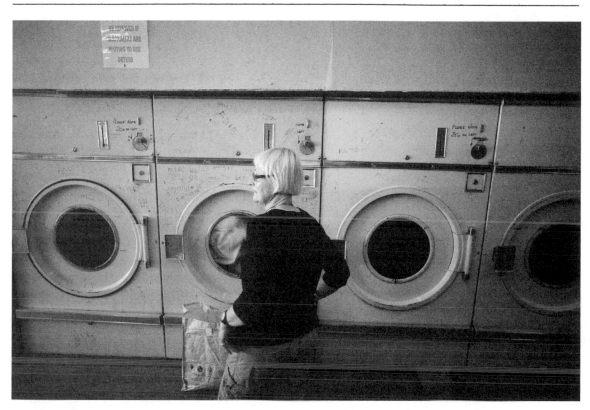

Woman doing laundry (*Christopher Furlong | Getty Images*)

Politics and the Economy

America's political scene in the 1970s was as tumultuous. President Richard Nixon began pulling troops out of Vietnam in the early years and began efforts to improve relations with China and the Soviet Union. These activities increased his popularity and helped him win reelection in 1972. By 1974, Nixon resigned over the Watergate scandal and Vice President Gerald Ford was sworn in as president. Ford was not a popular president, largely because he had pardoned Nixon, and he lost the 1976 election to Jimmy Carter whose problems with the Iranian hostage crisis served to point out the continuing discontent with American foreign policy.

The end of the decade saw America in economic and energy crisis, the foundation of which was the soaring cost of imported oil. Gasoline was rationed, and the country found itself in energy conservation mode, a huge factor in the rise of the environmental movement's activities. Inflation and recession both hurt economic growth.

Culture

As women gained more rights with the passing of federal legislation, social norms and laws were increasingly favorable to women. They became more visible outside the home and neighborhood and in the media as they broke traditional gender role expectations and blurred the lines of the social structure.

At home, American viewers enjoyed what became known as "social consciousness" programming. *All in the Family* was a comedy that explored controversial topics such as racism, feminism, poverty, and more and remained the highest-rated television series from 1971 through 1976. By the late 1970s, however, America was more interested in lighter-hearted series such as *Charlie's Angels* and *Three's Company*.

Art Mimics Life

All of these factors—social, political, economic, and cultural—influenced the arts of the 1970s. Whether art reflected life at the time or the other way around, one thing was certain: literature in the 1970s was all about self-exploration, mainly through poetry and primarily by women. Parallel to the increased exploration of racism and feminism was the rise in the interest of African American writers and their works. Popular poets of the decade include Maya Angelou, Nikki Giovanni, and Gwendolyn Brooks, each of whom wrote about women, their lives as African Americans, and the hardships experienced as both.

CRITICAL OVERVIEW

Maya Angelou is known and praised primarily for her autobiographical volumes. Her poem "Woman Work" was published in her third volume of poetry *And Still I Rise*. Of that collection, a *Publishers Weekly* critic writes, "Hers is not a major poetical voice.... But her warmth, honesty, strength and deep-rooted sense of personal pride—call it defiance—come through in almost every word she sets down."

Angelou's poetry written in the early 1970s focused on the role of African American women in the slave culture of the mid-nineteenth century through the more rebellious era of the 1960s. Though published in 1978, "Woman Work" is a poem that easily fits along that continuum. The thirty-two poems included in *And Still I Rise* include her oft-examined themes of love and its accompanying loneliness as well as the Southern oppression of African Americans. Yet this is the collection in which Angelou begins exploring other themes as well, including the nature of woman. Whether one considers "Woman Work" a slice-of-life portrayal of an African American slave woman or as a general commentary on the life of any woman in general, it is clear that Angelou is committing to print her thoughts on what it means to be a woman.

In the 1996 book, *Heart of a Woman, Mind of a Writer, and Soul of a Poet*, Lyman B. Hagen extols Angelou's gift as a natural storyteller saying, "She sometimes describes, sometimes narrates, but most often dramatizes." Angelou uses this gift in her prose and poetry alike.

In the twenty-first century, Angelou remains admired more for her prose than her poetry. Most of her poems are relatively short and rely on rhyme and simple language. Critical reception of her poetry has generally been more negative than positive, with critics unimpressed with the quality. Janet Blundell of *Library Journal* judged one poetry collection to be "no match

for Angelou's prose writings." Yet the author has a dedicated and loyal audience for her poetry as well as her prose.

Angelou's Random House editor, Robert Loomis, writes in a letter to the critic Lyman Hagen, "I've always believed that those who have reservations about Angelou's poetry simply don't understand what she's doing.... What she is writing is poetry that is very definitely in what I could call the oral tradition." This assessment goes hand-in-hand with Hagen's belief that Angelou is a storyteller. Stories in African American cultures were passed down orally; they rely on rhyme, rhythm, and sound for meaning and full appreciation.

CRITICISM

Rebecca Valentine

Valentine is a freelance writer and editor who holds a bachelor's degree in English with an emphasis on literary analysis. In this essay, she suggests that a feminist analysis of "Woman Work" supports the idea that the juxtaposition of nature and physical labor makes the poem a piece of protest literature.

The definition of protest literature is fluid and varies according to perspective. For example, social critics could insist that protest literature must include a specific political purpose. A feminist critic may look to protest literature to promote (or avoid promoting) a gender bias. The deconstructionist who is concerned only with language and definition and not at all with the author's intention may well argue that all literature is a form of protest. Whittled to the bare bones, any definition of protest literature must at least include the idea that the author is speaking against something. If we assume that "Woman Work" is written in the voice of a female slave, Angelou has written a poem in defiance of oppression. By essentially dividing the poem in half—the first half listing the speaker's chores, the second half reconnecting with nature—Angelou defends a woman's refusal to be only what she is socially allowed to be.

Lines 1–14 of "Woman Work" create a checklist of chores the speaker of the poem must do on a daily basis. She tends to children and the sick, shops for food and prepares it, cleans the house, mends and irons clothing, harvests crops and weeds gardens. The work is mundane and demanding; it is physically draining and mentally

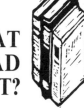

WHAT DO I READ NEXT?

- L. Patricia Kite's biography *Maya Angelou* (2006) is written for a young-adult audience. The book begins with Angelou being invited to read her poem at President Clinton's inauguration in 1993 and flashes back to her birth. From there, Kite works chronologically to present both personal and professional highlights.

- The Poetry Foundation's Web site at http://www.poetryfoundation.org provides visitors with full-text poems, biographies of poets, insightful articles, reading guides, the online edition of *Poetry* magazine, and much more.

- *Island: Poetry and History of Chinese Immigrants on Angel Island, 1910–1940* is a collection of poetry copied from the walls of Angel Island Immigration Station. Translated and published by Him Mark Lai, Genny Lim, and Judy Yung in 1999, these poems tell of the sad and lonely experiences of thousands of immigrant hopefuls who came to America only to be treated with disrespect.

- Twenty-five of Angelou's poems are collected in Edwin Graves Wilson's *Poetry for Young People: Maya Angelou* (2007), illustrated by award-winning artist Jerome Lagarrigue. Each poem is preceded by an introduction.

- A special edition of Angelou's *Phenomenal Woman* was published in 2000 and combines the poet's words with paintings of Paul Gaugin. The poem by the same title was written in 1978 and published in the same collection as "Woman Work."

- Young-adult author Anne Rinaldi has written a historical fiction novel about the slave poet Phillis Wheatley. *Hang a Thousand Trees with Ribbons: The Story of Phillis Wheatley* (1996) mixes fact with fiction to present the tale of America's first African American poet, who died at the age of 30.

unrewarding. It is the life that has been prescribed for the woman because she is a slave.

The tone of that stanza is depressing. There is no enthusiasm or interest in the voice of the speaker. She speaks in clipped phrases, using blunt words that reveal her world-weary attitude.

Compare that tone with that of the other half of the poem, in which the speaker reunites with nature and the elements that bring her peace and respite. These stanzas are created using imagery—icy kisses, curving sky—and words that roll off the tongue. Gone is the harshness of the first 14 lines; it has been replaced not with another list, but with a conversation—albeit one-sided—between the woman and nature.

Sociologists and cultural theorists alike have long purported that women are more earth centered than men. This is not to say that men do not appreciate and respect nature. But women, it is generally agreed upon, have a more reciprocal relationship with the earth. The work women have traditionally done—giving and nurturing life—is directly connected with nature and her cycles. This connection is more than just physical in nature; it is spiritual as well.

In the era of American slavery, African Americans were considered the property of their owners. They had no rights, no voice, no say. The first stanza of "Woman Work" reflects these imposed restrictions. The woman's life is filled with one chore, one responsibility, after another. Every waking moment is spent fulfilling the needs and wants of someone else; her own needs and desires go unattended. Her life is not her own.

These limitations would have been devastating for anyone, man or woman. But they arguably caused a greater sense of loss for women. In her book *Women, Earth, and Creator Spirit*, Elizabeth Johnson explores the idea that because of the way women have lived historically, they "tend to experience themselves as a self in fundamental embodied connection with others." Imagine, then, how crippling it must have been for African American women to lose their families and friends and be forced into bondage for people who cared not one bit for their well-being. Without that connection, this already marginalized group of women was pushed further to the outer banks of humanity.

Yet Angelou's poem suggests that no matter how merciless the master, no matter how back-breaking and tedious the labor, slave women refused to be oppressed to the point of nothingness. In "Woman Work," the speaker turns to the only option left: nature. In her workaday world, the woman has no power. But with nature, she still has the ability to make requests, to ask that her needs be fulfilled. She speaks to nature almost as if to a lover when she uses phrases such as "fall softly," "cover me," and "let me rest." Line 30 of the poem is especially pointed in its depiction of the woman's relationship with nature. She owns it, claiming its comfort for herself.

By depicting the woman's daily hardship in the first 14 lines of the poem and her communion with nature in the last 16 lines, Angelou has created a piece of protest literature. She tells the reader that life is one tedious chore after another for this slave. She is not appreciated or valued, but merely expected to perform duty upon duty. She is exploited to such an extent that she is left feeling empty, alone, without.

And yet this woman refuses to accept the life inflicted upon her as the only life she has. She turns and returns to nature and all her glorious gifts in search of comfort and solace. She makes requests and is honored with replies in the form of fiercely blowing winds, gently falling snowflakes, and endlessly curving skies. Despite the fact that the slave woman is ostracized, criticized, degraded, and nearly dehumanized, she retaliates—protests—by refusing to let those in power force her to a life of nothingness.

Rather than dominate nature as others dominate her, the woman seeks and builds connections with the natural world around her. She considers nature a friend. She will not become what she is believed to be. Through resistance and a resolute spirit, the woman retains her sense of dignity and worth. In her heart, she has not forgotten who she is.

Source: Rebecca Valentine, Critical Essay on "Woman Work," in *Poetry for Students*, Gale, Cengage Learning, 2010.

Cassandra Spratling

In the following interview, Spratling speaks with Angelou about her role as a woman.

If there is one thing women should do for their daughters, it is praise them and tell them that they are somebody special, says the celebrated author, singer and poet Maya Angelou.

"You tell them they're pretty," Angelou says. "You tell them they're beautiful. You tell them that their hair is nice. Make over her

because, know this, in the street there is somebody who's going to do that, and not to her benefit.

"Let her know that 'my mother thinks I'm the big cheese,' so that inside themselves they are secure that they are worthy to be treated well."

That's a lesson Angelou learned from her mother, and it's one described in her latest book, *Letter to My Daughter* (Random House).

Angelou's new book isn't actually a letter to her daughter. In fact, she has only one child, a son. But she has mothered and mentored many women, including Oprah Winfrey.

For twenty years, Angelou jotted down ideas, thoughts and snapshots of experiences — but never quite finished them. Last year she looked at what she had written and realized that she might have enough for a book. The result is a collection of reflections and insights that is part memoir, part prose, part poetry and all things Angelou.

It is writing that takes you to a place where you taste the red rice she writes about, sway to the music she talks about and feel the faith that caused her grandmother to trust God in the face of a devastating Depression.

Angelou says she didn't write the book to preach or to attach a lesson to every story.

"I try not to be that kind of teacher," she says. "I suggest the reader will know if there's a lesson in there for her, and it may be a different lesson than the one I extracted."

Born Marguerite Annie Johnson, Angelou was given the nickname Maya by her only sibling, her brother, Bailey. Her beloved grandmother raised her in Stamps, Ark., during her early childhood, although she later moved to California to live with her mother.

At age seven, she was sexually assaulted by her mother's boyfriend, and an uncle killed her attacker. She felt so responsible for the man's death that she stopped speaking for five years. She thought her naming him had killed him.

Her career began when she was given a scholarship to study dance and drama while in high school in San Francisco. It became her stepping stone to performing — singing, dancing, acting — and world travel, including a European tour in which she played Ruby in the opera "Porgy and Bess" in the 1950s.

After moving to New York in the early 1960s, she became part of a community of artists and writers whose words and work both reflected and inspired the growing civil rights movement.

She would eventually become most known for her writing. Her books include a series of biographical works, children's books, poetry, a line of greeting cards and a cookbook that re-creates many of her favorite foods.

She captured the world's attention when she read a poem she composed for President Bill Clinton's 1993 inauguration, "On the Pulse of the Morning."

Angelou teaches at Wake Forest University in Winston-Salem, N.C., where she lives. This semester, she's teaching a course on world poetry and dramatic performance.

During a recent telephone conversation, Angelou discussed subjects ranging from her latest book to Michelle Obama, the economy and aging.

People, she says, ought to look less at possessions and more toward one another for personal fulfillment.

"It's time for us to stop looking at things . . . and look at human beings. Look at the children. Look at the men. Look at the women."

She fondly recalls meeting Michelle Obama at a campaign fund-raiser in October, and describes her as genuine and graceful.

"She's the real deal. She has no pretense. No preening, no posturing," Angelou says. "She was exactly herself. I told her, 'I'm a 6-foot-tall, 80-year-old African-American woman and that brings me to certain things.' And she said to me, 'I expect to be able to say that myself.' . . .

"That's smart. That's very smart. She's very intelligent and knows where she is and who she is. She is a blessing."

As the nation's first lady, Obama presents a sense of grace and poise that others, regardless of race or gender, could learn from, Angelou says.

"It would behoove us all to learn some grace," she says. "Grace is not just posture. It really is civility and that's civil rights at the highest level. Civility, courtesy, well-chosen words, kindness, interest in other human beings, not just interest in one self."

That Angelou, who will turn 81 on April 4, is still teaching, writing, speaking and motivating women and men is a reflection of the poem that she has come to be known for, "Phenomenal Women."

Age shouldn't stop a woman — or anyone — from accomplishing all she can, she says. She mentions civil rights pioneer Dr. Dorothy Height, president emeritus of the National Council of Negro Women, as an example. The 95-year-old Height has invited Angelou to come to Washington, D.C., in April to speak at an event she is organizing.

"I'm a patsy for her and all older women... particularly older black women," says Angelou. "They clap their hands and I come running or walking as fast as I can."

Aging isn't an end point, she says.

"I can't run the 5K dash. There are certain constraints that prohibit me from reaching certain goals so I make goals that are within my reach," she says. "I don't ask myself to dance the jitterbug, but I still have rhythm."

Source: Cassandra Spratling, "Maya Angelou Reflects on Life, Grace, and Self-Esteem," in *Detroit Free Press*, March 18, 2009.

Cassandra Spratling
In the following article, Spratling writes about Angelou's ability to make even the most mundane task into poetry, as she does in "Woman Work."

Reading Maya Angelou's *Even the Stars Look Lonesome* (Random House) is almost like attending one of her soul-stirring readings: You get some poetry, some singing, some lecturing and a whole lot of earthy conversation about everything from Oprah and West African art to sexuality. And all of it's good, even the bad stuff.

Or, at least she makes it sound that way.

Take the story of her last marriage. It's a sad tale, really, because it's more about the love they lost than the ties that bound them together. But, Angelou makes it sound so sweet, you end up feeling as much joy as sorrow.

As usual, it's the most personal recollections that are the best in this collection. Angelou consistently is able to make even the most mundane topic warm and exciting. There is, for example, the description of her house in Winston-Salem, N.C., the one she moved to after another house made her heart crumble. In this essay about the power of houses to heal and hurt, she leads the reader to feel and understand how much her house means to her, how a house really can be a home. More than love at first sight, it was home upon entry.

Angelou ends with the tale of a woman who fails to find peace and joy within herself. But, again the reader isn't left feeling down. Angelou reminds us to find greatness in simple things, pleasure in plain pursuits and good company with ourselves. A good book wouldn't hurt either.

Source: Cassandra Spratling, "Maya Angelou Waxes Personal with Poetry," in *Detroit Free Press*, September 10, 2007.

SOURCES

Angelou, Maya, *Poems*, Bantam, 1993.

Blundell, Janet, Review of *Shaker, Why Don't You Sing?*, in *Library Journal*, Vol. 108, 1983, p. 746.

Casey, Erin, "Women of Influence: Shattering Stereotypes and Raising the Bar, These Women Are Shaping America's Future," in *Success Magazine*, May 2009, pp. 50–56.

"Global Renaissance Woman," in *MayaAngelou.com*, http://mayaangelou.com/bio/ (accessed August 4, 2009).

Hagen, Lyman B., *Heart of a Woman, Mind of a Writer, and Soul of a Poet: A Critical Analysis of the Writings of Maya Angelou*, University Press of America, 1996, p. 29, 118–36.

Johnson, Elizabeth A., *Women, Earth, and Creator Spirit*, Paulist Press, 1993, p. 25.

McGraw, Patricia Washington, "Maya Angelou," in *The Encyclopedia of Arkansas History & Culture*, http://www.encyclopediaofarkansas.net/encyclopedia/entry-detail.aspx?entryID=1085 (accessed August 4, 2009).

Mooney, Louise, "Maya Angelou," in *Newsmakers*, Gale Research, 1993, http://find.galegroup.com/srcx/basic Search (accessed November 17, 2009).

"1970s: Encyclopedia–1970s," in *Global Oneness*, http://www.experiencefestival.com/a/1970s/id/1900210 (accessed on July 31, 2009).

Plant, Judith, "Women and Nature," in *The Green Fuse*, http://www.thegreenfuse.org/plant.htm (accessed August 6, 2009).

Review of *Angelina of Italy* in *Publishers Weekly*, Vol. 251, No. 36, September 6, 2004, p. 62.

Soto, Kate, "American Poets in the 21st Century: The New Poetics," in *Artvoice*, http://artvoice.com/issues/v7 n4/american_poets_in_the_21st_century the new_poetics (accessed on July 31, 2009).

FURTHER READING

Angelou, Maya, *I Know Why the Caged Bird Sings*, Ballantine Books, 2009.

> Originally published in 1970, this is the first of five autobiographical works written by Angelou. This book recounts the author's abusive and frustrating childhood. Angelou shares her memories in an authentic and genuine voice as she takes the reader through the days of her early youth, which ended with an unwanted pregnancy that changed her life irrevocably.

Harper, Michael S., and Anthony Walton, *Every Shut Eye Ain't Asleep: An Anthology of Poetry by African Americans since 1945*, Back Bay Books, 1994.

> This anthology collects the poetry of 35 poets born between 1913 and 1962. Although some of the featured poets are well known—Gwendolyn Brooks and Rita Dove, for example—many are not. Taken together, the poetry provides a poignant look at life in America for African Americans.

Hughes, Langston, *The Collected Poems of Langston Hughes*, edited by Arnold Rampersad and David E. Roessel, Vintage, 1995.

> This collection includes 860 poems, more than any previous collection of Hughes's work. Readers will appreciate his humor and insight into the human condition.

Seager, Joni, *The Penguin Atlas of Women in the World: Fourth Edition*, 4th ed., Penguin, 2000.

> This updated edition provides a current analysis of key issues faced by women across the globe today: women at work, changing households, equality, motherhood, domestic violence, and more. Maps, graphics, and illustrations enrich the book for the more visual learner.

Glossary of Literary Terms

A

Abstract: Used as a noun, the term refers to a short summary or outline of a longer work. As an adjective applied to writing or literary works, abstract refers to words or phrases that name things not knowable through the five senses.

Accent: The emphasis or stress placed on a syllable in poetry. Traditional poetry commonly uses patterns of accented and unaccented syllables (known as feet) that create distinct rhythms. Much modern poetry uses less formal arrangements that create a sense of freedom and spontaneity.

Aestheticism: A literary and artistic movement of the nineteenth century. Followers of the movement believed that art should not be mixed with social, political, or moral teaching. The statement "art for art's sake" is a good summary of aestheticism. The movement had its roots in France, but it gained widespread importance in England in the last half of the nineteenth century, where it helped change the Victorian practice of including moral lessons in literature.

Affective Fallacy: An error in judging the merits or faults of a work of literature. The "error" results from stressing the importance of the work's effect upon the reader—that is, how it makes a reader "feel" emotionally, what it does as a literary work—instead of stressing its inner qualities as a created object, or what it "is."

Age of Johnson: The period in English literature between 1750 and 1798, named after the most prominent literary figure of the age, Samuel Johnson. Works written during this time are noted for their emphasis on "sensibility," or emotional quality. These works formed a transition between the rational works of the Age of Reason, or Neoclassical period, and the emphasis on individual feelings and responses of the Romantic period.

Age of Reason: See *Neoclassicism*

Age of Sensibility: See *Age of Johnson*

Agrarians: A group of Southern American writers of the 1930s and 1940s who fostered an economic and cultural program for the South based on agriculture, in opposition to the industrial society of the North. The term can refer to any group that promotes the value of farm life and agricultural society.

Alexandrine Meter: See *Meter*

Allegory: A narrative technique in which characters representing things or abstract ideas are used to convey a message or teach a lesson. Allegory is typically used to teach moral, ethical, or religious lessons but is sometimes used for satiric or political purposes.

Alliteration: A poetic device where the first consonant sounds or any vowel sounds in words or syllables are repeated.

Allusion: A reference to a familiar literary or historical person or event, used to make an idea more easily understood.

Amerind Literature: The writing and oral traditions of Native Americans. Native American literature was originally passed on by word of mouth, so it consisted largely of stories and events that were easily memorized. Amerind prose is often rhythmic like poetry because it was recited to the beat of a ceremonial drum.

Analogy: A comparison of two things made to explain something unfamiliar through its similarities to something familiar, or to prove one point based on the acceptedness of another. Similes and metaphors are types of analogies.

Anapest: See *Foot*

Angry Young Men: A group of British writers of the 1950s whose work expressed bitterness and disillusionment with society. Common to their work is an anti-hero who rebels against a corrupt social order and strives for personal integrity.

Anthropomorphism: The presentation of animals or objects in human shape or with human characteristics. The term is derived from the Greek word for "human form."

Antimasque: See *Masque*

Antithesis: The antithesis of something is its direct opposite. In literature, the use of antithesis as a figure of speech results in two statements that show a contrast through the balancing of two opposite ideas. Technically, it is the second portion of the statement that is defined as the "antithesis"; the first portion is the "thesis."

Apocrypha: Writings tentatively attributed to an author but not proven or universally accepted to be their works. The term was originally applied to certain books of the Bible that were not considered inspired and so were not included in the "sacred canon."

Apollonian and Dionysian: The two impulses believed to guide authors of dramatic tragedy. The Apollonian impulse is named after Apollo, the Greek god of light and beauty and the symbol of intellectual order. The

Dionysian impulse is named after Dionysus, the Greek god of wine and the symbol of the unrestrained forces of nature. The Apollonian impulse is to create a rational, harmonious world, while the Dionysian is to express the irrational forces of personality.

Apostrophe: A statement, question, or request addressed to an inanimate object or concept or to a nonexistent or absent person.

Archetype: The word archetype is commonly used to describe an original pattern or model from which all other things of the same kind are made. This term was introduced to literary criticism from the psychology of Carl Jung. It expresses Jung's theory that behind every person's "unconscious," or repressed memories of the past, lies the "collective unconscious" of the human race: memories of the countless typical experiences of our ancestors. These memories are said to prompt illogical associations that trigger powerful emotions in the reader. Often, the emotional process is primitive, even primordial. Archetypes are the literary images that grow out of the "collective unconscious." They appear in literature as incidents and plots that repeat basic patterns of life. They may also appear as stereotyped characters.

Argument: The argument of a work is the author's subject matter or principal idea.

Art for Art's Sake: See *Aestheticism*

Assonance: The repetition of similar vowel sounds in poetry.

Audience: The people for whom a piece of literature is written. Authors usually write with a certain audience in mind, for example, children, members of a religious or ethnic group, or colleagues in a professional field. The term "audience" also applies to the people who gather to see or hear any performance, including plays, poetry readings, speeches, and concerts.

Automatic Writing: Writing carried out without a preconceived plan in an effort to capture every random thought. Authors who engage in automatic writing typically do not revise their work, preferring instead to preserve the revealed truth and beauty of spontaneous expression.

Avant-garde: A French term meaning "vanguard." It is used in literary criticism to describe new writing that rejects traditional approaches to literature in favor of innovations in style or content.

B

Ballad: A short poem that tells a simple story and has a repeated refrain. Ballads were originally intended to be sung. Early ballads, known as folk ballads, were passed down through generations, so their authors are often unknown. Later ballads composed by known authors are called literary ballads.

Baroque: A term used in literary criticism to describe literature that is complex or ornate in style or diction. Baroque works typically express tension, anxiety, and violent emotion. The term "Baroque Age" designates a period in Western European literature beginning in the late sixteenth century and ending about one hundred years later. Works of this period often mirror the qualities of works more generally associated with the label "baroque" and sometimes feature elaborate conceits.

Baroque Age: See *Baroque*

Baroque Period: See *Baroque*

Beat Generation: See *Beat Movement*

Beat Movement: A period featuring a group of American poets and novelists of the 1950s and 1960s—including Jack Kerouac, Allen Ginsberg, Gregory Corso, William S. Burroughs, and Lawrence Ferlinghetti—who rejected established social and literary values. Using such techniques as stream of consciousness writing and jazz-influenced free verse and focusing on unusual or abnormal states of mind—generated by religious ecstasy or the use of drugs—the Beat writers aimed to create works that were unconventional in both form and subject matter.

Beat Poets: See *Beat Movement*

Beats, The: See *Beat Movement*

Belles- lettres: A French term meaning "fine letters" or "beautiful writing." It is often used as a synonym for literature, typically referring to imaginative and artistic rather than scientific or expository writing. Current usage sometimes restricts the meaning to light or humorous writing and appreciative essays about literature.

Black Aesthetic Movement: A period of artistic and literary development among African

Americans in the 1960s and early 1970s. This was the first major African-American artistic movement since the Harlem Renaissance and was closely paralleled by the civil rights and black power movements. The black aesthetic writers attempted to produce works of art that would be meaningful to the black masses. Key figures in black aesthetics included one of its founders, poet and playwright Amiri Baraka, formerly known as LeRoi Jones; poet and essayist Haki R. Madhubuti, formerly Don L. Lee; poet and playwright Sonia Sanchez; and dramatist Ed Bullins.

Black Arts Movement: See *Black Aesthetic Movement*

Black Comedy: See *Black Humor*

Black Humor: Writing that places grotesque elements side by side with humorous ones in an attempt to shock the reader, forcing him or her to laugh at the horrifying reality of a disordered world.

Black Mountain School: Black Mountain College and three of its instructors—Robert Creeley, Robert Duncan, and Charles Olson—were all influential in projective verse, so poets working in projective verse are now referred as members of the Black Mountain school.

Blank Verse: Loosely, any unrhymed poetry, but more generally, unrhymed iambic pentameter verse (composed of lines of five two-syllable feet with the first syllable accented, the second unaccented). Blank verse has been used by poets since the Renaissance for its flexibility and its graceful, dignified tone.

Bloomsbury Group: A group of English writers, artists, and intellectuals who held informal artistic and philosophical discussions in Bloomsbury, a district of London, from around 1907 to the early 1930s. The Bloomsbury Group held no uniform philosophical beliefs but did commonly express an aversion to moral prudery and a desire for greater social tolerance.

Bon Mot: A French term meaning "good word." A *bon mot* is a witty remark or clever observation.

Breath Verse: See *Projective Verse*

Burlesque: Any literary work that uses exaggeration to make its subject appear ridiculous, either by treating a trivial subject with profound seriousness or by treating a dignified subject frivolously. The word "burlesque" may also be used as an adjective, as in "burlesque show," to mean "striptease act."

C

Cadence: The natural rhythm of language caused by the alternation of accented and unaccented syllables. Much modern poetry—notably free verse—deliberately manipulates cadence to create complex rhythmic effects.

Caesura: A pause in a line of poetry, usually occurring near the middle. It typically corresponds to a break in the natural rhythm or sense of the line but is sometimes shifted to create special meanings or rhythmic effects.

Canzone: A short Italian or Provencal lyric poem, commonly about love and often set to music. The *canzone* has no set form but typically contains five or six stanzas made up of seven to twenty lines of eleven syllables each. A shorter, five- to ten-line "envoy," or concluding stanza, completes the poem.

Carpe Diem: A Latin term meaning "seize the day." This is a traditional theme of poetry, especially lyrics. A *carpe diem* poem advises the reader or the person it addresses to live for today and enjoy the pleasures of the moment.

Catharsis: The release or purging of unwanted emotions—specifically fear and pity—brought about by exposure to art. The term was first used by the Greek philosopher Aristotle in his *Poetics* to refer to the desired effect of tragedy on spectators.

Celtic Renaissance: A period of Irish literary and cultural history at the end of the nineteenth century. Followers of the movement aimed to create a romantic vision of Celtic myth and legend. The most significant works of the Celtic Renaissance typically present a dreamy, unreal world, usually in reaction against the reality of contemporary problems.

Celtic Twilight: See *Celtic Renaissance*

Character: Broadly speaking, a person in a literary work. The actions of characters are what constitute the plot of a story, novel, or poem. There are numerous types of characters, ranging from simple, stereotypical figures to intricate, multifaceted ones. In the techniques of anthropomorphism and personification, animals—and even places or things—can assume aspects of character. "Characterization" is the process by which an author creates vivid, believable characters in a work of art. This may be done in a variety of ways, including (1) direct description of the character by the narrator; (2) the direct presentation of the speech, thoughts, or actions of the character; and (3) the responses of other characters to the character. The term "character" also refers to a form originated by the ancient Greek writer Theophrastus that later became popular in the seventeenth and eighteenth centuries. It is a short essay or sketch of a person who prominently displays a specific attribute or quality, such as miserliness or ambition.

Characterization: See *Character*

Classical: In its strictest definition in literary criticism, classicism refers to works of ancient Greek or Roman literature. The term may also be used to describe a literary work of recognized importance (a "classic") from any time period or literature that exhibits the traits of classicism.

Classicism: A term used in literary criticism to describe critical doctrines that have their roots in ancient Greek and Roman literature, philosophy, and art. Works associated with classicism typically exhibit restraint on the part of the author, unity of design and purpose, clarity, simplicity, logical organization, and respect for tradition.

Colloquialism: A word, phrase, or form of pronunciation that is acceptable in casual conversation but not in formal, written communication. It is considered more acceptable than slang.

Complaint: A lyric poem, popular in the Renaissance, in which the speaker expresses sorrow about his or her condition. Typically, the speaker's sadness is caused by an unresponsive lover, but some complaints cite other sources of unhappiness, such as poverty or fate.

Conceit: A clever and fanciful metaphor, usually expressed through elaborate and extended comparison, that presents a striking parallel between two seemingly dissimilar things—for example, elaborately comparing a beautiful woman to an object like a garden or the sun. The conceit was a popular device throughout the Elizabethan Age and Baroque Age and was the principal technique of the seventeenth-century English metaphysical poets. This usage of the word conceit is unrelated to the best-known definition of conceit as an arrogant attitude or behavior.

Concrete: Concrete is the opposite of abstract, and refers to a thing that actually exists or a description that allows the reader to experience an object or concept with the senses.

Concrete Poetry: Poetry in which visual elements play a large part in the poetic effect. Punctuation marks, letters, or words are arranged on a page to form a visual design: a cross, for example, or a bumblebee.

Confessional Poetry: A form of poetry in which the poet reveals very personal, intimate, sometimes shocking information about himself or herself.

Connotation: The impression that a word gives beyond its defined meaning. Connotations may be universally understood or may be significant only to a certain group.

Consonance: Consonance occurs in poetry when words appearing at the ends of two or more verses have similar final consonant sounds but have final vowel sounds that differ, as with "stuff" and "off."

Convention: Any widely accepted literary device, style, or form.

Corrido: A Mexican ballad.

Couplet: Two lines of poetry with the same rhyme and meter, often expressing a complete and self-contained thought.

Criticism: The systematic study and evaluation of literary works, usually based on a specific method or set of principles. An important part of literary studies since ancient times, the practice of criticism has given rise to numerous theories, methods, and "schools," sometimes producing conflicting, even contradictory, interpretations of literature in general as well as of individual works. Even such basic issues as what constitutes a poem or a novel have been the subject of much criticism over the centuries.

D

Dactyl: See *Foot*

Dadaism: A protest movement in art and literature founded by Tristan Tzara in 1916. Followers of the movement expressed their outrage at the destruction brought about by World War I by revolting against numerous forms of social convention. The Dadaists presented works marked by calculated madness and flamboyant nonsense. They stressed total freedom of expression, commonly through primitive displays of emotion and illogical, often senseless, poetry. The movement ended shortly after the war, when it was replaced by surrealism.

Decadent: See *Decadents*

Decadents: The followers of a nineteenth-century literary movement that had its beginnings in French aestheticism. Decadent literature displays a fascination with perverse and morbid states; a search for novelty and sensation—the "new thrill"; a preoccupation with mysticism; and a belief in the senselessness of human existence. The movement is closely associated with the doctrine Art for Art's Sake. The term "decadence" is sometimes used to denote a decline in the quality of art or literature following a period of greatness.

Deconstruction: A method of literary criticism developed by Jacques Derrida and characterized by multiple conflicting interpretations of a given work. Deconstructionists consider the impact of the language of a work and suggest that the true meaning of the work is not necessarily the meaning that the author intended.

Deduction: The process of reaching a conclusion through reasoning from general premises to a specific premise.

Denotation: The definition of a word, apart from the impressions or feelings it creates in the reader.

Diction: The selection and arrangement of words in a literary work. Either or both may vary depending on the desired effect. There are four general types of diction: "formal," used in scholarly or lofty writing; "informal," used in relaxed but educated conversation; "colloquial," used in everyday speech; and "slang," containing newly coined words and other terms not accepted in formal usage.

Didactic: A term used to describe works of literature that aim to teach some moral, religious, political, or practical lesson. Although didactic elements are often found in artistically pleasing works, the term "didactic" usually refers to literature in which the message is more important than the form. The term may also be used to criticize a work that the critic finds "overly didactic," that is, heavy-handed in its delivery of a lesson.

Dimeter: See *Meter*

Dionysian: See *Apollonian and Dionysian*

Discordia concours: A Latin phrase meaning "discord in harmony." The term was coined by the eighteenth-century English writer Samuel Johnson to describe "a combination of dissimilar images or discovery of occult resemblances in things apparently unlike." Johnson created the expression by reversing a phrase by the Latin poet Horace.

Dissonance: A combination of harsh or jarring sounds, especially in poetry. Although such combinations may be accidental, poets sometimes intentionally make them to achieve particular effects. Dissonance is also sometimes used to refer to close but not identical rhymes. When this is the case, the word functions as a synonym for consonance.

Double Entendre: A corruption of a French phrase meaning "double meaning." The term is used to indicate a word or phrase that is deliberately ambiguous, especially when one of the meanings is risque or improper.

Draft: Any preliminary version of a written work. An author may write dozens of drafts which are revised to form the final work, or he or she may write only one, with few or no revisions.

Dramatic Monologue: See *Monologue*

Dramatic Poetry: Any lyric work that employs elements of drama such as dialogue, conflict, or characterization, but excluding works that are intended for stage presentation.

Dream Allegory: See *Dream Vision*

Dream Vision: A literary convention, chiefly of the Middle Ages. In a dream vision a story is presented as a literal dream of the narrator. This device was commonly used to teach moral and religious lessons.

E

Eclogue: In classical literature, a poem featuring rural themes and structured as a dialogue among shepherds. Eclogues often took specific poetic forms, such as elegies or love poems. Some were written as the soliloquy of a shepherd. In later centuries, "eclogue" came to refer to any poem that was in the pastoral tradition or that had a dialogue or monologue structure.

Edwardian: Describes cultural conventions identified with the period of the reign of Edward VII of England (1901-1910). Writers of the Edwardian Age typically displayed a strong reaction against the propriety and conservatism of the Victorian Age. Their work often exhibits distrust of authority in religion, politics, and art and expresses strong doubts about the soundness of conventional values.

Edwardian Age: See *Edwardian*

Electra Complex: A daughter's amorous obsession with her father.

Elegy: A lyric poem that laments the death of a person or the eventual death of all people. In a conventional elegy, set in a classical world, the poet and subject are spoken of as shepherds. In modern criticism, the word elegy is often used to refer to a poem that is melancholy or mournfully contemplative.

Elizabethan Age: A period of great economic growth, religious controversy, and nationalism closely associated with the reign of Elizabeth I of England (1558-1603). The Elizabethan Age is considered a part of the general renaissance—that is, the flowering of arts and literature—that took place in Europe during the fourteenth through sixteenth centuries. The era is considered the golden age of English literature. The most important dramas in English and a great deal of lyric poetry were produced during this period, and modern English criticism began around this time.

Empathy: A sense of shared experience, including emotional and physical feelings, with someone or something other than oneself. Empathy is often used to describe the response of a reader to a literary character.

English Sonnet: See *Sonnet*

Enjambment: The running over of the sense and structure of a line of verse or a couplet into the following verse or couplet.

Enlightenment, The: An eighteenth-century philosophical movement. It began in France but had a wide impact throughout Europe and America. Thinkers of the Enlightenment valued reason and believed that both the individual and society could achieve a state of perfection. Corresponding to this essentially humanist vision was a resistance to religious authority.

Epic: A long narrative poem about the adventures of a hero of great historic or legendary importance. The setting is vast and the action is often given cosmic significance through the intervention of supernatural forces such as gods, angels, or demons. Epics are typically written in a classical style of grand simplicity with elaborate metaphors and allusions that enhance the symbolic importance of a hero's adventures.

Epic Simile: See *Homeric Simile*

Epigram: A saying that makes the speaker's point quickly and concisely.

Epilogue: A concluding statement or section of a literary work. In dramas, particularly those of the seventeenth and eighteenth centuries, the epilogue is a closing speech, often in verse, delivered by an actor at the end of a play and spoken directly to the audience.

Epiphany: A sudden revelation of truth inspired by a seemingly trivial incident.

Epitaph: An inscription on a tomb or tombstone, or a verse written on the occasion of a person's death. Epitaphs may be serious or humorous.

Epithalamion: A song or poem written to honor and commemorate a marriage ceremony.

Epithalamium: See *Epithalamion*

Epithet: A word or phrase, often disparaging or abusive, that expresses a character trait of someone or something.

Erziehungsroman: See *Bildungsroman*

Essay: A prose composition with a focused subject of discussion. The term was coined by Michel de Montaigne to describe his 1580 collection of brief, informal reflections on himself and on various topics relating to human nature. An essay can also be a long, systematic discourse.

Existentialism: A predominantly twentieth-century philosophy concerned with the nature and perception of human existence. There are two major strains of existentialist thought: atheistic and Christian. Followers of atheistic existentialism believe that the individual is alone in a godless universe and that the basic human condition is one of suffering and loneliness. Nevertheless, because there are no fixed values, individuals can create their own characters—indeed, they can shape themselves—through the exercise of free will. The atheistic strain culminates in and is popularly associated with the works of Jean-Paul Sartre. The Christian existentialists, on the other hand, believe that only in God may people find freedom from life's anguish. The two strains hold certain beliefs in common: that existence cannot be fully understood or described through empirical effort; that anguish is a universal element of life; that individuals must bear responsibility for their actions; and that there is no common standard of behavior or perception for religious and ethical matters.

Expatriates: See *Expatriatism*

Expatriatism: The practice of leaving one's country to live for an extended period in another country.

Exposition: Writing intended to explain the nature of an idea, thing, or theme. Expository writing is often combined with description, narration, or argument. In dramatic writing, the exposition is the introductory material which presents the characters, setting, and tone of the play.

Expressionism: An indistinct literary term, originally used to describe an early twentieth-century school of German painting. The term applies to almost any mode of unconventional, highly subjective writing that distorts reality in some way.

Extended Monologue: See *Monologue*

F

Feet: See *Foot*

Feminine Rhyme: See *Rhyme*

Fiction: Any story that is the product of imagination rather than a documentation of fact. Characters and events in such narratives may be based in real life but their ultimate form and configuration is a creation of the author.

Figurative Language: A technique in writing in which the author temporarily interrupts the order, construction, or meaning of the writing for a particular effect. This interruption takes the form of one or more figures of speech such as hyperbole, irony, or simile. Figurative language is the opposite of literal language, in which every word is truthful, accurate, and free of exaggeration or embellishment.

Figures of Speech: Writing that differs from customary conventions for construction, meaning, order, or significance for the purpose of a special meaning or effect. There are two major types of figures of speech: rhetorical figures, which do not make changes in the meaning of the words, and tropes, which do.

Fin de siecle: A French term meaning "end of the century." The term is used to denote the last decade of the nineteenth century, a transition period when writers and other artists abandoned old conventions and looked for new techniques and objectives.

First Person: See *Point of View*

Folk Ballad: See *Ballad*

Folklore: Traditions and myths preserved in a culture or group of people. Typically, these are passed on by word of mouth in various forms—such as legends, songs, and proverbs—or preserved in customs and ceremonies. This term was first used by W. J. Thoms in 1846.

Folktale: A story originating in oral tradition. Folktales fall into a variety of categories, including legends, ghost stories, fairy tales, fables, and anecdotes based on historical figures and events.

Foot: The smallest unit of rhythm in a line of poetry. In English-language poetry, a foot is typically one accented syllable combined with one or two unaccented syllables.

Form: The pattern or construction of a work which identifies its genre and distinguishes it from other genres.

Formalism: In literary criticism, the belief that literature should follow prescribed rules of construction, such as those that govern the sonnet form.

Fourteener Meter: See *Meter*

Free Verse: Poetry that lacks regular metrical and rhyme patterns but that tries to capture the cadences of everyday speech. The form allows a poet to exploit a variety of rhythmical effects within a single poem.

Futurism: A flamboyant literary and artistic movement that developed in France, Italy, and Russia from 1908 through the 1920s. Futurist theater and poetry abandoned traditional literary forms. In their place, followers of the movement attempted to achieve total freedom of expression through bizarre imagery and deformed or newly invented words. The Futurists were self-consciously modern artists who attempted to incorporate the appearances and sounds of modern life into their work.

G

Genre: A category of literary work. In critical theory, genre may refer to both the content of a given work—tragedy, comedy, pastoral—and to its form, such as poetry, novel, or drama.

Genteel Tradition: A term coined by critic George Santayana to describe the literary practice of certain late nineteenth- century American writers, especially New Englanders. Followers of the Genteel Tradition emphasized conventionality in social, religious, moral, and literary standards.

Georgian Age: See *Georgian Poets*

Georgian Period: See *Georgian Poets*

Georgian Poets: A loose grouping of English poets during the years 1912-1922. The Georgians reacted against certain literary schools and practices, especially Victorian wordiness, turn-of-the-century aestheticism, and contemporary urban realism. In their place, the Georgians embraced the nineteenth-century poetic practices of William Wordsworth and the other Lake Poets.

Georgic: A poem about farming and the farmer's way of life, named from Virgil's *Georgics*.

Gilded Age: A period in American history during the 1870s characterized by political corruption and materialism. A number of important novels of social and political criticism were written during this time.

Gothic: See *Gothicism*

Gothicism: In literary criticism, works characterized by a taste for the medieval or morbidly attractive. A gothic novel prominently features elements of horror, the supernatural, gloom, and violence: clanking chains, terror, charnel houses, ghosts, medieval castles, and mysteriously slamming doors. The term "gothic novel" is also applied to novels that lack elements of the traditional Gothic setting but that create a similar atmosphere of terror or dread.

Graveyard School: A group of eighteenth-century English poets who wrote long, picturesque meditations on death. Their works were designed to cause the reader to ponder immortality.

Great Chain of Being: The belief that all things and creatures in nature are organized in a hierarchy from inanimate objects at the bottom to God at the top. This system of belief was popular in the seventeenth and eighteenth centuries.

Grotesque: In literary criticism, the subject matter of a work or a style of expression characterized by exaggeration, deformity, freakishness, and disorder. The grotesque often includes an element of comic absurdity.

H

Haiku: The shortest form of Japanese poetry, constructed in three lines of five, seven, and five syllables respectively. The message of a *haiku* poem usually centers on some aspect of spirituality and provokes an emotional response in the reader.

Half Rhyme: See *Consonance*

Harlem Renaissance: The Harlem Renaissance of the 1920s is generally considered the first significant movement of black writers and artists in the United States. During this period, new and established black writers published more fiction and poetry than ever before, the first influential black literary journals were established, and black authors and artists received their first widespread recognition and serious critical appraisal. Among the major writers associated with this period are Claude McKay, Jean Toomer, Countee Cullen, Langston Hughes, Arna Bontemps, Nella Larsen, and Zora Neale Hurston.

Hellenism: Imitation of ancient Greek thought or styles. Also, an approach to life that focuses on the growth and development of the intellect. "Hellenism" is sometimes used to refer to the belief that reason can be applied to examine all human experience.

Heptameter: See *Meter*

Hero/Heroine: The principal sympathetic character (male or female) in a literary work. Heroes and heroines typically exhibit admirable traits: idealism, courage, and integrity, for example.

Heroic Couplet: A rhyming couplet written in iambic pentameter (a verse with five iambic feet).

Heroic Line: The meter and length of a line of verse in epic or heroic poetry. This varies by language and time period.

Heroine: See *Hero/Heroine*

Hexameter: See *Meter*

Historical Criticism: The study of a work based on its impact on the world of the time period in which it was written.

Hokku: See *Haiku*

Holocaust: See *Holocaust Literature*

Holocaust Literature: Literature influenced by or written about the Holocaust of World War II. Such literature includes true stories of survival in concentration camps, escape, and life after the war, as well as fictional works and poetry.

Homeric Simile: An elaborate, detailed comparison written as a simile many lines in length.

Horatian Satire: See *Satire*

Humanism: A philosophy that places faith in the dignity of humankind and rejects the medieval perception of the individual as a weak, fallen creature. "Humanists" typically believe in the perfectibility of human nature and view reason and education as the means to that end.

Humors: Mentions of the humors refer to the ancient Greek theory that a person's health and personality were determined by the balance of four basic fluids in the body: blood, phlegm, yellow bile, and black bile. A dominance of any fluid would cause extremes in behavior. An excess of blood created a sanguine person who was joyful, aggressive, and passionate; a phlegmatic person was shy, fearful, and sluggish; too much yellow bile led to a choleric temperament characterized by impatience, anger, bitterness, and stubbornness; and excessive black bile created melancholy, a state of laziness, gluttony, and lack of motivation.

Humours: See *Humors*

Hyperbole: In literary criticism, deliberate exaggeration used to achieve an effect.

I

Iamb: See *Foot*

Idiom: A word construction or verbal expression closely associated with a given language.

Image: A concrete representation of an object or sensory experience. Typically, such a representation helps evoke the feelings associated with the object or experience itself. Images are either "literal" or "figurative." Literal images are especially concrete and involve little or no extension of the obvious meaning of the words used to express them. Figurative images do not follow the literal meaning of the words exactly. Images in literature are usually visual, but the term "image" can also refer to the representation of any sensory experience.

Imagery: The array of images in a literary work. Also, figurative language.

Imagism: An English and American poetry movement that flourished between 1908 and 1917. The Imagists used precise, clearly presented images in their works. They also used common, everyday speech and aimed for conciseness, concrete imagery, and the creation of new rhythms.

In medias res: A Latin term meaning "in the middle of things." It refers to the technique of beginning a story at its midpoint and then using various flashback devices to reveal previous action.

Induction: The process of reaching a conclusion by reasoning from specific premises to form a general premise. Also, an introductory portion of a work of literature, especially a play.

Intentional Fallacy: The belief that judgments of a literary work based solely on an author's stated or implied intentions are false and misleading. Critics who believe in the concept of the intentional fallacy typically argue that the work itself is sufficient matter for interpretation, even though they may concede that an author's statement of purpose can be useful.

Interior Monologue: A narrative technique in which characters' thoughts are revealed in a way that appears to be uncontrolled by the author. The interior monologue typically aims to reveal the inner self of a character. It portrays emotional experiences as they occur at both a conscious and unconscious level. Images are often used to represent sensations or emotions.

Internal Rhyme: Rhyme that occurs within a single line of verse.

Irish Literary Renaissance: A late nineteenth- and early twentieth-century movement in Irish literature. Members of the movement aimed to reduce the influence of British culture in Ireland and create an Irish national literature.

Irony: In literary criticism, the effect of language in which the intended meaning is the opposite of what is stated.

Italian Sonnet: See *Sonnet*

J

Jacobean Age: The period of the reign of James I of England (1603-1625). The early literature of this period reflected the worldview of the Elizabethan Age, but a darker, more cynical attitude steadily grew in the art and literature of the Jacobean Age. This was an important time for English drama and poetry.

Jargon: Language that is used or understood only by a select group of people. Jargon may refer to terminology used in a certain profession, such as computer jargon, or it may refer to any nonsensical language that is not understood by most people.

Journalism: Writing intended for publication in a newspaper or magazine, or for broadcast on a radio or television program featuring news, sports, entertainment, or other timely material.

K

Knickerbocker Group: A somewhat indistinct group of New York writers of the first half of the nineteenth century. Members of the group were linked only by location and a common theme: New York life.

Kunstlerroman: See *Bildungsroman*

L

Lais: See *Lay*

Lake Poets: See *Lake School*

Lake School: These poets all lived in the Lake District of England at the turn of the nineteenth century. As a group, they followed no single "school" of thought or literary practice, although their works were uniformly disparaged by the *Edinburgh Review*.

Lay: A song or simple narrative poem. The form originated in medieval France. Early French *lais* were often based on the Celtic legends and other tales sung by Breton minstrels—thus the name of the "Breton lay." In fourteenth-century England, the term "lay" was used to describe short narratives written in imitation of the Breton lays.

Leitmotiv: See *Motif*

Literal Language: An author uses literal language when he or she writes without exaggerating or embellishing the subject matter and without any tools of figurative language.

Literary Ballad: See *Ballad*

Literature: Literature is broadly defined as any written or spoken material, but the term most often refers to creative works.

Lost Generation: A term first used by Gertrude Stein to describe the post-World War I generation of American writers: men and women haunted by a sense of betrayal and emptiness brought about by the destructiveness of the war.

Lyric Poetry: A poem expressing the subjective feelings and personal emotions of the poet. Such poetry is melodic, since it was originally accompanied by a lyre in recitals. Most Western poetry in the twentieth century may be classified as lyrical.

M

Mannerism: Exaggerated, artificial adherence to a literary manner or style. Also, a popular style of the visual arts of late sixteenth-century Europe that was marked by elongation of the human form and by intentional spatial distortion. Literary works that are self-consciously high-toned and artistic are often said to be "mannered."

Masculine Rhyme: See *Rhyme*

Measure: The foot, verse, or time sequence used in a literary work, especially a poem. Measure is often used somewhat incorrectly as a synonym for meter.

Metaphor: A figure of speech that expresses an idea through the image of another object. Metaphors suggest the essence of the first object by identifying it with certain qualities of the second object.

Metaphysical Conceit: See *Conceit*

Metaphysical Poetry: The body of poetry produced by a group of seventeenth-century English writers called the "Metaphysical Poets." The group includes John Donne and Andrew Marvell. The Metaphysical Poets made use of everyday speech, intellectual analysis, and unique imagery. They aimed to portray the ordinary conflicts and contradictions of life. Their poems often took the form of an argument, and many of them emphasize physical and religious love as well as the fleeting nature of life. Elaborate conceits are typical in metaphysical poetry.

Metaphysical Poets: See *Metaphysical Poetry*

Meter: In literary criticism, the repetition of sound patterns that creates a rhythm in poetry. The patterns are based on the number of syllables and the presence and absence of accents. The unit of rhythm in a line is called a foot. Types of meter are classified according to the number of feet in a line. These are the standard English lines: Monometer, one foot; Dimeter, two feet; Trimeter, three feet; Tetrameter, four feet; Pentameter, five feet; Hexameter, six feet (also called the Alexandrine); Heptameter, seven feet (also called the "Fourteener" when the feet are iambic).

Modernism: Modern literary practices. Also, the principles of a literary school that lasted from roughly the beginning of the twentieth century until the end of World War II. Modernism is defined by its rejection of the literary conventions of the nineteenth century and by its opposition to conventional morality, taste, traditions, and economic values.

Monologue: A composition, written or oral, by a single individual. More specifically, a speech given by a single individual in a drama or other public entertainment. It has no set length, although it is usually several or more lines long.

Monometer: See *Meter*

Mood: The prevailing emotions of a work or of the author in his or her creation of the work. The mood of a work is not always what might be expected based on its subject matter.

Motif: A theme, character type, image, metaphor, or other verbal element that recurs throughout a single work of literature or occurs in a number of different works over a period of time.

Motiv: See *Motif*

Muckrakers: An early twentieth-century group of American writers. Typically, their works exposed the wrongdoings of big business and government in the United States.

Muses: Nine Greek mythological goddesses, the daughters of Zeus and Mnemosyne (Memory). Each muse patronized a specific area of the liberal arts and sciences. Calliope presided over epic poetry, Clio over history, Erato over love poetry, Euterpe over music or lyric poetry, Melpomene over tragedy, Polyhymnia over hymns to the gods, Terpsichore over dance, Thalia over comedy, and Urania over astronomy. Poets and writers traditionally made appeals to the Muses for inspiration in their work.

Myth: An anonymous tale emerging from the traditional beliefs of a culture or social unit. Myths use supernatural explanations for natural phenomena. They may also explain cosmic issues like creation and death. Collections of myths, known as mythologies, are common to all cultures and nations, but the best-known myths belong to the Norse, Roman, and Greek mythologies.

N

Narration: The telling of a series of events, real or invented. A narration may be either a simple narrative, in which the events are recounted chronologically, or a narrative with a plot, in which the account is given in a style reflecting the author's artistic concept of the story. Narration is sometimes used as a synonym for "storyline."

Narrative: A verse or prose accounting of an event or sequence of events, real or invented. The term is also used as an adjective in the sense "method of narration." For example, in literary criticism, the expression "narrative technique" usually refers to the way the author structures and presents his or her story.

Narrative Poetry: A nondramatic poem in which the author tells a story. Such poems may be of any length or level of complexity.

Narrator: The teller of a story. The narrator may be the author or a character in the story through whom the author speaks.

Naturalism: A literary movement of the late nineteenth and early twentieth centuries. The movement's major theorist, French novelist Emile Zola, envisioned a type of fiction that would examine human life with the objectivity of scientific inquiry. The Naturalists typically viewed human beings as either the products of "biological determinism," ruled by hereditary instincts and engaged in an endless struggle for survival, or as the products of "socioeconomic determinism," ruled by social and economic forces beyond their control. In their works, the Naturalists generally ignored the highest levels of society and focused on degradation: poverty, alcoholism, prostitution, insanity, and disease.

Negritude: A literary movement based on the concept of a shared cultural bond on the part of black Africans, wherever they may be in the world. It traces its origins to the former French colonies of Africa and the Caribbean. Negritude poets, novelists, and essayists generally stress four points in their writings: One, black alienation from traditional African culture can lead to feelings of inferiority. Two, European colonialism and Western education should be resisted. Three, black Africans should seek to affirm and define their own identity. Four, African culture can and should be reclaimed. Many Negritude writers also claim that blacks can make unique contributions to the world, based on a heightened appreciation of nature, rhythm, and human emotions—aspects of life they say are not so highly valued in the materialistic and rationalistic West.

Negro Renaissance: See *Harlem Renaissance*

Neoclassical Period: See *Neoclassicism*

Neoclassicism: In literary criticism, this term refers to the revival of the attitudes and styles of expression of classical literature. It is generally used to describe a period in European history beginning in the late seventeenth century and lasting until about 1800. In its purest form, Neoclassicism marked a return to order, proportion, restraint, logic, accuracy, and decorum. In England, where Neoclassicism perhaps was most popular, it reflected the influence of seventeenth- century French writers, especially dramatists. Neoclassical writers typically reacted against the intensity and enthusiasm of the Renaissance period. They wrote works that appealed to the intellect, using elevated language and classical literary forms such as satire and the ode. Neoclassical works were often governed by the classical goal of instruction.

Neoclassicists: See *Neoclassicism*

New Criticism: A movement in literary criticism, dating from the late 1920s, that stressed close textual analysis in the interpretation of works of literature. The New Critics saw little merit in historical and biographical analysis. Rather, they aimed to examine the text alone, free from the question of how external events—biographical or otherwise—may have helped shape it.

New Journalism: A type of writing in which the journalist presents factual information in a form usually used in fiction. New journalism emphasizes description, narration, and character development to bring readers closer to the human element of the story, and is often used in personality profiles and in-depth feature articles. It is not compatible with "straight" or "hard" newswriting, which is generally composed in a brief, fact-based style.

New Journalists: See *New Journalism*

New Negro Movement: See *Harlem Renaissance*

Noble Savage: The idea that primitive man is noble and good but becomes evil and corrupted as he becomes civilized. The concept of the noble savage originated in the Renaissance period but is more closely identified with such later writers as Jean-Jacques Rousseau and Aphra Behn.

O

Objective Correlative: An outward set of objects, a situation, or a chain of events corresponding to an inward experience and evoking this experience in the reader. The term frequently appears in modern criticism in discussions of authors' intended effects on the emotional responses of readers.

Objectivity: A quality in writing characterized by the absence of the author's opinion or feeling about the subject matter. Objectivity is an important factor in criticism.

Occasional Verse: poetry written on the occasion of a significant historical or personal event. *Vers de societe* is sometimes called occasional verse although it is of a less serious nature.

Octave: A poem or stanza composed of eight lines. The term octave most often represents the first eight lines of a Petrarchan sonnet.

Ode: Name given to an extended lyric poem characterized by exalted emotion and dignified style. An ode usually concerns a single, serious theme. Most odes, but not all, are addressed to an object or individual. Odes are distinguished from other lyric poetic forms by their complex rhythmic and stanzaic patterns.

Oedipus Complex: A son's amorous obsession with his mother. The phrase is derived from the story of the ancient Theban hero Oedipus, who unknowingly killed his father and married his mother.

Omniscience: See *Point of View*

Onomatopoeia: The use of words whose sounds express or suggest their meaning. In its simplest sense, onomatopoeia may be represented by words that mimic the sounds they denote such as "hiss" or "meow." At a more subtle level, the pattern and rhythm of sounds and rhymes of a line or poem may be onomatopoeic.

Oral Tradition: See *Oral Transmission*

Oral Transmission: A process by which songs, ballads, folklore, and other material are transmitted by word of mouth. The tradition of oral transmission predates the written record systems of literate society. Oral transmission preserves material sometimes over generations, although often with variations. Memory plays a large part in the recitation and preservation of orally transmitted material.

Ottava Rima: An eight-line stanza of poetry composed in iambic pentameter (a five-foot line in which each foot consists of an unaccented syllable followed by an accented syllable), following the abababcc rhyme scheme.

Oxymoron: A phrase combining two contradictory terms. Oxymorons may be intentional or unintentional.

P

Pantheism: The idea that all things are both a manifestation or revelation of God and a part of God at the same time. Pantheism was a common attitude in the early societies of Egypt, India, and Greece—the term derives from the Greek *pan* meaning "all" and *theos* meaning "deity." It later became a significant part of the Christian faith.

Parable: A story intended to teach a moral lesson or answer an ethical question.

Paradox: A statement that appears illogical or contradictory at first, but may actually point to an underlying truth.

Parallelism: A method of comparison of two ideas in which each is developed in the same grammatical structure.

Parnassianism: A mid nineteenth-century movement in French literature. Followers of the movement stressed adherence to well-defined artistic forms as a reaction against the often chaotic expression of the artist's ego that dominated the work of the Romantics. The Parnassians also rejected the moral, ethical, and social themes exhibited in the works of French Romantics such as Victor Hugo. The aesthetic doctrines of the Parnassians strongly influenced the later symbolist and decadent movements.

Parody: In literary criticism, this term refers to an imitation of a serious literary work or the signature style of a particular author in a ridiculous manner. A typical parody adopts the style of the original and applies it to an inappropriate subject for humorous effect. Parody is a form of satire and could be considered the literary equivalent of a caricature or cartoon.

Pastoral: A term derived from the Latin word "pastor," meaning shepherd. A pastoral is a literary composition on a rural theme. The conventions of the pastoral were originated by the third-century Greek poet Theocritus, who wrote about the experiences, love affairs, and pastimes of Sicilian shepherds. In a pastoral, characters and language of a courtly nature are often placed in a simple setting. The term pastoral is also used to classify dramas, elegies, and lyrics that exhibit the use of country settings and shepherd characters.

Pathetic Fallacy: A term coined by English critic John Ruskin to identify writing that falsely endows nonhuman things with human intentions and feelings, such as "angry clouds" and "sad trees."

Pen Name: See *Pseudonym*

Pentameter: See *Meter*

Persona: A Latin term meaning "mask." *Personae* are the characters in a fictional work of literature. The *persona* generally functions as a mask through which the author tells a story in a voice other than his or her own. A *persona* is usually either a character in a story who acts as a narrator or an "implied author," a voice created by the author to act as the narrator for himself or herself.

Personae: See *Persona*

Personal Point of View: See *Point of View*

Personification: A figure of speech that gives human qualities to abstract ideas, animals, and inanimate objects.

Petrarchan Sonnet: See *Sonnet*

Phenomenology: A method of literary criticism based on the belief that things have no existence outside of human consciousness or awareness. Proponents of this theory believe that art is a process that takes place in the mind of the observer as he or she contemplates an object rather than a quality of the object itself.

Plagiarism: Claiming another person's written material as one's own. Plagiarism can take the form of direct, word-for-word copying or the theft of the substance or idea of the work.

Platonic Criticism: A form of criticism that stresses an artistic work's usefulness as an agent of social engineering rather than any quality or value of the work itself.

Platonism: The embracing of the doctrines of the philosopher Plato, popular among the poets of the Renaissance and the Romantic period. Platonism is more flexible than Aristotelian Criticism and places more emphasis on the supernatural and unknown aspects of life.

Plot: In literary criticism, this term refers to the pattern of events in a narrative or drama. In its simplest sense, the plot guides the author in composing the work and helps the reader follow the work. Typically, plots exhibit causality and unity and have a beginning, a middle, and an end. Sometimes, however, a plot may consist of a series of disconnected events, in which case it is known as an "episodic plot."

Poem: In its broadest sense, a composition utilizing rhyme, meter, concrete detail, and expressive language to create a literary experience with emotional and aesthetic appeal.

Poet: An author who writes poetry or verse. The term is also used to refer to an artist or writer who has an exceptional gift for expression, imagination, and energy in the making of art in any form.

Poete maudit: A term derived from Paul Verlaine's *Les poetes maudits* (*The Accursed Poets*), a collection of essays on the French symbolist writers Stephane Mallarme, Arthur Rimbaud, and Tristan Corbiere. In the sense intended by Verlaine, the poet is "accursed" for choosing to explore extremes of human experience outside of middle-class society.

Poetic Fallacy: See *Pathetic Fallacy*

Poetic Justice: An outcome in a literary work, not necessarily a poem, in which the good are rewarded and the evil are punished, especially in ways that particularly fit their virtues or crimes.

Poetic License: Distortions of fact and literary convention made by a writer—not always a poet—for the sake of the effect gained. Poetic license is closely related to the concept of "artistic freedom."

Poetics: This term has two closely related meanings. It denotes (1) an aesthetic theory in literary criticism about the essence of poetry or (2) rules prescribing the proper methods, content, style, or diction of poetry. The term poetics may also refer to theories about literature in general, not just poetry.

Poetry: In its broadest sense, writing that aims to present ideas and evoke an emotional experience in the reader through the use of meter, imagery, connotative and concrete words, and a carefully constructed structure based on rhythmic patterns. Poetry typically relies on words and expressions that have several layers of meaning. It also makes use of the effects of regular rhythm on the ear and may make a strong appeal to the senses through the use of imagery.

Point of View: The narrative perspective from which a literary work is presented to the reader. There are four traditional points of view. The "third person omniscient" gives the reader a "godlike" perspective, unrestricted by time or place, from which to see actions and look into the minds of characters. This allows the author to comment openly on characters and events in the work. The "third person" point of view presents the events of the story from outside of any single character's perception, much like the omniscient point of view, but the reader must understand the action as it takes place and without any special insight into characters' minds or motivations. The "first person" or "personal" point of view relates events as they are perceived by a single character. The main character "tells" the story and may offer opinions about the action and characters which differ from those of the author. Much less common than omniscient, third person, and first person is the "second person" point of view, wherein the author tells the story as if it is happening to the reader.

Polemic: A work in which the author takes a stand on a controversial subject, such as abortion or religion. Such works are often extremely argumentative or provocative.

Pornography: Writing intended to provoke feelings of lust in the reader. Such works are often condemned by critics and teachers, but those which can be shown to have literary value are viewed less harshly.

Post-Aesthetic Movement: An artistic response made by African Americans to the black aesthetic movement of the 1960s and early '70s. Writers since that time have adopted a somewhat different tone in their work, with less emphasis placed on the disparity between black and white in the United States. In the words of post-aesthetic authors such as Toni Morrison, John Edgar Wideman, and Kristin Hunter, African Americans are portrayed as looking inward for answers to their own questions, rather than always looking to the outside world.

Postmodernism: Writing from the 1960s forward characterized by experimentation and continuing to apply some of the fundamentals of modernism, which included existentialism and alienation. Postmodernists have gone a step further in the rejection of tradition begun with the modernists by also rejecting traditional forms, preferring the anti-novel over the novel and the anti-hero over the hero.

Pre-Raphaelites: A circle of writers and artists in mid nineteenth-century England. Valuing the pre-Renaissance artistic qualities of religious symbolism, lavish pictorialism, and natural sensuousness, the Pre-Raphaelites cultivated a sense of mystery and melancholy that influenced later writers associated with the Symbolist and Decadent movements.

Primitivism: The belief that primitive peoples were nobler and less flawed than civilized peoples because they had not been subjected to the tainting influence of society.

Projective Verse: A form of free verse in which the poet's breathing pattern determines the lines of the poem. Poets who advocate projective verse are against all formal structures in writing, including meter and form.

Prologue: An introductory section of a literary work. It often contains information establishing the situation of the characters or presents information about the setting, time period, or action. In drama, the prologue is spoken by a chorus or by one of the principal characters.

Prose: A literary medium that attempts to mirror the language of everyday speech. It is distinguished from poetry by its use of unmetered, unrhymed language consisting of logically related sentences. Prose is usually grouped into paragraphs that form a cohesive whole such as an essay or a novel.

Prosopopoeia: See *Personification*

Protagonist: The central character of a story who serves as a focus for its themes and incidents and as the principal rationale for its development. The protagonist is sometimes referred to in discussions of modern literature as the hero or anti-hero.

Proverb: A brief, sage saying that expresses a truth about life in a striking manner.

Pseudonym: A name assumed by a writer, most often intended to prevent his or her identification as the author of a work. Two or more authors may work together under one pseudonym, or an author may use a different name for each genre he or she publishes in. Some publishing companies maintain "house pseudonyms," under which any number of authors may write installations in a series. Some authors also choose a pseudonym over their real names the way an actor may use a stage name.

Pun: A play on words that have similar sounds but different meanings.

Pure Poetry: poetry written without instructional intent or moral purpose that aims only to please a reader by its imagery or musical flow. The term pure poetry is used as the antonym of the term "didacticism."

Q

Quatrain: A four-line stanza of a poem or an entire poem consisting of four lines.

R

Realism: A nineteenth-century European literary movement that sought to portray familiar characters, situations, and settings in a realistic manner. This was done primarily by using an objective narrative point of view and through the buildup of accurate detail. The standard for success of any realistic work depends on how faithfully it transfers common experience into fictional forms. The realistic method may be altered or extended, as in stream of consciousness writing, to record highly subjective experience.

Refrain: A phrase repeated at intervals throughout a poem. A refrain may appear at the end of each stanza or at less regular intervals. It may be altered slightly at each appearance.

Renaissance: The period in European history that marked the end of the Middle Ages. It began in Italy in the late fourteenth century. In broad terms, it is usually seen as spanning the fourteenth, fifteenth, and sixteenth centuries, although it did not reach Great Britain, for example, until the 1480s or so. The Renaissance saw an awakening in almost every sphere of human activity, especially science, philosophy, and the arts. The period is best defined by the emergence of a general philosophy that emphasized the importance of the intellect, the individual, and world affairs. It contrasts strongly with the medieval worldview, characterized by the dominant concerns of faith, the social collective, and spiritual salvation.

Repartee: Conversation featuring snappy retorts and witticisms.

Restoration: See *Restoration Age*

Restoration Age: A period in English literature beginning with the crowning of Charles II in 1660 and running to about 1700. The era, which was characterized by a reaction against Puritanism, was the first great age of the comedy of manners. The finest literature of the era is typically witty and urbane, and often lewd.

Rhetoric: In literary criticism, this term denotes the art of ethical persuasion. In its strictest sense, rhetoric adheres to various principles developed since classical times for arranging facts and ideas in a clear, persuasive, appealing manner. The term is also used to refer to effective prose in general and theories of or methods for composing effective prose.

Rhetorical Question: A question intended to provoke thought, but not an expressed answer, in the reader. It is most commonly used in oratory and other persuasive genres.

Rhyme: When used as a noun in literary criticism, this term generally refers to a poem in which words sound identical or very similar and appear in parallel positions in two or more lines. Rhymes are classified into different types according to where they fall in a line or stanza or according to the degree of similarity they exhibit in their spellings and sounds. Some major types of rhyme are "masculine" rhyme, "feminine" rhyme, and "triple" rhyme. In a masculine rhyme, the rhyming sound falls in a single accented syllable, as with "heat" and "eat." Feminine rhyme is a rhyme of two syllables, one stressed and one unstressed, as with "merry" and "tarry." Triple rhyme matches the sound of the accented syllable and the two unaccented syllables that follow: "narrative" and "declarative."

Rhyme Royal: A stanza of seven lines composed in iambic pentameter and rhymed *ababbcc*. The name is said to be a tribute to King James I of Scotland, who made much use of the form in his poetry.

Rhyme Scheme: See *Rhyme*

Rhythm: A regular pattern of sound, time intervals, or events occurring in writing, most often and most discernably in poetry. Regular, reliable rhythm is known to be soothing to humans, while interrupted, unpredictable, or rapidly changing rhythm is disturbing. These effects are known to authors, who use them to produce a desired reaction in the reader.

Rococo: A style of European architecture that flourished in the eighteenth century, especially in France. The most notable features of *rococo* are its extensive use of ornamentation and its themes of lightness, gaiety, and intimacy. In literary criticism, the term is often used disparagingly to refer to a decadent or over-ornamental style.

Romance: A broad term, usually denoting a narrative with exotic, exaggerated, often idealized characters, scenes, and themes.

Romantic Age: See *Romanticism*

Romanticism: This term has two widely accepted meanings. In historical criticism, it refers to a European intellectual and artistic movement of the late eighteenth and early nineteenth centuries that sought greater freedom of personal expression than that allowed by the strict rules of literary form and logic of the eighteenth-century neoclassicists. The Romantics preferred emotional and imaginative expression to rational analysis. They considered the individual to be at the center of all experience and so placed him or her at the center of their art. The Romantics believed that the creative imagination reveals nobler truths—unique feelings and attitudes—than those that could be discovered by logic or by scientific examination. Both the natural world and the state of childhood were important sources for revelations of "eternal truths." "Romanticism" is also used as a general term to refer to a type of sensibility found in all periods of literary history and usually considered to be in opposition to the principles of classicism. In this sense, Romanticism signifies any work or philosophy in which the exotic or dreamlike figure strongly, or that is devoted to individualistic expression, self-analysis, or a pursuit of a higher realm of knowledge than can be discovered by human reason.

Romantics: See *Romanticism*

Russian Symbolism: A Russian poetic movement, derived from French symbolism, that flourished between 1894 and 1910. While some Russian Symbolists continued in the French tradition, stressing aestheticism and the importance of suggestion above didactic intent, others saw their craft as a form of mystical worship, and themselves as mediators between the supernatural and the mundane.

S

Satire: A work that uses ridicule, humor, and wit to criticize and provoke change in human nature and institutions. There are two major types of satire: "formal" or "direct" satire speaks directly to the reader or to a character in the work; "indirect" satire relies upon the ridiculous behavior of its characters to make its point. Formal satire is further divided into two manners: the "Horatian," which ridicules gently, and the "Juvenalian," which derides its subjects harshly and bitterly.

Scansion: The analysis or "scanning" of a poem to determine its meter and often its rhyme scheme. The most common system of scansion uses accents (slanted lines drawn above syllables) to show stressed syllables, breves (curved lines drawn above syllables) to show unstressed syllables, and vertical lines to separate each foot.

Second Person: See *Point of View*

Semiotics: The study of how literary forms and conventions affect the meaning of language.

Sestet: Any six-line poem or stanza.

Setting: The time, place, and culture in which the action of a narrative takes place. The elements of setting may include geographic location, characters' physical and mental environments, prevailing cultural attitudes, or the historical time in which the action takes place.

Shakespearean Sonnet: See *Sonnet*

Signifying Monkey: A popular trickster figure in black folklore, with hundreds of tales about this character documented since the 19th century.

Simile: A comparison, usually using "like" or "as," of two essentially dissimilar things, as in "coffee as cold as ice" or "He sounded like a broken record."

Slang: A type of informal verbal communication that is generally unacceptable for formal writing. Slang words and phrases are often colorful exaggerations used to emphasize the speaker's point; they may also be shortened versions of an often-used word or phrase.

Slant Rhyme: See *Consonance*

Slave Narrative: Autobiographical accounts of American slave life as told by escaped slaves. These works first appeared during the abolition movement of the 1830s through the 1850s.

Social Realism: See *Socialist Realism*

Socialist Realism: The Socialist Realism school of literary theory was proposed by Maxim Gorky and established as a dogma by the first Soviet Congress of Writers. It demanded adherence to a communist worldview in works of literature. Its doctrines required an objective viewpoint comprehensible to the working classes and themes of social struggle featuring strong proletarian heroes.

Soliloquy: A monologue in a drama used to give the audience information and to develop the speaker's character. It is typically a projection of the speaker's innermost thoughts. Usually delivered while the speaker is alone on stage, a soliloquy is intended to present an illusion of unspoken reflection.

Sonnet: A fourteen-line poem, usually composed in iambic pentameter, employing one of several rhyme schemes. There are three major types of sonnets, upon which all other variations of the form are based: the "Petrarchan" or "Italian" sonnet, the "Shakespearean" or "English" sonnet, and the "Spenserian" sonnet. A Petrarchan sonnet consists of an octave rhymed *abbaabba* and a "sestet" rhymed either *cdecde, cdccdc,* or *cdedce.* The octave poses a question or problem, relates a narrative, or puts forth a proposition; the sestet presents a solution to the problem, comments upon the narrative, or applies the proposition put forth in the octave. The Shakespearean sonnet is divided into three quatrains and a couplet rhymed *abab cdcd efef gg.* The couplet provides an epigrammatic comment on the narrative or problem put forth in the quatrains. The Spenserian sonnet uses three quatrains and a couplet like the Shakespearean, but links their three rhyme schemes in this way: *abab bcbc cdcd ee.* The Spenserian sonnet develops its theme in two parts like the Petrarchan, its final six lines resolving a problem, analyzing a narrative, or applying a proposition put forth in its first eight lines.

Spenserian Sonnet: See *Sonnet*

Spenserian Stanza: A nine-line stanza having eight verses in iambic pentameter, its ninth verse in iambic hexameter, and the rhyme scheme ababbcbcc.

Spondee: In poetry meter, a foot consisting of two long or stressed syllables occurring together. This form is quite rare in English verse, and is usually composed of two monosyllabic words.

Sprung Rhythm: Versification using a specific number of accented syllables per line but disregarding the number of unaccented syllables that fall in each line, producing an irregular rhythm in the poem.

Stanza: A subdivision of a poem consisting of lines grouped together, often in recurring patterns of rhyme, line length, and meter. Stanzas may also serve as units of thought in a poem much like paragraphs in prose.

Stereotype: A stereotype was originally the name for a duplication made during the printing process; this led to its modern definition as a person or thing that is (or is assumed to be) the same as all others of its type.

Stream of Consciousness: A narrative technique for rendering the inward experience of a character. This technique is designed to give the impression of an ever-changing series of thoughts, emotions, images, and memories in the spontaneous and seemingly illogical order that they occur in life.

Structuralism: A twentieth-century movement in literary criticism that examines how literary texts arrive at their meanings, rather than the meanings themselves. There are two major types of structuralist analysis: one examines the way patterns of linguistic structures unify a specific text and emphasize certain elements of that text, and the other interprets the way literary forms and conventions affect the meaning of language itself.

Structure: The form taken by a piece of literature. The structure may be made obvious for ease of understanding, as in nonfiction works, or may obscured for artistic purposes, as in some poetry or seemingly "unstructured" prose.

Sturm und Drang: A German term meaning "storm and stress." It refers to a German literary movement of the 1770s and 1780s that reacted against the order and rationalism of the enlightenment, focusing instead on the intense experience of extraordinary individuals.

Style: A writer's distinctive manner of arranging words to suit his or her ideas and purpose in writing. The unique imprint of the author's personality upon his or her writing, style is the product of an author's way of arranging ideas and his or her use of diction, different sentence structures, rhythm, figures of speech, rhetorical principles, and other elements of composition.

Subject: The person, event, or theme at the center of a work of literature. A work may have one or more subjects of each type, with shorter works tending to have fewer and longer works tending to have more.

Subjectivity: Writing that expresses the author's personal feelings about his subject, and which may or may not include factual information about the subject.

Surrealism: A term introduced to criticism by Guillaume Apollinaire and later adopted by Andre Breton. It refers to a French literary and artistic movement founded in the 1920s. The Surrealists sought to express unconscious thoughts and feelings in their works. The best-known technique used for achieving this aim was automatic writing—transcriptions of spontaneous outpourings from the unconscious. The Surrealists proposed to unify the contrary levels of conscious and unconscious, dream and reality, objectivity and subjectivity into a new level of "super-realism."

Suspense: A literary device in which the author maintains the audience's attention through the buildup of events, the outcome of which will soon be revealed.

Syllogism: A method of presenting a logical argument. In its most basic form, the syllogism consists of a major premise, a minor premise, and a conclusion.

Symbol: Something that suggests or stands for something else without losing its original identity. In literature, symbols combine their literal meaning with the suggestion of an abstract concept. Literary symbols are of two types: those that carry complex associations of meaning no matter what their contexts, and those that derive their suggestive meaning from their functions in specific literary works.

Symbolism: This term has two widely accepted meanings. In historical criticism, it denotes an early modernist literary movement initiated in France during the nineteenth century that reacted against the prevailing standards of realism. Writers in this movement aimed to evoke, indirectly and symbolically, an order of being beyond the material world of the five senses. Poetic expression of personal emotion figured strongly in the movement, typically by means of a private set of symbols uniquely identifiable with the individual poet. The principal aim of the Symbolists was to express in words the highly complex feelings that grew out of everyday contact with the world. In a broader sense, the term "symbolism" refers to the use of one object to represent another.

Symbolist: See *Symbolism*

Symbolist Movement: See *Symbolism*

Sympathetic Fallacy: See *Affective Fallacy*

T

Tanka: A form of Japanese poetry similar to *haiku*. A *tanka* is five lines long, with the lines containing five, seven, five, seven, and seven syllables respectively.

Terza Rima: A three-line stanza form in poetry in which the rhymes are made on the last word of each line in the following manner: the first and third lines of the first stanza, then the second line of the first stanza and the first and third lines of the second stanza, and so on with the middle line of any stanza rhyming with the first and third lines of the following stanza.

Tetrameter: See *Meter*

Textual Criticism: A branch of literary criticism that seeks to establish the authoritative text of a literary work. Textual critics typically compare all known manuscripts or printings of a single work in order to assess the meanings of differences and revisions. This procedure allows them to arrive at a definitive version that (supposedly) corresponds to the author's original intention.

Theme: The main point of a work of literature. The term is used interchangeably with thesis.

Thesis: A thesis is both an essay and the point argued in the essay. Thesis novels and thesis plays share the quality of containing a thesis which is supported through the action of the story.

Third Person: See *Point of View*

Tone: The author's attitude toward his or her audience may be deduced from the tone of the work. A formal tone may create distance or convey politeness, while an informal tone may encourage a friendly, intimate, or intrusive feeling in the reader. The author's attitude toward his or her subject matter may also be deduced from the tone of the words he or she uses in discussing it.

Tragedy: A drama in prose or poetry about a noble, courageous hero of excellent character who, because of some tragic character flaw or *hamartia*, brings ruin upon him- or herself. Tragedy treats its subjects in a dignified and serious manner, using poetic language to help evoke pity and fear and bring about catharsis, a purging of these emotions. The tragic form was practiced extensively by the ancient Greeks. In the Middle Ages, when classical works were virtually unknown, tragedy came to denote any works about the fall of persons from exalted to low conditions due to any reason: fate, vice, weakness, etc. According to the classical definition of tragedy, such works present the "pathetic"—that which evokes pity—rather than the tragic. The classical form of tragedy was revived in the sixteenth century; it flourished especially on the Elizabethan stage. In modern times, dramatists have attempted to adapt the form to the needs of modern society by drawing their heroes from the ranks of ordinary men and women and defining the nobility of these heroes in terms of spirit rather than exalted social standing.

Tragic Flaw: In a tragedy, the quality within the hero or heroine which leads to his or her downfall.

Transcendentalism: An American philosophical and religious movement, based in New England from around 1835 until the Civil War. Transcendentalism was a form of American romanticism that had its roots abroad in the works of Thomas Carlyle, Samuel Coleridge, and Johann Wolfgang von Goethe. The Transcendentalists stressed the importance of intuition and subjective experience in communication with God. They rejected religious dogma and texts in favor of mysticism and scientific naturalism. They pursued truths that lie beyond the "colorless" realms perceived by reason and the senses and were active social reformers in public education, women's rights, and the abolition of slavery.

Trickster: A character or figure common in Native American and African literature who uses his ingenuity to defeat enemies and escape difficult situations. Tricksters are most often animals, such as the spider, hare, or coyote, although they may take the form of humans as well.

Trimeter: See *Meter*

Triple Rhyme: See *Rhyme*

Trochee: See *Foot*

U

Understatement: See *Irony*

Unities: Strict rules of dramatic structure, formulated by Italian and French critics of the Renaissance and based loosely on the principles of drama discussed by Aristotle in his *Poetics*.

Foremost among these rules were the three unities of action, time, and place that compelled a dramatist to: (1) construct a single plot with a beginning, middle, and end that details the causal relationships of action and character; (2) restrict the action to the events of a single day; and (3) limit the scene to a single place or city. The unities were observed faithfully by continental European writers until the Romantic Age, but they were never regularly observed in English drama. Modern dramatists are typically more concerned with a unity of impression or emotional effect than with any of the classical unities.

Urban Realism: A branch of realist writing that attempts to accurately reflect the often harsh facts of modern urban existence.

Utopia: A fictional perfect place, such as "paradise" or "heaven."

Utopian: See *Utopia*

Utopianism: See *Utopia*

V

Verisimilitude: Literally, the appearance of truth. In literary criticism, the term refers to aspects of a work of literature that seem true to the reader.

Vers de societe: See *Occasional Verse*

Vers libre: See *Free Verse*

Verse: A line of metered language, a line of a poem, or any work written in verse.

Versification: The writing of verse. Versification may also refer to the meter, rhyme, and other mechanical components of a poem.

Victorian: Refers broadly to the reign of Queen Victoria of England (1837-1901) and to anything with qualities typical of that era. For example, the qualities of smug narrowmindedness, bourgeois materialism, faith in social progress, and priggish morality are often considered Victorian. This stereotype is contradicted by such dramatic intellectual developments as the theories of Charles Darwin, Karl Marx, and Sigmund Freud (which stirred strong debates in England) and the critical attitudes of serious Victorian writers like Charles Dickens and George Eliot. In literature, the Victorian Period was the great age of the English novel, and the latter part of the era saw the rise of movements such as decadence and symbolism.

Victorian Age: See *Victorian*

Victorian Period: See *Victorian*

W

Weltanschauung: A German term referring to a person's worldview or philosophy.

Weltschmerz: A German term meaning "world pain." It describes a sense of anguish about the nature of existence, usually associated with a melancholy, pessimistic attitude.

Z

Zarzuela: A type of Spanish operetta.

Zeitgeist: A German term meaning "spirit of the time." It refers to the moral and intellectual trends of a given era.

Cumulative Author/Title Index

Cumulative Nationality/Ethnicity Index

Subject/Theme Index

Cumulative Index of First Lines

A

A brackish reach of shoal off Madaket,— (The Quaker Graveyard in Nantucket) V6:158

"A cold coming we had of it (Journey of the Magi) V7:110

A few minutes ago, I stepped onto the deck (The Cobweb) V17:50

A gentle spring evening arrives (Spring-Watching Pavilion) V18:198

A line in long array where they wind betwixt green islands, (Cavalry Crossing a Ford) V13:50

A narrow Fellow in the grass (A Narrow Fellow in the Grass) V11:127

A noiseless patient spider, (A Noiseless Patient Spider) V31:190–91

A pine box for me. I mean it. (Last Request) V14: 231

A poem should be palpable and mute (Ars Poetica) V5:2

A stone from the depths that has witnessed the seas drying up (Song of a Citizen) V16:125

A tourist came in from Orbitville, (Southbound on the Freeway) V16:158

A wind is ruffling the tawny pelt (A Far Cry from Africa) V6:60

a woman precedes me up the long rope, (Climbing) V14:113

About me the night moonless wimples the mountains (Vancouver Lights) V8:245

About suffering they were never wrong (Musée des Beaux Arts) V1:148

Across Roblin Lake, two shores away, (Wilderness Gothic) V12:241

After the double party (Air for Mercury) V20:2–3

After the party ends another party begins (Social Life) V19:251

After you finish your work (Ballad of Orange and Grape) V10:17

Again I've returned to this country (The Country Without a Post Office) V18:64

"Ah, are you digging on my grave (Ah, Are You Digging on My Grave?) V4:2

All Greece hates (Helen) V6:92

All my existence is a dark sign a dark (A Rebirth) V21:193–194

All night long the hockey pictures (To a Sad Daughter) V8:230

All over Genoa (Trompe l'Oeil) V22:216

All winter your brute shoulders strained against collars, padding (Names of Horses) V8:141

Also Ulysses once—that other war. (Kilroy) V14:213

Always (Always) V24:15

Among the blossoms, a single jar of wine. (Drinking Alone Beneath the Moon) V20:59–60

Anasazi (Anasazi) V9:2

"And do we remember our living lives?" (Memory) V21:156

And God stepped out on space (The Creation) V1:19

And what if I spoke of despair—who doesn't (And What If I Spoke of Despair) V19:2

Animal bones and some mossy tent rings (Lament for the Dorsets) V5:190

Any force— (All It Takes) V23:15

April is the cruellest month, breeding (The Waste Land) V20:248–252

As I perceive (The Gold Lily) V5:127

As I walked out one evening (As I Walked Out One Evening) V4:15

As I was going down impassive Rivers, (The Drunken Boat) V28:83

As in an illuminated page, whose busy edges (Bonnard's Garden) V25:33

As virtuous men pass mildly away (A Valediction: Forbidding Mourning) V11:201

As you set out for Ithaka (Ithaka) V19:114

At five in the afternoon. (Lament for Ignacio Sánchez Mejías) V31:128–30

At noon in the desert a panting lizard (At the Bomb Testing Site) V8:2

At six I lived for spells: (What For) V33:266

Ay, tear her tattered ensign down! (Old Ironsides) V9:172

B

Back then, before we came (On Freedom's Ground) V12:186

The fiddler crab fiddles, glides and dithers, (Fiddler Crab) V23:111–112

The force that through the green fuse drives the flower (The Force That Through the Green Fuse Drives the Flower) V8:101

The grasses are light brown (September) V23:258–259

The green lamp flares on the table (This Life) V1:293

The house is crammed: tier beyond tier they grin ("Blighters") V28:3

The ills I sorrow at (Any Human to Another) V3:2

The instructor said (Theme for English B) V6:194

The king sits in Dumferling toune (Sir Patrick Spens) V4:177

The land was overmuch like scenery (Beowulf) V11:2

The last time I saw it was 1968. (The Hiding Place) V10:152

The Lord is my shepherd; I shall not want (Psalm 23) V4:103

The man who sold his lawn to standard oil (The War Against the Trees) V11:215

The moon glows the same (The Moon Glows the Same) V7:152

The old South Boston Aquarium stands (For the Union Dead) V7:67

The others bent their heads and started in ("Trouble with Math in a One-Room Country School") V9:238

The pale nuns of St. Joseph are here (Island of Three Marias) V11:79

The Phoenix comes of flame and dust (The Phoenix) V10:226

The plants of the lake (Two Poems for T.) V20:218

The poetry of earth is never dead: (On the Grasshopper and the Cricket) V32:161

The rain set early in to-night: (Porphyria's Lover) V15:151

The river brought down (How We Heard the Name) V10:167

The rusty spigot (Onomatopoeia) V6:133

The sea is calm tonight (Dover Beach) V2:52

The sea sounds insincere (The Milkfish Gatherers) V11:111

The slow overture of rain, (Mind) V17:145

The Soul selects her own Society— (The Soul Selects Her Own Society) V1:259

The summer that I was ten— (The Centaur) V30:20

"The sun was shining on the sea, (The Walrus and the Carpenter) V30:258–259

The surface of the pond was mostly green— (The Lotus Flowers) V33:107

The time you won your town the race (To an Athlete Dying Young) V7:230

The way sorrow enters the bone (The Blue Rim of Memory) V17:38

The whiskey on your breath (My Papa's Waltz) V3:191

The white ocean in which birds swim (Morning Walk) V21:167

The wind was a torrent of darkness among the gusty trees (The Highwayman) V4:66

The windows were open and the morning air was, by the smell of lilac and some darker flowering shrub, filled with the brown and chirping trills of birds. (Yet we insist that life is full of happy chance) V27:291

There are blows in life, so hard . . . I just don't know! (The Black Heralds) V26:47

There are strange things done in the midnight sun (The Cremation of Sam McGee) V10:75

There have been rooms for such a short time (The Horizons of Rooms) V15:79

There is a hunger for order, (A Thirst Against) V20:205

There is no way not to be excited (Paradiso) V20:190–191

There is the one song everyone (Siren Song) V7:196

There will come soft rains and the smell of the ground, (There Will Come Soft Rains) V14:301

There you are, in all your innocence, (Perfect Light) V19:187

There's a Certain Slant of Light (There's a Certain Slant of Light) V6:211

There's no way out. (In the Suburbs) V14:201

These open years, the river (For Jennifer, 6, on the Teton) V17:86

These unprepossessing sunsets (Art Thou the Thing I Wanted) V25:2–3

They eat beans mostly, this old yellow pair (The Bean Eaters) V2:16

They said, "Wait." Well, I waited. (Alabama Centennial) V10:2

They say a child with two mouths is no good. (Pantoun for Chinese Women) V29:241

they were just meant as covers (My Mother Pieced Quilts) V12:169

This girlchild was born as usual (Barbie Doll) V9:33

This is a litany of lost things, (The Litany) V24:101–102

This is my letter to the World (This Is My Letter to the World) V4:233

This is the Arsenal. From floor to ceiling, (The Arsenal at Springfield) V17:2

This is the black sea-brute bulling through wave-wrack (Leviathan) V5:203

This is the ship of pearl, which, poets feign, (The Chambered Nautilus) V24:52–53

This poem is concerned with language on a very plain level (Paradoxes and Oxymorons) V11:162

This tale is true, and mine. It tells (The Seafarer) V8:177

Thou still unravish'd bride of quietness (Ode on a Grecian Urn) V1:179

Three times my life has opened. (Three Times My Life Has Opened) V16:213

Time in school drags along with so much worry, (Childhood) V19:29

to fold the clothes. No matter who lives (I Stop Writimg the Poem) V16:58

To him who in the love of Nature holds (Thanatopsis) V30:232–233

To replay errors (Daughter-Mother-Maya-Seeta) V25:83

To weep unbidden, to wake (Practice) V23:240

Toni Morrison despises (The Toni Morrison Dreams) V22:202–203

Tonight I can write the saddest lines (Tonight I Can Write) V11:187

tonite, *thriller* was (Beware: Do Not Read This Poem) V6:3

Truth be told, I do not want to forget (Native Guard) V29:183

Turning and turning in the widening gyre (The Second Coming) V7:179

'Twas brillig, and the slithy toves (Jabberwocky) V11:91

'Twas mercy brought me from my pagan land, (On Being Brought from Africa to America) V29:223

Two roads diverged in a yellow wood (The Road Not Taken) V2:195

Tyger! Tyger! burning bright (The Tyger) V2:263

Cumulative Index of Last Lines

until at last I lift you up and wrap you within me. (It's like This) V23:138–139

Until Eternity. (The Bustle in a House) V10:62

unusual conservation (Chocolates) V11:17

Uttering cries that are almost human (American Poetry) V7:2

W

War is kind (War Is Kind) V9:253

watching to see how it's done. (I Stop Writing the Poem) V16:58

water. (Poem in Which My Legs Are Accepted) V29:262

We are satisfied, if you are; but why did I die?" (Losses) V31:167–68

we tread upon, forgetting. Truth be told. (Native Guard) V29:185

Went home and put a bullet through his head (Richard Cory) V4:117

Were not the one dead, turned to their affairs. (Out, Out—) V10:213

Were toward Eternity— (Because I Could Not Stop for Death) V2:27

What will survive of us is love. (An Arundel Tomb) V12:18

When I died they washed me out of the turret with a hose (The Death of the Ball Turret Gunner) V2:41

when they untie them in the evening. (Early in the Morning) V17:75

when you are at a party. (Social Life) V19:251

When you have both (Toads) V4:244

Where deep in the night I hear a voice (Butcher Shop) V7:43

Where ignorant armies clash by night (Dover Beach) V2:52

Which Claus of Innsbruck cast in bronze for me! (My Last Duchess) V1:166

Which for all you know is the life you've chosen. (The God Who Loves You) V20:88

which is not going to go wasted on me which is why I'm telling you about it (Having a Coke with You) V12:106

which only looks like an *l*, and is silent. (Trompe l'Oeil) V22:216

white ash amid funereal cypresses (Helen) V6:92

Who are you and what is your purpose? (The Mystery) V15:138

Why am I not as they? (Lineage) V31:145–46

Wi' the Scots lords at his feit (Sir Patrick Spens) V4:177

Will always be ready to bless the day (Morning Walk) V21:167

will be easy, my rancor less bitter . . . (On the Threshold) V22:128

Will hear of as a god." (How we Heard the Name) V10:167

Wind, like the dodo's (Bedtime Story) V8:33

windowpanes. (View) V25:246–247

With courage to endure! (Old Stoic) V33:144

With gold unfading, WASHINGTON! be thine. (To His Excellency General Washington) V13:213

with my eyes closed. (We Live by What We See at Night) V13:240

With silence and tears. (When We Two Parted) V29:297

with the door closed. (Hanging Fire) V32:93

With the slow smokeless burning of decay (The Wood-Pile) V6:252

With what they had to go on. (The Conquerors) V13:67

Without cease or doubt sew the sweet sad earth. (The Satyr's Heart) V22:187

Would scarcely know that we were gone. (There Will Come Soft Rains) V14:301

Y

Ye know on earth, and all ye need to know (Ode on a Grecian Urn) V1:180

You live in this, and dwell in lovers' eyes (Sonnet 55) V5:246

You may for ever tarry. (To the Virgins, to Make Much of Time) V13:226

you who raised me? (The Gold Lily) V5:127

You're all that I can call my own. (Woman Work) V33:289

you'll have understood by then what these Ithakas mean. (Ithaka) V19:114